W9-CKI-710

REICHEL'S CARE OF THE ELDERLY

The sixth edition of *Reichel's Care of the Elderly: Clinical Aspects of Aging* remains the pioneering text for the practicing physician confronted with the unique problems of an increasingly elderly population. Dr. William Reichel's formative text is designed as a practical and useful guide for health specialists from medical students to practicing physicians. This book is not a collection of subspecialty chapters but rather emphasizes the clinical management of the geriatric patient with simple to complex problems. The editors have reviewed every chapter and have included the most up-to-date advances in the care of the elderly. New topics include hormonal therapy in postmenopausal women, drug therapy for Alzheimer sufferers, alternative medicine, the chronic understaffing of nursing homes, management of delirium, and ethical issues. The targeted audience is not only the geriatric specialist, but also medical and allied health practitioners who need practical and relevant information in a comprehensive format.

Christine Arenson (MD, Jefferson Medical College) is Associate Professor of Family and Community Medicine, Director of the Division of Geriatric Medicine, and Co-Director of the Jefferson InterProfessional Education Center at Thomas Jefferson University, Philadelphia, Pennsylvania. Dr. Arenson is also the Director of the Eastern Pennsylvania–Delaware Geriatric Education Center. Dr. Arenson practices family and geriatric medicine at Jefferson Family Medicine Associates at the Philadelphia Senior Center.

Jan Busby-Whitehead (MD, University of Texas Medical Branch at Galveston) is Associate Director for Clinical Affairs and Co-Director of the Carolina Program for Healthcare and Aging at the University of North Carolina School of Medicine. She is also a Professor of Medicine and Director of the Center for Aging and Health there.

Kenneth Brummel-Smith (MD, University of Southern California School of Medicine) is Charlotte Edwards Maguire Professor and Chair of the Department of Geriatrics at Florida State University College of Medicine, Tallahassee, Florida. Dr. Brummel-Smith is past president of the American Geriatrics Society.

James G. O'Brien (MD, University College, Dublin, Ireland) is Professor and Margaret Dorward Smock Endowed Chair in Geriatric Medicine, Chair of the Department of Family Medicine and Geriatrics, and Medical Director of the Geriatric Medicine Center at the University of Louisville School of Medicine, Kentucky.

Mary H. Palmer (PhD, Johns Hopkins University School of Hygiene and Public Health; BSN, University of Maryland School of Nursing) is Professor and Helen W. and Thomas L. Umphlet Distinguished Professor in Aging at the University of North Carolina, Chapel Hill, School of Nursing. Dr. Palmer is also Co-Director of the Interdisciplinary Center for Aging Research: Uniting Scientists at the University of North Carolina.

William Reichel, MD, is Editor Emeritus of *Reichel's Care of the Elderly: Clinical Aspects of Aging, 6th edition*. Dr. Reichel is an affiliated scholar of the Center for Clinical Bioethics at Georgetown University School of Medicine, Washington, DC. Dr. Reichel has published extensively on geriatric and family medicine and is a pioneer of the study of aging.

Reichel's Care of the Elderly

Clinical Aspects of Aging

Sixth Edition

EDITED BY

Christine Arenson
Thomas Jefferson University

Jan Busby-Whitehead
University of North Carolina School of Medicine

Kenneth Brummel-Smith
Florida State University College of Medicine

James G. O'Brien
University of Louisville School of Medicine

Mary H. Palmer
University of North Carolina School of Nursing

William Reichel
Georgetown University School of Medicine

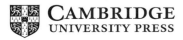

CAMBRIDGE
UNIVERSITY PRESS

CAMBRIDGE UNIVERSITY PRESS
Cambridge, New York, Melbourne, Madrid, Cape Town, Singapore, São Paulo, Delhi

Cambridge University Press
32 Avenue of the Americas, New York, NY 10013–2473, USA

www.cambridge.org
Information on this title: www.cambridge.org/9780521869294

First published 2009

Printed in the United States of America

A catalog record for this publication is available from the British Library.

Library of Congress Cataloging in Publication data

Reichel's care of the elderly : clinical aspects of aging. – 6th ed. / edited by Christine
Arenson . . . [et al.].
    p.; cm.
Includes bibliographical references and index.
ISBN 978-0-521-86929-4 (hardback)
1. Geriatrics.   2. Aging.   I. Reichel, William, 1937–   II. Arenson, Christine, 1964–
III. Title: Care of the elderly.
    [DNLM: 1. Geriatrics – methods.   2. Aging – physiology.   3. Health Services for the
Aged. WT 100 R349 2009]
RC952.C53   2009
618.97 – dc22   2008022701

ISBN   978-0-521-86929-4 hardback

Contents

Color plates appear after page 30

Editorial Advisory Committee

CONTRIBUTORS

1. William Reichel, MD
    Affiliated Scholar
    Center for Clinical Bioethics
    Georgetown University School of Medicine
    Washington, DC

    Christine Arenson, MD
    Associate Professor and Director
    Division of Geriatric Medicine
    Department of Family and Community
        Medicine
    Thomas Jefferson University
    Philadelphia, PA

    Joseph E. Scherger, MD, MPH
    Clinical Professor
    Department of Family and Preventive
        Medicine
    University of California
    San Diego School of Medicine
    Del Mar, CA

2. John D. Gazewood, MD, MSPH
    Associate Professor
    Residency Program Director
    Department of Family Medicine
    University of Virginia Health System
    Charlottesville, VA

3. Racquel Daley-Placide, MD
    Assistant Professor
    Division of Geriatric Medicine
    School of Medicine
    University of North Carolina at Chapel Hill
    Chapel Hill, NC

    Holly Jean Coward, MD
    Associate Professor of Medicine
    University of North Carolina School of Medicine
    Program on Aging
    Chapel Hill, NC

4. Laura Goldman, MD
    Assistant Professor of Family Medicine
    Director of Geriatrics
    Department of Family Medicine
    Boston University Medical Center
    Boston, MA

    Thomas C. Hines, MD
    Assistant Professor
    Department of Family Medicine
    Boston University Medical Center
    Boston, MA

    Ilona M. Kopits, MD, MPH
    Geriatrics Division
    Boston University Medical Center
    Boston, MA

5. Elena M. Umland, PharmD
    Associate Dean for Academic Affairs
    School of Pharmacy
    Thomas Jefferson University
    Philadelphia, PA

    Cynthia A. Sanoski, PharmD, BCPS, FCCP
    Chair
    Department of Pharmacy Practice
    School of Pharmacy
    Thomas Jefferson University
    Philadelphia, PA

Amber King, PharmD
Pharmacy Practice Resident
Thomas Jefferson University Hospital
Philadelphia, PA

6. Jacqueline Lloyd, MD
Department of Geriatrics
Florida State University College of Medicine
Tallahassee, FL

Randy Huffines, DDS
University of North Carolina School of Dentistry
James H. Quillen VA Medical Center
Mountain Home, TN

7. Maria A. Fiatarone Singh, MD, FRACP
John Sutton Chair of Exercise and Sport Science
Discipline of Exercise, Health and Performance
Professor of Medicine
University of Sydney
Faculty of Health Sciences
Lidcombe, Australia

8. Lisa B. Caruso, MD, MPH
Assistant Professor of Medicine
Boston University School of Medicine
Boston, MA

Rebecca A. Silliman, MD, PhD, MPH
Professor of Medicine and Public Health
Chief
Section of Geriatrics
Boston University Schools of Medicine and
    Public Health
Boston, MA

9. Phil Mendys, PharmD, CPP
University of North Carolina Hospitals
Chapel Hill, NC

Ross J. Simpson, Jr., MD, PhD
University of North Carolina School of Medicine
Department of Medicine
Division of Cardiology
Professor of Medicine
Clinical Professor of Epidemiology
School of Public Health
Director
Preventative Cardiology Clinic
Principal Clinical Coordinator
Medical Review of North Carolina
Chapel Hill, NC

10. B. Brent Simmons, MD
Assistant Professor
Department of Medicine

Section of Geriatrics
Temple University
Philadelphia, PA

Daniel DeJoseph, MD
Fellow in Geriatric Medicine
Department of Family and Community Medicine
Thomas Jefferson University
Philadelphia, PA

Christine Arenson, MD
Associate Professor and Director
Division of Geriatric Medicine
Department of Family and Community Medicine
Thomas Jefferson University
Philadelphia, PA

11. Joshua M. Stolker, MD
Assistant Professor of Medicine
Division of Cardiology
Washington University in St. Louis
St. Louis, MO

Michael W. Rich, MD
Associate Professor of Medicine
Division of Cardiology
Department of Medicine
Washington University in St. Louis
St. Louis, MO

12. Pushpendra Sharma, MD
Attending Geriatrician
Jewish Home and Hospital
Lifecare System
New York, NY

13. Kerri S. Remmel, MD, PhD
Assistant Professor of Neurology and Acting Chair
Director
University of Louisville Stroke Center
University of Louisville
Department of Neurology
Louisville, KY

14. Michele Zawora, MD
Instructor
Divison of Geriatric Medicine
Department of Family and Community
    Medicine
Thomas Jefferson University
Philadelphia, PA

Tsoa-Wei Liang, MD
Department of Neurology
Jefferson Hospital for Neurosciences
Philadelphia, PA

Hadijatou Jarra, MD
Attending Geriatrician
Gastonia, NC

15. James G. O'Brien, MD
Professor and Chair
The Margaret Dorward Smock Endowed Chair in
    Geriatric Medicine
Department of Family Medicine and Geriatrics
Medical Director of the Geriatric Medicine Center
University of Louisville School of Medicine
Louisville, KY

Stephanie Garrett, MD
Department of Family Medicine and Geriatrics
University of Louisville
Louisville, KY

16. Lauren G. Collins, MD
Assistant Professor
Division of Geriatric Medicine
Department of Family and Community Medicine
Thomas Jefferson University
Philadelphia, PA

Barry N. Rovner, MD
Professor and Director
Division of Geriatric Psychiatry
Department of Psychiatry
Jefferson Hospital for the Neurosciences
Philadelphia, PA

Marjorie M. Marenberg, MD, PhD, MPH
Assistant Professor
Division of Geriatric Medicine
Department of Family and Community Medicine
Thomas Jefferson University
Philadelphia, PA

17. John M. Tomkowiak, MD
Associate Dean for Curriculum
Rosalind Franklin University
Chicago Medical School
North Chicago, IL

18. Richard D. Blondell, MD
Director of Research in Addictions
Family Medicine Research Institute on Addictions
Department of Family Medicine
State University of New York, University at Buffalo
Buffalo, NY

Lynne M. Frydrych, MS
Family Medicine Research Institute on Addiction
State University of New York, University at Buffalo
Buffalo, NY

Rita M. Sawyer, MSN
Family Medicine Research Institute on Addiction
State University of New York, University at Buffalo
Buffalo, NY

19. Paula M. Minihan, MPH, PhD
Assistant Professor
Department of Public Health and Family Medicine
Tufts University School of Medicine
Boston, MA

20. David Defeo, MD
Fellow
Division of Pulmonary and Critical Care Medicine
University of North Carolina School of Medicine
Chapel Hill, NC

Shannon S. Carson, MD
Associate Professor of Medicine
Director
Pulmonary and Critical Care Fellowship Program
Associate Director
Medical Intensive Care Unit
Division of Pulmonary and Critical Care Medicine
University of North Carolina School of Medicine
Chapel Hill, NC

21. Christine Hsieh, MD
Instructor
Department of Family and Community Medicine
Thomas Jefferson University
Philadelphia, PA

Cuckoo Choudhary, MD
Assistant Professor
Division of Gastroenterology and Hepatology
Director of Medicine
Thomas Jefferson University
Philadelphia, PA

22. David Alain Wohl, MD
Associate Professor of Medicine
Division of Infectious Diseases
AIDS Clinical Trials Unit
University of North Carolina, Chapel Hill
Chapel Hill, NC

23. Karen Krigger, MD, MEd
Associate Professor
Department of Family and Geriatric Medicine
University of Louisville
Louisville, KY

Molly Rose, RN, PhD
Professor of Nursing and Coordinator
Community Systems Administration Master's Program
Department of Nursing
Co-Director
Jefferson Interprofessional Education Center
Thomas Jefferson University
Philadelphia, PA

24. Matthew Russell, MD, MSc
Division of Geriatrics
Boston University School of Medicine
Boston, MA

Rebecca A. Silliman, MD, PhD, MPH
Professor of Medicine and Public Health
Chief
Section of Geriatrics
Boston University Schools of Medicine and Public Health
Boston, MA

James Burke, MD
Professor
Division of Nephrology
Thomas Jefferson University
Philadelphia, PA

25. Tomas L. Griebling, MD, FACS, FGSA
Associate Professor and Vice Chair
Department of Urology
Faculty Associate, Center on Aging
University of Kansas Medical Center
Kansas City, KS

26. Jan Busby-Whitehead, MD
Professor of Medicine
Director, Program on Aging
Chief, Division of Geriatric Medicine
University of North Carolina, Chapel Hill
Chapel Hill, NC

Mary H. Palmer, PhD, RN-C, FAAN
Helen W. and Thomas L. Umphlet Distinguished
    Professor in Aging
School of Nursing
Co-Director
Interdisciplinary Center for Aging Research: Uniting
    Scientists
University of North Carolina, Chapel Hill
Chapel Hill, NC

Theodore N. Johnson, MD, MPH
Director of Geriatric Medicine
Emory University
Atlanta, GA

27. Carmen Sultana, MD
Assistant Professor
Director
Obstetrics and Gynecology Residency
Head of Education
Department of Obstetrics and Gynecology
Thomas Jefferson University
Philadelphia, PA

28. Matthew C. Leinung, MD
Director
Division of Endocrinology
Department of Medicine
Albany Medical College
Albany, NY

Paul J. Davis, MD
Senior Associate Dean for Research
Albany Medical College
Albany, NY

Faith B. Davis, MD
Senior Scientist
Ordway Research Institute
Staff Physician
Endocrinology
Stratton VA Medical Center
Albany, NY

29. Karen D. Novielli, MD
Associate Professor
Associate Dean for Faculty Affairs
Jefferson Medical College
Philadelphia, PA

30. Beth L. Jonas, MD
Clinical Assistant Professor of Medicine
Director
Rheumatology Fellowship Training Program
Division of Rheumatology
University of North Carolina School of
    Medicine
Chapel Hill, NC

31. Joseph D. Zuckerman, MD
Professor and Chairman
Department of Orthopaedic Surgery
New York University – Hospital for Joint Diseases
New York, NY

Aaron Schachter, MD
Chief Resident
Department of Orthopaedic Surgery
New York University – Hospital for Joint Diseases
New York, NY

32. Arthur E. Helfand, DPM
    Professor Emeritus
    School of Podiatric Medicine
    Temple University
    Narberth, PA

33. James Studdiford, MD
    Department of Family and Community Medicine
    Jefferson Medical College
    Philadelphia, PA

    Brooke E. Salzman, MD
    Assistant Professor
    Division of Geriatric Medicine
    Department of Family and Community Medicine
    Jefferson Medical College
    Thomas Jefferson University
    Philadelphia, PA

    Amber Tully, MD
    Assistant Professor
    Department of Family and Community Medicine
    Thomas Jefferson University Hospital
    Philadelphia, PA

34. Mary H. Palmer, PhD, RN-C, FAAN
    Professor and Helen W. and Thomas L. Umphlet
        Distinguished Professor in Aging
    School of Nursing
    Co-Director
    Interdisciplinary Center for Aging Research: Uniting
        Scientists
    University of North Carolina, Chapel Hill
    Chapel Hill, NC

    Jan Busby-Whitehead, MD
    Professor of Medicine
    Director
    Program on Aging
    Chief
    Division of Geriatric Medicine
    University of North Carolina, Chapel Hill
    Chapel Hill, NC

35. Inna Sheyner, MD
    Tampa, FL

    Karen Travis Stover, MPH, MSN, ARNP, CS
    Courtesy Faculty Appointment
    University of South Florida College of Medicine
    Tampa, FL

36. Danielle Snyderman, MD
    Instructor
    Department of Family and Community Medicine
    Thomas Jefferson University
    Philadelphia, PA

Christopher Haines, MD
Instructor
Department of Family and Community
    Medicine
Philadelphia, PA

Richard Wender, MD
Alumni Professor and Chair
Department of Family and Community
    Medicine
Thomas Jefferson University
Immediate Past President
American Cancer Society
Philadelphia, PA

37. Omesh P. Gupta, MD, MBA
    Chief Resident
    Wills Eye Hospital
    Philadelphia, PA

    William Tasman, MD
    Chair
    Department of Ophthalmology
    Jefferson Medical College
    Ophthalmologist-in-Chief
    Wills Eye Hospital
    Philadelphia, PA

38. Clarence (Fred) Gehris, MD
    Lutherville, MD

    Leonard Proctor, MD
    Associate Professor
    Department of Otolaryngology
    Johns Hopkins School of Medicine
    Baltimore, MD

    Lauren G. Collins, MD
    Assistant Professor
    Division of Geriatric Medicine
    Department of Family and Community
        Medicine
    Thomas Jefferson University
    Philadelphia, PA

39. Allen D. Samuelson, DDS
    Chapel Hill, NC

40. Susan Galandiuk, MD, FACS
    Department of Surgery and the Price Institute of
        Surgical Research
    Section of Colorectal Surgery
    University of Louisville School of Medicine
    Louisville, KY

Hiram C. Polk, Jr., MD, FACS
Professor of Surgery
Department of Surgery
School of Medicine
University of Louisville
Louisville, KY

41. Kenneth Brummel-Smith, MD
Charlotte Edwards Maguire Professor and
Chair
Department of Geriatrics
Florida State University College of Medicine
Tallahassee, FL

42. Nasiya N. Ahmed, MD
Geriatric Fellow
University of Arizona College of Medicine
Tucson, AZ

Randal W. Scott, MSW, MBA
Education Specialist
Arizona Center on Aging
University of Arizona
Tucson, AZ

Mindy J. Fain, MD
Director
Division of Geriatrics
Department of Medicine
University of Arizona
Tucson, AZ

43. Rebecca D. Elon, MD, MPH
Associate Professor of Medicine
Johns Hopkins University School of Medicine
Associate Professor of Medicine
University of Maryland School of Medicine
North Arundel Senior Care
Millersville, MD

Marshall B. Kapp, JD, MPH
Garwin Distinguished Professor of Law and
Medicine
Southern Illinois University School of Law
Carbondale, IL

44. Seema Modi, MD
Attending Geriatrician
RHD Senior Center
Dallas, TX

Terri Maxwell, MSN, PhD
Director of Research
ExcelleRX
Philadelphia, PA

45. Jeffrey Philip Spike, PhD
Associate Professor
Department of Medical Humanities and Social
Sciences
Florida State University College of Medicine
Tallahassee, FL

46. Amy R. Ehrlich, MD
Associate Professor of Clinical Medicine
Division of Geriatric Medicine
Department of Medicine
Albert Einstein College of Medicine
Montefiore Medical Center
Bronx, NY

Keiko Kimura, MD
Attending Japanese Medical Practice
Beth Israel Medical Center
Hartsdale, NY

Jody Rogers, MD
Assistant Professor
Department of Emergency Medicine
University of New Mexico
Albuquerque, NM

47. James G. O'Brien, MD,
Professor and Chair
The Margaret Dorward Smock Endowed Chair in
Geriatric Medicine
Department of Family Medicine and Geriatrics
Medical Director of the Geriatric Medicine Center
University of Louisville School of Medicine
Louisville, KY

48. Alice K. Pomidor, MD, MPH
Department of Geriatrics
Florida State University College of Medicine
Tallahassee, FL

Joanne Schwartzberg, MD
Director
Department of Aging and Community Health
American Medical Association
Chicago, IL

49. Joel S. Edman, DSc, FACN
Director of Integrative Nutrition
Myrna Brind Center for Integrative Medicine
Thomas Jefferson University Hospital
Philadelphia, PA

Bettina Herbert, MD
Department of Rehabilitation Medicine
Thomas Jefferson University
Philadelphia, PA

50. Thomas L. Edmondson, MD, CMD, AGSF
    Chief
    Section of Geriatrics
    Franklin Square Hospital System
    Clinical Assistant Professor of Medicine
    University of Maryland School of Medicine
    Baltimore, MD

    William Dean Charmak, PhD
    Employee Assistance Service
    Family and Children's Service of the Capital Region
    Albany, NY

51. Richard Falvo, PhD
    Adjunct Professor
    Department of Cell and Molecular Physiology
    School of Medicine
    University of North Carolina, Chapel Hill
    Chapel Hill, NC

52. Daniel Swagerty, MD, MPH
    Associate Professor
    Department of Family Medicine
    Director of Geriatric Education
    Landon Center on Aging
    Kansas City, KS

    Jonathan Evans, MD, MPH
    Associate Professor
    Department of Internal Medicine
    Director
    Section of Geriatrics and Palliative Medicine
    University of Virginia School of Medicine
    Charlottesville, VA

53. Fred Kobylarz, MD, MPH
    Associate Professor
    Department of Family Medicine
    University of Medicine and Dentistry, New Jersey–Robert
        Wood Johnson Medical School
    New Brunswick, NJ

    Gwen Yeo, PhD
    Co-Director
    Stanford Geriatric Education Center
    Director for Special Projects
    California Council on Gerontology and Geriatrics
    Stanford Geriatric Education Center
    Palo Alto, CA

54. Gordon F. Streib, PhD
    Professor Emeritus
    Department of Sociology
    College of Liberal Arts and Sciences
    University of Florida
    Gainesville, FL

55. Lisa Granville, MD
    Department of Geriatrics
    Florida State University College of Medicine
    Tallahassee, FL

    Karen Myers, ARNP
    Assistant Professor
    Family Medicine and Rural Health
    Florida State University College of Medicine
    Pensacola, FL

56. Susan Mockus Parks, MD
    Associate Professor and Director
    Geriatric Fellowship
    Division of Geriatric Medicine
    Department of Family Medicine
    Thomas Jefferson University
    Philadelphia, PA

    Laraine Winter, PhD
    Assistant Professor and Assistant Director
    Center for Applied Research on Aging and Health
    Thomas Jefferson University
    Philadelphia, PA

57. Jeanette Koran, BS, RN
    Quality Review Nurse
    Department of Health Policy
    Thomas Jefferson University
    Philadelphia, PA

    Amy Talati, PharmD
    Manager
    Oncology Strategic Analysis and Planning
    Cephalon, Inc.
    Frazer, PA

    Albert G. Crawford, PhD, MBA, MSIS
    Assistant Professor
    Department of Health Policy
    Thomas Jefferson University
    Philadelphia, PA

58. Peter Hollmann, MD
    Senior Medical Director
    Blue Cross and Blue Shield of RI
    Providence, RI

59. David J. Doukas, MD
    William Ray Moore Endowed Chair of Family Medicine
        and Medical Humanism
    Professor
    Department of Family Medicine and Geriatrics
    University of Louisville
    Louisville, KY

Laurence B. McCullough, PhD
Professor of Medicine and Medical Ethics
Center for Medical Ethics and Health Policy
Baylor College of Medicine
Houston, TX

Stephen S. Hanson, PhD
University of Louisville
Medical Center One
Louisville, KY

60. Brooke E. Salzman, MD
Assistant Professor
Division of Geriatric Medicine
Department of Family and Community Medicine

Thomas Jefferson University
Philadelphia, PA

Danielle Snyderman, MD
Instructor
Department of Family and Community Medicine
Jefferson Medical College
Thomas Jefferson University
Philadelphia, PA

Robert Perkel, MD
Professor
Department of Family and Community Medicine
Jefferson Medical College
Philadelphia, PA

ACKNOWLEDGMENTS

We would like to thank our family members and colleagues, without whose support this book would not have been possible. Special thanks to:

My husband, David Arenson, and children, Jacob and Rebecca, whose patience and support are boundless, and Catherine Mills, whose assistance in preparing this manuscript was priceless.

Christine Arenson

Delia Fleet, the grandmother who taught me that love and service are inextricably connected.

Ken Brummel-Smith

Dr. George Caransos, outstanding clinician, mentor, and friend.

Jan Busby-Whitehead

Dr. Sidney Katz, mentor, friend, and advocate.

James G. O'Brien

Dr. Edna Stilwell, pioneer in gerontological nursing.

Mary H. Palmer

Thanks also to Nat Russo, Marc Strauss, and Shelby Peak at Cambridge University Press and Larry Fox at Aptara for their advocacy and expertise in bringing this edition to fruition.

Finally, we want to thank our dear friend, William Reichel, MD. Dr. Reichel, Editor Emeritus of this text, has championed better care of older adults throughout his career. We are grateful for his wisdom, mentorship, and support. Thanks, Bill!

1

ESSENTIAL PRINCIPLES IN THE CARE OF THE ELDERLY

William Reichel, MD, Christine Arenson, MD, Joseph E. Scherger, MD, MPH

The world is aging. Already in 2003, the US Census Bureau reported that 35.9 million persons in the United States were 65 years or older, 12% of the population.[1] The first baby boomers turn 65 years old in 2011, and the next 25 years will witness the most rapid increase in the number of older adults. The oldest of the old, those aged 85 years and older, are the fastest-growing segment of the American population. This, coupled with further advances in chronic disease management, diffusion of "best practices," increased attention to maintaining physical, cognitive, and psychological function, and availability of improved treatments for the most common causes of death and disability, is likely to continue to extend both the average life expectancy and years of active life. Increasing awareness of persistent inequalities in our health care system, a decreasing ratio of working adults to support dependent children and retirees, and an increasing burden on family caregivers are just some of the countervailing forces that continue to limit the promise of healthy, productive aging.

We certainly want good health care waiting for us in our golden years, but what is good care? In the care of the elderly patient, there are 11 essential principles that should be considered: 1) the role of the physician as the integrator of the biopsychosocial–spiritual model; 2) continuity of care; 3) bolstering the family and home; 4) good communication skills; 5) building a sound doctor–patient relationship; 6) the need for appropriate evaluation and assessment; 7) prevention and health maintenance; 8) intelligent treatment with attention to ethical decision making; 9) interprofessional collaboration; 10) respect for the usefulness and value of the aged individual; and 11) compassionate care. These essentials are closely related to the six health system redesign imperatives identified by the Institute of Medicine in its landmark 2001 report, Crossing the Quality Chasm.[2] The embodiment of these eleven principles represents a standard of excellence to which we can all aspire.

THE PHYSICIAN AS INTEGRATOR OF THE BIOPSYCHOSOCIAL-SPIRITUAL MODEL

As medical care becomes more complex and specialized and relies more on technology, good care requires having a physician who provides leadership in the integration and coordination of the health care of the elderly patient. The current generation of older adults has witnessed amazing advances in research and great accomplishments in diagnostic and curative medicine, but, today, we are realizing that scientific reductionism is not enough. The reforms in medical education, care, and research over the past century have too often resulted in fragmentation of medical thought and care. It is imperative that the health care professional responsible for the care of older adults keep the "big picture" firmly in mind – we must never forget that the patient is so much more than the sum of his or her organ systems.[3,4]

Society is calling out for a physician with a commitment to the person and not just to a specific disease state or mechanism. The person is usually part of a family and a larger community, but, sadly, there are some elders who have no family and are isolated from the community. The first essential for the physician who cares for an elder is to act as an integrator of the biopsychosocial and, one can add, spiritual, model. To accomplish this, the physician must know the patient thoroughly. This is not to denigrate the excellence of the specialties and subspecialties that have achieved much over the past few decades. The ideal model of health care, however, will exist when the patient is seen not from a single specialty point of view but with the full appreciation of other organ systems, emotional or psychosocial factors, information based on the continuity of care over time, and knowledge of the patient's family and community.

Recent position statements of the Future of Family Medicine,[5] American Geriatrics Society,[6] and Society of General Internal Medicine[7] have all recognized this increasing fragmentation, and the resultant public demand for a rational, humanistic approach to care, especially of the older adult. All of these organizations and others have called for a system of primary care that provides a continuous, caring relationship and establishes a "medical home" in which patients can obtain the majority of their health care needs.[8] The primary care provider also must ensure the coordination, supervision, and interpretation that is vital for the older patient to navigate a complex system that often provides conflicting recommendations and in which the vested self-interest of the "system" is not always secondary to the needs of the individual patient. The primary physician, then, acts as advocate to obtain needed services, but also as advisor and confidant. At times, the best advice is to avoid tests or treatments that have little or no potential benefit but significant potential to harm. Perhaps most important, this physician will come to know the patient as an individual, within a family and a community, with particular values, beliefs, and priorities. Thus, the physician comes to serve as interpreter and integrator, helping the patient to obtain health care that is most consistent with his or her own preferences and needs. This role will most often be played by a family physician, general internist, geriatrician, or nurse practitioner. For some patients, it may be a trusted oncologist, cardiologist, or other specialist. The key factors are the interest and ability to see the patient as a whole person, not simply as the sum of his or her organ systems, and the clinician's time and expertise to serve in this critical role.

We can expect more evidence to accumulate in a wide variety of areas that will illustrate the relationship of the biological, psychological, social, and spiritual components in human problems. Clinical distrust, chronic stress, and depression have been linked with increased inflammatory markers that may result in higher rates of cardiovascular disease.[9] There is now overwhelming evidence that depression coexisting with diabetes leads to poor outcomes.[10] One study has demonstrated that social support may have a protective effect with respect to interleukin-6 elevation, and, thus, could potentially result in a survival benefit in patients with ovarian cancer.[11] We have much to learn about the dynamic relationships among wellness and disease, psychosocial factors, and the spiritual state. The practicing clinician is aware of the higher mortality in the first year of widowhood, more pronounced in the surviving widower than in the widow, and the higher morbidity and mortality seen in the elderly after a relocation has occurred.[12]

CONTINUITY OF CARE

The ideal situation may indeed be a warm and supportive relationship with the same personal physician serving as advisor, advocate, and friend as the patient moves through the labyrinth of medical care. The realities of today's complex medical environment, however, with the patient moving between office, home, hospital, specialized care units (coronary care units, intensive care units, stroke units, or oncology centers), nurs-

ing home, and hospice care, often make this ideal impossible. In fact, in many instances, patients receive the best care from physicians and other health professionals who focus their practice in these specialized environments. The medical intensivist provides the most up-to-date, skilled care in the intensive care unit; the physician in regular nursing home practice will be more available to patients, staff, and families than the one who has a few nursing home patients scattered among several facilities.

The failure of physicians to make visits as necessary in the home and in long-term care facilities is related to several factors in the United States, including training, physician attitudes, and reimbursement systems. Our medical schools and residencies for generalist physicians continue to struggle with incorporating excellence in house calls and nursing home care as part of their educational program. Although reimbursements for visits to the home and nursing home have generally improved in recent years, high office overhead and productivity expectations have continued to limit the ability of physicians to practice in these relatively time-inefficient sites. Physician attitudes have also been a problem, in that doctors in the health care system of the past few decades have been more interested in the acute aspects of care than in chronic and long-term care. These attitudes have been reinforced by the educational and reimbursement systems in place. We are just beginning to see research and education initiatives designed to address the gap in chronic care knowledge and attitudes of our students and residents.[13,14]

Nevertheless, continuity of care remains an essential principle in the care of the older patient.[15] Recently, a wealth of literature documenting the critical importance of adequate communication among health professionals around transitions in care[16,17] lends support to the notion that safe, effective, efficient, and patient-centered care can only occur when the in-depth knowledge and understanding of the personal physician is communicated to, and incorporated by, the specialized teams in the intensive care unit, general hospital setting, long-term care setting, and even hospice setting.

We must recognize that optimum health care can only be provided to the older adult by an ever-expanding team of professionals, including primary care and specialty physicians, hospitalists, nurses, therapists, and social workers. This does not mean we can abandon the concept of continuity. Rather, we must pay even more attention. Physicians, nurse practitioners, and others with a long-term relationship with a patient may remain active advocates and sounding boards, even when they are not the "provider of record" at a given time. Equally important, indeed critical, to the safety of patients is increased attention to continuity at transition points in the care of the older patient – from home to hospital, from hospital to rehab unit or nursing home. The physician responsible for the care of patients at each of these junctures must communicate fully and accurately with the patient, family, and receiving health care team to ensure that the patient's treatment plan, values, expectations, and preferences are known and honored at every step.

BOLSTERING FAMILY AND HOME

Every physician should enlist those means that would keep an elderly person either in the individual's own home or in an extended family setting. It should certainly be our goal to keep elderly persons functioning independently, preserving their lifestyles and self-respect as long as possible. The physician should use the prescription for a nursing home as specifically as a prescription for an antibiotic or an antihypertensive medication.

A number of forces have resulted in patients going to institutional settings when other alternatives might have been possible. Between 1960 and 1975, a massive push toward institutionalization took place, creating hundreds of thousands of nursing home beds. What are the forces that contributed to excessive institutional care? Funding mechanisms have been disproportionately directed toward reimbursement for institutional care rather than for other alternatives. With the increase in mobility of families, there simply may not be family members available in the community to participate in the elderly person's care. Homes are architecturally based on a small nuclear family and do not permit housing of an elderly patient. Finally, the movement of women into the work force has meant that fewer family members are available to remain home with the impaired or disabled elderly person. Despite these forces, rates of institutionalization have actually declined slightly in recent years; older adults and their families overcome amazing obstacles to keep loved ones at home whenever possible.

What alternative can the physician recommend to these caregivers? A simple list includes homemakers, home health aides, other types of home care, daycare, aftercare, specialized housing settings, visiting nurses, friendly visitors, foster home care, chore services, home renovation and repair services, congregate and home-delivered meal programs, transportation programs, and shopping services. Personal physicians should also understand and use legal and protective services for the elderly whenever indicated.

Publicly financed programs such as the Program for All Inclusive Care of the Elderly and home-based Medicaid waiver programs that support nursing home–eligible elders to remain in their homes have grown in recent years, as federal and state governments have recognized that supporting seniors' desire to stay in their own homes is not only better, but is actually less-expensive care.[18] States have explored options to provide services in the homes of nursing home–eligible patients through a combination of Medical Assistance waivers and other programs. In addition, a growing body of research demonstrates the benefits of home-based interventions that target patient and caregiver priorities and teach problem-solving skills to maintain physically frail[19] and demented[20] individuals in their homes.

Despite the pressure to contain institutional long-term care costs, funds have not been available for adequate expansion of publicly funded programs to support frail older adults in their own home. Further, many of the evidence-based interventions that might provide cost-effective strategies for supporting older persons in the community are not reimbursed by insurance. Thus, resources remain limited and disjointed. The role of health care providers is to facilitate referrals, coordinate services, and become knowledgeable about general resources available and appropriate referral sources (i.e., care manager, area agency on aging) with expertise to help patients and families navigate the system effectively.

Who are the caregivers in American society? Data from 2005[21] revealed that a majority (57%) of Americans are currently or have been in the past unpaid caregivers for an adult family member or friend. In 2005, 46 million Americans were actively providing care. Caregivers are a diverse group, with up to 44% of men in one recent survey. Nearly half (42%) are between the ages of 45 and 64 years, and 17% are aged 65 years and older. Caregivers provide an average of 21 hours of care per week, with 17% reporting 40 or more hours weekly. Many experience a significantly negative impact on their job performance, with up to $650,000 in wages, Social Security benefits, and pensions lost over a career as a caregiver. Family caregivers also experience negative health impacts, with nearly half of those caring for a person with dementia experiencing depression, 64% rating their emotional stress as 4 to 5 out of 5, and older spouses who are caregivers experiencing a 63% higher mortality risk than control subjects.

Many families feel the burden of caregiving today, sandwiched between the demands of their parents and their children and grandchildren. It has been said that the empty nest syndrome has been replaced by a crowded nest syndrome. Many caregivers experience extreme burden and stress, and sometimes the question is, who is the real patient – the patient or the caregiver? The physician will often see the caregiver who is in more distress than the patient, and who may, in fact, develop serious physical and emotional problems as a result of the burden and stress encountered.[22,23]

The belief that old people are rejected by their families is a much-exploited social myth. Many families are struggling to cope with the needs of parents who are frail and debilitated. The family member, friend, or neighbor is often the crucial link in guaranteeing that the dependent elder remains in the community. In repeated studies, the characteristics of the caregiver, more than those of the elderly patient, are essential in predicting institutional placement. Even when adult children and elderly parents are separated by distance, the quality of their relationship may be unaffected, maintaining cohesion despite limited face-to-face contact.

COMMUNICATION SKILLS

Specific communication skills are critical in good management of the care of the elderly patient. Most important in good communication is listening and allowing patients to express themselves. The physician should use an open-ended approach, interpreting what the patient is saying and reading between the lines. The physician can use intuition in deciding what the patient means. Why did the patient really come to see the physician? The elderly patient complaining of headache or backache may be expressing depression or grief. We should not miss important verbal clues when the patient tells us, "Doctor, I really think these headaches started when I lost my husband."

It is helpful to leave the door open for other questions or comments by the patient, both at the conclusion of the visit and in the future. It is always helpful to ask: "Are there other questions or concerns that you have at this time?" A physician anticipating a specific problem can make it easier for the patient to discuss this issue. For example, "You are doing well, but I know that you are concerned about your arthritis and whether you will be able to climb the stairs in your home. At some point, we may want to discuss the various alternatives that are open to you."

One important aspect of the aging of America is the increasing diversity of older adults.[1] In the past, white English-speaking individuals have comprised the majority of our older population. Increasingly, however, health care providers will need to be prepared to care for a racially, ethnically, and linguistically diverse population of elders. Physicians and other professionals caring for older patients will need to provide culturally sensitive care, recognizing the unique and varied cultural contexts of their patients. Further, groups, including the federal government, have recognized the critical role of health translators to provide appropriate care to patients who are not proficient in English. All of these issues may be magnified in the care of older patients.

Just as the physician providing care to pediatric patients must deal with the children's parents, the physician providing care to the elderly patient must be able to deal with their adult children. These children play a vital role in decision making and providing support, and the physician must, therefore, possess skills in communicating with them and in dealing with their emotional reactions, such as guilt or grief. The physician taking care of an elderly patient with cancer must be prepared when the adult daughter tells him: "Whatever you do, please do not tell my father that he has cancer," especially when it is apparent that the parent is totally and fully aware of all aspects of his problem.

The physician should be careful when meeting with an elderly patient who discusses his absent spouse or child, or when dealing with adult children or grandchildren who are discussing the parent or grandparent who is not present. The physician should not necessarily accept the assumptions that are stated about the absent family member. Physicians must be able to listen carefully, ask questions, and collect information; their opinion of the situation might be entirely different if they had an opportunity to hear the view of the absent family member.

Peabody[24] in 1927 said, "The good physician knows his patients through and through, and his knowledge is bought dearly. Time, sympathy and understanding must be lavishly dispensed, but the reward is to be found in that personal bond that forms the greatest satisfaction of the practice of medicine." The

physician who enters the patient's universe and understands the patient's perceptions, assumptions, values, and religious beliefs is a tremendous advantage. Frankl,[25] in *Man's Search for Meaning*, demonstrated how physicians can help patients understand the meaning and value of their lives. Of course, how elders find meaning in their lives is related to how they found meaning at other stages in their lives. It is therapeutic for the patient to feel that the physician cares enough about that individual to understand his life, particularly the meaning and purpose of his present existence. Frankl[26] stated in *The Doctor and the Soul* that human life can be fulfilled not only by creating and enjoying, but also by suffering. He provides examples in which suffering becomes an opportunity for growth, an achievement, a means for ennoblement. Frankl's existential psychiatry or logotherapy is a useful psychological method that helps the elderly patient appreciate the positive attributes, meanings, and purposes of his or her life.

Yalom[27] defines existential psychotherapy as "a dynamic approach to therapy which focuses on concerns that are rooted in the individual's existence." Many individuals are tormented by a crisis of meaning.[28] Many suffer an existential vacuum, experiencing a lack of meaning in life.[25–29] The patient experiencing an existential vacuum may demonstrate many symptoms that will rush in to fill it in the form of somatization, depression, alcoholism, and hypochondriasis. The physician recognizing an existential vacuum can help the patient find meaning. Frankl's main theme is that meaning is essential for life. Engagement or involvement in life's activities is a therapeutic answer to a lack of meaning in life. The physician can help guide the patient toward engagement with life, life's activities, other people, and other satisfactions.

Frankl[25,26] provides advice to all physicians in using hope as a therapeutic tool. The physician dealing with the elderly must focus on the significant role of hope in daily practice. As physicians, we must eventually understand the biological basis of hope. We do not understand sufficiently the biochemical, neurophysiological, and immunological concomitants of different attitudes and emotions and how they are affected by what is communicated from the physician. Physicians may worsen panic and fear; however, physicians also have an opportunity to create a state of confidence, calm, relaxation, and hope.

In this age of increasing technology and subspecialization, the patient's recovery may still depend on the physician's ability to reduce panic and fear and to raise the prospect of hope. Cousins[30] describes the "quality beyond pure medical competence that patients need and look for in their physicians. They want reassurance. They want to be looked after and not just over. They want to be listened to. They want to feel that it makes a difference to the physician, a very big difference, whether they live or die. They want to feel that they are in the physician's thoughts." For example, in building the doctor–elderly patient relationship, nothing is more effective than the physician picking up the phone and calling the patient and saying: "I was thinking about your problem. How are you doing?" This expression of interest by telephone represents a potent method for cementing the relationship between doctor and patient.

Jules Pfeiffer's cartoon character, the "modern Diogenes," carries on the following discourse upon meeting an inquisitive fellow traveler through the sands of time.

> "What are you doing with the lantern?" asks the traveler.
> "I'm searching," replies Diogenes.
> "For an honest man?" he asks.
> "I gave that up long ago!" exclaims Diogenes.
> "For hope?"
> "Lots of luck."
> "For love?"
> "Forget it!"
> "For tranquility?"
> "No way."
> "For happiness?"
> "Fat chance."
> "For justice?"
> "Are you kidding?"
> "Then what are you looking for?" he implores of Diogenes.
> "Someone to talk to."

Help comes from feeling that one has been heard and understood.[31]

DOCTOR–PATIENT RELATIONSHIP

What the Doctor and Patient Bring to Each Encounter

The physician must understand what both he or she and the patient bring to each interaction, including both positive and negative feelings. The patient's views of old age may be negative and fearful, believing illness signifies misery, approaching death, loss of self-esteem, loneliness, and dependency. The physician's own fears about aging and death may color the interview as well. The doctor may simply not view helping the older, impaired patient as worthwhile. The physician may have low expectations for success of treatment, writing off the elderly patient as "senile," "mentally ill," or "a hypochondriac." The doctor may have significant conflicts in his or her own relationship with parent figures or may feel threatened that the patient will die.

KNOWING THE PATIENT

Several steps are recommended in building a sound doctor–patient relationship, particularly applicable to the elderly patient.[24] The first rule is that the physician should know the patient thoroughly; the second rule is that the physician should know the patient thoroughly; and the third rule is that the physician should know the patient thoroughly. The interested physician performs the first step in building a sound doctor–patient relationship by gathering a complete history, including the personal and social history, and doing a complete physical. Ideally, the physician should be a good listener, warm and sensitive, providing the patient ample opportunity to express multiple problems and reflect on his or her life history and current life situation. Thus, the physician will be able to understand the meanings and purposes of the patient's present existence. Forces in the health care industry oftentimes prevent the physician from being a good listener, warm, and sensitive. The physician may not be listening as he or she is inputting information into an electronic health record system. The physician sadly may not be present for his or her patient.[32]

As stated previously, family and friends represent the principal support system for the elderly and usually call for nursing home placement only as a last resort, after all alternatives have failed; however, the physician must be able to recognize the dysfunctional family. There are elderly who have been rejected by children. There are elderly who have rejected a child for a variety of reasons, such as the adult child's same-sex relationship. There are families with members estranged from each other for many years. The patient may have had a stable and supportive marriage, but increasingly the rate of divorce has risen. Older adults may have relationships outside of marriage, including same-sex relationships. It is critical for the practitioner to have an accurate understanding of family dynamics and history to appropriately rally family support, and also to recognize when family dysfunction is harming their patient.

CREATING A PARTNERSHIP WITH THE PATIENT

In all dealings with the patient, the physician should be frank and honest and share information truthfully. The patient should feel a sense of partnership with the physician. In this partnership, the doctor first reviews his perception of the patient's problems. Then, for each problem, alternative choices are considered, and decision making is shared with the patient. Although there are situations in which frankness is counterproductive, with most patients, frankness is helpful. There are also situations in which the elderly patient does not want to share in decision making, but simply wants to surrender his or her autonomy to a relative such as a spouse or adult child, or to the physician. Again, in most cases, the physician should attempt to enter a partnership with the patient and share as much decision making as possible.

Discussions with the patient or family members should be presented in a hopeful manner. As discussed previously, it is important to offer a positive approach whenever possible. The physician's infusion of optimism and cheerfulness is therapeutic. The physician should help patients appreciate such positive attributes or purposes in their lives as religious beliefs, relationships with children and grandchildren, the enjoyment of friends, or the enjoyment of the relationship with doctors, nurses, and other health professionals in the immediate therapeutic environment.

The physician should be cautious that discussions with family members be held with the patient's consent. If the patient is sufficiently mentally impaired, then it might be appropriate to deal with the closest relative. Complex ethical and legal questions arise in the matter of confidentiality and decision making in regard to the elderly patient with partial mental impairment.

NEED FOR THOROUGH EVALUATION AND ASSESSMENT

The physician must avoid prejudging the patient. We must not allow preconceived notions of common patterns of illness to preclude the most careful individualized assessment of each patient. Conscientious history-taking and physical examination are essential. Treatment choices should be considered only following a thorough evaluation. Judicious consideration of all factors may result in a decision to treat or not to treat certain problems in certain patients. Attention to lesser problems may be postponed according to the priorities of the moment, rather than complicate an already complex therapeutic program.

Physicians must avoid wastebasket diagnoses. The past concept of "chronic brain syndrome" or "arteriosclerotic brain disease" is one such example. Not all mental disturbance in the elderly represents dementia; not all dementias in the elderly are arteriosclerotic. Neuropsychiatric disturbance in the elderly might be placed into a wastebasket and casually accepted as both expectable and untreatable when, in reality, a very treatable cause may be present. The physician must consider and seek out treatable disease.

For example, neuropsychiatric disturbance, including a dementia syndrome, may be caused by severe depression, which is a very treatable disorder. The most common types of dementia include Alzheimer's disease and vascular dementia. Other forms of dementia, potentially reversible, include myxedema, chronic drug intoxication, pernicious anemia, and chronic subdural hematoma. Neuropsychiatric disturbance may also include delirium secondary to many types of medical illness or drug toxicity. Such delirious states can be helped if the primary disorder is recognized and treated; failure to do so may in fact lead to hastened death of the patient.

It is often difficult to disentangle the physical from the emotional. Emotional disorder may present in the elderly as a physical problem, such as musculoskeletal tension being the principal manifestation of depression. Conversely, physical disease in the elderly might present as a mental disorder with confusion, disorientation, or delirium often being the first sign of many common medical ailments including myocardial infarction, pulmonary embolism, occult cancer, pneumonia, urinary tract infection, or dehydration (Table 1.1). For this reason, it cannot be emphasized too many times that proper diagnosis is essential to make specific treatment plans, such as the treatment of urinary tract infection in the case of an acute delirious state, or the treatment of thyroid deficiency in the case of a specific dementia or in the treatment of depression. Each of these is

Table 1.1. Characteristics of Elderly Patients

1. Physical disease might present as a mental disorder with confusion, disorientation, or delirium often being the first sign of many common medical ailments.

2. Functional or physiological capacities are diminished, for example, creatinine clearance declines with age; however, the rate of physiological decline varies between individuals.

3. Adverse effects of drugs are more pronounced and more likely.

4. Typical signs and symptoms of disease may be hidden or slight, for example, pain may be absent in myocardial infarction, fever may be minimal in pneumonia.

5. Multiple organic, psychological, and social problems are present.

very specific. Treatment in each case would be irrational if a specific diagnosis were not known.

It is often not sufficient to know the organic or anatomical or psychiatric diagnosis; rather, we should seek a more complete understanding of the elderly patient. At times, it is more important to assess the elderly patient's functional status, which might have greater significance than the diagnostic or anatomical label. For example, in the case of a cerebrovascular accident, knowledge of the precise anatomical lesion via magnetic resonance imaging angiography may not help the patient as much as understanding the patient's functional state. It may be more important to know whether the patient can walk or climb stairs, can handle his or her own bathing, eating, and dressing, whether he or she can get out of bed and sit in a chair, handle a wheelchair, or whether he or she requires a cane or walker. All these functional concerns must be considered in evaluating an elderly patient.

Affecting our diagnostic thinking in evaluating an elderly patient would be the consideration of what is physiological versus what is pathological. Aging itself can be defined as the progressive deterioration or loss of functional capacity that takes place in an organism after a period of reproductive maturity (Table 1.1). The Baltimore Longitudinal Study of Aging, since 1958, has studied this decline in each of several specific functional capacities, such as glucose tolerance and creatinine clearance. There is a progressive deterioration of glucose tolerance with each decade of life. Indeed, hyperglycemia is so common in the elderly that to avoid labeling a disquietly high proportion of people as diabetics, Elahi et al.[33] formulated a percentile system that ranks a subject with age-matched cohorts. (Some individuals, however, show no evidence of deterioration of glucose tolerance or insulin sensitivity with aging.) Although currently the accepted definitions allow the same diagnostic criteria to be applied at any age, it is recognized that treatment decisions must be individualized, especially for the frail or very old.[34] The rate of decline in creatinine clearance also accelerates with advancing age.[35] This phenomenon appears to represent true renal aging because it was seen in several hundred normal individuals who were free of specific diseases and not taking medications that might alter glomerular filtration rate.

In fact, two major conclusions from the Baltimore Longitudinal Study of Aging emerge. Even when specific functional capacities change with age, health problems need not be a consequence of aging. Many of the most common disorders of old age result from pathological processes and not from normal aging. The second important finding is that no single chronological timetable of normal aging exists. Even within one individual, the physiological capacities of organs show aging at different rates. Between individuals, more difference is noted in older people than in younger people.

Increased adverse effects of drugs are present in the elderly who often tolerate medications poorly (Table 1.1). Polypharmacy is a major problem in the care of the elderly patient. Not only do psychotropic medications cause an altered response of the central nervous system resulting in confusion and delirium, but also antibiotics or digitalis may cause these problems. Altered renal and hepatic functions may affect drug elimination. In general, the elderly demonstrate greater variability and idiosyncrasy in drug response in comparison to younger individuals.

Prudence is, therefore, extremely important in prescribing drugs for the elderly individual. The physician must determine if the patient's complaint is justification for treatment. Is this medication absolutely necessary? The skill of the physician is required in weighing benefit versus risk. The benefit–risk balance is more crucial in the elderly patient than in younger individuals. The physician must attempt to keep the total number of medications down to as small a number as possible. Tools such as the Beers Criteria for Potentially Inappropriate Medications in the Elderly[36] are available to assist the clinician.

Also affecting our diagnostic ability in the elderly is that signs and symptoms of disease in the aged may be slight or hidden. Pain, white blood cell response, and fever and chills are examples of defense mechanisms that may be diminished in older persons (Table 1.1). The aged person may have pneumonia or renal infection without chills or a rise in temperature. Myocardial infarction, ruptured abdominal aorta, perforated appendix, or mesenteric infarction may be present without pain in the elderly.[37]

Multiple clinical, psychological, and social problems (Table 1.1) are characteristic of the elderly.[37] Clinically and pathologically, an elderly patient may have 10 or 15 problems. Geriatric patients should benefit from the use of a problem-oriented approach to medical records. Medical records should include not only the medical problem, but should demonstrate an understanding of functional, psychological, social, and family problems as well. The key feature of the problem-oriented record is the problem list, which serves as a table of contents of the patient's total medical history. It behooves us to use a problem list as a minimal or core component of a problem-oriented system in caring for the elderly patient. Without a problem list, we can easily lose track over time of the elderly patient's multiple problems; for example, that the patient in 1975 was hospitalized for a psychiatric problem or that, in 1995, the patient suffered a compression fracture of the T-10 vertebra secondary to slipping on ice. These problems may be lost to memory without some form or problem-oriented system. In addition, care is enhanced by maintaining a medication list that is kept current at each patient visit.

PREVENTION AND HEALTH MAINTENANCE

A tremendous revolution is taking place in the United States with emphasis on prevention, health maintenance, and wellness. Unfortunately, the data for what constitutes the best care for the frail or extremely old is sparse, and clinicians must often make their best judgment, taking into consideration the wishes of the patient and family and extrapolating from evidence developed for younger patients. For example, less is known about primary and secondary prevention of heart disease and stroke for the elderly patient than for younger adults. Clinicians caring for these patients need to be prepared to discuss the relative risks and benefits of screening tests and preventive medicine in the context of the patient's overall health status and preferences.

More and more physicians and nurses are emphasizing health maintenance and wellness in their practice and in their community educational programs. The drive for wellness is coming not only from health professionals but also from the public itself. The personal physician has an opportunity in his practice to encourage preventive medicine and health maintenance at every age level and at each level of functional ability or disability.

A remarkable amount of new information is being discovered about the role of exercise and strength training in the prevention or reversibility of frailty and physiological decline.[38] It is expected that more will be learned and that the health of many elderly might be improved by exercise and physical activity. The next decade will see more advances in nutrition, exercise, and therapeutic measures to retard the aging process.

How do physicians and health professionals determine the standard for health screening and health promotion? The Guide to Clinical Preventive Services[39] represents one standard for health screening guidelines. Evidence for screening and prevention in older adults is still often lacking, or controversial. For instance, the Guide continues to conclude that there is insufficient evidence to recommend for or against screening for prostate cancer, in spite of clear recommendations to screen from the American Cancer Society and others. It is clear that each practicing physician will have to follow the medical literature and evaluate the algorithms and guidelines that unfold in the decade ahead. For each question, the evidence is being examined and reexamined.

We can expect that in each area of health screening and health promotion, guidelines will not be written in stone, but will be reconsidered and reevaluated in the years ahead, based on the evidence that is examined. Physicians and health professionals caring for the elderly will witness tension and debate as new guidelines are written. At any time, with the state of evidence-based knowledge that we do have in preventive medicine and health screening, there remains the differential between the physician's intellectual acceptance and awareness of these guidelines and the actual use of these guidelines on a regular, consistent basis. Increasingly, geriatric practice will rely on technology, such as electronic health records to ensure consistent application of prevention and wellness guidelines. Adoption of quality improvement strategies to provide consistent practice will continue to be driven both by the demands of our patients and, increasingly, the use of pay for performance strategies by insurers including Medicare.

INTELLIGENT TREATMENT WITH ATTENTION TO ETHICAL DECISION MAKING

The doctor should resist the temptation to treat a new problem that is poorly understood with still more medications. The question should be raised whether the present symptoms, such as confusion or depression, might be related to current drug use.

Therefore, the aphorism, "First, do no harm." A similar concept was stated by Seegal[40] as the "principle of minimal interference" in the management of the elderly patient. "First, do no harm" and the "principle of minimal interference" should be remembered when one reviews the abundant examples of iatrogenic problems that the elderly experience.[41,42]

The principle of minimal interference can be applied not only to drug therapy but also to other decisions, including the use of diagnostic tests (the principle of diagnostic parsimony), surgical intervention, and decision making in regard to hospitalization or placement in a long-term care facility. The principle of minimal interference may result in decisions that are both humanistic and cost-effective; for example, a decision that the patient should remain in his or her own home, despite limited access to medical therapy, rather than reside in a long-term care facility; or the decision not to do a gastrointestinal workup in the evaluation of anemia when the patient is terminal as a result of malignant brain tumor.

In the care of the elderly, there are times for minimal interference and there are times for maximal intervention. Again, certainly the patient with dementia caused by myxedema deserves every effort to replace the thyroid hormone carefully. The elderly patient with severe congestive heart failure secondary to rheumatic or congenital heart disease deserves full consideration for definitive treatment, including surgery, for his cardiac problems. The elderly patient with depression deserves specific treatment for this very treatable disorder.

In the future, we will be faced with more and more difficult decisions of an ethical nature. For example, an 80-year-old gentleman may present with a history of resection of an abdominal aneurysm 15 years ago, multiple myocardial infarctions, and multiple strokes causing severe dementia. His main problem on the current hospitalization is pneumonia causing a worsening of his confused state. Because of periods of sinus arrest, a pacemaker is considered. Should a pacemaker be placed in patients with significant dementia? Should pneumonia be treated in patients with severe dementia or terminal carcinoma? Difficult and ambiguous clinical problems such as these will face the personal physician with increasing frequency. The physician in the future will be called on to make complex decisions according to the accepted traditions and values of the specific religion, nation, and society or culture, with major guidance from the patient's stated wishes that were affirmed at a time when the patient was fully competent.

In regard to all therapeutic decisions, a personal physician is at an advantage if his or her understanding of the patient is based on continuity of care. The physician then can consider the patient in totality including psychological, spiritual, social, family, and environmental factors. To recommend intelligently any treatment plan, it is beneficial to have the knowledge of home or institutional environment, the family constellation, the availability of friends, access to transportation, and the economic situation of the patient. Also, as the physician grapples with complex decisions of an ethical nature, specific knowledge of the patient's value systems and beliefs is critically important.

INTERPROFESSIONAL COLLABORATION

The physician must understand when to call on other health professionals, such as nutrition education, visiting home nurses, social workers, psychologists, or representatives of community agencies. One must know when to call for legal or financial counseling. All physicians would do well to work in closer harmony with the patient's or family's clergy or pastor.

The physician should know when to recommend specific rehabilitative therapies. Specific use of physical, occupational, recreational, and speech therapies are vital for the proper care of certain problems. For example, the elderly patient with diabetic neuropathy and flapping gait might benefit from bilateral leg braces. Another patient recovering from stroke might benefit from occupational therapy that should be used as a reintroduction of the patient to the activities of normal daily living, and not simply as a recreational or diversionary therapy.

The improvement in health care of the chronically ill elderly requires that health professionals work together for the best interest of the patient. What is required is a genuine collaborative effort to act in a unified fashion to bring about a system that will best meet the needs of the frail elderly. This collaboration will be even more important as more community-based, long-term care options involving home care, home hospice care, and other services, and as care of patients with multiple, complex comorbidities becomes the norm.

RESPECT FOR THE USEFULNESS AND VALUE OF THE AGED INDIVIDUAL

Much in our society works to reject or devalue the aged. We are certainly living in a youth-oriented era and a physician must guard against viewing the elderly as useless, insignificant, or worthless. This lack of respect and devaluation occurs in society at large, in the workplace, in the family, in the entertainment media, but it should not occur in the doctor's office or other clinical settings. The anthropologist knows other cultures and societies in which the elders of the community are most valued. An hour of watching American television is instructive to witness the youth orientation of our society. It is unfortunate that many elderly patients report that previous physicians treated them poorly because the patient was old.

An exceptional book, although not actively directed to the elderly, is *Respectful Treatment: A Practical Handbook of Patient Care.*[43] The author, Martin Lipp, describes the therapeutic benefit of respect in the doctor–patient relationship, especially in dealing with those we consider problem patients: In the angry patient; the dependent, passive patient; the complaining, demanding patient; the denying patient; the overly affectionate patient; the mentally ill patient; and so on, respect is therapeutic. Many patients feel weak, vulnerable, and demonstrate low self-esteem by virtue of age, illness, and various psychological and personality factors. Respect is a message to the patient that quickly brings about a sounder doctor–patient relationship.

Discussions are held on the subject of calling patients, and elderly patients in particular, by their first name or by their last name proceeded by Mr., Mrs., or Ms. An immediate demonstration of respect is to call the elderly patient by their family name with Mr., Mrs., or Ms. used appropriately.

The next 20 years will see considerable social change with redefinition of the age for retirement and other entitlement plans. We hope that social and economic changes will allow the elderly to function as a continuing resource in our society. We can expect to see reduced restrictions on older workers with particular reference to mandatory retirement. We can also expect to see more educational programs that will provide skilled training, job counseling, and placement for older men and women to initiate, enhance, and continue their voluntary participation in the workforce. We should anticipate the breakdown of stereotypes and greater recognition of the value of the elderly as a human resource.

There are many social forces at play. In 1930, 54% of men aged 65 years and older were in the work force. Then in 1960, 31% were working. Compare this to 2003 when 18.6% of men and 10.6% of women were working. Interestingly, participation in the workforce by men aged 65 years and older had declined steadily from the 1950s through the 1980s, because of improved pension and Social Security benefits. Participation leveled off in the 1990s, and has actually increased slightly since 1993. Meanwhile, women aged 65 years and older have had a steady 10% employment rate since 1950. As the Baby Boomers begin to reach 65 years in 2011, it remains to be seen what decisions they will make about employment beyond the age of 65 years.[1]

Evaluation of workers aged 51–56 years in 1992 and 2004 as part of the Health and Retirement Study suggests that lower rates of retiree health insurance from employers, higher levels of educational attainment, and lower rates of defined benefit pension coverage have led significantly more workers from the 2004 cohort to expect to work past the age of 65 years, compared to the 1992 cohort.[44] Many older workers indicate that they would prefer phasing down and continuing to do some paid

work when they retire. Others approaching retirement or in retirement opt for a retirement career. There are many in good health, who have financial stability or a satisfactory pension, who would prefer to pursue a retirement career with passion. This may be part-time or full-time. The person retiring today at age 65 years or younger may enjoy a retirement career that might span 10–20 years. Society must allow elders to fulfill such roles and to retain the wisdom that has accumulated with time. At the same time, there are those approaching retirement who would not want or be able to continue employment, whether in their former role or in new roles that could be created. All of these variations need to be considered in counseling our patients.

COMPASSIONATE CARE

In an increasingly technological society, caring and compassion must be foremost in the practice of medicine. We must avoid the possible dehumanization that takes place when patients simply become subjects for study and treatment. Every year in the United States, we are seeing new accomplishments in medical technology and specialization. Computed tomography, computerized nuclear medicine, magnetic resonance imaging, positron emission tomography, organ transplants, achievements in cardiovascular surgery, achievements in hemodialysis, and achievement in intensive and critical care all have become part of our routine medical environment. In such a medical world, it is imperative that compassionate care not be lost in daily encounters between health professionals and elderly patients.

In all the great religions, various forms of a Golden Rule are stated. Many religions teach "You must love your neighbor as you do yourself," and, "What you do not want done to yourself, do not do to others." Surpassing new technical achievements and new specialized knowledge is the need to express compassion.[45] The physician's duty is "to cure sometimes, to comfort always."

Critically important is the attitude of the doctor toward the elderly patient. Is the physician willing to spend time with the patient? Is the physician willing to be involved in the chronic and long-term aspects of the patient as well as in the acute illness? Is the physician concerned with the social, psychological, and family aspects of the patient, in addition to clinical and organic aspects?

Care and compassion mean that the physician must dispense sufficient time in her encounters with elderly patients. There is evidence in one study[46] that physicians spend less time with elderly patients than with younger ones. Fifteen to 20 minutes may be minimal time to conduct a visit in the office, home, hospital or long-term care facility. A total of 1.5 hours, not necessarily in one sitting, may be required to complete an examination of a new patient, particularly in the presence of multiple complex problems. More time will be required in each encounter if the various functions of counseling, psychological support, health maintenance, and prevention are to be accomplished, in addition to making decisions about treatment and possible rehabilitation.

Examples of failure in caring and compassion include the physician who waves at the door of the patient's room; the physician who quickly resorts to psychotropic drugs in the office, rather than taking the time to listen; and the physician on teaching rounds who never sees the patient and who limits her discussion to laboratory studies or some specific, interesting aspect of the case in a nearby conference room.

The physician should be a good listener and read between the lines what the patient is saying. Often, by nonverbal means, the physician can express warmth, understanding, or sympathy. Staying close to the patient and maintaining eye contact is helpful. Sitting adjacent to the patient's bed or sitting on the edge of the bed in the hospital or long-term care facility brings the doctor right into the patient's small universe. The physician might put a hand on the patient's shoulder and pat or touch the patient or hold hands at appropriate points during the visit. As previously stated, however, the physician faced with increasing pressures, may not be present for the patient.[32]

As the revered physician, Eugene Stead, Jr., would say: "What this patient needs is a doctor."[47] Our elderly patients, and in fact, all of our patients are yearning for a physician who will listen and understand. Again, we remember Peabody's words,[24] "The good physician knows his patients through and through, and his knowledge is bought dearly. Time, sympathy, and understanding must be lavishly dispensed, but the reward is to be found in that personal bond that forms the greatest satisfaction of the practice of medicine. One of the essential qualities of the clinician is interest in humanity, where the secret of the care of the patient is in caring for the patient."

CHANGING TIMES IN HEALTH CARE

In the performance of these essential aspects of care of the elderly patient, the physician may be distraught that these are difficult times and a revolution in health care is looming. Physicians and other health professionals may feel discouraged during this period of cost-containment, evolving pay for performance rules, increased competition, the malpractice threat, and other forces in health care reform taking place today. The physician may be disheartened by a system that frequently rewards performing a procedure over talking to the patient; that excessively scrutinizes and profiles the physician in the hospital; and that may often seem to emphasize the financial bottom line rather than excellence of patient care. Despite this tug of war, the physician must simply have faith that patient care that is compassionate and humane, care that is characterized by continuity, care that is sensitive to psychosocial and family issues, and care that is characterized by all the other essential principles will endure. Although the organization of health care delivery will undoubtedly change, we can expect that society will ultimately demand a quality of care that we would each want for ourselves. The authors can visualize that social pressure will enforce the maintenance of quality of care, patient satisfaction, and the fulfillment of the professional ethic of medicine and the other health care professions. The example of the Federal Aviation Agency to the aviation industry (that is characterized in this country by high standards of safety and quality) has been cited as one model that the current changing health care system might follow.

We have discussed previously the work of Frankl[25,26] and Yalom,[27] and the presence of an existential vacuum. The physician caring for 80- and 90-year-old patients must be prepared to hear the patient utter, "I do not know why I'm still here" or, "I do not know why God does not take me away. I have lived long enough." The physician must be alert to the presence of depression and suicidal ideation. If the physician's assessment is that these statements do not represent suicidal thoughts, then the physician must be prepared to respond to ruminations about death that are heard commonly in the very elderly. Without entering too much into the world of theology, it might be appropriate for the physician to say such things as, "That is not for you to decide or ponder. There must be a reason you are still here. Apparently, God must want you here for some reason. There is the friendship that you and I still enjoy, and the friendship that you enjoy with the visiting nurse (or home health aide). You have your nephew in New Hampshire and his family. You may see him only three or four times per year, but I know that you both care about each other. Again, your being here is not really for you or me to decide. All of us must make the best of each day while we are still here."

What about the extraordinarily independent patient who is feisty and maybe a bit eccentric? The patient will not accept what seems to be needed treatment or will refuse home health aides or daycare. Others have divorced themselves from the medical system, at least for the present time, because of past experience that was burdensome, expensive, and seemingly unnecessary. Some will refuse supports such as having health aides because they do not want the burden of strangers in the home or the expense of this assistance (even though they can afford it). They do not want to divert their savings in case they need it in the future, or not to reduce an inheritance to a loved one. They may recall bad experiences with a series of dentists whose bills ran into thousands of dollars. The patient may be wary of the medical system that, each time she suffered a fractured vertebra related to her osteoporosis, kept her in the hospital emergency room for 12–36 hours where she underwent repeated bone scans and other seemingly needless tests. It would seem prudent to state the case for what is reasonable, but to allow as much self-determination and autonomous action as possible. This respect for the patient's autonomy may help cement or enhance the doctor–patient relationship. Many elderly who exhibit extraordinary independence appear to do well despite their selective lack of participation in medical care or other support systems. Segerberg in *Living To Be 100* describes anecdotally manifestations of exceptional independence in 1,200 centenarians.[48] Extraordinary independence needs to be studied more as a positive factor in successful aging, at least in some individuals.

HELPING THE DISCONNECTED FAMILY

Although there are American families that resemble the Norman Rockwell portrait, there are many others that do not. Many teenagers and young adults are thinking of the future and are not able to identify with their parents or grandparents. Many middle-aged people are still thinking of the future, and still unable to identify with their elderly parents. Each is in a separate compartment and has difficulty with the cultural diversity that exists between generations. The members of each generation may have their own dress and hair code, music, values, religious beliefs, friends, and traditions. If they gather for Thanksgiving or a wedding, it may be an ordeal. The parents may not want the grandparents to know that the grandchild is having problems with drugs. The parents may have moved away from a faith community that was of great meaning to the grandparents. Secrets may be commonplace between members or branches of a family about marital status or financial problems. In fulfillment of independent living with each generation determining its own existence, there is a disconnectedness, separation, isolation, and loneliness that each generation feels, particularly the elderly who are not busy with work or child-raising, and are disappointed over their lack of connection with their children and grandchildren. Elders may feel dejected, wishing for more contact with their family members, their community, or other people, and the elders simply may not be able to make these connections. They may especially be separated from young people who have chosen a new direction for their lives. The physician caring for the elderly must be prepared to deal with distant children, family estrangements, families rocked by divorce recently or 30 years ago, and, in general, the lack of a support system. Understanding of principles of family systems and family therapy is necessary. Whether it is in caring for the frail, disabled elder who suddenly cannot take care of herself, or whether it is in providing end-of-life care, the physician must be able to deal with these complexities.

END-OF-LIFE CARE: DYING WELL

As a society, we are beginning to realize that dying in America is often not optimal, and there is a crying-out that end-of-life care must be improved. The negative aspects of how the dying process is handled by the medical profession and by families and their community has created a demand for assisted suicide. Nonetheless, there are many alternatives to assisted suicide that can improve the care of the dying patient. The greatest danger of assisted suicide or euthanasia in the era of cost-cutting is that society or patients themselves will decide that their lives are not worth living.[49,50] Woody Allen said, "Think of death as cutting down on your expenses." At a time when cost containment is paramount, we must fear for the frail, debilitated elderly, those who have been marginalized as a result of Alzheimer's disease and other major disorders.

There are many initiatives in medical care, teaching, and research that are focusing on improving the care of the dying.[51] This has been called "dying well,"[49,52,53] "living while dying," and "physician-assisted living." At first, we thought that there was a rising interest in living wills and other advance directives to be made with fully informed consent by a competent patient. Many elderly have witnessed burdensome, expensive, and what appeared to be futile care provided to their friends and loved ones, and this has led to the importance of these health care directives, supported by the Cruzan Supreme Court decision and the Patient Self-Determination Act.[54] Although many still are lacking in the use of advance directives, the sad case of Terri Schiavo has led many to take the step of preparing an advance directive.

Society is crying out for a paradigm shift in which people can "die well" or continue to enjoy their family and loved ones and other treasures until their death. Pain must be alleviated, and we are near a point where all pain in the dying will be manageable. All physicians need to understand and use palliative care appropriately.

The paradigm shift calls for a change not only in physician practices but also in the public's thinking. The patient dying well at home need not be required to go to the hospital for the final moments. We can expect that more terminally ill patients will choose to be at home to die with proper care from family, aides, caregivers, and volunteers, and as a profession we should respect and support the terminally ill patient's wish to die at home.[53,56] Doctors and health professionals and patients and families will have to speak more openly about what is occurring and what options are available, particularly offering the possibility of comfort care and hospice principles. Home care, whether the patient will be taken care of at home or participating in a home hospice program, will be a choice that our patients will make with greater frequency, and we can anticipate a marked increase in attention to home care in our health care system in the years ahead.

Byock[53] speaks of the prospect for growth at the end of life. Dying can represent a time of love and reconciliation, a time of transcendence of suffering. We can expect a new era in care at the end of life.[53,56] We must ensure greater continuity of care for dying patients. We must provide greater support to those caring for the dying and their family members. Again, we must provide more information about treatment choices to dying patients and their families. As stated previously, doctors and hospitals must treat their patients' pain. We must translate to the American people what Dyck and Lynn and Byock and others have been proposing: that the possibility of dying well exists and that Americans should not be separated by a curtain from the dying process. Americans can more frequently die at home or in other care settings where they are surrounded by loved ones, and without the sword of pain as a threat. The patient's family and friends, the patient's faith community, the patient's doctor and the entire hospice team are all there while the patient lives to provide comfort, love, support, and spiritual counseling, and they will also be there in the bereavement period. America is crying out for this change to take place. We can expect that this will be the role of all primary care doctors as well as other health professionals in the years ahead.

REFERENCES

1. Wan H, Sengupta M, Velkoff VA, DeBarros KA. *US Census Bureau, Current Population Reports, P23–209, 65+ in the United States: 2005*. Washington, DC: US Government Printing Office; 2005.
2. Institute of Medicine. *Crossing the Quality Chasm: A New Health System for the 21st Century*. Washington, DC: National Academy Press; 2001.
3. Engel GL. The need for a new medical model: a challenge for biomedicine. *Science*. 1977;196:129–136.
4. Fava GA and Sonino N. The biopsychosocial model thirty years later. *Psychother Psychosom*. 2008;77:1–2.
5. Future of Family Medicine Project Leadership Committee. The future of family medicine: a collaborative project of the family medicine community. *Ann Fam Med*. 2004;2:S3–S32.
6. American Geriatrics Society Core Writing Group of the Task Force on the Future of Geriatric Medicine. Caring for older Americans: the future of geriatric medicine. *JAGS*. 2005;3:S245–S256.
7. Larson EB, Fihn SD, Kirk LM, et al. The future of general internal medicine. Report and recommendations from the Society of General Internal Medicine (SGIM) Task Force on the Domain of General Internal Medicine. *J Gen Intern Med*. 2004;19(1):69–77.
8. American Academy of Family Physicians, American Academy of Pediatrics, American College of Physicians, American Osteopathic Association. Joint Principles of the Patient-Centered Medical Home 2007. Available at: http://www.aafp.org/pcmh/principles.pdf,. Accessed May 14, 2008.
9. Ranjit N, Diez-Roux AV, Shea S, et al. Psychosocial factors and inflammation in the multi-ethnic study of atherosclerosis. *Arch Intern Med*. 2007;167:174–181.
10. Egede LE. Disease-focused or integrated treatment: diabetes and depression. *Med Clin N Am*. 2006;90:627–646.
11. Costanzo ES, Lutgendorf SK, Sood AK, Anderson B, Sorosky J, Lubaroff DM. Psychosocial factors and interleukin-6 among women with advanced ovarian cancer. *Cancer*. 2005;104(2):305–313.
12. Holmes TH, Rahe RH. The Social readjustment rating scale. *J Psychosom Res*. 1967;11:213–218.
13. Wagner EH, Ausin BT, Davis C, Hindmarsh M, Schaefer J, Bonomi A. Improving chronic illness care: translating evidence into action. *Health Aff (Millwood)*. 2001;20:64–78.
14. Curran VR, Sharpe D. A framework for integrating interprofessional education curriculum in the health science. *Ed Health*. 2007;20(3):93.
15. Reichel W. The continuity imperative. *JAMA*. 1981;246:2065.
16. Coleman EA, Smith JD, Frank JC, Min SJ, Parry C, Dramer AM. Preparing patients and caregivers to participate in care delivered across settings: the care transitions intervention. *JAGS*. 2004; 52(11):1817–1825.
17. Clancy CM. Care transitions: a threat and an opportunity for patient safety. *Am J Med Qual*. 2006;21:415–417.
18. Wieland D, Lamb VL, Sutton SR, et al. Hospitalization in the Program of All-Inclusive Care for the Elderly (PACE): rates, concomitants, and predictors. *JAGS*. 2000;48(11):1373–1380.
19. Gitlin LN, Winter L, Dennis MP, Corcoran M, Schinfeld S, Hauck WW. Randomized trial of a multicomponent home intervention to reduce functional difficulties in older adults. *JAGS*. 2006; 54(5):809–816.
20. Belle SH, Burgio L, Burns R, et al. Resources for enhancing Alzheimer's Caregiver Health (REACH) II Investigators. Enhancing the quality of life of dementia caregivers from different ethnic or racial groups: a randomized, controlled trial. *Ann Intern Med*. 2006; 145(10):727–738.
21. The Caregiver Initiative. Attitudes and beliefs about caregiving in the US: findings of a national opinion survey. Johnson & Johnson Consumer Products Company, 2005. Available at: http://www.strengthforcaring.com/util/press/research/index.html. Accessed May 14, 2008.
22. Pinuart M, Sorensen S. Correlates of physical health of informal caregivers: a meta-analysis. *J Gerontol Series B: Pysch Sci Social Sci*. 2007;62(2):P126–137.
23. Parks SM, Novielli KD. A practical guide to caring for caregivers. *Am Fam Physician*. 2000;62(12):2613–2622.
24. Peabody FW. The care of the patient. *JAMA*. 1927;88:877–882.
25. Frankl VE. *Man's Search for Meaning*. Boston: Beacon Press; 1959.
26. Frankl VE. *The Doctor and the Soul*. New York: AA Knopf; 1955.
27. Yalom ID. *Existential Psychotherapy*. New York: Basic Books, Inc.; 1980.
28. Cassel EJ. The nature of suffering and the goals of medicine. *NEJM*. 1982;306:639–645.
29. Kushner H. *When All You've Ever Wanted Isn't Enough*. New York: Summit Books; 1986.
30. Cousins N. The physician as communicator. *JAMA*. 1982; 248:587–589.
31. Frank JD, Frank JB. *Persuasion and Healing: A Comparative Study of Psychotherapy*. Third Ed. Baltimore: The Johns Hopkins University Press; 1991.
32. Elon R. Personal communication.
33. Elahi D, Clark B, Andres R. Glucose tolerance, insulin sensitivity and age. In: Armbracht HJ, Coe RM, Wongsurawat N, eds. *Endocrine Function and Aging*. New York: Springer-Verlag; 1990:48–63.
34. California Healthcare Foundation/American Geriatrics Society Panel on Improving Care for Elders with Diabetes. Guidelines for improving the care of the older person with diabetes mellitus. *JAGS*. 2003;51:S265–S280.
35. Rowe JW, Andres R, Tobin JR, Norris AH, Shock NW. The effect of age on creatinine clearance in men: a cross-sectional and longitudinal study. *J Gerontol*. 1976;31:155–163.
36. Flick DM, Cooper JW, Wade WE, Waller JL, Maclean R, Beers MH. Updating the Beers criteria for potentially inappropriate medication use in older adults. *Arch Intern Med*. 2003;163:2716–2724.
37. Reichel W. Multiple problems in the elderly. In Reichel, W, ed. *The Geriatric Patient*. New York: Hospital Practice, 1978;17–22.
38. Evans WJ, Effects of exercise on body composition and functional capacity of the elderly. *J Gerontol Series A: Bio Med Sci*. 1995; 50:147–150.
39. Guide to Clinical Preventive Services, 2007, AHRQ Publication No. 07–05100, September 2007. Agency for Healthcare Research and Quality, Rockville, MD. Available at: http://www.ahrq.gov/clinic/pocketgd.htm.
40. Seegal D. The principle of minimal interference in the management of the elderly patient. *J Chron Dis*. 1964;17:299–300.
41. Reichel W. Complications in the care of 500 elderly hospitalized patients. *JAGS*. 1965;13:973–981.
42. Steel K, Gertman PM, Crescenzi C, Anderson J. Iatrogenic illness on a general medical service at a university hospital. *NEJM*. 1981; 304:638–642.

43. Lipp MR. *Respectful Treatment: A Practical Handbook of Patient Care.* Second Ed. New York: Elsevier; 1986.

44. Mermin GB, Johnson RW, Murphy DP. Why do boomers plan to work longer? *J Gerontol Series B: Psych Social Sci.* 2007;625:S286–S294.

45. Glick S. Humanistic medicine in a modern age. *NEJM.* 1981; 304:1036–1038.

46. Keeler EB, Solomon DH, Beck JC, Mendenhall RC, Kane RL. Effect of patient age on duration of medical encounters with physicians. *Med Care.* 1982;20:1101–1108.

47. Wagner GS, Cebe B, Rozear MP (eds). *E. A. Stead, Jr., What This Patient Needs Is a Doctor.* Durham, NC: Carolina Academic Press; 1978.

48. Segerberg O. *Living to Be 100.* New York: Charles Scribners Sons, 1982.

49. Reichel W, Dyck AJ. Euthanasia; a contemporary moral quandary. *Lancet.* 1989;2(8675):132–133.

50. Lynn J, Cohn F, Pickering JH, Smith J, Stoeppelwerth, JD. The American Geriatrics Society on physician-assisted suicide: brief to the U.S. Supreme Court. *JAGS.* 1997;45:489–499.

51. Horgan J. Seeking a better way to die. *Sci Am.* 1997;276(5):100–105.

52. Dyck AJ. An alternative to the ethic of euthanasia. In Williams RH, ed. *To Live and to Die: When, Why, and How?* New York: Springer Verlag, 1973:98–112.

53. Byock I. *Dying Well: The Prospect for Growth at the End of Life.* New York: Riverhead Books/GP Putnam's Sons; 1997.

54. Doukas DJ, Reichel W. *Planning for Uncertainty: Living Wills and Other Advance Directives for You and Your Family.* Second Ed. Baltimore: The Johns Hopkins University Press; 2007.

55. Sankar A. *Dying at Home: A Family Guide for Caregiving.* Baltimore: The Johns Hopkins University Press; 1991.

56. Lynn J. Caring at the end of our lives. *NEJM.* 1996;335:201–202.

2

ASSESSMENT OF THE OLDER PATIENT

John D. Gazewood, MD, MSPH

Function is the filter through which physicians and others caring for older patients must view them to provide optimal care. Assessing function is necessary for a number of reasons – older adults are more heterogeneous in their functional capacities than younger adults, functional capacity correlates highly with quality of life,[1] and function in and of itself is an important outcome in older patients. Functional status is also an important predictor of outcomes, such as mortality and institutionalization, in a variety of settings,[2,3] and changes in functional capacity frequently signal changes in an individual's health. Unfortunately, physicians are frequently unaware of or underestimate their patients' functional limitations.[4] Limiting the approach to older patients to a biomedical or even biopsychosocial approach is likely to result in care that at best fails to meet the needs of an older patient, and at worst may cause harm.

COMPREHENSIVE GERIATRIC ASSESSMENT

Comprehensive geriatric assessment (CGA) is "a multidisciplinary evaluation in which the multiple problems of older persons are uncovered, described, and explained, if possible, and in which the resources and strengths of the person are catalogued, need for services assessed, and a coordinated care plan developed to focus interventions on the person's problems."[5] The goals of CGA are to improve diagnostic accuracy, optimize medical treatment and outcomes, improve functional status, recommend the most appropriate living environment, and minimize unnecessary use of services.[6] While investigators continue to refine the model of CGA, principles of geriatric care garnered from these trials have become more widely adopted in a variety of clinical settings.

The process of CGA involves a team of health care providers, often a geriatrician, a nurse practitioner, and a medical social worker. Geriatric psychiatry, pharmacy, nutrition, and physical and occupational therapy are other disciplines that may participate in CGA in some settings. This multidisciplinary team uses a systematic approach that incorporates validated assessment tools to assess multiple domains of function, including the physical, mental, social, functional, and environmental.[5] The team meets and develops recommendations based on results of the evaluation – the integration of information and the multidisciplinary perspectives brought to bear on this information facilitate its translation into a rational plan of care.[5]

This multidisciplinary approach to CGA has been rigorously evaluated in a variety of settings, including the home, outpatient clinic, inpatient consultation services, and inpatient geriatric units,[6] and the evidence that incorporating functional assessment improves patient outcomes is derived from these studies. In a landmark meta-analysis, Stuck et al.[7] obtained original data from the authors of 28 randomized controlled trials with a total of 4,959 patients in intervention groups and 4,912 patients in control groups. The meta-analysis authors combined data and evaluated both the combined data and the data based on the site of the CGA intervention, separately evaluating CGA in geriatric evaluation and management units (GEMU), inpatient geriatric consultation services (IGCS), home assessment (HAS), home assessment following hospital discharge (HHAS), and in outpatient clinic settings (OAS). Overall, the mortality rate was reduced by 14% at 12 months, hospital admission rate was reduced by 12%, institutionalization reduced by 26% and there was no effect on functional status. In the site-based analysis, GEMU, HAS, and IGCS-based interventions reduced mortality; GEMU, HAS, and HHAS decreased institutionalization, HAS reduced hospitalization, and GEMU and IGCS improved cognitive status. Interestingly, outpatient CGA had no positive effect on any of the measured outcomes.[7] Stuck and associates examined the effects of characteristics of the various interventions on outcomes and found that four covariates influenced effectiveness. Programs that excluded either the very healthy or the very ill were more likely to show benefit, as were programs that maintained control over implementation of recommendations and programs that provided long-term ambulatory follow-up of patients.[7] This analysis confirmed earlier hypotheses that targeting of CGA intervention to a population likely to benefit was important and that control of implementing CGA recommendations and follow-up was also important for benefit.[5]

Additional studies examining functional interventions have continued to show both the promise and limitations of incorporating functional assessment into care of elders. In a meta-analysis of home visit programs, Stuck et al.[8] showed that programs including CGA improved functional status, whereas those that did not had no effect on functional status. A large multicenter Veterans' Administration trial in which inpatient and outpatient geriatric clinic care were compared with regular inpatient and outpatient care showed that inpatient geriatric care resulted in better functional status at discharge, and outpatient geriatric care resulted in better mental health at 1 year.[9] The authors speculate that the diffusion of geriatric care principles into general medical inpatient wards and outpatient clinics may have lessened the effect of the intervention in this trial.

EVIDENCE SUPPORTING FUNCTIONAL ASSESSMENT IN PRIMARY CARE SETTINGS

Several CGA trials were performed in primary care settings or incorporated delivery of interventions in primary care settings into their design. A trial in community-dwelling elders coupled the use of CGA with an intervention to empower patients to speak to their primary care physicians, and close communication of the CGA team with the primary care physician improved mortality, function, emotional well-being, mental health, and pain outcomes. This study demonstrated that treatment recommendations provided in primary care settings can be effective.[10] A 2-year randomized trial of interdisciplinary primary care in a group of veterans showed that a multidisciplinary intervention that included an interdisciplinary assessment improved functional status, health perception, social activity, depression, life satisfaction, cognitive function, and lessened clinic visits.[11]

Several groups have investigated the effectiveness of coupling brief educational interventions by physicians with brief functional screenings and focused physician feedback. In a study conducted in a general medicine training practice, patients completed a brief functional assessment tool that was used to generate computerized feedback reports listing functional deficits, linking them to the patient's medical problems and suggesting management interventions. After 6 months, patients in the intervention group had better emotional well-being and fewer limitations in social activities.[12] Moore et al.[13] studied the effectiveness of a 10-minute office staff–administered screening. Physicians received brief, written evidence-based intervention recommendations for patients with identified conditions. At 6 months, patients in the study group were more likely to have hearing impairment identified

and evaluated, but there were no differences in health status. Both office staff and physicians found the brief screening instrument useful and feasible. In a large trial in Great Britain, community-dwelling elders were randomized to a universal indepth in-home evaluation or to a brief screening followed by an indepth evaluation if targeting criteria were met. Participants were then randomized to follow-up by their general practitioner or a local geriatrician. The study showed a trend toward lower rates of institutionalization in the universal evaluation group and slight improvement in social interaction among the group followed-up by the geriatrician.[14] The basically equivalent outcomes between the general practitioner and geriatrician groups suggest that general practitioners are capable of managing functional deficits and medical problems in patients once these problems have been identified.[15]

TARGETING COMPREHENSIVE GERIATRIC ASSESSMENT

Targeting CGA to the appropriate patient is key to its effectiveness,[6,7] and no benefit has been shown in studies that have included elders who were too well or too ill.[16] Most frequently, CGA is targeted at older patients at risk for progressive disability. These individuals exhibit decline in physiological reserve in a number of organ systems, making it harder for them to respond to intrinsic (disease) or extrinsic (environmental) challenges to their physiological or functional status – they are "frail." If individuals progress along this pathway of physiological and functional decline, they may pass a "point of no return," where continued physiological and functional decline leading to disability and death is inevitable; CGA will not help these patients. It is important to keep in mind that progressive decline is not inevitable. Many elderly who are at risk for frailty and functional decline frequently transition between states of functional impairment and disability.[17] Individuals who have longer or more frequent episodes of disability are at greater risk for recurrent, prolonged, or inevitable functional decline.[18] On the other hand, individuals who are not frail may be too healthy to garner benefit from CGA.

The purpose of targeting is to identify elders at risk for progressive disability. Targeting criteria, tested empirically in a number of studies, include diseases that serve as markers for physiological impairment, evidence of functional impairment or disability, and geriatric syndromes that may be markers for underlying frailty (Table 2.1). Targeting criteria include exclusionary criteria that identify individuals who are too ill or too severely impaired to benefit from a comprehensive multi-dimensional assessment.[11,19,20]

INSIDE THE BLACK BOX: WHAT HAPPENS IN CGA PROCESSES?

What happens in CGA? What problems are discovered? How are they addressed? A few studies provide some insight into the

Table 2.1. Targeting Criteria

Age ≥75 years

Functional status: ≥1 ADL deficiency; falls; poor self-rated health

Medical utilization: ≥1 hospital admission in past year; ≥6 physician visits in past year; ≥5 prescription medications

Medical conditions: coronary artery disease; diabetes mellitus; depression; urinary incontinence

Social: absence of a caregiver

CGA process. In a pilot study in which outpatient CGA was assessed, 528 interventions were developed for 139 patients. Prioritization of these interventions by the CGA team geriatrician resulted in 139 "most important" recommendations: general medical problems (30%); depression (21%); incontinence (19%); musculoskeletal problems (12%); hypertension (8%); functional impairment (6%); and falls, visual and hearing problems, and other problems (5% or less).[21] In a 3-year study of home-based CGA, geriatric nurse practitioners identified an average of 19.2 problems/patient and made 5,694 specific recommendations. Approximately, 66% of patients had a medical problem, 23% a mental health problem, 19.8% a social problem, and 17% a functional problem. Slightly over 50% of the recommendations involved self-care activities, such as performing Kegel exercises or increasing fluid intake; 29% involved referral to a physician, most commonly to change a medication, discuss an examination finding or functional problem, or to request a treatment or procedure; and 20% involved referral to a nonphysician health professional or community service.[22] Repeated annual assessments yielded an average of two new medical problems and one new psychosocial problem per patient each year.[23] The variable rates of problems found in these studies likely relate to heterogeneity between patient populations and the intensity and comprehensiveness of the intervention.

Another important consideration in achieving success in CGA settings is the degree of adherence to the recommendations generated in the process.[10] Physicians, family members, and patients often have widely divergent goals.[24] A cohort study of caregivers of patients who underwent CGA found higher rates of adherence to treatment recommendations if caregivers agreed with them.[25]

FUNCTIONAL ASSESSMENT IN PRIMARY CARE SETTINGS: MAKING IT WORK

CGA is not widely available and there will not be enough geriatricians to provide care to an aging populace.[26,27] Most older adults will continue to obtain most of their care from family physicians, general internists, or mid-level providers working in collaboration with physicians.[27,28] These professionals must be competent in comprehensive evaluation and management

of most of the older adults for whom they care. The evidence presented thus far allows for some broad recommendations to be made on how to perform a comprehensive evaluation in a busy primary care setting. First, not all patients require a comprehensive evaluation. Using a brief screening tool based on targeting criteria can identify patients who may benefit from a more comprehensive evaluation and will help practices to focus limited resources toward patients most likely to benefit (Grade A).* Second, a systematic process should be used when performing either a screening assessment or a comprehensive assessment (Grade A). This will ensure that important aspects of the evaluation are not overlooked. Third, validated instruments should be used whenever available (Grade A). Fourth, the physician does not have to obtain all of the information needed to complete either a screening evaluation or a comprehensive evaluation. Patients and their caregivers can complete some instruments, medical assistants or nurses can complete other assessment instruments, and the physician can use outside resources for other parts of the assessment (Grade B). For example, a referral to a home health agency can help the physician in obtaining assessment from a home health nurse, a physical therapist, and a social worker. Finally, working with the patient, family, and caregivers, physicians and patients should develop a prioritized list of goals that will make patient and family adherence to interventions more likely (Grade A).

MAKING FUNCTIONAL ASSESSMENT WORK: PICKING AN INSTRUMENT

There are a plethora of instruments available to assess functional domains. Characteristics to consider in selecting an instrument include its validity, reliability, responsiveness, and ease of administration. Of course, the most important consideration in choosing an instrument is that its use will lead to improved outcomes for patients. Because all CGA trials use assessment instruments, it is reasonable to believe that their use leads to better patient outcomes.[7,23]

A valid instrument measures what it is intended to measure. Validity is typically assessed using content, construct, and criterion validity. A measure with content validity makes sense to experts and to patients who take it: It looks like it addresses the area of concern. Construct validity refers to how well the instrument measures the theoretical construct underlying the instrument. Predictive validity is one way that construct validity is assessed. For example, an instrument measuring functional

---

*Grades of Recommendation are those developed by the Centre for Evidence-Based Medicine, Oxford, and are available at: www.cebm.net/levels_of_evidence.asp

Grade A: consistent level 1 studies
Grade B: consistent level 2 or 3 studies or extrapolations from level 1 studies
Grade C: level 4 studies or extrapolations from level 2 or 3 studies
Grade D: level 5 evidence or troublingly inconsistent or inconclusive studies of any level.

Table 2.2. Sources of Electronic Instruments

Product/Site	Assessment Tool	Comments
InfoRetriever	MMSE	Subscription only.
Available from Infopoems.com	GDS (5 question) Fall Risk Calculator	Desktop version available
GeriatricWeb, available at: geriatricweb.sc.edu/	MMSE Depression Scale BMI calculator	Web site with links to instruments (online and PDA) on other sites
Geriatrics at Your Fingertips, available at: www.geriatricsatyourfingertips.org/ default.asp	Mini-cog GDS (5 question) Lawton IADL scale ADL scale Reuben hearing screen	Available in web-based version, and PDA version. PDA version automates instrument scoring

impairment should be associated with outcomes, such as nursing home placement, that would arise from functional impairment. Criterion validity measures how well an instrument compares with a criterion or gold standard. Sensitivity, specificity, and predictive value are how criterion validity is typically measured in the clinical literature. Diagnostic accuracy of instruments is also measured and compared by using a receiver-operating curve. By plotting the true-positive rate (sensitivity) against the false-positive rate (1-specificity) a curve is constructed. Instruments with a larger area under the curve (AUC) are more accurate.

A reliable instrument measures in a reproducible fashion. Reliability requires internal consistency and reproducibility. Internal consistency, usually measured with the Cronbach alpha statistic, is a measure of how closely different items in an instrument relate to each other. A Cronbach alpha value of 0.7 or greater indicates acceptable internal consistency. A reproducible measure shows good interrater, intrarater, and test–retest reliability, that is, results within and between observers and results for the same patient when a test is repeated over a short period of time, are stable.

Responsiveness indicates how well an instrument can determine meaningful changes over time. Ceiling and floor effects, which indicate the upper and lower limits of an instrument's measurement range, limit instrument responsiveness. For example, an activities of daily living (ADLs) scale is not likely to give a meaningful picture of a functionally independent person, as this person's function is above the ability of the instrument to discriminate meaningful changes (ceiling effect).

The properties of functional assessment instruments can be affected by characteristics of the population in which they are developed. Language, culture, education, socioeconomic status, and severity of a condition can all affect the performance of an assessment tool, either changing the scoring or rendering the instrument altogether useless in a given population. In general, it is best to use only instruments that have been validated in a population that is similar to the intended target population (Grade D).

It is also important to consider more practical aspects of instrument administration. Functional assessment tools can be completed by the patient, a proxy, or through direct observation. Patients overestimate their functional capacity in comparison to proxy measures or direct measurement.[29] It may sometimes be necessary to assess certain aspects of function with several different instruments or sources of information, particularly if an individual's reported functional status is not congruent with other measures or one's general clinical impression. Ease of use is, from a practical standpoint, one of the most important considerations in selecting a functional assessment instrument. Instruments should not take too much time to administer, they should not impose too great a burden on a patient or caregiver, and they should be fairly easy to score. Many instruments are available that can be filled out by the patient or caregiver. Office staff or other health personnel can complete others. None require that a physician administer them, although clinicians can find observation of the patient during instrument completion helpful in formulating clinical impressions. Many instruments are now available in electronic format for personal digital assistants or via the Internet. These programs allow for automated scoring and make some instruments easier to use (Table 2.2).

MAKING GERIATRIC ASSESSMENT WORK: PUTTING IT TOGETHER

The components of geriatric assessment are listed in Table 2.3. Although the physician or mid-level provider will complete the history and physical examination, much of the information can be obtained before the appointment through use of a questionnaire. Because the presence of known functional or other deficits may affect the examination process, exploring this information before performing the history and physical examination will increase efficiency (Grade D). A highly capable office assistant can perform a detailed assessment. For example, in one family medicine office, a 22-minute assessment performed by

Table 2.3. Domains of Geriatric Assessment

Physical health

Traditional history and physical examination

Hearing and vision screen

Oral and dental health

Continence assessment

Gait, mobility, and falls risk assessment

Nutrition assessment

Functional ability

ADLs

IADLs

Performance measures

Mental status

Cognitive function

Depression screening

Social support

Social history

Advanced directive

Caregiver burden

Finances

Environment

an office assistant identified at least one new or incompletely treated geriatric problem in 68% of patients.[30]

History and Physical Examination

As in all medical endeavors, a thorough history is necessary to ensure diagnostic accuracy. Accommodations must be made for barriers to communication. Having a pocket talker available and speaking clearly in a low-pitched voice while looking directly at the patient will improve communication with a hearing impaired person. Providers must also be prepared to provide interpreters for patients with limited English proficiency. Many older patients will be accompanied by a caregiver, often a spouse or adult child. Incorporating this third party into the encounter, while maintaining primary focus on the patient is a necessary skill. The caregiver can corroborate and expand on a patient's history and will provide important historical information when the patient has cognitive impairment. Establishing rapport and a good working relationship with the caregiver will also be helpful in maximizing the therapeutic effect of your relationship with the patient.

The history should explore acute and subacute problems, with a particular focus on problems that have affected function. In the patient with a recent functional decline, delineating the impairments contributing to the decline will help determine

prognosis and therapy. For example, difficulty dressing could result from cognitive impairment, weakness secondary to a stroke, or a frozen shoulder. The history includes a review of chronic medical conditions, resulting end-organ damage, and the medical, surgical, psychiatric, and obstetric history, including immunizations. The history should also review episodes of disability and length of disability, because both increase future risk of disability.[18]

A substance use history, including tobacco, alcohol, and other drugs should be obtained. Inquire about all forms of tobacco use, not just cigarettes. Screening for alcohol use should be done using items derived from the AUDIT tool and should address both frequency and intensity of drinking (Grade A). The first question is "How often do you have a drink containing alcohol, including any beer, wine, or liquor/spirits?" Follow-up questions are 1) On average, how many days per week do you drink alcohol? 2) On a typical day when you drink, how many drinks do you have? and 3) How often do you have three or more drinks on one occasion? A positive screen is more than one drink a day or more than three drinks on any occasion.[31]

Thorough review of the patient's medications may be one of the most important components of a thorough assessment. Outpatient CGA programs were found to reduce the risk of serious adverse drug reactions in a recent randomized trial. The most commonly implicated classes of medications were cardiovascular, central nervous system, antimicrobials, hormones, and blood modifying agents.[32] Patients should be asked to bring all of their medications, including vitamins and supplements. Every medication should have an appropriate indication for its use, the dose should be appropriate for the patient, and potential drug interactions should be identified. Based on a recent comparison of commercially available products, Epocrates Pro has the most accurate drug interaction program.[33] The social history should elucidate the patient's sources of support, including emotional, spiritual, physical, and financial sources. Understanding the patient's educational, occupational, and avocational history will provide a richer picture of the patient. The family history, although perhaps less important than in younger patients, can still provide useful information regarding the longevity and late-life health of the patient's parents and siblings, as well as information that may influence screening decisions for certain cancers.

The review of systems should address changes in hearing and vision, oral, and dental problems. The review of systems should also include questions targeting geriatric syndromes. The review of systems is one aspect of the history that could be efficiently obtained in questionnaire format, assuming that the patient or caregiver is functionally literate.

Physical Examination

Vital signs should include supine and standing pulse and blood pressure, weight and height, and determination of body mass index (BMI). If a patient is unable to stand, height can be estimated using the length of the patient's lower leg.[*,34] Office staff can assess vision using a Snellen or a handheld chart. Hearing is best assessed using a handheld audiometer, the Audio-Scope (Welch Allyn, Inc., Skaneateles Falls, NY). This audioscope is easy to use, and office staff can screen the patient for hearing loss by setting the sound intensity to 40 dB. The audioscope delivers a pretone at 60 dB, and then delivers 40-dB tones at 500, 1,000, 2,000 and 4,000 Hz. Patients fail the screen if they are unable to hear either the 1,000 or 2,000 Hz frequency in both ears, or cannot hear both the 1,000 and 2,000 Hz frequency in one ear. The sensitivity of this test ranges from 94% to 97%, with specificity values of 69% to 80%. Alternatively, a brief self-response questionnaire, the Hearing Handicap Inventory for the Elderly-Screening version can be used. With a cut-off of 10 points, the sensitivity ranges from 63% to 80%. The whisper test, although easy to perform, has uncertain reliability and accuracy.[35]

Examination of the head and neck should include assessment of oral and dental health. Oral and dental problems are highly predictive of poor outcomes. Poorly fitting dentures, broken teeth, missing teeth, carious teeth, gingivitis, and periodontitis can all contribute to poor oral intake, and the latter three may produce inflammatory mediators that can lead to functional decline.[36] Thorough musculoskeletal and neurological examinations are especially important in the presence of functional impairment.

All elderly patients who are targeted for a geriatric assessment should undergo systematic assessment of cognition, affect, functional status, falls, continence, nutrition, environment, and social support, based on incorporation of assessment of these domains in multiple CGA trials (Grade A). Selected instruments available in the public domain are listed in Table 2.4, along with web addresses.

Cognitive Assessment

Cognitive impairment can be secondary to dementia, delirium, depression, and aphasia, among others. A complete assessment of mental status includes evaluation of attention, executive function, memory, orientation, language, visuospatial abilities, psychomotor speed, and intelligence. None of the instruments typically used in primary care office settings addresses all of these domains.

Many of the instruments used for mental status testing in the office setting have low sensitivities and high specificities, meaning that in a population of older patients in whom dementia is prevalent, a positive test is likely to be true, and a negative test may frequently miss a patient with cognitive impairment.

The widely used and well-validated Mini-Mental State Examination (MMSE) evaluates orientation, memory, calculation, language, and visuospatial orientation. It has 30 items and takes approximately 10 minutes to administer. The cut-off score is 24, the sensitivity ranges from 0.7 to 0.9, and the specificity ranges from 0.56 to 0.96.[37] Sensitivity is lower for mild dementia. The score must be adjusted for age and educational level.[38] A low score on the MMSE reliably identifies patients with cognitive impairment and usually obviates the need for further neuropsychiatric evaluation. A normal score, however, does not rule out cognitive impairment.

Short screening tests have been developed in an effort to lessen the burden of dementia screening. The Time and Change test requires the patient to tell the time given on a large clockface diagram and make 1 dollar's worth of change from a standard amount of change. Both tests are timed, and an individual who fails either is positive for dementia. The Time and Change test has a sensitivity of 0.86 and a specificity of 0.71, and takes 23 seconds to complete.[39] The Mini-Cog combines three-item recall with a clock-drawing test. Individuals are given three items to remember, are asked to draw a clock, and then are asked to recall the three items. A positive test is either failure to recall all items, or failure to recall one or two items and failure on the clock-drawing test (CDT).[40] In a large, population-based cohort study, the Mini-Cog had a sensitivity of 0.76 and a specificity of 0.84. The MMSE in this same study had a sensitivity of 0.71 and a specificity of 0.94.[41] Other short mental status tests, including the Memory Impairment Screen, the Short Portable Mental Status Questionnaire, the Hopkins Verbal Learning Test, and the 7-Minute Screen, have been shown to be accurate in detection of dementia in small samples, but have not been validated widely enough to warrant routine use.[37]

Executive function involves integration of all cognitive functions and is used in planning and problem solving. It can be impaired in the presence of normal memory and normal basic cognitive processes.[42] Decline in executive function may be among the earliest changes in patients with dementia. Several simple tests can assess executive function. The CDT has been shown to correlate well with a valid test of executive function, the Executive Interview.[43,44] Although a grossly abnormal clock is easily recognized, the use of a validated scoring system is necessary to improve the sensitivity of the CDT in detecting early changes in executive function.

Several informant-based tests for cognitive impairment may be more sensitive than the MMSE for detection of dementia. The functional activities questionnaire (FAQ) can be filled out by caregivers in less than 5 minutes and asks about changes in the patient's ability to perform instrumental ADLs (IADLs), and reportedly has a sensitivity and specificity of 0.9 with a cut-off score of 9.[45] The Informant Questionnaire for Cognitive Decline in the Elderly (IQCODE) is filled out by an informant, who compares the patient's current functional state to 10 years ago by using a Likert scale. The long time scale may cause difficulties for some respondents.[37] When cognitive impairment is identified by an MMSE score below 24, and an

---

[*]Alternative height calculations using knee-to-heel measurements:

with knee at 90° angle (foot flexed or flat on floor or bed board), measure from bottom of heel to top of knee.

Men: Ht (cm) = $(2.02 \times \text{knee height, cm}) - (0.04 \times \text{age}) + 64.19$
Women: Ht (cm) = $(1.83 \times \text{knee height, cm}) - (0.24 \times \text{age}) + 84.8834$.

Table 2.4. Online Sources for Assessment Instruments

Instrument	Available at URL
Functional Assessment Instruments	
Katz Activities of Daily Living Scale	www.hartfordign.org/resources/education/tryThis.html
Lawton Instrumental Activities of Daily Living	www.abramsoncenter.org/PRI/scales.htm
Cognitive Scales	
Mini-Mental State Exam	www.chcr.brown.edu/MMSE.PDF
Mini-Cog	www.hospitalmedicine.org/geriresource/toolbox/mini_cog.htm
IQCODE	www.anu.edu.au/iqcode/
FAQ	www.alz.org/coordinated_care.asp, Via link "Tools for Early Identification, Assessment and Treatment for People with Alzheimer's Disease and Dementia"
Depression Scales	
GDS	www.stanford.edu/~yesavage/GDS.html
CES-D	www.chcr.brown.edu/pcoc/cesdscale.pdf
Nutrition	
MNA-SF	www.asaging.org/CDC/module8/phase5/phase5_6.cfm
Subjective Global Assessment	www.hospitalmedicine.org/geriresource/toolbox/subjective_global_assessmen.htm
Social Assessment	
Caregiver Burden Scale	www.fpnotebook.com/GER6.htm
Lubben Social Network Scale	www2.bc.edu/~norstraj/default.html
Brief Abuse Screen for the Elderly	www.vchreact.ca/attachments/BASE.pdf
Elder Assessment Instrument	www.uihealthcare.com/depts/med/familymedicine/research/geriatrics/eldermistreatment/index.html
Urinary Incontinence	
Incontinence Severity Index	www.aodgp.gov.au/internet/wcms/publishing.nsf/Content/3B2396DB310243ABCA25717700110DEE/$File/isi.pdf
King's Health Questionnaire	www.nice.org.uk/page.aspx?o=379021-

IQCODE score greater than 4, the sensitivity of this combination is 0.93 with a specificity of 0.81.[46]

Assessment of Affect

The U.S. Preventive Services Task Force recommends screening for depression in all adults if treatment can be offered to those identified as having depression (Grade A).[47] Many older adults do not display symptoms of depression, and instruments can be helpful in identifying these patients. There are a number of validated instruments available for screening and diagnosis of depression, although only a few have been adequately validated in older individuals.

A recent systematic review identified three instruments with proven validity for diagnosis of major depression in the elderly; each instrument takes 2 to 3 minutes to administer.[48] The widely used Geriatric Depression Scale (GDS) consists of 30 or 15 questions. It is a self-rating scale that asks respondents to answer yes or no to a series of questions.[49] It can also be administered in an interview format. The cut-off score on the 15-item GDS is 3 to 5 for depression, the sensitivity ranges from 0.79 to 1.00, and the specificity ranges from 0.68 to 0.8. The 15-item and 30-item GDS have similar test characteristics.[48] One study has shown that a 5-item GDS performs similarly to the 15-item GDS; however, this sample had a very high prevalence (48%) of depression, and it is unclear how the 5-item test would perform in a more representative population.[50] The Center for Epidemiologic Studies Depression Scale (CES-D) is a 20-item self-report depression scale that requires respondents to rate how frequently they experienced depressive symptoms over the past week. Sensitivities of the CES-D, with cut-off scores ranging from 9 to 21, were 0.75 to 0.93 in five studies.[48] The SelfCARE (D) consists of 12 questions, with scoring based on a Likert scale, asking respondents to answer based on symptoms over the past month. In three studies, the sensitivity of the SelfCARE (D) was 0.9. Specificities in outpatient clinics were 0.7 to 0.86, but, in one study in a homecare setting, it was 0.53.[48] In a large cohort study, the 10-item CES-D was found to have the best sensitivity in the outpatient setting, and the 15-item GDS was best in a nursing home population.[51]

The Cornell Scale for Depression was validated for identification of depression among patients with dementia and relies on patient observation and caregiver report. In hospital and outpatient settings, it has a reported sensitivity of 0.9 and a specificity of 0.75.[48]

Functional Assessment

Assessing functional status requires evaluation of the domains of physical activity necessary for independent living in modern society. These domains include basic ADLs, IADLs, and mobility. Typical facets of these domains are listed in Table 2.5. These measures typically scale responses from complete independence in an activity to complete dependence. Numeric scoring systems are useful in identifying individuals at risk for poorer outcomes for purposes of research or management of populations. In the clinical setting, these scales are more typically used to identify specific functional deficits to develop specific interventions. All of these instruments suffer from both floor and ceiling effects. Supplementing these largely self-reported measures of function with physical performance measures can help identify those highly functioning individuals at risk for functional decline.[52]

Activities of Daily Living

ADL instruments measure basic functioning and in the outpatient setting are typically completed by self-report. In home, inpatient, or rehabilitation settings they can also be completed by direct observation. The Katz Index of Independence in Activities of Daily Living is the prototypic ADL scale, assessing function in the basic activities noted in Table 2.5.[53] The Katz index is a hierarchical scale, that is, more advanced functions such as bathing are lost before the most basic function, such as eating. The Katz index, although frequently used in clinical settings, lacks the validity and reliability for use in research or health administration.[54] The Barthel Index[55] and the Functional Independence Measure (FIM) are ADL tools that are frequently used in rehabilitation settings. The FIM was derived from the Barthel Index and is valid, reliable, and widely used in rehabilitation settings. In addition to measures of basic physical function, it also includes basic assessment of communication and cognitive skills necessary for daily functioning.[54]

Instrumental Activities of Daily Living

IADL scales measure more advanced functions that require intact cognitive and executive function, in addition to intact physical function. Impairment in IADLs can be an early indicator of conditions affecting cognitive function, such as dementia. In the outpatient setting, these are almost always completed by self- or informant-report. Lawton and Brody's IADL scale asks about the respondent's ability to perform eight items necessary for independent living in the community.[56] The FAQ is similar to the Lawton and Brody scale in the activities assessed, but it is completed by an informant instead of the patient.[57]

Table 2.5. Functional Assessment Domains

ADLs	Bathing
	Dressing
	Grooming
	Toileting
	Transferring
	Eating
	Continence
IADLs	Food preparation
	Housekeeping
	Laundry
	Shopping
	Managing personal finances
	Administration of medications
	Use of transportation
	Use of telephone
Mobility	Walking
	Transferring
	Balance
	Stairs

Selection of Scales

There are not enough data from studies that directly compare the performance of the various ADL and IADL scales to show the superiority of any given instrument.[54] Katz's ADL index and Lawton's IADL scale have both been used in successful randomized trials of CGA, and this evidence, coupled with their widespread use and ease of administration, supports their use in the outpatient and homecare settings (Grade B).[11,58–61] Other instruments used to measure function in successful trials of CGA include the Functional Status Questionnaire,[10] the Barthel Index of Disability,[62] and the FIM.[63]

Physical Performance Measures

Physical performance measures can identify individuals at risk of functional decline and other poor outcomes who are not identified by ADL and IADL measures.[64] Their use when a patient is dependent in an ADL does not improve ability to predict poor outcomes.[52] In patients who are impaired, however, physical performance measures may help identify treatable functional impairments. These instruments typically require direct observation of the patient performing a simple task and may require timing, subjective assessment (by the observer) of the difficulty the patient encounters when performing the task, or more sophisticated measurement using calibrated instruments of subject performance.[65] For example, the Get-up and Go test is a widely used physical performance measure that requires the observer to evaluate subjectively the patient's ability to rise from a chair, walk 3 m, turn around, walk back,

Table 2.6. Determination of Gait Speed [70]

Test Administration

Patient instructed to "walk at your own speed"

1-m start up

4-m timed distance

Test Interpretation

<0.6 m/s	High risk
0.6 m/s to 1 m/s	Intermediate risk
>1 m/s	Low risk

and sit down.[66] It can identify patients at risk for falls and can identify specific physical impairments, such as proximal muscle weakness. The timed up and go test, which was found to have good sensitivity and specificity for identifying fallers in a small sample of patients,[67] has demonstrated poor test–retest reliability in the large Canadian Study of Health and Aging,[68] and a smaller study of adults in a physical therapy setting,[69] and, therefore, cannot be recommended for routine clinical use.

Gait speed has demonstrated AUC values for identification of highly functioning older adults at risk of functional decline that are comparable to the AUC of the well-validated EPESE (Established Populations for Epidemiologic Studies of the Elderly) physical performance test battery in a large and ethnically diverse group of older patients.[64] In another study examining predictors of functional decline among a population of veterans and health maintenance organization enrollees, a gait speed of less than 0.6 m/sec was found to have an AUC value similar to that of the EPESE test battery for identifying residents at risk of functional decline.[70] This study measured walking distance of 4 m with an instruction to participants to "walk at your normal speed." This measurement typically took less than 2 minutes and was found acceptable by a large majority of personnel in both outpatient and home settings (Table 2.6).[70] Another study examining performance measures among highly functioning Japanese-Americans found that the EPESE 10-ft walk and rapid 10-ft walk had moderate reliability, the EPESE timed chair rises and hand held grip strength had high reliability, and all of these measures had the ability to discriminate functional differences in this population, while being easily administered in a clinic or home setting.[65]

There is also growing evidence that simple questions can identify highly functioning individuals at risk of functional decline and disability.[71] For example, in a study of independent older women, a report of slowed walking was associated with new onset of difficulty walking at 1 year.[72] Patients who used a cane and reported no walking difficulty were more likely to develop new mobility problems at 2 years than patients who did not use a cane.[73] Asking highly functioning patients about task modification, as manifested by slower walking or use of assistive devices, is recommended to identify a subset at increased risk of functional decline (Grade B).

Falls

Falls are an important cause of morbidity and mortality in older adults and can be prevented.[74,75] All elderly patients should be asked about the occurrence of falls in the past year and should perform a Get-up and Go test (Grade A).[74] Patients who present for evaluation after a fall, or who have recurrent falls, or who have an abnormal Get-up and Go test require further evaluation.[74] Much of this evaluation would be included in a typical CGA (e.g., orthostatic vitals signs, review of medications, musculoskeletal and neurological evaluation, and a home safety assessment).[74]

Incontinence

CGA includes an assessment of continence. Routine use of questionnaires is recommended (Grade D).[76] A systematic review has identified three well-validated tools for both men and women that address all forms of incontinence.[77] The King's Health Questionnaire is available in the public domain but has 29 items. The short form of the Urinary Distress Inventory has 6 items, but is not in the public domain. The International Consultation on Incontinence developed and validated a brief, 3-item instrument that assesses incontinence and its effect on quality-of-life.

Evaluation of patients with incontinence includes exploration of the effect of functional status on incontinence, toilet access, fecal incontinence, sexual dysfunction, the effect of incontinence on quality-of-life and pelvic floor assessment. Post-void residual should be measured in patients with symptoms of voiding dysfunction or frequent urinary tract infections. Finally, patients with incontinence should be given a voiding diary.[76]

Nutrition

Malnutrition in older patients is associated with increased risks of functional decline, hospitalization, and death. Rates of malnutrition vary in the elderly population: 1% to 5% of community-dwelling elders are malnourished, compared to at least 20% of those admitted to the hospital and 37% residing in long-term care facilities.[78] The Nutrition Screening Initiative developed a multitiered approach to screening, beginning with a self-administered questionnaire, followed by a provider-administered instrument for patients identified at increased risk. In a prospective study, the instrument's summary score was not associated with mortality, indicating that it is not an optimal tool for nutrition screening.[79] The Mini-Nutritional Assessment (MNA) is a well-validated tool[78,80]; however, its 20 minute administration time makes it impractical in most outpatient assessment settings. The Mini-Nutritional Assessment Short Form (MNA-SF) is a 6-item instrument derived from the MNA that combines historical items with the BMI. It correlates very well with the MNA, with an AUC of 0.96, a sensitivity of 0.979, and specificity of 1.00 for patients with malnutrition.[81] In hospital settings, the Subjective Global Assessment predicts poor outcomes.[82] This instrument has been used in randomized trials of patients undergoing elective surgery, and, in combination with nutritional interventions, has resulted in improved outcomes.[83] The Geriatric Nutrition Risk Index uses a combination of albumin level and weight to identify malnourished hospitalized patients and has demonstrated validity.[84] The simplified nutritional appetite questionnaire is a 4-item appetite assessment tool that can predict significant weight loss among elders who reside in either the community or nursing home.[85] The Geriatric Nutrition Risk Index and simplified nutritional appetite questionnaire, although promising, have not been widely validated. Based on the limited data available, use of the MNA-SF for outpatients and the Subjective Global Assessment for patients undergoing elective surgery is reasonable (Grade B).

Environment

The goals of environmental assessment in the geriatric assessment are to ensure that an older person lives safely in a home that maximizes functional independence.[86] Many trials to prevent falls in older persons include interventions to improve home safety, and these interventions are effective in reducing falls.[87,88] Common fall-related hazards in homes include low ambient lighting, slippery surfaces in bathrooms, throw-rugs, stopovers, stairs, absence of railings and trailing cords.[89–91] Safety assessment also includes attention to fire safety, such as the presence of smoke detectors, fire extinguishers, carbon monoxide detectors, and use of portable heaters.[92,93] Assessing the presence and storage of firearms, as well as crime safety is also necessary. Assessment of accessibility and supportiveness includes queries about the use of adaptive equipment, such as grab-bars, in the home, and how readily a patient that requires a mobility aid, such as a wheelchair or walker, can access and move about in their home.

Should the assessment process include a home visit? Some successful randomized trials of geriatric assessment have not included a home visit.[10,11,59,63] Fall-reduction trials typically include an in-home environmental assessment,[75] as do a number of successful trials of geriatric assessment.[23,58,61] A trial examining the effectiveness of providing home safety checklists showed no difference between the intervention and control groups in the rate of home safety improvements.[94] If an elderly patient is at risk to fall, an in-home environmental assessment should be a part of the evaluation (Grade A). This assessment could be conducted by a variety of health care professionals, including home health nurses or therapists for homebound patients, or adult social service workers for at-risk elders. For patients not at risk to fall, an in-home environmental assessment is preferred but not mandated by the available evidence.

Social Assessment

Assessing an elder's social situation includes assessment of social support, caregiver stress, and risk for elder abuse. Social support refers to friends, family, and other persons who are available to provide care for the elderly person, and includes an assessment of the number available for crises and long-term care.[95] The Lubben Social Network Scale-6 is an abbreviated version of the widely used Lubben Social Network Scale that has been shown to have good internal reliability and validity.[96] The authors suggest a cut-off score of 12 for identifying elderly persons at risk of social isolation.[96] Evaluation of financial resources can help the older patient and their caregivers plan for in-home or institutional long-term care needs.

Caring for an impaired elderly person can be stressful, and caregiver burden has been associated with increased mortality,[97] and with institutionalization of patients with dementia.[98,99] Although there are several theoretical frameworks to guide assessment of caregiver stress, most of the available validated instruments measure caregiving burden.[100] These scales, although developed for use in research, can be used clinically; however, their length may preclude their routine use.[100] The Zarit Burden Interview has good reliability and validity and has been widely used. It consists of 22 items scored from "never" to "nearly always" that can be self-administered or completed during an interview.[101] The 7-item version of the Screen for Caregiver Burden also has good reliability and validity and is easy to administer but has not been widely used.[102] The currently available data do not allow for a specific recommendation to choose any one scale over another.

Elder mistreatment encompasses elder abuse, neglect, exploitation, and abandonment, and affects up to 5% of older Americans. Frail elders, who are more likely to undergo geriatric assessment, are at increased risk of elder mistreatment. Because older adults are unlikely to report mistreatment, clinicians interested in identifying elder mistreatment must ask older adults about mistreatment and should do so without the caregiver present. The authors of a recent systematic review of instruments to screen for elder mistreatment recommend three instruments for clinical use (Grade B). The Brief Abuse Screen for the Elderly is a 5-item questionnaire that takes 1 minute to complete. The Elder Assessment Instrument has good inter-rater reliability, a sensitivity of 0.71, and specificity of 0.93 for identifying mistreatment in an emergency room population. It consists of an easily administered 42-item checklist. The Conflict Tactics Scale is a 19-item self-report or interview instrument that assesses physical and verbal abuse. It has good psychometric properties and has been the most widely used.[103]

OPTIONAL ASSESSMENT

Systematic assessments of health literacy, spirituality, driving ability, and pain have not been routinely included in CGA trials. Although the available evidence does not require their inclusion in the comprehensive assessment of an older patient, many geriatricians include assessment of these domains (Grade D).

Health Literacy

Health literacy describes a basic mathematical, reading, and communication skill set that allows patients to function in the health care system and to use health information.[104] Low levels of health literacy are associated with lower functional status,[105] more comorbidities and poorer access to health care,[106] and higher health care costs.[107] Low health literacy is common, affecting 30% of well-educated community-dwelling elders.[108] Understanding the ability of an elderly patient or their primary caregiver to use health information is important to help provide appropriate health education and supporting materials.

Assessing the ability of a patient to understand and use health care information obviously involves assessment of functional domains such as hearing, sight, and cognition that are a routine part of geriatric assessment,[109] as well as a literacy assessment. The Test of Functional Health Literacy in Adults is a well-validated instrument, but it is not suitable for an outpatient setting because of its administration length of 18 to 22 minutes.[110] The Rapid Estimate of Adult Literacy in Medicine consists of a list of 66 medical terms and can take as long as 5 or 6 minutes to adminster.[111] One question, "How often do you have someone help you read hospital materials" (responses – never, occasionally, sometimes, often, always) had an AUC of 0.87, in comparison to a version of the Test of Functional Health Literacy in Adults, and a sensitivity of 0.8 and specificity of 0.77 for low health literacy with a response of "sometimes" as the cut-off point.[112] In another clinic population, the question "How confident are you filling out medical forms by yourself" (extremely, quite a bit, somewhat, a little bit, not at all) had an AUC of 0.82, in comparison to the Rapid Estimate of Adult Literacy in Medicine, and a sensitivity of 0.83 and specificity of 0.65 for impaired health literacy with a cut-off point of "somewhat."[113] Using one of these questions is a quick and reasonably accurate way to screen for impaired health literacy.

Spirituality and Religiosity

Religious beliefs and practice become more important as people age.[114] Religiosity and spirituality are also associated with improved psychosocial and cognitive function and better health.[115] Patients' desire to have physicians ask about their spiritual or religious believe seems to depend on their health status: in one multicenter study, only 33% felt that their physician should routinely inquire about spiritual beliefs, but fully 70% responded that they would want their physicians to ask about spiritual beliefs if they were seriously ill.[116]

Because older patients are likely to turn to spiritual or religious beliefs to make sense of the many losses they experience, physicians have a responsibility, derived from the principles of beneficence and fidelity to the patient, to assess spirituality.[117,118] Appropriate times to assess spirituality includes during discussion of support systems, advanced directive discussions, discussions of coping with chronic pain and illness, new diagnoses of serious or terminal illness, and end-of-life care planning.[119] There are no brief instruments that have been validated for use in clinical settings, although several have been developed and validated for research purposes.[120] Several authors have proposed brief mnemonics, which have not been validated, to guide clinicians.[117,119] A common sense approach to spiritual assessment involves informal exploration of patients' sources of hope, belief, support, and meaning in their lives. Further exploration of a patient's spirituality or religiosity can be guided by their initial response to these queries.

Driving

Most elderly patients continue to rely on driving for transportation. Unfortunately, they have the highest fatality rate per mile driven of any age group, other than drivers younger than 25 years.[121] Older drivers are both more likely to have accidents, and their increased frailty increases their susceptibility to fatal injury.[121] A number of factors are associated with increased accident risk, including age, medical conditions, dementia, and polypharmacy.[121] All older patients should be asked if they drive, and about accidents, near misses, or driving citations (Grade D). Driving errors most frequently associated with unsafe driving include problems negotiating an intersection, poor gap estimate in lane change or merging, and failure to maintain appropriate speed.[122]

In the outpatient setting, assessments normally included in a geriatric assessment can identify patients requiring further evaluation. Patient's with decreased visual acuity; with strength less than 4/5 in either upper or the right lower extremity, with a decreased range of motion or with a full range of motion performed slowly or with pain; and those patients who walk 10 ft up and back in more than 9 sec are more likely to have motor vehicle accidents.[121] A score of 4 or less on the CDT when using the Freund scoring system was 0.64 sensitive and 0.98 specific for identifying individual's who were unsafe drivers (Table 2.7).[123] Abnormal performances on the Trail-making

Table 2.7. Freund Method of Scoring CDT [123]

Characteristic	Points
One hand points to 2 (or symbol representative of 2)	1
Exactly two hands	1
Absence of intrusive marks	1
Numbers are inside the clock circle	1
All numbers 1–12 are present, no duplicates or omissions	1
Numbers spaced equally or nearly equally from each other	1
Numbers spaced equally, or nearly equally, from edge of circle	1
Cut-off score	4

part B test also predict unsafe driving.[121] If individuals at risk for unsafe driving want to continue to drive, they should be referred for formal driving assessment.

Pain

The prevalence of important pain in community-dwelling elderly ranges from 25% to 50%.[124] Evaluation of pain includes assessment of its intensity, duration, frequency, location, quality, and alleviating and precipitating factors. Older patients may deny the presence of pain, but may acknowledge discomfort, hurting, or aching. The effects of pain on, and pain's relationship to, performance of ADLs and IADLs should be assessed, as should the use the analgesic medications and the patient's and caregiver's attitudes and beliefs regarding pain.[124]

A validated scale should be used to measure pain intensity.[124] A number of scales are available, including visual analog scales (VAS), numeric rating scales, which add numbered gradations to a VAS, verbal descriptor scales (VDS), the familiar "0 to 10" verbal numeric scales, and face pain scales. Several studies have compared the performance of these scales directly and found that the VDS may be the best scale for use in the elderly population, although all of these scales, apart from the VAS, are acceptable.[54,125] The VDS consists of seven adjectival descriptions, "no pain," "mild pain," "moderate pain," "severe pain," "extreme pain," and "the most intense pain imaginable."[126]

Pain assessment in patients with dementia is more difficult, as patients have less cognitive capability to process and communicate their experience of pain. Nonetheless, more than 80% of communicative demented individuals with MMSE scores in a moderate to severe range can locate pain on themselves[127] and complete a pain intensity scale if given enough time.[128] For patients with advanced dementia who are unable to communicate, a number of pain-rating scales that use observable behaviors, such as grimacing and moaning, have been developed.[129] Most are not suitable for clinical use because of their length and the extensive training required for proper administration. A recent systematic review of available instruments rated them using comprehensive, validated criteria.[130] The three highest scoring instruments in this review that are suitable for clinical use are the DOLOPLUS-2,[131] the Pain Assessment Checklist for Seniors with Limited Ability to Communicate (PACSLAC),[132] and the Pain Assessment in Advanced Dementia (PAINEAD). Of these, the DOLOPLUS-2, developed for use among French speakers, but with an available (but unvalidated) English language version (available at www.doloplus.com) has been the most widely used.[130] The PAINEAD is the shortest, with five items rated on a 3-point scale.[133] One recent study that compared these three items among Dutch speaking subjects found that the PACSLAC had good reliability and validity and was the most clinically useful, whereas the DOLOPLUS-2 was the least useful.[134] Based on the limited data available, either the PACSLAC or PAINEAD appear to be the most useful tools for pain assessment among elderly patients with dementia (Grade B).

GERIATRIC ASSESSMENT IN VARIOUS SETTINGS

Home visits offer insights important in the care of the older patient. In a study of dementia patients evaluated in both the home and the clinic, 81% had a problem identified at home, but not in the clinic.[135] Home visits are also effective: A meta-analysis of 18 trials with 13,347 older adults showed that geriatric assessment in the home improved function and decreased mortality among those younger than 80 years and decreased nursing home admission if the home visit program included comprehensive geriatric assessment and multiple visits.[8] These interventions could be led by a physician or a nurse practitioner.[23,136] Teleconferencing extends the reach of geriatricians to isolated rural elders and is a promising use of technology.[137] Assessment instruments used in outpatient settings can be readily used in the home setting as well.

CGA in the hospital can be done by an inpatient geriatric consult team or on a unit designed for the care of the older patient. Inpatient consultations teams are effective if they have control over implementation of management recommendations.[7] Geriatric evaluation and management (GEM) units have been shown to reduce functional decline at discharge[9] and can improve long-term function and reduce institutionalization if coupled with long-term follow-up.[7] GEM units utilize a multidisciplinary approach and assessment of the usual functional domains, including assessment of caregiver capabilities and the patient's social situation.[9] Acute Care for the Elderly units combine environmental modifications with protocol-driven functional interventions and a geriatrician-led review of medications and care aimed at minimizing harm. They have been shown to improve functional status at discharge and increase rates of discharge to home settings.[138] Targeting these interventions to the appropriate patient is important for their success. The assessment instruments used in outpatient settings can also be used in hospital settings.

All patients cared for in nursing homes that receive Medicare or Medicaid payment undergo assessment using the Minimum Data Set (MDS).[139] The MDS addresses multiple domains of function and is targeted to the frail elderly. The original MDS and the revised 1996 version of the MDS have been shown to have good interrater reliability.[139] The ADL long-scale component has good validity and is able to detect clinically meaningful changes in patients.[140] MDS cognitive scales have good correlation with the MMSE,[141] and the MDS incontinence measures have proved usefulness in incontinence management.[142] The MDS does not perform as well as the GDS in detection of depression,[143] and the 15-item GDS should be used for assessment of depression in this population.[48] The MDS also underreports disruptive behaviors.[144] The MDS fall indicator underreports falls,[145] and the MDS is insensitive to the presence of pain.[146] Pain in this population should be assessed using tools appropriate for a patient's level of cognitive functioning.

CONCLUSION

The evidence that functional assessment of elderly patients at risk of decline is effective is strong enough that physicians who want to provide the best care to their patients need to find ways to incorporate a systematic approach to functional assessment into their practice. Although few trials of CGA have been done in circumstances identical to the busy outpatient settings in which most primary care physicians find themselves, enough is known about comprehensive approaches to geriatric assessment to guide practitioners. In brief, assessments should be comprehensive, should include use of validated assessment instruments, and should include the patient and family in goal setting. Assessment can be spread out over several visits, and the assessment process is more practical and more enjoyable if done in collaboration with other health care professionals. By developing a process of functional assessment that works in their practice, physicians will be able to improve the quality of care that they provide to their older patients.

REFERENCES

1. Ferrucci L, Baldasseroni S, Bandinelli S. Disease severity and health-related quality of life across different chronic conditions. *J Am Geriatr Soc.* 2000;48:1490–1495.
2. Reuben D, Rubenstein LV, Hirsch SH, Hays RD. Value of functional status as a predictor of mortality: results of a prospective study. *Am J Med.* 1992;93:663–669.
3. Satish S, Winograd CH, Chavez C, Bloch DA. Geriatric targeting criteria as predictors of survival and health care utilization. *J Am Geriatr Soc.* 1996;44(8):914–921.
4. Nelson E, Conger B, Douglass R, et al. Functional health status levels of primary care patients. *JAMA.* 1983;249(24):3331–3338.
5. Anonymous. National Institutes of Health Consensus Development Conference Statement: geriatric assessment methods for clinical decision-making. *J Am Geriatr Soc.* 1988;36(4):342–347.
6. Rubenstein LZ, Joseph T. Freeman award lecture: comprehensive geriatric assessment: from miracle to reality. *J Gerontol Series A-Biol Sci Med Sci.* 2004;59(5):473–477.
7. Stuck AE, Siu AL, Wieland GD, Adams J, Rubenstein LZ. Comprehensive geriatric assessment: a meta-analysis of controlled trials. *Lancet.* 1993;342(8878):1032–1036.
8. Stuck AE, Egger M, Hammer A, Minder CE, Beck JC. Home visits to prevent nursing home admission and functional decline in elderly people: systematic review and meta-regression analysis. *JAMA.* 2002;287(8):1022–1028.
9. Cohen HJ, Feussner JR, Weinberger M, et al. A controlled trial of inpatient and outpatient geriatric evaluation and management. *NEJM.* 2002;346(12):905–912.
10. Reuben DB, Frank JC, Hirsch SH, McGuigan KA, Maly RC. A randomized clinical trial of outpatient comprehensive geriatric assessment coupled with an intervention to increase adherence to recommendations. *J Am Geriatr Soc.* 1999;47(3):269–276.
11. Burns R, Nichols LO, Martindale-Adams J, Graney MJ. Interdisciplinary geriatric primary care evaluation and management: Two-year outcomes. *J Am Geriatr Soc.* 2000;48:8–13.
12. Rubenstein LV, McCoy JM, Cope DW, et al. Improving patient quality of life with feedback to physicians about functional status. *J Gen Int Med.* 1995;10(11):607–614.
13. Moore AA, Siu A, Partridge JM, Hays RD, Adams J. A randomized trial of office-based screening for common problems in older persons. *Am J Med.* 1997;102(4):371–378.
14. Fletcher AE, Price GM, Ng ESW, et al. Population-based multidimensional assessment of older people in UK general practice: a cluster-randomised factorial trial. *Lancet.* 2004;364(9446):1667–1677.
15. Stuck AE, Beck JC, Egger M. Preventing disability in elderly people.[comment]. *Lancet.* 2004;364(9446):1641–1642.
16. Reuben DB, Borok GM, Wolde-Tsadik G, et al. A randomized trial of comprehensive geriatric assessment in the care of hospitalized patients. *NEJM.* 1995;332(20):1345–1350.
17. Gill TM, Allore HG, Hardy SE, Guo Z. The dynamic nature of mobility disability in older persons. *J Am Geriatr Soc.* 2006;54(2):248–254.
18. Hardy SE, Allore HG, Guo Z, Dubin JA, Gill TM. The effect of prior disability history on subsequent functional transitions. *J Gerontol Series A-Biol Sci Med Sci.* 2006;61(3):272–277.
19. Pacala JT, Boult C, Boult L. Predictive validity of a questionnaire that identifies older persons at risk for hospital admission. *J Am Geriatr Soc.* 1995;43(4):374–377.
20. Rubenstein LZ, Goodwin M, Hadley E, et al. Working group recommendations: targeting criteria for geriatric evaluation and management research. *J Am Geriatr Soc.* 1991;39(9 Pt 2):37S–41S.
21. Reuben DB, Maly RC, Hirsch SH, et al. Physician implementation of and patient adherence to recommendations from comprehensive geriatric assessment. *Am J Med.* 1996;100(4):444–451.
22. Alessi CA, Stuck AE, Aronow HU, et al. The process of care in preventive in-home comprehensive geriatric assessment. *J Am Geriatr Soc.* 1997;45(9):1044–1050.
23. Stuck AE, Aronow HU, Steiner A, et al. A trial of annual in-home comprehensive geriatric assessments for elderly people living in the community. *NEJM.* 1995;333(18):1184–1189.
24. Glazier SR, Schuman J, Keltz E, Vally A, Glazier RH. Taking the next steps in goal ascertainment: a prospective study of patient, team, and family perspectives using a comprehensive standardized menu in a geriatric assessment and treatment unit. *J Am Geriatr Soc.* 2004;52(2):284–289.
25. Bogardus ST, Jr., Bradley EH, Williams CS, Maciejewski PK, Gallo WT, Inouye SK. Achieving goals in geriatric assessment: role of caregiver agreement and adherence to recommendations. *J Am Geriatr Soc.* 2004;52(1):99–105.
26. Reuben DB, Zwanziger J, Bradley TB, et al. How many physicians will be needed to provide medical care for older persons? Physician manpower needs for the twenty-first century. *J Am Geriatr Soc.* 1993;41(4):444–453.
27. Besdine R, Boult C, Brangman S, et al. Caring for older Americans: the future of geriatric medicine. *J Am Geriatr Soc.* 2005;53(6 Suppl):S245–256.
28. Reuben DB, Bradley TB, Zwanziger J, Beck JC. Projecting the need for physicians to care for older persons: effects of changes in demography, utilization patterns, and physician productivity. *J Am Geriatr Soc.* 1993;41(10):1033–1038.
29. Rubenstein LZ, Schairer C, Wieland GD, Kane R. Systematic biases in functional status assessment of elderly adults: effects of different data sources. *J Gerontol.* 1984;39(6):686–691.

30. Miller DK, Brunworth D, Brunworth DS, Hagan R, Morley JE. Efficiency of geriatric case-finding in a private practitioner's office. *J Am Geriatr Soc.* 1995;43(5):533–537.

31. Moore AA. Clinical guidelines for alcohol use disorders in older adults. Available at: http://www.americangeriatrics.org/products/positionpapers/alcohol.shtml. Accessed May 5, 2008.

32. Schmader KE, Hanlon JT, Pieper CF, et al. Effects of geriatric evaluation and management on adverse drug reactions and suboptimal prescribing in the frail elderly. *Am J Med.* 2004;116(6):394–401.

33. Perkins NA, Murphy JE, Malone DC, Armstrong EP. Performance of drug-drug interaction software for personal digital assistants. *Ann Pharmacother.* 2006;40(5):850–855.

34. Chumlea WC, Roche AF, Steinbaugh ML. Estimating stature from knee height for persons 60 to 90 years of age. *J Am Geriatr Soc.* 1985;33:116–120.

35. Yueh B, Shapiro N, Maclean CH, Shekelle PG. Screening and management of adult hearing loss in primary care: scientific review. *JAMA.* 2003;289(15):1976–1985.

36. Hamalainen P, Rantanen T, Keskinen M, Meurman JH. Oral health status and change in handgrip strength over a 5-year period in 80-year-old people. *Gerodontology.* 2004;21(3):155–160.

37. Boustani M, Peterson B, Hanson LC, Harris R, Lohr KN. U.S. Preventive Services Task Force. Screening for dementia in primary care: a summary of the evidence for the U.S. preventive services task force. *Ann Int Med.* 2003;138:927–937.

38. Tombaugh TN, McIntyre NJ. The Mini-mental State Examination: a comprehensive review. *J Am Geriatr Soc.* 1992;40(9):922–935.

39. Inouye SK, Robison JT, Froehlich TE, Richardson ED. The Time and Change Test: a simple screening test for dementia. *J Gerontol: Med Sci.* 1998;53A(4):M281–M286.

40. Borson S, Scanlan J, Brush M, Vitaliano P, Dokmak A. The Mini-Cog: a cognitive "vital signs" measure for dementia screening in multi-lingual elderly. *Int J Geriatr Psych.* 2000;15:1021–1027.

41. Borson S, Scanlan JM, Chen P, Ganguli M. The Mini-Cog as a screen for dementia: validation in a population-based sample. *J Am Geriatr Soc.* 2003;51:1451–1454.

42. Cooney LM, Jr., Kennedy GJ, Hawkins KA, Hurme SB. Who can stay at home? Assessing the capacity to choose to live in the community. *Arch Int Med.* 2004;164(4):357–360.

43. Juby A, Tench S, Baker V. The value of clock drawing in identifying executive cognitive dysfunction in people with a normal Mini-Mental State Examination score. *CMAJ.* 2002;167(8):859–864.

44. Royall DR, Mulroy AR, Chiodo LK, Polk MJ. Clock drawing is sensitive to executive control: a comparison of six methods. *J Gerontol Series B-Psychol Sci Soc Sci.* 1999;54(5):P328–333.

45. Costa PJ, Williams TF, Somerfield M, et al. Recognition and Initial Assessment of Alzheimer's Disease and Related Dementias. Clinical Practice Guideline. Guideline no. 19. In: Department of Health and Human Services PHS, Agency for Health Care Policy and Research, ed: AHCPR, Rockville, MD, 1996.

46. MacKinnon A, Mulligan R. Combining cognitive testing and informant report to increase accuracy in screening for dementia. *Am J Psych.* 1998;155:1529–1535.

47. U.S. Preventive Services Task Force. Screening for depression: recommendations and rationale. *Ann Int Med.* 2002;136:760–764.

48. Watson LC, Pignone MP. Screening accuracy for late-life depression in primary care: a systematic review. *J Fam Pract.* 2003;52(12):956–964.

49. Yesavage JA, Brink TL, Rose TL, et al. Development and validation of a geriatric depression screening scale: a preliminary report. *J Psych Res.* 1983;17:37–49.

50. Rinaldi P, Mecocci P, Benedetti C, et al. Validation of the five-item geriatric depression scale in elderly subjects in three different settings. *J Am Geriatr Soc.* 2003;51(5):694–698.

51. Blank K, Gruman C, Robison JT. Case-finding for depression in elderly people: balancing ease of administration with validity in varied treatment settings. *J Gerontol Series A-Biol Sci Med Sci.* 2004;59(4):378–384.

52. Reuben DB, Seeman TE, Keeler E, et al. Refining the categorization of physical functional status: the added value of combining self-reported and performance-based measures. *J Gerontol Series A-Biol Sci Med Sci.* 2004;59(10):1056–1061.

53. Katz S, Akpom CA. A measure of primary sociobiological functions. *Int J Health Serv.* 1976;6:493–507.

54. McDowell I. *Measuring Health: A Guide to Rating Scales and Questionnaires.* 3rd ed. New York: Oxford University Press; 2006.

55. Mahoney F, Barthel D. Functional evaluation: the Barthel Index. *Maryland State Med J.* 1965;14(2):61–65.

56. Lawton MP, Brody EM. Assessment of older people: self-maintaining and instrumental activities of daily living. *Gerontologist.* 1969;9:179–186.

57. Pfeffer RI, Kurosaki TT, Harrah CH, et al. Measurement of functional activities in older adults living in the community. *J Gerontol.* 1982;37:323–329.

58. Fabacher D, Josephson K, Pietruszka F, Linderborn K, Morley JE, Rubenstein LZ. An in-home preventive assessment program for independent older adults: a randomized controlled trial. *J Am Geriatr Soc.* 1994;42(6):630–638.

59. Burns R, Nichols LO, Graney MJ, Cloar FT. Impact of continued geriatric outpatient management on health outcomes of older veterans. *Arch Int Med.* 1995;155(12):1313–1318.

60. Hendriksen C, Lund E, Stromgard E. Consequences of assessment and intervention among elderly people: a three year randomised controlled trial. *Br Med J Clin Res.* 1984;289(6457):1522–1524.

61. Boult C, Boult L, Murphy C, Ebbitt B, Luptak M, Kane RL. A controlled trial of outpatient geriatric evaluation and management. *J Am Geriatr Soc.* 1994;42(5):465–470.

62. Hughes S, Weaver FM, Giobbie-Hurder A, et al. Effectiveness of team-managed home-based primary care: a randomized multicenter trial. *JAMA.* 2000;284(22):2877–2885.

63. Engelhardt JB, Toseland RW, O'Connell, JC, Richie JT, Jue D, Banks S. The effectiveness and efficiency of outpatient geriatric evaluation and management. *J Am Geriatr Soc.* 1996;44(7):847–856.

64. Guralnik JM, Ferrucci L, Pieper CF, et al. Lower extremity function and subsequent disability: consistency across studies, predictive models, and value of gait speed alone compared with the short physical performance battery. *J Gerontol Series A-Biol Sci Med Sci.* 2000;55(4):M221–M231.

65. Curb JD, Ceria-Ulep CD, Rodriguez BL, et al. Performance-based measures of physical function for high-function populations. *J Am Geriatr Soc.* 2006;54:737–742.

66. Mathias S, Nayak US, Isaacson A. Balance in elderly patients: the "get-up and go" test. *Arch Phys Med Rehabil.* 1986;67(6):387–389.

67. Shumway-Cook A, Brauer S, Woollacott M. Predicting the probability for falls in community-dwelling older adults using the Timed Up & Go Test. *Phys Ther.* 2000;80(9):896–903.

68. Rockwood K, Awalt E, Carver D, MacKnight C. Feasibility and measurement properties of the functional reach and the timed

up and go tests in the Canadian study of health and aging. *J Gerontol Series A-Biol Sci Med Sci.* 2000;55(2):M70–M73.

69. Nordin E, Rosendahl E, Lundin-Olsson L. Timed "Up & Go" test: reliability in older people dependent in activities of daily living–focus on cognitive state. *Phys Ther.* 2006;86(5):646–655.

70. Studenski S, Perera S, Wallace D, et al. Physical performance measures in the clinical setting. *J Am Geriatr Soc.* 2003;51(3):314–322.

71. Chaves PH, Garrett ES, Fried LP. Predicting the risk of mobility difficulty in older women with screening nomograms: the Women's Health and Aging Study II. *Arch Int Med.* 2000;160(16):2525–2533.

72. Pine ZM, Gurland B, Chren MM. Report of having slowed down: evidence for the validity of a new way to inquire about mild disability in elders. *J Gerontol Series A-Biol Sci Med Sci.* 2000;55(7):M378–M383.

73. M Pine Z, Gurland B, Chren M-M. Use of a cane for ambulation: marker and mitigator of impairment in older people who report no difficulty walking. *J Am Geriatr Soc.* 2002;50(2):263–268.

74. American Geriatrics Society, British Geriatrics Society, and American Academy of Orthopaedic Surgeons Panel on Falls Prevention. Guideline for the prevention of falls in older persons. *J Am Geriatr Soc.* 2001;49(5):664–672.

75. Gillespie LD, Gillespie WJ, Robertson MC, Lamb SE, Cumming RG, Rowe BH. Interventions for preventing falls in elderly people. *Cochrane Database of Systematic Reviews.* 2006;4.

76. Scottish Intercollegiate Guidelines Network. Management of urinary incontinence in primary care: a national clinical guideline. 2005. Available at: http://www.sign.ac.uk/guidelines/published/index.html#Other. Accessed May 5, 2008.

77. Donovan JL, Badia X, Corcos J, et al. Symptom and quality of life assessment. In Abrams P, Cardozo L, Khoury S, Wein A, eds. *Incontinence: 2nd International Consultation on Incontinence, Paris, July 1–3, 2001.* Plymouth: Health Publications, Ltd; 2002:267–314.

78. Guigoz Y, Lauque S, Vellas B. Identifying the elderly at risk for malnutrition: the Mini Nutritional Assessment. *Clin Ger Med.* 2002;18(4):737–757.

79. Sahyoun NR, Jacques PF, Dallal GE, Russell RM. Nutritional Screening Initiative checklist may be a better awarenesss/educational tool than a screening one. *J Am Diet Assoc.* 1997;97:760–764.

80. Van Nes MC, Herrmann FR, Gold G, Michel JP, Rizzoli R. Does the mini nutritional assessment predict hospitalization outcomes in older people? *Age Ageing.* 2001;30(3):221–226.

81. Rubenstein LZ, Harker JO, Salva A, Guigoz Y, Vellas B. Screening for undernutrition in geriatric practice: developing the short-form mini-nutritional assessment (MNA-SF). *J Geront Series A-Biol Sci MedSci.* 2001;56(6):M366–M372.

82. Covinsky KE, Martin GE, Beyth RJ, Justice AC, Sehgal AR, Landefeld CS. The relationship between clinical assessments of nutritional status and adverse outcomes in older hospitalized medical patients. *J Am Geriatr Soc.* 1999;47(5):532–538.

83. Detsky AS, Smalley PS, Chang J. The rational clinical examination. Is this patient malnourished? *JAMA.* 1994;271(1):54–58.

84. Bouillanne O, Morineau G, Dupont C, et al. Geriatric Nutritional Risk Index: a new index for evaluating at-risk elderly medical patients. *Am J Clin Nutr.* 2005;82(4):777–783.

85. Wilson M-MG, Thomas DR, Rubenstein LZ, et al. Appetite assessment: simple appetite questionnaire predicts weight loss in community-dwelling adults and nursing home residents. *Am J Clin Nutr.* 2005;82(5):1074–1081.

86. Cutler LJ. Assessment of physical environments of older adults. In Kane RL, Kane RA, eds. *Assessing Older Persons: Measures, Meaning, and Practical Applications.* Oxford: Oxford University Press; 2000:360–379.

87. Close J, Ellis M, Hooper R, Glucksman E, Jackson S, Swift C. Prevention of falls in the elderly trial (PROFET): a randomized controlled trial. *Lancet.* 1999;353(9147):93–97.

88. Nikolaus T, Bach M. Preventing falls in community-dwelling frail older people using a home intervention team (HIT): results from the randomized Falls-HIT trial. *J Am Geriatr Soc.* 2003;51(3):300–305.

89. Stevens M, Holman CD, Bennett N. Preventing falls in older people: impact of an intervention to reduce environmental hazards in the home. *J Am Geriatr Soc.* 2001;49(11):1442–1447.

90. van Bemmel T, Vandenbroucke JP, Westendorp RGJ, Gussekloo J. In an observational study elderly patients had an increased risk of falling due to home hazards. *J Clin Epidemiol.* 2005;58(1):63–67.

91. Marshall SW, Runyan CW, Yang J, et al. Prevalence of selected risk and protective factors for falls in the home. *Am J Prev Med.* 2005;28(1):95–101.

92. Runyan CW, Johnson RM, Yang J, et al. Risk and protective factors for fires, burns, and carbon monoxide poisoning in U.S. households. *Am J Prev Med.* 2005;28(1):102–108.

93. Tanner EK. Assessing home safety in homebound older adults. *Geriatr Nurs.* 2003 2002;24(4):250–254.

94. Gerson LW, Camargo CA, Jr., Wilber ST. Home modification to prevent falls by older ED patients. *Am J Emerg Med.* 2005;23(3):295–298.

95. Lubben JE, Gironda M. Social support networks. In Osterweil D, Brummel-Smith K, Beck JC, eds. *Comprehensive Geriatric Assessment.* New York: McGraw-Hill; 2000:121–138.

96. Lubben J, Blozik E, Gillmann G, et al. Performance of an abbreviated version of the Lubben Social Network Scale among three European community-dwelling older adult populations. *Gerontologist.* 2006;46(4):503–513.

97. Schulz R, Beach SR. Caregiving as a risk factor for mortality: the Caregiver Health Effects Study. *JAMA.* 1999;282(23):2215–2219.

98. Gilley DW, McCann JJ, Bienias JL, Evans DA. Caregiver psychological adjustment and institutionalization of persons with Alzheimer's disease. *J AgingHealth.* 2005;17(2):172–189.

99. Yaffe K, Fox P, Newcomer R, et al. Patient and caregiver characteristics and nursing home placement in patients with dementia. *JAMA.* 2002;287(16):2090–2097.

100. Gaugler JE, Kane RA, Langlois JA. Assessment of family caregivers of older adults. In Kane RL, Kane RA, eds. *Assessing Older Persons.* Oxford: Oxford University Press; 2000:320–359.

101. Zarit SH, Reever KE, Bach-Peterson J. Relatives of the impaired elderly: correlates of feelings of burden. *Gerontologist.* 1980;20:649–655.

102. Hirschman KB, Shea JA, Xie SX, Karlawish JHT. The development of a rapid screen for caregiver burden. *J Am Geriatr Soc.* 2004;52(10):1724–1729.

103. Fulmer T, Guadagno L, Bitondo Dyer C, Connolly MT. Progress in elder abuse screening and assessment instruments. *J Am Geriatr Soc.* 2004;52(2):297–304.

104. Berkman ND, DeWalt DA, Pignone MP, et al. *Literacy and Health Outcomes. Summary, Evidence Report/Technology Assessment No. 87.* Rockville, MD: Agency for Healthcare Research and Quality; January, 2004 2004. AHRQ Publication No. 04-E007-1.

105. Wolf MS, Gazmararian JA, Baker DW. Health literacy and functional health status among older adults. *Arch Intern Med.* 2005;165(17):1946–1952.

106. Howard DH, Sentell T, Gazmararian JA. Impact of health literacy on socioeconomic and racial differences in health in an elderly population. *J Gen Intern Med.* 2006;21(8):857–861.

107. Howard DH, Gazmararian J, Parker RM. The impact of low health literacy on the medical costs of Medicare managed care enrollees. *Am J Med.*2005;118(4):371–377.

108. Gausman Benson J, Forman WB. Comprehension of written health care information in an affluent geriatric retirement community: use of the Test of Functional Health Literacy. *Gerontology.* 2002;48(2):93–97.

109. Kobylarz FA, Pomidor A, Heath JM. SPEAK. A mnemonic tool for addressing health literacy concerns in geriatric clinical encounters. *Geriatrics.* 2006;61(7):20–26.

110. Parker RM, Baker DW, Williams MV, Nurss JR. The test of functional health literacy in adults: a new instrument for measuring patients' literacy skills. *J Gen Intern Med.* 1995;10(10):537–541.

111. Davis TC, Crouch MA, Long SW, et al. Rapid assessment of literacy levels of adult primary care patients. *Fam Med.* 1991;23(6):433–435.

112. Chew LD, Bradley KA, Boyko EJ. Brief questions to identify patients with inadequate health literacy. *Fam Med.* 2004;36(8):588–594.

113. Wallace LS, Rogers ES, Roskos SE, Holiday DB, Weiss BD. Brief report: screening items to identify patients with limited health literacy skills. *J Gen Intern Med.* 2006;21(8):874–877.

114. Saad L. Religion is very important to majority of Americans. December 5, 2003. http://brain.gallup.com/content/default.aspx?ci=9853. Accessed October 23, 2006.

115. Koenig HG, George LK, Titus P. Religion, spirituality, and health in medically ill hospitalized older patients. *J Am Geriatr Soc.* 2004;52(4):554–562.

116. MacLean CD, Susi B, Phifer N, et al. Patient preference for physician discussion and practice of spirituality. *J Gen Intern Med.* 2003;18(1):38–43.

117. Post SG, Puchalski CM, Larson DB. Physicians and patient spirituality: professional boundaries, competency, and ethics. *Ann Intern Med.* 2000;132(7):578–583.

118. Daaleman TP. Religion, spirituality, and the practice of medicine. *J Am Board Fam Pract.* 2004;17(5):370–376.

119. Anandarajah G, Hight E. Spirituality and medical practice: using the HOPE questions as a practical tool for spiritual assessment. *Am Fam Phys.* 2001;63(1):81–89.

120. Daaleman TP, Frey BB. The Spirituality Index of Well-Being: a new instrument for health-related quality-of-life research. *Ann Fam Med.* 2004;2(5):499–503.

121. Wang CC, Kosinski CJ, Schwartzberg JG, Shanklin AV. *Physician's Guide to Assessing Counseling Older Drivers.* Washington, DC: National Highway Traffic Safety Administration; 2003.

122. Di Stefano M, Macdonald W. Assessment of older drivers: relationships among on-road errors, medical conditions and test outcome. *J Safety Res.* 2003;34(4):415–429.

123. Freund B, Gravenstein S, Ferris R, Burke BL, Shaheen E. Drawing clocks and driving cars. *J Gen Intern Med.* 2005;20(3):240–244.

124. Persons APoPPiO. The management of persistent pain in older persons. *J Am Geriatr Soc.* 2002;50:S205–224.

125. Herr KA, Spratt K, Mobily PR, Richardson G. Pain intensity assessment in older adults: use of experimental pain to compare

126. Herr KA, Garand L. Assessment and measurement of pain in older adults. *Clin Geriatr Med.* 2001;17(3):457–478.

127. Wynne CF, Ling SM, Remsburg R. Comparison of pain assessment instruments in cognitively intact and cognitively impaired nursing home residents. *Geriatr Nurs.* 2000;21(1):20–23.

128. Ferrell BA, Ferrell BR, Rivera L. Pain in cognitively impaired nursing home patients. *J Pain Symp Management.* 1995;10(8):591–598.

129. Stolee P, Hillier LM, Esbaugh J, Bol N, McKellar L, Gauthier N. Instruments for the assessment of pain in older persons with cognitive impairment. *J Am Geriatr Soc.* 2005;53(2):319–326.

130. Zwakhalen SMG, Hamers JPH, Abu-Saad HH, Berger MPF. Pain in elderly people with severe dementia: a systematic review of behavioural pain assessment tools. *BMC Geriatr.* 2006;6(3).

131. DOLOPLUS-2: Behavioral pain assessment scale for elderly subjects with verbal communication disorders. March, 2004. http://www.doloplus.com/versiongb/index.htm. Accessed May 5, 2008.

132. Fuchs-Lacelle S, Hadjistavropoulos T. Development and preliminary validation of the pain assessment checklist for seniors with limited ability to communicate (PACSLAC). *Pain Manag Nurs.* 2004;5(1):37–49.

133. Warden V, Hurley AC, Volicer L. Development and psychometric evaluation of the Pain Assessment in Advanced Dementia (PAINAD) scale. *J Am Med Dir Assoc.* 2003;4(1):9–15.

134. Zwakhalen SMG, Hamers JPH, Berger MPF. The psychometric quality and clinical usefulness of three pain assessment tools for elderly people with dementia. *Pain.* 2006;126(1–3):210–220.

135. Ramsdell JW, Jackson JE, Guy HJB, Renvall MJ. Comparison of clinic-based home assessment to a home visit in demented elderly patients. *Alz DisAssoc Disorders.* 2004;18(3):145–153.

136. Bula CJ, Berod AC, Stuck AE, et al. Effectiveness of preventive in-home geriatric assessment in well functioning, community-dwelling older people: secondary analysis of a randomized trial. *J Am Geriatr Soc.* 1999;47(4):389–395.

137. Cravens DD, Mehr DR, Campbell JD, Armer J, Kruse RL, Rubenstein LZ. Home-based comprehensive assessment of rural elderly persons: the CARE project. *J Rur Health.* 2005;21(4):322–328.

138. Landefeld CS, Palmer RM, Kresevic DM, Fortinsky RH, Kowal J. A randomized trial of care in a hospital medical unit especially designed to improve the functional outcomes of acutely ill older patients. *NEJM.* 1995;332(20):1338–1344.

139. Mor V. A comprehensive clinical assessment tool to inform policy and practice: applications of the minimum data set. *Med Care.* 2004;42(4 Suppl):III50–III59.

140. Carpenter GI, Hastie CL, Morris JN, Fries BE, Ankri J. Measuring change in activities of daily living in nursing home residents with moderate to severe cognitive impairment. *BMC Geriatr.* 2006;6:7.

141. Gruber-Baldini AL, Zimmerman SI, Mortimore E, Magaziner J. The validity of the minimum data set in measuring the cognitive impairment of persons admitted to nursing homes.[see comment]. *J Am Geriatr Soc.* 2000;48(12):1601–1606.

142. Resnick NM, Brandeis GH, Baumann MM, Morris JN. Evaluating a national assessment strategy for urinary incontinence in nursing home residents: reliability of the minimum data set and validity of the resident assessment protocol. *Neurourol Urodynamics.* 1996;15(6):583–598.

143. McCurren C. Assessment for depression among nursing home elders: evaluation of the MDS mood assessment. *Geriatr Nurs.* 2002;23(2):103–108.

144. Horgas AL, Margrett JA. Measuring behavioral and mood disruptions in nursing home residents using the Minimum Data Set. *Outcomes Manag Nurs Pract.* 2001;5(1):28–35.

145. Hill-Westmoreland EE, Gruber-Baldini AL. Falls documentation in nursing homes: agreement between the minimum data set and chart abstractions of medical and nursing documentation. *J Am Geriatr Soc.* 2005;53(2):268–273.

146. Lin W-C, Lum TY, Mehr DR, Kane RL. Measuring pain presence and intensity in nursing home residents. *J Am Med Dir Assoc.* 2006;7(3):147–153.

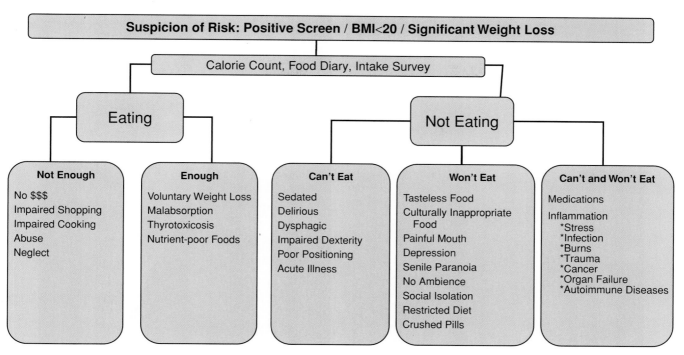

Suspicion of Risk: Positive Screen / BMI<20 / Significant Weight Loss

Calorie Count, Food Diary, Intake Survey

Eating

Not Eating

Not Enough	**Enough**	**Can't Eat**	**Won't Eat**	**Can't and Won't Eat**

Not Enough

No $$$
Impaired Shopping
Impaired Cooking
Abuse
Neglect

Enough

Voluntary Weight Loss
Malabsorption
Thyrotoxicosis
Nutrient-poor Foods

Can't Eat

Sedated
Delirious
Dysphagic
Impaired Dexterity
Poor Positioning
Acute Illness

Won't Eat

Tasteless Food
Culturally Inappropriate
  Food
Painful Mouth
Depression
Senile Paranoia
No Ambience
Social Isolation
Restricted Diet
Crushed Pills

Can't and Won't Eat

Medications

Inflammation
  *Stress
  *Infection
  *Burns
  *Trauma
  *Cancer
  *Organ Failure
  *Autoimmune Diseases

Plate 6.1. Practical approach to undernutrition.

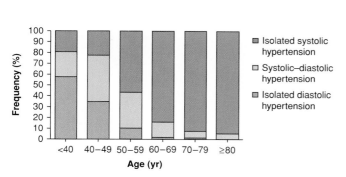

Plate 10.1. Isolated systolic hypertension (used with permission of N Eng J Med Aug 21, 2007; Vol 357(8): 791).

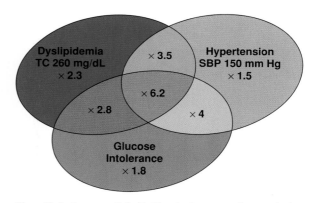

Plate 11.2. Impact of dyslipidemia, hypertension, and glucose intolerance on cardiovascular risk.*

*Compared with risk for a 40-year-old male nonsmoker with total cholesterol = 185 mg/dL, systolic blood pressure = 120 mm Hg, no glucose intolerance, and no electrocardiographic LV hypertrophy, whose probability of developing CVD is 15/1000 (1.5%) in 8 years.

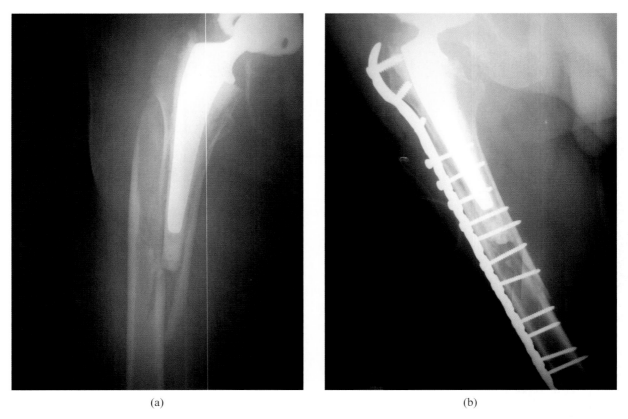

(a)   (b)

Plate 31.1. Preoperative (a) and postoperative (b) AP radiographs of a displaced periprosthetic fracture of the femur distal to a total hip replacement. The implant was stable in the femur and the decision was made to proceed with open reduction and internal fixation of the fracture while retaining the implant in the stable position.

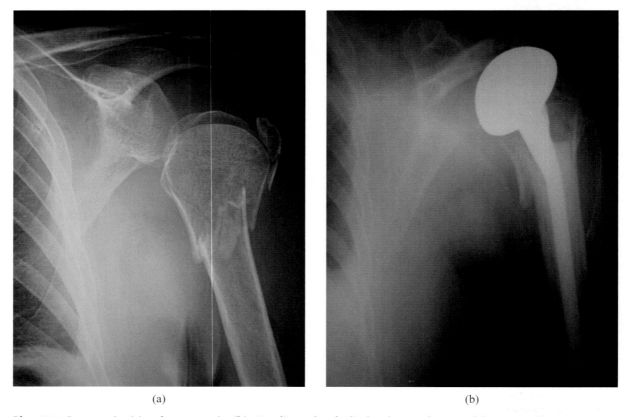

(a)   (b)

Plate 31.7. Preoperative (a) and postoperative (b) AP radiographs of a displaced 3-part fracture of the proximal humerus treated with prosthetic replacement.

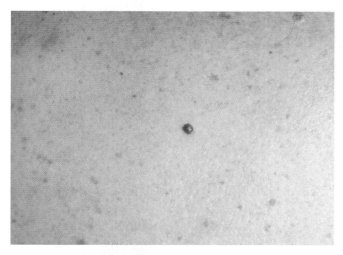

Plate 33.2. Cherry Angioma. Symetrical erythematous benign vascular lesion found on this patient's trunk.

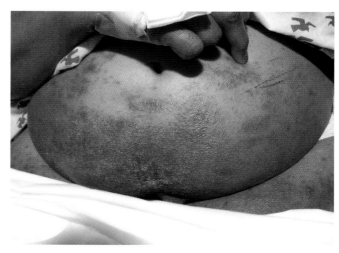

Plate 33.5. Lichen Simplex Chronicus. Hyperpigmented, scaly, pruritic plaques on the patient's abdomen.

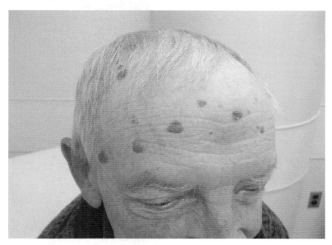

Plate 33.3. Seborrheic keratosis. Hyperpigmented, cratered plaque with a classic "stuck on" appearance on this patient's forehead.

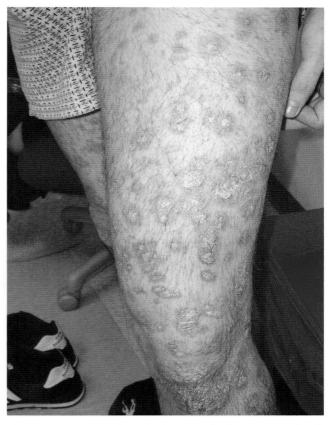

Plate 33.6. Psoriasis. Inflamed, edematous skin lesions covered with a thick silvery white scale.

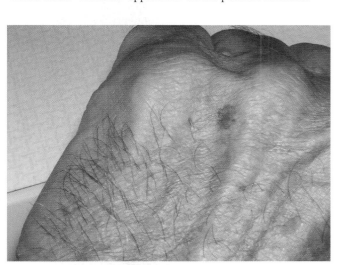

Plate 33.4. Solar lentigo. Localized proliferation of melanocytes caused by chronic sun exposure, expressed as a circumscribed brown macule on the dorsal surface of the hand.

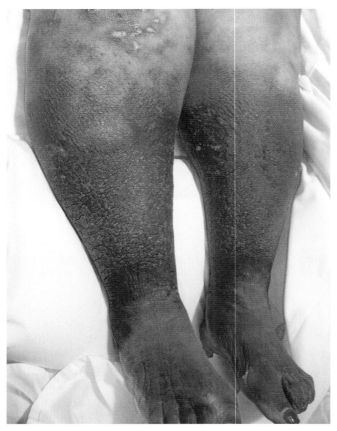

Plate 33.7. Stasis Dermatitis. Hyperpigmented, thickened, edematous skin and subcutaneous tissue bilaterally on this patient's lower extremities.

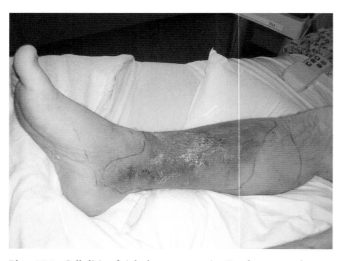

Plate 33.8. Cellulitis of right lower extremity. Erythematous, hyperpigmented, edematous, tender, warm pretibial skin in a patient with venous insufficiency. Pen lines indicate original and current border of infection.

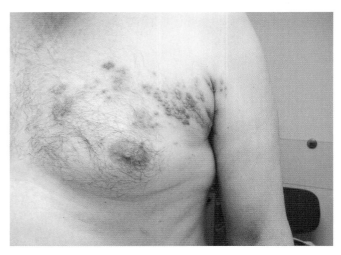

Plate 33.9. Herpes zoster of the left T2 and T3 dermatomes. Groups and clusters of vesicles on an erythematous, edematous base.

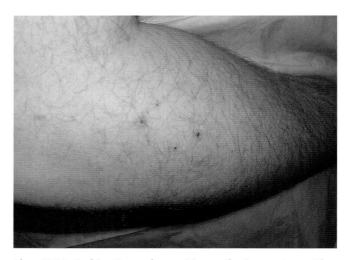

Plate 33.10. Scabies. Intensely pruritic papules in a patient with a prolonged scabies infestation.

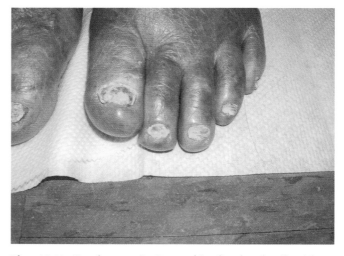

Plate 33.11. Onychomycosis. Dystrophic, discolored nails with an accumulation of white keratinaceous debris under the distal and lateral nail plate.

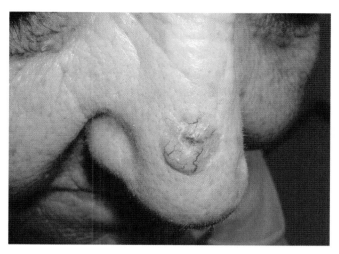

Plate 33.12. Basal cell carcinoma. Pearly, erythematous papule with raised edges and telangectasias on the surface.

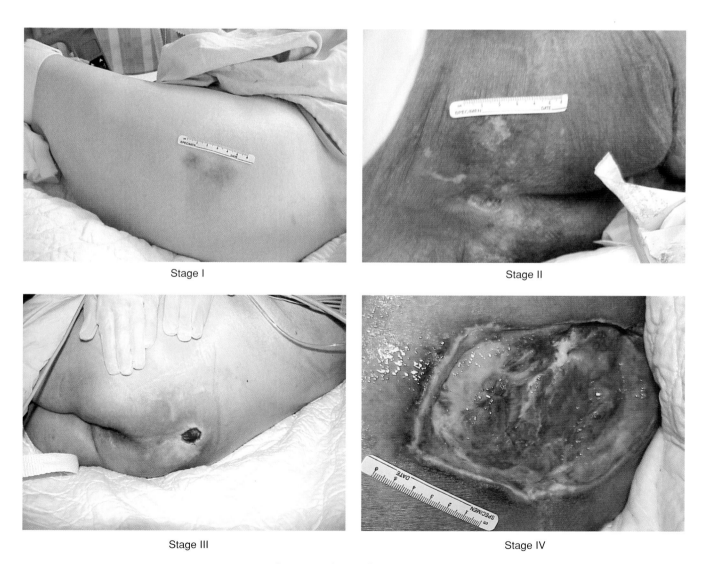

Stage I

Stage II

Stage III

Stage IV

Plate 34.1. Photos of stages I to IV.

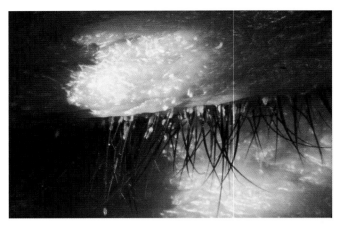

Plate 37.2. Anterior blepharitis. Clinical external photograph demonstrating crusting on eyelids and collarettes on eyelashes.

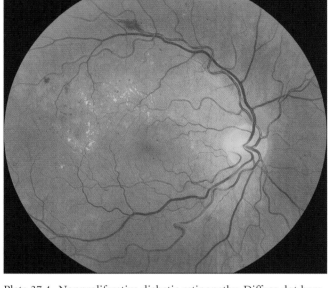

Plate 37.4. Nonproliferative diabetic retinopathy. Diffuse dot hemorrhages, microaneurysms, and hard exudate are noted throughout the fundus.

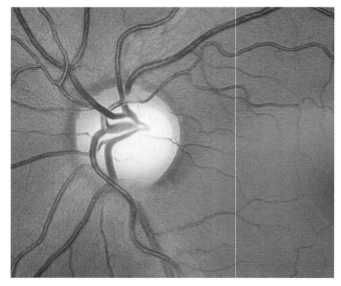

Plate 37.3. Glaucomatous cupping of the optic nerve. A thin rim is noted along the inferior portion of the optic nerve. An associated nerve fiber layer defect also is present.

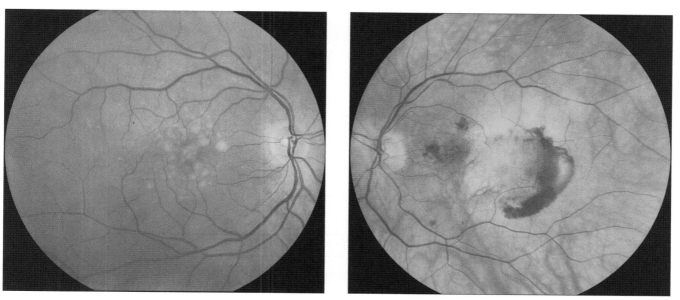

Plate 37.5. A and B. Dry AMD (left).: Hard and soft drusen are noted in the center of the macula. Exudative AMD (right): Subretinal hemorrhage and exudate denote a choroidal neovascularization.

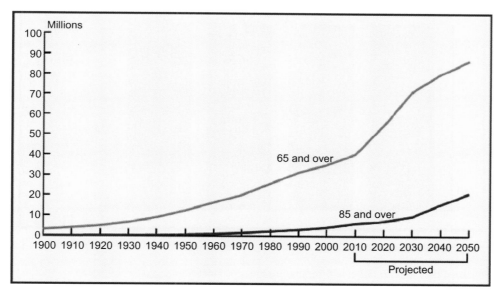

Plate 52.1. Number of people age 65 and over, by age group, selected years 1900–2000. *Note:* Data for 2010–2050 are projections of the population. *Reference population:* These data refer to the resident population. *Source:* U.S. Census Bureau, Decennial Census and Projections.

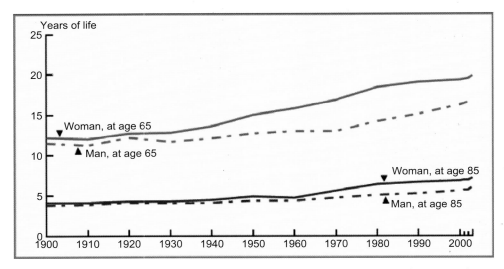

Plate 52.2. Life expectancy at ages 65 and 85, by sex, selected years 1900–2003. *Reference population:* These data refer to the resident population. *Source:* Centers for Disease Control and Prevention, National Center for Health Statistics, National Vital Statistics System.

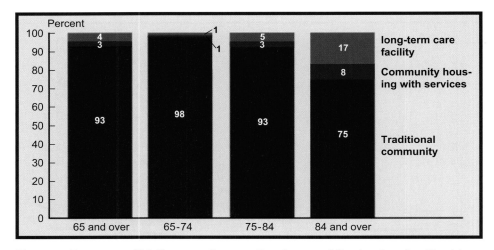

Plate 52.3. Percentage of Medicare enrollees age 65 and over residing in selected residential settings, by age group, 2003. *Note:* Community housing with services applies to respondents who reported they lived in retirement communities or apartments, senior citizen housing, continuing care retirement facilities, assisted living facilities, staged living communities, board and care facilities/homes, and other similar situations, AND who reported they had access to one or more of the following services through their place of residence: meal preparation, cleaning or housekeeping services, laundry services, help with medications. Respondents were asked about access to these services but not whether they actually used the services. A residence is considered a long-term care facility if it is certified by Medicare or Medicaid; or has 3 or more beds and is licensed as a nursing home or other long-term care facility and provides at least one personal care service, or provides 24-hour, 7-day-a-week supervision by a caregiver. *Reference population:* These data refer to Medicare enrollees. *Source:* Centers for Medicare & Medicaid Services. Medicare Current Beneficiary Survey.

3

PREVENTION FOR OLDER ADULTS

Racquel Daley-Placide, MD, Holly Jean Coward, MD

INTRODUCTION

For many clinicians, the time taken to care for the immediate needs of elders seems to preclude the ability to address preventive care issues. For others, lack of a perceived benefit may result in missed opportunities to offer preventive care. The clinician who is motivated to learn and apply screening measures in this population will find that most studies and clinical guidelines exclude elders or make no specific recommendation for them. This chapter attempts to help the clinician identify which elders may benefit from screening and current recommendations for implementing these measures; conversely, we also attempt to advise when it is prudent to avoid screening. These recommendations have been obtained primarily from the U.S. Preventive Services Task Force (USPSTF); we also compiled evidence from the medical literature including documentation provided by the Centers for Disease Control and Prevention (CDC).

Recognizably, there are significant time pressures related to patient care. Because of the frequent impracticality of addressing all screening issues at once, the authors would like the reader to consider performing ongoing assessments of their elderly patients by choosing one specific preventive measure to address at each visit.

IMMUNIZATIONS

Immunization efforts in children have been highly successful. In fact, in 1998, the CDC reported that the childhood immunization initiative goals had been met or exceeded during the previous year.[1] Among adults, immunization efforts have been less successful; however, recently the rates of immunization in older adults have been improving significantly. The CDC reported that from 1989 to 2003 rates of vaccination increased from 15% to 64.5% for pneumococcal vaccine and 33% to 69.9% for annual influenza vaccination[2] among adults aged 65 years and older. The success of immunization efforts in older adults ultimately lies in the hands of the knowledgeable clinician who ensures that the vaccine is administered and documented in the medical record. Table 3.1 provides a brief summary of immunizations recommended for adults (aged 60 years and older). Further information on immunizations can be obtained from the CDC's Advisory Committee on Immunization Practices (www.cdc.gov/nip/).

BLOOD PRESSURE

The prevalence of hypertension increases with age and the end result of long-standing hypertension is well established – increased risk of cardiovascular disease.[3] The diagnosis and treatment of hypertension in elders (including isolated systolic hypertension) reduces the risk of cardiovascular endpoints and mortality.[4] Blood pressure screening is typically done each office visit in a primary care setting. The Seventh Report of the Joint National Committee on Prevention, Detection, Evaluation, and Treatment of High Blood Pressure[5] provides recommended intervals for follow up of a patient's blood pressure based on the measurement obtained (Table 3.2).

Geriatrics Pearl

Ask patients on antihypertensive therapy about symptoms consistent with orthostasis at each interaction. Medications should be titrated so as to avoid postural hypotension and, therefore, falls. Recall that to determine blood pressure most accurately, appropriate cuff size needs to be determined – very thin elders may require a child-sized cuff.

Table 3.1. Immunization Schedule for Adults 60 Years and Older

	Not Routinely Recommended	Once	Yearly	Other
Tetanus booster[a]				✓
Human papilloma virus	✓			
Measles, mumps, and rubella[b]	✓			
Varicella[c]	✓			
Shingles[d]		✓		
Influenza[e]			✓	
Pneumococcal (polysaccharide)[f]		✓		
Hepatitis A[g]				✓
Hepatitis B[h]				✓
Meningococcal[i]				✓

[a] Tetanus/diphtheria (Td) booster once every 10 years.

[b] Those born before 1957 are considered immune to measles, mumps, and rubella.

[c] Those born before 1966, with a self-reported history of chicken pox, or with a physician diagnosis of herpes zoster (shingles) are considered immune to varicella.

[d] Once at age 60 years or older.

[e] Once yearly for all adults aged 65 years and older. For adults younger than 65 years, immunize annually if the person has any chronic illness, is a health care worker, lives in a long-term care or assisted living facility, is likely to infect persons at high risk for influenza, or any person who desires vaccination.

[f] Once at age 65 years or older. Revaccinate once after the age of 65 years if the first vaccine was administered 1) 5 or more years previously and 2) the patient was younger than 65 years old.

[g] One 2-dose regimen if at high risk for hepatitis A infection (e.g., clotting factor disorders, chronic liver disease, men who have sex with men, illegal drug users, persons working with hepatitis A–infected primates or with hepatitis A in a research setting, persons working or traveling in countries with high or intermediate endemicity of hepatitis A, or any person who wishes to receive the vaccine).

[h] One 3-dose regimen if at risk for hepatitis B infection (e.g., patients on hemodialysis, patients who receive clotting factor concentrates, health care workers [students and clinicians] and public-safety workers who have exposure to blood in the workplace, illegal drug users, persons with one or more sexual partners in the past 6 months, men who have sex with men, persons with a recently acquired sexually transmitted disease, household contacts and sexual partners of persons with chronic hepatitis B infection, persons traveling to countries with high or intermediate prevalence of chronic hepatitis B infection).

[i] One or more doses if at risk for meningococcal infection (e.g., anatomical or functional asplenia, persons with terminal complement component deficiencies, or those traveling to countries where meningococcal disease is highly endemic).

Table and footnotes adapted from the CDC's Advisory Committee on Immunization Practices (www.cdc.gov/nip/).

Table 3.2. Joint National Committee on Prevention, Detection, Evaluation, and Treatment of High Blood Pressure Recommendations for Blood Pressure Follow-up

Initial Blood Pressure (Systolic/Diastolic)	Follow-up Recommendations
≤120/80	Recheck in 2 y
120–139/80–89	Recheck in 1 y
140–159/90–99	Confirm within 2 mo
≥160/100	Confirm within 1 mo
>180/110	Evaluate/treat immediately or within 1 wk based on the clinical scenario

Note: If the systolic and diastolic readings are in different categories use the shorter follow-up interval. An average reading of ≥140/90 on two or more separate occasions meets criteria for the diagnosis of hypertension.

LIPID DISORDERS

There is a paucity of data regarding the effectiveness of treating dyslipidemia to prevent coronary heart disease in the elderly; however, the literature available suggests that elders benefit from treatment just as much as their younger counterparts.[6–8] The current recommendation is to screen men 35 years or older and women 45 years or older for lipid disorders by obtaining a lipid profile that includes a total cholesterol level and a high-density lipoprotein cholesterol level.[9] Combine this information with the person's mean 10-year risk of a coronary heart disease event (using the Framingham risk equations[9,10]) to determine what therapies are appropriate for each patient. Individuals with previously normal results should be screened every 5 years and those with borderline or higher results more frequently.[11]

Geriatrics Pearl

It takes up to 5 years to see a full benefit from lipid-lowering therapy.[8] It is, therefore, not advisable to screen a person or initiate lipid-lowering medications if his or her life expectancy is less than 5 years; in this scenario, the risk of adverse drug effects will likely exceed its benefit.

OSTEOPOROSIS

Osteoporosis is characterized by a decrease in bone mineral density and bone mass. In the United States, it is estimated that 4–6 million women and 1–2 million men have osteoporosis.[12] The prevalence of osteoporosis increases with age and men tend to be at lower risk than women until approximately the age of 80 years when their risk of developing osteoporosis begins to rise. Risk factors are female sex, Caucasian or Asian heritage, a diet low in calcium and/or vitamin D, sedentary lifestyle, smoking, alcohol, family history, certain medications (e.g., steroids, gonadotropin-releasing hormone analogs, phenytoin) and diseases (e.g., Cushing's disease, hyperparathyroidism, hyperthyroidism).

All women should be screened for osteoporosis starting at age 65 years. Additionally, screening should begin at age 60 years for women who are at increased risk for developing osteoporosis.[13] Men are not routinely screened and there exists no formal recommendation for them at this time.

When screening for osteoporosis one should also consider that subclinical vitamin D deficiency is quite common in postmenopausal women who have osteoporosis.[14] Vitamin D is necessary for the absorption of calcium from the gastrointestinal tract and a deficiency may contribute to the development of osteoporosis.[15] Risk factors for the development of a vitamin D deficiency include older age, insufficient oral vitamin D intake, and lack of sunlight exposure (resulting from the winter season or confinement indoors). Consider checking a serum 25-hydroxyvitamin D level in patients who have or are at risk for osteoporosis as this deficiency can be treated relatively easily with high-dose vitamin D.

Geriatrics Pearl

Measuring (not asking) and recording your patients' height intermittently can help detect persons who develop loss of height from vertebral compression fractures. In men, risk factor assessment and change in height can guide who should have bone mineral density testing; a loss of height of 1.5 inches or more may be an indication that vertebral compression fractures have already occurred.

Proton pump inhibitors and histamine-2 receptor antagonists will prevent absorption of many calcium preparations (because of the altered pH of the stomach); consider using a calcium citrate preparation in such patients.

WEIGHT AND PHYSICAL ACTIVITY

Screening for obesity involves calculating a patient's body mass index. Intensive counseling is recommended for those with a body mass index ≥ 30 kg/m^2 (obesity). Counseling should focus on increasing physical activity and eating a healthy diet to glean benefits such as improved glucose metabolism, lipid profiles, and blood pressure[16,17]; a healthy diet and regular physical activity benefit patients at any age. Physical activity decreases the risk of death at all ages and, in the elderly, decreases the incidence of CHD and diabetes mellitus.[18] Furthermore, one should recommend aerobic activity as well as resistance, balance, and flexibility training to achieve benefits such as blood pressure lowering,[19] decreased spinal bone loss,[20] and decreased incidence of falls.[21]

Geriatrics Pearl

Even frail, sedentary elders can benefit from physical therapy and a program of regular exercise.

HEARING

Hearing impairment affects approximately 40%–50%[22] of adults between the ages of 48 and 92 years. For frail elders, hearing impairment is associated with isolation and depression. All older adults should be screened periodically for hearing impairment. The gold standard for detecting hearing loss is audiometric testing, but according to the USPSTF, there is currently insufficient evidence to recommend for or against routinely screening older adults for hearing impairment with audiometric testing. There are, however, other screening tools that one can use in the office to assess who may need referral to an audiologist. They include simply asking the patient whether he believes he currently has a hearing problem, completing a questionnaire (such as the Hearing Handicap Inventory for the Elderly-Screening questionnaire[23]), performing the *whisper test, or using special equipment (such as a handheld otoscope with audiometer). Of the screens mentioned, the latter two have the highest sensitivity and specificity.[24,25] Referral is warranted for those with abnormal findings who are willing and able to purchase a hearing aid if indicated.

Geriatrics Pearl

A thorough examination of the internal and external structures of the auricles is an integral part of assessing a person for hearing impairment because up to 30% of elderly patients with hearing loss have chronic otitis media or cerumen impaction as the cause.[25,26]

VISION

In 2004, the National Institutes of Health reported that 3.3 million Americans aged 40 years and older were affected by blindness or low vision and the number was projected to increase to 5.5 million by 2020. They also reported that although those aged 80 years or older made up 8% of the population they accounted for 69% of the cases of blindness.[27] Poor vision is associated with increased risk of depression, physical disability (including falls and hip fractures[28]), and poorer performance in basic and instrumental activities of daily living.[29] One study found that impaired depth perception, low-contrast visual acuity, and contrast sensitivity may play a role in visually impaired persons who fall repeatedly.[30] Additionally, elders with impaired peripheral vision are at increased risk of being involved in a motor vehicle collision. The most common causes of vision impairment in elders include age-related macular degeneration (the leading cause of blindness), glaucoma, and cataracts (the leading cause of low vision).

The American Academy of Ophthalmology recommends a comprehensive eye examination every 1–2 years for persons

---

* Whisper test – stand one arm's length behind the patient and occlude one ear by pressing on the tragus. At the end of full expiration, whisper a short phrase or sequence of letters and numbers and then ask the patient to repeat it to you; alternatively, whisper a short, easily answered question. Repeat the test, this time occluding the other ear and releasing the first.

65 years and older and glaucoma screening every 1–2 years for persons aged 50 years and older. People with Type 2 diabetes are recommended to have a comprehensive eye examination by an ophthalmologist once diagnosed and at least annually thereafter. The USPSTF recommendation is to screen older adults for vision impairment with a Snellen visual acuity chart. The optimal screening interval is not known and, therefore, left to the practitioner's judgment.

Geriatrics Pearl

Think about poor vision as a possible culprit in elders who are having gait abnormalities or frequent falls.

ABDOMINAL AORTIC ANEURYSM

There are two groups of people for whom abdominal aortic aneurysm (AAA) screening (with ultrasonography) is recommended: 1) one-time screening for AAA in men 65 to 75 years old who have a history of smoking; and 2) men with a family history of AAA.[31] The USPSTF recommends against routine screening for AAA in women.

Geriatrics Pearl

There has been a recent trend in radiological screening to market tests, such as carotid ultrasounds or whole-body computed tomography scans, directly to the patient without a physician referral. This is worrisome as most (if not all) the services being rendered are too inaccurate to screen for disease among those at low risk.[32] Particularly concerning is what to do with results the patients bring in, especially in light of the fact that a false-positive result could mean significant morbidity for an individual. It is the authors' opinion that these tests are in need of more rigorous evaluation before they can be recommended as a means of screening in low-risk individuals.

CANCER

Cancer screening will be covered in the chapter 36 of this book, "Cancer in the Elderly." A comprehensive review of cancer screening in the elderly is also covered in Walter LC, Covinsky KE. Cancer screening in elderly patients: a framework for individualized decision making. *JAMA*. 2001;285(21):2750–2756.

DEPRESSION

Diagnosing depression in elders frequently poses a challenge to clinicians as they are less likely to endorse having a depressed mood. In this population, depression typically manifests as symptoms or signs such as anxiety, anhedonia, memory impairment, or multiple somatic complaints. Appropriate identification and treatment of these persons is imperative as, in the elderly, depression is associated with declining physical function[33] and increased mortality.[34] Additionally, treatment

is effective as long as therapy is tailored to the individual and comorbid conditions are addressed.

There are several validated instruments available to screen for depression.[35–37] Among them is the Geriatrics Depression Scale – a self-report questionnaire with three versions, all of which have been validated.[38] The screening interval is left to the clinician's judgment.

Geriatrics Pearl

The utility of depression screening instruments that require self-reporting may be limited in persons who prefer to minimize their complaints. It is, therefore, important to work with caregivers to obtain further information about changes in mood, loss of interest in activities or self-care, sadness, tearfulness, or any other clues that may be indicators of depression.

DEMENTIA

Dementia is a gradual and progressive decline in cognitive function: specifically, memory and at least one other cognitive domain (including language disturbance, inability to execute skilled motor activities (in the absence of motor weakness), disturbance of visual processing, or a disturbance of executive function). In general, there is insufficient evidence to recommend for or against routine screening for dementia in older adults. Screening should therefore occur on a case-by-case basis. A geriatric clinician typically determines screening is necessary based on key history (usually from caregivers) or signs that the person's cognitive impairment is affecting daily function. Some examples include forgetfulness for things that ought to be familiar, paranoia, repeating questions, or a personality change. Assessment frequently begins with a Mini-Mental State Examination[39] and a depression screen as part of a complete history and physical examination. Laboratory and radiological testing is guided by the history and physical, but should include a thyroid-stimulating hormone, chemistry, complete blood count, folate, vitamin B12 levels and, in select patients, syphilis testing. Genetic testing for Alzheimer's disease is not currently recommended.

Geriatrics Pearl

Please note that the Mini-Mental State Examination is most sensitive for Alzheimer's disease; other types of dementias will require different methods of assessment. Referral to a neurologist or neuropsychologist can help elucidate the cause of the memory impairment.

ELDER MISTREATMENT

Elder abuse and neglect or "elder mistreatment" is an intentional act that results in intentional or unintentional harm (or threatened harm) to the health/welfare of an elder. It occurs when a vulnerable elder relies on assistance from a caregiver who does not appropriately provide the elder's basic needs or take measures to protect him/her from danger. Mistreatment includes not just physical or psychological abuse; it also includes neglect (intentional or unintentional), abandonment, and misuse of an elder's finances. Mistreatment can occur within a family, the community at large, or in institutions such as long-term care facilities. Although the exact prevalence of elder mistreatment remains unknown, it is estimated that between 1 and 2 million Americans aged 65 years or older have been mistreated by someone on whom they depended for care.[40]

There are several screening tools available to help identify elder mistreatment. Unfortunately, there is currently not enough evidence to verify whether they are accurate or effective.[41,42]

Geriatrics Pearl

If you suspect an elder is being mistreated, the following web site provides state-specific guidance on how to proceed with reporting the problem to an adult protective service program – www.elderabusecenter.org. If you suspect that the elder's life is in jeopardy, it is necessary to report this to the authorities by calling 911 immediately.

FALLS/INJURY PREVENTION

Falls are associated with increased morbidity and mortality in the elderly. The incidence varies by living situation and age. Thirty to 40% of community-dwelling elders over the age of 65 years will fall in any given year. Fifty percent of those in long-term care facilities and approximately 60% of those with a history of falling the previous year are likely to fall in the upcoming year. Additionally, the incidence of falls increases with age. Of those older adults who fall, 20%–30% will suffer a severe injury (e.g., fracture or head trauma) that will result in decreased mobility and independence and increased risk of premature death.[43]

Risk factors for falling include postural hypotension, use of psychoactive medications (e.g., benzodiazepines, anticholinergics, opioids), use of four or more prescription drugs, environmental hazards, gait impairment (e.g., undiagnosed Parkinson's disease), balance impairment, and impairment of muscle strength and/or range of motion of the joints. Measures to help decrease an elder's risk of falling are targeted at assessing a patient for and managing these risk factors. A useful screen to identify elders at risk for falls is the *Timed Up and Go test.[44]

Other considerations for injury prevention include counseling patients on the necessity of properly functioning smoke

---

* Timed Up and Go test:

- Have the patient sit in a standard height chair.
- Ask the patient to stand up, walk 3 m (10 ft), turn around, walk back to the chair, and sit.
- Start timing upon the attempt to rise from the chair and stop timing when the patient returns to a seated position after completing the task.
- If this process takes longer than 14 seconds the patient is at an increased risk of falling and referral to colleagues such as a physical therapist to help improve strength, balance, and/or mobility may be warranted.

detectors in the home. Carbon monoxide detectors are recommended for those who use liquid-fueled space heaters, a wood stove, oil heat, gas appliances, or have a garage that is attached to the home.

Geriatrics Pearl

Occupational therapists are able to perform home-safety evaluations and make recommendations to adapt the home to a patient's needs. Their services are available through the Medicare home health services benefit if another skilled need is in place (such as nursing or physical therapy). Alternatively, your area agency on aging may have an occupational therapist on staff who is able to perform this service (usually free of charge to the patient).

ALCOHOLISM

Approximately one-half of older adults (aged ≥65 years) report drinking alcohol at least on occasion. The prevalence of alcohol use and alcoholism among older adults depends on the population sampled. In general, samples that include more people over age 75 years show less alcohol use and alcoholism. It is important to remember that as adults age and their total body water decreases they achieve higher blood alcohol levels per drink than their younger counterparts. Additionally, persons with even mild memory impairment have even less tolerance for alcohol. For this reason, the National Institute on Alcohol Abuse and Alcoholism recommends that older men and women limit themselves to one drink per day[45] (barring contraindications).

Assessing whether an elder has a problem drinking can be difficult. In fact, the definitions of alcohol abuse and dependence include many criteria (such as failed work obligations) that would be difficult to observe in seniors who are isolated and at risk for problem drinking.

The CAGE questionnaire[46] is applicable in an older patient population. A positive answer to any of the questions should raise the clinician's suspicion for problem drinking.

C-have you ever felt the need to **cut** back on drinking?
A-have you ever felt **annoyed** by people complaining about your drinking?
G-have you ever felt **guilty** about your drinking?
E-have you ever had an **eye-opener** to get moving in the morning?

The American Geriatrics Society holds the position that all persons 65 years of age and older should be asked about their use of alcohol at least yearly.

Geriatrics Pearl

Late-life onset problem drinking may occur in elders who previously had no history of alcoholism. The typical scenario involves an elder who begins to use alcohol to self-medicate health problems such as chronic pain, insomnia, or depression. Additionally, recall that when combined with psychoactive medications, alcohol can have an additive effect, worsening cognitive and motor functioning.

DRIVING

Motor vehicle collisions are the second leading cause of injury-related deaths (after falls) in 75- to 84-year-olds and the number one cause of injury-related deaths among 65- to 74-year-olds.[47] Older drivers are involved in more collisions per mile driven and are more likely to die as a result of a collision than their younger counterparts. Several age-related changes have been implicated as playing roles in this problem. These include changes in vision, hearing, slower reaction times, and musculoskeletal changes (e.g., decreased joint range of motion). Furthermore, the development of chronic illnesses may also affect one's ability to drive safely either from the underlying disease itself (e.g., Parkinson's disease) or because of medication side effects. Despite many self-imposed safety measures by older adults (like avoiding highways, inclement weather, or night driving) the crash rate per mile begins to increase at the age of 65 years.[48]

There is currently no consensus on what constitutes appropriate screening in older drivers; however, in 2003 the U.S. Department of Transportation National Highway Traffic Safety Administration published a study of older drivers. They examined data from 2,508 drivers aged 55 years and older over a 3-year period and concluded that the loss of certain functional abilities (especially poor performance on the motor-free visual perception test* and Trail-making part B**) may predict an increased risk of impaired driving and crash involvement.[49] They further relay that poor performance does not necessarily mean that the person's driving privilege should be withdrawn – evaluation and treatment by a physician may, in fact, allow some individuals to continue driving safely.

Geriatrics Pearl

Issues surrounding the cessation of driving can be very emotional for elders and should be approached with care. It should be stressed that referral to a driver screening program (such as those provided by some specially trained occupational therapists) is an effort to identify reversible problems that may hinder safe driving. If it is clear that the patient must stop driving, be prepared to provide information about alternative modes of transportation.

The American Medical Association and the National Highway Traffic Safety Administration have published a tool to help physicians assess and counsel older drivers. See the

following Web site for details: www.ama-assn.org/ama/pub/category/10791.html.

SMOKING CESSATION

Approximately 33% of all cancer deaths are directly attributable to smoking.[50] Additionally, cigarette smoking is a predecessor to tens of thousands of cases of coronary heart disease, strokes, and chronic lung diseases every year. According to the CDC smoking results in serious illness in 8.6 million people and causes approximately 440,000 deaths per year. All adults should be screened for tobacco use and provided with tools to help them quit. Screening involves simply asking the patient about his or her history of tobacco use and asking whether he or she is ready to quit. It is important to convey the message that ceasing tobacco use is of benefit to an individual at any age. In fact, smoking cessation substantially decreases the risk of dying even among persons who quit after age 70.[50] Elders benefit from combined modalities of smoking cessation such as patches, medications, and support groups.

Geriatrics Pearl

Advise all patients (and especially smokers) to have working smoke detectors in the home. Severely addicted patients with dementia should smoke only under supervision.

REFERENCES

1. Centers for Disease Control and Prevention National, state, and urban area vaccination coverage levels among children aged 19–35 months – United States, July 1996–June 1997. *MMWR.* 1998;47(6):108–116.
2. Centers for Disease Control and Prevention Influenza and pneumococcal vaccination coverage among persons. Aged ≥65 Years and Persons Aged 18–64 Years with Diabetes or Asthma – United States, 2003. *MMWR.* 2004;53(43):1007–1012.
3. Padwal R, Straus SE, McAlister FA. Cardiovascular risk factors and their effects on the decision to treat hypertension: evidence based review. *BMJ.* 2001;322(7292):977–980.
4. Gueyffier F, Froment A, Gouton M. New meta-analysis of treatment trials of hypertension: improving the estimate of therapeutic benefit. *J Hum Hypertens.* 1996;10(1):1–8.
5. Chobanian AV, Bakris GL, Black HR, et al. The Seventh Report of the Joint National Committee on Prevention, Detection, Evaluation, and Treatment of High Blood Pressure. *JAMA.* 2003; 289:2560–2571.
6. The Long-Term Interventions with Pravastatin in Ischaemic Disease (LIPID) Study Group. Prevention of cardiovascular events and death with pravastatin in patients with coronary heart disease and a broad range of initial cholesterol levels. *NEJM.* 1998;339:1349–1357.
7. Lewis SJ, Moye LA, Sacks FM, et al. Effect of pravastatin on cardiovascular events in older patients with myocardial infarction and cholesterol levels in the average range: results of the Cholesterol and Recurrent Events (CARE) trial. *Ann Intern Med.* 1998;129(9):681–689.
8. Law MR, Wald NJ, Thompson SG. By how much and how quickly does reduction in serum cholesterol concentration lower

---

* The motor-free visual perception test assesses visual perception without reliance on a person's motor skills. It is useful in children and adults (up to approximately 85 years of age) who may have cognitive or physical disabilities.
** The Trail-making part B test assesses executive function and requires both attention and motor control.

risk of ischaemic heart disease? *BMJ.* 1994; 308(6925):367–372.

9. Pignone MP, Phillips CJ, Lannon CM, et al. Screening for Lipid Disorders, Systematic Evidence Review No. 4 (Prepared by the Research Triangle Institute – University of North Carolina Evidence-based Practice Center, under contract No. 290–98–0011). AHRQ Publication No. AHRQ 01-S004. Rockville, MD: Agency for Healthcare Research and Quality. April 2001.

10. Wilson PW, D'Agostino RB, Levy D, et al. Predication of coronary heart disease using risk factor categories. *Circulation.* 1998;97:1837–1847.

11. Grundy SM, Cleeman JI, Rifkind BM, Kuller LH. Cholesterol lowering in the elderly population: Coordinating Committee of the National Cholesterol Education Program. *Arch Intern Med.* 1999;159:1670–1678.

12. Looker AC, Orwoll ES, Johnston CC Jr, et al. Prevalence of low femoral bone density in older U.S. adults from NHANES III. *J Bone Miner Res.* 1997;12:1761–1768.

13. Nelson HD, Helfand M, Woolf SH, Allan JD. Screening for post-menopausal osteoporosis: a summary of the evidence. *Ann Intern Med.* 2002;137(6):529–541.

14. Holick MF, Siris ES, Binkley N, et al. Prevalence of vitamin inadequacy among postmenopausal North American women receiving osteoporosis therapy. *J Clin Endocrinol Metab.* 2005;90(6):3215–3224.

15. Mezquita-Raya P, Muñoz-Torres M, Luna JD, et al. Relation between vitamin D insufficiency, bone density, and bone metabolism in healthy postmenopausal women. *J Bone Min Res.* 2001;16(8):1408–1415.

16. McTigue KM, Harris R, Nemphill B, et al. Screening and interventions for obesity in adults: summary of the evidence for the U.S. Preventive Services Task Force. *Ann Intern Med.* 2003;139(11):933–949.

17. Eden KB, Orleans CT, Mulrow CD, Pender NJ, Teutsch SM. Does counseling by Cclinicians improve physical activity? A summary of the evidence. *Ann Intern Med.* 2002;137(3):208–215.

18. U.S. Department of Health and Human Services. Physical Activity and Health: A Report of the Surgeon General. Atlanta, GA: U.S. Department of Health and Human Services, Centers for Disease Control and Prevention, National Center for Chronic Disease Prevention and Health Promotion, The President's Council on Physical Fitness and Sports, 1996. http://www.cdc.gov/nccdphp/sgr/sgr.htm.

19. Cononie CC, Graves JE, Pollock ML, Phillips MI, Sumners C, Hagberg JM. Effect of exercise training on blood pressure in 70- to 79-yr-old men and women. *Med Sci Sports Exerc.* 1991;23:505–511.

20. Bérard A, Bravo G, Gauthier P. Meta-analysis of the effectiveness of physical activity for the prevention of bone loss in postmenopausal women. *Osteoporos Int.* 1997;7:331–337.

21. American Geriatrics Society, British Geriatrics Society, and American Academy of Orthopedic Surgeons Panel on Falls Prevention. Guideline for the prevention of falls in older persons. *J Am Geriatr Soc.* 2001;49(5):664–672.

22. Cruickshanks KJ, Wiley TL, Tweed TS, et al. Prevalence of hearing loss in older adults in Beaver Dam, Wisconsin. The epidemiology of hearing loss study. *Am J Epidemiol.* 1998; 148(9):879–886.

23. Gates GA, Murphy M, Rees TS, Fraher A. Screening for handicapping hearing loss in the elderly. *J Fam Pract.* 2003; 52(1):56–62.

24. Pirozzo S, Papinczak T, Glasziou P. Whispered voice test for screening for hearing impairment in adults and children: systematic review. *BMJ.* 2003;327(7421):967.

25. Yueh B, Shapiro N, MacLean CH, et al. Screening and management of adult hearing loss in primary care: scientific review. *JAMA.* 2003;289(15):1976–1985.

26. Lewis-Culinan C, Janken J. Effect of cerumen removal on the hearing ability of geriatric patients. *J Adv Nursing.* 1990;15(5):594–600.

27. The Eye Diseases Prevalence Research Group. Causes and prevalence of visual impairment among adults in the United States. *Arch Ophthalmol.* 2004;122:477–485.

28. Felson DT, Anderson JJ, Hannan MT, Milton RC, Wilson PW, Kiel DP. Impaired vision and hip fracture. The Framingham Study. *J Am Geriatr Soc.* 1989;37(6):495–500.

29. Keller BK, Morton JL, Thomas VS, et al. The effect of visual and hearing impairments on functional status. *J Am Geriatr Soc.* 1999;47:1319–1325.

30. Lord SR, Dayhew J. Visual risk factors for falls in older people. *J Am Geriatr Soc.* 2001;49:508–515.

31. Fleming C, Whitlock EP, Beil TL, Lederle FA. Screening for abdominal aortic aneurysm: a best-evidence systematic review for the U.S. Preventive Services Task Force. *Ann Intern Med.* 2005;142:203–211.

32. Fenton JJ, Deyo RA. Patient self-referral for radiologic screening Tests: clinical and ethical concerns. *J Am Board Fam Pract.* 2003;16:494–501.

33. Penninx BW, Guralnik JM, Ferrucci L, Simonsick EM, Deeg DJ, Wallace RB. Depressive symptoms and physical decline in community-dwelling older persons. *JAMA.* 1998; 279(21):1720–1726.

34. Denihan A, Kirby M, Bruce I, Cunningham C, Coakley D, Lawlor BA. Three-year prognosis of depression in the community-dwelling elderly. *Br J Psychiatry.* 2000;176(5):453–457.

35. Löwe B, Spitzer RL, Gräfe K, et al. Comparative validity of three screening questionnaires for DSM-IV depressive disorders and physicians' diagnoses. *J Affect Disord.* 2004; 78(2):131–40.

36. Montoria I, Izal M. The Geriatric Depression Scale: a review of its development and utility. *Int Psychogeriatr.* 1996;8(1):103–112.

37. See www.stanford.edu/~yesavage/GDS.html for long and short forms of the Geriatric Depression Scale.

38. Rinaldi P, Mecocci P, Benedetti C, et al. Validation of the five-item geriatric depression scale in elderly subjects in three different settings. *J Am Geriatr Soc.* 2003;51(5):694–698.

39. Crum RM, Anthony SS, Folstein MF. Population-based norms for the Mini-Mental State Examination by age and educational level. *JAMA.* 1993;269(18):2386–2391.

40. Elder mistreatment: abuse, neglect and exploitation in an aging America. 2003. Washington, DC: National Research Council Panel to Review Risk and Prevalence of Elder Abuse and. Neglect.

41. Several elder mistreatment screening tools have been placed in PDF format and compiled by the University of Iowa. The web address is as follows: www.uihealthcare.com/depts/med/familymedicine/research/geriatrics/eldermistreatment/index.html.

42. Information about the utility and limitations of some of the screening tools in reference number 2 above can be found in Fulmer, T et al. Progress in elder abuse screening and assessment instruments. *J Am Geri Soc.* 2004;52:297–304.

43. Sterling DA, O'Connor JA, Bonadies J. Geriatric falls: injury severity if high and disproportionate to mechanism. *J Trauma-Injury Infect Crit Care.* 2001;50(1):116–119.

44. Shumway-Cook A, Brauer S, Woollacott M. Predicting the probability for falls in community-dwelling older adults using the timed up & go test. *Phys Ther.* 2000;80(9):896–903.

45. The National Institute on Alcohol Abuse and Alcoholism defines one drink to be: 0.5 oz (15 ml) ethanol = 12 oz beer = 5 oz wine =

1.5 oz 80 proof whiskey; however, there is no formally established standard for what constitutes one alcoholic drink.

46. Ewing JA. Detecting alcoholism: the CAGE Questionnaire. *JAMA.* 1984;252(14):1905–1907.

47. Ten leading causes of injury deaths, United States, 1999, All races, both sexes. Office of Statistics and Programming, National Center for Disease Control. Data Source: National Center for Health Statistics Vital Statistics System. You may submit an online request for a customized report at: http://webappa.cdc.gov/sasweb/ncipc/leadcaus10.html.

48. Li G, Braver ER, Chen LH. Fragility versus excessive crash involvement as determinants of high death rates per vehicle-mile of travel among older drivers. *Accident Anal Prevent.* 2003;35(2): 227–235.

49. Staplin L, Gish KW, Wagner EK. Model driver screening and evaluation program final technical report volume II: Maryland Pilot Older Driver Study (2003). U.S. DOT/NHTSA Publication no. DOT HS 809 583, Washington, DC.

50. United States Department of Health and Human Services. The health benefits of smoking cessation: a report of the Surgeon General. DHHS Pub. No. (CDC) 90-8416. Washington, DC: Public Health Service, Centers for Disease Control, Center for Health Promotion and Education, Office on Smoking and Health, 1990.

4

COMMON COMPLAINTS IN THE ELDERLY

Laura Goldman, MD, Thomas C. Hines, MD, Ilona M. Kopits, MD, MPH

As patients cope with the burden of often multiple chronic conditions, they present their physicians with common complaints that may have a disproportionate impact on their quality of life. These complaints may have multiple causes, and management needs to take into account the multifactorial nature of the cause. Sometimes treating underlying causes can relieve symptoms, but often the symptoms must be managed independently. We have included in this chapter several of the most common complaints that may have dire consequences if left untreated, and outlined an approach to diagnosis and management.

INSOMNIA

As many as 50% of older adults suffer from insomnia.[1] Patients may complain of difficulty falling asleep, frequent nocturnal or early morning awakening, or not feeling rested after sleep. Insomnia may have severe consequences: Studies have shown increased risk of cognitive impairment, poor self-perceived health, falls, and depression.[2–5] Prevalence is higher in women, especially women who are divorced or widowed, as well as nursing home residents, demented individuals, and elders with psychiatric illness.[6–8] Insomnia is usually chronic: Most of those affected will still have insomnia in 2 years.[9] On the other hand, there is evidence that healthy elders have little or no increase in prevalence over the general population.[1]

Sleep architecture changes with age. Stages 3 and 4, or deep sleep, almost disappear, replaced by lighter Stage 1. Circadian rhythm is shifted earlier, so that older adults may fall asleep early in the evening and awaken at 3 or 4 AM. The actual number of hours of sleep does not change,[10] but nighttime awakenings are more frequent and last longer. These changes are seen in both good and bad sleepers, and, most likely, have limited causal contribution to insomnia.[11]

Common causes of insomnia are listed in Table 4.1. Half of patients will have chronic medical illness. Identifying and treating the underlying illness may produce relief. If not, insomnia should be treated separately.

Insomnia is associated with a mental disorder in 33% of cases. All patients should be screened for depression, which is by far the most common disorder. Up to 80% of patients with major depression will complain of insomnia.[1] When treating depression, it is important to address and treat sleep disturbances. There is some evidence that insomnia is an independent risk factor for relapse after treatment as well as a risk of suicide in depressed patients.[12,13]

Medications and use of other substances are a third major cause, and a complete medication review is an important part of the evaluation. Several studies show a positive relationship between smoking and sleeping difficulties.[1]

Caffeine has a half-life of 3–5 hours, but, in some individuals, may be as long as 10 hours. It has been shown to disrupt sleep and should be avoided after lunch. Despite the common belief that alcohol promotes sleep, drinking before bed causes awakening during sleep when blood levels drop. Alcohol has also been shown to exacerbate obstructive sleep apnea.[14]

Sleep disorders include sleep disordered breathing, periodic limb movement in sleep, advanced sleep phase syndrome, and rapid eye movement sleep behavior disorder. All are more common in the elderly. Patients may not be aware of snoring, apnea, or abnormal limb movements, thus interviewing the bed partner becomes essential to detection. Excessive daytime sleepiness and snoring are the most common symptoms of sleep-disordered breathing. Treatment options are a continuous positive airway pressure device, uvulopharyngopalatoplasty, weight loss, and oral appliances.[14] Patients with periodic limb movement in sleep experience leg kicks or leg jerks every 20–40 seconds causing brief awakenings for periods throughout the night. This condition has been associated with anemia, uremia, and peripheral neuropathy. Most common complaints are

Table 4.1. Common Causes of Insomnia in the Elderly

Medical illness

− Angina, asthma, arthritis, congestive heart failure, chronic obstructive pulmonary disease, dementia, gastroesophageal reflux disease, nocturia, peptic ulcer disease, stroke

Psychiatric illness

− Depression, anxiety, bipolar disorder, psychosis, eating disorders

Medications/alcohol/nicotine

− Antidepressants, beta-blockers, bronchodilators, caffeine, calcium channel blockers, decongestants, thyroid hormones, H_2-blockers, theophylline, hydrochlorothiazide, furosemide, anti-Parkinsonian drugs

− Benzodiazepines, antihistamines, analgesics (by causing daytime sleepiness)

Sleep disorders

− Sleep disordered breathing (sleep apnea, obesity hypoventilation syndrome)

− Periodic limb movement disorder (includes restless leg syndrome)

− REM sleep behavior disorder

− Advanced sleep phase syndrome (circadian rhythm change)

Poor behaviors

− Lack of exercise

− Lack of light exposure

− Large meals before bedtime

− Caffeine, smoking

− Excessive daytime napping

− Misconceptions about sleep

Environmental or psychosocial factors

− Recent lifestyle changes: divorce, widowhood, retirement, bereavement

− Extreme ambient light and noise

− Stress

Table 4.2. Sleep Hygiene Recommendations

1. No caffeine or nicotine 4–6 hr before bed
2. Avoid heavy meals and alcohol before bed
3. Leave bed if unable to sleep, use bed only for sleep and sex
4. Maintain a regular sleep wake cycle
5. Limit naps to 30 minutes/day
6. Light exercise daily, but not too close to bedtime
7. Avoid liquids in the evening
8. Avoid light and noise in bedroom, use earplug, mask if necessary

difficulty falling asleep, maintaining sleep, and daytime sleepiness. There is good evidence that use of a dopaminergic agent promotes sleep.[12]

Insomnia is usually diagnosed based on a detailed medical, psychiatric, and sleep history. Polysomnography, which entails an overnight study in a sleep laboratory, is indicated when sleep disordered breathing or periodic limb movement disorder is suspected, the initial diagnosis is uncertain, treatment fails, or there is violent or injurious behavior during sleep.[15] It is not recommended for routine evaluation.

Following assessment and treatment of associated medical, psychiatric, medication, and substance-related conditions, the primary care physician can offer practical advice for behavior change. The term for this advice has been coined "sleep hygiene." Table 4.2 lists some recommendations, and there are many other examples in the literature. Studies have found,

however, that adherence is often not achieved and counseling alone is rarely enough to treat insomnia effectively.

Treatment for insomnia is most commonly pharmacological; however, six trials, which included 282 elderly participants, have demonstrated the effectiveness of cognitive-behavioral treatment (CBT).[16] Methods include stimulus control, restricted sleep therapy, and CBT. A typical behavioral program takes 4–6 hours.[17,18] CBT should be considered in patients in whom hypnotic medication is contraindicated, not effective, or not desired.

There is limited evidence to support the benefit of exercise on sleep in older patients. One trial, with 43 participants, showed exercise consisting of four 30-minute sessions of brisk walking or low impact aerobics a week improved time to sleep onset, total sleep duration, and sleep satisfaction.[19] There is no evidence to support the use of bright light therapy,[20] and insufficient evidence on effectiveness and safety of valerian and melatonin.[21]

An ideal hypnotic is one that has a rapid onset, duration of action that lasts through the night, but not longer, and no side effects. Antihistamines, tricyclic antidepressants, or trazodone are often used, despite the lack of data on effectiveness and their significant side effects. Diphenhydramine, frequently used in over-the-counter preparations, should be avoided. It is associated with daytime sedation and cognitive impairment. Antidepressants are recommended only when there is coincident depression. Amitriptyline, in particular, should not be used in the elderly.[21]

Benzodiazepines (most commonly, temazepam), and the newer benzodiazepine receptor agonists are often prescribed. The melatonin receptor agonist, ramelteon, recently received Food and Drug Administration (FDA) approval. This drug works to correct circadian rhythm disturbance and has been shown to improve sleep in elderly patients with difficulty falling asleep. For all of these classes of medications, there are few trials in elderly patients, and most trials are limited to 2–8 weeks.

Selection of medication is based on pharmacokinetics and symptoms: Temazepam has a half-life of 8–20 hours and may be suited for patients with sleep maintenance insomnia, whereas zaleplon (half-life 1 hour) and zolpidem (half-life 2.5 hours) are shorter acting and may be better for difficulty falling asleep. Prescribers must be aware that all sedative hypnotics can increase risk of falls, slow reaction time, and cause anterograde amnesia. The lowest doses should be used and drugs should be tapered off gradually.[22] Flurazepam has a long half-life. It accumulates in the elderly and should not be used. Estazolam and quazepam are newer benzodiazepines; both also have long half-lives in older patients (18 hours and 39 hours, respectively).

Epidemiological studies have shown tolerance to hypnotics and anxiolytics.[1] Rebound insomnia has also been reported with temazepam and zolpidem. Despite common long-term use of hypnotics, there are insufficient data to support this practice.[21,23,24] There is one study demonstrating effectiveness and safety with zaleplon used for 6–12 months.[25] Ramelteon and eszopiclone are the only sleep medications FDA approved for long-term use.

Persistent Pain

Twenty-five percent to 50% of community-dwelling older adults suffer from pain that interferes with daily functioning. The prevalence is even higher in the nursing home, where up to 80% has been found in studies. Undertreatment is a well-recognized problem, especially in the elderly. In fact, in one study, the major risk factor for undertreatment was age older than 70 years.[26] In the SUPPORT study involving 9,000 adults hospitalized with life-threatening conditions, half suffered moderate to severe pain in the last days of life as reported by family members.[27] There are many barriers to adequate pain relief. One is lack of knowledge on the part of the physician in the safe and effective use of analgesics.

It is useful to categorize pain as nociceptive or neuropathic. Nociceptive pain is caused by the injury of soft tissues, joints, and organs. It is either somatic pain, which is well localized, or it is visceral, which is often poorly localized or referred. Nociceptive pain is described subjectively as dull, aching, throbbing or stabbing, and responds to common analgesics.

Neuropathic pain is caused by disease of the nervous system, either central or peripheral. It is described subjectively as shooting, burning, or numbness. Diabetic neuropathy is a common example. This type of pain does not respond to usual analgesics, and tricyclic antidepressants, anticonvulsants, or antiarrhythmic drugs are effective. Amitriptyline and imipramine should be avoided because of significant adverse effects including falls.[28] Nortriptyline and desipramine are better choices. Gabapentin or other anticonvulsants may have fewer adverse effects than tricyclics.[26]

Affective factors contribute greatly to the perception of pain. Treatment of depression has been shown to improve pain management. Similarly, there is fair evidence that treatment of anxiety can improve outcomes.[26]

The most accurate assessment of pain is by patient report. History includes onset and duration, precipitating and relieving factors, and type of pain and localization. Intensity should be measured by using a pain scale. Several are in common use: A verbally administered 0–10 scale has been recommended by the American Geriatric Society Panel on Persistent Pain in Older Adults. In some patients, including the cognitively impaired, pain thermometers or faces pain scales are accepted alternatives. A scale should be chosen for each patient, and the results recorded with every reevaluation. A complete physical examination is important, but clinicians should keep in mind that physical findings in older individuals may be subtle, even in the face of significant disease.[28]

Treatment of the underlying condition may result in relief; however, pain treatment should not be deferred during work-up or treatment. Acute pain in a patient with chronic pain should trigger an investigation of a new condition or adverse effect of treatment. Only after this is done should it be considered worsening of the underlying disease or tolerance to medication.

The World Health Organization has advocated a three-step approach to pain management in cancer, which can be applied to other types of pain. The first step is a nonopioid, such as acetaminophen or nonsteroidal antiinflammatory drug (NSAID). If pain persists, the second step is an opioid for moderate pain, such as oxycodone. In Step 3, for persistent pain, an opioid for severe pain, most commonly morphine, is substituted. In severe pain, it is reasonable to begin at Step 3. Acceptable pain relief should be achievable with this approach. If it is not, other conditions should be considered such as metastatic bone pain, which responds to bisphosphonates; compression fractures, in which calcitonin has been shown to be effective; or vitamin D deficiency. Consultation with an appropriate specialist may result in nerve blocks or other modalities and should be obtained if needed.

Nonpharmacological therapies, including heat, cold, transcutaneous electrical nerve stimulation, acupuncture, relaxation techniques, biofeedback, exercise, and physical or occupational therapy have all been shown to aid in pain relief. They may be used alone or in conjunction with analgesics at any step in the ladder.[26]

Experts have elucidated general principles of pharmacological management in the literature. They include discussing goals for pain relief with patients, as complete relief may be unrealistic. Pain regimens should be individually tailored. Primary sleep disturbances should be treated.

Unfortunately, few studies evaluating pain treatment have included older adults. There is fair evidence that older patients are more sensitive to opioids. They achieve more pain relief and longer duration of action with lower doses than younger adults. Adverse effects are more than twice as common,[29] and anticipated problems such as constipation and nausea should be managed prospectively.

Frequent monitoring is important, and unneeded medications should be stopped in light of increased drug–drug interactions in this group. Begin with low doses, even less than recommended, and titrate with an eye on adverse reactions and treatment goals. Medications that do not meet goals in a few days should be discontinued.

Round-the-clock dosing achieves better results than "as needed" use. The maximal daily dose of acetaminophen is 4,000 mg, less in patients with hepatic or renal dysfunction or alcohol use. Combination drugs, such as acetaminophen/oxycodone, if given every 4 hours, may result in higher than recommended doses and should be avoided. Frail elders are more likely to suffer from gastrointestinal (GI) bleeding with NSAIDs even when used with a proton pump inhibitor. NSAIDs have also been associated with hypertension, renal failure, and exacerbation of congestive heart failure and, therefore, are contraindicated in many elders. There is little benefit to using both NSAIDs and acetaminophen.[29]

Using opioids for noncancer pain is becoming more acceptable and considering common adverse effects in the elderly with other analgesics, many experts in pain management advocate their use.[26,29] In addition to scheduled doses, many patients require additional medication for breakthrough pain or before activities that may exacerbate pain; however, the evidence to support this common approach is limited. Only four studies in which oral fentanyl was used were found in a recent Cochrane Abstract.[30] Short-acting opiates should be converted to controlled-release equivalents for better pain relief and fewer side effects. Physical dependence is a consequence of long-term use, and tapering should be done over days to weeks if the painful condition is resolved. True addiction is unlikely, and tolerance is likely slow to develop.[29]

Certain analgesics are best avoided in the elderly. These include propoxyphene, which may cause unacceptable ataxia or dizziness, and is only as effective as aspirin or acetaminophen alone in studies.[31] Methadone and levorphanol are not recommended because of a long and variable half-life. Meperidine has been linked to increased sedation and risk of falls and should not be used. Selective serotonin reuptake inhibitors are important antidepressants, but have not been shown to relieve pain.[26] Adverse effects from NSAIDs have been mentioned previously.

UNINTENTIONAL WEIGHT LOSS

Weight loss has been recognized in 5%–15% of community-dwelling older adults and in 25% of frailer adults who are using home care services.[32] Numerous studies have documented an association of weight loss and increased mortality, decreased functional status, and increased risk of hospitalization.[32–35] Weight loss may result from starvation from reduced caloric intake or from chronic systemic inflammation seen with cachexia. Cachexia, unlike starvation, is associated with increases in metabolic function and muscle wasting and may be resistant to refeeding. Medically significant weight loss has been defined as 5% loss over 6–12 months.[33]

Weight loss may be a marker for disease, or it may exist independently. A review of six studies demonstrated the three most common causes are cancer (most often GI or lung), benign GI disease (motility disorders and peptic ulcer disease most commonly), and depression. In these studies, the cancers were not occult. Basic evaluation, described later, can be expected to uncover a cause in 75% of cases.[33]

The physician should perform a complete history and physical examination, and tailor the work-up to symptoms or positive physical findings. History should pay particular attention to GI symptoms, symptoms of depression, and functional issues related to acquisition of food and preparation of meals. Alcohol use should be explored. Social and economic factors may be important: Recent widowhood or change in caregiver can make eating less pleasurable. Eating with family and friends results in 23% more calories consumed than when eating alone.[36] Abuse, neglect, or social isolation may also result in poor intake.

A physical examination, including mental status, may uncover problems with the oral cavity, thyroid disease, cardiopulmonary or GI disease, cognitive impairment, mood, or mobility problems. Laboratory analysis of complete blood count, electrolytes, glucose, renal, liver and thyroid function, stool for occult blood, and urinalysis is advised; a chest x-ray should be obtained.[33] Medications should be reviewed: Some such as digoxin and fluoxetine can cause anorexia; psychotropic medication can cause over sedation; NSAIDs, iron, and bisphosphonates can cause nausea and dysphagia; anticholinergics can cause xerostomia.[32] Anorexia and weight loss have been reported in up to 17% of patients with dementia who were taking cholinesterase inhibitors.[37]

If no cause is apparent on this initial work-up, it is reasonable to assess adequacy of caloric intake, supplement if needed, and follow weights over time. There is some evidence that as many as 50% of patients reporting weight loss have normal weights in their medical charts.[33] In those with normal physical examinations and laboratory analysis, serious illness is rare. If there is persistent weight loss and no apparent cause, upper GI series or upper endoscopy has been advocated by some experts.[32]

Treatment should be based on underlying cause. Medications not needed should be withdrawn. Restrictive diets, which may be unpalatable, should be removed, and patients should be encouraged to eat foods they prefer. Nutrition and/or speech therapy referral for swallowing evaluation may provide essential information for designing an individual treatment plan, which may include pureed foods or thickened liquids.

High-calorie liquid supplements are most often prescribed. There is good evidence that supplements can be effective in achieving weight gain; however, the exact timing (with or between meals) and correct amounts are unknown. Nutritional supplements cannot compensate for the lack of assistance that many cognitively or functionally disabled patients require to eat. The physician should ensure that patients are not malnourished because of inadequate help.[38] In one descriptive study of six nursing homes, only 10% of patients received oral supplements as ordered. Multiple studies have shown that nursing home staff spend significantly less time feeding patients than required for adequate intake.[39]

Successful treatment of depression may be beneficial. There are limited data that mirtazapine may increase appetite and promote weight gain.[35]

There are few trials of medications in the elderly to promote weight gain. None has been labeled for this use by the FDA.

Megestrol has been shown to effect weight gain in patients with acquired immunodeficiency syndrome or cancer, but there are limited data in the elderly. In one randomized controlled trial in which elderly patients received megestrol, 800 mg daily, appetite and well-being improved in 3 months and significant weight gain was achieved after 3 months.[40] Use may be limited by significant side effects of delirium, constipation, and edema. Megestrol increases the risk of thromboembolism and should be avoided in bed-bound patients. Use of lower doses has not been studied.

Dronabinol is a cannabinoid that has been used in patients with acquired immunodeficiency syndrome. It has been studied in patients with Alzheimer's disease, but there is insufficient evidence to recommend its use in the elderly. Significant side effects including dizziness, confusion, and somnolence make it less than ideal.

There is insufficient evidence to recommend the use of cyproheptadine, metoclopramide, or anabolic steroids.

Use of feeding tubes in the face of continued weight loss is a complex issue that cannot be addressed in this chapter. There is good evidence for their use with short-term problems such as hip fracture.[32] Multiple studies have shown that tube feeding in patients with advanced dementia does not prevent aspiration, promote weight gain, or lengthen life. The American Geriatric Society does not recommend tube feeding this group.[41]

CONSTIPATION

Constipation is by far one of the most common complaints of the elderly population. The incidence in acute geriatric wards is 41% and over 80% in nursing homes and extended care facilities. This leads to significant morbidity among elderly patients, resulting in high costs of prevention, diagnosis, and treatment. Constipation is defined as two or less bowel movements in 1 week, straining at defecation, hard stools, or a feeling of incomplete evacuation.[42] The Rome II criteria developed at the International Congress of Gastroenterology define chronic constipation as two or more of the following symptoms for 12 weeks in the past year: straining; lumpy, hard stools; sensation of incomplete evacuation; sensation of anorectal obstruction; or manual maneuvers in >25% of bowel movements; and/or less than three bowel movements per week.[44]

A thorough history and physical examination are the first steps in identifying the cause of constipation. General common causes are identified as medications, medical conditions, diet, dehydration, and immobility.[43] First, it is important to determine whether the complaints are acute or chronic in nature. Once the potential catastrophic causes of acute constipation have been eliminated, a more comprehensive, individual work-up can be initiated. Certain accompanying signs and symptoms, such as weight loss, anemia, persistent abdominal pain, gross/occult rectal bleeding, family history of colon cancer, or refractory constipation, may indicate need for referral to a gastroenterologist.[43,44]

In addition to acute versus chronic, constipation is classified into primary versus secondary.[45] Causes of primary constipation include normal transit constipation, slow transit constipation, and anorectal dysfunction. Secondary causes refer to those listed previously, particularly medications and medical conditions leading to constipation. Medications include anticholinergics, antidepressants, antihistamines, calcium channel blockers, clonidine, iron, diuretics, levodopa, narcotics, NSAIDs, and opioids. When the causative medication is identified, often times the medication is necessary to treat another comorbid condition. For example, in the case of opioids, the extent of constipation as a side effect varies among opiates.[45] Physicians may consider a different form of the medication or prescribe a prophylactic laxative for patients who require chronic pain treatments.

Many medical conditions are also potential causes of constipation. Some of these include metabolic/endocrine disorders such as diabetes, hypothyroidism, hypercalcemia, and neurological diseases such as autonomic neuropathy, cerebrovascular disease, and Parkinson's disease.

If no secondary cause is identified, treatment can begin with various nonpharmacological and pharmacological options. Nonpharmacological methods should always be initiated first. These include bowel training, dietary intake, fluid intake, and exercise.[45] Patients should be educated about the gastrocolic reflex and attempt to have a bowel movement in the morning, 30 minutes following a meal and, preferably, at the same time every day.[45,46]

The American diet is lacking in fiber for all adults, especially the elderly. Studies show that an increase in fiber intake leads to bulky stools and decreased transit time. Keeping a dietary journal helps determine a patient's daily intake and how much more they should add to their diet. Good sources of dietary fiber are bran, fruit and vegetables and prune juice. Increase in fiber intake may be poorly tolerated if given in large doses; therefore treatment should start with small amounts.[43]

Fluid intake is also a concern among the elderly and can lead to constipation. Although few studies have shown a cause–effect relationship between dehydration and constipation, fecal impaction can result from low fluid intake.[47] Elderly patients need reminders to maintain fluid intake regardless.

Lastly, decreased activity and sedentary lifestyle are associated with higher risk for constipation. These options provide more reasons to encourage exercise and a healthy diet among elderly patients.

No evidence-based consensus exists on the order of initiation of pharmacological agents to treat constipation. The five categories include bulk laxatives, stool softeners, osmotic laxatives, stimulant laxatives, and prokinetic agents. Psyllium, a bulk laxative, does increase stool frequency but large amounts can lead to bloating and increased flatulence. Bulking agents help relieve abdominal pain and improve stool consistency. Stool softeners are shown to be less helpful in elderly with chronic constipation and are better for patients with fissures or painful defecation.

Studies have shown osmotic laxatives to be effective in increasing stool frequency and consistency, with the most effective being polyethylene glycol and lactulose.[44] These agents should be used cautiously in patients with congestive heart failure and renal insufficiency because of potential hypokalemia, fluid and salt overload, and diarrhea.[45]

Stimulant laxatives increase intestinal motility and can relieve constipation within hours; however, few studies show any significant difference between these and other types of laxatives.

Lastly, few prokinetic agents are FDA approved for use for treatment of constipation in the elderly. Although colchicine has been shown in several small studies to be an effective agent, larger trials are needed to examine long-term efficacy and safety.[45]

DIZZINESS

Another frequent presenting complaint in elderly patients in the primary care clinic is dizziness. The estimated prevalence ranges from 13% to 38% and increases with age.[48] Dizziness should not be taken lightly as it is associated with increased risk of falls, syncope, stroke, and functional disability. A recent study also shows that 47% of those with dizziness report a fear of falling. This often leads to patients becoming homebound and isolated, as well as more sedentary.

No single definition for dizziness exists. Some investigators categorize by duration or a type of sensation, such as vertigo, presyncope, disequilibrium and "other."[49] Others propose that because the types and causes are so varied and so many, one could consider dizziness to be a geriatric syndrome that is a result of the cumulative effect of many impairments and diseases leading to a multifactorial health condition.[50]

Using a categorical approach can be helpful in identifying an underlying cause. Vertigo is a rotational sensation, often described as "the room spinning" and has an element of motion perception.[51] Vestibular abnormalities often, but not always, lead to vertigo. These can be classified as peripheral or central. Peripheral disorders include benign positional vertigo, labyrinthitis, and Ménière's disease. Central causes are less frequent and include cerebrovascular disease, brain tumors, and multiple sclerosis. These disorders are usually accompanied by other neurological deficits as well.[48,51]

The term "presyncope" refers to the feeling of lightheadedness that precedes a syncopal episode. Patients describe decreased vision and "almost passing out." Presyncope results from hypoperfusion of the brain.[51] Orthostatic presyncope occurs only in an upright position, whereas symptoms resulting from cardiovascular disease can occur in any position. Hypoglycemia is also a common reason for episodes of presyncope.[49]

The third category of dizziness is disequilibrium. There are no symptoms of abnormal head sensations, rather a sense of imbalance or unsteadiness particularly when standing or walking.[51] The cause tends to be of neuromuscular origin, and

it is important to determine if the episodes occur in isolation or with other type of dizziness.[52]

Lastly, there is the "other" category of dizziness, which includes all types of sensations other than those already listed. Idiopathic and psychiatric causes tend to fall under this heading, particularly in patients with comorbid anxiety disorders.[53]

What are the causes leading to the types of dizziness described here? In the geriatric population, rarely will a clinician find a single cause leading to a single type of dizziness. As with most geriatric syndromes, symptoms result from the accumulation of several impairments and risk factors involving multiple systems. This places dizziness among syndromes such as delirium and falls that affect primarily the elderly population.[50]

Of the many disorders causing dizziness, more than 90% of cases are from seven common areas or disease processes. These include peripheral vestibular disorders, hyperventilation syndrome, multisensory dizziness, psychiatric disorders, brainstem cerebrovascular accidents, neurological disorders, and cardiovascular disorders.[49] One study identified patients taking more than five medications to be a characteristic of the elderly patient with dizziness.[50] As expected, a patient will often have more than one cause of dizziness.[49]

What is the best approach to the elderly patient with dizziness? The evaluation begins with a thorough history to determine the type of dizziness. Four questions help to narrow down the possibilities. What type of dizziness does the patient have? How old is the patient? What is the relation of dizziness to position or motion? What is the course of the dizziness?[49] A stepwise approach helps to focus the examination and workup, without subjecting the patient to a battery of expensive and extensive testing.[54] The physical examination also helps elicit the possible cause. Key parts should include measuring orthostatic blood pressures; ear, hearing, eye, heart, and neurological examinations; and testing the neck range of motion. Provocative tests, such as, Dix-Hallpike, done at the bedside can be used to evaluate the vestibular system, with particular attention to various types of nystagmus.[48]

Laboratory tests should only be used in settings of significant medical disease. Brain imaging is reserved for patients with neurological deficits, progressive unilateral hearing loss, or major risk factors for cerebrovascular disease.[49] Cardiovascular testing such as electrocardiography, Holter and event monitors, tilt tables, and electrophysiology studies have not been useful in the evaluation of isolated dizziness.[51]

There are no well-tested, evidence-based therapies for dizziness. Often times the symptoms will resolve on their own, but specific strategies do exist for some treatable causes. Acute vertigo attacks may be treated with meclizine or a benzodiazepine, although meclizine is often overprescribed for chronic and nonvertigo dizziness. Patients with benign positional vertigo benefit from home exercises and repositioning techniques. Disequilibrium can be corrected with simple fall prevention protocols and use of an assistive device. Dizziness in the setting of anxiety disorders may resolve with a trial of selective serotonin reuptake inhibitors.[55] As with other syndromes, it is important to use multifactorial interventions to target the various associated risk factors that lead to dizziness in the elderly patient.[55]

HEARING LOSS

Hearing loss has long been recognized as one of the most frequently encountered problems worldwide in the elderly. In the United States, it stands as the third most common chronic medical problem in the geriatric population, surpassed only by hypertension and arthritis.[56] The consequences of hearing loss are significant. Chronic hearing impairment has been associated with decreased functional capacity, depression, and social isolation.[57,58] These sequelae are particularly notable in older patients. Effective treatment of hearing impairment has been shown to mitigate these problems.[59,60]

The prevalence of hearing loss increases with age, with a 25% prevalence between the ages of 50 and 65 years, over 33% by age 65 years, and over 50% by the age of 85 years.[59] Although presbycusis, or age-related sensorineural hearing loss, is the condition that accounts for most of this observed increase, hearing impairment in the elderly is often multifactorial, including conductive mechanisms such as cerumen impaction and chronic otitis media with effusion, and sensorineural factors such as noise-related hearing loss and ototoxicity from medications.

Multiple strategies have been proposed for the screening of older patients for hearing loss. The simplest method is merely to inquire about the presence of hearing loss during routine history taking. Although acknowledging the utility of this approach, some have questioned its value in detecting subtle or gradual deficits, and note that the reluctance of some patients to admit to a hearing disability might limit its effectiveness.[56] Other screening techniques in common use include qualitative measures of hearing such as the whispered voice test or finger-rub test, use of standardized questionnaires, and use of hand-held audiometric equipment.[60,61]

Evaluation and management of the elderly patient with hearing loss varies depending on the specific clinical setting. Sudden-onset hearing loss in the absence of an easily observable cause such as cerumen impaction should prompt consideration of urgent referral to specialty care. Several causes of such sudden hearing loss, including ototoxicity from medication and idiopathic sudden sensorineural hearing loss, are potentially treatable and should be thoroughly evaluated. Other indications for early referral include hearing loss with evidence of trauma and asymmetrical hearing loss.[56]

For the majority of older patients with hearing loss requiring treatment, hearing amplification remains the principle option. For these individuals, referral to an audiologist for evaluation and, as needed, hearing aid fitting is appropriate. For patients with severe sensorineural hearing deficits, cochlear implants have increasingly been recognized as a viable option.[61,62]

Primary care physicians play an essential role in the detection, evaluation, and management of hearing loss in the elderly.

In the process of providing ongoing medical care to older patients, primary care physicians are in an ideal position to screen for hearing loss. In cases of hearing loss amenable to simple interventions, primary care physicians may be able to offer definitive treatment. In situations requiring specialty referral, they play an important role in facilitating referral in an appropriate timeframe. In patients who are fitted for hearing aids, primary care physicians may serve as a useful resource in identifying barriers to effective use and assisting patients and families in overcoming such obstacles as they arise.

VISUAL IMPAIRMENT

More than 3 million Americans suffer from low vision and almost 1 million are legally blind, making visual impairment 1 of the 10 most prevalent causes of disability in America.[64] Individuals older than 65 years of age make up 66% of the total number of those with visual impairment. It has been estimated that over 10% of individuals aged 55–84 years, and over 20% of individuals aged 85 years and older, suffer from visual impairment.[64] Low vision is particularly prevalent in the nursing home population.[65–67]

In many countries, the most common causes of visual impairment are uncorrected refractive error and cataracts, both of which are reversible causes of vision loss.[68–71] In the United States, the most common causes of visual impairment in the elderly are age-related macular degeneration, cataract, diabetic retinopathy, and glaucoma. Although age-related macular degeneration is the most common cause of blindness in white Americans, cataract, a treatable condition, remains the leading cause of blindness in African Americans.[72]

Visual impairment is associated with various morbidities, including cognitive and functional decline[73,74] and increased risk of falls.[75] Even mild visual impairment increases an individual's risk of death.[76,77] Combined sensory deficits involving visual and hearing impairment are very strongly associated with cognitive and functional decline.[73,77]

Screening for visual impairment in the primary care setting most commonly involves use of standardized tools such as the Snellen visual acuity chart. Various visual function questionnaires have been developed, but their value compared with more direct measurement of visual acuity has been questioned.[58]

Low vision rehabilitation has been shown to improve many although not all aspects of vision-related quality of life.[78–80] A variety of assistive low vision devices and environmental adaptations are available.[81,82] Despite this, available services are often underutilized, apparently because, at least in part, of the lack of understanding on the part of both patients and professionals as to the benefits of these programs.[83]

The primary care physician has an important role in approaching the patient with low vision. Effective screening for visual acuity and referral as appropriate to low vision clinical specialists and rehabilitation programs have the potential for positive impact on the quality of life of individuals. Awareness of available local resources for low vision evaluation and rehabilitation can facilitate efforts by the physician in dealing with this significant disability.

REFERENCES

1. Ohayon MM. Epidemiology of insomnia: what we know and what we still need to learn. *Sleep Med Rev.* 2002;6:97–111.
2. Brassington GS, King, AC, Bliwise DL. Sleep problems as a risk factor for falls in a sample of community-dwelling adults aged 64–99 years. *JAGS.* 2000;48(10):1234–1240.
3. Jacobs MB, Cohen A, Hammerman-Rozenberg R, Stessman J. Global sleep satisfaction of older people: the Jerusalem Cohort study. *JAGS.* 2006;54:325–329.
4. Newman AB, Enright PL, Manolio TA, Haponik EF, Wahl PW. Sleep disturbance, psycho social correlates, and cardiovascular disease in 5201 older adults: the cardiovascular health study. *JAGS.* 1997;45(1):1–7.
5. Newman AB, Spiekerman CF, Enright P, et al. Daytime sleepiness predicts mortality and cardiovascular disease in older adults: the Cardiovascular Health Study Research Group. *JAGS.* 2000;48(2):115–123.
6. Shubert CR, Cruickshanks KJ, Dalton DS, Klein BE, Klein R, Nondalh DM. Prevalence of sleep problems and quality of life in an older population. *Sleep.* 2002;25(8):889–893.
7. Maggi S, Langlois JA, Minicuci N, et al. Sleep complaints in community-dwelling older persons: prevalence, associated factors and reported causes. *JAGS.* 1998;46(2):161–168.
8. Johnson F, Stevens T. Pharmacological interventions for sleep disorder in people with dementia. *Cochrane Collaboration* 2006;1.
9. Ganguli M, Reynolds CF, Gilby JE. Prevalence and persistence of sleep complaints in a rural older community sample: the MoVIES project. *JAGS.* 1996;44(7):778–784.
10. Ohayon MM, Vecchierini MF. Normative sleep data, cognitive function and daily living activities in older adults in the community. *Sleep.* 2005;28(8):981–989.
11. Campbell SS, Murphy PJ. Relationships between sleep and body temperature in middle-aged and older subjects. *JAGS.* 1998;46(4):458–462.
12. Ancoli-Israel A, Cooke JR. Prevalence and comorbidity of insomnia and effect on functioning in elderly populations. *JAGS.* 2005;53:S264–S271.
13. Krystal AD. The effect of insomnia definitions, terminology and classifications on clinical practice. *JAGS.* 2005;53:S258–S263.
14. Martin J, Sochat T, Ancoli-Israel S. Assessment and treatment of sleep disturbances in older adults. *Clin Psychol Rev.* 2000;20:783–805.
15. Littner M, Hirshkowitz M, Kramer M, et al. Practice Parameters for using polysomnography to evaluate insomnia: an update. *Sleep.* 26;2003:754–760.
16. Montgomery P, Dennis J. Cognitive behavioral interventions for sleep problems in adults aged 60+. *Cochrane Database System Rev.* 2006;1.
17. Morin CM, Mimeault V, Gagne A. Non-pharmacologic treatment of late-life insomnia. *J Psychosomat Res.* 1999;46:103–116.
18. Morin CM, Colecchi C, Stone J, Sood R, Brink D. Behavioral and pharmacologic therapies for late-life insomnia: a randomized control trial. *JAMA.* 1999;281(11):991–999.
19. Montgomery P, Dennis J. Physical exercise for sleep problems in adults aged 60+. *Cochrane Database of System Rev.* 2006;1.
20. Montgomery P, Dennis J. Bright light therapy for sleep problems in adults aged 60+ *Cochrane Database of System Rev.* 2006;1.
21. Ancoli-Israel S. Insomnia in the elderly: a review for the primary care practitioner. *Sleep.* 2000;23(Supp 1):s23–s30.
22. McCall WV. Diagnosis and management of insomnia in older people. *JAGS.* 2005;53:S272–S277.
23. Krystal AD, Walsh JK, Laska E, et al. Sustained efficacy of eszopiclone over 6 months of nightly treatment: results of a randomized, double-blind, placebo controlled study in adults with chronic insomnia. *Sleep.* 2003;26:793–799.
24. Roth T, Krystal A, Walsh J, Roehrs T, Wessel T, Caron J. Twelve months of nightly eszopiclone treatment in patients with chronic insomnia: assessment of long-term efficacy and safety. *Sleep.* 2004;27(Suppl):A260.
25. Ancoli-Israel S, Richardson GS, Mangano RM, et al. Long-term exposure to zaleplon is safe and effective in younger-elderly and older-elderly patients with primary insomnia. *Sleep.* 2003;26(Suppl):A77.
26. Gloth MF. Pain management in older adults: prevention and treatment. *JAGS.* 2001;49:188–199.
27. The Support Principle Investigators. A controlled trial to improve care for the seriously ill hospitalized patients. *JAMA.* 1995;274(20):1591–1598.
28. Beers MH. Explicit criteria for determining potentially inappropriate medication for use by the elderly: an update. *Arch Intern Med.* 1997;157(14):1531–1536.
29. AGS Panel on Persistent Pain in Older Persons. The management of persistent pain in older persons. *JAGS.* 2002;50:S205–S224.
30. Potter MB. Opioids for management of breakthrough pain in cancer patients. *Am Fam Physician.* 2006;74(11):1855–1857.
31. Hanlon JT, Schmader KE, Ruby CM, Weinberger M. Suboptimal prescribing in older inpatients and outpatients. *JAGS.* 2001;49:200–209.
32. Gazewood JD, Mehr R. Diagnosis and management of weight loss in the elderly. *J Fam Pract.* 1998;47(1):19–25.
33. Wallace JI, Scwartz RS. Epidemiology of weight loss in humans with special reference to wasting in the elderly. *Int J Cardiol.* 2002;85:15–21.
34. Enis BW, Saffel-Shrier S, Verson H. Diagnosing malnutrition in the elderly. *Nurse Prac.* 2001;26(3):52–54.
35. Huffman GB. Evaluating and treating unintentional weight loss in the elderly. *Am Fam Physician.* 2002;65(4):640–650.
36. ADA. Position paper of the American Dietetic Association: nutrition across the spectrum of aging. *J Am Dietetic Assoc.* 2005;105(4):616–633.
37. Stewart JT, Gorelik AR. Involuntary weight loss associated with cholinesterase inhibitors in dementia. Letter to the editor. *JAGS.* 2006;54(6):1013.
38. Kayser-Jones JS. Use of oral supplements in nursing homes: remaining questions. *JAGS.* 2006;54:1463–1464.
39. Simmons SF, Patel AV. Nursing home staff delivery of oral liquid nutritional supplements to residents at risk for unintentional weight loss. *JAGS.* 2006;54:1372–1376.
40. Yeh SS, Wu SY, Lee TP, et al. Improvement in quality of life measures and stimulation of weight gain after treatment with megestrol acetate oral suspension in geriatric cachexia: results of a double blind placebo controlled study. *JAGS.* 2000;48:485–492.
41. McCann RM, Judge J. Feeding tube placement in elderly patients with advanced dementia. AGS Clinical Practice Committee Guideline. 2005. www.american geriatrics.org.
42. De Lillo AR, Rose S. Functional bowel disorders in the geriatric populations: constipation, fecal impaction, and fecal incontinence. *Am J Gastroenterol.* 2000;95:901–905.

43. Brandt LJ, Schoenfeld P, Prather CM, Quigley EMM, Schiller LR, Talley NJ. Evidence-based approach to the management of chronic constipation in North America. *Am J Gastroenterol.* 2005;100:S1.

44. Hsieh C. Treatment of constipation in older adults. *Am Fam Physician.* 2005;72:2277–2284.

45. Romero Y, Evans JM, Fleming KC, Phillips SF. Constipation and fecal incontinence in the elderly population. *Mayo Clin Proc.* 1996;71:81–92.

46. Lindeman RD, Romero LJ, Liang HC, et al. Do elderly persons need to be encouraged to drink more fluids? *J Gastroenterol.* 2000;55(7):m361–m365.

47. Nanda A, Tinetti ME. Chronic dizziness and vertigo. *Geriatric Medicine: An Evidence Based Approach.* 4th ed. New York: Springer-Verlag; 2003.

48. Drachman D. A 69 year-old man with chronic dizziness. *JAMA.* 1998;280:2111–2118.

49. Tinetti ME, Williams CS, Gill TM. Dizziness among older adults: a possible geriatric syndrome. *Ann Intern Med.* 2000;132:337–344.

50. Kroenke K. Dizziness (ch 23). Geriatric Review Syllabus. Available at www.americangeriatrics.org/directory/ABIM/GRS? Dizz5_m.htm/.

51. Sloane PD, et al. Dizziness: state of the science. *Ann Intern Med.* 2001;134 S1:823–832.

52. Nages N, Ip J, Bou-Haidar P. The vestibular dysfunction and anxiety disorder interface: a descriptive study with special reference to the elderly. *Arch Gerontol Geriatr.* 2005;40:253–264.

53. Colledge NR, Barr-Hamilton RM, Lewis SJ, Sellar RJ, Wilson JA. Evaluation of investigations to diagnose the cause of dizziness in elderly people: a community based controlled study. *BMJ.* 1996;313:788–792.

54. Khan A, Kroenke K. Diagnosis and treatment of the dizzy patient. *Prim Care Case Rev.* 1999; 2:9.

55. Kao AC, Nanda A, Williams CS, Tinetti ME. Validation of dizziness as a possible geriatric syndrome. *J Am Geriatr Soc.* 2001;49:72–75.

56. Bogardus ST, Yueh B, Shekelle PG. Screening and management of adult hearing loss in primary care: clinical applications. *JAMA.* 2003;289:1986–1990.

57. Tay T, Kifley A, Lindley R, et al. Are sensory and cognitive declines associated in older persons seeking aged care services? *Ann Acad Med (Singapore).* 2006;35:254–259.

58. U.S. Preventive Service Task Force. *Guide to Clinical Preventive Services.* 2nd ed. Baltimore: Williams & Wilkins; 1996.

59. Stark P, Hickson L. Outcomes of hearing aid fitting for older people with hearing impairment and their significant others. *Int J Audiol.* 2004;43:390–398.

60. Yueh B, Shapiro N, MacLean C, Shekelle PG. Screening and management of adult hearing loss in primary care: scientific review. *JAMA.* 2003;289:1976–1985.

61. Mo B, Lindbaek M, Harris S. Cochlear implants and quality of life: a prospective study. *Ear Hear.* 2005;26:186–194.

62. Vermeire K, Brokx JP, Wuyts FL, et al. Quality-of-life benefit from cochlear implantation in the elderly. *Otol Neurootol.* 2005;26:188–195.

63. U.S. Department of Health and Human Services. Vision Research A National Plan 1999–2003: NIH Publication No. 98–4120. Bethesda: National Eye Institute; 1998:117–130.

64. Watson G. Low vision in the geriatric population: rehabilitation and management. *J Am Geriatr Soc.* 2001;49:317–330.

65. Friedman D, West S, Munoz B, et al. Racial variations in causes of vision loss in nursing homes. *Arch Ophthalmol.* 2004;122:1019–1024.

66. Brezin AP, Lafuma A, Fagnani F, et al. Blindness, low vision, and other handicaps as risk factors attached to institutional residence. *Br J Ophthalmol.* 2004;88:1330–1337.

67. de Winter LJ, Hoyng CB, Froeling PG, et al. Prevalence of remedial disability due to low vision among institutionalised elderly people. *Gerontology.* 2004;50:96–101.

68. Saw S, Foster PJ, Gazzard G, Seah S. Causes of blindness, low vision, and questionnaire-assessed poor visual function in Singaporean Chinese adults. *Ophthalmology.* 2004;111:1161–1168.

69. Buch H, Vinding T, la Cour M, et al. Prevalence and causes of visual impairment and blindness among 9980 Scandinavian adults. *Ophthalmology.* 2004;111:53–61.

70. Thulsiraj RD, Nirmalan PK, Ramakrishnan R, et al. Blindness and vision impairment in a rural South Indian population: the Aravind comprehensive eye survey. *Ophthalmology.* 2003;110:1491–1498.

71. Saw S, Husain R, Gazzard GM, et al. Causes of low vision and blindness in rural Indonesia. *Br J Ophthalmol.* 2003;87:1075–1078.

72. The Eye Diseases Prevalence Research Group. Causes and prevalence of visual impairment among adults in the United States. *Arch Ophthalmol.* 2004;122:477–485.

73. Lin M, Gutierrez PR, Stone KL, et al. Vision impairment and combined vision and hearing impairment predict cognitive and functional decline in older women. *J Am Geriatr Soc.* 2004;52:1996–2002.

74. Reyes-Ortiz CA, Kuo YF, DiNuzzo AR, et al. Near vision impairment predicts cognitive decline: data from the Hispanic Established Populations for Epidemiologic Studies of the Elderly. *J Am Geriatr Soc.* 2005;53:681–686.

75. Buckley JG, Heasley KJ, Twigg P, Elliot DB. The effects of blurred vision on the mechanics of landing during stepping down by the elderly. *Gait Posture.* 2005;21:65–71.

76. McCarty CA, Nanjan MB, Taylor HR. Vision impairment predicts 5 year mortality. *Br J Ophthalmol.* 2001;85:322–326.

77. Lam BL, Lee DL, Gomez-Marin O, et al. Concurrent visual and hearing impairment and risk of mortality: the National Health Interview Survey. *Arch Ophthalmol.* 2006;124:95–101.

78. Hinds A, Sinclair A, Park J, et al. Impact of an interdisciplinary low vision service on the quality of life of low vision patients. *Br J Ophthalmol.* 2003;87:1391–1396.

79. Brody BL, Roch-Levecq AC, Gamst AC, et al. Self-management of age-related macular degeneration and quality of life. *Arch Ophthalmol.* 2002;120:1477–1483.

80. McCabe P, Nason F, Demers Turco P, et al. Evaluating the effectiveness of a vision rehabilitation intervention using an objective and subjective measure of functional performance. *Ophthalmic Epidemiol.* 2000;7:259–270.

81. Culham LE, Chabra A, Rubin GS. Clinical performance of electronic, head-mounted, low-vision devices. *Ophthal Physiol Opt.* 2004;24:281–290.

82. Brunnstrom G, Sorensen S, Alsterstad K, Sjostrand J. Quality of light and quality of life – the effect of lighting adaption among people with low vision. *Ophthal Physiol Opt.* 2004;24:274–280.

83. Pollard TL, Simpson JA, Lamourex EL, Keeffe JE. Barriers to accessing low vision services. *Ophthal Physiol Opt.* 2003;23:321–327.

5

Appropriate Use of Medications in the Elderly

Elena M. Umland, PharmD, Cynthia A. Sanoski, PharmD, BCPS, FCCP, Amber King, PharmD

INTRODUCTION

Thirty-five million people, 12% of the population of the United States, are older than the age of 65 years.[1] These individuals consume 25% of all prescription medications.[1] Being such large consumers of prescription medications as well as being at increased risk for adverse drug reactions (ADRs) from their use, this population is in need of heightened diligence in prescribing. Some reasons for the increased attention to prescribing in the elderly population include but are not limited to: 1) the increased sensitivity to drug effects that this patient population experiences secondary to pharmacokinetic and pharmacodynamic changes that naturally occur with aging; 2) the less than optimal medication adherence rates that have been observed within this patient population; 3) the current state of not fully following and applying treatment guidelines to these patients; and 4) the high incidence of both underprescribing and polypharmacy among these patients. Furthermore, this increased diligence is necessary, as this population is medically more complicated with the usual presence of several concomitant disease states. Addressing such issues by using an interdisciplinary team–based approach should aid in reducing medication errors.

Although the reduction in medication errors in all patients is of extreme importance, the gravity of the importance in those patients older than the age of 65 years is indisputable when more than 800,000 preventable adverse drug events (ADEs) are projected to occur in long-term care settings.[2] These projected events do not include errors of omission. In addition to the humanistic burden of ADEs via a reduction (either temporary or permanent) in quality of life, the occurrence of ADEs also carries a huge financial burden. The calculated annual cost of each preventable ADE among Medicare patients older than 65 years in 2000 was $1,983 with the national annual cost estimated at $887 million.[2]

PHARMACOKINETIC AND PHARMACODYNAMIC CHANGES IN THE ELDERLY

There are a number of age-related changes in drug pharmacokinetics (Table 5.1) and pharmacodynamics that occur in the elderly population. Pharmacokinetics describes how the body handles a drug in terms of absorption, distribution, metabolism, and elimination. Pharmacodynamics refers to the effects that a drug has on the body. Although all of the changes described herein may potentially occur in the elderly, it is important to remember that these age-related physiological changes do not occur uniformly in every patient in this particular population. Although many of these changes may be attributed to the aging process alone, many may also result from the combined effects of age and other factors such as concomitant disease states, polypharmacy, genetics, and environment.

Pharmacokinetic Changes in the Elderly

Absorption and Bioavailability

Absorption appears to be the least affected of all the pharmacokinetic processes in the elderly. There are several age-related physiological changes that could affect the absorption of drugs in the elderly, including an increase in gastric pH and reductions in gastric motility, mucosal absorptive surface in the small intestine, and gastrointestinal blood flow.[3–6] These potential alterations are more likely to lead to a slight delay in the rate of drug absorption and usually do not have significant impact on the overall extent of absorption of drugs.

The bioavailability of certain drugs may also be affected by age-related physiological changes. Because of a reduction in liver mass and hepatic blood flow, the clearance of drugs that would normally be subject to extensive first-pass metabolism (e.g., propranolol, verapamil, and amitriptyline) may be impaired.[7,8] Consequently, this reduction in first-pass

Table 5.1. Potential Age-related Physiological Changes that can Affect Drug Pharmacokinetics in the Elderly

Absorption	Metabolism
↑ gastric pH	↓ hepatic mass/hepatic blood flow
↓ gastric motility	↓ activity of CYP1A2, CYP2C9, CYP2C19, and CYP3A4 enzymes
↓ surface area of small intestine	
↓ gastrointestinal blood flow	
↓ hepatic mass/hepatic blood flow	
Distribution	**Elimination**
↑ total body fat	↓ kidney size
↓ lean body mass and total body water	↓ renal blood flow
↓ albumin concentrations	↓ glomerular filtration
↑ α-1 acid glycoprotein concentrations	↓ tubular secretion

metabolism may increase the bioavailability of those drugs subject to that process. The function of P-glycoprotein, which normally acts as an efflux pump and serves as a barrier for drug absorption, does not appear to be significantly altered by the aging process.[9] Additionally, the bioavailability of drugs administered via the transdermal route does not appear to be affected by age.[1]

Distribution

The distribution of drugs appears to be affected to a greater extent when compared with absorption in the elderly population. Several alterations occur in the elderly that may affect the distribution of drugs including changes in body composition and protein binding. With regard to body composition, the elderly generally experience an increase in total body fat and reductions in lean body mass and total body water. In fact, it is estimated that lean body mass may be reduced by as much as 15% whereas total body fat may be increased by as much as 40% in the elderly.[10] As a result of this change in body composition, drugs that are more water soluble (hydrophilic) or that distribute primarily to muscle (e.g., digoxin, aminoglycosides, theophylline) may have a reduced volume of distribution that results in increased plasma concentrations.[11] Consequently, for digoxin in particular, if loading doses are going to be used in elderly patients, the dose should be calculated using the ideal rather than the actual body weight. In contrast, drugs that are more fat soluble (lipophilic) may have an increased volume of distribution (e.g., diazepam, oxazepam) that leads to an increase in tissue concentrations and duration of action.

In the elderly, plasma albumin concentrations are reduced by 15%–20%.[12] Although this reduction in albumin may be attributed, in part, to age-related physiological changes, it may also be from malnutrition and/or comorbid disease states (e.g., heart failure, chronic kidney disease, rheumatoid arthritis, or cancer). Acidic drugs (e.g., phenytoin, sulfonylureas, warfarin, and levothyroxine) primarily bind to albumin. The reduction in plasma albumin concentrations causes an increase in

the free (unbound) concentration of these drugs, which may lead to an increased risk of toxicity. For phenytoin, in particular, free phenytoin concentrations should be monitored in this population to evaluate appropriately whether the patient is within the therapeutic range and if dosage adjustments need to be made. Basic drugs (e.g., lidocaine, propranolol) primarily bind to α-1 acid glycoprotein, which is an acute-phase reactant protein. Concentrations of this protein are believed to increase with aging, or when the body encounters a stress such as following a myocardial infarction, in chronic inflammatory disease states, and in malignancies.[13] Consequently, plasma binding of these basic drugs may be increased, leading to a reduction in their free plasma concentrations. The alteration that can develop with basic drugs is considered to be relatively minor and to have much less clinical significance than with acidic drugs.

Metabolism

Drug metabolism primarily takes place in the liver. Several changes that occur in the elderly may account for a decline in drug clearance, which could lead to an increased risk of drug toxicity. Age-related declines in liver mass and hepatic blood flow are known to occur in the elderly.[14] In fact, it is estimated that hepatic blood flow decreases by up to 40% in this population.[8] As a result of this change, the hepatic clearance of drugs that have a high hepatic extraction ratio (e.g., lidocaine, propranolol, verapamil) may be decreased, which results in increased plasma concentrations.

The age-related hepatic changes that occur in the elderly also affect the liver enzymes responsible for the metabolism of drugs. In general, drug metabolism can be categorized into phase I and phase II reactions; however, only phase I reactions appear to be significantly affected by age.[15,16] Phase I reactions include the processes of oxidation, reduction, and hydrolysis. Most of the oxidative reactions involve the cytochrome P-450 (CYP) enzyme system. Although numerous CYP isoenzymes have been identified, those that have been shown to have the most significant role in drug metabolism include CYP1A2, CYP2C9, CYP2C19, CYP2D6, and CYP3A4. Drugs that induce or inhibit certain isoenzymes act to decrease or increase, respectively, the plasma concentration of certain drugs (substrates) metabolized by this particular isoenzyme. Although the results of various studies have shown inconsistent effects of age on CYP isoenzyme activity, in general, it appears that a decline in the activity of the CYP1A2, CYP2C9, CYP2C19, and CYP3A4 enzymes can occur in the elderly.[17] The clearance of substrates of the CYP2D6 isoenzyme has not been shown to be significantly affected in the elderly.[17] Because of the complexity of potential drug interactions that can occur through the CYP enzyme system, it is essential for practitioners to become familiar with common drugs that serve as substrates, inhibitors, or inducers of this system (Table 5.2). Phase II reactions, which involve the processes of glucuronidation, acetylation, and sulfation, are not significantly affected by age.[16] Certain benzodiazepines such as oxazepam, lorazepam, and temazepam are subject only to phase II metabolism; therefore, the metabolism of these drugs is unchanged in the elderly. Other benzodiazepines such as chlordiazepoxide and diazepam undergo both phase I and II metabolism and may have impaired clearance in the elderly.[18] Consequently, selecting a benzodiazepine that exclusively undergoes phase II metabolism may be more prudent in an elderly patient.

Renal Elimination

The renal clearance of many drugs may be decreased in the elderly. Age-related reductions in kidney size, renal blood flow, glomerular filtration, and tubular secretion appear to contribute to this decline in drug clearance.[16] Renal blood flow decreases by approximately 10% each decade after the age of 40 years.[19] These age-related physiological changes may also be compounded by certain disease states (e.g., hypertension, diabetes) that are frequently present in the elderly and that may also have an adverse effect on renal function. As a result of these alterations, the clearance of those drugs that are primarily excreted unchanged by the kidneys (Table 5.3) may be significantly reduced in the elderly.

Serum creatinine (SCr) alone should not be used to estimate the patient's renal function, as the amount of lean body mass decreases with aging. Instead, to provide a more accurate approximation, the serum creatinine should be assessed along with the age and weight to calculate the creatinine clearance (CrCl). Creatinine is a byproduct of muscle breakdown. The age-related reduction in muscle mass that tends to occur in the elderly subsequently leads to less production of creatinine. Therefore, even in the presence of renal dysfunction, an elderly patient's SCr may appear to be "normal" (i.e., less than 1 mg/dl). The Cockcroft–Gault formula, which incorporates SCr as well as age and weight to estimate CrCl, can be used in elderly patients:

$$CrCl (ml/min) = (140 - age) * weight (kg) 72 * serum creatinine (mg/dl).$$

In women, the calculated value should then be multiplied by a factor of 0.85. In elderly patients with an SCr less than 1 mg/dl, to avoid overestimating CrCl in these individuals, a value of "1" should be used for the SCr in this equation. Although the Cockcroft–Gault formula is frequently used to both assess renal function and to make dosage adjustments of renally excreted drugs, it is important for clinicians to be aware that this equation tends to overestimate the glomerular filtration rate (GFR), because creatinine is also secreted in the proximal tubule.[20] Most recently, the Modification of Diet in Renal Disease (MDRD) equation is being advocated as an alternative method for assessing renal function because it appears to have a better correlation with GFR when compared with the Cockcroft–Gault formula.[20,21] Although the MDRD equation was derived from patients with chronic kidney disease, it has been shown to provide a more accurate estimate of renal function in the elderly when compared with the Cockcroft–Gault formula.[22] Because the MDRD equation has not been validated for use in adjusting drug dosages, health care providers should continue to use the Cockcroft–Gault formula for this purpose. The MDRD formula is as follows:

$$GFR (ml/min)$$
$$= 186 * (SCr)^{-1.154} * (age)^{-0.203}$$
$$* 0.742 (if female) * 1.212 (if African American).$$

Pharmacodynamic Changes in the Elderly

A number of age-related physiological changes may occur that could cause the elderly to exhibit either increased or decreased sensitivity to a drug. This altered sensitivity usually occurs in the absence of any change in the drug's metabolism or plasma concentrations. Because of the decline in β-receptor activity that occurs with age, a decline in β-adrenergic responsiveness may occur that could minimize the heart rate response that the elderly exhibit toward both β-agonists and β-blockers. For example, the bradycardic response to labetalol has been shown to be reduced in the elderly.[23] Additionally, blunting of the baroreceptor reflex can occur with aging, thereby resulting in the development of exaggerated postural hypotensive effects during therapy with drugs such as nitrates, diuretics, calcium channel blockers, and $α_1$ blockers.[24] Changes in the pharmacodynamics of benzodiazepines may also occur in the elderly, including an alteration in the permeability of the blood–brain barrier as well as an increase in the binding to, or functionality of, the benzodiazepine receptor.[25] Overall, these changes result in the elderly exhibiting an increased sensitivity to the effects of benzodiazepines. Although no significant differences in the pharmacokinetics of warfarin have been demonstrated between younger and elderly patients, the pharmacodynamics of this drug may be altered in the elderly population, potentially resulting in an enhanced anticoagulant effect and an increased risk of bleeding.[26] Consequently, it may be prudent for health care providers to use lower initial and maintenance doses of warfarin in these patients.

Table 5.2. Select Substrates, Inducers, and Inhibitors of CYP Isoenzymes

	CYP1A2	*CYP2C9/10*	*CYP2C19*	*CYP2D6*	*CYP3A4*
Substrates	Acetaminophen	Fluoxetine	Cilostazol	Amitriptyline	Amiodarone
	Caffeine	Fluvastatin	Citalopram	Carvedilol	Atorvastatin
	Clozapine	Ibuprofen	Omeprazole	Codeine	Calcium-channel blockers
	Fluvoxamine	Losartan	Phenobarbital	Dextromethorphan	Carbamazepine
	Imipramine	Phenytoin	Phenytoin	Flecainide	Clarithromycin
	Mirtazapine	S-warfarin	Sertraline	Fluoxetine	Cyclosporine
	Olanzapine			Fluvoxamine	Diazepam
	R-warfarin			Haloperidol	Erythromycin
	Ropinirole			Metoprolol	Estrogens
	Theophylline			Paroxetine	Ketoconazole
				Propafenone	Lidocaine
				Propranolol	Lovastatin
				Risperidone	Methadone
				Tramadol	Midazolam
					Protease inhibitors
					Quinidine
					R-warfarin
					Sildenafil
					Simvastatin
					Tacrolimus
					Tadalafil
					Vardenafil
Inhibitors	Amiodarone	Amiodarone	Cimetidine	Amiodarone	Amiodarone
	Cimetidine	Sertraline	Fluoxetine	Cimetidine	Cimetidine
	Ciprofloxacin		Fluvoxamine	Citalopram	Clarithromycin
	Erythromycin		Isoniazid	Fluoxetine	Diltiazem
	Fluoxetine		Sertraline	Haloperidol	Erythromycin
	Fluvoxamine			Paroxetine	Grapefruit juice
				Propafenone	Ketoconazole
				Quinidine	Ritonavir
				Ritonavir	Sertraline
				Sertraline	Verapamil
					Voriconazole
Inducers	Phenobarbital	Phenobarbital	Phenobarbital		Carbamazepine
	Phenytoin	Phenytoin	Rifampin		Phenobarbital
	Rifampin	Rifampin			Phenytoin
	Smoking				Rifampin
					St. John's wort

Table 5.3. Select Drugs with Reduced Renal Clearance in the Elderly

Drug Class	Drugs Affected
Angiotensin-converting enzyme inhibitors	Benazepril, captopril, enalapril, lisinopril, moexipril, perindopril, quinapril, ramipril
Antiarrhythmics	Digoxin, disopyramide, dofetilide, procainamide, sotalol
Antibiotics	Aminoglycosides, cephalosporins, fluoroquinolones, penicillins, sulfonamides, vancomycin
Anticoagulants	Dalteparin, enoxaparin, fondaparinux
Antiepileptics	Gabapentin, levetiracetam, pregabalin
Antiplatelets	Eptifibatide, tirofiban
Antivirals	Acyclovir, amantadine, ganciclovir, valacyclovir
β-blockers	Acebutolol, atenolol, bisoprolol, nadolol
Gout drugs	Allopurinol, colchicine
H_2-receptor antagonists	Cimetidine, famotidine, nizatidine, ranitidine
Opioid analgesics	Meperidine, morphine (both have renally eliminated metabolites)

BEERS CRITERIA

Potentially inappropriate drug prescribing refers to a circumstance when the risk of an ADR outweighs the drug's potential clinical benefit. The elderly are particularly susceptible to inappropriate drug use because of age-related pharmacokinetic and pharmacodynamic changes, increased comorbidities, and increased risk for drug interactions, polypharmacy, and ADRs. To help guide drug selection in the elderly, Beers et al. developed a list of potentially inappropriate drugs based on consensus methodology. The initial criteria were developed in 1991 and included medications that generally should be avoided in elderly nursing home residents.[27] In 1997, these criteria were updated to include drugs that were considered to be potentially inappropriate in all elderly persons regardless of whether they were residing in the community or in a nursing home.[28] The most recent version of these criteria was developed in 2003 and includes 48 medications or drug classes that should generally be avoided in elderly patients as well as a list of medications or drug classes that should be avoided in 20 specific disease states/conditions in this patient population.[29] Numerous studies have been conducted to evaluate the health care outcomes associated with the use of the potentially inappropriate drugs included in the various versions of the criteria developed by Beers et al. Although these studies have been conducted in a variety of environments, including the community, nursing home, and hospital settings, the results demonstrate that use of these drugs in the elderly population is consistently associated with an increased risk of ADRs and health care costs.[30] In addition, inappropriate medication use was associated with an increased risk of hospitalization in the elderly living in community settings.

Although the Beers' criteria have been increasingly used as quality-of-care measures in the nursing home and managed care settings (as evidenced by the Beerslike list of inappropriate drugs adopted by the 2006 Health Plan Employer and Data and Information Set), this list of drugs has also been criticized for potentially creating a checklist approach for assessing the appropriateness of drug therapy in the elderly. Therefore, there has been concern that the presence of at least one of these drugs in an elderly patient's medication profile may automatically prompt a health care provider to discontinue the drug(s) without considering the patient's overall clinical scenario. Consequently, drugs that were intended to be considered potentially inappropriate could evolve into being absolutely inappropriate with such a checklist approach. Concern that the Beers criteria could be translated into a list of definitely inappropriate medications prompted the American Medical Directors Association and the American Society of Consultant Pharmacists to release a position statement to provide guidance, not only on the appropriate use of these criteria, but also on the appropriate prescription and management of medication regimens in the elderly.[31] Based on this position statement, the Beers criteria should not be used as the sole measure of determining the potential inappropriateness of drug therapy. Rather, the patient's medical history, medication history, functional status, and prognosis should be taken into consideration before determining whether a drug from this list should be discontinued.

ADVERSE DRUG REACTIONS IN THE ELDERLY: AN OVERVIEW

An ADR is a harmful, unpleasant, or unwanted effect of a medication that requires treatment of the effect, modification of the drug regimen, or cessation of treatment.[32] There are four classes of ADRs, types A–D. Type A ADRs are predictable because their mechanism is related to the pharmacological activity of the drug. They are the most common and are often dose related.[33] Examples of Type A ADRs include cough associated with an angiotensin-converting enzyme (ACE) inhibitor or somnolence secondary to morphine administration. Type B reactions are less predictable and are not related to a particular drug's pharmacology or dose dependent. These reactions include hypersensitivity reactions, such as anaphylaxis on penicillin administration, that occur when the body mounts an immune-mediated response to a medication.[18,32] Type C ADRs result from long-term use of a medication, such as development of myelosuppression in patients taking linezolid for longer than 2 weeks.[34] Finally, Type D ADRs can occur many years after medication administration.[33] Doxorubicin-associated cardiomyopathy and thalidomide-induced birth defects are examples of Type D ADRs.

A landmark trial found that approximately 6.5% of all hospital admissions were from ADRs, many of which were avoidable.[35] Furthermore, ADRs were responsible for the death of 0.15% of all patients admitted to the hospital. Patients admitted because of an ADR were an average of 76 years old, significantly older than the median age (66 years) of patients admitted without ADRs. Other studies estimate that the incidence of hospital admissions caused by ADRs ranges from 3% to 30.4%.[36,37] A large meta-analysis that examined the incidence of ADRs in hospital inpatients found that 2.1% of inpatients experience an ADR.[38] Smaller studies estimate the incidence of ADRs in hospital inpatients to range from 6.6% to 60.7%.[39–42]

Changes in pharmacokinetics and pharmacodynamics, along with the presence of decreased mobility and multiple disease states contribute to the increased incidence of ADRs in the elderly. Polypharmacy, the use of multiple medications, increases the risk of ADRs because of drug interactions, synergistic toxic effects of medications, or nonadherence because of complicated or expensive medication regimens. In addition, ADRs such as memory impairment, confusion, and anorexia may be inappropriately attributed to the normal aging process as opposed to potential side effects from drug therapy.[18] Documented risk factors for the development of ADRs in the elderly include polypharmacy, the presence of multiple comorbid disease states, renal or hepatic dysfunction, female sex, low body weight, and a history of ADRs.[33]

To prevent the occurrence of ADRs in the elderly population, it is imperative that health care providers pay close attention to their patients' medication regimens and weigh the risk versus benefit profile of each medication. When starting a new medication, the lowest dose should be chosen, and increased as needed.[43] Medications should be used for the shortest time possible. For chronic therapy, practitioners should choose the agent least likely to cause an ADR. This may involve taking into consideration the drug's half-life, its level of renal elimination, and/or the extent to which it relies on hepatic metabolism. Medication side effects are frequently attributed to a patient's concomitant disease states or to aging. Therefore, when searching for the cause of a patient's new complaints, the physician should consider the possibility that the complaint could be related to the patient's medications.[18] Finally, medication regimens must be individualized for elderly patients. A medication recommended in evidence-based guidelines may not necessarily be appropriate for individual patients.

Common ADRs in the elderly include an increased risk of falls, changes in mental status, and effects on urinary continence. Each of these will be discussed in further detail later. Table 5.4 identifies some of the common pharmacological agents that may cause each of these ADRs.

Adverse Drug Reactions: Falls in the Elderly

Falls in the elderly are concerning because of their associated significant morbidity and mortality. Approximately 30% of noninstitutionalized people older than 65 years fall at least once per year.[55] With each fall, a patient is at risk of fractures; hip fractures are particularly problematic. In one study, 20% of elderly patients who experienced a hip fracture died within a year of the fracture.[56] Furthermore, elderly people who do experience hip fractures are more likely to be hospitalized, disabled, or placed in a nursing home when compared with their peers.[56]

The risk of falling increases as one ages. Cognitive impairment, visual problems, gait or balance disturbances, decreased muscle strength, joint pain or stiffness, orthostatic hypotension, and dizziness are all factors that may increase a person's likelihood of falling.[57–59] In addition, falls are more common in elderly patients who take more than four drugs per day, regardless of whether the agent(s) are considered to be high risk or not.[59] Certain medication classes, when used alone or in combination with other medications, can increase an elderly patient's risk of falling.[59] Adverse effects of medications, including sedation, dizziness, orthostasis, or hypotension can increase the risk of falls.

Psychotropic medications are often used in the elderly to treat depression, psychosis, and insomnia. These medications increase a patient's risk of falling, particularly if the patient takes other medications that are associated with a high risk of falling. Antipsychotic medications can cause many adverse effects, including extrapyramidal symptoms, orthostasis, and cognitive impairment. These effects, which can increase a patient's risk of falls, are more commonly associated with the typical antipsychotics, (e.g., haloperidol, thiothixene, droperidol), but have been documented with the newer atypical agents (e.g., quetiapine, risperidone, olanzapine).[45,49] Antidepressants are also associated with an increased fall risk.[44–46] It was originally thought that tricyclic antidepressants, which can cause sedation, orthostatic hypotension, and confusion, were more likely to be associated with falls than selective SSRIs, which do not typically cause these adverse effects. Studies have shown, however, that selective SSRIs are associated with fall rates similar to the tricyclic antidepressants.[44,46]

Any medication that causes sedation can increase the likelihood of falling in an elderly patient.[45] In particular, benzodiazepines have been implicated in increasing the fall risk of elderly patients. Although short-acting benzodiazepines are commonly used in and considered to be safe for the elderly, both long- and short-acting benzodiazepines have been associated with an increased fall risk.[44,45] It is likely that the risk

Table 5.4. Adverse Drug Reactions in the Elderly

	Increased Fall Risk	Mental Status Changes	Urinary Incontinence	Urinary Retention
Prescription Agents (by class)	Antidepressants[44–46]	Amphetamines[29]	Dopamine antagonists (thioridazine, clozapine, haloperidol)[47]	Tricyclic antidepressants[47]
	Anticonvulsants[44]	Opioid analgesics[29]	α-blockers[47,48]	Antispasmodics[47]
	Antipsychotics[45,49]	Antipsychotics[49,50]	Reserpine[47]	Anticholinergics (antipsychotics, antispasmodic, antiparkinson)[48]
	Sedative/hypnotics[51]	Antispasmodics[52,53]	Misoprostol[47]	
	Benzodiazepines[44,45]	Bronchodilators[52,53]	Diuretics[47,48]	
	Type Ia antiarrhythmics[54]	Antiarrhythmics[52,53]	Selective serotonin reuptake inhibitors[48]	
	Digoxin[54]	Antiparkinson[52,53]		
	Diuretics[54]	Skeletal muscle relaxants[52,53]		
	Antihypertensives[51]	Psychotropics[52,53]		
	Opioid analgesics[51]	Antidepressants[52,53]		
	Hypoglycemics[51]	Antidiarrheals[52]		
	α_1 blockers[51]			
Over the Counter Agents	Laxatives[51]	Antihistamines[52,53]		Antihistamines[48]
		Antiemetics[52,53]		
Herbal Agents		Herbane[52]		
		Deadly nightshade[52]		

increases with increasing dose; therefore, if benzodiazepines must be used, the lowest dose should be used for the shortest duration possible.[44,45] Opioid analgesics also cause sedation and, therefore, have the theoretical potential to increase an elderly patient's fall risk.[51] A large meta-analysis of trials conducted in elderly patients, however, did not find an association between narcotic analgesics and falls.[54]

Agents that cause hypotension or dizziness may promote falls in the elderly. Agents, such as α_1 blockers, which can be used to treat benign prostatic hypertrophy, commonly cause dizziness.[51] Evidence regarding the risk of falls associated with antihypertensive agents, however, is mixed. Some studies show that elderly patients have an increased fall risk with these agents, but others do not.[54] It has been demonstrated in observational studies that type Ia antiarrhythmics, digoxin, and diuretics are associated with increased fall rates in the elderly.[54] Because these agents are commonly used, it is important to educate patients about the risk of falls because of hypotension or dizziness, as well as steps to take in preventing falls. Whenever possible, antihypertensives and other agents known to cause dizziness should be dosed at bedtime to decrease the risk of falling.

At times, the intended effect of a medication may increase a patient's likelihood of falling. In addition to increasing risk of falling because of orthostasis, diuretics can also precipitate an urgent need to urinate, thus increasing a patient's risk of falling. Similarly, laxatives can cause an urgent need to defecate. Patient education can decrease the likelihood of these types of falls.

The risks of medication-related falls can be mitigated through patient education, slow dose titration, and avoiding high-risk medications, when possible. Physicians must remember, however, that polypharmacy itself is a risk factor for falls, particularly when elderly patients take more than one high-risk medication. Medication regimens should be reviewed regularly to assess the risks and benefits of each medication a patient takes.

Adverse Drug Reactions: Cognitive Impairment in the Elderly

Cognitive impairment is common in the elderly and ranges from forgetfulness occurring as a natural part of the aging process, to confusion and agitation associated with dementia and Alzheimer's disease.[49] Patients with acute illnesses, such as urinary tract infections, or worsening chronic illnesses, such as heart failure, can present with cognitive dysfunction in the form of confusion or mental status changes.[60,61] Many commonly used medications can also precipitate or contribute to the development of cognitive disturbances in elderly patients. It can be difficult for the practitioner to distinguish between cognitive impairment secondary to a disease process versus a medication. It is, therefore, important to consider the possibility that changes in cognitive function may be partially or wholly from ADRs.

Any medication with central nervous system (CNS) effects has the potential to cause cognitive dysfunction. Opioid analgesics, in particular pentazocine, can cause sedation, confusion, and even hallucinations.[29] Alternately, amphetamines cause CNS stimulation and excitation, effects that are often exaggerated in the elderly.[29]

Anticholinergic agents are frequently responsible for causing CNS disturbances. Confusion, excitement, disorientation, and delirium have been reported with their use, particularly in the elderly.[51] Many commonly used medications, including over-the-counter antihistamines (e.g., diphenhydramine, chlorpheniramine), as well as prescription-only antidepressants (e.g., amitriptyline, doxepin, imipramine) skeletal muscle relaxants (e.g., cyclobenzaprine, orphenadrine) and bronchodilators (atropine and ipratropium) have anticholinergic actions.[49,52,53] Antipsychotics, which can cause anticholinergic-associated cognitive impairment, are used to treat psychotic disorders or behavioral problems in the elderly.[49] A small observational trial found that use of neuroleptic agents in patients with dementia was associated with a significant cognitive decline when compared with patients not taking neuroleptic agents.[50]

A patient's risk of developing cognitive impairment increases with the number of medications, particularly anticholinergic agents.[29,49] Furthermore, anticholinergic-associated cognitive dysfunction is more likely to occur in patients with preexisting cognitive impairment, as anticholinergic use can exacerbate that impairment.[49,52] Physicians must be aware of an agent's potential to cause cognitive dysfunction when prescribing a new medication. They must also consider the "anticholinergic burden" of a patient's medication regimen, knowing that, although a single medication may not result in anticholinergic-associated cognitive changes, the use of multiple drugs with such effects may increase that risk.[52]

Adverse Drug Reactions: Continence Issues in the Elderly

Although most cases of drug-induced bladder and urinary disorders are idiosyncratic, populations who are at risk for their occurrence are identifiable and include the elderly. There are also drugs commonly known for their contribution to these disorders, and as such, should be used with caution.[47] The effects of agents causing or exacerbating urinary retention are more pronounced when there is preexisting bladder outflow obstruction.[47]

The aging process has an impact on all the various forms of incontinence, and they may be exacerbated by certain pharmacological agents. Sphincter weakness that increases with increasing age leads to stress incontinence. Drugs that relax the sphincter, such as calcium channel blockers, may worsen stress incontinence. Overflow incontinence results from an inability of the bladder to contract. Bladder contraction requires cholinergic parasympathetic stimulation; therefore, the use of any agent with anticholinergic effects may contribute to urinary retention and subsequently, overflow incontinence. Functional incontinence often results from conditions that occur commonly in the elderly population such as dementia, stroke, and arthritis. Therefore, the agents that can negatively affect mental status as noted in the previous section, may also contribute to functional incontinence.[48] Other agents that may contribute to urinary incontinence include diuretics that increase urinary output. The combined effects of increased urinary output and impaired functional ability to reach the toilet in a timely manner contribute further to incontinence.[48] When the use of agents that may cause or exacerbate incontinence is unavoidable, behavioral therapy that includes bladder-sphincter biofeedback, bladder training, and pelvic floor exercises may be considered.[48]

POLYPHARMACY AND THE UNDERUTILIZATION OF DRUG THERAPY IN THE ELDERLY

The interconnectedness of polypharmacy and undertreatment has been repeatedly illustrated.[62,63] In studies of patients whose mean ages ranged from 75 to 80 years, the simultaneous presence of drug underuse and inappropriate use has been observed in approximately 43% of the population.[62,63] Although it is known that the number of medications used is associated with an increased risk of an ADR ($p < 0.001$), and that the mean number of events per patient increases by 10% for each additional medication,[64] undertreatment is still a large problem.

Despite receiving five or more medications, undertreatment has been observed to occur in 64%–83% of elderly patients.[62,63] The highest incidence of undertreatment has been observed with laxatives to prevent constipation in patients receiving chronic opioids, and ACE inhibitor and β-blocker use for patients with cardiovascular disease.[62,65] Other agents that are underused among the geriatric population include antihypertensives, aspirin, antihyperlipidemics, oral hypoglycemic agents, and calcium supplements.[63,65] In a study of patients with coronary artery disease in an academic nursing home, only 62% received aspirin, 58% received an ACE inhibitor or an angiotensin II receptor blocker, 57% received a β-blocker, 27% received a calcium channel blocker, and 21% received a statin.[65] None of these patients had a contraindication to the agent(s) with which they were not treated.

A similar trend was observed in a chart review of 144 patients (average age 61.6 years) with New York Heart Association functional class III-IV heart failure who were admitted for an exacerbation.[66] During their admission, ACE inhibitor and aldosterone antagonist use was 93.1% and 58.3%, respectively. At home, only 75% received an aldosterone antagonist and 38.2% received an ACE inhibitor or angiotensin II receptor blocker.

Another disease state that appears to be undertreated in the geriatric population is osteoporosis. In a Japanese study of 422 patients with osteoporosis-related fractures (299 were hip fractures), only 13% received antiosteoporosis medication following their fracture.[67] Of the 55 patients who did receive treatment, 5 received a bisphosphonate, 11 received vitamin D, 6 received a bisphosphonate plus vitamin D, and 33 received calcium, vitamin K, or calcitonin.

In evaluating ways to minimize both polypharmacy and the underutilization of well-studied and supported therapeutic initiatives in the elderly population, a collaborative approach has been observed.[68] When the addition of a clinical pharmacist to the geriatric team (Geriatric Evaluation and Management [GEM] care) was compared to the use of the GEM alone, the intervention patients (stratified by age and number of medications) were more likely to experience improvement in receiving appropriate medications.

DRUG ADHERENCE IN THE ELDERLY POPULATION

The true rate of medication adherence is estimated to be 50%, and it ranges from 26% to 59% in patients age 60 years and older.[69] Among the elderly population, as many as 10% of hospital admissions and 23% of nursing home admissions may be attributed to medication nonadherence.[69] Seventy-five percent of hospital admissions related to nonadherence involved cardiovascular and CNS medications. The most frequent manifestations of nonadherence in this population were falls, postural hypotension, heart failure, and delirium.[69]

Factors Affecting Drug Adherence

Once an optimal therapeutic regimen is determined for a patient, with the issues of both inappropriate medication use and undertreatment addressed, adherence becomes a key component to therapeutic success. Adherence is a preferred term to compliance as it implies a collaborative relationship between the patient and/or caregiver(s) and the health care provider(s). Compliance, in comparison, implies a one-way relationship wherein the health care provider makes all decisions and provides "directions" independent of the wants and needs of the patient.

In optimizing medication adherence, identifying the most common reasons for nonadherence is important. The reasons frequently cited by patients admitted to the hospital are economic factors and adverse effects.[69] Some general aspects observed to affect adherence include demographics (e.g., occupation, educational level, health literacy), medical factors (e.g., type, severity, and duration of disease/illness), medication profile (e.g., complexity of regimen and total number of prescriptions), behavioral factors (including interaction with the provider and the health beliefs of the patient), and economic facets (e.g., type of insurance, cost of medication, and patient income). The elderly, in particular, are at high risk of nonadherence secondary to medical factors.

Improving Drug Adherence

Improving adherence to drug therapy is both a public health and individual patient issue. In assessing individual patient adherence, self-report, pill counts, and medication profile reviews all are felt to overestimate adherence. Furthermore, no one way of evaluating adherence is superior to another. Rather, using a combination of such methods, along with an openly communicative relationship among the patient, pharmacist, and health care provider(s) may aid in improving overall medication adherence. Other methods for improving adherence include automated refill reminders, pill boxes, and the involvement of family members. High-tech devices that can be used include the Medication-Events-Monitoring System (MEMS®), MDILog™ (metered dose inhaler adherence measuring device), CompuMed® weekly pill box that automatically dispenses medication at programmed intervals, and the Health Buddy® pagerlike device.[69]

In addition to utilizing devices to help improve compliance, the use of fixed-dose medication combinations has also been observed to have a positive impact. These products typically contain two active agents, each at a particular dose. Such agents currently exist for the disease states of hypertension (i.e., Zestoretic® 10–12.5 that contains 10 mg of lisinopril and 12.5 mg of hydrochlorothiazide), human immunodeficiency virus, tuberculosis, and diabetes. A meta-analysis showed that the use of these products resulted in a significant overall 26% decrease in the risk of noncompliance compared with single-drug component regimens.[70] A 24% reduction in the risk of noncompliance was noted for hypertension in particular.[70]

CONCLUSION

The safe, effective, and optimal use of medications in the elderly requires heightened diligence in comparison to other patient populations. The issues of increased sensitivity to drug effects (both desired and adverse), the underuse of proved drug therapies, and a high incidence of medication nonadherence, increase the need for due diligence in prescribing and monitoring drug therapy in this patient population. The use of a multidisciplinary approach to patient care as well as the use of known methods for improving medication adherence are key to long-term success in the medical management of the elderly patient.

REFERENCES

1. Schwartz JB. The current state of knowledge on age, sex, and their interactions on clinical pharmacology. *Clin Pharmacol Ther.* 2007;82:87–96.
2. National Academy of Sciences Committee on Identifying and Preventing Medication Errors. Executive Summary of Preventing Medication Errors: Quality Chasm Series. Available at: http://books.nap.edu/catalog/11623.html. Accessed May 9, 2008.
3. Kekki M, Samloff IM, Ihamaki T, et al. Age- and sex-related behaviour of gastric acid secretion at the population level. *Scand J Gastroenterol.* 1982;17:737–743.
4. Orr WC, Chen CL. Aging and neural control of the GI tract: IV. Clinical and physiological aspects of gastrointestinal motility and aging. *Am J Physiol.* 2002;283:G1226–G1231.
5. Corazza GR, Frazzoni M, Gatto MR, et al. Aging and small-bowel mucosa: a morphometric study. *Gerontology.* 1986;32:60–65.
6. Bender AD. The effect of increasing age on the distribution of peripheral blood flow in man. *J Am Geriatr Soc.* 1965;13:192–198.
7. Anantharaju A, Feller A, Chedid A. Aging liver: a review. *Gerontology.* 2002;48:343–353.
8. Le Couteur DG, McLean AJ. The aging liver: drug clearance and an oxygen diffusion barrier hypothesis. *Clin Pharmacokinet.* 1998;34:359–373.
9. Brenner SS, Klotz U. P-glycoprotein function in the elderly. *Eur J Clin Pharmacol.* 2004;60:97–102.
10. Beaufrere B, Morio B. Fat and protein redistribution with aging: metabolic considerations. *Eur J Clin Nutr.* 2000;54:S48–53.
11. Cusack B, Kelly J, O'Malley K, et al. Digoxin in the elderly: pharmacokinetic consequences of old age. *Clin Pharmacol Ther.* 1979;25:772–776.
12. Campion EW, deLabry LO, Glynn RJ. The effect of age on serum albumin in healthy males: report from the Normative Aging Study. *J Gerontol.* 1988;43:M18–M20.
13. Verbeeck RK, Cardinal JA, Wallace SM. Effect of age and sex on the plasma binding of acidic and basic drugs. *Eur J Clin Pharmacol.* 1984;27:91–97.
14. Wynne HA, Cope LH, Mutch E, et al. The effect of age upon liver volume and apparent liver blood flow in healthy man. *Hepatology.* 1989;9:297–301.
15. Schmucker DL. Liver function and phase I drug metabolism in the elderly: a paradox. *Drugs Aging.* 2001;18:837–851.
16. Hammerlein A, Derendorf H, Lowenthal DT. Pharmacokinetic and pharmacodynamic changes in the elderly: clinical implications. *Clin Pharmacokinet.* 1998;35:49–64.
17. Benedetti MS, Whomsley R, Canning M. Drug metabolism in the pediatric population and in the elderly. *Drug Discov Today.* 2007;12:599–610.
18. Bressler R, Bahl JJ. Principles of drug therapy for the elderly patient. *Mayo Clin Proc.* 2003;78:1564–1577.
19. Muhlberg W, Platt D. Age-dependent changes of the kidneys: pharmacological implications. *Gerontology.* 1999;45:243–253.
20. Stevens LA, Coresh J, Greene T, Levey AS. Assessing kidney function: measured and estimated glomerular filtration rate. *NEJM.* 2006;354:2473–2483.
21. Levey AS, Bosch JP, Lewis JB, et al. A more accurate method to estimate glomerular filtration rate from serum creatinine: a new prediction equation. Modification of Diet in Renal Disease Study Group. *Ann Intern Med.* 1999;130:461–470.
22. Verhave JC, Fesler P, Ribstein J, du Cailar G, Mimran A. Estimation of renal function in subjects with normal serum creatinine levels: influence of age and body mass index. *Am J Kidney Dis.* 2005;46:233–241.
23. Abernethy DR, Schwartz JB, Plachetka JR, Todd EL, Egan JM. Comparison in young and elderly patients of pharmacodynamics and disposition of labetalol in systemic hypertension. *Am J Cardiol.* 1987;60:697–702.
24. Schwartz JB, Gibb WJ, Tran T. Aging effects on heart rate variation. *J Gerontol.* 1991;46:M99–M106.
25. ElDesoky ES. Pharmacokinetic-pharmacodynamic crisis in the elderly. *Am J Ther.* 2007;14:488–498.
26. Jacobs LJ. Warfarin pharmacology, clinical management, and evaluation of hemorrhagic risk for the elderly. *Clin Geriatr Med.* 2006;22:17–32.
27. Beers MH, Ouslander JG, Rollingher J, Reuben DB, Beck JC. Explicit criteria for determining inappropriate medication use in nursing home residents. *Arch Intern Med.* 1991;151:1825–1832.
28. Beers MH. Explicit criteria for determining potentially inappropriate medication use by the elderly. *Arch Intern Med.* 1997;157:1531–1536.
29. Fick DM, Cooper JW, Wade WE, et al. Updating the Beers criteria for potentially inappropriate medication use in older adults. *Arch Intern Med.* 2003;163:2716–2724.
30. Jano E, Aparasu RR. Healthcare outcomes associated with Beers' criteria: a systematic overview. *Ann Pharmacother.* 2007;41:438–448.
31. Swagerty D, Brickley R. American Medical Directors Association and American Society of Consultant Pharmacists joint position statement on the Beers list of Potentially Inappropriate Medications in Older Adults. *J Am Med Dir Assoc.* 2005;6:80–86.
32. Edwards IR, Aronson JK. Adverse drug reactions: definitions, diagnosis, and management. *Lancet.* 2000;356:1255–1259.
33. Atkin PA, Veitch PC, Veitch EM, et al. The epidemiology of serious adverse drug reactions among the elderly. *Drugs Aging.* 1999;14:141–152.
34. Pfizer, Inc. Zyvox (linezolid) package insert. New York; 2007.
35. Pirmohamed M, James S, Meakin S, et al. Adverse drug reactions as cause of admission to hospital: prospective analysis of 18,820 patients. *Br Med J.* 2004;329:15–19.
36. Veehof LJG, Stewart RE, Meyboom-deJong B, Haaijer-Ruskamp FM. Adverse drug reactions and polypharmacy in the elderly in general practice. *Eur J Clin Pharmacol.* 1999;55:533–536.
37. Chan M, Nicklason F, Vial JH. Adverse drug events as a cause of hospital admission in the elderly. *Intern Med J.* 2001;31:199–205.
38. Lazarou J, Pomeranz BH, Corey PN. Incidence of adverse drug reactions in hospitalized patients: a meta-analysis of prospective studies. *JAMA.* 1998;279:1200–1205.
39. Egger T, Dormann H, Ahne G, et al. Identification of adverse drug reactions in geriatric inpatients using a computerized drug database. *Drugs Aging.* 2003;20:769–776.
40. Davies EC, Green CF, Mottram DR, Pirmohamed M. Adverse drug reactions in hospital in-patients: a pilot study. *J Clin Pharm Ther.* 2006;31:335–341.
41. Hardmeier B, Braunschweig S, Cavallaro M, et al. Adverse drug events caused by medication errors in medical inpatients. *Swiss Med Wkly.* 2004;134:664–670.
42. Moore N, Lecointre D, Noblet C, Mabille M. Frequency and cost of serious adverse drug reactions in a department of general medicine. *Br J Clin Pharmacol.* 1998;45:301–308.
43. Routledge PA, O'Mahony MS, Woodhouse KW. Adverse drug reactions in elderly patients. *Br J Clin Pharmacol.* 2003;57:121–126.

44. Ensrud DE, Blackwell TL, Mangione CM, et al. Central nervous system-active medications and risk for falls in older women. *J Am Geriatr Soc.* 2002;50:1629–1637.

45. Leipzig RM, Cumming RG, Tinetti ME. Drugs and falls in older people: a systematic review and meta-analysis: I. Psychotropic drugs. *J Am Geriatr Soc.* 1999;47:30–39.

46. Thapa PB, Gideon P, Cost TW, Milam AB, Ray WA. Antidepressants and the risk of falls among nursing home residents. *NEJM.* 1998;339:875–882.

47. Drake MJ, Nixon PM, Crew JP. Drug-induced bladder and urinary disorders: incidence, prevention and management. *Drug Safety.* 1998;19:45–55.

48. Wagg A. Managing special populations: the elderly. *Eur Urol.* 2006;Suppl 5:866–870.

49. Maixner SM, Mellow AM, Tandon R. The efficacy safety and tolerability of antipsychotics in the elderly. *J Clin Psychiatry.* 1999;60:29–41.

50. McShane R, Keene J, Gedling K, Fairburn C, Jacoby R, Hope T. Do neuroleptic drugs hasten cognitive decline in dementia? *Br Med J.* 1997;314:266–270.

51. McEvoy GK, editor. AHFS Drug Information 2007. Bethesda, MD: ASHP; 2007.

52. Mintzer J, Burns A. Anticholinergic side-effects of drugs in elderly people. *J R Soc Med.* 2000;93:457–462.

53. Ancelin ML, Artero S, Portet F, et al. Non-degenerative mild cognitive impairment in elderly people and use of anticholinergic drugs: longitudinal cohort study. *Br Med J.* 2006;332:455–459.

54. Leipzig RM, Cumming RG, Tinetti ME. Drugs and falls in older people: a systematic review and meta-analysis: II. Cardiac and analgesic drugs. *J Am Geriatr Soc.* 1999;47:40–50.

55. Tinetti ME, Speechley M, Ginter SF. Risk factors for falls among elderly persons living in the community. *NEJM.* 1988;319:1701–1707.

56. U.S. Department of Health and Human Services. Bone health and osteoporosis a report of the Surgeon General–2004. Available at: http://www.surgeongeneral.gov/library/bonehealth/content.html. Accessed October 5, 2007.

57. Ganz DA, Bao Y, Shekelle PG, Rubenstein LZ. Will my patient fall? *JAMA.* 2007;297;77–86.

58. Fuller GF. Falls in the elderly. *Am Fam Physician.* 2000;61:2159–2174.

59. Zeire G, Dieleman JP, Hofman A, et al. Polypharmacy and falls in the middle age and elderly population. *Br J Clin Pharmacol.* 2005;61:218–223.

60. Liang SY, Mackowiak PA. Infections in the elderly. *Clin Geriatr Med.* 2007;23:441–456.

61. Cohen MB, Mather PJ. A review of the association between congestive heart failure and cognitive impairment. *Am J Geriatr Cardiol.* 2007;16:171–174.

62. Kuijpers MAJ, vanMarum RJ, Egberts ACG, Jansen PAF. Relationship between polypharmacy and underprescribing. *Br J Clin Pharmacol.* 2008;65:130–133.

63. Steinman MA, Landefeld, CS Rosenthal, et al. Polypharmacy and prescribing quality in older people. *J Am Geriatr Soc.* 2006;54:1516–1523.

64. Ghandi TK, Weingart SN, Borus J, et al. Adverse drug events in ambulatory care. *NEJM.* 2003;348:1556–1564.

65. Ghosh S, Ziesmer V, Aronow WS. Underutilization of aspirin, beta blockers, angiotensin-converting enzyme inhibitors, and lipid-lowering drugs and overutilization of calcium channel blockers in older persons with coronary artery disease in an academic nursing home. *J Gerontol.* 2002;57A:M398–M400.

66. Guglin M, Awad KE, Polavaram L, et al. Aldosterone antagonists – the most underutilized class of heart failure medications. *Am J Cardiovasc Drugs.* 2007;7:75–79.

67. Iba K, Takada J, Hatakeyama N, et al. Underutilization of antiosteoporotic drugs by orthopedic surgeons for prevention of a secondary osteoporotic fracture. *J Orthop Sci.* 2006;11:446–449.

68. Spinewine A, Swine C, Dhillon S, et al. Effect of a collaborative approach on the quality of prescribing for geriatric inpatients: a randomized, controlled trial. *J Am Geriatr Soc.* 2007;55:658–665.

69. MacLaughlin EJ, Raehl CL, Treadway AK, et al. Assessing medication adherence in the elderly – which tools to use in clinical practice? *Drugs Aging.* 2005;22:231–255.

70. Bangalore S, Kamalakkannan G, Parkar S, et al. Fixed-dose combinations improve medication compliance: a meta-analysis. *Am J Med.* 2007;120:713–719.

6

NUTRITION AND AGING

Jacqueline Lloyd, MD, Randy Huffines

INTRODUCTION

Hippocrates said, "If we could give every individual the right amount of nourishment and exercise, not too little and not too much, we would have found the safest way to health. Let your food be your medicine, and your medicine be your food." Scientific research continues to confirm the wisdom of Hippocrates, as it has significantly expanded our knowledge of the "right" nutrition for the older adult. Indirect evidence is accumulating that indicates optimal nutrition contributes to the prevention of diseases associated with "aging" such as coronary heart disease, stroke, and type 2 diabetes mellitus. Increased intake of certain nutrients can reduce the risks of falls and fractures among older adults and thus retard the development of frailty.[1] The interaction among nutrient status, deficiency states, and disease suggests new opportunities for primary and secondary preventive care for older adults. This chapter presents an updated review of what constitutes optimal nutrition for the older adult, a practical and evidence-based approach to assessment of nutrition, and discusses available nutritional therapies to optimize the experience of aging and to reduce the morbidity and mortality associated with malnutrition in the older adult.

NUTRITION AND OPTIMAL AGING

Aging might be seen as the process by which the human organism continues its maturation and development by adapting and compensating to changes in its internal and external environment over time. It is characterized by progressive reduction of reserve capacity in most organ systems and results in progressively increasing morbidity and eventual mortality. Optimal aging implies that adaptation to these changes takes place in ways that maintain the best possible functioning of the organism and the highest possible quality of life for the individual.[3]

Nutrition certainly plays a crucial role in the ability of the older adult to age optimally.

Physiological changes in each organ system with age can have an impact on the nutritional status of the older adult in numerous ways. The loss of lean body mass at approximately 0.3 kg/yr, consisting mostly of skeletal muscle, begins as early as the third decade of life and continues into old age.[2,3] This change, called sarcopenia, occurs even in healthy older adults living independently and is accompanied by a relative increase in adiposity resulting in preservation of body weight. Adipose tissue is much less metabolically active than muscle and, therefore, a resultant decreased requirement for energy intake occurs as age advances. There may additionally be a relative decrease in physical activity occurring with aging, which acts as both a cause and a consequence of sarcopenia because decreased activity results in corresponding decrements in appetite and food intake.[1]

In the healthy older adult, total body weight usually peaks in the 6th decade, and then remains stable until approximately 70 years of age, after which it begins to very slowly decrease. After the age of 75 years, those older adults who have maintained high levels of physical activity experience minimal weight loss.[4,5] Significant weight loss in the older adult is defined as 5% or more of body weight in 1 month or 10% or more over 6 months. Weight loss of this magnitude should never be ignored or dismissed as "normal aging."[6]

Age-related reduction in sense of smell and sensitivity of taste, especially to sweet and salty flavors, occurs.[7] An intact sense of smell is directly connected to food consumption; pleasant food odors enhance intake. The decrease in appetite and intake that occurs with age, however, does not appear to result from changes in special senses alone. Central changes in the perception of hunger and the regulation of the feeding response and peripheral changes in gastric- and duodenal-mediated satiation responses contribute to reduction in food consumption and weight as well.[7]

Alterations occurring in the oral cavity are frequent concomitants of advancing age and can have a significant impact on the desire for food as well as oral functions of ingestion and digestion. Good oral health and oral comfort are prerequisites for effective masticatory function.[8] The decrease in lean body mass that occurs with aging includes a decrease in the mass of the muscles of mastication and of the tongue that results in less efficient chewing and intraoral manipulation of the food bolus, especially if the person is missing teeth, edentulous, or wears dentures.[9] This problem is further exacerbated when the older adult wears full dentures, ill-fitting dentures, or has loose teeth or periodontal disease because impaired chewing has an impact on the types and consistencies of food that the older adult is able to ingest.[10] Affected older adults often avoid or eliminate foods that are difficult to chew such as tough, stringy meats and crunchy high-fiber foods like fresh fruits and vegetables.

The occurrence of xerostomia, or dry mouth, results from a change in the composition, production, or flow of saliva. Xerostomia complicates chewing, increases the possibility of mucosal trauma during mastication, impairs the ability to taste, and retards bolus formation and swallowing in approximately 40% of older people. Xerostomia is not a normal consequence of aging, as stimulated salivary flow is unchanged with physiological aging. Medical diseases, numerous common medications, decreased fluid intake, and frank dehydration are all potential contributors to dry mouth. Saliva has a rich chemistry consisting of lubricants, antimicrobial properties, minerals, and pH buffering for maintaining mineralization of tooth surfaces and digestive enzymes. In the absence of sufficient salivary flow, food loses much of its taste because the tasteants cannot be delivered to the taste buds unless they are in salivary solution.

Oral pain from dentures that no longer fit properly, or from untreated endodontic, periodontal, or mucosal disease, is an under recognized cause of older persons refusing to eat, especially for cognitively impaired individuals who may be unable to verbalize their discomfort or identify its source. Cognitively impaired older adults are often subject to impairment of the flavor of their food because of poor oral care. Mouth hygiene may be overlooked. Retention of particles in the mouth from receiving suspensions of crushed medications can result in hours of bitter and metallic tastes in their mouths and refusal of food in spite of an intact appetite. Clearly, maintaining oral health is a requirement for optimal aging. Unfortunately, far too many older adults or their caregivers consider basic dental care to be luxuries they simply cannot afford.

NUTRITIONAL REQUIREMENTS OF OLDER ADULTS

The new Dietary Reference Intakes (DRIs) have been developed by the Institute of Medicine's Food and Nutrition Board to expand and enhance the former system of Recommended Dietary Allowances (RDAs). The DRIs provide quantitative estimates of necessary nutrient intakes across the lifespan utilizing "life stage groups," which are subsets of the population by age and sex. The new DRIs take into account current

evidence for the role nutrients and food components play in maintaining health, preventing onset of disease, and treating disease states, thus expanding their usefulness far beyond simply defining nutritional deficiency states. For example, the DRIs for calcium and vitamin D were increased above previously recommended levels to levels appropriate to prevent and/or treat osteoporosis. In a recent study of the diets of healthy independently living elderly subjects in the southwest, 80% of study participants reported inadequate intakes of vitamin D and calcium.[11] Recent studies have also shown that bisphosphonates are ineffective in treating osteoporosis in the absence of adequate calcium intake.[12] The DRI for folate has been increased to reflect evidence that folate can lower the atherogenic rise in plasma homocysteine associated with aging and, thus, may be effective in helping to prevent cardiovascular disease.[11]

There are four types of reference intakes that together comprise the DRIs.

1. RDAs: established based on evidence of level of nutrient intake at which the needs of 97%–98% of all healthy individuals in a life stage group are met. It is useful in assessing the adequacy of an individual's nutrient intake.
2. *Tolerable Upper Intake Level*: advises an individual of the maximum intake of a given nutrient that may be safely ingested if adverse effects are to be avoided.
3. *Estimated Average Requirement* (EAR): the intake level at which 50% of healthy individuals in that life stage group meet their nutritional needs. It is useful in assessing the adequacy of intake of population groups and to determine the RDA (EAR + 2 standard deviations = RDA).
4. *Adequate Intake*: is the nutrient level deemed by the review panel experts to meet the needs of all individuals in a group, but which is not supported by the same level of evidence as the EAR or RDA.

All of the macro- and micronutrients were divided into groups based on type and function, and a panel of experts was assigned to a comprehensive review of existing evidence for all nutrients in that particular group. The nutrient groups included in the DRIs include:

1. *Calcium, vitamin D, phosphorus, magnesium, and fluoride;*
2. *Folate and other B vitamins;*
3. *Antioxidants – vitamins C and E, selenium;*
4. *Macronutrients – protein, fat, carbohydrates;*
5. *Trace elements – vitamins A and K, iron, zinc;*
6. *Electrolytes and water.*

The complete set of DRI tables may be found at www.iom.edu/CMS/54133/54377.aspx.

There is an abundance of recent evidence to suggest that the old "food pyramid" in the original or the modified version has been ineffective in promoting improved nutrition. One reason for this lack of efficacy in improving the health and nutritional status of the U.S. population is likely the tendency of the pyramids to "lump" all foods into categories without emphasizing significant differences in health benefits and risks associated with specific foods within certain groups. Not all "fats" are "bad," requiring severe limitation of intake, and not all "vegetables" or "breads/cereals" are "good."[13] The new DRI tables, which include recommended intakes for individuals based on age and sex, require adjustment for the level of activity of the person so that energy intake does not exceed average daily energy utilization. This approach is obviously different from the old food pyramid that suggested a specific number of servings from each food group each day for all adults, regardless of age or activity level.

To respond, in part, to criticism of the food pyramid and its modifications, the U.S. Department of Agriculture has published "Dietary Guidelines for Americans 2005,"[14] which is a detailed review of current evidence by the government, the intention being to serve as a guide for policy makers and others in assisting those who provide nutrition advice and counseling. The goal of the guideline is to promote health and reduce risk for major chronic diseases. Some selected "key recommendations" from this guideline relating to dietary intake for all age groups include:

1. Consume a variety of nutrient-dense foods and beverages from the basic food groups, and while limiting intake of saturated and "*trans* fats," cholesterol, add sugars, salt and alcohol;
2. Consume sufficient quantities of fruits and vegetables while staying within energy needs. This may be especially difficult for the older adult because the quantity of food required to meet energy needs may be significantly less than that to supply vitamin and other micronutrient needs;
3. Choose a variety of fruits and vegetables each day;
4. Consume 3 or more ounce-equivalents of whole grain products per day;
5. Consume 3 cups per day of fat-free or low fat milk or equivalent milk products;
6. Consume <10% of calories from saturated fatty acids and <300 mg/day cholesterol, keeping trans fatty acid consumption as low as possible;
7. Choose fiber-rich fruits, vegetables, and whole grains often.

Adapted from Dietary Guidelines for Americans 2005 www.health.gov/dietaryguidelines/dga2005/document/default.htm.

The new guideline eliminates the oversimplified recommendations of the pyramid for lay public use by targeting nutrition and health professionals instead, and is much more discriminating in recommending health-promoting intake of polyunsaturated and omega 3-fatty acids while limiting trans fatty acids and saturated fats.[1]

Willett and Skerrett have published a "healthy eating pyramid" in their book, *Eat, Drink and be Healthy: The Harvard Medical School Guide to Healthy Eating*, in which they advocate eating only as many servings, that is, calories, as required for energy on a daily basis. Whole grain foods and plant oils are recommended to become the base of the diet along with an

abundance of brightly colored vegetables and fruits at least two to three times per day. Legumes (beans) and nuts are touted as the mainstay of protein in the diet with supplementation with fish, poultry and eggs – zero to two times per day. Their new "pyramid" is then topped-off with either calcium supplements or no more than two daily servings of dairy. Alcohol, if not otherwise contraindicated, in moderation is encouraged for most individuals as is a daily multivitamin supplement. They suggest that red meat, butter, white rice, potatoes, white bread, pastas, and sweets be consumed very sparingly or eliminated altogether.[13]

NUTRITION SCREENING AND ASSESSMENT

Malnutrition is common in the geriatric age group and is most often not attributable to a single cause, but rather to multiple predisposing risk factors. As with most geriatric syndromes, it requires interaction among the environment, physiological changes of aging, and impairment or disease in multiple systems for this syndrome to be manifest. The interactions that occur among risk factors tend to reinforce each other in an escalating vicious cycle. For example, reduced muscle mass leads to decreased physical activity, which leads to physical deconditioning, which in turn leads to decreased tolerance for shopping in the "supermarket," where prices are lowest and merchandise aisles are longest. Corner groceries are hard to find and tend to be prohibitively expensive for many older adults on a fixed income. Inability to grocery shop leads to the "empty refrigerator" and impaired exercise tolerance predisposes to impaired tolerance for food preparation. Hence, the stage is now set for undernutrition, with resultant impaired protein synthesis and weight loss, nutrient deficiency, impaired immune function, increased likelihood of infection, and, therefore, acute illness that may present nonspecifically with decreased appetite. All clinicians caring for older adults in every setting where geriatric care is undertaken must be prepared to assess patients for risk of protein-energy undernutrition and be able to detect it in its earliest stage. To recommend "screening" all older adults for malnutrition syndromes, certain criteria must be applicable. First, the condition to be screened for must have negative outcomes. There is significant evidence of the outcomes of malnutrition in older adults that are independent of any underlying illness, disease state, or disability. There is increased risk of falls, increased duration of hospital and rehabilitation stay, increased need for institutionalization, increased postoperative complications, increased infections, increased incidence of pressure ulcers, poorer wound healing, impaired muscle and respiratory function, and death as a result of undernutrition.

Second, simple, reliable, cost-effective screening tests must be available with a reasonable degree of patient acceptability. Tests must have reasonable sensitivity to be able to identify persons at risk of malnutrition before clinical consequences are obvious. Finally, intervention at the preclinical level must improve outcomes. There must be some treatment, which if rendered, reduces negative consequences for the patient.

The first level of screening can be accomplished with some simple preliminary queries.

- Have you lost 10 lb in the past 6 months without trying to do so?[15]
- Is your current weight? <100 lb[15]
- Has there been any change to your *appetite* or to your usual eating habits?

An affirmative response to any of these questions would justify the further investigation beginning with objective observation and documentation of change in weight. When weight loss is suspected or confirmed, a number of tests for further assessment and quantification of changes in nutritional status are available, including the body mass index (BMI), anthropometrics, and assay of biochemical markers. Each of these tools has distinct advantages and limits to its usefulness.

- **BMI** (weight [kg]/height [m^2]) is predictive of disease risk in those who are underweight, but can fail to detect significant involuntary weight loss especially in the obese. It is also unreliable in the presence of edema or ascites. Accurate measurement of height is fraught with error in the older adult because of vertebral compression, loss of muscle tone, and arthritic or postural change such as kyphosis. BMI does not meet criteria to be an optimal screen because a significant reduction would mean that significant change in weight/nutrition has already taken place.[16]
- **Anthropometrics**, which include measurement of skinfold thickness and mid–upper arm circumference, are simple and inexpensive to obtain but require training and skilled technique to administer as well as to interpret results, which vary with the age, sex, and ethnic makeup of the individual.
- **Biochemical markers** include serum proteins manufactured by the liver such as albumin, transferrin, and prealbumin.[17] Albumin levels are predictive of mortality and other outcomes but are not dependent solely on nutritional status. Total lymphocyte count signifies a poor prognosis and is independent of albumin. Low total cholesterol also correlates with risk of malnutrition; however, most biochemical markers are affected by other disease states such as infection, inflammation, and organ impairment, that is, liver disease, and therefore, as individual tests, have low specificity for screening malnutrition. Prealbumin has been found to have some efficacy as a screening test in hospitalized patients.[17]

Formal malnutrition assessment tools comprise combinations of individual screening items and have been developed to overcome the various inadequacies of the individual tests described previously. Two such tools that have been widely used and very well validated are the Malnutrition Universal Screening Tool (MUST)[18] and the Mini Nutritional Assessment (MNA).[19]

- **MUST** was developed in the UK primarily for screening in the community setting and consists of the BMI, history of unexplained weight loss, and survey of acute illness effects. MUST has been shown to have high predictive validity in the hospital environment as well. It can be completed in 3 to 5 minutes.[18]
- **MNA** Stage 1 is a screening questionnaire consisting of six components: survey of food intake in past 3 months, weight loss in past 3 months, mobility status, psychological stress or acute disease in the past 3 months, neuropsychological problems, and BMI. It was designed for screening patients in home care, nursing facilities, and hospitals, and is able to detect risk of malnutrition before change in other parameters occurs, such as BMI or albumin. It is a fairly sensitive screen; a score of 11 or more indicates strong evidence that malnutrition is *absent*. The MNA assessment tool contains 12 items. The maximum possible score is 16. Scores >12 indicate satisfactory nutritional status with no need to proceed further. Once the assessment stage is completed, its score is added to the screening score to obtain the total assessment score or malnutrition indicator score. A total score of 17–23.5 indicates risk of malnutrition, whereas a score of <17 indicates existing malnutrition.[19]

Comprehensive assessment of nutritional status is most thoroughly done by a combination of modalities including careful, focused history and physical (including oral/dental) examination, detailed medication review, social and psychological assessment, anthropometrics, and laboratory studies. This complete data set is most efficiently compiled and assessed with management plans developed, implemented, and monitored with the assistance of a multidisciplinary team.

In addition to quantitative assessment for malnutrition, a number of tools are also available for qualitative assessment of dietary intake to counsel older adults on how to modify their risk of developing certain chronic and or acute diseases. A brief assessment could be accomplished using the Food Frequency Screening Questionnaire,[20] or a 24-hour dietary recall for older adults living independently. Forty-eight or 72-hour calorie counts are commonly used in inpatient and other institutional settings.

MALNUTRITION SYNDROMES

There are several types of malnutrition syndromes that occur in the older adult. Protein-energy undernutrition is a state of impaired homeostasis that occurs as a result of insufficient intake of basic macronutrients or inability to absorb or utilize ingested nutrients. As a result of energy, protein, and other micronutrient needs of the body not being met, both structure and function of tissues and organs are impaired. The reported prevalence of undernutrition in the geriatric adult varies from study to study, but has been estimated at approximately 14% for independent community dwellers, and perhaps as high as

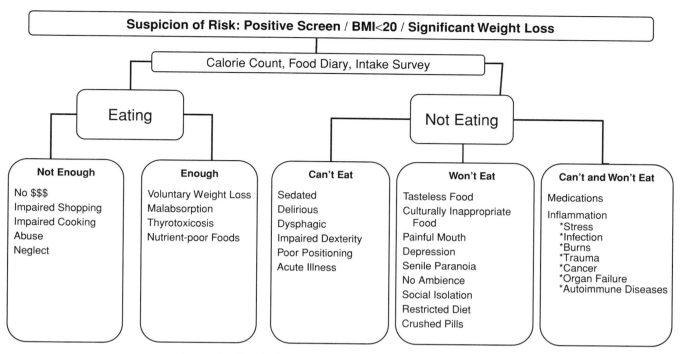

Figure 6.1. Practical approach to undernutrition. See color plates.

27% among *high-risk* community-dwelling older adults.[21] High-risk older adults are those with cognitive impairment, multiple medical comorbidities, disability, low socioeconomic status, low education level, and/or low baseline body weight. Up to 50% of hospitalized acutely ill older adults are considered to be undernourished.[22] Among nursing facility and other institutionalized residents, 25%–85% show evidence of protein calorie undernutrition.[7,23] This devastating syndrome is so common that the terms undernutrition and malnutrition are frequently used synonymously, ignoring the other malnutrition syndromes. The causes of undernutrition in the older adult are myriad. It is important to recognize that the causes are not mutually exclusive, but commonly a number of factors contribute to the occurrence of the syndrome of undernutrition in the geriatric patient. Loss of appetite with or without resulting weight loss is often a key component of the nonspecific presentation of disease so that evaluation of a patient with a recent change in appetite for an acute illness is an important task for the clinician caring for any older adult. If the older adult is not eating (starvation), the question to be asked is whether they cannot eat or they will not eat sufficient quantities. Neurological or gastrointestinal dysfunction as well as oral problems can all result in a patient who is unable to eat. Inappropriate mealtime ambience, anorexia, social isolation, certain oral problems, depression, paranoia, and other psychiatric disorders might cause a patient to refuse to eat. A practical approach to conceptualizing causes and contributors to undernutrition in the older adult is illustrated in Figure 6.1. Undernutrition is the major cause for concern in the population older than

65 years because protein-calorie undernutrition results in a greater increase in morbidity and mortality in this population cohort than overnutrition.[24] Some of the adverse outcomes of undernutrition that occur independently of underlying conditions or comorbidities include increased fall risk, complicated postoperative courses, longer hospital stays, increased infection rates, increased susceptibility to pressure sores, impaired respiratory function, deconditioning, markedly impaired quality of life, and even death.

The other major malnutrition syndrome is that of overnutrition, which results from the consistent consumption of excess calories or nutrients above the actual needs of the individual. Overweight is defined as a BMI of 25–29.9 and obesity is defined as a BMI of 30 or above; these conditions occur when more calories are consistently consumed on a daily basis than are utilized for energy. Treatment for overweight and obesity in geriatric adults should be carefully considered because of the frequency with which they impair function and diminish quality of life. Disability appears approximately 10 years earlier in obese persons than in persons of recommended weight, and obesity may in fact predispose the geriatric adult to "frailty."[25] With regard to morbidity and mortality resulting from overweight and obesity in the geriatric individual, there is considerable controversy and relationships are not clear-cut or straightforward. It has been suggested that in persons older than 85 years, overweight is not a mortality risk factor and mild overweight may even be "protective" against death.[26] Although high BMI is a strong indicator of risk for disability in older women, BMI alone is insufficient as an indicator of negative obesity-related effects.[26,27] BMI is less accurate in predicting the actual percentage of body fat present in older persons because of changes in height resulting from vertebral compression, kyphosis, and other degenerative skeletal conditions.[16] Potentially beneficial effects of increased body weight have been noted in older adults, including increased bone mineral density and a "cushioning" effect around the greater trochanter. These benefits of adiposity may, in some cases, result in decreased incidence of hip fracture. A decrease of one standard deviation in fat mass has been shown to be associated with a 30% increase in risk of hip fracture.[28] In older geriatric patients, weight loss has been found to be associated with increased rather than decreased mortality in women regardless of whether that loss was intentional or unintentional.[28] Perhaps that is because intentional weight loss results in loss of both fat mass (75%) and fat-free or lean body mass (25%), which might exacerbate the sarcopenia already present as a result of normal or obligatory aging.

Overnutrition in specific micronutrients can result in toxicity states. The new DRI tables now categorize the maximum safe intake levels for specific nutrients known to have potential toxicities or adverse effects when taken in excess. For older adult men and women, these micronutrients include vitamins A, C, D, E, niacin, B6, folate, and choline, and the minerals include calcium, iodine, iron, magnesium, manganese phosphorus, and potassium.[29]

NUTRITIONAL THERAPIES FOR UNDERNUTRITION

Oral Liquid Nutritional Supplementation may be the most common treatment offered nursing facility residents with unintentional weight loss, with a number of studies showing variable results on weight gain in these patients. A study by Simmons and Patel showed that fewer than 10% of patients with orders for oral nutritional supplements actually received and ingested the supplement as ordered and positive results were very staff dependent.[30,31] Efficacy of oral supplementation very much depends on the cause of the protein-energy undernutrition, the functioning of the gastrointestinal tract, and the severity of the nutritional deficits. Systemic inflammation is a major cause of failure of nutritional therapy to improve nutritional status. Research provides insight into the role of inflammation and inflammatory mediators in chronic disease, offering new opportunities for pharmacological use of nutrients in treating certain diseases. Weight loss mediated by an inflammatory state (cachexia) is a hypermetabolic condition, often unresponsive to increasing nutrient intake. Pharmacological modulation of the inflammatory process with a number of agents including megestrol acetate, thalidomide, pentoxifylline, and dronabinol can stimulate appetite and promote conversion from a catabolic state to an anabolic condition in certain cases. Increased physical exercise and growth hormone may augment this change to anabolism.[32]

Temporary or episodic nutritional supplementation of undernourished older adults also has the potential for positive or negative outcome. Some individuals respond to supplementation by decreasing their intake of regular meals. When supplementation is no longer provided, individuals may not respond with a return to pre-supplementation intake at mealtime. When individuals maintain steady intake of regular meals, whether supplemented or not, more lasting and beneficial "boosting" effects of nutritional therapy result.[31] Nutritional supplementation can have a positive impact on organ function more quickly than improvements in weight and certain biochemical markers tend to occur.

NUTRITIONAL THERAPY FOR UNDERNUTRITION IN SELECTED DISEASE STATES

Cardiovascular Disease is the leading cause of death in industrialized nations. There is good evidence that management of cardiovascular disease in patients with hyperlipidemias, diabetes mellitus, and other risk factors can be made more efficacious by appropriately intensive dietary counseling therapy delivered by a multidisciplinary team including a primary care provider, and a dietician and/or a nutritionist.[20] Such counseling should focus on identifying and changing excessive or deficient dietary patterns to patterns more consistent with "Key Recommendations" from "Dietary Guidelines for Americans 2005" and current DRI recommendations.

Congestive Heart Failure is a leading cause of acute hospitalization in adults 65 years or older in the United States and is associated, in severe cases, with cytokine-mediated (inflammatory) catabolism. This state, often termed "cardiac cachexia" is defined by body fat less than 27%–29% in an adult who also weighs less than 80%–90% of their ideal body weight. Watson et al.[33] have found that cytokines regulate the structure and function of the heart. Certain cytokines, which increase with advancing age, seem to mediate abnormal function of cardiac fibroblasts resulting in changes in collagen. It is believed that the inflammatory cytokines interleukin-6 and tumor necrosis factor-α (TNF-α), which are elevated in congestive heart failure, are increased by high fat and high simple carbohydrate diets, inducing a dilated cardiomyopathy.[34] The significance of these cytokines is that they also seem to mediate cardiac cachexia, characterized by significant negative nitrogen balance. Although it is often unresponsive to nutritional supplementation, overfeeding, or even enteral or parenteral nutrition, cardiac cachexia may be amenable to dietary treatment with n-3 polyunsaturated fatty acids or pharmacological treatment with megestrol.[33] As a consequence of nutritional therapy, these homeostatically fragile patients are sometimes placed at risk of a "refeeding syndrome," a potentially lethal symptom complex of electrolyte and fluid disturbances and other metabolic abnormalities including thiamine deficiency, hypokalemia, hypomagnesemia, and hypophosphatemia.[35]

Some **stroke** patients show evidence of protein-energy undernutrition at the time of presentation and others have an impact during the post stroke interval. As with the general undernutrition syndrome in the older adult, multiple factors have an impact on the increased risk of malnutrition for the stroke patient. Dysphagia plays a significant role for 35%–40% of all stroke patients in the post stroke interval, but 87% of these regain swallow function in the first 2 weeks poststroke.[36] Clinical signs indicative of potential swallowing problems include wet, "congested" voice, weak cough that does not fully clear airway, drooling, and dysarthria indicating poor control of the muscles of speech. Bedside clinical screening for swallowing efficacy should therefore include evaluation of the patient's level of consciousness and ability to follow instructions, assessment of control of posture and of oral secretions, and water swallow test if appropriate. Videofluoroscopic studies of swallow or modified barium swallow can be very helpful in revealing aspiration risk in stroke patients with and without obvious clinical signs and in formulating management strategies for speech and swallow therapy. The modified barium swallow is considered the "gold standard" in assessing dysphagia; on the other hand, the presence or absence of a gag reflex reveals little about the efficacy of the pharyngeal swallow mechanism. When the patient has been shown to aspirate during the swallow, placement of a percutaneous endoscopic gastrostomy (PEG) tube is often the route chosen for nutritional therapy. The ability to eat also has a negative impact from deficits in communication, perception, and coordination. Many of these deficits, if recognized, may be responsive to speech/swallow and occupational therapies. A full spectrum of nutritional therapy modalities including oral, nasogastric tube, PEG, or jejunostomy PEG tube–administered supplementation are available. Artificial feeding should be used only after realistic and achievable goals, consistent with the informed wishes of the patient, have been established. The patient's wishes may be expressed by the patient or the appropriate surrogate or proxy. Although some immediate benefits of PEG nutritional therapy have clearly been shown, a long-term benefit of improved mortality after continued PEG therapy has not been as evident.[37,38] In fact, PEG feeding may serve to prolong the time of poor function and poor quality of life for stroke patients who would have likely succumbed to their disease earlier but for the artificial feeding provided by the PEG.

Protein-energy undernutrition has a prevalence of 20%–70% in patients with ***chronic obstructive pulmonary disease***, which is also a chronic inflammatory state.[32] In these patients, an increased basal metabolic rate may be associated with elevated TNF-α concentrations in the patient's blood. The resulting catabolic state causes loss of lean body mass including diaphragmatic muscle mass, resulting in reduced capacity for physical activity and reduced pulmonary function capacity. Although some studies have shown a positive effect of nutritional supplementation therapy on body composition, muscle strength, and respiratory function in patients with chronic obstructive pulmonary disease, patients with very high levels of TNF-α may be less responsive to nutritional supplement therapy.[32]

Protein-energy undernutrition commonly occurs in patients suffering from **dementia**. Within 8 years of the diagnosis of Primary Degenerative Dementia of the Alzheimer type, 50% of patients require assistance with feeding or artificial nutrition.[32] Anorexia, dyspraxias, apraxias, altered taste and smell, and paranoia with refusal to eat may all contribute to symptomatic weight loss in Alzheimer's disease. A retrospective study of nursing home residents with severe cognitive impairment found there to be no survival advantage to tube feeding among demented patients with tubes compared with those without tubes. Dementia, in its end stage, can be considered to be "brain failure" and comparable to end-stage organ failure of any other major organ, ultimately representing terminal collapse of that individual's homeostatic integrity.[39] Finucane's review concluded that evidence was entirely lacking that tube feeding could achieve the therapeutic goals of preventing aspiration, improving pressure sore outcome, and/or decreasing risk of infection in dysphagic dementia patients.[37] A recent literature review and meta-analysis by Stratton suggests that high-protein oral nutritional supplements compared with routine care are associated with a 25% reduction in pressure ulcer development in at risk patients, but this review was inclusive of all "at risk" patients, not strictly dementia patients, and insufficient data were available to make conclusions about healing already existing pressure sores.[40]

Because protein-energy undernutrition is in and of itself a risk factor for **hip fracture**, it is not surprising that up to 50% of patients with hip fracture are found to be malnourished.[32] Such undernutrition is associated with longer hospital stays and longer rehabilitation stays. There is evidence that treatment of the undernutrition is associated with shorter hospitalizations, fewer postoperative complications, and perhaps even a demonstrable beneficial effect on mortality.[41]

Thurston Thomas Thurber Jr., in his tongue-in-cheek book on old age comments on diet and nutrition: "Doing everything right offers no guarantees, but it increases your chances and if you feel better, that in itself is worth the hassle."[42] Research and continued clinical investigation offer tremendous promise in helping us determine not only what is possible to do, but what is right to do in optimizing the nutrition, and ultimately the quality of life of the older adult individual. It becomes more and more of a reality that optimized nutrition can help the older adult not only to feel better, but to be healthier. That is, indeed, worth the hassle.

REFERENCES

1. Bischoff HA, Staehelin HB, Willett WC. The effect of undernutrition in the development of frailty in older persons. *J Gerontol.* 2006;61(6):585–589.
2. Gallagher D, Ruts E, Visser M, et al. Weight stability masks sarcopenia in elderly men and women. *Am J Physiol Endocrinol Metab.* 2000;279(2):E366–E375.
3. Bozzetti F. Nutritional issues in the care of the elderly patient. *Crit Rev Oncol Hematol.* 2003;48(2):113–121.
4. Morley JE. Anorexia, body composition, and ageing. *Curr Opin Clin Nutr Metab Care.* 2001;4(1):9–13.

5. Mott JW, Wang J, Thornton JC, Allison DB, Heymsfield SB, Pierson RN, Jr. Relation between body fat and age in 4 ethnic groups. *Am J Clin Nutr.* 1999;69(5):1007–1013.

6. Wallace JI, Schwartz RS. Epidemiology of weight loss in humans with special reference to wasting in the elderly. *Int J Cardiol.* 2002;85(1):15–21.

7. Morley JE. Anorexia, sarcopenia, and aging. *Nutrition.* 2001;17(7–8):660–663.

8. Walls AW, Steele JG. The relationship between oral health and nutrition in older people. *Mech Ageing Dev.* 2004;125(12):853–857.

9. Budtz-Jorgensen E, Chung JP, Rapin CH. Nutrition and oral health. *Best Pract Res Clin Gastroenterol.* 2001;15(6):885–896.

10. Jensen GL, McGee M, Binkley J. Nutrition in the elderly. *Gastroenterol Clin North Am.* 2001;30(2):313–334.

11. Foote JA, Giuliano AR, Harris RB. Older adults need guidance to meet nutritional recommendations. *J Am Coll Nutr.* 2000;19(5):628–640.

12. Sunyecz JA, Weisman SM. The role of calcium in osteoporosis drug therapy. *J Womens Health.* 2005;14(2):180–92.

13. Willett WC, Skerrett PJ Eat, drink and be healthy: the Harvard Medical School guide to healthy eating. New York: Simon & Schuster. 2001;21–22.

14. U.S. Department of Agriculture. Dietary Guidelines for Americans 2005: Executive summary. Available at: http://www.health.gov/dietaryguidelines/dga2005/document/html/executivesummary.htm. Accessed May 12, 2008.

15. Moore AA, Siu A, Partridge JM, Hays RD, Adams J. A randomized trial of office-based screening for common problems in older persons. *Am J Med.* 1997;102(4):371–378.

16. Cook Z, Kirk S, Lawrenson S, Sandford S. Use of BMI in the assessment of undernutrition in older subjects: reflecting on practice. *Proc Nutr Soc.* 2005;64(3):313–317.

17. Robinson MK, Trujillo EB, Mogensen KM, Rounds J, McManus K, Jacobs DO. Improving nutritional screening of hospitalized patients: the role of prealbumin. *J Parenter Enteral Nutr.* 2003;27(6):389–395; quiz 439.

18. Stratton RJ, Hackston A, Longmore D, et al. Malnutrition in hospital outpatients and inpatients: prevalence, concurrent validity and ease of use of the 'malnutrition universal screening tool' ('MUST') for adults. *Br J Nutr.* 2004;92(5):799–808.

19. A guide to completing the mini nutritional assessment MNA. Nestle. Accessed 2006, at http://www.mna-elderly.com/.

20. Olendzki B, Speed C, Domino FJ. Nutritional assessment and counseling for prevention and treatment of cardiovascular disease. *Am Fam Physician.* 2006;73(2):257–264.

21. Alibhai SM, Greenwood C, Payette H. An approach to the management of unintentional weight loss in elderly people. *CMAJ.* 2005;172(6):773–780.

22. Powers JS. Facilitated feeding in disabled elderly. *Curr Opin Clin Nutr Metab Care.* 2002;5(3):315–319.

23. Thomas DR, Ashmen W, Morley JE, Evans WJ. Nutritional management in long-term care: development of a clinical guideline. Council for Nutritional Strategies in Long-Term Care. *J Gerontol.* 2000;55(12):M725–734.

24. Stratton RJ, King CL, Stroud MA, Jackson AA, Elia M. 'Malnutrition Universal Screening Tool' predicts mortality and length of hospital stay in acutely ill elderly. *Br J Nutr.* 2006;95(2):325–330.

25. Ferraro KF, Su YP, Gretebeck RJ, Black DR, Badylak SF. Body mass index and disability in adulthood: a 20-year panel study. *Am J Public Health.* 2002;92(5):834–840.

26. Inelmen EM, Sergi G, Coin A, Miotto F, Peruzza S, Enzi G. Can obesity be a risk factor in elderly people? *Obes Rev.* 2003;4(3):147–155.

27. Sharkey JR, Ory MG, Branch LG. Severe elder obesity and 1-year diminished lower extremity physical performance in homebound older adults. *J Am Geriatr Soc.* 2006;54(9):1407–1413.

28. Villareal DT, Apovian CM, Kushner RF, Klein S. Obesity in older adults: technical review and position statement of the American Society for Nutrition and NAASO, The Obesity Society. *Obes Res.* 2005;13(11):1849–1863.

29. Food and Nutrition Board, Institute of Medicine, National Academies. Dietary reference intakes (DRIs): recommended intakes for individuals, Electrolytes and Water Table http://www.iom.edu/CMS/54133/54377.aspx.

30. Simmons SF, Patel AV. Nursing home staff delivery of oral liquid nutritional supplements to residents at risk for unintentional weight loss. *J Am Geriatr Soc.* 2006;54(9):1372–1376.

31. Parrott MD, Young KW, Greenwood CE. Energy-containing nutritional supplements can affect usual energy intake post-supplementation in institutionalized seniors with probable Alzheimer's disease. *J Am Geriatr Soc.* 2006;54(9):1382–1387.

32. Akner G, Cederholm T. Treatment of protein-energy malnutrition in chronic nonmalignant disorders. *Am J Clin Nutr.* 2001;74(1):6–24.

33. Watson RR, Zibadi S, Vazquez R, Larson D. Nutritional regulation of immunosenescence for heart health. *J Nutr Biochem.* 2005;16(2):85–87.

34. Kornman KS. Interleukin 1 genetics, inflammatory mechanisms, and nutrigenetic opportunities to modulate diseases of aging. *Am J Clin Nutr.* 2006;83(2):475S–483S.

35. Crook MA, Hally V, Panteli JV. The importance of the refeeding syndrome. *Nutrition.* 2001;17(7–8):632–637.

36. Scottish Intercollegiate Guidelines Network. Management of patients with stroke: identification and management of dysphagia. Available at: http://www.sign.ac.uk/pdf/sign78.pdf. Accessed May 12, 2008.

37. Finucane TE, Christmas C, Travis K. Tube feeding in patients with advanced dementia: a review of the evidence. *JAMA.* 1999;282(14):1365–1370.

38. McMahon MM, Hurley DL, Kamath PS, Mueller PS. Medical and ethical aspects of long-term enteral tube feeding. *Mayo Clin Proc.* 2005;80(11):1461–1476.

39. Chouinard J, Lavigne E, Villeneuve C. Weight loss, dysphagia, and outcome in advanced dementia. *Dysphagia.* 1998;13(3):151–155.

40. Stratton RJ, Ek AC, Engfer M, et al. Enteral nutritional support in prevention and treatment of pressure ulcers: a systematic review and meta-analysis. *Ageing Res Rev.* 2005;4(3):422–450.

41. Avenell A, Gillespie WJ, Gillespie LD, O'Connell DL. Vitamin D and vitamin D analogues for preventing fractures associated with involutional and post-menopausal osteoporosis. *Cochrane Database Syst Rev.* 2005(3):CD000227.

42. Thurber TTJ. *Old Age 101.* Gillett, PA: Methuselah Press; 2000.

7

USING EXERCISE AS MEDICINE FOR OLDER ADULTS

Maria A. Fiatarone Singh, MD, FRACP

AGING AND PHYSICAL ACTIVITY PATTERNS

Currently, disparities exist among population groups in habitual physical activity patterns that exaggerate the negative health consequences of a sedentary lifestyle. Unchanged from the 1996 Surgeon General's Report on Physical Activity and Health,[1] demographic groups still at highest risk for inactivity are the elderly, women, minorities, those with low income or educational background, and those with disabilities or chronic health conditions. As might be expected, these are the same demographic groups that both bear a large burden of the diseases amenable to prevention and treatment with exercise, and, yet, often have the least access and opportunity for health promotion efforts related to physical activity. Therefore, all health care providers should identify and understand barriers to physical activity faced by these population groups and utilize programs and tools that address these barriers.

Previous objectives for middle-aged and older adults have primarily focused on physical activities designed to improve cardiorespiratory fitness and prolong life. It is now recognized, however, that older adults can benefit from physical activities designed to maintain or improve functional independence as well. The specific physical fitness components that provide continued physical function as individuals age include muscle strength, cardiovascular and muscular endurance, balance, and flexibility.[2] The problems of mobility impairment, falls, arthritis, osteoporotic fractures, and functional status are clearly related in part to muscle strength and mass,[3,4] characteristics that are amenable to intervention even in frail elders,[5,6] and thus strengthening activities, although important for all age groups, are particularly important for older adults. Additionally, the metabolic benefits of retention and activation of muscle mass are now increasingly recognized as an important facet of the epidemic of age- and obesity-related insulin resistance and type 2 diabetes.[5] Age-related loss of strength, muscle mass (sarcopenia), and bone density, which are most dramatic in women,

may be attenuated by strengthening exercises.[6,7] and improved even in late life with appropriate resistance training.[8,9] Unfortunately, U.S. survey and other data indicate that women in general report lower than average adult participation levels for strength training (11% vs. 16%).[10] Additionally, despite the evidence on safety and efficacy in even frail elders,[11–13] the prevalence rate for resistive exercise is even lower among the old (6% at ages 65–74 years) or the very old (4% older than age 75 years). Individuals in this latter age group, particularly those older than the age of 85 years, are primarily women, making an understanding of the risks and benefits of exercise in this population a priority.[14]

Rationale for the Integration of Exercise Prescription into Geriatric Care

The rationale for the integration of a physical activity prescription into geriatric health care is based on four essential concepts.[15] First, there is a great similarity between the physiological changes that are attributable to disuse (sarcopenia, osteopenia, central and generalized adiposity, low fitness, insulin resistance, etc.) and those that have been typically observed in aging populations, leading to the speculation that the way in which we age may in fact be greatly modulated with attention to activity levels.[16] Second, chronic diseases increase with age, and exercise has now been shown to be an independent risk factor and/or potential treatment for most of the major causes of morbidity and mortality in western societies (see Table 7.1), a potential that is, currently, vastly underutilized. Third, traditional medical interventions do not typically address disuse syndromes accompanying chronic disease, which may be responsible for much of their associated disability. Exercise is particularly good at targeting these syndromes of disuse. Finally, many pathophysiological aberrations that are central to a disease or its treatment are better addressed by exercise than by pharmacological therapy (e.g., the visceral adiposity of

Table 7.1. Benefits of Exercise in Older Adults

Physiological Adaptations	Disease Prevention	Disease Treatment
Increased bone density	Cancer (breast, colon, endometrial, prostate)	Arthritis
		Insomnia
Decreased total body and visceral adipose tissue, decreased intramuscular and hepatic lipid accumulation	Coronary artery disease	Coronary artery disease
	Dementia	Congestive heart failure
Decreased fibrinogen levels	Depression	Dementia
Decreased sympathetic and hormonal response to exercise	Disability	Depression
Decreased LDL, increased HDL levels, increased fat oxidation	Hyperlipidemia	Disability
	Hypertension	Hyperlipidemia
Improved cognitive function and brain volume	Impotence	Hypertension
Decreased postural blood pressure response to stressors	Obesity	Obesity
	Osteoporosis	Osteoporosis
Decreased HR/blood pressure/perceived exertion response to submaximal exercise	Stroke	Peripheral vascular disease
	Type 2 diabetes mellitus	Parkinson's disease
Increased oxygen extraction by skeletal muscle		Stroke
Increased HR variability		Type 2 diabetes mellitus
Increased neural reaction time		
Increased blood volume and hematocrit		
Increased energy expenditure		
Increased glycogen storage in skeletal muscle		
Increased oxidative enzyme capacity in skeletal muscle		
Increased glucose disposal rate, decreased postprandial dysmetabolism		
Increased mitochondrial volume density in skeletal muscle		
Decreased resting HR and blood pressure		
Increased GLUT-4 receptors in skeletal muscle, insulin sensitivity, glucose tolerance		
Decreased arterial stiffness		
Increased maximal aerobic capacity		
Increased stroke volume during exercise*		
Increased capillary density in skeletal muscle		
Increased cardiac contractility during exercise*		
Decreased systemic inflammation		
Improved endothelial cell function		
Improved baroreceptor function, decreased orthostasis		

* Observed only in older endurance-trained men thus far.

metabolic syndrome), which, therefore, deserves a place in the mainstream of medical care, not as an optional adjunct.

It is clear that the optimum approach to "successful aging" or to health care in the older population cannot ignore the overlap of these areas. In some cases, exercise can be used to avert "age-related" decrements in physiological function and thereby maximize function and quality of life in the elderly. On the other hand, the combination of exercise and sound nutrition, particularly in relation to favorable alterations in body composition, will have numerous important effects on risk factors for chronic disease as well as the disability that accompanies such conditions. Therefore, understanding the effects of aging on exercise capacity and how habitual physical activity can modify this relationship in the older adult, including its specific utility in treating medical diseases, is critical for health care practitioners of all disciplines.

Monitoring the Benefits of Exercise

Most health outcomes appear to be related to the accumulated volume and intensity of exercise, and so monitoring compliance will theoretically provide evidence that the benefits are occurring. There may, however, be benefit also in monitoring the improvements in cardiovascular fitness from training, as aerobic capacity itself has an even stronger relationship to mortality than level of physical activity.[17] Documenting improvements in fitness or function may have a reinforcing effect on long-term behavioral adaptations as well. Improved fitness/function across the multiple domains of exercise capacity may be shown by:

- Improved measurements of peak aerobic capacity;
- Decreased heart rate and blood pressure response to a fixed submaximal workload;
- Decreased rating of perceived exertion for a fixed submaximal workload;
- Improved muscle strength, endurance, or power;
- Ability to lift a submaximal load more times;
- Ability to withstand postural stress or negotiate obstacles;
- Improved joint range of motion;
- Improved functional performance (e.g., gait speed, chair stand time, stair climbing, etc.).

Exercise Testing for Older Adults

Cardiovascular Endurance

Because treadmill testing and indirect calorimetry are not always available or feasible, particularly in frail adults older than 75 years of age, field estimates of aerobic capacity and cardiovascular responses are usually substituted. A simple way to do this in clinical practice that requires minimal equipment is the 6-minute walk test.[18] This test has been used as an index of rehabilitation in cardiac and pulmonary patients and is known to improve with effective interventions. With training, pulse and blood pressure at 6 minutes should decrease and distance covered should increase. Alternatives to the 6-minute walk are walking a fixed distance (e.g., 400 m) climbing multiple flights of stairs as rapidly as possible, or stepping up and down a single step for several minutes, followed by the measurements above. Availability of stairs and the potential for musculoskeletal injury because of balance, hip and knee arthritis, or vision problems make rapid stepping tests less desirable in the older adult, however. The 6-minute walk tests reflects not only aerobic capacity, but contributions from gait stability, muscle strength, pain, body composition, and neuropsycho-

logical function, and thus is a good overall index of exercise capacity (not simply aerobic capacity) and has direct clinical relevance to ambulatory function in daily life.[19]

Strength Testing

If maximal strength itself cannot be measured, or measurement is not considered safe or feasible in an elderly individual, there is an option that is commonly used to rate effort during a lift, using a scale of perceived exertion, such as the Borg Rating of Perceived Exertion (RPE) scale.[20] On this scale from 6–20, a rating of 15–18 (hard to very hard) is equivalent to 70%–80% of maximum lifting capacity in studies conducted in young and older adults, and is, therefore, an appropriate training goal for a resistance training prescription.[5,14]

Preexercise Assessment in Older Adults

Most older adults, despite the presence of chronic diseases and disabilities, are able to undertake and benefit from an exercise prescription that is tailored to their physiological capacities, comorbidities, and neuropsychological and behavioral needs.[15] The relatively few permanent exclusions to any structured exercise are generally severe irreversible conditions that are obvious exclusions because of the nature of the specific exercise prescription under consideration or the risk the exercise would impose on the health status of the individual. There may be some forms of exercise in which even permanently bed-bound patients or those with severe behavioral problems may engage, but they are not able to participate in the usual aerobic, resistive, or balance exercises described later. For some older adults, such as those with critical aortic stenosis, cardiac or peripheral vascular ischemia at rest, or an enlarging aortic aneurysm or known cerebral aneurysm (when surgery is not an option because of other medical considerations or very advanced age), any exercise that significantly elevates cardiac workload or blood pressure is considered high risk, and, therefore, is not recommended.[5,14] It is anticipated that relatively few older adults (even those in long-term care) would be excluded from all exercise programs based on items in this category (see Table 7.2) outside of those with severe forms of dementia or terminal illness.

The majority of questions about exercise prescription eligibility will be because of items in the "temporary exclusion" or WAIT category (see Table 7.2), so judgments must be made based on the severity of the diagnosis, timing of the event in question, and reevaluation after a diagnostic work-up or adjustment of medications is made. Most older adults in this category will be able to be reclassified as appropriate for exercise once their condition has been treated or stabilized. Notably, these are all conditions that require stabilization or medical attention *regardless* of the intent to begin exercise, so a review of exercise eligibility also serves as a check for optimal control of most acute and chronic health conditions.

Notably, the majority of chronic illnesses (GO category, Table 7.2) are *indications for*, rather than *contraindications to*, regular exercise. Thus, if a patient with osteoporosis, chronic

Table 7.2. Screening Older Adults for an Exercise Prescription

I. STOP! Permanent Exclusion	*II. WAIT! Temporary Exclusion*	*III. GO! Exercise Recommended*
If any boxes in this column are checked, individual is ineligible for any exercise prescription at this time.	If any boxes in this column are checked, follow protocols for further evaluation of these concerns with medical personnel prior to reevaluating for appropriateness/modification of exercise prescription.	If only boxes in this column are checked, individual is suitable for exercise prescription without additional evaluation by medical personnel at this time.
a. ☐ End-stage congestive heart failure	**a.** ☐ Acute change in mental status or delirium, psychosis	**a.** ☐ Arthritis, stable
b. ☐ Permanent bed-bound status	**b.** ☐ Cerebral hemorrhage within the past 3 mo	**b.** ☐ Chronic obstructive pulmonary disease, asthma
c. ☐ Severe cognitive impairment or behavioral disturbance	**c.** ☐ Exacerbation of chronic inflammatory joint disease or osteoarthritis	**c.** ☐ Congestive heart failure, stable
d. ☐ Unstable abdominal, thoracic, or cerebral aneurysm	**d.** ☐ Eye surgery within the past 6 wk	**d.** ☐ Coronary artery disease, stable
e. ☐ Untreated severe aortic stenosis	**e.** ☐ Fracture in healing stage	**e.** ☐ Chronic renal failure
f. ☐ Other	**f.** ☐ Hernia, symptomatic (abdominal or inguinal), or bleeding hemorrhoids	**f.** ☐ Cancer (history or current)
	g. ☐ Myocardial infarction or cardiac surgery within past 3 mo	**g.** ☐ Chronic liver disease
	h. ☐ Other acute illness or change in symptoms	**h.** ☐ Chronic venous stasis
	i. ☐ Proliferative diabetic retinopathy or severe nonproliferative retinopathy	**i.** ☐ Dementia, cognitive impairment
	j. ☐ Pulmonary embolism or deep venous thrombosis within 3 mo	**j.** ☐ Depression, anxiety, low morale
	k. ☐ Soft tissue injury, healing	**k.** ☐ Diabetes
	l. ☐ Active suicidality or suicidal ideation	**l.** ☐ Drugs causing muscle wasting (steroids)
	m. ☐ Systemic infection	**m.** ☐ Frailty
	n. ☐ Uncontrolled blood pressure (>160/100)	**n.** ☐ Falls, history of hip fracture
	o. ☐ Uncontrolled diabetes mellitus (FBS >200 mg/dl)	**o.** ☐ Gait and balance disorders, mobility impairment
	p. ☐ Uncontrolled malignant cardiac arrhythmia (ventricular tachycardia, complete heart block, atrial flutter, symptomatic bradycardia)	**p.** ☐ Hypertension
	q. ☐ Unstable angina (at rest or crescendo pattern, ECG changes)	**q.** ☐ HIV infection
	r. ☐ Other	**r.** ☐ Hyperlipidemia
		s. ☐ Malnutrition, poor appetite
		t. ☐ Neuromuscular disease
		u. ☐ Obesity
		v. ☐ Osteoporosis
		w. ☐ Parkinson's disease
		x. ☐ Peripheral vascular disease
		y. ☐ Stroke, stable

renal failure, and depression is *not* exercising, their medical management can be seen as suboptimal, as regular exercise is, in fact, additive to the benefits of usual medical care in these and all of the other chronic conditions listed. Therefore, screening a patient for exercise should be seen as an opportunity to "screen in" those sedentary adults who have exercise-responsive diseases, rather than primarily as a task of "screening out" those

few adults with conditions that absolutely preclude exercise of any sort.

Exercise Prescription in Older Adults

It is quite likely that after initial screening, many barriers and difficulties with adherence will be identified in the typically sedentary older individual. Therefore, it becomes important to know how to deliver the prescription in logical stages that are palatable and feasible and have some likelihood of successful implementation. Current position stands[2] generally recommend a multimodal exercise prescription including aerobic, strengthening, balance, and flexibility training, via a combination of structured and incidental (lifestyle integrated) activities. It is usually best to start with only one mode of exercise and let the older adult get used to the new routine of exercise before adding other components, or optimal adherence and adaptation may be compromised.[21] This approach obviously requires attention to risk factors, medical history, physical examination findings, and personal preferences, to prioritize prescriptive elements; these will be different for each individual. There are, however, a few generalizations that can be made.

- If significant deficits in muscle strength or balance are identified, these should be addressed prior to the initiation of aerobic training. Prescribing progressive aerobic training in the absence of sufficient balance or strength is likely to result in knee pain, fear of falling, falls, and limited ability to progress aerobically, and is not recommended. Attempting to ambulate those who cannot lift their body weight out of a chair or maintain standing balance is a suboptimal approach.
- Paying attention to the physiological determinants of transfer ability and ambulation, and targeting these specifically with the appropriate exercise prescription when reversible deficits are uncovered is most likely to succeed.
- In some cases, a chronic health condition may benefit equally from resistance or aerobic training (as in the treatment of depression for example[22]), but the decision is made based on ability to tolerate one form of exercise over another. Severe osteoarthritis of the knee, recurrent falls, and a low threshold for ischemia may make resistance training safer than aerobic training as an antidepressant treatment in this case.
- Prioritization requires careful consideration of the risks and benefits of each mode of activity, as well as the current health status and physical fitness level.
- Patient preference for group versus individual exercise, structured versus lifestyle physical activity, level of supervision desired, and attraction or aversion to specific modalities of exercise must be considered to optimize behavioral change and long-term adherence.

Aerobic Activity

Cardiovascular endurance training refers to exercise in which large muscle groups contract many times (thousands of times at a single session) against little or no resistance other than that imposed by gravity.[5] The purpose of this type of training is to increase the maximal amount of aerobic work that can be performed, as well as to decrease the physiological response and perceived difficulty of submaximal aerobic workloads. Exten-

sive adaptations in the cardiopulmonary system, peripheral skeletal muscle, circulation, and metabolism are responsible for these changes in exercise capacity and tolerance. Many different kinds of exercise fall into this category, including walking and its derivatives (hiking, running, dancing, stair climbing, biking, swimming, ball sports, etc.). The key distinguishing feature between activities that are primarily aerobic versus resistive in nature is the much larger degree of overload to the muscle in resistance training. Obviously, there may be some overlap if aerobic activities are altered to increase the loading to muscle, as in resisted stationary cycling or stair climbing machines. Such activities are still primarily aerobic in nature, as they do not cause fatigue within a very few contractions as resistance training does, and they therefore do not cause the kinds of adaptations in the nervous system and muscle that lead to marked strength gain and hypertrophy.

Modes of Aerobic Exercise

There are many more kinds of cardiovascular exercise available than is the case for strengthening exercise. The decision about how to train aerobically depends on factors such as preference, access, likelihood of injury, and health-related restrictions or desired benefits. In general, although there are differences in oxygen consumption among various kinds of aerobic exercise, unless one is training for a particular sport, personal preference can provide much of the direction in this regard, as long-term compliance will require that an enjoyable pursuit has been selected. Given attention to the intensity and volume requirements described later, most activities can contribute to improvements in cardiovascular efficiency, reduction of metabolic risk factors, and reduced risk of many chronic diseases.

Two other factors assume importance in older adults and older women in particular. The first is the beneficial effects of weight-bearing aerobic activities on bone density. The loading of bone is critical to this outcome, so that nonweight-bearing aerobic activities (such as swimming and biking) have not been shown to maintain or increase bone density, whereas walking, jogging, and stepping have positive effects in cross-sectional and longitudinal studies. Second, high-impact activities such as skipping rope, hopping and plyometrics (jumping), although exceptionally beneficial for bone formation in animal models, children, and premenopausal women,[9] have been associated with significant rates of knee and ankle injuries, even in healthy older adults, and have generally not been shown to increase bone density by themselves in this age group.[9] In older adults with preexisting arthritis or fall risk, such high-impact activities are neither feasible nor recommended, as they are even more likely to result in injuries and exacerbations of arthritis in this cohort. Balancing the skeletal need for weight-bearing or high-impact loading and the safety requirements of the joints and connective tissues for low-impact loading, one would favor exercises such as walking, dancing, hiking, or stair climbing over running, step aerobics, or jumping rope in most older adults. Men and women without underlying arthritis or balance disorders may generally perform higher-impact activities safely, as long as muscle and ligament strength and joint structure are normal, and such exercise should improve muscle power as well as bone strength.

Overall, walking and its derivations surface as the most widely studied, feasible, safe, accessible, and economical mode of aerobic training for men and women of most ages and states of health. This does not require special equipment or locations and does not need to be taught or supervised (except in the cognitively impaired, very frail, or medically unstable individual). Walking bears a natural relationship to ordinary activities of daily living, making it easier to integrate into lifestyle and functional tasks than any other mode of exercise. Therefore, it is theoretically more likely to translate into improved functional independence and mobility than other types of aerobic exercise.

Intensity of Aerobic Exercise

The intensity of aerobic exercise refers to the amount of oxygen consumed (VO_2) or energy expended per minute while performing the activity, which will vary from approximately 5 kcal/min for light activities; 7.5 kcal/min for moderate activities, and 10 to 12 kcal/min for very heavy activities.[5] Energy expenditure increases with increasing body weight for weight-bearing aerobic activities, as well as with inclusion of larger muscle mass, and increased work (force × distance) and power output (work/time) demands of the activity. Therefore, the most intensive activities are those that involve the muscles of the arms, legs, and trunk simultaneously, necessitate moving the full body weight through space, and are done at a rapid pace (e.g., cross-country skiing). Adding extra loading to the body weight (backpack, weight belt, wrist weights) increases the force needed to move the body part through space, and, therefore, increases the aerobic intensity of the work performed. Biomechanical inefficiency (e.g., gait disorder, arthritis pain, use of an assistive device) increases the oxygen demands of a given task, which must be considered when prescribing aerobic exercise to adults with such impairments.

The rise in heart rate is directly proportional in normal individuals in sinus rhythm to the increasing oxygen consumption or aerobic workload. Thus, monitoring heart rate has traditionally been a primary means of prescribing appropriate intensity levels as well as following training adaptations when direct measurements of oxygen consumption are not available. The heart rate reserve (HRR) method is the most useful estimate of intensity based on heart rate (HR),[2] calculated as:

$$\text{HRR} = \text{Relative Percent} \times [\text{Maximal HR-Resting Heart Rate}] + \text{Resting Heart Rate}$$

Maximal HR can be taken from a maximal treadmill test or roughly estimated as (220-age). Training intensity is normally recommended at a moderate (40%–59% HRR) level,[2,23] although vigorous (60%–84% HRR) training levels may be used in selected individuals and may provide increased adaptation or health benefits for some disease outcomes.

Difficulties with an intensity prescription based on HR in the older adult include inaccurate pulse recording during exercise, and the presence of arrhythmias, pacemakers, or β-blockers (systemic or ophthalmological) that will alter the HR response to exercise. Therefore, a more easily obtainable and reliable estimate of aerobic intensity is to prescribe a moderate level as 12–14 or a vigorous level as 15–17 on the RPE scale, which runs from 6–20.[23] At a moderate level, the exerciser should note increased pulse and respiratory rate but still be able to talk. This scale has been validated for use in men and women, young and old, those with coronary disease as well as healthy adults, and is therefore of widespread applicability. It is easy to teach and is a means to "supervise" training intensity from afar through written diaries or telephone calls, making it cost-effective in community programs and health care settings. Usually a visual representation of the RPE scale is used to increase accuracy, but assessment can even be done without this prop in patients who are blind or cannot read.

As is the case with all other forms of exercise, to maintain the same relative training intensity over time, the absolute training load must be increased as fitness improves. In younger individuals, typically walking may be changed to jogging and then running to increase intensity as needed. More appropriate in older or frail adults are progressive alterations in workload that increase energy expenditure without converting to a high-impact form of activity. Examples of how to prescribe such progression for various modes of aerobic exercise are given in Table 7.3. The workloads should be progressed based on ratings of effort at each training session. Once the perceived exertion slips below 12 on the RPE scale, the workload should be increased to maintain the physiological stimulus for continued cardiovascular adaptation. As with resistance training, the most common error in aerobic training is a *failure to progress*, which results in an early suboptimal plateau in cardiovascular and metabolic improvement.

Volume of Aerobic Exercise

In most older adults, 60 to 150 minutes of aerobic exercise each week will be sufficient to provide benefits in the domains of improved maximal and submaximal cardiovascular efficiency, psychological well being, and control of chronic diseases such as arthritis, diabetes, peripheral vascular disease, chronic lung disease, coronary artery disease, and congestive heart failure, for example. Higher volumes of exercise generally result in greater fitness adaptations[24] and health benefits,[25] and 200 to 300 min/wk are recommended for treatment of obesity.[26] It should be noted, however, that very little research on aerobic training in very old or frail adults has actually been conducted, and most recommendations are simply extrapolated from studies in younger individuals.

It has been shown that aerobic exercise does not need to be performed at a single session to provide training effects and may be broken up into increments of 10 minutes to reach the

Table 7.3. Increasing the Intensity of Aerobic Exercise

Mode of Exercise	Ways to Increase Intensity
Walking	Add small weights around wrists
	Swing arms
	Use "race walking" style
	Add inclines, hills, stairs
	Carry weighted backpack or waist belt*
	Push a wheelchair or stroller (with someone in it)
Cycling	Increase pedaling speed
	Increase resistance to pedals
	Add hills
	Add backpack*
	Add child carrier to back of bike
Water activities	Use arms and legs in strokes
	Add resistive equipment for water
	Increase pace
Tennis	Convert from doubles to singles game
Golf	Carry clubs*
	Eliminate golf cart
Dance	Increase pace of movements
	Add more arm and leg movements

* Avoid flexing the spine when doing this to prevent excessive compressive forces on the thoracic spine.

desired volume of training.[5] Shorter-duration sessions than this have not been evaluated for efficacy, although public health recommendations for integrating short bouts of even 5 minutes into the daily routine have been made recently. Very frail adults may only tolerate 2–5 minutes of walking or other aerobic activities initially, and a reasonable goal is to increase tolerance for longer workloads until 10–20 minutes of exercise can be sustained without resting. This would provide substantial functional benefit in the nursing home, as walking for 20 minutes would likely enable the older adult to get to almost any location in the home without having to stop and rest.

Overall, a session or sessions of aerobic exercise performed at least once every 3 days adding up to at least 60 minutes per week appears to be the minimal prescription for health and longevity justifiable based on the currently available literature. Higher volumes of exercise than this (e.g., 30 min/day, most days per week, or 150 min/wk) are generally associated with greater health-related outcomes and improvements in fitness.[5] It is not recommended to exercise in very long bouts once or twice a week as an alternative to several shorter sessions, as this is likely to result in overuse muscle soreness and injuries. The risk of sudden death during physical activity appears to be limited to those who do not exercise on a regular basis (at least 1 h/wk), which is another reason for advocating regular, moderate doses of exercise rather than periodic high-volume training.

Benefits of Aerobic Exercise

The benefits of aerobic exercise have been extensively studied over the past 50 years, and the most important of these for older adults are listed in Table 7.1. They include a broad range of physiological adaptations that are, in general, opposite to the effects of aging on most body systems, as well as major health-related clinical outcomes.[27] The health conditions that are responsive to aerobic exercise include most of those of concern to older adults: osteoporosis, heart disease, stroke, breast cancer, diabetes, obesity, hypertension, arthritis, depression, memory loss, and insomnia.[25] These physiological and clinical benefits form the basis for the inclusion of aerobic exercise as an essential component of the overall physical activity prescription for healthy aging.[28]

Risks of Aerobic Exercise

The major potential risks of exercise are listed in Table 7.4. Most of these adverse events are preventable with attention to the underlying medical conditions present, making appropriate choices of exercise modality, avoiding exercise during extreme environmental conditions, wearing proper footwear and clothing, and minimizing or avoiding exercise during acute illness or in the presence of new, undefined symptoms. Most fluid balance problems can be handled by exercising in reasonable temperature and humidity only and drinking extra fluid on exercise days.

All older adults should have yearly ophthalmological examinations for glaucoma and retinal changes, and, therefore, exercise programming should be delayed until this routine health screen has been completed to avoid complications. If someone has had recent ophthalmological surgery, exercise is contraindicated for several weeks to avoid raising intraocular pressure, and the exact recommendations should be obtained from the ophthalmologist in these cases.

Metabolic complications are rare unless diabetes is out of control at the time exercise is initiated, or dehydration or acute illnesses are present. The improvement in insulin sensitivity at the initiation of regular exercise may require modification of insulin and oral hypoglycemic medications to prevent hypoglycemia. Exercising in the 1–2 hour period after meals should both prevent hypoglycemia as well as minimize the postprandial rise in serum glucose, which is an independent risk factor for cardiovascular events, even in nondiabetics.[29] This cardiovascular toxicity is mediated by oxidant stress, which triggers inflammation, endothelial dysfunction, hypercoagulability, sympathetic hyperactivity, and other atherogenic changes. Exercise has been shown to attenuate this postprandial dysmetabolism, which may mediate some of the cardioprotective effects of exercise.[29,30]

Cardiovascular complications are most likely if ischemic heart disease is not well controlled medically or surgically prior to exercise initiation, if warning signs are ignored, or if sudden, vigorous exercise is tried in a previously completely sedentary individual. When properly prescribed and monitored, both

Table 7.4. The Risks of Exercise in Older Adults

Musculoskeletal	Cardiovascular	Metabolic
Falls	Arrhythmia	Dehydration
Foot ulceration or laceration	Cardiac failure	Electrolyte imbalance
Fracture, osteoporotic or traumatic	Hypertension	Energy imbalance
Hemorrhoids*	Hypotension	Heat stroke
Hernia*	Ischemia	Hyperglycemia
Joint or bursa inflammation, exacerbation of arthritis	Pulmonary embolism	Hypoglycemia
Ligament or tendon strain or rupture	Retinal hemorrhage or detachment, lens detachment	Hypothermia
Muscle soreness or tear	Ruptured cerebral or other aneurysm	Seizures
Stress incontinence	Syncope or postural symptoms	

* Primarily associated with increased intraabdominal pressure during resistive exercise, but may occur if Valsalva maneuver occurs during aerobic activities.

aerobic and resistance training have been shown to reduce the incidence of angina and medication use in cardiac rehabilitation settings and are indicated as part of standard medical management of coronary artery disease.[14] Although claudication is mentioned as a possible adverse side effect of exercise in those with peripheral vascular disease, there is an important treatment caveat here. It has been shown that aerobic exercise significantly increases exercise tolerance in patients with peripheral vascular disease (i.e., time to claudication), and resistance training has some benefit as well. Exercise works optimally when continued if possible for approximately 30–90 seconds after the onset of claudication. This is different from angina or any of the other symptoms listed in,Table 7.4 for which exercise should be stopped immediately if they occur.

Musculoskeletal problems are more common than any other risk of aerobic or resistive exercise, particularly in the novice or very frail adults, and those with underlying joint disease. Often if significant weakness or balance impairment is present, it is best to avoid aerobic exercise altogether until strength and balance have been improved sufficiently with specific training, so as to allow safe weight-bearing exercise such as walking. If this is not done, falls, arthritis pain, fear of falling, and muscle fatigue will be so limiting that effective aerobic training is precluded. Warming up muscles gently with slow movements prior to aerobic routines is important to avoid soft tissue injury. The most important point is to avoid high-impact activities (such as jumping, step aerobics, and jogging) in those with preexisting arthritis or weak muscles and ligaments, as this is a principle cause of sports-related injury.

Muscle Strengthening Activity

Progressive resistance training (PRT) is one of the four basic modalities of exercise that are recommended for older adults as part of a balanced physical activity program, whether this is formalized as an exercise prescription or integrated into lifestyle changes.[28] PRT is the process of challenging the skeletal muscle with an unaccustomed stimulus, or load, such that neural and muscle tissue adaptations take place, leading ultimately to increased muscle force producing capacity (strength) and muscle mass.[5] In this kind of exercise, the muscle is contracted slowly just a few times in each session against a relatively heavy load. Any muscle may be trained in this way, although usually 8–10 major muscle groups with clinical relevance are trained, for a balanced and functional outcome.

Equipment

There are many ways to conduct PRT. Equipment may range from only body weight to technologically sophisticated pneumatic or hydraulic resistance training machines. In general, in the older adult, machine-based training allows the most robust adaptations to be achieved, offers maximum safety, and requires less technique to be learned. Free weights, on the other hand, offer significant advantages in terms of cost and flexibility in programming and may provide a better stimulus for motor coordination and balance; they are the only option in most home and limited-space settings.

Intensity

Virtually all of the randomized controlled trials of resistance training in the elderly that have resulted in large gains in strength have used an intensity of approximately 70%–80% of maximum strength as the training intensity (a level of 15–17 on the RPE scale[31] can be used to prescribe the proper intensity if strength cannot be measured). There is no evidence that this intensity is unsafe or poorly tolerated in men or women, healthy or frail, as old as 100 years of age, or even those in early outpatient cardiac rehabilitation for example. By contrast, low-intensity training results in negligible or modest gains in strength and associated clinical benefits and cannot therefore be recommended if the primary intent of training is to increase muscle size and strength.[32]

Volume

The volume of resistance training refers to the frequency of sessions, and the number of sets and repetitions (lifts) performed during each session for each muscle group. It is most effective to recommend training frequencies of 2–3 days per week in the older adult, with at least a day of rest between sessions. There is no consistent evidence that multiple sets (two–three) are substantially superior to one set (8–10 repetitions) in terms of strength gain, so if time is a barrier to implementation, one-high intensity set will provide good clinical benefits most efficiently.[28] Increased volume of low-intensity repetitions will not provide the musculoskeletal adaptations associated with high-intensity training.

Benefits

Increases in muscle size and strength following appropriate PRT are not seen with other forms of exercise and are not obtainable with low-intensity PRT. Therefore, if a primary goal of exercise is to prevent or treat sarcopenia, then there is no effective substitute for this modality of exercise. The hypertrophic response to training does appear to be affected by health status, anabolic hormonal milieu, nutritional substrate availability, changes in protein synthesis with age, genetic profile, and other factors yet to be identified. It is clear that exogenous anabolic steroids can augment the hypertrophic response to resistive exercise in young men and appears to have the same effect in older men as well. Trials with growth hormone or its secretagogues, or estrogen, have, however, thus far largely failed to show benefit in terms of muscle mass or strength in older adults when given alone or in combination with resistance training.

The benefits of PRT extend beyond the prevention and treatment of sarcopenia itself.[9,33] Resistance training has now been shown to have benefit for the treatment of type 2 diabetes, obesity, depression, osteoporosis, frailty, falls, hip fracture, joint replacement, arthritis, insomnia, coronary artery disease, peripheral vascular disease, congestive heart failure, chronic obstructive pulmonary disease, cancer cachexia, human immunodeficiency virus wasting, end-stage renal failure, and neuromuscular disease, and efficacy in other conditions is emerging as well.[14] This broad spectrum of benefit places PRT within the mainstream of treatment options for older adults.

Risks

PRT has been thought of as a risky form of exercise in the past and has therefore been sometimes avoided by health care professionals in their counseling of older adults. A wealth of literature over the past 20 years indicates that this modality of

exercise is in fact quite safe and is more feasible in many groups of patients and frail elders than is cardiovascular exercise.[14] There are relatively few absolute medical contraindications to PRT, such as unstable coronary disease, unrepaired aneurysms, malignant arrhythmias, symptomatic hernias, or critical aortic stenosis. Apart from these specific circumstances, PRT is a realistic option even in very frail elderly individuals. Frailty is not a contraindication to strength training, but conversely one of the most important reasons to prescribe it.[15]

The potential risks of PRT are primarily musculoskeletal injury and cardiovascular events. Musculoskeletal injury is largely preventable with attention to the following points:

- adherence to proper form;
- isolation of the targeted muscle group;
- slow velocity of lifting;
- limitation of range of motion to the pain-free arc of movement;
- avoidance of use of momentum and ballistic movements to complete a lift;
- use of machines or chairs with good back support;
- observation of rest periods between sets and rest days between sessions.

In patients with preexisting arthritis, there may be intermittent exacerbation of joint symptoms or inflammation with the initiation of PRT; however, the overall effect of training is the moderate decrease of chronic arthritis pain and disability over time.[34] During periods of disease flare-up, it may be necessary to switch to isometric contractions, lower the weight lifted, limit the range of motion through which the load is lifted, or insert additional days of rest between training sessions. It is advisable to continue isometric contractions if nothing else, as this will prevent loss of strength, and will not further increase pain. Once the symptoms have lessened, normal exercise sessions may resume.

Blood pressure changes are difficult to measure during PRT because of the transient nature of the rises, and the fact that blood pressure falls almost immediately after a repetition is completed. This makes monitoring of intraarterial pressure the only accurate way to gather such information. The HR response to PRT is in general lower than that from aerobic exercise such as walking up an incline or stair climbing, whereas the increase in systolic blood pressure tends to be intermediate between walking and stair climbing. Diastolic pressure elevations are greater with PRT than aerobic exercise, thus increasing mean arterial pressure to a greater degree. The double product (the product of systolic blood pressure and HR), which is thought to be representative of myocardial oxygen demand, is greatest for stair climbing, followed by weight lifting and walking.

In the largest series of maximum strength tests yet reported, in 26,000 individuals undergoing testing, not a single cardiovascular event occurred.[35] Additionally, the literature suggests a reduction in ischemic signs and symptoms after PRT in cardiac patients, attesting to the safety of this form of exercise even in individuals with heart disease.

Table 7.5. Factors Related to Increased Circulatory Stress During Resistance Training

- Higher relative intensity of load lifted
- Static contractions
- Early phase of concentric contraction
- Greater muscle mass used
- Performance of a Valsalva maneuver during lifts
- Increasing number of repetitions
- Fatigue of muscles (performing a set "to failure")

Circulatory stress = increase of HR and blood pressure in response to resistive exercise.

Patients with unstable cardiovascular signs and symptoms should not begin any exercise regimen, including weight lifting, without medical evaluation. Cardiovascular stress is minimized with attention to the factors listed in Table 7.5.

Balance Exercises for Fallers or Individuals with Mobility Problems

Balance training is probably the least well defined of the various exercise modalities. Despite the use of balance-enhancing modalities for decades by physical therapists and others working with adults and children with developmental or degenerative neurological diseases affecting balance, only recently have there been well-controlled formalized studies of techniques and outcomes. The recognition that balance impairment is a risk factor for falls and hip fracture even in adults without identifiable neurological disease has expanded the potential target population for balance training to the general aging cohort. The pressing need for definitive outcome data on feasibility and efficacy of various intervention techniques has stimulated quantitative research that will assist in the development of clinical protocols. In the meantime, the balance prescription must be formulated from a variety of evidence collected in epidemiological studies, experimental trials, and clinical practice. It should be noted that, in many cases, it is difficult to compare the results across trials, as investigators have used unique training interventions and different outcome measures.

Any activity that increases one's ability to maintain balance in the face of a threat to stability may be considered a balance-enhancing activity. Common stressors include:

- narrowing of the base of support;
- perturbation of the ground support;
- decrease in proprioceptive sensation;
- diminished or misleading visual inputs;
- disturbed vestibular system input;
- increased compliance of the support surface;
- movement of the center of mass of the body away from the vertical;
- addition of a cognitive distractor or "dual tasking" while practicing balance.

In real life, stressors may also include things such as environmental hazards to traverse, postural hypotension, and drugs that affect central nervous system function. The plethora of conditions that contribute to gait and balance abnormalities in older adults require a multifactorial approach to balance enhancement and falls prevention.[4,36] What is presented herein is a summary of exercise techniques that have favorable effects on this physiological capacity, and, therefore, form an important part of the exercise prescription for older adults.

General Technique

Balance-enhancing activities have an impact on the central nervous system control of balance and coordination of movement, or augment the peripheral neuromuscular system response to signals that balance is threatened. The general approach to the enhancement of balance should rely on theoretical principles that are designed to elicit adaptations in the central neurological control of posture and equilibrium. The basic idea is to challenge progressively the system with stressors of increasing difficulty in four different domains:

1. narrowing the base of support for the body;
2. displacing the center of mass to the limits of tolerance;
3. removing or minimizing contributions of visual, vestibular, and proprioceptive pathways to balance;
4. adding simultaneous cognitive tasks such as set tests (animal naming) or calculations (serial 7s, etc.) during balance exercises.

All balance movements should be done slowly and with deliberation, as this stresses the control systems more and produces better physiological adaptation. It can be seen, for example, that an exercise such as heel walking is actually easier when done rapidly rather than slowly, so the challenge and adaptation will be greater when the slow speed is practiced. Balance training may also be prescribed as structured exercise forms such as Tai chi[37] or yoga, or may be incorporated into resistance training during one-legged standing movements.[38]

Intensity

Intensity in balance training refers to the degree of difficulty of the postures, movements, or routines practiced. *The appropriate level of difficulty or "intensity" for any balance-enhancing exercise is the highest level that can be tolerated without inducing a fall or near-fall.* In a supervised session, the individual can be pushed to the limits of such tolerance, as safety is assured by the physical presence of the trainer. In an unsupervised setting, the person should be told to try movements only up to the level that they fail to master completely. For example, if the goal is to hold the heel-to-toe stand for 15 seconds, then if someone can only hold the posture for 10 seconds before grabbing the wall for support, this is the appropriate initial training intensity. Progression in intensity is the key to improvement, as in other exercise domains, but this concept of mastery of the previous level before progression must be adhered to for safety. This is particularly important in frail elders, who are at highest risk of falls, osteoporotic fractures, and other injuries.

Volume and Frequency

No definite statement can be made at this time about the minimum effective dose of balance training techniques described previously. Regimens have ranged from 1 to 7 days per week, and from once a day to several times per day. A reasonable recommendation would appear to be 2–3 days per week, but it is noted that this is more a matter of convention rather than an evidence-based recommendation. It is likely that as with other forms of training, a dose–response relationship exists, although thresholds have not been defined. There is no evidence that any negative effects are seen with high-volume training. Therefore, for adults with significant balance impairments that require intervention, training 3–7 days per week may be advantageous. On the other hand, healthy, normal adults may require only preventive practice 1 day a week for maintenance of mobility and function. Many more studies are needed in this area to define the recommendation further.

Benefits

Balance training has been shown to result in improved balance performance, decreased fear of falling, decreased incidence of falls, and increased ability to participate in other activities that may have been limited by gait and balance difficulties.[4] It is expected, although not proved, that such changes would ultimately lead to improvements in functional independence and reduced hip fractures, and other serious injuries, and improved overall quality of life. Such long-term outcomes will require larger studies of longer duration than those that have been reported to date. In particular, there is a need for data on the feasibility and efficacy of balance training in the very old and frail, in whom deficits are larger, fall risk is usually multifactorial, and cognitive impairments or degenerative neurological diseases exist. All of these factors may alter the robustness of the physiological adaptation achieved with training.

Balance training does not generally result in increased strength or aerobic capacity by itself, whereas resistance training in some cases may improve balance.[38] There may, however, be some maintenance of muscle strength from the isometric contractions that occur during many of the balance-enhancing and one-legged postures and the bent knee stance during Tai chi.[37] In addition, to the extent that balance training results in increased overall physical activity and mobility, these other activities may lead to improvements in strength and endurance.

Risks

The only real risk of balance training is actual or threat of loss of balance, resulting in a fall or injury or increased fear of falling. This is preventable with attention to the previously discussed factors governing progression, intensity, setting, and supervision. There is little or no elevation in pulse or blood pressure during these kinds of exercises, so that cardiovascular events are not an expected or reported consequence. Musculoskeletal injury, other than that resulting from a fall, would also be unlikely.

It should be noted that there might be exacerbation of preexisting arthritic pain or inflammation of the knee during prolonged one-legged standing, Tai chi, or yoga postures requiring a semicrouched stance. These positions may have to be adapted or avoided in those with significant weight-bearing pain in the joint. Once quadriceps muscle strength improves with appropriate resistive exercises (as noted) these kinds of movements may be tolerable. Impaired flexibility may initially limit some Tai chi or yoga postures and may lead to injury if range of motion is forced in the beginning. Gradual progression in the complexity of postures should prevent most injuries to soft tissues.

Summary

Exercise is integral to the prevention, treatment, and rehabilitation strategies necessary for the care of the geriatric patient. Exercise should be prescribed, as is all other medical treatment, with consideration of patient risks and benefits, knowledge of appropriate modality and dose (intensity, frequency, and volume), monitoring for drug interactions, benefits and adverse events, and utilization of the strongest possible behavioral medicine techniques known to optimize adoption and adherence. There is no age above which physical activity ceases to have benefits across a wide range of diseases and disabilities. Sedentariness is a lethal condition; physical activity is the antidote, and health care practitioners should be well-educated leaders and role models in the effort to enhance functional independence, psychological well-being, and quality of life through promotion of exercise for the aged, both fit and frail.

REFERENCES

1. U.S. Dept of Health and Human Services. Physical Activity and Health: A Report of the Surgeon General. Atlanta: US Dept of Health and Human Services, Centers for Disease Control and Prevention, National Center for Chronic Disease Prevention and Health Promotion; 1996.
2. Nelson ME, Rejeski WJ, Blair SN, et al. Physical activity and public health in older adults: recommendation from the American College of Sports Medicine and the American Heart Association. *Med Sci Sports Exerc.* 2007;39(8):1435–1445.
3. Newman AB, Kupelian V, Visser M, et al. Sarcopenia: alternative definitions and associations with lower extremity function. *J Am Geriatr Soc.* 2003;51(11):1602–1609.
4. Rubenstein LZ. Falls in older people: epidemiology, risk factors and strategies for prevention. *Age Ageing.* 2006;35 Suppl 2:ii37–ii41.
5. Haskell WL, Lee IM, Pate RR, et al. Physical activity and public health: updated recommendation for adults from the American

College of Sports Medicine and the American Heart Association. *Med Sci Sports Exerc.* 2007;39(8):1423–1434.

6. Mazzeo R, Cavanaugh P, Evans W, et al. Exercise and physical activity for older adults. *Med Sci Sports Exerc.* 1998;30(6):992–1008.

7. Nelson M, Fiatarone M, Morganti C, Trice I, Greenberg R, Evans W. Effects of high-intensity strength training on multiple risk factors for osteoporotic fractures. *JAMA.* 1994;272:1909–1914.

8. Pu C, Johnson M, Forman D, Piazza L, Fiatarone M. High-intensity progressive resistance training in older women with chronic heart failure. *Med Sci Sports Exerc.* 1997;29(5):S148.

9. Suominen H. Muscle training for bone strength. *Aging Clin Exp Res.* 2006;18(2):85–93.

10. Azevedo MR, Araujo CL, Reichert FF, Siqueira FV, da Silva MC, Hallal PC. Gender differences in leisure-time physical activity. *Int J Public Health.* 2007;52(1):8–15.

11. Fiatarone MA, Marks EC, Ryan ND, Meredith CN, Lipsitz LA, Evans WJ. High-intensity strength training in nonagenarians. Effects on skeletal muscle. *JAMA.* 1990;263:3029–3034.

12. Fiatarone MA, O'Neill EF, Ryan ND, et al. Exercise training and nutritional supplementation for physical frailty in very elderly people. *NEJM.* 1994;330:1769–1775.

13. Morris J, Fiatarone M, Kiely D, et al. Nursing rehabilitation and exercise strategies in the nursing home. *J Gerontol.* 1999;54A(10):M494–M500.

14. Williams MA, Haskell WL, Ades PA, et al. Resistance exercise in individuals with and without cardiovascular disease: 2007 update: a scientific statement from the American Heart Association Council on Clinical Cardiology and Council on Nutrition, Physical Activity, and Metabolism. *Circulation.* 2007;116(5):572–584.

15. Fiatarone Singh M. Exercise comes of age: Rationale and recommendations for a geriatric exercise prescription. *J Gerontol Med Sci.* 2002;57(A):M262–M82.

16. Bortz WM. Redefining human aging. *J Am Geriatr Soc.* 1989;37(11):1092–1096.

17. Blair SN, Kampert JB, Kohn HW, et al. Influences of cardiovascular fitness and other precursors on cardiovascular disease and all-cause mortality in men and women. *JAMA.* 1996;276(3):205–210.

18. Guyatt G, Thompson P, Berman L, et al. How should we measure function in patients with chronic heart and lung disease? *J Chronic Dis.* 1985;38:517–528.

19. Boxer RS, Wang Z, Walsh SJ, Hager D, Kenny AM. The utility of the 6-minute walk test as a measure of frailty in older adults with heart failure. *Am J Geriatr Cardiol.* 2008;17(1):7–12.

20. Borg G, Linderholm H. Perceived exertion and pulse rate during graded exercise in various age group. *Acta Med Scand.* 1970;472(Suppl):194–206.

21. Baker MK, Atlantis E, Fiatarone Singh MA. Multi-modal exercise programs for older adults. *Age Ageing.* 2007;36(4):375–381.

22. Singh NA, Stavrinos TM, Scarbek Y, Galambos G, Liber C, Fiatarone Singh MA. A randomized controlled trial of high versus low intensity weight training versus general practitioner care for clinical depression in older adults. *J Gerontol A Biol Sci Med Sci.* 2005;60(6):768–776.

23. Borg G, Linderholme H. Exercise performance and perceived exertion in patients with coronary insufficiency, arterial hypertension and vasoregulatory asthenia. *Acta Med Scand.* 1970;187:17–26.

24. Church TS, Earnest CP, Skinner JS, Blair SN. Effects of different doses of physical activity on cardiorespiratory fitness among sedentary, overweight or obese postmenopausal women with elevated blood pressure: a randomized controlled trial. *JAMA.* 2007;297(19):2081–2091.

25. Pedersen BK, Saltin B. Evidence for prescribing exercise as therapy in chronic disease. *Scand J Med Sci Sports.* 2006;16(s1):3–63.

26. Jakicic JM, Clark K, Coleman E, et al. American College of Sports Medicine position stand. Appropriate intervention strategies for weight loss and prevention of weight regain for adults. *Med Sci Sports Exerc.* 2001;33(12):2145–2156.

27. Paterson DH, Jones GR, Rice CL. Ageing and physical activity: evidence to develop exercise recommendations for older adults. *Can J Public Health.* 2007;98 Suppl 2:S69–S108.

28. Nelson ME, Rejeski WJ, Blair SN, et al. Physical activity and public health in older adults: recommendation from the American College of Sports Medicine and the American Heart Association. *Circulation.* 2007;116(9):1094–1105.

29. O'Keefe JH, Bell DS. Postprandial hyperglycemia/hyperlipidemia (postprandial dysmetabolism) is a cardiovascular risk factor. *Am J Cardiol.* 2007;100(5):899–904.

30. Rizvi AA. Management of diabetes in older adults. *Am J Med Sci.* 2007;333(1):35–47.

31. Lagally KM, Amorose AJ. The validity of using prior ratings of perceive exertion to regulate resistance exercise intensity. *Percept Mot Skills.* 2007;104(2):534–542.

32. Seynnes O, Fiatarone Singh M. Relationship between resistance training intensity and physiological and functional adaptation in frail elders. *J Gerontol A Biol Sci Med Sci.* 2004;59(4):33–39.

33. Taaffe DR. Sarcopenia–exercise as a treatment strategy. *Aust Fam Physician.* 2006;35(3):130–134.

34. Conn VS, Hafdahl AR, Minor MA, Nielsen PJ. Physical activity interventions among adults with arthritis: meta-analysis of outcomes. *Semin Arthritis Rheum.* 2008;37:307–316.

35. Gordon N, Kohl H, Pollock M, Vaandrager H, Gibbons S, Blair S. Cardiovascular safety of maximal strength testing in healthy adults. *Am J Cardiol.* 1995;76:851–853.

36. Oliver D, Connelly JB, Victor CR, et al. Strategies to prevent falls and fractures in hospitals and care homes and effect of cognitive impairment: systematic review and meta-analyses. *BMJ.* 2007;334(7584):82.

37. Tsang WW, Hui-Chan CW. Comparison of muscle torque, balance, and confidence in older tai chi and healthy adults. *Med Sci Sports Exerc.* 2005;37(2):280–289.

38. Orr R, Raymond J, Fiatarone Singh M. Efficacy of progressive resistance training on balance performance in older adults: a systematic review of randomized controlled trials. *Sports Med.* 2008;38(3):1–51.

8

Diabetes Mellitus in the Older Adult

Lisa B. Caruso, MD, MPH, Rebecca A. Silliman, MD, PhD, MPH

INTRODUCTION

Diabetes mellitus (DM) is a dominant chronic disease of older adults in the United States as well as in many other countries of the world. The prevalence of DM in the future is only expected to grow with the increase in the population of older adults, the prevalence of obesity, and physical inactivity. Clinicians will be faced with many unique challenges when caring for this older diabetic population. The clinician's major challenges are 1) to avoid symptoms and complications of hyper- and hypoglycemia, 2) to minimize or delay micro- and macrovascular complications, if possible, and 3) to maximize daily functioning. Underlying these challenges is the realization that the geriatric population is a heterogeneous one. Goals of care and treatment decisions may vary. These may depend less on the chronological age of the patient, although issues of life expectancy must be considered especially in the very old, but more so on the patient's functional abilities and on other comorbidities or coexisting geriatric syndromes. This chapter will focus on specific aspects of diabetes care in the older adult.

EPIDEMIOLOGY

An estimated 10.3 million people, or 20.9% of those 60 years of age or older, in the United States are afflicted with DM, the majority of whom have type 2 disease.[1] Approximately half of Americans with diabetes are 60 years of age or older with an approximately even split between men and women. DM is more prevalent in minority groups. After adjusting for population age differences, Native Americans are 2.2 times as likely, African-Americans are 1.8 times as likely, and Hispanic/Latino Americans are 1.7 times as likely to have DM as non-Hispanic whites. The costs of medical care are great with almost $48 billion being spent in 2002 on medical care for older adults with

DM.[2] The majority of this expense is for inpatient costs, with most being attributed to the care of cardiovascular complications. The absolute number of older persons with diabetes will continue to rise in the foreseeable future for at least two reasons: 1) the rate of diagnosed diabetes in persons 65–74 years of age and >75 years has increased approximately 2.5 times in the past 30 years, and 2) the number of older persons at risk is growing. Because approximately half of all cases in older persons are undiagnosed, if methods of detection improve, the numbers of clinically recognized cases could rise even further.[3]

DIAGNOSIS

Although the "poly" symptoms (polydipsia, polyuria, and polyphagia) are considered by many to be pathognomonic of diabetes, for several reasons this is often not true in older persons. First, these symptoms are nonspecific and may result from other conditions, such as urinary difficulties or diuretic use. Second, they may not be present because of age-related or disease-related changes in organ function. For example, thirst mechanisms often become impaired with age. Third, they may be masked by other conditions. Thus, relying on them will result in both false positives and false negatives. The challenge to the clinician is to maintain a high level of suspicion, yet be prudent with glucose testing.

To improve the predictive power of glucose testing, criteria for the diagnosis of diabetes were revised by the Expert Committee on the Diagnosis and Classification of Diabetes Mellitus in 1997.[4] The criteria are: 1) symptoms of diabetes and a random glucose level of >200 mg/dL, **or** 2) a fasting plasma glucose level of 126 mg/dL or greater, **or** 3) an elevation in plasma glucose to ≥200 mg/dL 2 hours following a 75-g oral glucose tolerance test. The diagnosis must be confirmed by abnormal glucose levels on a different day unless the patient has obvious hyperglycemia.

The majority of elderly diabetics are classified as either type 1 or type 2. Type 1 diabetics require insulin and are ketosis prone. Type 2 diabetics are insulin resistant and ketosis resistant. Many elderly type 1 diabetics who started insulin in the 1930s are still alive, therefore when caring for a diabetic patient, it is important to establish when and how the diagnosis of diabetes was made to institute proper therapy and to anticipate the types of complications that are likely to develop.

SCREENING

As with other conditions, screening for diabetes would be indicated if the treatment of asymptomatic patients resulted in better outcomes, if the burden of suffering associated with it were high, and if the screening test were sensitive and specific, simple and inexpensive, safe, and acceptable for both patients and practitioners.[5] Although no one would argue that the burdens associated with diabetes are great, there is insufficient evidence that early detection and treatment improve outcomes for patients with type 2 disease.[6] The value of screening for diabetes has been evaluated with mixed results, although one study showed more cost-effectiveness in people with hypertension and those aged 55–75 years.[7] The U.S. Preventive Services Task Force (USPSTF) suggests that clinicians may wish to screen adults who are at increased risk for cardiovascular disease (CVD), mainly those with hypertension or hyperlipidemia (the grade of evidence is B; the U.S. Preventive Services Task Force found at least fair evidence that [the service] improves important health outcomes and concludes that benefits outweigh harms).[8] Once diabetes has been detected clinically, screening for complications, specifically for retinopathy and foot lesions, can be effective in reducing morbidity, as will be discussed later.

MANAGEMENT

To the elderly person, receiving the diagnosis of diabetes may evoke multiple emotions including dread, fear, and sadness. Not only are complications devastating but following complex dietary, medication, and monitoring regimens can be overwhelming. Daily functional, nutritional, and medical assistance from professional and lay caregivers is often necessary when patients are physically and/or cognitively impaired. When developing a treatment plan with the older diabetic patient, it is important to involve the patient in her own self-care, to the extent that this is possible, and to be sensitive to the patient's perception of her quality of life, as it is affected by various therapeutic interventions.

Recently, the concept of *collaborative management* has received attention as a mechanism to better care for patients with chronic diseases such as diabetes. Collaborative management consists of 1) defining problems from the perspective of the patient and physician, 2) targeting key problems, goal setting, and planning methods to achieve goals, 3) creating patient education and support services, and 4) evaluating

Table 8.1. Summary of Key Recommendations[12]

- Older persons with diabetes should be offered individualized therapy that takes into consideration life expectancy, functional status, the presence of cognitive impairment, social support, and patient preferences.

- Care should be kept simple and inexpensive, wherever possible.

- Older persons with diabetes are likely to benefit greatly from cardiovascular risk reduction; therefore, monitor and treat hypertension and dyslipidemias.

- For many older persons, treatment of hypertension may require more than one medication to achieve adequate control. Treatment should be gradual, if possible, and persons should be monitored for drug interactions and side effects.

- Monitor and treat hyperglycemia, with a target A1C of 7%, but less stringent goals of therapy may be appropriate once patient preferences, diabetes severity, life expectancy, and functional status have been considered.

- Encourage diabetes education and make patients and their families aware that it is a covered benefit under Medicare.

- Dilated eye examinations should be performed every 2 years at a minimum, and more often if there are additional risk factors for diabetic eye disease or evidence of age-related eye disease.

- Maintain an updated medication list and evaluate the patient regularly for adverse medication effects.

- Older persons with diabetes should be screened for depression, and, if depression is identified, therapy should be offered and response to therapy monitored.

- Persons should also be screened annually for cognitive impairment, urinary incontinence, injurious falls, and persistent pain because these conditions are more prevalent among older persons with diabetes.

patient progress in a frequent and regular follow-up plan.[9] These elements can be implemented in a variety of practice models from the small group practice to the large health maintenance organization. It is important for all the members of the health care team to provide as much education to the patient as possible to make the patient an active participant in his own diabetic management. Evidence suggests that interventions targeted at improving the diabetes care delivery system and promoting diabetes self-management lead to improved patient outcomes and metabolic control.[10,11]

In 2003, the first guidelines for improving the care of the older adult with diabetes were created by the California Healthcare Foundation and the American Geriatrics Society.[15] These published guidelines were the first to stress the importance of setting individualized goals of care by using the best evidence available for the very heterogeneous group of older adults with diabetes. The guidelines also included recommendations for the management of six geriatric syndromes, or conditions, for which there is evidence or strong consensus opinion that persons with diabetes are at greater risk. The syndromes include polypharmacy, depression, cognitive impairment, urinary incontinence, injurious falls, and pain. Table 8.1 summarizes the recommendations.

The remaining sections of this chapter will elaborate on diet and weight loss, exercise, glucose-lowering therapy, managing cardiovascular risk factors, eye disease, and foot care. More specific information on managing the aforementioned geriatric syndromes can be found in other chapters of this book.

Diet and Weight Loss

In general, diabetes is closely related to being overweight or obese, although a subset of older patients is either of normal weight or underweight.[13] What constitutes an optimal diabetic diet for older persons has not yet been determined, but weight loss, even if modest, in obese older persons can improve metabolic control, thereby reducing symptoms of hyperglycemia.

Achieving weight loss and metabolic control is not easy. Lifelong dietary habits are difficult to change, as are notions of what constitutes a "healthy" diet. This may be compounded by the fact that older patients frequently must rely on someone else for food acquisition and preparation. They may live in households where food preferences are disparate. Furthermore, limited financial resources may interfere with patients' procuring appropriate foods, such as fresh fruits and vegetables.

Weight loss in obese diabetics should be attempted to improve insulin sensitivity. A registered dietitian or nutritionist should be an active member of the diabetes management team to assist the patient and/or caregiver in creating an individualized diet plan. For many patients, for a variety of reasons, when weight loss is not possible, the best strategy should be to help them achieve a balanced diet that includes fruit and legume sources of carbohydrates, restricts the amount of animal fat to <7% of total calories, maintains the intake of protein at 0.8–1 g/kg of body weight, and incorporates fiber in moderate amounts.[14] Adequate fluid intake of nonsucrose-containing beverages is also important. This alone may help to reduce glucose levels and will correct mild volume contraction related to osmotic diuresis.

Older diabetics living in long-term care facilities must have diets appropriate to prevent or correct malnutrition. The American Diabetes Association recommends serving regular, unrestricted meals to institutionalized older adults with diabetes.[13] It is important for such patients to enjoy meal time to satisfy nutritional needs as well as to contribute to their quality of life.

Exercise

If the elderly diabetic is able to exercise regularly, specifically with resistance training exercise, weight maintenance and glycemic control may be added benefits. Physical activity has been found to increase insulin sensitivity of muscle and other tissues that have insulin receptors. Other cardiovascular risk factors, such as hyperlipidemia and hypertension, may be reduced by regular exercise as well. Self-esteem and quality of life may also improve. Exercise in the older diabetic may not be without substantial risk, however. Exercise can exacerbate angina or ischemia in a patient with underlying cardiovascular disease (CVD). The presence of peripheral neuropathy may result in soft tissue or musculoskeletal injuries. Symptomatic hypoglycemia can also occur, especially in patients taking oral hypoglycemic drugs. The American Diabetes Association recommends that type 2 diabetics who want to begin an exercise program "more vigorous than brisk walking" undergo an assessment for CVD and other conditions, such as uncontrolled hypertension, neuropathy, and retinopathy, which may increase the risks of harm from the exercise program.[15] Older adults with diabetes should also monitor their glucose levels following any workout.

Glucose-Lowering Therapy

Unless the patient has significant symptoms of hyperglycemia, a 3-month trial of dietary modifications, exercise, and weight loss should be undertaken. As lifestyle modification is often difficult especially for the clinically complex older adult, engaging the help of a Certified Diabetes Educator, specialty physician care, or group adult education classes can improve the patient's chances for success. Individualized education may be especially helpful for non-English-speaking and culturally diverse older adults.[16] Drug therapy is warranted if the combination of diet, exercise, and weight loss are not successful in eliminating symptomatic hyperglycemia.

Establishing individualized goals of therapy is of great importance when treating older adults with diabetes. In certain patients, such as the frail, demented nursing home resident with sporadic eating habits, controlling the symptoms of hyperglycemia is more important than preventing macrovascular and microvascular complications of diabetes. Other older, more active patients with longer life expectancies may benefit from tighter glucose control. The benefits of improved glycemic control in reducing microvascular complications of diabetes, such as retinopathy and nephropathy, are seen at approximately 8 years.[17]

Multiple oral hypoglycemic agents are currently available including: 1) the sulfonylureas, such as glipizide, glyburide, and glimepiride; 2) the biguanide, metformin; 3) the α-glucosidase inhibitors acarbose and miglitol; 4) the meglitinides, nateglinide and repaglinide; 5) the thiazolidinediones (TZDs), pioglitazone and rosiglitazone; and 6) the dipeptidyl peptidase-IV (DPP-IV) inhibitor, sitagliptin. Oral agents are easy to use and are frequently preferred by patients. Multiple types of insulin are also available, giving clinicians even more tools to individualize therapy for older adults. Pramlintide, an amylin mimetic, and exenatide, an incretin mimetic, both decrease postprandial plasma glucose and suppress glucagon secretion and are administered subcutaneously before meals. These will not be discussed here given their limited use.

Sulfonylureas

The sulfonylurea drugs are the most frequently prescribed agents for treating hyperglycemia. They are generally efficacious especially in patients who are not obese and in the first

2–5 years after diagnosis. Given that their mechanism of action is to stimulate the β cells to produce more insulin, their loss of efficacy with time is probably from a progressive diminution in pancreatic β cell function and increased insulin resistance. The choice of sulfonylurea should take into account the following considerations. First, because all are metabolized at least in part by the liver, they should be used with care in patients with severe liver disease. Second, renal insufficiency will prolong the half-lives of the sulfonylureas. Third, because of its long half-life (36 hours), a risk factor for hypoglycemia, and its propensity to cause hyponatremia, chlorpropamide should be avoided in older persons. Fourth, longer-acting sulfonylureas, such as glyburide, have the highest risk of hypoglycemia in older adults, and should be used with caution. Glipizide is preferable because it does not have any active metabolites and has a half-life of 2–5 hours. It must be taken 30 minutes before meals so as not to delay absorption. The sulfonylureas may contribute to modest weight gain probably resulting from the effect of increased circulating insulin. All sulfonylureas are now available in generic form and are reasonably priced.

Biguanides

The only biguanide currently available in the United States is metformin. It is approved for oral treatment of type 2 diabetes, either alone or in combination with a sulfonylurea, a TZD, sitagliptin, or insulin. Metformin is a unique treatment for diabetes in that it suppresses hepatic glucose production and improves insulin sensitivity to promote glucose uptake at the cellular level. Therefore, the drug alone does not cause hypoglycemia. It also has a positive effect on lipids by lowering triglycerides and low-density lipoprotein (LDL) cholesterol and does not contribute to weight gain in the obese patient, and in fact, may assist with weight loss. After 10 years of follow-up, data from the United Kingdom Prospective Diabetes Study showed a decrease in macrovascular complications of diabetes and in overall mortality in obese patients with newly diagnosed diabetes taking metformin independent of glucose control compared with patients on only dietary changes and with patients taking a sulfonylurea.[18]

Its current contraindications are drug hypersensitivity, administration of iodinated contrast dye in radiological studies, metabolic acidosis, and renal impairment (in men, a serum creatinine concentration >1.5 mg/dL and in women, a serum creatinine concentration >1.4 mg/dL) including that caused by other conditions.

The most serious potential side effect of metformin is lactic acidosis but this is a much less common problem than with the biguanide phenformin, which is no longer available. Because the biguanides inhibit lactate metabolism, increased concentrations of the drug because of renal insufficiency can cause lactic acidosis. A recent Cochrane Collaboration meta-analysis found that lactic acidosis occurs as often in patients with diabetes who are metformin users as in those nonmetformin users.[19] The trials combined were both prospective, comparative and observational cohorts. Twenty-four percent of patients were older than age 65 years, and 46% of the trials allowed inclusion of patients with renal insufficiency, defined as a creatinine >1.5 mg/dL. No trial listed any cases of lactic acidosis, but it was not clear how many patients with standard contraindications were included in the trials. A separate trial reported no cases of lactic acidosis in 393 diabetic patients taking metformin with at least one contraindication to its use who were followed for 4 years. All participants in this trial had creatinine levels of 1.5–2.5 mg/dL.[20]

Given the cardiovascular benefits of the drug and that it does not cause hypoglycemia, it is an excellent choice for the management of diabetes in the older adult. Although age should not be a contraindication to the use of metformin, renal function should be monitored closely during treatment. Metformin therefore should probably be avoided in patients with conditions associated with renal insufficiency (e.g., hepatic or cardiac failure) and in patients with renal failure who are more susceptible to lactic acidosis. It should be used with caution in patients with impaired glomerular filtration rates, probably less than 30–60 ml/min, although there is no evidence to support a specific cutoff. Drug clearance decreases with increases in age independent of renal function,[21] so low to moderate doses, 500–2000 mg/day, should be used in older adults. Side effects include nausea, vomiting, anorexia, diarrhea, most of which resolve within a few weeks and can be avoided with slowly titrating up the dose. The drug should be stopped 2 days prior to radiological procedures involving contrast dyes.

α-Glucosidase Inhibitors

Acarbose and miglitol reversibly bind to α-glucosidases on the upper intestinal brush border. This delays the digestion of disaccharides and complex carbohydrates and, hence, the absorption of glucose and other monosaccharides. In a recent meta-analysis, acarbose, in addition to lowering the risk of any cardiovascular event, also was shown to lower fasting glucose levels, postprandial glucose levels, and hemoglobin A1c values compared to placebo.[22] It can be used alone with diet therapy or in addition to other hypoglycemics. Unfortunately, its gastrointestinal side effects may be prohibitive to the older diabetic patient. Flatulence, bloating, and diarrhea are common at higher doses because of fermentation of unabsorbed carbohydrates in the large bowel.

Meglitinides

Nateglinide and repaglinide act similarly to the sulfonylureas in stimulating the pancreatic insulin release but are very short acting, with half-lives of 1–1.5 hours. These agents can be used when patients have erratic eating habits. The medication can be administered with a meal or held if the meal is not eaten. The most common adverse events of this class include hypoglycemia, diarrhea, and weight gain.

Thiazolidinediones

The agents rosiglitizone and pioglitizone are peroxisome proliferator-activated receptor-γ agonists. Activation of peroxisome proliferator-activated receptor-γ receptors regulates gene transcription involved in lipid metabolism and in glucose production, transport, and utilization, thus decreasing peripheral insulin resistance.

The pharmacokinetics of these drugs do not appear to be altered by age. The TZDs have been used in trials alone as well as in combination with sulfonylureas or insulin. They have been shown to improve glucose control significantly in older patients with diabetes.[23] These drugs do increase the risk of fluid retention and should not be used in patients with New York Heart Association Class III or IV heart failure.[24] Troglitazone, the first of these agents to be approved for use in the United States, was removed from the market because of its association with hepatic failure. Therefore, serum transaminase levels should be checked at the start of therapy and periodically thereafter. Therapy should be stopped if the patient exhibits signs or symptoms of liver disease or if the transaminases are elevated to three times normal level.

Recently, there has been some controversy as to the safety of the TZDs. The TZDs have been associated with macular edema,[25] bone loss,[26] and increased fracture risk in women.[27] Rosiglitazone has been implicated in increasing the risk of myocardial infarction and death from cardiovascular causes in a meta-analysis of 42 randomized, controlled trials.[28] Methodological limitations of the study somewhat weaken the conclusions, but this preliminary evidence should stimulate further review of original source data. Pioglitazone, on the other hand, may have a protective effect in reducing the risk of myocardial infarctions in patients with diabetes and existing macrovascular disease.[29] Although the use of the TZDs in combination with other oral agents may delay the transition to or addition of insulin therapy, each individual's risks for known side effects of this class of agents must be weighed against potential benefits.

Insulins

Insulin therapy may be needed to achieve metabolic control and may be preferable to oral agents in some patients. The decision to treat with insulin must include an assessment of patients' beliefs about insulin and the potential for its safe use. For example, because most older patients have type 2 disease, they are likely to have had experiences with other family members or friends with diabetes. Insulin therapy is frequently instituted after several years of diagnosed disease duration, at a time when disease complications may be manifest. Thus, the development of worsening complications may be falsely attributed to the insulin itself. This and other fears should be explored with patients. In addition, visual and cognitive function and manual dexterity require careful evaluation if patients will be administering the insulin themselves. If not, the adequacy of informal or formal supports to manage insulin therapy consistently and safely must be evaluated.

Dipeptidyl-Peptidase-IV Inhibitors

Sitagliptin, a very recently approved oral agent for the treatment of type 2 diabetes, inhibits DPP-IV, an enzyme that metabolizes glucagon-like peptide-1 and glucose-dependent insulinotropic peptide, which are the dominant incretins of glucose homeostasis.[30] It is administered once daily and has a half-life of approximately 12 hours. Its excellent side-effect profile and its complementary action with metformin may increase the use of this agent in the future for older adults with diabetes.

Insulin therapy is frequently instituted in the hospital setting, when a diagnosis of diabetes is first made in conjunction with an admission for an acute infectious illness or for a complication, or when a patient is admitted for complicated hyperglycemia (e.g., for the diabetic hyperosmolar state or ketoacidosis). Even patients admitted to the hospital on oral agents may be transitioned to insulin to achieve better glycemic control. Randomized, controlled trials have shown that intensive glucose control in critically ill adults requiring intensive care unit settings decreases mortality, sepsis, new dialysis, blood transfusions, and critical illness-related polyneuropathy.[31] Observational studies of general medical and surgical patients have found an association between hyperglycemia and poor clinical outcomes,[32] making glycemic control with insulin the standard of care in many hospital settings. Given the differences in diet, physical activity, and stress levels that exist in the hospital compared with the home setting, particular attention should be paid to monitoring the transition from hospital to home. This is a time when serious hyperglycemia or hypoglycemia is likely to occur, either because of changes in these factors or because of misunderstandings about dosing and the technical aspects of insulin administration.

When exogenous insulin is used as sole therapy for older diabetics, its dosage and injection schedule should be individualized to each patient's needs. The ideal insulin regimen should have a low risk of hypoglycemia while still controlling symptoms of hyperglycemia. Newer basal insulins, such as glargine and detemir, have no peak and a duration of action of 24 hours. When these are combined with rapid-acting insulin, such as lispro or aspart, prior to meals, glycemic goals for fasting and postprandial states can be achieved. Older adults with physical and cognitive impairments may not be able to monitor plasma glucose and/or self-administer different types and doses of insulin reliably. A starting dose of 0.25 units/kg/day of intermediate-acting insulin (NPH) minimizes the risk of hypoglycemia. Adding a dose before dinner or at bedtime will help to lower fasting blood glucose values. Additional doses of short-acting insulin can be given with or between the NPH to control hyperglycemia. Insulin regimens should be tailored according to the individual patient's response as well as to her acceptance of the regimen.

Monitoring

Although self-monitoring of blood glucose is safe and relatively easy for most patients to manage, its use has not been studied systematically in older persons. The main reasons to consider glucose monitoring in older patients are 1) to prevent the development of hypoglycemia in patients treated with hypoglycemic medications, particularly during times of illness or when medication changes are planned, and 2) to guide adjustments of hypoglycemic therapy in conjunction with hemoglobin A1c levels. The hemoglobin A1c reflects glucose levels over the previous 8–12 weeks and is therefore useful in monitoring glycemic control over time.

Cardiovascular Risk Factors

Although diabetes was ranked as the sixth leading cause of death in American adults in 2002, approximately 65% of deaths in adults with diabetes result from heart disease or stroke.[33] Mutable risk factors for CVD include hypertension, hyperlipidemia, smoking, and obesity. Embedded in the known CVD risk factors is the insulin resistance syndrome, otherwise known as the *metabolic syndrome,* which is a group of conditions that collectively increases an individual's risk of developing coronary artery disease and diabetes. The syndrome includes the presence of three of the five following conditions: abdominal obesity, elevated triglycerides, low high-density lipoprotein, hypertension, and higher than normal fasting glucose.[34] The underlying defect in the metabolic syndrome is insulin resistance in adipose and muscle tissue resulting in high circulating insulin levels.

Evidence suggests that older adults with diabetes are less likely to meet recommended glycemic, blood pressure, and cholesterol goals than older adults without diabetes.[35] The question remains for the older adult with diabetes, what are the specific goals of care or target outcomes? Specific guidelines regarding aspirin use, smoking cessation, hypertension management, glycemic control, and lipid management in the older person with diabetes can be found in *Guidelines from the California Healthcare Foundation/American Geriatrics Society Panel on Improving Care for Elders with Diabetes* from 2003.[15] The guidelines recommend a target blood pressure of less than 140/80 mmHg if tolerated, and less than 130/80 mmHg may provide further benefit, although the evidence for this target is less strong. Although many studies showing the benefits of blood pressure reduction on cardiovascular events and mortality enrolled middle-aged and "younger" older adults, older adults as a group may be most likely to benefit in terms of decreased CVD morbidity and mortality given their decreased life expectancy compared with persons of the same age without diabetes. Reductions in macrovascular endpoints from treating hypertension in controlled studies are seen at approximately 2–5 years.[36,37]

The choice of antihypertensive therapy should be guided by side-effect profile, ease of administration, and cost, as diuretics, angiotensin-converting enzyme (ACE) inhibitors, angiotensin-receptor blockers (ARBs), β-blockers, and calcium channel blockers are comparable in their impact on reducing cardiovascular morbidity and mortality. The ACE inhibitors and the ARBs have the added benefit of delaying the progression of proteinuria and the decline in renal function.[15,38,39] This is an important consideration because at least 20% of type 2 patients will develop nephropathy. Careful attention should be paid to electrolyte, renal function, and potassium levels when beginning therapy or changing doses with diuretics, ACE inhibitors, and ARBs. An additional advantage of using ACE inhibitors or ARBs is that they do not cause or exacerbate urinary incontinence, constipation, lipid abnormalities, or hyperglycemia.

It is recommended that all adults with diabetes be considered for aggressive treatment of dyslipidemia with the goal of LDL <100 mg/dL in those without overt CVD and <70 mg/dL in those with overt CVD.[15] Further review of lipid abnormalities in the elderly can be found in Chapter 9. Once nutrition therapy and weight reduction therapy have been attempted, drug therapy is indicated. The 3-hydroxy-3-methylglutaryl coenzyme A reductase inhibitors (statins) have some gastrointestinal side effects, but minimal drug–drug interactions. Liver transaminases and creatinine kinase levels should probably be checked 3 months after starting therapy or after a dose change, and every 9–12 months while on therapy. Niacin should be avoided because it can worsen glycemic control.

Finally, although rates of cigarette smoking decline with age, an important subset of smokers survives to old age. Recent evidence suggests that the hazards of cigarette smoking for men and women, particularly with respect to cardiovascular mortality, extend into later life. Furthermore, the risk of death from CVD for former smokers is similar to that of never smokers, independent of age at which people quit.[40] Taken together, these data should compel clinicians to work with their older diabetic smokers to help them to quit.

Eye Disease

Given the critical importance of visual function to overall functional independence, eye disease in older diabetics deserves critical attention by clinicians. Data from the 1989 National Health Interview Survey indicate that among diabetics aged 65 years and older, approximately 16% have serious trouble seeing, even with glasses.[41] This is from not only the ravages of diabetic retinopathy; older diabetics are likely to have comorbid eye conditions, namely cataracts and glaucoma. The risk of developing diabetic retinopathy increases with duration of disease. Nearly all of type 1 diabetics and more than 60% of type 2 diabetics have retinopathy after 20 years. Because patients with type 2 disease frequently have had their disease for some time prior to diagnosis, over one third may already have retinopathy at the time they are diagnosed.[42] Poor glucose control, higher blood pressure, and abdominal obesity are also risk factors for developing retinopathy, and the progression of retinopathy has been associated with male sex, older age, and higher hemoglobin A1c.[43,44] Studies are ongoing to determine the impact of smoking on diabetic retinopathy.

Retinopathy may be manifested by preproliferative background changes, nonproliferative retinopathy, or by more severe proliferative changes. Because of the high likelihood of finding preexisting retinopathy, all newly diagnosed diabetics should be referred for ophthalmological evaluation, not only for the presence of retinopathy, but also for the presence of cataracts and glaucoma. This evaluation should include a comprehensive and dilated-eye examination by an ophthalmologist or an optometrist, because even in the best hands, dilated ophthalmoscopy only has a sensitivity of approximately 80% for detecting proliferative retinopathy.[45] In addition, there is strong evidence from two randomized, controlled trials showing that diagnosis and treatment of diabetic retinopathy reduces its progression and visual loss.[46,47] The American College of Physicians and the American Diabetes Association have published guidelines stating that if initial stereoscopic screening is normal, the frequency of eye examinations should be every 2–3 years. This strategy, of course, demands that careful attention be given to ensuring that older patients are followed carefully 1) to avoid missing vision changes because of other eye diseases common in this group, and 2) to monitor blood pressure and hemoglobin A1c.

Foot Care

For diabetic patients advancing in age, the risk of amputation increases. In 2003, the lower extremity amputation rate per 1,000 persons with diabetes was 3.9 among persons younger than 65 years, 6.6 among persons aged 65–74 years, and 7.9 among persons 75 years or older.[48] The rate of amputation for people with diabetes is 10 times higher than for people without diabetes. Of those with diabetes, Mexican Americans are 1.8 times as likely, non-Hispanic Blacks are 2.7 times as likely, and American Indians are 3–4 times as likely as Whites to undergo a lower extremity amputation. Amputation rates are 1.4–2.7 times higher in men than women with diabetes.[49] In addition to the monetary costs of amputations, they obviously have a profound effect on patients' mobility and may precipitate institutionalization.

Older adults with diabetes are at increased risk of developing foot ulcers due to peripheral arterial disease, sensory neuropathy, and joint malformations. Resulting gait abnormalities from these problems can lead to falls and trauma. Prevention of diabetic foot ulcers would lead to reductions in amputation rates. One case-controlled study demonstrated that lack of patient education is an additional important risk factor for amputation.[50] It is well-known that patients do not engage in preventive care of their feet and that physicians infrequently examine diabetics' feet. Improved self-care and physician attention to foot abnormalities, however, can be achieved relatively easily and inexpensively, with resulting reductions in foot lesions in one randomized, controlled trial,[51] but a recent Cochrane Collaboration review found mixed results on the effect of patient education for the prevention of diabetic foot ulceration.[52] Even without better evidence, patients should be instructed in self-examination methods, nail and callous care, washing techniques, and what constitutes appropriate footwear. Because many older persons have fungal infections of their nails and may not be able to safely cut them, referral to a podiatrist is a prudent strategy.

For their part, physicians should examine diabetic feet at each patient visit, although there is no evidence to support this interval of screening. The foot examination can be used to reinforce important patient foot care behaviors. Again, by consensus opinion, at least annually, diabetics should also have a thorough vascular examination, which includes palpation of the lower extremity pulses, a neurological examination to assess sensorimotor deficits by using the Semmes–Weinstein 5.07 (10-g) monofilament, an assessment of skin integrity, and a musculoskeletal examination to evaluate range of motion of the foot and ankle as well as bony abnormalities.[15,16] Although there is still much to learn about the prevention and treatment of diabetic foot lesions, successful implementation of these strategies is a place to start.

Cognitive Function

There is evidence that compared with age-matched controls, older adults with diabetes are more likely than their nondiabetic counterparts to perform poorly on cognitive tests.[53,54] A recent literature review found consistent deficits in verbal memory in diabetics compared to nondiabetics despite significant heterogeneity among the methods of the studies reviewed.[55] These changes are similar to those associated with normal aging, but whether they are manifestations of an accelerated aging process or occur via other mechanisms is not clear. Older diabetics are also more likely to have strokes and may experience adverse effects on cognition from hyperglycemia and hypoglycemia and hyperosmolar and hypoosmolar states. These are additional reasons for treating hypertension and for maintaining metabolic stability. Indeed, recent studies suggest that improved glycemic control improves some aspects of cognitive function in older patients with type 2 disease.[56]

Because of diabetes-related changes in cognitive function and the increased likelihood of dementia, both age- and diabetes-related periodic assessment of cognitive function in older diabetics is essential. This can serve to reassure the "worried well" who may have concerns about memory problems and to identify early those beginning to experience subtle difficulties. Careful attention to these issues may uncover adverse drug effects, other metabolic derangements (e.g., hypothyroidism), or depression and will identify those who may need additional help from clinicians and family or friends in adhering to complex treatment regimens.

Comorbidity

By virtue of their having diabetes and having manifestations of the complications described previously, as well as by virtue of being older, older type 2 diabetic patients are likely to have considerable coexisting disease. Because of the fact that these patients take several medications and the likelihood that they may have diminished organ function (especially renal function) and decreased physiological reserve together mean that they are at an increased risk of adverse drug effects. Careful attention therefore needs to be paid to avoiding drug–drug interactions.

In addition, because compliance with medications is known to diminish as the number of medications and the complexity of the regimen increases, thought needs to be given to ways of decreasing the total number of medications (e.g., using one medication for multiple indications).

Other Considerations

There is growing evidence that families play significant roles in the management of older persons with chronic disease in addition to the well-known role that they play in the general daily care of frail older persons.[57] A study of 357 family members of diabetic patients 70 years of age or older demonstrated that over half (71% were spouses) participated in the patient's diabetes care.[58] If patients are having difficulty adhering to treatment regimens, if they rely on family members for certain activities (e.g., food preparation, managing medications), or if they have functional disabilities, their family members or other informal care providers need to be educated about diabetes and receive instruction and support in methods of management.

There is some evidence that group visits, defined as several patients with a chronic illness meeting together with the provider at the same time, for older adults with diabetes, may reduce emergency department utilization, reduce hospital admissions, improve vaccination rates, and improve patient and physician satisfaction.[59,60] The group visit is billable under Medicare if the patient has appropriate physician supervision (i.e., face-to-face contact at some point during the visit.) The structure and implementation of the group visit, however, varies greatly among citations in the medical literature, and the impact of group visits on reducing macro- or microvascular complications of diabetes has not been evaluated. The organization of such groups requires a new process to be implemented into an existing care delivery system, which may or may not be feasible given the resources available within an individual system of care. In addition, it is not clear that group visits reduce costs.[61] Although in need of more study, the group visit model may be an effective and efficient way of improving care for motivated older adults with diabetes.

SUMMARY AND CONCLUSIONS

Diabetes is a common condition in older persons and is associated with considerable economic and personal costs. Attention to the prevention and management of cardiovascular, eye, and foot disease is, therefore, critical. The risks and benefits of tight glycemic control will vary for a given individual depending on cognitive status, functional status, and life expectancy. Although reducing blood glucose levels to values that eliminate hyperglycemic symptoms while minimizing the potential for hypoglycemic reactions should be attempted, and cardiovascular risk factors treated, equal attention should be given to preventing eye and foot complications, where screening and treatment interventions also have known efficacy.

REFERENCES

1. Centers for Disease Control and Prevention. National Diabetes Fact Sheet: General Information and National Estimates on Diabetes in the United States, 2005. Atlanta: US Department of Health and Human Services, Centers for Disease Control and Prevention, 2005.
2. American Diabetes Association. Economic costs of diabetes in the US in 2002. *Diabetes Care.* 2003;26:917–932.
3. Harris MI. Epidemiology of diabetes mellitus among the elderly in the United States. *Clin Geriatr Med.* 1990;6:703–719.
4. The Expert Committee on the Diagnosis and Classification of Diabetes mellitus. Report of the Expert Committee on the Diagnosis and Classification of Diabetes Mellitus. *Diabetes Care.* 1997;20:1183–1197.
5. Fletcher RH, Fletcher SW, Wagner EH. *Clinical Epidemiology – The Essentials.* Baltimore: Williams & Wilkins; 1982.
6. US Preventive Services Task Force. Screening for type 2 diabetes mellitus in adults: recommendations and rationale. *Ann Intern Med.* 2003;138:212–214.
7. Heorger TJ, Harris R, Hicks KA, et al. Screening for type 2 diabetes mellitus: a cost-effectiveness analysis. *Ann Intern Med.* 2004;140:689–699.
8. US Preventive Services Task Force. Screening for Diabetes Mellitus, Adult type 2. February 2003. Available at: http://www.ahrq.gov/clinic/uspstf/uspsdiab.htm. Accessed May 13, 2008.
9. Von Korff M, Gruman J, Schaefer J, et al. Collaborative management of chronic illness. *Ann Intern Med.* 1997;127:136–145.
10. Renders, CM, Valk GD, Griffin SJ, et al. Interventions to improve the management of diabetes in primary care, outpatient, and community settings; a systematic review. *Diabetes Care.* 2001;24:1821–1833.
11. Caruso LB, Clough-Gorr KM, Silliman RA. Improving quality of care for urban older people with diabetes and mellitus and cardiovascular disease. *J Am Geriatr Soc.,* 2007;55(10):1656–1662.
12. American Geriatrics Society. *AGS Clinical Practice Guideline: Guidelines for Improving the Care of the Older Person with Diabetes Mellitus.* Available at: http://www.americangeriatrics.org/education/diabetes_executive_summ.shtml. Accessed May 13, 2008.
13. National Heart, Lung, and Blood Institute. *Clinical Guidelines on the Identification, Evaluation and Treatment of Overweight and Obesity in Adult.* Bethesda, MD: National Institutes of Health, 1998.
14. American Diabetes Association. Position statement: nutrition recommendations and interventions for diabetes. *Diabetes Care.* 2007;30:S48–S65.
15. American Diabetes Association. Position statement: standards of medical care in diabetes – 2007. *Diabetes Care.* 2007;30:S4–S41.
16. California Healthcare Foundation/American Geriatrics Society Panel on Improving Care for Elders with Diabetes. Guidelines for improving the care of the older person with diabetes mellitus. *J Am Geriatr Soc.* 2003;51:S265–S280.
17. United Kingdom Prospective Diabetes Study (UKPDS) Group. Intensive blood-glucose control with sulphonylureas or insulin compared with conventional treatment and risk of complications in patients with type 2 diabetes (UKPDS 33). *Lancet.* 1998;352:837–853.
18. United Kingdom Prospective Diabetes Study (UKPDS) Group. Effect of intensive blood-glucose control with metformin on complications in overweight patients with type 2 diabetes (UKPDS 34). *Lancet.* 1998;352:854–865.

19. Salpeter S, Greyber E, Pasternak G, et al. Risk of fatal and non-fatal lactic acidosis with metformin use in type 2 diabetes mellitus. *Cochrane Database Syst Rev.* 2006;(1):CD002967 [update of *Cochrane Database Syst Rev.* 2003;(2):CD002967; PMID: 12804446].

20. Rachmani R, Slavachevski I, Levi Z, et al. Metformin in patients with type 2 diabetes mellitus: reconsideration of traditional contraindications. *Eur J Int Med.* 2002;13:428–433.

21. Sambol NC, Chiang J, Lin ET, et al. Kidney function and age are both predictors of pharmacokinetics of metformin. *J Clin Pharmacol.* 1995;35:1094–1102.

22. Hanefelda M, Cagatayb M, Petrowitsch T, et al. Acarbose reduces the risk for myocardial infarction in type 2 diabetic patients: meta-analysis of seven long-term studies. *Eur Heart J.* 2004;25:10–16.

23. Rajagopalan R, Perez A, Ye Z, et al. Pioglitazone is effective therapy for elderly patients with type 2 diabetes mellitus. *Drugs Aging.* 2004;21:259–271.

24. Nesto RW, Bell D, Bonow RO, et al. Thiazolidinedione use, fluid retention and congestive heart failure; a consensus statement from the American Heart Association and American Diabetes Association. *Diabetes Care.* 2004;27:256–263.

25. Kendall C, Wooltorton E. Rosiglitazone (Avandia) and macular edema. *CMAJ.* 2006;174:623.

26. Schwartz AV, Sellmeyer DE, Vittinghoff E, et al. Thiazolidinedione use and bone loss in older diabetic adults. *J Clin Endocrinol Metab.* 2006;91:3349–3354.

27. Kahn SE, Haffner SM, Heise MA, et al. Glycemic durability of rosiglitazone, metformin, or glyburide monotherapy. *NEJM.* 2006;355:2427–2443.

28. Nissen SE, Wolski K. Effect of rosiglizaone on the risk of myocardial infarction and death from cardiovascular causes. *NEJM.* 2007;356 (page numbers not available yet.)

29. Dormandy JA, Charbonnel B, Eckland J, et al. Secondary prevention of macrovascular events in patients with type 2 diabetes in the PROactive Study (Prospective pioglitazone clinical trial in macrovascular events): a randomized trial. *Lancet.* 2005;366:1279–1289.

30. Goldstein BJ, Feinglos MN, Lunceford JK, et al. Sitagliptin 036 Study Group. Effect of initial combination therapy with sitagliptin, a dipeptidyl peptidase-4 inhibitor, and metformin on glycemic control in patients with type 2 diabetes. *Diabetes Care.* 2007;30:1979–1987.

31. Van den Berghe G, Wouters p, Weekers F, et al. Intensive insulin therapy in the critically ill patients. *NEJM.* 2001;345:1359–1367.

32. ACE/ADA Task Force on Inpatient Diabetes: American College of Endocrinology and American Diabetes Association Consensus Statement on Inpatient Diabetes and Glycemic Control. *Diabetes Care.* 2006;29:1955–1962.

33. National Institute of Diabetes and Digestive and Kidney Diseases. *Deaths Among People with Diabetes, United States, 2002.* Available at: http://diabetes.niddk.nih.gov/dm/pubs/statistics/index.htm#12. Accessed May 13, 2008.

34. Executive summary of the third report of the National Cholesterol Education Program (NCEP) Expert Panel on Detection, Evaluation, and Treatment of High Blood Cholesterol in Adults (Adult Treatment Panel III). *JAMA.* 2001;285:2486–2497.

35. Smith NL, Savage PJ, Heckbert SR, et al. Glucose, blood pressure, and lipid control in older people with and without diabetes mellitus: the Cardiovascular Health Study. *J Am Geriatr Soc.* 2002;50:416–423.

36. Curb JD, Pressel SL, Cutler JA, et al. Effect of diuretic-based antihypertensive treatment on cardiovascular disease risk in older diabetic patients with isolated systolic hypertension. Systolic Hypertension in the Elderly Program Cooperative Research Group. *JAMA.* 1996;276:1886–1892.

37. United Kingdom Prospective Diabetes Study (UKPDS) Group. Tight blood pressure control and risk of macrovascular and microvascular complications in type 2 diabetes (UKPDS 38). *BMJ.* 1998;317:703–713.

38. Ravid M, Lang R, Rachmani R, et al. Long-term renoprotective effect of angiotensin-converting enzyme inhibition in non-insulin-dependent diabetes mellitus: a 7-year follow-up study. *Arch Intern Med.* 1996;156:286–289.

39. Brenner BM, Cooper ME, de Zeeuw D, et al. Effects of losartan on renal and cardiovascular outcomes in patients with type 2 diabetes and nephropathy. *NEJM.* 2001;345:861–869.

40. LaCroix AZ, Lang J, Scherr P, et al. Smoking and mortality among older men and women in three communities. *NEJM.* 1991;324:1619–1625.

41. National Diabetes Data Group. *Diabetes in America.* 2nd ed. Bethesda: National Institutes of Health; 1995.

42. Kohner EM, Aldington SJ, Stratton IM, et al. United Kingdom Prospective Diabetes Study, 30: Diabetic retinopathy at diagnosis of non-insulin-dependent diabetes mellitus and associated risk factors. *Arch Ophthalmol.* 1998;116:297–303.

43. van Leiden HA, Dekker JM, Moll AC, et al. Risk factors for incident retinopathy in a diabetic and nondiabetic population: the Hoorn study. *Arch Ophthalmol.* 2003;121:245–251.

44. Stratton IM, Kohner EM, Aldington SJ, et al. UKPDS 50. Risk factors for incidence and progression of retinopathy in type II diabetes over 6 years from diagnosis. *Diabetologia.* 2001;44:156–163.

45. Singer DE, Nathan DM, Fogel HA, et al. Screening for diabetic retinopathy. *Ann Intern Med.* 1992;116:660–671.

46. Early Treatment Diabetic Retinopathy Study Research Group. Photocoagulation treatment of proliferative diabetic retinopathy: the second report of diabetic retinopathy study findings. *Ophthalmology.* 1978;85:82–106.

47. Early Treatment Diabetic Retinopathy Study Research Group. Photocoagulation for diabetic macular edema. Early Treatment Diabetic Retinopathy Study report number 1. *Arch Ophthalmol.* 1985;103:1796–1806.

48. Centers for Disease Control and Prevention. *Hospital Discharge Rates for Nontraumatic Lower Extremity Amputation per 1,000 Diabetic Population, by Age, United States, 1980–2003.* Available at: http://www.cdc.gov/diabetes/statistics/lea/fig4.htm. Accessed May 13, 2008.

49. American Diabetes Association. Complications of Diabetes in the United States. Available at: http://www.diabetes.org/diabetes-statistics/complications.jsp. Accessed May 13, 2008.

50. Reiber GE, Pecoraro RE, Koepsell TD. Risk factors for amputation in patients with diabetes mellitus: a case-control study. *Ann Inter Med.* 1992;117:97–105.

51. Litzelman DK, Slemenda CW, Langefeld CD, et al. Reduction of lower extremity clinical abnormalities in patients with non-insulin-dependent diabetes mellitus: a randomized, controlled trial. *Ann Intern Med.* 1993;119:36–41.

52. Valk GD, Kriegsman DM, Assendelft WJ. Patient education for preventing diabetic foot ulceration [update of *Cochrane Database Syst Rev.* 2001;(4):CD001488;PMID:11687114]. *Cochrane Database Syst Rev.* (1):CD001488, 2005.

53. Logroscino G, Kang, JH, Grodstein F. Prospective study of type 2 diabetes and cognitive decline in women aged 70–81 years. *BMJ*. 2004;328:548.

54. Bent N, Rabbitt P, Metcalfe D. Diabetes mellitus and the rate of cognitive ageing. *Br J Clin Psychol*. 2000;39:349–362.

55. Strachan MWJ, Deary IJ, Ewing FME, et al. Is type II diabetes associated with an increased risk of cognitive dysfunction? *Diabetes Care*. 1997;20:438–445.

56. Meneilly GS, Cheung E, Tessier D, et al. The effect of improved glycemic control on cognitive functions in the elderly patient with diabetes. *J Gerontol Med Sci*. 1993;48:M117–M121.

57. Wolff JL, Kasper JD. Caregivers of frail elders: updating a national profile. *Gerontologist*. 2006;46:344–356.

58. Silliman RA, Bhatti S, Khan A, et al. The care of older persons with diabetes mellitus: families and primary care physicians. *J Am Geriatr Soc*. 1996;44:1314–1321.

59. Coleman EA, Eilertsen, TB, Kramer AM, et al. Reducing emergency visits in older adults with chronic illness. A randomized, controlled trial of group visits. *Eff Clin Pract*. 2001;4:49–57.

60. Beck A, Scott J, Williams P, et al. A randomized trial of group outpatient visits for chronically ill older HMO members: the Cooperative Health Care Clinic. *J Am Geriatr Soc*. 1997;45:543–549.

61. Jaber R, Braksmajer A, Trilling JS. Group visits: a qualitative review of current research. *J Am Board Fam Med*. 2006;19:276–290.

9

LIPID MANAGEMENT IN OLDER PATIENTS

Phil Mendys, PharmD, CPP, Ross J. Simpson, Jr., MD, PhD

OVERVIEW

This chapter will introduce issues related to management of lipid disorders in older patients to reduce the risk of atherosclerosis and cardiovascular disease (CVD). Because lipid metabolism and regulation do not vary greatly between younger and older people, age-related influences on cardiovascular risk and lipoprotein-mediated disease processes will be our central theme. In addition, aspects of appropriate pharmacotherapy and support of treatment adherence will balance out the overall review.

AGE AND CARDIOVASCULAR RISK

Clinicians typically approach the task of assessing cardiovascular risk by focusing on patient age as an obvious "nonmodifiable risk factor." The Framingham risk score estimates 10-year absolute risk for CVD events and age contributes enormously to the end result, given that indeed age is the greatest contributor to absolute cardiovascular risk. This may be related to the multiple observations that have concluded atherosclerosis as a process that begins early in life.[1,2] Advanced age reflects an increased duration of exposure to various risk factors and an accumulation of coronary disease burden.[3] The Framingham Risk Score is less robust in the elderly (age >70 years) as this group has already had their "age-based" exposure. A comparison of the risk factor counting method as outlined in the National Cholesterol Education Program Guidelines to a multivariate analysis demonstrated that these guidelines underestimate risk among more than 5 million persons with fewer than two risk factors. Compared to individuals whose classification was unchanged, those *misclassified* as low risk were older and more likely to be male.[4] Therefore, recognizing that age is such a powerful predictor for risk of heart disease, clinicians should address common modifiable risk factors in older

patients – including low-density lipoprotein (LDL) cholesterol – to slow the development of subclinical disease. As many elderly are eligible for secondary prevention and many others qualify as "high risk" primary prevention. Treatment of the elderly has been summarized as follows:

- The purpose of treating risk factors is to prevent morbid and mortal cardiovascular events and to decrease the disease burden of atherosclerosis in individuals and in communities.
- Current guidelines on pharmacological therapy of hypertension and hypercholesterolemia are based on algorithms estimating the 5- or 10-year absolute risk of morbid and mortal events.
- Age is the strongest determinant of absolute risk. The algorithms underemphasize modifiable risk factors by emphasizing age.
- Functional and structural cardiovascular abnormalities are caused by risk factors and precede the occurrence of morbid and mortal events.
- Prevention of these asymptomatic functional and structural abnormalities by controlling all risk factors will result in the prevention of cardiovascular events.
- Age should be removed from the algorithms used to decide whether to treat risk factors.[5]

It is clear from clinical trials that both younger and older patients benefit from intensive lipid-lowering therapy when at risk for atherosclerotic events, either deemed primary or secondary prevention. Ultimately treatments should be based on a comprehensive assessment of overall cardiovascular risk, not chronological age.

Lessons from Observational Data

The incidence of coronary disease in individuals older than 65 years is high. In the middle of the 1990s, there were numerous analyses published questioning the predictive value of cholesterol in determining cardiovascular risk in older patients. As reported in the 52 nations INTERHEART study, however, the two most important predictors of coronary disease mortality were total cholesterol and smoking. In fact, abnormal lipid profiles, as determined by an ApoB/ApoA1 ratio, was the most important population-attributable risk in both younger and older individuals.[6]

The basis for the Cardiovascular Health Study (CHS) was to address the uncertainty of the risk of smoking and cholesterol in predicting risk in older patients. The CHS reported that in patients with subclinical disease, the following criteria served as significant predictors of CHD in both men and women: ankle brachial blood pressure, carotid artery stenosis and wall thickness, electrocardiographic and echocardiographic abnormalities, and positive responses to the rose angina and claudication questionnaire. At present, these measures are readily accessible to clinicians and can add greatly to the assessment of patients at risk for cardiovascular events.[7] As these assessments are combined with the demonstrated benefit of current preventive therapies, we can now support an effective strategy to reduce the incidence of and mortality associated with CVD in older patients.

CURRENT GUIDELINES FOR MANAGING LIPID DISORDERS

National Cholesterol Education Panel Adult Treatment Panel

Numerous clinical trials demonstrate benefits of LDL cholesterol lowering in older persons with established coronary heart disease (CHD). Increased levels of LDL cholesterol carry predictive power for the development of CHD in older persons as well as younger individuals. Implications from several recent clinical studies with an even broader range of baseline risk of cardiovascular disease influenced the National Cholesterol Education Panel (NCEP) panel to revise thinking on the intensity of treatment.[8] The NCEP ATP III reaffirms their position that older persons who are at higher risk of CHD and who are otherwise in good health are candidates for cholesterol-lowering therapy.[3] As reported in the CHS in 2002, the baseline use of statin therapy in study participants who were 65 years or older and free of CVD resulted in a 56% lower risk of cardiovascular events and 44% lower all-cause mortality.[9] Taken together with the evidence of the value of lipid lowering in older patients with known coronary disease, the benefits of lipid lowering should not be denied to individuals at risk solely on the basis of age.

Primary Prevention in Older Patient Groups

Persons older than 65 years of age account for approximately two of three first-time major coronary events. Many older persons with advanced coronary atherosclerosis are asymptomatic and require further assessment – as well as clinical judgment – to determine a proper risk/benefit estimate. In older persons, CHD deaths account for one-half of all CHD events. Given the assumption that statin therapy reduces risk for all CHD categories by approximately one third, the likely mortality benefits of lipid lowering of 50% in older patients appears reasonable.[3] Based on this construct, the prospects for reducing clinical CHD in the older patients by intensive LDL lowering are good.

Prevention Trials in Older Patients

The first specific prevention trial to evaluate the role of lipid lowering with statins in older patients (aged 70–82 years) was the Prospective Study of Pravastatin in the Elderly. This trial looked at both older men (n = 2,804) and women (n = 3,000) at high risk of developing CVD and stroke. Once randomized to placebo or 40 mg pravastatin, the patients were evaluated over an average of 3.2 years and assessed based on a composite endpoint of major coronary events, including nonfatal myocardial infarction and CHD death. Each endpoint was reduced with treatment by 19% and 24%, respectively. Although no reduction in stroke occurred in the treatment group, there was a 25% reduction in transient ischemic events. As concluded by the authors of the study, the results support the notion that the benefits of statin therapy could be safely extended to older persons.[10]

A more contemporary trial evaluating the possible role of lipid lowering in an "at risk" population was completed in a large population of patients with hypertension. The Anglo-Scandinavian Cardiac Outcomes Trial – Lipid-Lowering Arm program evaluated more than 10,000 patients aged 40–79 (average age 63) years with at least three risk factors beyond high blood pressure who were randomized to receive either atorvastatin (10 mg) or placebo. The primary endpoint of the study was a composite of nonfatal myocardial infarction and fatal CHD. The average baseline LDL cholesterol at study entry was 132 mg/dL, which was reduced an average of 29% by the end of the trial. The original study design was to provide follow up for an average of 5 years; however, the trial was stopped at a median follow up of 3.3 years because of a marked reduction of events in the treatment group. Treatment with atorvastatin resulted in a reduction in the incidence of fatal and nonfatal stroke by 27% (P = 0.024), total cardiovascular events by 21% (P = 0.0005), and total coronary events by 29% (P = 0.0005). The authors concluded that LDL lowering with statin therapy has considerable potential to reduce risk for CVD in primary prevention in patients with multiple CVD risk factors. The results of both the Prospective Study of Pravastatin in the Elderly and the Anglo-Scandinavian Cardiac Outcomes Trial support the efficacy of statin therapy in older, high-risk persons without established CVD.[8]

Trials in Older Persons with Established CVD

Early landmark trials in which both simvastatin (Scandinavian Simvastatin Survival Study) and pravastatin (Cholesterol and Recurrent Events) were used helped to establish the benefit of cholesterol lowering in a wide range of patients with established coronary disease.[10,11] Both of these studies, which looked at patients with a background of coronary disease, but at different baselines levels of cholesterol, demonstrated a treatment benefit in patients older than 60 years of age. In the Long-term Intervention with Pravastatin in Ischemic Disease Study, an analysis was performed of the comparative effects of pravastatin on CVD outcomes in patients with CHD who were 65 years or older with those in patients 31–64 years of age. Although older patients were at greater risk for death, myocardial infarction, unstable angina, and stroke than younger patients, pravastatin reduced risk for all cardiovascular events in a similar relative manner. For every 1,000 older patients treated over 6 years, pravastatin prevented 45 deaths and 133 major cardiovascular events, compared with 22 deaths and 107 major cardiovascular events per 1,000 younger patients. In older patients with CHD, statin therapy reduced the risk for all major cardiovascular events and all-cause mortality.[12] Given that older patients are at greater risk than younger patients for these events, the absolute benefit of treatment is significantly greater in older patients.

The Heart Protection Study documented risk reduction with statin therapy in patients at high risk, including those with coronary disease, other vascular disease, or diabetes and a baseline LDL cholesterol level of 131 (by direct measurement). After assignment to either 40 mg simvastatin or placebo, all-cause mortality was significantly reduced by 13% (P = 0.0003). In addition, major vascular events were reduced by 24%, coronary death rate by 18%, nonfatal myocardial infarction plus coronary death by 27%, nonfatal or fatal stroke by 25%, and cardiovascular revascularization by 24%. The reduction in the event rate was similar for men and women and for participants either younger or older than 70 years of age at entry. Older persons tolerated statin therapy well. Taken together with the findings from other statin trials, strong justification exists for intensive LDL-lowering therapy in older persons with established CVD.[8]

Studies in patients with acute coronary syndromes (ACS) have also supported intensity of treatment as outlined in the 2004 NCEP consensus statement. As compared with individuals with stable coronary disease, patients with ACS are at particularly high risk of recurrent events. In an analysis from the Pravastatin or Atorvastatin Evaluation and Infection Therapy – Thrombolysis in Myocardial Infarction 22 study, the relationship between LDL cholesterol at 30 days after ACS and subsequent clinical outcomes were compared among elderly patients (aged ≥70 years) and younger counterparts by using the composite endpoint of death, myocardial infarction, or unstable angina. Among 634 elderly patients, the achievement of the NCEP goal was associated with an 8% absolute and a 40% relative lower risk of events. Based on the achievement of these goals the estimated number of events preventable among the elderly was 80 events at 2 years for every 1,000 patients at goal versus those not at goal, compared with 23 events potentially prevented in younger patients. The occurrence of major side effects among the older patients was similar to that in younger patients and did not differ with the intensity of the statin regimen.[13]

BEYOND CORONARY DISEASE

Peripheral Arterial Disease

Peripheral arterial disease (PAD) has become an established CHD equivalent as outlined in various epidemiological studies as well as represented in the current NCEP treatment guidelines. Given the increased risk for all-cause and cardiovascular mortality, individuals with PAD – regardless of age – should be aggressively managed with respect to coexisting risk factors. In addition, as demonstrated in three separate studies, the use of statins improved walking performance in people with PAD. In summary, older persons with hypercholesterolemia and PAD should be managed with statins not only to reduce the risk of cardiovascular events, but also to have a favorable impact on the progression of PAD.[14]

Cholesterol and Stroke

Clear benefits of cholesterol lowering on coronary disease events have been established; however, cholesterol was traditionally considered a poor predictor of stroke. Moreover, the results of treatment studies in the pre–statin era were inconclusive. Recently, high serum cholesterol was identified as a predictor of risk in patients with ischemic stroke.[15] Given that almost 30% of the 700,000 strokes that occur each year are recurrent events, it is critical that we identify the risk and determinants of recurrent stroke and review the evidence base to support improved outcomes in this patient population. Recent studies, such as the Heart Protection Study, have been encouraging in reducing the risk of coronary events in this patient group; however, among those patients with preexisting cerebrovascular disease, the incidence of stroke was not significantly reduced. The first trial to demonstrate a reduction in stroke risk in noncoronary disease patients with a history of cerebrovascular events (stroke, transient ischemic attack [TIA]) associated with statin therapy has been published. The Stroke Prevention by Aggressive Reduction in Cholesterol Levels study included more than 4,700 patients with a history of stroke or TIA within 6 months before study entry. These individuals had no known history of CHD and baseline LDL between 100 and 190 mg/dL. After treatment assignment to either placebo or atorvastatin (80 mg), patients were followed for a median of 4.9 years. In patients with a recent stroke or TIA, treatment with atorvastatin (80 mg/day) decreased the risk of stroke, major coronary events, and revascularization procedures. These results support the initiation of atorvastatin treatment soon after a stroke or TIA.[16]

THERAPY DIRECTED AT DYSLIPIDEMIA

Therapeutic Lifestyle Changes

The current treatment guidelines to reduce coronary disease risk endorse a comprehensive lifestyle management approach, including weight reduction goals as appropriate and increased physical activity as practical for individual patients.[3]

These guidelines are referred to as Therapeutic Lifestyle Changes, and patients are encouraged to reduce intake of saturated fats (7% of total calories) and cholesterol (200 mg/day). This Step I diet is generally preferred for use in older patients, as the more restricted Step II diet may not provide adequate nutrition. Although the guidelines for most patient groups support a dietary trial of up to 6 months, the clinician may consider drug therapy at a period of 4 to 6 weeks in older patients who are not approaching their respective treatment goal.[17] Plant stanols/sterols (2 g/day) and up to 25 mg of soluble fiber can aid in lowering LDL cholesterol, which can be used alone or in conjunction with appropriate pharmacotherapy.

Pharmacological Therapy for Lipid Management in Older Patients

We have established that the decision to treat a patient should be predicated on the assessment of baseline risk. LDL cholesterol has been established as the primary target in reducing cardiovascular risk. Although the use of therapeutic lifestyle changes, including LDL-lowering dietary options (plant stanols/sterols and increased viscous fiber), will achieve the therapeutic goal in many at risk persons, drug treatment options add greatly to our ability to achieve treatment goals, reduce cardiovascular risk, and improve patient outcomes.

Statins

A number of agents/classes have an impact on the lipid profile, allowing for adjustment of the regimen if treatment goals are not met or if tolerability is an issue. Only the statin class, however, has evidence to support a reduction in morbidity and mortality, and the statins should remain first line treatment per the NCEP guidelines. The availability of the statins, which have been used clinically for more than 20 years, allows attainment of the LDL goal in most high-risk persons, including those with known coronary disease. Currently statins are considered as first line treatment because of their ability to safely and effectively lower LDL cholesterol up to 60%. Initiation of treatment is made on risk assessment and determination of identified treatment targets.[3] Currently available statins allow for a flexible starting dose to achieve individual patient goals. Onset of effect is generally within 4–6 weeks, which allows a reasonable time for patient follow up. Treatment with statins is generally safe, although rarely persons experience myopathy. Serious muscular adverse events are infrequent, and the incidence of myopathy is 1.2 per 10,000 person-years, similar to the rate of 0.2 observed in the general population. Presentation of statin-associated myopathy is more likely in persons with complex medical problems or in those who are taking multiple medications. Among several factors that may predispose patients to increased risk of myopathy is age. This may result from a number of features such as comorbidities, polypharmacy, or an age-related decline in renal function. Despite the fact that statins may differ in their ability to lower LDL cholesterol levels and inhibit hydroxymethylglutaryl–coenzyme A reductase, the risk

of severe myotoxic events does not appear to be associated with LDL cholesterol effect.[18] The most comprehensive age-based analysis of safety for a statin was published as a pooled analysis of more than 50 clinical trials of atorvastatin. The analysis compared four doses of active drug to placebo in 5,437 patients older than 65 years (range of mean age, 71–74 years), of whom almost half were women (42%). This included a large number of individuals on both the 10-mg (n = 2,042) and the 80-mg dosage (n = 1,698), along with a comparison of almost 1,000 placebo-treated individuals. Serious adverse events were rare (≤1%) and rates of discontinuation because of treatment adverse events were low between treatment doses and placebo (2.1% vs 1.7%). At the maximum dose, elevations of liver enzymes (aspartate aminotransferase/alanine aminotransferase) were higher than placebo (3.2 vs ≤0.9%). Treatment associated myalgia was low, and no patient experienced persistent elevated creatine kinase of greater than 10 times the upper limits of normal.[19]

Frequently in clinical practice, statins have been discontinued for suspected myopathy, which is, in fact, not present. It may be useful in clinical practice to make a baseline estimate of muscle symptoms prior to initiating treatment and then compare the assessment at follow up with the patient. Ultimately, as supported by the American Heart Association/American College of Cardiology position statement on the use of statins, the incidence of severe statin-induced myopathy, as well as other adverse events, is low and does not outweigh the benefits of risk reduction of coronary events.[18]

Cholesterol Absorption Inhibitors

The newest class of agents available for cholesterol lowering is represented by ezetimibe, a cholesterol absorption inhibitor. The drug is given once daily, and the kinetic profile does not appear to be dependent on age, renal, or hepatic function. Ezetimibe undergoes rapid and extensive glucuronidation in the intestinal wall and the liver and should not be recommended in patients with moderate or severe liver dysfunction. The lipid-lowering effect of ezetimibe correlates well with dose and plasma concentration. Ezetimibe is given in a 10-mg dosage and has been shown to reduce the fractional cholesterol absorption by 54% compared with placebo, which correlated with a decrease in LDL cholesterol of 20.4%. Because ezetimibe has rather modest lipid-lowering effects compared with statins and lacks long-term outcomes data, it is generally reserved for statin-intolerant patients or as an add-on treatment to optimize LDL cholesterol lowering.[20] The Ezetimibe Add on to Statin for Effectiveness study, a recent study in which the safety of ezetimibe when added to current statin therapy, was evaluated in more than 3,000 patients aged older than 65 years with LDL cholesterol exceeding NCEP treatment goals. Although this was not an actual outcomes trial, the investigators were able to assess both the percentage of LDL cholesterol reduction and proportion of patents achieving target LDL cholesterol. The results of the 6-week study proved the ability of ezetimibe to provide additional LDL cholesterol lowering (22%–25%) on top of baseline statin and an increase in the number of patients achieving respective NCEP targets. The safety of the add-on therapy appeared to be similar to that of placebo plus statin with discontinuation rates from adverse events of approximately 1%.[21]

Bile Acid Sequestrants/Resins

Bile acid sequestrants or resins (cholestyramine, colestipol, colesevelam) have been available for many years. They were the first drugs to have suggested benefits in lowering LDL cholesterol, as demonstrated in the Lipid-Lowering Coronary Primary Prevention Trail primary prevention study. Like the aforementioned cholesterol absorption inhibitor, ezetimibe, this class of agents has modest effects on LDL cholesterol, in the range of 15%–30%. Bile acid resins are poorly tolerated and have limitations because of potential drug–drug interactions. Because they lack systemic toxicity, they may be used as alternatives to statins in younger persons or women considering pregnancy. They can be useful as add-on therapy to statins for high-risk individuals. Bile acid resins should not be used in patients with elevated triglycerides above 200 mg/dL and are contraindicated in patients with triglyceride levels higher than 400 mg/dL.[3]

Nicotinic Acid

Nicotinic acid has been available for many years as an agent to modify lipid profiles, which is currently available as crystalline nicotinic acid, sustained-release (or timed-release) nicotinic acid, or extended-release nicotinic acid (Niaspan®) Niacin can lower LDL cholesterol up to 25%, raise high-density lipoprotein up to 35%, and lower triglycerides up to 50%. Despite its ability to modify each lipid parameter in a positive direction, the evidence base for niacin therapy to have an impact on cardiovascular outcomes is diffuse and currently limited compared to the statin class. Common side effects, such as flushing and itching of the skin, gastrointestinal distress, and glucose intolerance may limit patient acceptance. Niacin should be used with caution in patients with active liver disease, recent peptic ulcer, and hyperuricemia/gout. Niacin may be considered for patients with an atherogenic profile that is characterized by limited LDL cholesterol elevations or in combination with other agents in patients with high LDL cholesterol.[3]

Fibrates

Fibric acid derivatives, which include gemfibrozil, fenofibrate, and clofibrate, are agents that have primary utility in the management of hypertriglyceridemia. They may be combined with other lipid-lowering drugs to impact an atherogenic profile associated with combined dyslipidemia. Fibrates may have beneficial effects in conjunction with their high-density lipoprotein–elevating capacity as demonstrated in the Veterans Affairs High Density Lipoprotein Intervention Trial study; however, the overall evidence base for fibrates is limited. They are generally poor treatments for the management of LDL cholesterol with effects in the 5%–25% range. Although they are generally well tolerated, fibrates may produce a variety of adverse gastrointestinal events, from bloating to increased risk of gallstones. The combination of fibrate and statin should be carefully monitored as concomitant use imparts an increased risk for myopathy.[3]

Limitations of Treatment in the Older Patient

Older patients generally do not receive evidence-based therapies for atherosclerosis-related disease on par with their younger counterparts. That being said, there are certainly real limitations of treatment in this age group. Statins, for example, are contraindicated in patients with active liver disease or unexplained persistent elevations of serum transaminases. Although cases of rhabdomyolysis with statin therapy are rare, patients should promptly report muscle pain, tenderness, or weakness. The clinician should review these patients carefully for possible concomitant physiological compromise, including renal status, and the potential for drug–drug interactions as a contribution to risk for rhabdomyolysis. Other pharmacological approaches as well have specific limitations in this age group. Bile acid resins often interfere with absorption of other drugs and are difficult to dose. Fibrates carry warnings on their use in patients with compromised renal function, as well as distinct risk/benefit considerations when used in combinations with statins. Sound judgment and a review of specific agents should be made in all patients, particularly older patients who are likely to be on multiple medications and may have age-related physiological compromise.

There are certain conditions in which the benefits of intensive LDL cholesterol lowering are unclear. Two examples come to mind. In the case of aortic stenosis, particularly calcific aortic stenosis, the benefits of intensive lipid lowering are not well documented. Often this patient population may have concomitant atherosclerosis risk and indeed evidence of aortic atherosclerosis. Treatment, however, in small studies has not been proved to benefit this patient group.[22] Patients on dialysis, also a very high-risk group for cardiovascular events, have not shown clear benefit with concurrent lipid management in reducing cardiovascular events.[23] Beyond risk assessment, there may be other factors that come into play in older persons that affect the decision to prescribe LDL-lowering drugs. These include coexisting diseases, social and economic considerations, and functional age. Ultimately, as with patients of any age, individualized therapy should match the needs of each specific patient.

ADHERENCE

Official guidelines offer a framework to address many specific patient care challenges, yet there are often issues up to and beyond the patient–physician encounter that have an impact on the optimization of outcomes and quality of care. Adherence to treatment is one such issue. Poor adherence to all therapies across all age groups represents a significant challenge to the health care system, leading to suboptimal outcomes and increased costs from additional emergency room visits and hospitalizations. In 2001, the costs associated with nonadherence were estimated at $300 billion. Nonadherence in the elderly is estimated at between 14% and 77% in association with numerous age-related chronic conditions such as hypertension, diabetes, and CVD. These conditions frequently place this age group on complex regimens and an average of five to eight medications daily.[24]

Considerations for Adherence in Older Patients

Older patients may require additional support for medication management and monitoring. Based on a study of elders enrolled in two separate managed care plans, the primary challenges were related to the failure to prescribe appropriate medications, monitoring treatment, providing adequate education, and supporting continuity of treatment among providers. Quality improvement in this regard should focus on errors of omission in which the underuse of potentially beneficial medications manifests potential harm. These omissions may arise from the provider belief that there is insufficient evidence of clinical benefit associated with underrepresentation of older patients in clinical trials, concerns regarding polypharmacy, and substantial financial barriers with insufficient insurance coverage of outpatient prescription drugs.[25]

Underutilization and Nonadherence with Lipid-Lowering Therapies

The beneficial role of statins in secondary prevention is well documented for patients of all age groups; however, in a recently published retrospective, cohort study of more than 75,000 patients older than 65 years, the use of statin therapy declined with increasing age. This treatment paradox suggested that despite an annual 1% increase of mortality risk, there was a great than 6% decline in the use of preventive therapy. Other reviews have commented on the relative "clinical inertia" with respect to using statins in older patients.[26–28]

Additional studies have been completed to assess the specific challenges in using statins in older patients. Brenner and colleagues[29] described a rapid decline in statin persistence in older patients from a retrospective cohort analysis of more than 34,000 New Jersey Medicaid patients. Unlike data as reported in clinical trial experiments, these data suggested that after 5 years, only 26% of patients were still taking their prescribed medications. Several predictors of poor persistence were identified as age (>75 years), socioeconomic disparities, issues of ethnicity, and depression. These findings supported the concept that strategies for improved adherence require early intervention and specific targeting of high-risk groups.

Using a different methodological approach, Jackevicius and colleagues evaluated 2-year adherence in three distinct patient cohorts – those with recent ACS, those with chronic coronary artery disease, and those at high risk of disease. From 1994 through 1998 the population, aged older than 66 years, was fol-

lowed for 2 years after their first prescription for a statin. A total of more than 140,000 patients were included in the analysis. Two-year adherence rates were higher in the ACS group (40.1%), followed by 36.1% in the chronic coronary artery disease catchment, and only 25.4% in the at risk cohort. Although those with evident CHD fared better than primary prevention patients, the adherence of less than 50% suggests that many patients who are started on statin therapy receive limited benefits because of premature discontinuation.[30]

These analyses of nonadherence leave care providers with the challenge of improving adherence in the elderly as well as in all patient groups. A recent series of articles support the Institute of Medicine report that states that much of the care gap between recommended care and actual levels of chronic disease is attributable to medication nonadherence. Although a systems approach must be recognized and acted on by providers, payers, insurers, and policy makers, there are steps individual clinicians and team can take to improve adherence.[31]

For example, providers should acknowledge self-efficacy, or the awareness that an individual patient has the confidence and belief in their ability to take medicine properly. This is related to the issue of a patient's knowledge of their disease and in the case of CVD, an awareness of risk factors. Patients who understand the benefits/necessity of their treatment and have fewer concerns about the risk of prescribed drugs have better self-reported adherence rates. Lastly, there is a clear benefit of a trusting patient–provider relationship, in which the patient has trust in the care decisions being provided by the clinician. At the time of the patient visit, providers should learn to identify specific patient characteristics including age, number and complexities of regimen, motivation, and knowledge. If clinical judgment suggests a risk for nonadherence, caregivers should attempt to intervene early and establish continuity within the practice as well as among providers.[24,31]

CONCLUSION

Appropriate cholesterol management in older patients provides an important opportunity to address cardiovascular risk. As health care providers acknowledge the higher absolute risk of CVD in older patients, they should also acknowledge the benefits of currently available diagnostic and treatment modalities. Implementation of processes that translate the benefits of clinical trials into clinical practice – including adherence – is an urgent priority that requires personal and systematic endorsement.

REFERENCES

1. Enos WF, Holmes RH, Beyer J. Coronary disease among United States soldiers killed in action in Korea. *JAMA.* 1953;152:1090–1093.
2. Berenson GS, Wattigney WA, Tracy RE, et al. Atherosclerosis of the aorta and coronary arteries and cardiovascular risk factors in

persons ages 6 to 30 years and studied at necropsy (the Bogalusa Heart Study). *Am J Cardiol.* 1992;70:851–858.

3. Detection, Evaluation, and Treatment of High Blood Cholesterol in Adults (Adult Treatment Panel III) Full Report; Final Report; National Cholesterol Education Program, National Heart, Lung, and Blood Institute, National Institutes of Health NIH Publication No. 02-5215, September 2002. URL: http://www.nhlbi.nih.gov/guidelines/cholesterol/atp3_rpt.htm, accessed August 8, 2006.

4. Persell SD, Lloyd-Jones DM, Baker DW. National Cholesterol Education Program risk assessment and potential for risk misclassification. *Prevent Med.* 2006;43(5):368–371.

5. Kostis JB. Disputation on the use of age in determining the need for treatment of hypercholesterolemia and hypertension. *J Clin Hypertens.* 2006;8(7):519–520.

6. Yusuf S, Hawken S, Ôunpuu S, et al. on behalf of the INTERHEART Study Investigators. Effect of potentially modifiable risk factors associated with myocardial infarction in 52 countries (the INTERHEART study): case-control study. *Lancet.* 2004;364:937–952

7. Kuller LH, Arnold AM. 10-Year follow-up of subclinical cardiovascular disease and risk of coronary heart disease in the Cardiovascular Health Study. *Arch Intern Med.* 2006;166:71–78.

8. Grundy SM, Cleeman JI. Implications of recent clinical trials for the National Cholesterol Education Program Adult Treatment Panel III Guidelines. *J Am Coll Cardiol.* 2004;44:720–732.

9. Lemaitre RM, Psaty BM, Heckbert SR, Kronmal RA, Newman AB, Burke GL. Therapy with hydroxylmethylglutaryl coenzyme A reductase inhibitors (statins) and associated risk of incident cardiovascular events in older adults – evidence from the Cardiovascular Health Study. *Arch Intern Med.* 2002;162:1395–1400.

10. Scandinavian Simvastatin Survival Study Group. Randomised trial of cholesterol lowering in 4444 patients with coronary heart disease: the Scandinavian Simvastatin Survival Study (4S). *Lancet.* 1994;344:1383–1389.

11. Sacks FM, Pfeffer MA, Moye LA, et al for the Cholesterol and Recurrent Events Trial Investigators. The effect of pravastatin on coronary events after myocardial infarction in patients with average cholesterol levels. *NEJM.* 1996;335:1001–1009.

12. Hunt D, Young P, Simes J, et al. Benefits of pravastatin on cardiovascular events and mortality in older patients with coronary heart disease and equal to or exceed those seen in younger patients; Results from the LIPID Trial. *Ann Intern Med.* 2001;134:931–940.

13. Ray KK, Bach RG, Cannon CP, et al for the PROVE IT-TIMI 22 Investigators. Benefits of achieving the NCEP optional LDL-C goal among elderly patients with ACS. *Eur Heart J.* 2006;27(19):2310–2316.

14. Aronow WS. Drug treatment of peripheral arterial disease in the elderly. *Drugs Aging.* 2006;23(1):1–12.

15. Guidelines for Prevention of Stroke in Patients With Ischemic Stroke or Transient Ischemic Attack. A Statement for Healthcare Professionals From the American Heart Association/American Stroke Association Council on Stroke Co-Sponsored by the Council on Cardiovascular Radiology and Intervention. The American Academy of Neurology affirms the value of this guideline. *Stroke.* 2006;37:577–617.

16. Amarenco P, Bogousslavsky J, Callahan A 3rd, et al for The Stroke Prevention by Aggressive Reduction in Cholesterol Levels (SPARCL) Investigators. High-dose atorvastatin after stroke or transient ischemic attack. *NEJM.* 2006;355:549–559.

17. Davidson MH, Kurlandsky SB, Kleinpell RM, Maki KC. Lipid Management and the Elderly. *Prevent Cardiol.* 2003;6(3):128–133.

18. Rosenson RS. Current overview of statin-induced myopathy. *Am J Med.* 2004;116:408–416.

19. Hey-Hadavi JH, et al. Tolerability of atorvastatin in a population aged ≥65 years: a retrospective pooled analysis of results from fifty randomized clinical trials. *Am J Geriatr Pharmacother.* 2006;4:112–122.

20. Bruckert E, Giral P, Tellier P. Perspectives in cholesterol-lowering therapy. The role of ezetimibe, a new selective inhibitor of intestinal cholesterol absorption. *Circulation.* 2003;107:3124–3128.

21. Pearson T. Effectiveness of the addition of ezetimibe to ongoing statin therapy in modifying lipid profiles and attaining low-density lipoprotein cholesterol goals in older and elderly patients: subanalyses of data from a randomized, double-blind, placebo-controlled trial. *Am J Geriatr Pharmacother.* 2005;4:218–228.

22. Cowell SJ, Newby DE, Prescott RJ, et al. A randomized trial of intensive lipid-lowering therapy in calcific aortic stenosis. *NEJM.* 2005;352:2389–2397.

23. Wanner C, Krane V, März W, et al for the German Diabetes and Dialysis Study Investigators. Atorvastatin in patients with type 2 diabetes mellitus undergoing hemodialysis. *NEJM.* 2005;353:238–248.

24. Chia L, Schlenk EA. Effect of personal and cultural beliefs on medication adherence in the elderly. *Drugs Aging.* 2006;23(3):191–202.

25. Higashi T, Shekelle PG, Solomon DH, et al. The quality of pharmacologic care for vulnerable older patients. *Ann Intern Med.* 2004;140:714–720.

26. Ayanian JZ, Landrum MB, McNeil BJ. Use of cholesterol-lowering therapy by elderly adults after myocardial infarction. *Arch Intern Med.* 2002;162:1013–1019.

27. Ko DT, Mamdani M, Alter D. Lipid-lowering therapy with statins in high-risk elderly patients: the treatment risk paradox. *JAMA.* 2004;291:1864–1870.

28. Dewilde S, Carey IM, Bremner SA, Hilton SR, Cook DG. Evolution of statin prescribing 1994–2001: a case of ageism but not sexism? *Heart.* 2003;89:417–421.

29. Brenner JS, Glynn RJ, Mogen H, et al. Long term persistence in use of statin therapy in elderly patients. *JAMA.* 2002;288:445–456.

30. Jackevicius C, Mamdami M, Tu J. Adherence to statin therapy in elderly patients with and without acute coronary syndromes. *JAMA.* 2002;288:463–467.

31. O'Connor PJ. Improving medication adherence: challenges for physicians, payers, and policy makers. *Arch Intern Med.* 2006;166:1802–1804.

32. Osterberg L, Blaschke T. Adherence to medication. *NEJM.* 2005;353:487–497.

10

HYPERTENSION

B. Brent Simmons, MD, Daniel DeJoseph, MD, Christine Arenson, MD

INTRODUCTION

Hypertension is the single most common outpatient diagnosis in the United States, and older Americans have the highest prevalence of any age group. Therefore, it is vital for clinicians to be comfortable with the classification, treatment, and circumstances unique to the geriatric patient. Adequately treated hypertension has been well documented to help prevent adverse outcomes such as kidney failure, stroke, myocardial infarction, ventricular hypertrophy, and heart failure. Special consideration in older patients, especially those with multiple comorbid illnesses, and frail elders require individualized therapy.

EPIDEMIOLOGY

More than 65 million American adults have hypertension, creating a large public health burden. The overall prevalence of hypertension in the United States is approximately 25%; however, the prevalence for people 60 years or older is much higher at 66%. The Framingham Heart Study indicated the lifetime risk of developing hypertension in this age group to be 90%. The most recent data indicate for patients 60 years and older, 81% of people with hypertension are aware of their diagnosis and approximately 73% of them were treated. Of those treated, only approximately 50% achieved target blood pressure goals. Framingham calculated the lifetime probability of being on antihypertensive medications for patients aged 55–65 years to be 60%. For all people older than 60 years with hypertension, including those not treated, only 36% were at goal, well short of the Healthy People 2010 goal of 50%. Although these statistics are dire, there has been increasing control of hypertension since 1999. Furthermore, the geriatric population is most likely to be aware of their diagnosis, most likely to be treated, and most likely to be at goal. There has also been a trend of increasing use of antihypertensive medication based on compelling

indications (e.g., diabetic on an angiotensin-converting enzyme [ACE] inhibitor).[1,2]

HYPERTENSION AND RISK

Risk Factors for Developing Hypertension

The Strong Heart Study identified multiple metabolic factors as independent risk factors for developing hypertension. Trend analysis showed normotensive patients who, at baseline, were obese, had central fat distribution, high–normal blood pressure, hyperglycemia, or diabetes, were more likely to develop hypertension in the future. Patients with unfavorable lipid profiles were also more likely to develop hypertension.[3] Other risk factors for the development of hypertension include family history, cigarette smoking, black race, high sodium intake, low socioeconomic status, and alcohol intake.

Hypertension as a Risk Factor

Hypertension is an important cardiovascular risk factor, and given its prevalence, one of the most common. Hypertension has well-documented relationship to myocardial infarction and stroke. The stresses hypertension puts on various organ systems can lead to an array of target organ damage such as left ventricular hypertrophy, heart failure, renal insufficiency, and retinopathy. These endpoints seem to be more severe depending on the level of hypertension. One large meta-analysis showed that for patients between the ages of 40 and 70 years, for every decrease of 20 mm Hg in systolic blood pressure (SBP), there was more than a twofold decrease in the incidence of stroke death rate between the ranges of 115/75 to 185/115.[4] Antihypertensive therapy has been shown in multiple trials to be associated with lowering the risk of these cardiovascular endpoints. Therapy results in 30%–40% reductions in stroke, 20%–25% reductions in myocardial infarction, and up to 50% reduction in heart failure.[5]

Table 10.1. JNC Recommended Classification and Management of Hypertension

BP Classification	Systolic BP, mm Hg*		Diastolic BP, mm Hg*	Lifestyle Modification	Initial Drug Therapy Without Compelling Indication	Initial Drug Therapy With Compelling Indications
Normal	<120	and	<80	Encourage		
Prehypertension	120–139	or	80–89	Yes	No antihypertensive drug indicated	Drug(s) for the compelling indications[‡]
Stage 1 hypertension	140–159	or	90–99	Yes	Triazide-type diuretics for most; may consider ACE inhibitor, ARB, β-blocker, CCB, or combination	Drug(s) for the compelling indications Other antihypertensive drugs (diuretics, ACE inhibitor, ARB, β-blocker, CCB) as needed
Stage 2 hypertension	≥160	or	≥100	Yes	2-Drug combination for most (usually thiazide-type diuretic and ACE inhibitor or ARB or β-blocker or CCB)[§]	Drug(s) for the compelling indications Other antihypertensive drugs (diuretics, ACE inhibitor, ARB, β-blocker, CCB) as needed

Abbreviations: ACE, angiotensin-converting enzyme; ARB, angiotensin receptor blocker; BP, blood pressure; CCB, calcium channel blocker.

* Treatment determined by highest BP category.

[‡] Treat patients with chronic kindney disease or diabetes to BP goal of less than 130/80 mm Hg.

[§] Initial combined therapy should be used cautiously in those at risk for orthostatic hypotension.

Table used with permission of JAMA, May 21, 2003; Vol 289(9): 2561.

DIAGNOSIS

The U.S. Preventive Services Task Force recommends routine in-office blood pressure screening for all adults. For the physician to diagnose hypertension confidently, patients must have blood pressures of greater than or equal to 140 systolic or greater than or equal to 90 diastolic on two or more blood pressure readings on at least two different office visits. Diagnostic class is based on the Seventh Report of the Joint National Committee on Prevention, Detection, Evaluation, and Treatment of High Blood Pressure (JNC 7) report classification system (see Table 10.1). Normal is defined as less than 120 systolic blood pressure (SBP) and less than 80 diastolic blood pressure (DBP).

Prehypertension is defined as SBP between 120 and 139 or DBP between 80 and 89. Above these levels, the diagnosis of hypertension is made, starting with Stage 1, which is within the range of 140–159 SBP or 90–99 DBP. Finally, Stage 2 hypertension is defined as SBP greater than or equal to 160 or DBP greater than or equal to 100. These classes all pertain to in-office measurements. Home and ambulatory measurements typically are lower than blood pressures obtained in the office. Because of this phenomenon, JNC 7 further defines self-measurements greater than 135/85 to be considered hypertensive.[6]

Appropriate blood pressure measurement technique involves a seated patient with both feet on the ground and the arm should be supported at the level of the patient's heart. The patient should be seated quietly for at least 5 minutes prior to measurement. It is equally important to be sure the cuff fits the patient's arm correctly because a cuff that is too small or too large will affect the reading and lead to inaccurate results.[6]

Further Evaluation

Further physical examination of the hypertensive patient should include neck, abdominal, and femoral auscultation to detect possible bruits. Careful auscultation of heart and lungs should be conducted. Palpation of the abdomen is recommended to detect possible enlarged kidneys or pulsatile abdominal masses. Lower extremities should be examined for edema and pulses. Neurological examination and examination of optic fundi are also recommended. All patients should undergo an electrocardiogram, both as a baseline tracing, which can be vital for future comparison, and to detect any possible pathology such as ventricular hypertrophy. Blood glucose and lipid profiles should be obtained to determine further cardiac risk factors. Creatinine is an important element of the workup to determine if the patient has any evidence of hypertensive nephropathy and to have a baseline to monitor kidney function over time. Serum electrolytes should be obtained for a baseline

Table 10.2. Initial Evaluation of Hypertension

1. Serum electrolytes
2. Serum creatinine
3. Fasting glucose
4. Lipid panel
5. Electrocardiogram
6. Thyroid-stimulating hormone
7. Complete blood count
8. Urine microalbumin
9. Microscopic urinalysis

measurement, especially because many antihypertensives can alter electrolyte balance.[6] In addition, thyroid-stimulating hormone, complete blood count, microalbumin, and microscopic urinalysis should be included (Table 10.2).

Secondary causes of hypertension should be investigated if the patient is refractory to treatment or if there is concern over a specific cause. Identifiable secondary causes include sleep apnea, renal artery stenosis, and thyroid disease, or, less frequently, primary hyperaldosteronism, Cushing's syndrome, and pheochromocytoma.[6]

TREATMENT

When individualizing treatment decisions in a geriatric population, consideration must be given to the overall health of the patient. A general definition stratifying older patients into "well" and "frail" has been proposed. A "well" elderly patient has a life expectancy of more than 5 years, no deficits in activities of daily living (ADLs) and limited deficits in instrumental activities of daily living (IADLs), and fewer than two comorbid medical conditions, none of which is severe. A "frail" elderly patient has a life expectancy of less than 5 years, significant deficits in ADLs and IADLs, and more than two comorbid medical conditions, one of which is in the severe range.[7]

The treatment of hypertension in frail older adults should be considered on an individual basis. The clinician must give significant thought to potential drug–drug interactions and adverse drug reactions in this population. Some patients and families may have strong health beliefs that favor treating risk factors. Thus, the decision to treat, and how, must be individualized, and based on discussion with the patient or surrogate decision maker, in the overall context of the patient's health, life expectancy, and quality of life. If treatment is instituted, specific medications should be picked based on minimizing risk, and dosages titrated with great care. If the decision is made to not treat, reasoning should be carefully documented in the medical record. In any event, these patients require frequent monitoring and reevaluation of the treatment plan.

The goal of antihypertensive therapy in well elders is to reduce cardiovascular and renal morbidity and mortality. This goal can be accomplished by keeping the blood pressure under 140/90 mm Hg in patients without diabetes or renal disease. For patients with these conditions, blood pressure should be kept below 130/80 mm Hg.

Lifestyle Modification

Treatment should begin with a discussion of lifestyle modifications. All patients with abnormal blood pressure, including those in the prehypertension category, should be encouraged to make specific lifestyle changes (see Table 10.3), in particular, weight reduction in obese patients, adoption of the Dietary Approaches to Stop Hypertension eating plan, sodium reduction, increased physical activity, and moderate alcohol consumption. All patients should be encouraged to stop cigarette smoking. These modifications have been shown to be as effective as single-drug therapy for some patients. In addition to lowering blood pressure, adopting a healthy lifestyle improves overall cardiovascular health. Also, dietary sodium reduction potentiates the efficacy of most antihypertensive medications.

Pharmacotherapy

In patients whose blood pressure is not at goal despite an adequate trial of lifestyle modifications (usually 6 months in a nondiabetic patient, Stage 1 hypertensive) or in patients with Stage 2 hypertension, pharmacological therapy should be offered. The general approach to selecting pharmacotherapy for older adults is based on the guidelines presented in the JNC 7. Special consideration must be given to the very elderly hypertensive patient (>85 years old), because to date few have participated in any randomized controlled trials. Recently, the Hypertension in the Very Elderly Trial (HYVET) demonstrated that treating stage 2 hypertension in patients older than 80 has beneficial effects, including reductions in stroke, cardiovascular death, and heart failure.[8] Initiating or maintaining pharmacotherapy in this population, as with younger frail elders, should be discussed on an individual basis.

There are several classes of drugs commonly prescribed for treating hypertension in the elderly patient, and all are supported by excellent clinical data for reducing cardiovascular endpoints. The most common are thiazide-type diuretics, ACE inhibitors, angiotensin receptor blockers (ARBs), β-blockers, and calcium channel blockers (CCBs). Alpha-blockers are also prescribed, but they should generally be avoided in the elderly because of increased risk of orthostatic hypertension. Alpha-blockers are usually used in combination with another agent for men with prostatism. Most patients are started on a thiazide-type diuretic for first-line therapy. Patients in whom diuretics are contraindicated or with a compelling indication (e.g., diabetics) may be started on a different drug for first-line therapy.

Thiazides

Thiazide-type diuretics are effective, inexpensive, and well tolerated when used at low doses (hydrochlorothiazide ≤25 mg).

Table 10.3. Lifestyle Modifications to Manage Hypertension *†

Modification	Recommendation	Approximate SBP Reduction (Range)
Weight reduction	Maintain normal body weight (body mass index 18.5–24.9 kg/m²).	5–20 mm Hg/10 kg weight loss
Adopt DASH eating plan	Consume a diet rich in fruits, vegetables, and low-fat dairy products with a reduced content of saturated and total fat.	8–14 mm Hg
Dietary sodium reduction	Reduce dietary sodium intake to no more than 100 mmol/day (2.4 g sodium or 6 g sodium chloride).	2–8 mm Hg
Physical activity	Engage in regular aerobic physical activity such as brisk walking (at least 30 min/day, most days of the week).	4–9 mmHg
Moderation of alcohol	Limit consumption to no more than 2 drinks (1 oz or 30 mL ethanol; e.g., 24 oz beer, 10 oz wine, or 3 oz 80-proof whiskey) per day in most men and to no more than 1 drink per day in women and lighter weight persons.	2–4 mmHg

DASH=Dietary Approaches to Stop Hypertension.

* For overall cardiovascular risk reduction, stop smoking.

† The effects of implementing these modifications are dose and time dependent and could be greater for some individuals.

Source: JAMA. 2003;289(9):2564.

When used as a single agent, lower doses exert as much antihypertensive effect as higher doses, with significantly fewer side effects. Most patients can expect a 10–15 mm Hg lowering in blood pressure, so combining a thiazide diuretic with another agent is usually necessary for patients with stage 2 hypertension. Thiazide-type diuretics can cause hypokalemia and hyponatremia, impair glucose tolerance, increase serum lipid concentration, and increase uric acid concentration. They should be used with caution in people with gout. Again, using low doses minimizes most of these side effects.

Angiotensin-Converting Enzyme (ACE) Inhibitors

ACE inhibitors can be used as first-line therapy in diabetics, especially those with microalbuminuria. The Second Australian National Blood Pressure trial reported slightly better outcomes in white men started on an ACE inhibitor than a diuretic as first-line therapy.[9] Other compelling indications for using ACE inhibitors are found in patients with heart failure, high coronary disease risk, chronic kidney disease, postmyocardial infarction, and for recurrent stroke prevention. ACE inhibitors are generally well tolerated but can cause a cough in 5%–10% of patients, hyperkalemia in patients with renal insufficiency, and angioedema. Both ACE inhibitors and ARBs can cause a rise in creatinine as high as 35% above the patient's baseline, but this rise is not a reason to stop therapy unless accompanied by hyperkalemia.

Angiotensin Receptor Blockers

ARBs have a similar use profile to ACE inhibitors, although they are generally not used as first-line agents for lack of adequate randomized, controlled trials with older adults. A recent meta-analysis comparing ACE inhibitors and ARBs in the treatment of hypertension showed no difference in blood pressure control.[10] ARBs cause less coughing than ACE inhibitors. Incidence of hyperkalemia is similar to that of ACE inhibitors.

Calcium Channel Blockers

CCBs have been shown to reduce cardiovascular disease and stroke incidence in patients with diabetes, and the dihydropyridine (i.e., amlodipine) class of CCBs has been shown to reduce stroke risk in older hypertensive patients. They are often used in combination with diuretics. The Beers Criteria for potentially inappropriate medication use in older adults lists short-acting nifedipine as a medication to be avoided in the elderly because of the potential for hypotension.[11] In general, short-acting CCBs should not be used. As a class, CCBs can cause peripheral edema and can exacerbate constipation and gastroesophageal reflux symptoms.

Beta-Blockers

Beta-blockers are generally not considered first-line agents in older adults. A recent meta-analysis showed an increased risk of stroke for patients taking β-blockers when compared with patients taking other antihypertensive agents, although still lower than patients not receiving therapy.[12] Compelling indications for β-blocker therapy are found in patients with heart failure, postmyocardial infarction, high coronary disease risk, and diabetes. Beta-blockers should be used with caution in patients with chronic obstructive pulmonary disease and asthma, particularly propranolol.

After initiating treatment, patients should return monthly for medication adjustments, with the goal of achieving blood pressure control while minimizing dosages and the number of medicines used. Once blood pressure is controlled, patients

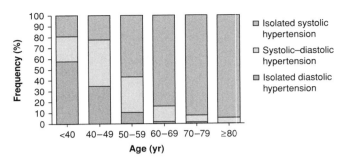

Figure 10.1. Isolated systolic hypertension (used with permission of N Eng J Med Aug 21, 2007; Vol 357(8): 791). See color plates.

can return for medication adjustments every 3–6 months, depending on their comorbidities. After baseline laboratory tests have been obtained, patients should have at least their sodium, potassium, and creatinine monitored every 6–12 months depending on their medication regimen and their stability. Two-thirds of patients will require a second agent to achieve goal blood pressure. This agent can come from any of the other classes and should be chosen based on the patient's other comorbidities.

Palliative Care

There are no specific guidelines for treating hypertension in patients on comfort measures such as hospice patients. When deciding whether to continue or discontinue a specific antihypertensive, it is important to keep in mind that if a patient develops symptoms from elevated blood pressure (i.e., headache), continuing the antihypertensive should be considered a palliative measure. However, if the patient or health care proxy desires to cease antihypertensive treatment, it is appropriate to do so.

ISOLATED SYSTOLIC HYPERTENSION AND PULSE PRESSURE

In the elderly population, elevated SBP has been found to be a more important risk factor than DBP.[13] This represents an ongoing reassessment over the past several decades. Many patients are unaware of this shift and still believe DBP to be the more important factor. SBP increases steadily with age while DBP increases steadily and parallel to SBP up to approximately the age of 50 years; after 60 years, it begins to decease while SBP continues to increase leading to an overwhelming preponderance of isolated systolic hypertension in the geriatric population (Figure 10.1).[14] The National Health and Nutrition Examination Survey study reported isolated systolic hypertension to be present in 65% of all hypertensive patients older than 60 years, regardless of sex.[15]

This phenomenon is explained by the decrease in compliance and increase of stiffness that accompanies the aged arterial vessels. The increase in SBP and decrease in DBP also result in

increased pulse pressure (PP), which is the difference between SBP and DBP and is considered to be an independent risk factor for coronary artery disease (CAD). Framingham Heart Study data were used to study the effects of increased PP and CAD risk. The results of this analysis showed that for any given SBP, the risk for CAD increased as DBP decreased. In other words, patients with a blood pressure of 160/70 mm Hg consistently showed higher CAD risk than patients with blood pressures of 160/100 mm Hg. Alternatively, for any given DBP, increasing the SBP leads to incrementally higher CAD risk. This observation of risk inversely related to DBP for a specific SBP supports the hypothesis that PP is an independent risk factor. Increasing PP is believed to reflect increased calcification and stiffening of the large arteries, and, therefore, serves as a proxy for more severe atherosclerotic burden.[14] It is not totally clear if this increased risk is caused by higher PP or if the higher PP is simply a marker for more severe cardiovascular disease. What is clear is that SBP is the more important risk factor in elderly patients and that clinicians should not necessarily be reassured by DBP at goal if SBP is elevated.

J-Curve Hypothesis

Understanding the relationship between SBP, DBP, PP, and cardiac risk is vital to understand the so-called "J-Curve Hypothesis." The term J-Curve refers to the "J" shape of the mortality curve for DBP. As DBP decreases, so does mortality until it hits a nadir, and then as DBP continues to drop, mortality increases incrementally. This phenomenon led to concern that treating isolated SBP would lead to a concurrent drop in DBP and would paradoxically increase mortality. Evidence has shown DBP less than 60 to be potentially harmful, especially in patients with documented CAD; however, this risk is independent of treatment with antihypertensive medication. A study published in 2002 addressed this issue and demonstrated that there was in fact a higher risk for fatal events at lower DBP; however, this observation was consistent among patients receiving antihypertensive medications and those who did not. There was no evidence of increasing cardiovascular death by treating systolic hypertension. The conclusion of this study was that the J-shaped mortality curve is independent of antihypertensive treatment and is most likely explained by other factors, such as low DBP acting as a marker for overall poorer health.[16]

SUMMARY

Hypertension is a very common morbidity among elderly patients. It is a significant risk factor leading to the most common causes of death in the United States, namely myocardial infarction and stroke. Treating patients to JNC 7 goals has shown significant reductions in morbidity and mortality. Special consideration needs to be given to frail elderly, and those over the age of 85 years. Multiple medications are available, each with its own benefits, adverse effects, and compelling indications, leading to each patient needing their own individualized treatment plan. Isolated systolic blood pressure is an important subgroup of hypertensives most commonly seen in the elderly which represents decreased compliance of arterial vasculature. A normal DBP should not be reassuring in these patients, and they should be treated to JNC 7 goals.

REFERENCES

1. Ong KL, Gheung BMY, Yu BM, et al. Prevalence, awareness, treatment, and control of hypertension among United States adults 1999–2004. *Hypertension.* 2007;49:69–75.
2. Vasan, RS, Beiser A, Seshadri S, et al. Residual lifetime risk for developing hypertension in middle-aged women and men, The Framingham Heart Study. *JAMA.* 2002;287:1003–1010.
3. DeSimone G, Devereux RB, Chinali M, et al. Risk factors for arterial hypertension in adults with initial optimal blood pressure: the Strong Heart Study. *Hypertension.* 2006;47:162–167.
4. Lewington S, Clarke R, Qizilbash N, et al. Age specific relevance of usual blood pressure to vascular mortality: a meta-analysis of individual data for one million adults in 61 prospective studies. *Lancet.* 2002;360:1903–1913.
5. Neal B, MacMahon S, Chapman N. Effects of ACE inhibitors, calcium antagonists, and other blood pressure lowering drugs: results of prospectively designed overviews of randomized trials. *Lancet.* 2000;355:1955–1964.
6. Chobanian AV, Bakris GL, Black HR, et al. The seventh report of the joint national committee on prevention, detection, evaluation, and treatment of high blood pressure, The JNC 7 Report. *JAMA.* 2003;289:2560–2572.
7. Parks SM, Hsieh C. Preventive health care for older patients. *Prim Care Clin Office Pract.* 2002;29:599–614.
8. Beckett NS, Peters R, Fletcher AE, et al. Treatment of hypertension in patients 80 years of age or older. *NEJM.* 2008; 358:1887–1898.
9. Wing LMH, Reid CM, Ryan P, et al. for Second Australian National Blood Pressure Study Group. A comparison of outcomes with angiotensin-converting-enzyme inhibitors and diuretics for hypertension in the elderly. *NEJM.* 2003;348:583–592.
10. Matchar DB, McCrory DC, Orlando LA, et al. Systematic review: comparative effectiveness of angiotensin-converting enzyme inhibitors and angiotensin II receptor blockers for treating essential hypertension. *Ann Intern Med.* 2008;148:16–29.
11. Fick DM, Cooper JW, Wade WE, Waller JL, Maclean JR, Beers MH. Updating the Beers Criteria for Potentially Inappropriate Medication Use in Older Adults: results of a US consensus panel of experts. *Arch Intern Med.* 2003;163:2716–2724.
12. Lindholm LH, Carlberg B, Samuelsson O. Should Beta-blockers remain first choice in the treatment of primary hypertension? A meta-analysis. *Lancet.* 2005;366:1545–1552.
13. Chobanian AV. Isolated systolic hypertension in the elderly. *NEJM.* 2007;357:789–796.
14. Frankin SS, Khan SA, Wong ND, et al. Is pulse pressure useful in predicting risk for coronary heart disease? The Framingham Heart Study. *Circulation.* 1999;100:354–360.
15. Izzo JL, Levy D, Black HR. Importance of systolic blood pressure in older Americans. *Hypertension.* 2000;35:1021–1024.
16. Boutitie F, Gueyffier F, Pocock S, et al. J-shaped relationship between blood pressure and mortality in hypertensive patients: new insights from a meta-analysis of individual patient data. *Ann Intern Med.* 2002;136:438–448.

11

Diagnosis and Management of Heart Disease in the Elderly

Joshua M. Stolker, MD, Michael W. Rich, MD

SIGNIFICANCE OF GERIATRIC CARDIOLOGY

As the leading cause of death and major disability in the United States, cardiovascular disease (CVD) has become a modern epidemic resulting in part from the aging of our population. Nearly two-thirds of all cardiovascular hospitalizations occur in patients aged 65 years and older, more than 83% of cardiovascular deaths occur in geriatric individuals, and an estimated 70% of Americans older than the age of 70 years have clinically recognized cardiovascular diagnoses.[1] For these reasons, both geriatric and nongeriatric practitioners should become familiar with strategies for CVD prevention and management in older individuals.

EFFECTS OF AGING ON THE CARDIOVASCULAR SYSTEM

Aging is associated with many alterations of cardiovascular structure and function (Table 11.1).[2] Some of the most clinically relevant changes include increasing vascular stiffness, impaired endothelial function, impaired left ventricular relaxation and compliance, diminished responsiveness to neurohormonal signals such as β-adrenergic stimulation, and degeneration of the sinus node and electrical conduction system. These factors contribute to the development of medical conditions such as hypertension, coronary artery disease (CAD), and heart failure (HF), and many components of these aging processes also modulate clinical presentations and responses to cardiovascular therapies in the geriatric population. Similarly, aging affects other organ systems (Table 11.2), which frequently interact with CVDs and therapeutics. Other influences related to medical comorbidities, absorptive and metabolic alterations, behavioral or neuropsychiatric changes, and financial issues frequently play a role in modulating cardiovascular prognosis in older individuals as well.[3]

ISCHEMIC HEART DISEASE

Epidemiology and Primary Prevention

In 2002, 58% of all Americans discharged with a first-listed diagnosis of CAD were aged 65 years or older.[1] The incidence of acute myocardial infarction (MI) increases with age (Figure 11.1), and more than 83% of people who die from atherosclerotic CAD are aged 65 years and older.[4] Importantly, whereas younger patients with MI tend to be male, in the geriatric population the number of men and women with CAD is nearly equal.

Increasing age is the strongest predictor of CAD, a fact that is emphasized in risk assessment tools such as the Framingham Risk Score.[5] Age-related changes in the arterial wall and prolonged exposure to other risk factors contribute to the paramount importance of advancing age as a predictor of ischemic cardiovascular events. Apart from age, other major risk factors for CAD include hypertension, dyslipidemia, tobacco use, family history (with incompletely defined genetic factors), and environmental contributions such as atherogenic diet and sedentary lifestyle.[5] Diabetes is considered a CAD risk-equivalent, because diabetics without CAD experience 7-year rates of MI that are similar to patients with known CAD.[6] Although these risk factors are discussed in detail elsewhere, it is important to note that their prevalence is accentuated in the geriatric population. For example, 58.9% of men and 72.5% of women between the ages of 65 and 74 years have hypertension, and at older ages these numbers increase to 68.4% of men and 82.8% of women. Similarly, among Americans aged 60–79 years, more than 50% of men and more than 70% of women have borderline high or high-risk cholesterol levels by current guidelines.[1] Importantly, these risk factors often cluster in individual patients,[7] with additive or multiplicative effects on the risk of future CAD and ischemic cardiovascular events (Figure 11.2).[8–11] In addition, subclinical CVD is highly prevalent

Table 11.1. Effects of Aging on the Cardiovascular System

Gross anatomy

- Increased LV wall thickness
- Decreased LV cavity size
- Endocardial thickening and sclerosis
- Increased left atrial size
- Valvular fibrosis and sclerosis
- Increased epicardial fat

Histology

- Increased lipid and amyloid deposition
- Increased collagen degeneration and fibrosis
- Calcification of fibrous skeleton, valve rings, and coronary arteries
- Shrinkage of myocardial fibers with focal hypertrophy
- Decreased mitochondria, altered mitochondrial membranes
- Decreased nucleus: myofibril size ratio

Biochemical changes

- Decreased protein elasticity
- Numerous changes in enzyme content and activity affecting most metabolic pathways, but no change in myosin adenosine triphosphatase activity
- Decreased catechol synthesis, especially norepinephrine
- Decreased acetylcholine synthesis
- Decreased activity of nitric oxide synthase

Conduction system

- Degeneration of sinus node pacemaker and transition cells
- Decreased number of conducting cells in the AV-node and HIS–Purkinje system
- Increased connective tissue, fat, and amyloid
- Increased calcification around conduction system

Vasculature

- Decreased distensibility of large- and medium-sized arteries
- Impaired endothelial function
- Aorta and muscular arteries become dilated, elongated, and tortuous
- Increased wall thickness
- Increased connective tissue and calcification

Autonomic nervous system

- Decreased responsiveness to β-adrenergic stimulation
- Increased circulating catecholamines, decreased tissue catecholamines
- Decreased α-adrenergic receptors in left ventricle
- Decreased cholinergic responsiveness
- Diminished response to Valsalva and baroreceptor stimulation
- Decreased heart rate variability

Table 11.2. Effects of Aging on Other Organ Systems

Kidneys

- Gradual decline in glomerular filtration rate, ~8 cc/min/decade
- Impaired fluid and electrolyte homeostasis

Lungs

- Reduced ventilatory capacity
- Increased ventilation/perfusion mismatching

Neurohumoral system

- Reduced cerebral perfusion autoregulatory capacity
- Diminished reflex responsiveness
- Impaired thirst mechanism

Hemostatic system

- Increased levels of coagulation factors
- Increased platelet activity and aggregability
- Increased inflammatory cytokines and C-reactive protein
- Increased inhibitors of fibrinolysis and angiogenesis

Musculoskeletal system

- Decreased muscle mass (sarcopenia)
- Decreased bone mass (osteopenia), especially in women

in the geriatric population[12] and magnifies the risk of developing CAD.

Clinical Presentation

Whereas substernal chest pain or pressure is considered the hallmark of obstructive CAD, geriatric individuals frequently present without symptoms of classic angina. Elderly patients may experience dyspnea, nausea or gastrointestinal distress, presyncope or syncope, generalized malaise or fatigue, diaphoresis, altered mental status, or even no symptoms at all when experiencing acute coronary syndromes (ACS). Overall, the proportion of patients with acute MI who present with chest pain decreases with age,[13] although dyspnea remains a prominent presenting symptom. Exertional angina may not occur because of sedentary lifestyle or limited functional capacity in frail individuals, so the diagnosis of CAD may be delayed.

Physical findings are variable; however, subacute or late presentations in the geriatric population with MI may lead to more profound cardiovascular deterioration and associated signs of HF, pericarditis, acute mitral regurgitation, hypotension, or shock. Other findings may include pallor, confusion, tachycardia, low-grade fever, leukocytosis, or elevated sedimentation rate. Bradycardia is common with inferior MI, resulting from ischemia of the sinoatrial or atrioventricular node and vagal nerve input related to the Bezold–Jarisch reflex. Individuals presenting with hypotension, HF, prolonged ischemia,

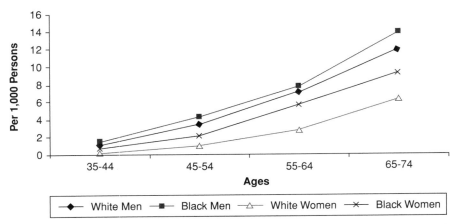

Figure 11.1. Annual rate of first heart attacks by age, sex, and race in the Atherosclerosis Risk In Communities (ARIC) Study, 1987–2000

or life-threatening arrhythmias have a markedly increased risk of death, and the mortality rate following acute MI increases exponentially with age (Figure 11.3).[14]

Diagnosis of Myocardial Infarction

The electrocardiogram (ECG) is the first step in evaluating a patient with a potential ACS, with ST-segment deviations signaling myocardial ischemia or MI. ST-segment *elevation* of 1 mm or greater in two or more contiguous ECG leads suggests myocardial injury and requires immediate evaluation for reperfusion therapy (see later). These infarctions are often associated with the development of Q-waves and deep, symmetrical T-wave inversions. New left bundle branch block at presentation is considered equivalent to ST-elevation MI in terms of urgency and management strategy. ST-segment *depression*

of at least 1 mm in two or more contiguous leads suggests coronary ischemia, and this clinical scenario also should be treated urgently in a hospital setting. Of note, many patients with ACS do not have diagnostic ECG findings, and the proportion of such patients increases progressively with age because of pre-existing conduction system disease (e.g., left bundle branch block), ventricular pacemakers, left ventricular hypertrophy, prior MI, metabolic and electrolyte abnormalities, or drugs affecting the ST-segment, including digoxin and antiarrhythmic agents.

The diagnosis of MI is confirmed when serum biomarkers of myocardial necrosis are elevated. Troponin-I and troponin-T offer the best combination of sensitivity and specificity for diagnosing acute MI. Troponin levels peak by approximately 24 hours after the onset of infarction and may remain elevated for several days to weeks. Importantly, serum troponin levels may be mildly elevated in the presence of renal insufficiency, which can confound the diagnosis of acute MI, especially in older patients who often have impaired renal function. Although

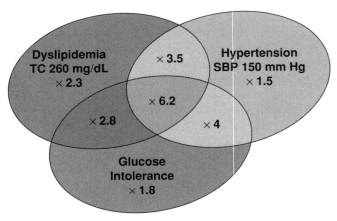

Figure 11.2. Impact of dyslipidemia, hypertension, and glucose intolerance on cardiovascular risk.*

*Compared with risk for a 40-year-old male nonsmoker with total cholesterol = 185 mg/dL, systolic blood pressure = 120 mm Hg, no glucose intolerance, and no electrocardiographic LV hypertrophy, whose probability of developing CVD is 15/1000 (1.5%) in 8 years. See color plates.

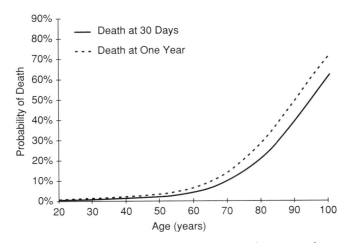

Figure 11.3. Probability of mortality at 30 days and 1 year as a function of age in the GUSTO-I trial (N = 41,021).

less reliable than the troponins, the MB isoenzyme of creatine kinase (CK-MB) is also elevated in patients with significant myocardial injury. CK-MB levels usually return to normal within 72 hours of MI, a feature that may aid in determining MI acuity in patients with elevated troponins of uncertain duration.

The high prevalence of atypical presentations and nondiagnostic ECG findings in the geriatric population requires a higher index of suspicion for acute MI in elderly patients. Delayed diagnosis is common in older patients, reducing the "window of opportunity" for implementing appropriate treatment and limiting the extent of ischemic damage. Treatment delays also increase the risk for complications, including HF, arrhythmias, hypotension, myocardial rupture, and shock.

Other cardiovascular and medical conditions with similar symptom complexes should be included in the differential diagnosis for MI, especially because many of these diseases also occur more frequently in elderly individuals. Chest pain without ECG changes could signify unstable angina, but other life-threatening conditions such as pulmonary embolus, aortic dissection, acute pericardial disease, pneumonia, severe peptic ulcer disease, cholecystitis, pancreatitis, or esophageal rupture must also be considered.

Pharmacological Management of Myocardial Infarction

Acute MI with ST-segment elevation usually involves atherosclerotic plaque rupture and associated thrombotic occlusion of an epicardial coronary artery. A large proportion of infarctions in the geriatric population, however, occur without ST-segment elevation and arise because of a mismatch between oxygen supply and demand in the setting of fixed coronary obstruction. For this reason, acute MI in the elderly often occurs in association with an infection (e.g., pneumonia or sepsis), significant hypertension or hypotension, anemia, perioperative volume shifts, or other systemic illness such as thyroid disease. Therapies are directed toward improving coronary blood flow, reducing myocardial oxygen demand, reducing the risk of coronary thrombosis, correcting the precipitating illness (e.g., infection), reducing sympathetic tone, and preventing adverse remodeling of hypoperfused myocardium.

The major therapeutic options for acute MI are listed in Table 11.3. All patients should be supported initially with supplemental oxygen to improve oxygen-carrying capacity to ischemic myocardium. Intravenous access and telemetry monitoring are imperative to identify and treat potential complications of MI. Morphine and nitroglycerin should be administered as needed to control pain and dyspnea.

Antiplatelet Therapy

Aspirin 160–325 mg should be administered immediately and continued indefinitely at a dose of 75–325 mg/day.[15,16] Aspirin reduces mortality in patients with unstable angina or acute MI, and the benefit of aspirin therapy increases with age, from a 1% absolute mortality reduction for those younger than age 60 years to a 4.7% absolute mortality reduction for those

Table 11.3. Management of Acute MI

- General measures
    - Oxygen to maintain arterial saturation ≥90%
    - Telemetry monitoring
    - Morphine for pain and dyspnea
    - Nitroglycerin for ischemia and HF
- Antiplatelet and antithrombotic therapy
    - Aspirin
    - Clopidogrel (withhold if bypass surgery indicated)
    - Glycoprotein IIb/IIIa inhibitors
    - Unfractionated or low-molecular-weight heparin
- Beta-blockers
- ACEIs
- Other agents
    - ARBs (if ACEIs contraindicated)
    - Eplerenone (if reduced LV systolic function)
    - Lipid-lowering agents (i.e., statin drugs)
- With compelling indications
    - Calcium channel blockers (immediate-release nifedipine contraindicated)
    - Antiarrhythmic agents
- Reperfusion therapy
    - Fibrinolysis (ST-elevation or new left bundle branch block only)
    - Primary coronary angioplasty and/or stenting
    - Urgent coronary bypass surgery in selected cases
- Prior to hospital discharge
    - Measurement of serum lipid levels
    - Assessment of LV function
    - Tobacco cessation counseling
    - Nutritional evaluation
    - Exercise counseling and consideration for cardiac rehabilitation

aged 70 years and older.[17] Clopidogrel is a reasonable alternative (300–600 mg loading dose followed by 75 mg/day) in individuals unable to take aspirin, and aspirin plus clopidogrel reduces the risk of death or reinfarction after MI by approximately 20% when compared with aspirin alone.[18] Despite this benefit, the use of clopidogrel is controversial because of its high cost and incremental bleeding risks (especially during surgical procedures), and it should be withheld in patients potentially needing immediate bypass surgery. In addition, although improvement in cardiovascular outcomes has been demonstrated for patients older and younger than the age of 65 years, the utility of clopidogrel in patients older than the age of 75 years is unknown.

Glycoprotein IIb/IIIa inhibitors (eptifibatide, tirofiban, abciximab) block the final common pathway of platelet aggregation and improve clinical outcomes in patients with non-ST-elevation ACS. High-risk patients tend to benefit most, particularly when undergoing percutaneous coronary intervention (PCI), but the risk of bleeding increases with age. Few studies have enrolled individuals older than the age of 75 years, and one study demonstrated higher event rates in patients older than the age of 80 years receiving eptifibatide,[19] so the value of these agents in the elderly remains unclear. Abciximab should only be used in conjunction with planned PCI, whereas eptifibatide or tirofiban may be used even with conservative therapeutic approaches.[16] Because of a high risk of hemorrhage, glycoprotein IIb/IIIa inhibitors are contraindicated in patients older than the age of 75 years who are receiving thrombolytic therapy for ST-elevation MI,[15] and their incremental benefit in older patients receiving clopidogrel remains unclear.

Antithrombotic Therapy

In patients with acute MI, unfractionated or low-molecular-weight heparin should be administered immediately in addition to the antiplatelet agents described previously, particularly in patients with high-risk features such as large anterior MI, associated atrial fibrillation (AF), or recurrent ischemia.[15,16] Intravenous unfractionated heparin is also required with certain thrombolytics (e.g., alteplase, reteplase, tenecteplase). The value of routine unfractionated heparin therapy in elderly patients has been questioned based on an analysis suggesting increased bleeding and longer hospital length-of-stay in Medicare beneficiaries receiving heparin in the setting of acute MI.[20] The newer low-molecular-weight heparins (i.e., enoxaparin, dalteparin) offer more predictable degrees of anticoagulation with easier subcutaneous administration and monitoring, but declining renal function and increasing age are associated with increased rates of hemorrhagic complications. Nevertheless, the combined endpoint of death, MI, and recurrent angina is reduced,[21] with significant benefits in older patients.[22] Thus, administration of low-molecular-weight heparin is preferable to unfractionated heparin, but these agents must be used with caution, if at all, in patients with severe renal insufficiency (creatinine clearance <30 mL/min) and should be avoided when coronary bypass surgery is planned within 24 hours.[16]

Patients with large anterior MI or evidence for a left ventricular thrombus should be treated with warfarin for 3 months after MI to maintain an international normalized ratio of 2.0–3.0. Long-term therapy with warfarin is indicated in patients with AF, mechanical prosthetic heart valves, or other conditions requiring systemic anticoagulation. Older patients are at increased risk for warfarin-associated bleeding complications, especially when warfarin is used in combination with aspirin or clopidogrel.

Beta-Blockers

Beta-blockers reduce mortality, recurrent ischemia, and arrhythmias in patients with acute MI.[15,16] Contraindications include bradyarrhythmias, hypotension, moderate or severe HF

during MI, or active bronchospasm. A history of obstructive lung disease alone should not preclude β-blocker therapy. In a pooled analysis of several clinical trials, early treatment with β-blockers reduced mortality by 23% in older patients with ACS, but had no effect in younger patients.[3] In addition, long-term β-blocker treatment after MI is associated with 6 lives saved per 100 older patients treated, compared with only 2.1 lives saved per 100 younger patients. Intravenous metoprolol and atenolol are approved for treatment of acute MI in the United States. Metoprolol, propranolol, and timolol are approved for long-term use after MI, and carvedilol is approved for use after MI in patients with left ventricular (LV) ejection fractions less than 40%.

Angiotensin and Aldosterone Inhibition

Angiotensin-converting enzyme inhibitors (ACEIs) reduce mortality in MI, particularly in geriatric individuals aged 65–74 years[23] and in the setting of HF, LV dysfunction, or anterior ST-elevation MI. In geriatric patients, ACEIs reduce mortality by 17%–34%, with an absolute benefit that is three times greater than in younger individuals.[24–26] Angiotensin receptor blockers ([ARBs] e.g., candesartan or valsartan) are suitable alternatives for ACEI-intolerant patients, but head-to-head trials have confirmed that ACEIs are the preferred medications in patients with MI.[27] Serious potential adverse effects with both classes of drugs include hypotension, renal failure, and hyperkalemia – initiation and up-titration of these medications must be performed with caution in elderly patients with renal dysfunction or low blood pressure in the MI setting. Many authorities recommend starting therapy with captopril or enalapril, which have short half-lives, followed by conversion to a longer-acting agent once tolerance is confirmed.

Eplerenone is a selective aldosterone antagonist that reduces mortality and cardiovascular hospitalizations at 2 years in acute MI patients with LV systolic dysfunction (ejection fraction <40% at time of event) and either HF or diabetes.[28] Like spironolactone, eplerenone requires close monitoring of renal function and serum potassium levels after initiation and during follow-up.

Statins

Statin therapy improves clinical outcomes after acute MI and should be initiated in all patients prior to hospital discharge.[5] The benefits of statin treatment have been verified in geriatric patients with known CAD or vascular disease,[29–32] with one study demonstrating a 15% reduction in recurrent MI, stroke, or cardiovascular death in patients aged 70–82 years.[32] Intensive statin treatment after MI has been shown to reduce further the risk of recurrent events,[33–35] and observational data suggest that an aggressive approach to lipid therapy may benefit elderly patients as well.[36] Higher statin doses are, however, associated with an increased risk of adverse effects such as myalgias and myopathy; statin therapy must, therefore, be titrated carefully in elderly patients to achieve an optimal reduction in low-density lipoprotein (LDL) cholesterol without precipitating side effects.

Other Agents

Nitrates[24] and intravenous morphine are recommended for reducing ischemia and ongoing angina, but neither agent has been shown to reduce mortality or recurrent cardiovascular events. Similarly, long-acting calcium channel blockers are safe in select individuals with ongoing ischemia and either hypertension or supraventricular tachyarrhythmias (SVTs) in the setting of MI, but these agents have no demonstrated mortality benefit and short-acting dihydropyridines (e.g., nifedipine) are detrimental.[16] Empiric antiarrhythmic drugs (e.g., lidocaine or amiodarone), magnesium therapy, and glucose-insulin-potassium infusions are not recommended in acute MI in the absence of a specific indication.

Reperfusion in Acute Myocardial Infarction

Multiple clinical trials have demonstrated the efficacy of reperfusion therapy for acute MI associated with ST-segment elevation or new left bundle branch block, with reductions in morbidity and mortality if the occluded artery is recanalized within 6–12 hours.[15,16] Therefore, these patients should undergo thrombolytic or catheter-directed reperfusion therapy without delay. Selected patients with left main involvement or multivessel CAD may require urgent bypass surgery. The absolute mortality benefit of thrombolysis in patients older than 75 years is nearly double that in patients younger than 55 years despite a significant increase in hemorrhagic complications.[37,38] The risk of intracranial hemorrhage is 1%–2% in elderly individuals receiving thrombolytic therapy, so many authorities recommend judicious use of these agents in patients older than 75 (Table 11.4).[15] Catheter-based PCI is associated with better outcomes and fewer major complications than thrombolytic therapy,[39,40] although frail elderly patients with multiple medical comorbidities are markedly underrepresented in all trials evaluating PCI. Nonetheless, PCI is the preferred method of reperfusion for elderly patients with ST-elevation MI if readily available. For patients who experience clinical reperfusion after thrombolytic therapy (i.e., resolution of chest pain and ST-elevations), routine coronary angiography is not indicated unless additional high-risk features are present. At any age, in-hospital revascularization appears to benefit patients with recurrent ischemic episodes, pulmonary edema, hemodynamic instability, ventricular arrhythmias, or high-risk findings on a stress test performed prior to discharge.

In elderly patients with ACS without ST-segment elevation, thrombolytic therapy is contraindicated and the role of PCI is unclear. Investigators from the Thrombolysis in Myocardial Infarction (TIMI) group have identified seven variables that identify high-risk individuals presenting with unstable angina or non-ST-elevation MI (Table 11.5).[41] This TIMI risk score may aid in triaging patients to an early invasive (i.e., coronary angiography) versus early conservative strategy (i.e.,

Table 11.4. Criteria for Fibrinolytic Therapy in Older Adults

Indications

- Symptoms of acute myocardial infarction within 6–12 hours of onset*

- ST-elevation ≥1 mm in 2 or more contiguous limb leads, or ≥2 mm in 2 or more contiguous precordial leads, or left bundle branch block not known to be present previously

Contraindications (absolute)

- Any prior intracranial hemorrhage or hemorrhagic stroke

- Ischemic stroke within the past 3 months (except if occurring within 3 hours)

- Known malignant intracranial neoplasm or structural vascular lesion

- Active internal bleeding (excluding menses)

- Suspected aortic dissection

- Significant closed head or facial trauma within 3 months

Contraindications (relative)

- Blood pressure ≥180/110 mm Hg on presentation, not readily controlled

- Prior ischemic stroke (>3 mo ago)

- Advanced dementia, other intracranial pathology not described in contraindications

- Traumatic or prolonged cardiopulmonary resuscitation (>10 min)

- Recent major trauma, surgery, or internal bleeding (within 2–4 wk)

- Noncompressible vascular puncture (e.g., subclavian intravenous line)

- Active peptic ulcer

- Pregnancy

- For streptokinase/anistreplase: prior exposure or allergic reaction to these agents

- Systemic anticoagulation with warfarin or heparin products prior to MI presentation (greater coagulopathy = greater hemorrhagic risk)

* Within 6 hours in patients ≥75 years of age.

medical therapy, with invasive assessment only for patients with recurrent ischemia or other clinical indications), and a similar approach is recommended by national guidelines for acute MI.[16] Several of the most important discriminators – including increasing age, elevated cardiac proteins, and ST-segment deviation at presentation – have also been associated with higher rates of in-hospital mortality in large observational databases.[42] Because older age is associated with worse outcomes in acute MI, early coronary angiography is recommended in geriatric patients with recurrent ischemia, HF, or hemodynamic instability who are suitable candidates for percutaneous or surgical revascularization.[43]

Table 11.5. TIMI Risk Score Variables for Predicting Adverse Clinical Outcomes in Non-ST-Elevation ACS*

- Age ≥65 y
- ≥3 risk factors for CAD
- Prior coronary stenosis of ≥50%
- ST-segment deviation on presenting ECG
- At least 2 anginal events in the prior 24 h
- Use of aspirin in prior 7 d
- Elevated serum cardiac markers

* The combined endpoint of mortality, myocardial infarction, and urgent revascularization increases in linear fashion, with Risk Scores 0–1 associated with a 4.7% risk of events at 2 weeks, versus 8.3% for Risk Score 2, 13.2% for Risk Score 3, 19.9% for Risk Score 4, 26.2% for Risk Score 5, and 40.9% for Risk Scores 6–7.

Patients with acute MI at highest risk for death are those presenting with cardiac arrest, HF, hypotension, or significant tachycardia, and the in-hospital mortality rate approaches 50% for patients with cardiogenic shock.[44] Although early coronary revascularization is beneficial in patients up to the age of 75 years presenting with acute MI complicated by cardiogenic shock, the value of this approach in patients older than 75 years is less clear.[45,46] Nevertheless, urgent revascularization is a reasonable option in selected elderly patients in the absence of other life-threatening conditions.

Complications of Myocardial Infarction

HF occurs in up to 50% of older patients with acute MI and is the most common cause of in-hospital death. Treatment includes diuretics and vasodilator therapy, especially nitroglycerin and ACEIs. In mild cases, β-blockers should be administered. In more advanced HF, inotropic agents may be required transiently until the patient stabilizes (e.g., dopamine, dobutamine – see Heart Failure later).

Clinically significant right ventricular (RV) infarction occurs in 10%–20% of patients with acute inferior MI and portends an ominous prognosis in the elderly.[47] Manifestations of RV infarction include hypotension and signs of right-sided HF. Treatment involves intravenous fluid administration to maintain RV filling pressure and inotropic therapy if needed.

Life-threatening mechanical complications of MI occur in 1%–2% of all patients and appear to be decreasing in incidence since the advent of reperfusion therapy. Mechanical complications include LV free wall rupture with pericardial tamponade, papillary muscle dysfunction or rupture with severe acute mitral regurgitation, rupture of the interventricular septum, and aneurysm or pseudoaneurysm formation. Advanced age is a potent risk factor for each of these catastrophic consequences of acute MI.[48] Care should be individualized; however, all forms of rupture require urgent attention and surgical repair, if at all

possible. Management of ventricular aneurysm depends on size and degree of hemodynamic instability; in most cases, smaller aneurysms can be managed medically whereas surgical repair should be considered for large aneurysms associated with HF or thromboembolic complications. LV pseudoaneurysm refers to a situation in which a free wall rupture has been locally contained by adherent pericardium. Pseudoaneurysms are prone to expand, leading to pericardial tamponade, so surgical repair is recommended.

Sustained ventricular tachyarrhythmias are generally treated with direct-current cardioversion or defibrillation, β-blocker therapy, and correction of electrolyte abnormalities and ischemia. Selected individuals may require antiarrhythmic therapy or implantable defibrillators, particularly if new life-threatening ventricular arrhythmias occur more than 48 hours after MI, but these approaches are not indicated for routine management or for prophylactic purposes.[15] Supraventricular arrhythmias such as AF should be treated according to standard recommendations (see Arrhythmias later). Bradyarrhythmias frequently resolve spontaneously once ischemia has been treated, but patients may occasionally require temporary transvenous or transcutaneous pacing. Permanent pacing may be necessary in patients with persistent high-grade heart block (e.g., Mobitz type II second degree atrioventricular block or complete heart block in the setting of anterior MI).

Diagnosis and Management of Chronic Coronary Disease

After experiencing MI, all patients should be counseled in conjunction with their families or caregivers regarding the medication regimen, diet, and long-term recommendations for CAD management. This is particularly important in elderly patients, for whom sensory or memory deficits may combine with polypharmacy to affect adversely medication compliance. Assessment of risk factors should be targeted during the convalescent phase after MI, with nutritional counseling and tobacco cessation efforts addressed prior to discharge.[15,16] Systolic blood pressure should be kept below 140 mm Hg (<130 mm Hg in patients with diabetes or chronic kidney disease), lipid therapy should be initiated or titrated appropriately, diabetes management should be intensified if indicated, and medical follow-up should be arranged. Cardiac rehabilitation reduces mortality and improves quality of life after MI, with similar benefits in younger and older patients. Cardiac rehabilitation is, however, significantly underutilized in the geriatric population relative to younger patients.[49]

Chronic CAD, with or without prior MI, increases in prevalence with age – likely as a result of prolonged exposure to multiple cardiac risk factors in conjunction with structural and metabolic changes related to vascular aging. Atherosclerotic changes tend to be more diffuse in older adults, with a higher likelihood of left main and multivessel CAD. Compared with younger patients, geriatric patients tend to present with more advanced disease and fewer or no anginal symptoms because of comorbidities (e.g., diabetes), neuropsychiatric changes, and more sedentary lifestyles. Indications for stress testing are similar to those for younger individuals; however, clinicians should carefully screen geriatric patients prior to stress testing, taking into consideration whether the patient is a suitable candidate for coronary angiography and revascularization in the event the stress test is abnormal. Often, elderly patients are unable to perform an exercise stress test; in such cases, a pharmacological test such as an adenosine nuclear scan or dobutamine echocardiogram is appropriate.[50]

Medical management of chronic stable angina includes aspirin, β-blockers, nitrates, and calcium channel blockers – with β-blockers being the antiischemic agents of first choice unless contraindicated.[51] Recently, ranolazine (a drug that improves myocardial substrate utilization) was approved for treatment of chronic stable angina in patients who do not respond to conventional antianginal agents.[52] As with most medications, side effects from ranolazine (including syncope) are more common in older patients, especially at higher dosages.

Compared with medical management, coronary revascularization with PCI or coronary artery bypass graft (CABG) surgery reduces symptoms and improves quality of life, although the effect on mortality is unclear.[53] Coronary angiography, PCI, and CABG in the geriatric population are associated with higher complication rates than in younger patients,[54–59] with in-hospital mortality in octogenarians averaging 3%–4% following elective PCI and 7%–10% following isolated CABG. Higher mortality in the elderly results in part from more advanced and diffuse CAD, worse LV function resulting from prior MI, and diminished cardiac reserve related to aging itself. Comorbidities play an important role as well, with vascular and renal disease contributing to procedural difficulty, bleeding complications, and contrast nephropathy. Stroke and other thromboembolic events, as well as HF, occur more commonly after either percutaneous or surgical revascularization in older patients. In addition, older patients undergoing CABG experience higher rates of arrhythmias (particularly AF), cognitive dysfunction,[60] and pulmonary complications than younger patients, and these adverse events contribute to increased duration of hospital stay and mortality. Despite the attendant risks, outcomes following PCI and CABG in older adults are generally favorable and more than 50% of patients undergoing these procedures in the United States are older than the age of 65 years.[1]

In patients with persistent chest pain despite medical treatment who are not candidates for PCI or CABG, another option is enhanced external counterpulsation. With enhanced external counterpulsation, patients undergo a series of treatments with sequential lower extremity blood pressure cuff inflations designed to improve coronary collateral circulation and perhaps activate components of natural fibrinolytic or vasodilatory pathways.[61] Several trials have demonstrated improved symptoms after several weeks of therapy but limb compression may be problematic in geriatric patients.

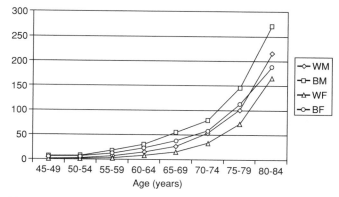

Figure 11.4. HF mortality rates Per 100,000 persons in the United States by age, sex, and race in 1990.

HEART FAILURE AND CARDIOMYOPATHY

Epidemiology and Pathophysiology

More than 5 million Americans have HF, with more than 1 million hospitalizations for HF as a primary diagnosis each year.[62] HF increases in both incidence and prevalence with increasing age, with close to 80% of HF hospitalizations occurring in patients aged 65 years and older and more than 50% occurring in patients older than 75 years. In addition, HF is the most costly Medicare diagnosis-related group by a factor of almost two, and mortality from HF rises exponentially with age (Figure 11.4).[63,64] Age-related changes in cardiovascular structure and function – including increased arterial stiffness, impaired LV diastolic relaxation and compliance, diminished responsiveness to β-adrenergic stimulation, and dysfunction of the sinus node – all contribute to a marked reduction in cardiovascular reserve, predisposing older adults to the development of HF. In addition, increased vascular stiffness leads to a progressive rise in systolic blood pressure, which is a major risk factor for the development of HF in geriatric patients. Indeed, approximately 75% of HF patients have antecedent hypertension, although the increasing prevalence rates of CAD, diabetes, and valvular disease also contribute to the exponential rise in geriatric HF.

Cause and Prevention

Most HF in the geriatric population is related to hypertension and/or CAD, including improved survival from acute MI, which often results in residual LV dysfunction. Other common causes include nonischemic dilated cardiomyopathy, valvular disease, and hypertrophic cardiomyopathy. Less common etiologies include myocarditis, constrictive pericarditis, thyroid disease, high-output states such as an arteriovenous fistula or anemia, and infiltrative diseases such as amyloid or hemochromatosis. Individuals with exposure to certain drugs, such as cocaine or chemotherapeutic agents (e.g., anthracyclines and trastuzumab), are also at risk for developing LV dysfunction.

Clinical guidelines emphasize prevention in high-risk populations – especially in patients with multiple cardiovascular risk factors – and more aggressive titration of therapies in the presence of asymptomatic LV dysfunction, significant valvular disease, or symptomatic HF.[62] Large-scale clinical trials have verified that lowering blood pressure reduces the risk of developing HF,[65] and the greatest benefit is derived from control of systolic hypertension in patients older than 80 years.[66] In patients with MI, the syndrome of HF may be delayed for months or years through implementation of the secondary prevention therapies described earlier. In the geriatric population, deconditioning and pulmonary disease may contribute to exercise intolerance, for which rehabilitation and lifestyle modifications are beneficial. Exercise training in particular is recommended in patients with asymptomatic LV dysfunction or chronic HF in the absence of severe symptoms.[62] Pharmacological regression of LV hypertrophy in hypertensive patients also reduces the incidence of HF and cardiovascular events.[67] Dietary counseling, including sodium restriction and avoidance of excessive fluid intake, may help reduce fluid retention and subsequent HF exacerbations. Medication compliance should be discussed early after diagnosing HF because rebound effects may occur after sudden withdrawal of therapies, and medication nonadherence is a leading cause of rehospitalization for HF.

Clinical Features and Diagnosis

Classic symptoms of HF include shortness of breath (especially with exertion), exercise intolerance, orthopnea, paroxysmal nocturnal dyspnea, lower extremity edema, fatigue, and weakness. Elderly patients with HF also commonly experience anorexia, bloating, psychomotor slowing, lethargy, altered sensorium, and gastrointestinal disturbances. Because elderly persons are often sedentary, exertional symptoms may be less prominent than in younger patients. Conversely, "atypical" symptoms such as anorexia and altered cognition become increasingly prevalent.

Assessing symptom severity in patients with HF is useful for identifying therapeutic goals, monitoring disease progression, and determining prognosis. Although there are several metrics available, the New York Heart Association (NYHA) functional classification is the most widely used (Table 11.6).[68] Nearly 70% of patients with HF are in class I or II, with minimal or mild limitations to routine physical activities. Approximately 25% of patients experience more severe activity limitations (class III), whereas only 5% of patients are class IV, with symptoms during minimal exertion (e.g., going to the bathroom) or at rest. Patients with class IV HF have a 1-year mortality rate of 25%–50% – worse than for many forms of metastatic cancer.[69]

Initial assessment should include a detailed history and physical examination. This is of vital importance in the geriatric population because patients may not present with typical symptoms or signs, and other medical conditions such as pulmonary disease or deconditioning may confound the clinical picture. Common precipitants of HF exacerbations in the elderly include medication or dietary noncompliance,

Table 11.6. New York Heart Association Functional Classification

Class	General Characteristics
I	Cardiac disease does not limit physical activity.
	Ordinary physical activity does not cause undue fatigue, palpitation, dyspnea, or anginal pain.
II	Cardiac disease results in slight limitation of physical activity. Patients are comfortable at rest.
	Ordinary physical activity results in fatigue, palpitation, dyspnea, or anginal pain.
III	Cardiac disease results in marked limitation of physical activity.
	Patients are comfortable at rest.
	Less than ordinary physical activity causes fatigue, palpitation, dyspnea, or anginal pain.
IV	Cardiac disease results in inability to carry on any physical activity without discomfort.
	Symptoms of cardiac insufficiency or anginal syndrome may be present even at rest.
	If any physical activity is undertaken, discomfort is increased.

ischemia, uncontrolled hypertension, new arrhythmias (especially AF), infection, volume overload (e.g., perioperatively or with blood transfusions), anemia, and drug interactions that adversely affect renal or cardiac function. Vital signs and volume status should be evaluated, and complete examination of the neck, chest, cardiovascular system, abdomen, and extremities should be performed. Routine laboratory studies include an assessment of electrolytes and renal function, and a complete blood count.[62] Select patients may require thyroid hormone assessment. An ECG is imperative because HF is often precipitated by ischemia or arrhythmia. Chest radiography may be useful for diagnosing volume overload. Echocardiography should be performed at the time of initial diagnosis or when there is unexplained clinical deterioration to assess LV systolic and diastolic function and to identify other structural abnormalities that may be contributing to the HF syndrome.

A recently developed diagnostic tool is B-type natriuretic peptide (BNP), which is released into the circulation by myocardium when ventricular filling pressures are elevated, and which can easily be measured in peripheral blood. One large trial demonstrated the utility of BNP for distinguishing cardiac from noncardiac causes of dyspnea in the emergency department.[70] BNP levels increase with age and female,[71,72] and other common disorders in the geriatric population may also contribute to higher BNP levels, including AF, renal dysfunction, and pulmonary hypertension. The predictive accuracy of BNP therefore declines with increasing age.[71] Nonetheless, BNP frequently adds useful diagnostic and prognostic information to the evaluation of patients with suspected

HF. Levels must be interpreted cautiously in elderly patients with concurrent renal dysfunction or other factors that affect BNP.

Therapy of Systolic Heart Failure

Initial goals of therapy for acute HF exacerbations include hemodynamic stabilization and correction of volume overload. Care for elderly patients must be individualized, with comorbid conditions, functional limitations, and personal preferences being taken into consideration in designing a therapeutic plan. In addition, because few clinical trials have included many patients older than 75 years, most HF therapies are of unproved benefit in older patients.[73] Multidisciplinary programs that provide individualized patient education and close follow-up have been shown to reduce hospitalizations and improve quality of life in elderly HF patients.[74,75]

Diuretics

Loop diuretics are an essential component of the acute management of HF with volume overload. These agents intravenously administered promote rapid natriuresis and increased urine output. Older patients are more sensitive to diuretic-induced electrolyte disturbances and volume shifts than younger patients, so close monitoring is imperative in conjunction with regular assessments of renal function and electrolytes. Although loop diuretics have not been shown to improve survival and there are conflicting data concerning the short- and long-term benefits of these agents,[76–79] relief of congestion is a primary goal of initial HF therapy.[62] In patients who do not respond adequately to loop diuretics, the addition of metolazone (usually administered 30–60 minutes before the loop diuretic) may facilitate diuresis, but renal and electrolyte disturbances are common. Dietary sodium restriction helps prevent fluid retention, and patients should be counseled to avoid salty foods and limit sodium intake to no more than 2 g/day. Patients should also be instructed to monitor daily weights at home. A baseline "dry weight" should be defined, and patients should be advised to adjust their diuretic dosage or contact their health care provider if their weight varies by more than 2 lb from baseline.

Angiotensin-Converting Enzyme Inhibitors

In patients with systolic HF, ACEIs reduce HF hospitalizations, improve quality of life, and decrease mortality by approximately 25%–30% – with similar effects in older and younger patients.[80,81] Older patients experience higher rates of hypotension, hyperkalemia, and renal dysfunction during ACEI titration than younger individuals; close monitoring of these parameters is warranted. Up to 20% of patients may experience cough and a small percentage may experience angioedema from ACEIs, but these side effects do not appear to increase in frequency with advancing age. In the absence of adverse effects, ACEI dosages should be titrated to those studied in clinical trials (e.g., captopril 50 mg three times daily, enalapril 10 mg two times daily, lisinopril 20–40 mg/day, ramipril 10 mg/day). In addition, ACEI therapy in patients with asymptomatic LV dysfunction reduces progression to clinical HF,[82] so ACEIs are indicated in patients with LV systolic dysfunction (LV ejection fraction <40%–45%) regardless of NYHA functional class.

Angiotensin Receptor Blockers

ARBs have not been shown to be as effective as ACEIs in patients with systolic HF,[27] but they are suitable alternatives in individuals intolerant to ACEIs because of cough or angioedema.[83,84] The addition of an ARB to an ACEI may provide additional benefit in patients with advanced HF.[85,86] The effects of ARBs are similar in older and younger patients, but as with ACEIs, older patients are at increased risk for hypotension, renal dysfunction, and hyperkalemia with these agents.

Other Oral Vasodilators

The combination of hydralazine and nitrates improves clinical outcomes in systolic HF,[87] although mortality reduction is less than with ACEI therapy.[88] Nevertheless, this combination remains useful in patients with renal dysfunction or hyperkalemia that precludes the use of ACEIs or ARBs. Recently, the African-American Heart Failure Trial showed that the addition of a fixed combination of hydralazine and isosorbide dinitrate (taken three times per day) improves clinical outcomes in class III–IV HF patients already treated with standard therapies including ACEIs and β-blockers.[89] All patients in this trial were African American and the mean age was only 57 years, so the role of these vasodilators in older patients and other racial/ethnic groups remains to be determined. In addition, side effects are common with both hydralazine and nitrates, and the need for multiple daily doses of both agents is a disadvantage.

Beta-Blockers

Although β-blockers were once considered contraindicated in HF patients, multiple, large, randomized trials have now confirmed improvements in LV function, decreased hospitalizations, and reduced mortality with β-blocker therapy in class I–IV HF patients.[90,91] Patients with class III–IV HF require meticulous and slow titration because of transient worsening of symptoms that may occur with increasing doses of β-blockers. Beta-blockers are beneficial in elderly patients, including those older than 75 years, with improvements in hospitalization rates, mortality, and LV ejection fraction.[92] Geriatric patients frequently are sensitive to β-blockade, so initiation at a low dose with slow upward titration over time is imperative to avoid bradycardia, heart block, hypotension, or worsened HF. Nevertheless, like ACEI, β-blocker doses should be titrated to those proved to be effective in clinical trials.[93] Active bronchospasm is a contraindication to β-blocker therapy, but chronic pulmonary disease does not preclude use of these drugs. Other contraindications include marked bradycardia, advanced heart block, hypotension, and severe decompensated HF.

Digoxin

Digitalis has been used for centuries to improve HF symptoms, but a large clinical trial failed to demonstrate a reduction in mortality from routine use.[94] Digoxin, however, reduces HF hospitalizations and improves symptoms, and the benefits are similar in older and younger patients – including those older than 80 years.[95] Moreover, a recent retrospective analysis suggests that when the serum digoxin level is maintained at less than 1.0 ng/mL, digoxin reduces the risk of mortality.[96] In geriatric patients with persistent HF symptoms despite other therapeutic measures, digoxin should be initiated at a low dose (0.125 mg/day in the absence of renal dysfunction) with close monitoring for side effects such as bradycardia, heart block, arrhythmias, gastrointestinal distress, and mental status changes or visual disturbances. Digoxin toxicity occurs more frequently in the setting of hypokalemia, hypomagnesemia, hypercalcemia, and concurrent use of common cardiovascular drugs, including amiodarone and verapamil.

Spironolactone

Spironolactone is an aldosterone antagonist with weak diuretic potency but with antifibrotic properties and other beneficial cardiovascular effects. When added to other therapies in class III–IV systolic HF patients, low doses of spironolactone reduce mortality risk by approximately 25%.[97] Older and younger patients gain similar benefits, but spironolactone also adversely affects creatinine and potassium levels in many patients. In one study, an increase in hospitalizations for renal failure and hyperkalemia was reported after spironolactone became standard HF therapy.[98] This finding is particularly relevant in elderly patients given the worsening of renal function with age. Meticulous electrolyte and renal surveillance is, therefore, required in geriatric HF patients treated with spironolactone. Up to 10% of individuals may also develop gynecomastia and breast tenderness with prolonged therapy, although these side effects may be avoided by using eplerenone (indicated for LV systolic dysfunction after MI, as described earlier).

Anticoagulant and Antiinflammatory Drugs

Although the thromboembolic risk associated with chronic systolic HF approaches that seen in AF, no clinical trial has demonstrated benefit from therapeutic anticoagulation in HF patients. Warfarin or other anticoagulant treatment should therefore be reserved for patients with mechanical heart valves, AF, or other compelling indications.[62] Aspirin should be prescribed in patients with CAD, peripheral arterial disease, diabetes, or other indications for antiplatelet therapy. The value of aspirin in HF patients without clear indications for its use is controversial, because it may interact adversely with ACEI therapy. Other nonsteroidal antiinflammatory medications – commonly used to treat arthritis and chronic pain in older individuals – should be avoided whenever possible because these agents promote sodium and water retention, antagonize ACEIs and other HF medications, and may worsen renal function.

Inotropic Agents and Intravenous Vasodilators

With the exception of digoxin, inotropic therapy has not been shown to improve clinical outcomes, and several randomized trials have demonstrated higher mortality rates with these agents (Table 11.7).[99–103] Nevertheless, many clinicians utilize intravenous inotropes in patients with severe, intractable HF or cardiogenic shock unresponsive to standard therapies.[62] The three agents licensed for use in the United States – dobutamine, dopamine, and milrinone – may also be used in select patients awaiting heart transplantation or ventricular assistive devices – an uncommon scenario in elderly patients. Nesiritide, a recombinant form of BNP administered intravenously, has been shown to reduce LV filling pressures more effectively than intravenous nitrates or standard therapy (including diuretics), although morbidity and mortality benefits have not been demonstrated.[104] Nesiritide may promote diuresis even in patients with reduced renal function, but the infusion (and the initial bolus in particular) often precipitates hypotension. Judicious selection of elderly patients is therefore imperative, as these individuals are often sensitive to rapid reductions in LV preload – particularly in the setting of diastolic HF. Long-term nesiritide therapy outside of the acute setting is not recommended, as it may be associated with worsening renal function and increased mortality,[105] although additional trials investigating this treatment approach are in progress.

Diastolic Heart Failure

Approximately half of HF cases in the elderly occur in the context of normal or near-normal LV systolic function.[64,106–108] Observational studies have demonstrated nearly identical hospitalization and mortality rates in systolic and diastolic HF patients,[109,110] with increasing age and medical comorbidities (e.g., worsening renal function in the elderly) likely contributing to adverse outcomes in diastolic HF. Very few trials have evaluated HF with preserved LV systolic function, despite the high prevalence of this syndrome in the geriatric population. One trial demonstrated reductions in HF hospitalizations with the ARB candesartan (mean age 67 years, class II–IV HF), but there was no effect on mortality.[111] Similarly, digoxin has a favorable effect on HF hospitalizations, but not all-cause hospitalizations or mortality.[112]

Current guidelines for managing diastolic HF recommend empiric control of heart rate, blood pressure, and volume status. Hypertension, in particular, needs to be treated aggressively. Treatment of precipitating factors such as ischemia or arrhythmia remains important, with judicious diuresis as needed and close monitoring of blood pressure and renal function because of the preload-dependent state of the left ventricle with impaired diastolic filling. Important differential diagnostic considerations in HF with preserved LV systolic function include valvular heart disease, pericardial constriction, restrictive cardiomyopathy (e.g., amyloid deposition, hemochromatosis, sarcoidosis), and noncardiac causes such as pulmonary disease with right heart failure. Hypertrophic cardiomyopathy may also mimic diastolic HF and is commonly

Table 11.7. Inotropic Agents and Mortality in HF

Agent	No. Patients	Mortality Study	Mortality Placebo (%)	Result Inotrope (%)	P Value
Digoxin	6,800	Yes	35.1	34.8	0.80
Dobutamine	60	Yes	17	41	0.15
Amrinone	99	No	4	4	NS
Enoximone	102	No	6	20	<0.05
Enoximone	164	No	5	7	NS
Milrinone	1,088	Yes	24	30	0.04
Xamoterol	516	No	4	9	0.02
Flosequinan	422	Yes	15	21	<0.01
Vesnarinone	3,833	Yes	18	21.3	0.02
Dobutamine	471	Yes	37	71	0.0001
Dobutamine	199	Yes	28	42	0.03
Milrinone	951	Yes	2.3	3.8	0.19
TOTAL:	14,705				

associated with exertional chest pain and syncope. Advanced hypertrophic cardiomyopathy with LV outflow tract obstruction may require surgical myectomy or percutaneous alcohol septal ablation to reduce the severity of outflow tract obstruction.

Device Therapy and Prognosis in Advanced Heart Failure

Implantable Devices

Although pharmacological and behavioral therapies are the cornerstones of HF management, implantable devices are playing an increasingly important role in the treatment of HF patients. Advanced HF frequently is associated with dyssynchronous LV contraction related to abnormalities of electrical conduction, and biventricular pacemaker implantation improves symptoms in systolic HF patients with wide QRS durations on ECG.[113,114] Mortality benefits also have been demonstrated when biventricular pacing is combined with an implantable cardioverter-defibrillator (ICD).[114] ICD therapy alone for primary prevention of sudden death may benefit select patients with either ischemic or nonischemic cardiomyopathy who are in NYHA class II–III HF with an LV ejection fraction below 30%–35%.[115,116] The mortality benefit of an ICD accrues over 3–5 years following implantation. For this reason, and in consideration of the high cost and potential complications related to ICD placement, ICD use in the very elderly (i.e., older than 75–80 years) should be reserved for carefully selected patients with few comorbidities and a relatively favorable long-term prognosis.

Although most geriatric patients with severe HF are not considered candidates for "heroic" measures such as heart transplantation, a select few with reversible or surgically correctable HF may be considered for ventricular assistive devices. These devices are bulky and prone to hemorrhagic and infectious complications, but newer assistive devices are being evaluated in clinical trials for both surgical and percutaneous implantation.

Prognosis

The prognosis for elderly patients with HF remains poor, with 5-year survival rates of 20%–25%. Factors associated with worsened prognosis include older age, more severe symptoms (NYHA functional class III–IV), ischemic origin, renal insufficiency, hyponatremia, peripheral arterial disease, and dementia.[117] Patients with diastolic HF have a somewhat better short-term prognosis than patients with systolic HF, but long-term prognosis is similar. Older patients who elect to undergo ICD placement should be counseled about long-term prognosis, with options for future ICD reprogramming if HF becomes severe or refractory. Many patients who have experienced ICD shocks have indicated the desire to avoid recurrences, and discussions about deactivating the device may provide clinicians with an opportunity to review other end-of-life issues, including preferences for cardiopulmonary resuscitation, pharmacological and mechanical life support, and durable power-of-attorney.

VALVULAR HEART DISEASE

Aortic Stenosis

Aortic stenosis (AS) is the most common valvular abnormality requiring surgical intervention in older adults. In the geriatric population, most AS is related to progressive calcific and fibrotic changes of the valve leaflets. Classic symptoms of AS include chest pain, shortness of breath, and light-headedness or syncope. Physical examination findings include a harsh systolic ejection murmur that tends to peak later in systole as the degree of stenosis worsens, and delayed and low-amplitude carotid arterial pulses. Once symptoms attributable to AS develop, the prognosis is poor, with an average survival of 2–3 years without surgical intervention.[118] As with CAD and HF, the presentation of severe AS may be delayed in the geriatric population because of reduced physical activity levels. Symptoms may not be evident until another medical illness or need for surgery arises, at which time stenosis may be more advanced than in younger patients at the time of diagnosis.

An aortic valve (AV) area of 1.0 cm^2 or less is generally considered severe stenosis, whereas a valve area of 1.0–1.5 cm^2 defines moderate stenosis and a valve area of 1.5–2.0 cm^2 is considered mild stenosis.[118] LV hypertrophy commonly results from chronic LV pressure overload, and conduction system disease may be present as a result of concurrent calcium deposition. CAD frequently coexists in calcific AS because of the related underlying pathophysiology and the increasing age of the patient population affected.

Treatment of AS is almost exclusively surgical, as medical therapy does not delay disease progression or improve outcomes, and percutaneous valvuloplasty is ineffective. AV replacement is indicated in symptomatic patients with severe AS, as determined by echocardiography or cardiac catheterization. In older individuals, coronary angiography is warranted prior to surgery to assess whether there is concomitant CAD. In geriatric patients, bioprosthetic valves are preferred over mechanical valves because they offer satisfactory durability while avoiding the need for long-term systemic anticoagulation. Operative mortality is less than 5% for isolated AV replacement, and somewhat higher if combined with coronary bypass surgery. Postoperative quality of life is substantially improved, and long-term survival is excellent – even in octogenarians. Lifelong endocarditis prophylaxis is indicated for dental or surgical procedures in all patients with prosthetic heart valves.

Aortic Insufficiency

Chronic regurgitation at the AV is often well tolerated for many years, as the LV can effectively compensate for chronic volume overload. Common geriatric causes of chronic AV insufficiency include long-standing hypertension, myxomatous degeneration of the AV leaflets, and disorders of the ascending aorta (e.g., aneurysmal dilation). Other causes include rheumatic valve disease, other rheumatological conditions, prior endocarditis, and tumors. Many patients are asymptomatic but may exhibit findings of increased stroke volume such as increased pulse pressure or prominent arterial pulsations ("bounding pulses"). A decrescendo diastolic murmur is usually heard along the left sternal border. LV hypertrophy is often present on the ECG.

Optimal medical therapy for severe chronic AV regurgitation is undefined. Vasodilators such as ACEIs or nifedipine are often prescribed, but the value of such treatment in delaying surgery and improving clinical outcomes remains unproved.[119,120] Progressive exertional dyspnea or HF signifies a failing LV and necessitates AV replacement.[118] Other indications for surgery include increasing LV dilation or a reduction in LV systolic function with exercise. Operative mortality in geriatric patients undergoing AV replacement is acceptable, and long-term outcomes are generally favorable.

Mitral Stenosis

In younger patients, stenosis of the mitral valve (MV) is almost always rheumatic in origin, although rare inflammatory or infectious processes may result in MV scarring and narrowing. In older individuals, calcification of the MV annulus with impingement into the valve orifice is the most common cause of MV stenosis, although it is rarely severe enough to warrant surgery. Mitral stenosis in older patients usually runs an indolent course, with gradual progression over several decades. Common symptoms include exertional dyspnea and fatigue. In advanced cases, signs of biventricular failure and pulmonary hypertension are evident. The left atrium is often markedly enlarged, increasing the risk of AF and systemic thromboembolism. Pulmonary hypertension is also common, which contributes to the development of right-sided HF. Classic physical findings include an early diastolic opening snap and a mid-diastolic low-pitched rumbling murmur best heard at the cardiac apex, often with presystolic accentuation. An MV area less than 1.0 cm^2 is considered severely stenotic, with valve areas of 1.0–1.5 cm^2 and 1.6–2.0 cm^2 indicating moderate and mild stenosis, respectively.

Diuretics and sodium restriction are recommended to maintain euvolemia in patients with MV stenosis. If AF is present, anticoagulation with warfarin should be initiated, and the resting heart rate should be maintained in the range of 60–90 beats/min.[118] Endocarditis prophylaxis is indicated for dental work and other surgical procedures. Unlike AV stenosis, the MV can be dilated via percutaneous valvuloplasty with good intermediate-to-long-term success, provided there is no significant MV regurgitation or other technical factors such as heavy valvular calcification. As these contraindications to valvuloplasty are more common in older than in younger patients, most elderly patients with severe symptomatic MV stenosis will require MV replacement. As with AV surgery, bioprosthetic valves are generally recommended in geriatric patients, although many older patients will still require anticoagulation for AF. Operative mortality is generally higher with MV replacement than with AV replacement, ranging from 5% to 15% depending on age, functional status, prevalent comorbidities, and the experience of the surgical team. The risk of developing AF after surgery increases with age and is particularly high after MV surgery;[121,122] however, preoperative β-blocker or amiodarone therapy reduces postoperative morbidity from AF.[122,123] Recovery following MV surgery may be slow, often requiring prolonged rehabilitation.

Mitral Regurgitation

MV regurgitation can occur as a result of CAD, myxomatous degeneration, rheumatic MV disease, or stretching of the MV annulus from progressive LV dilation and HF. All of these processes occur more commonly in the elderly, and the majority of MV surgeries are performed in the Medicare population. Severe chronic MV regurgitation is usually asymptomatic until the left ventricle begins to fail, leading to HF symptoms such as exertional dyspnea, fatigue, orthopnea, and edema. An apical holosystolic murmur with radiation to the axilla is usually present, occasionally accompanied by an S3 gallop. Echocardiography – especially transesophageal echocardiography – is useful for defining the severity of MV regurgitation and identifying other structural abnormalities.

Medical therapy has not been shown to reduce progression of MV regurgitation, although many physicians recommend empiric afterload reduction with ACEIs or other vasodilators. Endocarditis prophylaxis should be prescribed for patients with chronic MV disease.[118] Symptomatic patients with severe MV regurgitation and an LV ejection fraction of 30% or higher should be referred for MV surgery. Surgery should also be considered in asymptomatic individuals with LV dilation and/or mild-to-moderate LV dysfunction, as early intervention has been associated with improved long-term outcomes in these patients.[124] MV repair, when feasible, is preferable to MV replacement.[125] Operative mortality and long-term outcomes following MV repair for nonischemic regurgitation are generally good in patients with preserved LV systolic function, but are less favorable in patients with an ischemic etiology or with impaired LV systolic function.[118,126] Because elderly patients often have other comorbid conditions that may affect postoperative outcomes and long-term prognosis, the decision to proceed with MV surgery must be individualized.

Tricuspid and Pulmonic Valve Disease

In geriatric patients, the right-sided heart valves generally become dysfunctional as a consequence of left heart problems or cor pulmonale from acute or chronic lung disease. Tricuspid regurgitation often results from RV dilation and dysfunction in the setting of pulmonary hypertension or HF. Symptoms and signs reflect right-sided HF and may include dyspnea, elevated jugular venous pressure, a murmur of tricuspid regurgitation, hepatic congestion, and lower extremity edema. Tricuspid repair (i.e., annuloplasty) is occasionally performed at the time of cardiac surgery for other reasons, but tricuspid regurgitation rarely is the primary indication for heart surgery. Similarly, pulmonic insufficiency may result from left-sided HF but usually does not require surgical intervention.

Endocarditis

Age-associated valvular degeneration and stenosis increase the risk for infective endocarditis in older adults. The risk is further compounded by higher rates of blood-borne infection in older patients, as conditions such as cancer, dental disease, pneumonia, indwelling catheters, pacemakers, and noncardiac surgery provide common sources for prolonged bacteremia. Management of endocarditis includes intensive antibiotic therapy and consideration of valve repair or replacement in patients with high-risk features such as embolic phenomena, large vegetations (>1 cm), perivalvular abscess, hemodynamic instability, or failure to respond to antibiotics.[118] All patients with prior endocarditis should receive prophylactic antibiotics prior to major surgery or dental procedures.

PERICARDIAL AND VASCULAR DISEASES

Pericarditis

Acute pericarditis usually presents as pleuritic chest pain that is worse in the supine position and improved with sitting. Fever and leukocytosis are common with infectious causes, which represent the majority of cases worldwide. Additional causes in the geriatric population include recent MI, hypothyroidism, uremia, recent cardiac or thoracic surgery, malignancy, and prior radiation therapy to the chest. The ECG may show diffuse ST-segment elevation with PR-segment depression. Sinus tachycardia is common, but new pathological Q-waves are absent. The cardinal sign is a pericardial friction rub, although this may be transient or absent. Serum troponin levels may be slightly elevated, indicating myocardial involvement. Echocardiography may demonstrate a pericardial effusion, but the absence of an effusion does not preclude the diagnosis of pericarditis. Nonsteroidal anti-inflammatory drugs are recommended for initial therapy. Corticosteroids and colchicine may be effective in refractory or relapsing cases. Anticoagulation should be avoided due to the risk of hemorrhagic transformation.

Pericardial Effusion and Tamponade

Common causes of pericardial effusion are similar to those for pericarditis but also include HF, hypoalbuminemia, rheumatologic disorders, hemorrhage, and certain medications (e.g., minoxidil). Although most pericardial effusions do not progress to tamponade, patients with malignant or infectious causes are at increased risk. Clinical manifestations of pericardial tamponade include dyspnea, tachycardia, hypotension, and pulsus paradoxus (although the latter is not always present). In addition to a moderate or large pericardial effusion, echocardiographic features of tamponade include respiratory variability to ventricular inflow, right atrial or ventricular compression by the effusion, and a dilated inferior vena cava. Treatment of tamponade involves percutaneous pericardiocentesis (preferably with echocardiographic or hemodynamic guidance) or surgical drainage with creation of a pericardial "window" – the therapy of choice when the effusion is likely to recur (e.g., with malignancy).

Pericardial Constriction

Pericardial constriction is a late complication of an inflammatory or infectious pericarditis. The pericardium becomes thickened and scarred, inhibiting ventricular filling. In the past, tuberculous pericarditis was the most commonly identified cause of constriction. Currently, most cases occur following radiation therapy for thoracic cancer or after open heart surgery; as a result, the diagnosis is becoming more common in the geriatric population. The clinical course is usually one of biventricular HF, manifested by exertional dyspnea and fatigue, lower extremity edema, ascites, hepatic congestion, and bowel edema leading to bloating and anorexia. Cirrhosis of the liver may occur in long-standing cases. Inspiratory expansion of the jugular veins (Kussmaul sign) is a hallmark of pericardial constriction. Echocardiographic findings include small ventricular cavities with normal systolic function but restrictive filling, biatrial enlargement, and a thickened pericardium. Chest imaging may reveal pericardial thickening or calcification. Simultaneous right and left heart catheterization demonstrates equalization of diastolic pressures throughout all chambers with an early plateau in the RV and LV diastolic wave forms ("square root sign"). Constriction must be differentiated from restrictive cardiomyopathy, which presents a similar clinical and hemodynamic picture. The only effective treatment is surgical pericardiectomy, which is associated with substantial morbidity and mortality and may not be feasible for elderly patients with advanced comorbidities.

ARRHYTHMIAS AND CONDUCTION DISTURBANCES

All forms of arrhythmia and conduction system disease increase with age, and more than 85% of pacemakers and two-thirds of ICDs are placed in patients 65 years of age or older.[127] Aging is associated with fibrosis and calcification throughout the cardiac skeleton, leading to a slowing in impulse generation and conduction, with an increased frequency of atrial and ventricular premature depolarizations. In the absence of symptoms, most age-associated bradyarrhythmias, conduction abnormalities, and nonsustained tachyarrhythmias do not require treatment.

Bradycardia

Sick sinus syndrome is a collection of disorders related to impaired function of the sinus node and supraventricular conduction system. Sinus node pacemaker cells degenerate with age, and only approximately 10% of these cells continue to function normally by the age of 75 years. Similarly, conduction of the sinus impulse to atrial tissue (sinus node exit block) or to the ventricles (atrioventricular nodal block) may become impaired as well. Age-related stiffening of the carotid arteries also predisposes elderly individuals to carotid sinus hypersensitivity and associated vagally mediated bradyarrhythmias. Potential symptoms from bradycardia include dizziness and lightheadedness, angina, dyspnea, exercise intolerance, impaired mental function, fatigue, and syncope. Symptoms may occur at rest, upon standing, with positional changes of the head or neck (e.g., in patients with carotid sinus hypersensitivity), or during exertion (e.g. chronotropic incompetence, the inability to increase heart rate commensurate with increased metabolic demands). Often a 24-hour Holter or 30-day event monitor is required to diagnose correctly symptomatic bradycardia.

Acute bradycardia is treated with atropine but the effect is short-lived. Reversible causes such as CAD (especially inferior ischemia), autonomic dysfunction, hypothyroidism, and electrolyte abnormalities should be treated if possible. Beta blockers, certain calcium channel blockers (diltiazem, verapamil), digoxin, and many antiarrhythmic drugs may also precipitate symptomatic bradycardia, and a reduction in dosage or discontinuation of these agents may be required. Pacemaker implantation is indicated for nonreversible symptomatic bradycardia.[128] A prophylactic pacemaker is occasionally recommended in asymptomatic patients with severe bradycardia (heart rate <35–40 beats/min) or high-degree atrioventricular block. In sick sinus syndrome, dual-chamber pacing is associated with lower risks of developing AF or requiring hospitalization compared with single-chamber pacing, but this does not reduce the risk of mortality.[129]

Supraventricular Tachycardias

SVTs increase in prevalence with advancing age. In many cases, brief episodes of SVT respond to β-blockers or calcium channel blockers. Some individuals may require digoxin, antiarrhythmic drugs, or radiofrequency ablation, but these approaches (especially ablation) are usually reserved for more refractory arrhythmias. Of note, termination of SVT may be associated with prolonged sinus pauses and syncope in elderly patients ("tachy-brady syndrome"), occasionally requiring pacemaker placement to enable suppression of the tachyarrhythmia with medications. Multifocal atrial tachycardia (MAT) is an irregular SVT characterized by three or more P-wave morphologies on the ECG. MAT is most commonly seen in patients with severe chronic lung disease and often responds to treatment of the underlying lung disease in conjunction with diltiazem, verapamil, or a β-blocker (if tolerated).

The most common sustained tachyarrhythmia in the geriatric population is AF. Nearly 20%–25% of individuals will develop either AF or atrial flutter during their lifetime,[1] with a prevalence under 1% in people younger than the age of 40 years and increasing to approximately 10% in those older than age 80 years (Figure 11.5).[130] Most AF arises in the context of preexisting CVD, as fibrosis and hemodynamic changes in the atria lead to adverse remodeling and electrical abnormalities. The arrhythmia may also be precipitated by uncontrolled hypertension, ischemia or acute MI, hyperthyroidism, alcohol excess, HF, progressive valvular disease, acute or chronic lung conditions (e.g., pulmonary embolus or pneumonia), hypokalemia, cardiac or noncardiac surgery, and chemotherapy for cancer.

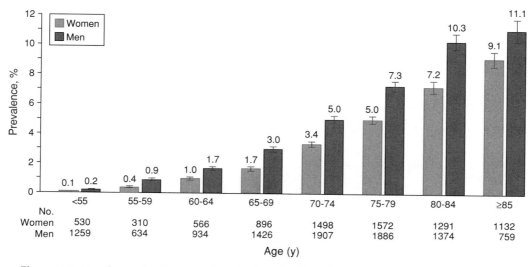

Figure 11.5. Prevalence of AF by age and sex in a large health maintenance organization in 1996–1997.

Echocardiography is indicated in patients with new AF to evaluate whether there is structural heart disease or pulmonary hypertension.[131] Electrolyte and thyroid hormone levels should be assessed as well. Patients with acute or chronic AF may be asymptomatic or experience palpitations, chest discomfort, effort intolerance, lightheadedness, syncope, or symptoms of HF. Occasionally elderly patients with acute-onset AF present with pulmonary edema due to the sudden loss of the atrial contribution to LV filling (the "atrial kick") and associated fall in cardiac output. Some elderly patients present with bradycardia in the setting of AF, resulting from underlying conduction system disease or therapy with AV nodal blocking agents. Unfortunately, in some cases AF is first diagnosed after a thromboembolic event, such as a stroke, has occurred.

Postoperative AF occurs in up to 30% of older patients undergoing major cardiac surgery. Beta-blockers, sotalol, and amiodarone reduce the risk of AF after cardiac surgery in the geriatric population.[132,133] Although no mortality benefit has been demonstrated with these perioperative interventions, duration of hospital stay is reduced relative to patients experiencing postoperative AF.

Management of acute AF requires rate control and prevention of thromboembolism. Most patients presenting in AF have a rapid heart rate that is irregularly irregular, so therapy is directed toward slowing the ventricular rate with a β-blocker or calcium channel blocker (i.e., diltiazem or verapamil). Digoxin is less effective than other agents but may be used as adjunctive therapy or when β-blockers and calcium channel blockers are contraindicated (e.g., due to hypotension). Concurrent HF should be treated with diuretics, and hemodynamically unstable patients should undergo immediate electrical cardioversion. In hemodynamically stable patients, the need for and timing of pharmacological or electrical cardioversion is unclear because clinical trials indicate that cardioversion of asymptomatic or mildly symptomatic patients with AF does not improve quality of life or reduce mortality or stroke risk compared with a strategy of rate control and long-term anticoagulation.[134,135] Most clinicians recommend at least one attempt to restore sinus rhythm for patients with recent-onset AF. In patients in whom AF has clearly been present for less than 48 hours (e.g., in the postoperative setting), the risk of thromboembolism is low, so pharmacological or electrical cardioversion (if necessary) can be safely undertaken. In patients with AF of longer or unknown duration, elective cardioversion should be preceded by 3–4 weeks of systemic anticoagulation. Alternatively, in selected cases transesophageal echocardiography may be performed, and if no atrial thrombus is demonstrated, electrical cardioversion can then be undertaken. In either case, systemic anticoagulation is essential for a minimum of 4 weeks following cardioversion, and, as discussed later, long-term anticoagulation is warranted for most patients.[131] In patients who remain highly symptomatic despite efforts to control rate and/or maintain sinus rhythm with antiarrhythmic drug therapy, additional therapeutic options include pulmonary vein isolation, ablation of the atrioventricular node with pacemaker implantation, and the surgical "Maze" procedure.

Long-term prevention of thromboembolic complications from AF usually requires warfarin therapy in geriatric patients, because increasing age is a potent risk factor for stroke in this population. In the Framingham Heart Study, the proportion of strokes related to AF increased from 1.5% for patients in their 50s to 23.5% for patients older than 80 years.[136] Additional risk factors for stroke in AF patients include a prior thromboembolic event, structural heart disease including valvular problems, and coexisting hypertension or diabetes.[137] Warfarin to maintain an international normalized ratio of 2.0–3.0 reduces stroke risk by approximately two-thirds, and the absolute benefit is greater in the elderly than in younger patients. In the absence of major contraindications – such as prior intracranial hemorrhage, known intracranial tumor, potentially life-threatening bleeding disorders, or frequent injurious falls – warfarin therapy is recommended for all geriatric patients with paroxysmal or chronic AF.[131] Aspirin (or clopidogrel in aspirin-intolerant patients) is much less effective than warfarin, reducing stroke risk by 20%–25%, but is a reasonable alternative when warfarin is contraindicated.

Because AF and atrial flutter frequently coexist in the same patient, atrial flutter is managed using the same approach as that for AF. In an occasional patient with isolated atrial flutter, radiofrequency ablation of the reentrant pathway may be curative.

Ventricular Arrhythmias

Ventricular arrhythmias, both isolated ventricular premature depolarizations (VPDs) and ventricular tachycardia (VT), increase in frequency with age – in part from age-related changes in the cardiac conduction system and in part from the higher prevalence of cardiac disease in older age (especially CAD and hypertensive heart disease). In general, management of ventricular arrhythmias is similar in older and younger individuals and is dependent on symptoms, hemodynamic impact, and the severity of underlying heart disease. CAD, hypertension, and valvular heart disease should be treated as previously discussed. Electrolyte abnormalities, including hypokalemia, hyperkalemia, and hypomagnesemia, should be corrected. Isolated VPDs require no specific therapy unless the patient experiences disabling symptoms, in which case β-blockers are first-line treatment, followed by antiarrhythmic drugs, if needed.

In the absence of HF or LV systolic dysfunction, asymptomatic nonsustained VT does not require treatment, and symptomatic patients should be managed in the same manner as for symptomatic VPDs. Sustained VT in geriatric patients almost always occurs in the context of advanced structural heart disease and portends an increased risk for sudden death. Acute sustained VT with hypotension or hypoperfusion should be treated with immediate electrical cardioversion, followed by an evaluation for precipitating causes. Recurrent sustained VT, whether symptomatic or asymptomatic, usually warrants consideration of antiarrhythmic drug therapy and implantation of an ICD.[138,139] Finally, as noted previously, patients with NYHA class II–III HF and an LV ejection fraction of 35% or lower should be considered for an ICD on an individual basis,[115,116] in the absence of very advanced age, frailty, or other major life-limiting comorbidities. In this context, patients with CAD and documented VT (sustained or non-sustained) are at greatest risk for sudden cardiac death – a factor that should be taken into account in the decision-making process.

SUMMARY

Aging is associated with diffuse changes throughout the cardiovascular system as well as increasing prevalence of most forms of CVD. As a result, the majority of men and women over the age of 65 years have clinically manifest cardiovascular disorders, and such disorders are the leading cause of death and a major source of disability and impaired quality of life in older adults. In general, the diagnosis and treatment of CVDs are similar in older and younger patients. However, most cardiovascular therapies have been less well studied in elderly patients, especially women and individuals with multiple comorbid conditions. As a result, treatment of the older patient with cardiac disease must be individualized, taking into consideration each patient's unique set of circumstances, needs, and personal preferences. Finally, as the population ages, there is a clear need for additional research focusing specifically on the prevention and management of CVDs in the geriatric age group.

REFERENCES

1. American Heart Association. Statistical Fact Sheet: Older Americans and Cardiovascular Diseases, 2006 Update. Dallas, TX: American Heart Association; 2006.
2. Lakatta EG. Age-associated cardiovascular changes in health: impact on cardiovascular disease in older persons. *Heart Fail Rev.* 2002;7:29–49.
3. Rich MW. Heart Disease in the Elderly. In: Rosendorff C, ed. *Essential Cardiology: Principles and Practice.* 2nd ed. Totowa, NJ: Humana Press, Inc.; 2005:705–727.
4. American Heart Association. Heart disease and stroke statistics–2006 Update. *Circulation.* 2006;113:85–151.
5. Expert Panel on Detection, Evaluation, and Treatment of High Blood Cholesterol in Adults. Executive summary of the third report of the National Cholesterol Education Program (NCEP). *JAMA.* 2001;285:2486–2497.
6. Haffner SM, Lehto S, Ronnemaa T, et al. Mortality from coronary heart disease in subjects with type 2 diabetes and in nondiabetic subjects with and without prior myocardial infarction. *NEJM.* 1998;339:229–234.
7. MacMahon SW, Macdonald GJ, Blacket RB. Plasma lipoprotein levels in treated and untreated hypertensive men and women: the National Heart Foundation of Australia Risk Factor Prevalence Study. *Arterioscler Thromb Vasc Biol.* 1985;5:391–396.
8. Neaton JD, Wentworth D. Serum cholesterol, blood pressure, cigarette smoking, and death from coronary heart disease: overall findings and differences by age for 316,099 white men, Multiple Risk Factor Intervention Trial (MRFIT) Research Group. *Arch Intern Med.* 1992;152:56–64.
9. Isomaa B, Almgren P, Tuomi T, et al. Cardiovascular morbidity and mortality associated with the metabolic syndrome. *Diabetes Care.* 2001;24:683–689.
10. Wilson PWF, Kannel WB, Silbershatz H, D'Agostino RB. Clustering of metabolic factors and coronary heart disease. *Arch Intern Med.* 1999;159:1104–1109.
11. Poulter N. Coronary heart disease is a multifactorial disease. *Am J Hypertens.* 1999;12:92S95S.
12. Kuller LH, Arnold AM, Psaty BM, et al. Ten-year follow-up of subclinical cardiovascular disease and risk of coronary heart disease in the Cardiovascular Health Study. *Arch Intern Med.* 2006;166:71–78.
13. Rich MW. Cardiac Disease. In: Landefeld CS, et al. eds. *Current Geriatric Diagnosis and Treatment.* New York: Lange Medical Books/McGraw-Hill; 2004:156–182.
14. White HD, Barbash GI, Califf RM, et al. Age and outcome with contemporary thrombolytic therapy: results from the GUSTO-I trial. *Circulation.* 1996;94:1826–1833.

15. American College of Cardiology/American Heart Association. Management of patients with STEMI: executive summary. *J Am Coll Cardiol.* 2004;44:671–719.

16. American College of Cardiology/American Heart Association. Management of patients with unstable angina and non-ST-segment elevation myocardial infarction. Executive summary. *J Am Coll Cardiol.* 2002;40:1366–1374.

17. ISIS-2 (Second International Study of Infarct Survival) Collaborative Group. Randomised trial of intravenous streptokinase, oral aspirin, both, or neither among 17187 cases of suspected acute myocardial infarction: ISIS-2. *Lancet.* 1988;332:349–360.

18. The Clopidogrel in Unstable Angina to Prevent Recurrent Events Trial Investigators. Effects of clopidogrel in addition to aspirin in patients with acute coronary syndromes without ST-segment elevation. *NEJM.* 2001;345:494–502.

19. The PURSUIT Trial Investigators. Inhibition of platelet glycoprotein IIb/IIIa with eptifibatide in patients with acute coronary syndromes. *NEJM.* 1998;339:436–443.

20. Krumholz HM, Hennen J, Ridker PM, et al. Use and effectiveness of intravenous heparin therapy for treatment of acute myocardial infarction in the elderly. *J Am Coll Cardiol.* 1998;31:973–979.

21. Antman EM, Cohen M, Radley D, et al. Assessment of the treatment effect of enoxaparin for unstable angina/non-Q-wave myocardial infarction: TIMI 11B-ESSENCE meta-analysis. *Circulation.* 1999;100:1602–1608.

22. Fragmin and Fast Revascularization during Instability in Coronary artery disease (FRISC II) Investigators. Long-term low-molecular-mass heparin in unstable coronary-artery disease: FRISC II prospective randomised multicentre study. *Lancet.* 1999;354:701–707.

23. ACE Inhibitor Myocardial Infarction Collaborative Group. Indications for ACE inhibitors in the early treatment of acute myocardial infarction: systematic overview of individual data from 100,000 patients in randomized trials. *Circulation.* 1998;97:2202–2212.

24. Gruppo Italiano per lo Studio della Sopravvivenza nell'Infarto Miocardico. GISSI-3: effects of lisinopril and transdermal glyceryl trinitrate singly and together on 6-week mortality and ventricular function after acute myocardial infarction. *Lancet.* 1994;343:1115–1122.

25. Ambrosioni E, Borghi C, Magnani B, for the Survival of Myocardial Infarction Long-Term Evaluation (SMILE) Study Investigators. The effect of the angiotensin-converting-enzyme inhibitor zofenopril on mortality and morbidity after anterior myocardial infarction. *NEJM.* 1995;332:80–85.

26. The Acute Infarction Ramipril Efficacy (AIRE) Study Investigators. Effect of ramipril on mortality and morbidity of survivors of acute myocardial infarction with clinical evidence of heart failure. *Lancet.* 1993;342:821–828.

27. Dickstein K, Kjekshus J. Effects of losartan and captopril on mortality and morbidity in high-risk patients after acute myocardial infarction: the OPTIMAAL randomised trial. *Lancet.* 2002;360:752–760.

28. Pitt B, Remme W, Zannad F, et al. Eplerenone, a selective aldosterone blocker, in patients with left ventricular dysfunction after myocardial infarction. *NEJM.* 2003;348:1309–1321.

29. Miettinen TA, Pyorala K, Olsson AG, et al. Cholesterol-lowering therapy in women and elderly patients with myocardial infarction or angina pectoris: findings from the Scandinavian Simvastatin Survival Study (4S). *Circulation.* 1997;96:4211–4218.

30. Lewis SJ, Moye LA, Sacks FM, et al. Effect of pravastatin on cardiovascular events in older patients with myocardial infarction and cholesterol levels in the average range: results of the Cholesterol and Recurrent Events (CARE) trial. *Ann Intern Med.* 1998;129:681–689.

31. The Long-Term Intervention with Pravastatin in Ischaemic Disease (LIPID) Study Group. Prevention of cardiovascular events and death with pravastatin in patients with coronary heart disease and a broad range of initial cholesterol levels. *NEJM.* 1998;339:1349–1357.

32. Shepherd J, Blauw GJ, Murphy MB, et al. Pravastatin in elderly individuals at risk of vascular disease (PROSPER): a randomised controlled trial. *Lancet.* 2002;360:1623–1630.

33. Schwartz GG, Olsson AG, Ezekowitz MD, et al. for the Myocardial Ischemia Reduction with Aggressive Cholesterol Lowering (MIRACL) Study Investigators. *JAMA.* 2001;285:1711–1718.

34. Cannon CP, Braunwald E, McCabe CH, et al. for the Pravastatin or Atorvastatin Evaluation and Infection Therapy – Thrombolysis in Myocardial Infarction 22 (PROVE IT-TIMI 22) Investigators. Intensive versus moderate lipid lowering with statins after acute coronary syndromes. *NEJM.* 2004;350:1495–1504.

35. Stenestrand U, Wallentin L for the Swedish Register of Cardiac Intensive Care (RIKS-HIA). *JAMA.* 2001;285:430–436.

36. Aronow WS, Ahn C. Incidence of new coronary events in older persons with prior myocardial infarction and serum low-density lipoprotein cholesterol ≤125 mg/dL treated with statins versus no lipid-lowering drug. *Am J Cardiol.* 2002;89:67–69.

37. White HD. Thrombolytic therapy in the elderly. *Lancet.* 2000;356:2028–2030.

38. The GUSTO Investigators. An international randomized trial comparing four thrombolytic strategies for acute myocardial infarction. *NEJM.* 1993;329:673–682.

39. The Global Use of Strategies to Open Occluded Coronary Arteries in Acute Coronary Syndromes (GUSTO IIb) Angioplasty Substudy Investigators. A clinical trial comparing primary coronary angioplasty with tissue plasminogen activator for acute myocardial infarction. *NEJM.* 1997;336:1621–1628.

40. de Boer MJ, Ottervanger JP, van't Hof AW, et al. Reperfusion therapy in elderly patients with acute myocardial infarction: a randomized comparison of primary angioplasty and thrombolytic therapy. *J Am Coll Cardiol.* 2002;39:1723–1728.

41. Antman EM, Cohen M, Bernink PJLM, et al. The TIMI risk score for unstable angina/non-ST elevation MI: a method for prognostication and therapeutic decision making. *JAMA.* 2000;284:835–842.

42. Granger CB, Goldberg RJ, Dabbous O, et al. Predictors of hospital mortality in the Global Registry of Acute Coronary Events (GRACE). *Arch Intern Med.* 2003;163:2345–2353.

43. FRagmin and Fast Revascularization during InStability in Coronary artery disease (FRISC II) Investigators. Invasive compared with non-invasive treatment in unstable coronary-artery disease: FRISC II prospective randomised multicentre study. *Lancet.* 1999;354:708–715.

44. Hochman JS. Cardiogenic shock complicating acute myocardial infarction: expanding the paradigm. *Circulation.* 2003;107:2998–3002.

45. Hochman JS, Sleeper LA, White HD, et al for the SHOCK Investigators. One-year survival following early revascularization for cardiogenic shock. *JAMA.* 2001;285:190–192.

46. Dzavik V, Sleeper LA, Cocke TP, et al for the SHOCK Investigators. Early revascularization is associated with improved survival in elderly patients with acute myocardial infarction complicated by cardiogenic shock: a report from the SHOCK Trial Registry. *Eur Heart J.* 2003;24:828–837.

47. Bueno H, Lopez-Palop R, Perez-David E, et al. Combined effect of age and right ventricular involvement on acute inferior myocardial infarction prognosis. *Circulation.* 1998;98:1714–1720.

48. Hasdai D, Topol EJ, Califf RM, et al. Cardiogenic shock complicating acute coronary syndromes. *Lancet.* 2000;356:749–756.

49. Witt BJ, Jacobsen SJ, Weston SA, et al. Cardiac rehabilitation after myocardial infarction in the community. *J Am Coll Cardiol.* 2004;44:988–996.

50. American College of Cardiology/American Heart Association Task Force on Practice Guidelines (Committee to Update the 1997 Exercise Testing Guidelines). ACC/AHA 2002 guidelines update for exercise testing. *Circulation.* 2002;106:1883–1892.

51. American College of Cardiology/American Heart Association Task Force on Practice Guidelines. ACC/AHA 2002 guideline update for the management of patients with chronic stable angina. *J Am Coll Cardiol.* 2003;41:159–168.

52. Chaitman BR. Ranolazine for the treatment of chronic angina and potential use in other cardiovascular conditions. *Circulation.* 2006;113:2462–2472.

53. The TIME Investigators. Trial of invasive versus medical therapy in elderly patients with chronic symptomatic coronary-artery disease (TIME): a randomised trial. *Lancet.* 2001;358:951–957.

54. Shaw RE, Anderson HV, Brindis RG, et al. Development of a risk adjustment mortality model using the American College of Cardiology-National Cardiovascular Data Registry (ACC-NCDR) experience: 1998–2000. *J Am Coll Cardiol.* 2002;39:1104–1112.

55. Hannan EL, Racz M, Ryan TJ, et al. Coronary angioplasty volume-outcome relationships for hospitals and cardiologists. *JAMA.* 1997;277:892–898.

56. Ellis SG, Weintraub W, Holmes D, et al. Relation of operator volume and experience to procedural outcome of percutaneous coronary revascularization at hospitals with high interventional volumes. *Circulation.* 1997;95:2479–2484.

57. O'Connor GT, Malenka DJ, Quinton H, et al. Multivariate prediction of in-hospital mortality after percutaneous coronary interventions in 1994–1996. *J Am Coll Cardiol.* 1999;34:681–691.

58. Hannan EL, Burke J. Effect of age on mortality in coronary artery bypass surgery in New York, 1991–1992. *Am Heart J.* 1994;128:1184–1191.

59. Vaccarino V, Abramson JL, Veledar E, Weintraub WS. Sex differences in hospital mortality after coronary artery bypass surgery. *Circulation.* 2002;105:1176–1181.

60. Newman MF, Kirchner JL, Phillips-Bute B, et al for the Neurological Outcome Research Groups and the Cardiothoracic Anesthesiology Research Endeavors Investigators. Longitudinal assessment of neurocognitive function after coronary-artery bypass surgery. *NEJM.* 2001;344:395–402.

61. Shea ML, Conti CR, Arora RR. An update on enhanced external counterpulsation. *Clin Cardiol.* 2005;28:115–118.

62. American College of Cardiology/American Heart Association. ACC/AHA 2005 guideline update for the diagnosis and management of chronic heart failure in the adult. *J Am Coll Cardiol.* 2005;46:1116–1143.

63. Gillum RF. Epidemiology of heart failure in the United States. *Am Heart J.* 1993;126:1042–1047.

64. Gottdiener JS, Arnold AM, Aurigemma GP, et al. Predictors of congestive heart failure in the elderly: the Cardiovascular Health Study. *J Am Coll Cardiol.* 2000;35:1628–1637.

65. The ALLHAT Collaborative Research Group. Major outcomes in high-risk hypertensive patients randomized to angiotensin-converting enzyme inhibitor or calcium channel blocker versus diuretic: the Antihypertensive and Lipid-Lowering Treatment to Prevent Heart Attack Trial (ALLHAT). *JAMA.* 2002;288:2981–2997.

66. Moser M, Hebert PR. Prevention of disease progression, left ventricular hypertrophy and congestive heart failure in hypertension treatment trials. *J Am Coll Cardiol.* 1996;27:1214–1218.

67. Okin PM, Devereux RB, Jern S, et al. Regression of electrocardiographic left ventricular hypertrophy during antihypertensive treatment and the prediction of major cardiovascular events. *JAMA.* 2004;292:2343–2349.

68. Goldman L, Hashimoto B, Cook EF, Loscalzo A. Comparative reproducibility and validity of systems for assessing cardiovascular functional class: advantages of a new specific activity scale. *Circulation.* 1981;64:1227–1234.

69. Hunt SA, Baker DW, Chin MH, et al. ACC/AHA guidelines for the evaluation and management of chronic heart failure in the adult. *J Am Coll Cardiol.* 2001;38:2101–2113.

70. Maisel AS, Krishnaswamy P, Nowak RM, et al. for the Breathing Not Properly Multinational Study Investigators. Rapid measurement of B-type natriuretic peptide in the emergency diagnosis of heart failure. *NEJM.* 2002;347:161–167.

71. Redfield MM, Rodeheffer RJ, Jacobsen SJ, et al. Plasma brain natriuretic peptide concentration: impact of age and gender. *J Am Coll Cardiol.* 2002;40:976–982.

72. Wang TJ, Larson MG, Levy D, et al. Impact of age and sex on plasma natriuretic peptide levels in healthy adults. *Am J Cardiol.* 2002;90:254–258.

73. Heiat A, Gross CP, Krumholz HM. Representation of the elderly, women, and minorities in heart failure clinical trials. *Arch Intern Med.* 2002;162:1682–1688.

74. McAlister FA, Lawson FME, Teo KK, Armstrong PW. A systematic review of randomized trials of disease management programs in heart failure. *Am J Med.* 2001;110:378–384.

75. Rich MW, Beckham V, Wittenberg C, et al. A multidisciplinary intervention to prevent the readmission of elderly patients with congestive heart failure. *NEJM.* 1995;333:1190–1195.

76. Faris R, Flather M, Purcell H, et al. Current evidence supporting the role of diuretics in heart failure: a meta analysis of randomised controlled trials. *Int J Cardiol.* 2002;82:149–158.

77. Domanski M, Norman J, Pitt B, et al. Diuretic use, progressive heart failure, and death in patients in the Studies of Left Ventricular Dysfunction (SOLVD). *J Am Coll Cardiol.* 2003;42:705–708.

78. Cooper HA, Dries DL, Davis CE, et al. Diuretics and risk of arrhythmic death in patients with left ventricular dysfunction. *Circulation.* 1999;100:1311–1315.

79. Neuberg GW, Miller AB, O'Connor CM, et al. Diuretic resistance predicts mortality in patients with advanced heart failure. *Am Heart J.* 2002;144:31–38.

80. Flather MD, Yusuf S, Kober L, et al. for the ACEI-Inhibitor Myocardial Infarction Collaborative Group. Long-term ACEI-inhibitor therapy in patients with heart failure or left-ventricular dysfunction: a systematic overview of data from individual patients. *Lancet.* 2000;355:1575–1581.

81. Garg R, Yusuf S for the Collaborative Group on ACE Inhibitor Trials. Overview of randomized trials of angiotensin-converting enzyme inhibitors on mortality and morbidity in patients with heart failure. *JAMA.* 1995;273:1450–1456.

82. The SOLVD Investigators. Effect of enalapril on mortality and the development of heart failure in asymptomatic patients with reduced left ventricular ejection fraction. *NEJM.* 1992;327:685–691.

83. Maggioni AP, Anand I, Gottlieb SO, et al. Effects of valsartan on morbidity and mortality in patients with heart failure not

receiving angiotensin-converting enzyme inhibitors. *J Am Coll Cardiol.* 2002;40:1414–1421.

84. Granger CB, McMurray JJV, Yusuf S, et al. Effects of candesartan in patients with chronic heart failure and reduced left-ventricular systolic function intolerant to angiotensin-converting-enzyme inhibitors: the CHARM-Alternative trial. *Lancet.* 2003;362:772–776.

85. Cohn JN, Tognoni G, and the Valsartan Heart Failure Trial Investigators. A randomized trial of the angiotensin-receptor blocker valsartan in chronic heart failure. *NEJM.* 2001;345:1667–1675.

86. McMurray JJV, Ostergren J, Swedberg K, et al. Effects of candesartan in patients with chronic heart failure and reduced left-ventricular systolic function taking angiotensin-converting-enzyme inhibitors: the CHARM-Added trial. *Lancet.* 2003;362:767–771.

87. Cohn JN, Archibald DG, Ziesche S, et al. Effect of vasodilator therapy on mortality in chronic congestive heart failure: results of a Veterans Administration Cooperative Study. *NEJM.* 1986;314:1547–1552.

88. Cohn JN, Johnson G, Ziesche S, et al. A comparison of enalapril with hydralazine-isosorbide dinitrate in the treatment of chronic congestive heart failure. *NEJM.* 1991;325:303–310.

89. Taylor AL, Ziesche S, Yancy C, et al for the African-American Heart Failure Trial Investigators. Combination of isosorbide dinitrate and hydralazine in blacks with heart failure. *NEJM.* 2004;351:2049–2057.

90. MERIT-HF Study Group. Effect of metoprolol CR/XL in chronic heart failure: Metoprolol CR/XL Randomised Intervention Trial in Congestive Heart Failure (MERIT-HF). *Lancet.* 1999;353:2001–2007.

91. Packer M, Coats AJS, Fowler MB, et al. for the Carvedilol Prospective Randomized Cumulative Survival Study Group. Effect of carvedilol on survival in severe chronic heart failure. *NEJM.* 2001;344:1651–1658.

92. Deedwania PC, Gottlieb S, Ghali JK, et al. Efficacy, safety and tolerability of beta-adrenergic blockade with metoprolol CR/XL in elderly patients with heart failure. *Eur Heart J.* 2004;25:1300–1309.

93. Gullestad L, Wikstrand J, Deedwania P, et al. for the MERIT-HF Study Group. What resting heart rate should one aim for when treating patients with heart failure with a beta-blocker? *J Am Coll Cardiol.* 2005;45:252–259.

94. The Digitalis Investigation Group. The effect of digoxin on mortality and morbidity in patients with heart failure. *NEJM.* 1997;336:525–533.

95. Rich MW, McSherry F, Williford WO, Yusuf S for the Digitalis Investigation Group. Effect of age on mortality, hospitalizations and response to digoxin in patients with heart failure: the DIG study. *J Am Coll Cardiol.* 2001;38:806–813.

96. Ahmed A, Rich MW, Love TE, et al. Digoxin and reduction in mortality and hospitalization in heart failure: a comprehensive post hoc analysis of the DIG trial. *Eur Heart J.* 2006;27:178–186.

97. Pitt B, Zannad F, Remme WJ, et al. for the Randomized Aldactone Evaluation Study Investigators. The effect of spironolactone on morbidity and mortality in patients with severe heart failure. *NEJM.* 1999;341:709–717.

98. Juurlink DN, Mamdani MM, Lee DS, et al. Rates of hyperkalemia after publication of the Randomized Aldactone Evaluation Study. *NEJM.* 2004;351:543–551.

99. Amidon TM, Parmley WW. Is there a role for positive inotropic agents in congestive heart failure: focus on mortality. *Clin Cardiol.* 1994;17:641–647.

100. Ewy GA. Inotropic infusions for chronic congestive heart failure: medical miracles or misguided medicinals? *J Am Coll Cardiol.* 1999;33:572–575.

101. O'Connor CM, Gattis WA, Uretsky BF, et al. Continuous intravenous dobutamine is associated with an increased risk of death in patients with advanced heart failure: Insights from the Flolan International Randomized Survival Trial (FIRST). *Am Heart J.* 1999;138:78–86.

102. Coletta AP, Cleland JGF, Freemantle N, et al. Clinical trials update from the European Society of Cardiology Heart Failure meeting: SHAPE, BRING-UP 2 VAS, COLA II, FOSIDIAL, BETACAR, CASINO and meta-analysis of cardiac resynchronisation therapy. *Eur J Heart Fail.* 2004;6:673–676.

103. Cuffe MS, Califf RM, Adams KFJ, et al. Short-term intravenous milrinone for acute exacerbation of chronic heart failure: a randomized controlled trial. *JAMA.* 2002;287:1541–1547.

104. Publication Committee for the VMAC Investigators (Vasodilation in the Management of Acute CHF). Intravenous nesiritide vs nitroglycerin for treatment of decompensated congestive heart failure: a randomized controlled trial. *JAMA.* 2002;287:1531–1540.

105. Sackner-Bernstein JD, Kowalski M, Fox M, Aaronson K. Short-term risk of death after treatment with nesiritide for decompensated heart failure: a pooled analysis of randomized controlled trials. *JAMA.* 2005;293:1900–1905.

106. Kitzman DW, Gardin JM, Gottdiener JS, et al. for the Cardiovascular Health Study Research Group. Importance of heart failure with preserved systolic function in patients > or = 65 years of age. *Am J Cardiol.* 2001;87:413–419.

107. Vasan RS, Larson MG, Benjamin EJ, et al. Congestive heart failure in subjects with normal versus reduced left ventricular ejection fraction. *J Am Coll Cardiol.* 1999;33:1948–1955.

108. Devereux RB, Roman MJ, Liu JE, et al. Congestive heart failure despite normal left ventricular systolic function in a population-based sample: the Strong Heart Study. *Am J Cardiol.* 2000;86:1090–1096.

109. Bhatia RS, Tu JV, Lee DS, et al. Outcome of heart failure with preserved ejection fraction in a population-based study. *NEJM.* 2006;355:260–269.

110. Owan TE, Hodge DO, Herges RM, et al. Trends in prevalence and outcome of heart failure with preserved ejection fraction. *NEJM.* 2006;355:251–259.

111. Yusuf S, Pfeffer MA, Swedberg K, et al. for the CHARM investigators and Committees. Effects of candesartan in patients with chronic heart failure and preserved left-ventricular ejection fraction: the CHARM-Preserved Trial. *Lancet.* 2003;362:777–781.

112. Ahmed A, Rich MW, Fleg JL, et al. Effects of digoxin on morbidity and mortality in diastolic heart failure: the Ancillary Digitalis Investigation Group Trial. *Circulation.* 2006;114:397–403.

113. Bristow MR, Saxon LA, Boehmer J, et al. for the Comparison of Medical Therapy, Pacing, and Defibrillation in Heart Failure (COMPANION) Investigators. Cardiac-resynchronization therapy with or without an implantable defibrillator in advanced chronic heart failure. *NEJM.* 2004;350:2140–2150.

114. Cleland JGF, Daubert JC, Erdmann E, et al. for the Cardiac Resynchronization-Heart Failure (CARE-HF) Study Investigators. The effect of cardiac resynchronization on morbidity and mortality in heart failure. *NEJM.* 2005;352:1539–1549.

115. Moss AJ, Zareba W, Hall WJ, et al. for the Multicenter Automatic Defibrillator Implantation Trial II Investigators. Prophylactic implantation of a defibrillator in patients with myocardial

infarction and reduced ejection fraction. *NEJM*. 2002;346:877–883.

116. Bardy GH, Lee KL, Mark DB, et al. for the Sudden Cardiac Death in Heart Failure Trial (SCD-HeFT) Investigators. Amiodarone or an implantable cardioverter-defibrillator for congestive heart failure. *NEJM*. 2005;352:225–237.

117. Huynh BC, Rovner A, Rich MW. Long-term survival in elderly patients hospitalized for heart failure: 14-year follow-up from a prospective randomized trial. *Arch Intern Med*. 2006;166:1892–1898.

118. American College of Cardiology/American Heart Association. ACC/AHA 2006 guidelines for the management of patients with valvular heart disease. *J Am Coll Cardiol*. 2006;48:e1–e148.

119. Scognamiglio R, Rahimtoola SH, Fasoli G, et al. Nifedipine in asymptomatic patients with severe aortic regurgitation and normal left ventricular function. *NEJM*. 1994;331:689–694.

120. Evangelista A, Tornos P, Sambola A, et al. Long-term vasodilator therapy in patients with severe aortic regurgitation. *NEJM*. 2005;353:1342–1349.

121. Mathew JP, Fontes ML, Tudor IC, et al. A multicenter risk index for atrial fibrillation after cardiac surgery. *JAMA*. 2004;291:1720–1729.

122. Crystal E, Connolly SJ, Sleik K, et al. Interventions on prevention of postoperative atrial fibrillation in patients undergoing heart surgery: a meta-analysis. *Circulation*. 2002;106:75–80.

123. Mitchell LB, Exner DV, Wyse DG, et al. Prophylactic oral amiodarone for the prevention of arrhythmias that begin early after revascularization, valve replacement, or repair – PAPABEAR: a randomized controlled trial. *JAMA*. 2005;294:3093–3100.

124. Enriquez-Sarano M, Avierinos JF, Messika-Zeitoun D, et al. Quantitative determinants of the outcome of asymptomatic mitral regurgitation. *NEJM*. 2005;352:875–883.

125. Enriquez-Sarano M, Schaff HV, Orszulak TA, et al. Valve repair improves the outcome of surgery for mitral regurgitation: a multivariate analysis. *Circulation*. 1995;91:1022–1028.

126. Grigioni F, Enriquez-Sarano M, Zehr KJ, et al. Ischemic mitral regurgitation: long-term outcome and prognostic implications with quantitative Doppler assessment. *Circulation*. 2001;103:1759–1764.

127. American Heart Association. Heart disease and stroke statistics–2003 update. Dallas, TX: American Heart Association; 2003.

128. American College of Cardiology/American Heart Association. ACC/AHA/NASPE 2002 guidelines update for implantation of cardiac pacemakers and antiarrhythmia devices: summary article. *Circulation*. 2002;106:2145–2161.

129. Lamas GA, Lee KL, Silverman R, et al. Ventricular pacing or dual-chamber pacing for sinus-node dysfunction. *NEJM*. 2002;346:1854–1862.

130. Go AS, Hylek EM, Phillips KA, et al. Prevalence of diagnosed atrial fibrillation in adults: national implications for rhythm management and stroke prevention: the AnTicoagulation and Risk factors In Atrial fibrillation (ATRIA) study. *JAMA*. 2001;285:2370–2375.

131. American College of Cardiology/American Heart Association. ACC/AHA/ESC 2006 guidelines for management of patients with atrial fibrillation. *J Am Coll Cardiol*. 2006;48:854–906.

132. Coleman CI, Perkerson KA, Gillespie EL, et al. Impact of prophylactic beta blockade on post-cardiothoracic surgery length of stay and atrial fibrillation. *Ann Pharmacother*. 2004;38:2012–2016.

133. Kluger J, White CM. Amiodarone prevents symptomatic atrial fibrillation and reduces the risk of cerebrovascular events and ventricular tachycardia after open heart surgery: results of the Atrial Fibrillation Suppression Trial (AFIST). *Card Electrophysiol Rev*. 2003;7:165–167.

134. Wyse DG, Waldo AL, DiMarco JP, et al. A comparison of rate control and rhythm control in patients with atrial fibrillation. *NEJM*. 2002;347:1825–1833.

135. The AFFIRM Investigators. Quality of life in atrial fibrillation: the Atrial Fibrillation Follow-up Investigation of Rhythm Management (AFFIRM) study. *Am Heart J*. 2005;149:112–120.

136. Wolf PA, Abbott RD, Kannel WB. Atrial fibrillation as an independent risk factor for stroke: the Framingham Study. *Stroke*. 1991;22:983–988.

137. Gage BF, Waterman AD, Shannon W, et al. Validation of clinical classification schemes for predicting stroke: results from the National Registry of Atrial Fibrillation. *JAMA*. 2001;285:2864–2870.

138. The Antiarrhythmics Versus Implantable Defibrillators (AVID) Investigators. A comparison of antiarrhythmic-drug therapy with implantable defibrillators in patients resuscitated from near-fatal ventricular arrhythmias. *NEJM*. 1997;337:1576–1583.

139. Buxton AE, Lee KL, Fisher JD, et al. For the Multicenter Unsustained Tachycardia Trial Investigators. A randomized study of the prevention of sudden death in patients with coronary artery disease. *NEJM*. 1999;341:1882–1890.

12

Peripheral Arterial Disease in the Elderly

Pushpendra Sharma, MD

INTRODUCTION

Peripheral arterial disease (PAD) is a common, age-related, chronic arterial occlusive disease caused by atherosclerosis, resulting in a narrowing of the arteries in the lower extremities and sometimes in the upper extremities. The disease process begins gradually, many years before clinical findings are apparent, and parallels the atherosclerosis of the coronary and cerebral vessels associated with a high mortality rate secondary to cardiovascular and cerebrovascular ischemic events.[1] Cigarette smoking and diabetes are the most common exacerbating factors.[2] Most of the patients with PAD of the lower extremities are asymptomatic. A thorough physical examination is the key to evaluation and treatment. Laboratory tests help confirm the diagnosis and quantify the extent of the disease.

Absence of palpable peripheral arteries and symptomatic intermittent claudication, which are usually present only in the late stages of the disease, are relatively insensitive tools for the diagnosis of atherosclerosis in the peripheral arteries. With the availability of better diagnostic testing, especially the noninvasive methods such as measurement of ankle and brachial blood pressures, and the increasing prevalence in our aging population, PAD is now being identified at an earlier stage. Despite this, there remains a substantial percentage of patients who are not diagnosed with this disorder, especially in the elderly population. These patients continue to have increased morbidity and mortality, largely because of progressive atherosclerosis in multiple vascular beds. The Ankle Brachial Index (ABI) is an important cost-effective, noninvasive tool for assessment of PAD and systemic atherosclerotic disease overall. The ABI measurement in the elderly should be performed by primary care physicians to screen for PAD. Identification of this disease at an early stage may improve the health and life expectancy of our elderly population.

In 2003, The Executive Committee of the Prevention of Atherothrombotic Disease Network issued a "call to action"

citing critical issues in PAD detection and management and recommended the following five measures to address PAD as a significant global public health concern[3]:

1. Increase awareness of PAD and its consequences;
2. Improve the identification of patients with symptomatic PAD;
3. Initiate a screening protocol for patients with high risk for PAD;
4. Improve treatment rates for patients diagnosed with symptomatic PAD;
5. Increase the rates of early detection among the asymptomatic population.

EPIDEMIOLOGY

The incidence of PAD is 3–8 cases/1,000 persons and the prevalence is 2%–4% in the general population. The disease may be more common than the estimates of 8–12 million Americans.[3] It largely remains underdiagnosed and undertreated.[4] The disease tends to be overlooked by physicians because most of the patients with PAD of the lower extremities are asymptomatic. The symptoms may be present in only 10% of individuals with this disease and they include intermittent claudication or rest pain with or without tissue loss or critical limb ischemia. Attention to the risk factors combined with measurement of ABI by the primary care physician can lead to a more frequent diagnosis of the disease.

The prevalence of PAD depends on the method of diagnosis, the patient's age, sex, race, and the geographical area. A U.S. study found that approximately 30% of patients older than 70 years of age and those older than 50 years with history of smoking or diabetes mellitus had PAD,[5] whereas a survey of French cardiologists showed that 10% of their patients had PAD. Using intermittent claudication as a marker of PAD highly results in underestimation the prevalence because more than 70% of the patients with PAD are asymptomatic.[6] The occurrence of intermittent claudication is much lower in younger age groups and increases significantly with older age, from 1% in 55–60 years age group to 4.6% in 80–85 years age group.[7] An ABI of less than 0.9 can be considered the best indicator for estimating the prevalence of PAD. Based on this criterion approximately 27 million people in Europe and North America are presumed to have PAD, with 8–12 million people in United States.[3]

PAD is more prevalent in African American patients compared with white or Hispanic populations and in patients with chronic renal failure.[8] Although the disease may have a more asymptomatic course in women, the prevalence of PAD is similar in women and men, contrary to some earlier beliefs.[9] D-Dimer and markers such as soluble intercellular adhesion molecules–1 correlate significantly with the development of the disease,[10] whereas high-sensitivity C-reactive protein has a strong association with poorer lower extremity functioning in PAD patients.[11] Other factors that have been reported to be associated with development of PAD are use of oral contraceptive agents[12] and depression.[13] Multivessel coronary artery disease (CAD) is more common in patients with both CAD and PAD compared with those with CAD only.[14] Approximately 30% of these patients have left ventricular systolic dysfunction[15] and 22% have a 70% or greater carotid artery stenosis.[16] The risk for ischemic cardiovascular events in patients with PAD is further enhanced by atherosclerosis in other vascular beds, increased prothrombotic state secondary to platelet activation,[17] and perhaps inflammation, as evidenced by a strong relationship between interleukin-6 gene polymorphism and PAD.[18]

PATHOPHYSIOLOGY, RISK FACTORS, AND SCREENING

PAD is a slow atherosclerotic process beginning with injury to the endothelial lining of the arteries, especially the bifurcation of arteries and areas that undergo increased stress from turbulent flow, high pressure, or torsion. This leads to atherosclerotic plaque formation and ultimately the occlusion of major arteries. This may result from thrombosis, embolism, trauma, or a combination thereof. When the artery fails to meet the metabolic requirements of the limb, the symptoms of PAD appear, in the form of intermittent claudication, usually on exertion but it may also occur at rest in cases of severe disease. PAD usually affects three distinct segments in the lower limbs and the disease in each segment produces a distinct pattern of claudication

1. the aortoiliac (infrarenal abdominal aorta and common iliac arteries)
2. the femoropopliteal (superficial femoral artery in the abductor canal)
3. the peroneotibial (below the knee)

Risk factors for PAD include tobacco consumption,[19] diabetes mellitus,[19] hyperlipidemia,[19] hyperhomocysteinemia,[20] hypertension,[19] polycythemia, hypothyroidism,[21] age,[7,22] family history, obesity, stress, and depression[13] and early hysterectomy and oophorectomy and use of oral contraceptive agents[12] in women. Tobacco consumption, especially smoking, damages the arteries by the toxic effect of carbon monoxide and other metabolites of smoke components on the intima as well as the direct arterial vasoconstrictor effect of nicotine that decreases the distal blood flow. Cigarette smoking is the most important factor in determining the disease progression. The incidence of limb amputation is 10 times higher in those who continue to smoke after developing arterial occlusion than in those who quit. Poorly controlled diabetes mellitus leads to intimal injury and atheroma formation. Hyperlipidemia augments plaque formation. High levels of homocysteine directly injure the vessel wall. High blood pressure may lead to initial intimal injury. Polycythemia increases the hematocrit, thereby increasing the resistance to blood flow and the shearing force against vessel walls, resulting in intimal injury and atheroma formation.

Poor prognostic features in patients with PAD that correlate with increased incidence of future ischemic events are:

1. ABI of less than 0.4;[23]
2. Abnormal endothelium dependent flow-mediated vasodilation;[24]
3. Elevated D-dimer levels;[25]
4. Low adenosine diphosphate–induced platelet aggregation;[25]
5. Prothrombin G20210A mutation.[26]

Screening for PAD is frequently overlooked during a general medical checkup. It may have serious implications for the health of elderly patients, especially those with cardiovascular risk factors who may benefit from an early intervention.[27] Screening with an ABI can detect asymptomatic PAD, but whether early detection leads to better outcomes is debatable. The U.S. Preventive Services Task Force recommends against routine screening for PAD.[28] Although there is little evidence that routine screening for PAD with ABI in asymptomatic elderly improves outcome and screening may produce false-positive results, a careful history and physical examination along with ABI can prove to be an effective tool especially in patients at high risk for PAD.[4]

CLINICAL PRESENTATION

Most patients with PAD including the elderly are asymptomatic. The symptoms of classic claudication are present only in a minority of patients with PAD.[4] Over two-thirds of a vessel's lumen must be occluded before the disease can be clinically recognized. The most common clinical symptoms of PAD are aching pain and cramping or numbness in the affected limb. These symptoms are induced by activities such as exercise and

Table 12.1. Symptoms of PAD According to the Site of Occlusion

Occlusion Site	Symptoms
Abdominal aorta	Foot pain at rest, erectile dysfunction in men
Distal to common iliac artery	Buttock, thigh, and calf pain
Aortoiliac artery	Pain in the hips and buttocks
Iliac arteries	Pain in calf and thighs
Common femoral artery	Pain in thighs
Superficial femoral artery	Pain in upper calf
Popliteal artery	Pain in lower calf
Tibial or peroneal artery	Pain in foot

walking that increase the oxygen and blood demand of the lower extremities and they are usually relieved by rest. The cardinal symptom of PAD is intermittent claudication that refers to pain, tightness, or weakness in an exercising muscle brought on by exertion and relieved with rest. The primary cause of claudication is atherosclerosis with subsequent stenosis of peripheral vessels and inability to supply blood to working muscles. It is not present at rest, but occurs during walking, forcing the person to stop because of severe pain, and is relieved by a few minutes of rest. The distance at which claudication occurs is usually constant but may shorten over time with disease progression and during windy and cold weather, inclines, and rapid walking. Use of assistive devices does not improve walking distance.

Potentially serious ischemia in PAD is best described as the six Ps, consisting of pain, paresthesia, pulselessness, paralysis, poikilothermia, and pallor. The pain occurs because of the ischemia resulting from reduced blood flow. Paresthesia results from the death of nerve tissue supplying the diseased segment. Pulselessness leading to the absence of distal pulses and paralysis of the lower extremity usually occurs in advanced disease or with severe occlusion. Poikilothermia relates to a change in the temperature between the unaffected and the affected segments. The pallor results from the paleness of the color of the skin, subcutaneous tissue, and the affected muscle caused by lack of blood supply.

The pain is most often described as squeezing and usually occurs in the calf, but occlusion of specific arterial segments gives rise to particular patterns as shown in Table 12.1.

The common physical findings in PAD are diminished pulses; bruits over the distal aorta, iliac, or femoral arteries; pallor of the distal extremities on elevation; rubor with prolonged capillary refill on dependency; cool skin temperature; trophic changes of hair loss and muscle atrophy and nonhealing ulcers; and necrotic tissue and gangrene.

Less specific symptoms of peripheral atherosclerosis that are caused by defective cutaneous circulation of the foot are numbness, paresthesias, coldness, and pain during rest. Foot or toe numbness during walking and new onset or a recently increased sense of coldness in only one limb that persists after

sleep indicates an arterial disease. The paresthetic, burning foot pain at rest, most severe distally and typically worse at night, preventing sleep, is an extreme symptom, which indicates that blood flow capacity is reduced to less than 10% of normal. The gangrene starts as ecchymosis that develops into ischemic ulcers followed by blackening and mummification of the affected part. The dependent rubor and subsequent gangrene may be painless in patients with peripheral neuropathy or diabetes. The skin is prone to breakdown progressing rapidly to cellulitis and deeper infections that often heal poorly.

PAD results in a functional decline in the elderly. Older patients may use alternative means of ambulation such as a wheelchair or they may stay away from walking altogether to avoid the pain of claudication. Some older patients may not report the symptoms because of impaired cognitive status, fear, anxiety, and financial or caregiver issues. Atypical presentation of PAD in elderly is in the form of acute agitation or worsening evening confusion. Sedentary elderly or those with concurrent pulmonary, arthritic, or cardiovascular conditions, who do not walk far enough to evoke claudication may present with foot pain at rest or even gangrene.

DIAGNOSIS

The diagnosis of PAD can presumptively be established with an accurate history and a thorough physical examination. The history should focus not only on symptoms related to the lower extremity arterial circulation, but also the circulation in other parts of the body including the carotids, coronaries, and the renal arteries. The physical examination should be able to differentiate acute physical findings requiring immediate attention from chronic and nonvascular etiologies from vascular ones.

Assessment of the peripheral pulses is the most basic step in detecting PAD. Absence of peripheral pulses, especially the posterior tibial pulse, strongly suggests peripheral atherosclerosis. It may be difficult to feel whether the patient has edema or prominent malleoli and so the area under the medial malleolus is best palpated with the patient supine and the examiner on the same side as the pulse, with the foot dorsiflexed and everted. The dorsalis pedis artery pulse is easily palpated but may be absent in some healthy individuals. The popliteal artery pulse is the most difficult to palpate and may require the patient to be supine and relaxed with the knee slightly flexed. Obese patients may require very deep palpation in the popliteal space. In addition to examiner's sensitivity, the evaluation of pulses depends on the pulse pressure, thickness of the limb, and the age of the patient. In elderly the pulses tend to become more prominent as the media loses smooth muscle and elastic tissue, predisposing the arteries to ectasia.

Temperature differences between the toes of each foot and skin color changes are also significant. To evaluate the color changes, the foot is elevated above heart level for 20 seconds and then lowered to the dependent position. Pallor lasting more than 30 seconds or rubor appearing after 20 seconds signifies that normal blood flow capacity has declined to less than 10%. Rubor is more pronounced in the toes extending proximally and may require a few minutes to reach its maximum. A severely ischemic foot may appear pale even when flat. Prolonged pallor and rubor associated with pain at rest suggest serious disease. Skin ulceration or frank gangrene of the toes, heels, and lateral malleoli is indicative of extensive disease.

Doppler ultrasonography can be used to assess pulses, but it cannot be used to confirm the adequacy of the flow. It can help to locate the occluded areas and assess the patency of the distal arterial system or a previously treated arterial segment, such as a stented superficial femoral artery or a bypass graft. Blood pressure in the leg is considered low if it is lower than the pressure in the upper extremities or if it decreases during exercise.[4] Its utility in assessment of the entire lower extremity arterial system is highly imprecise despite the use of new ultrasound contrast agents, which have improved the diagnostic ability.

Noninvasive vascular testing helps to confirm the clinical impression of claudication and to locate major occlusive sites. It uses continuous-wave Doppler for measuring systolic arterial pressures to calculate the ABI and segmental pressures as well as the Doppler waveforms.[4] The ABI, which is the ratio of the systolic ankle pressure to the systolic brachial pressure and is usually about 1, is the most efficient, objective, and practical means of documenting presence and severity of PAD. It ranges from 0.5 to 0.8 in claudication and ≤ 0.3 in patients with resting pain or impending limb loss. Segmental systolic pressures objectively define the level of involvement and are usually measured from the upper thigh, above the knee, below the knee and the ankle. Normally there should not be more than 20 mm Hg gradient in pressures between the adjacent segments. A difference of more than 20 mm Hg indicates significant narrowing in the intervening segments. Both ABI and segmental pressures can be done before and after exercise. A resting ABI of less than 0.9 is considered abnormal and has a sensitivity of 95% and specificity of 100% for the detection of PAD, far superior to many other popular screening tests such as Pap smear, fecal occult blood, or mammography.[3] It is also a useful prognostic indicator correlating well with mortality rate over 5 and 10 years.[23] ABI also correlates highly with the severity of PAD. ABI values of 0.5–0.9 are usually seen in patients with claudication and values below 0.5 are usually seen in patients with rest pain or tissue loss.[29] Exercise ABI increases the sensitivity for detection of PAD in patients with high-grade aortoiliac stenosis or occlusion associated with large arterial collaterals, who have normal ABI but still experience intermittent claudication and have a higher mortality risk. On the other hand, ABI may be falsely elevated in patients with diabetes mellitus and renal failure because of noncompressible and calcified lower extremity arteries. An alternate approach in these patients is photoplethysmography to measure the toe brachial index by using a small toe cuff. Transcutaneous oxygen tension can also be used to assess the severity and response to various revascularization therapies, especially in patients with critical limb ischemia, and

it has proved useful in predicting the most appropriate level of amputation.[30]

Angiography remains the gold standard for imaging peripheral arterial occlusions. It should only be performed if surgical reconstruction is being considered because complications can occur during the procedure. Unlike the traditional catheter-based angiography, magnetic resonance angiography and spiral computed tomography are noninvasive imaging methods used to demonstrate the peripheral arteries in patients with PAD. Contrast-enhanced magnetic resonance angiography is superior to duplex ultrasonography in sensitivity and specificity and is as good as standard angiography. In one study, computed tomography angiography when compared with digital subtraction angiography yielded a sensitivity of 91% and a specificity of 92% for lesions with greater than 50% arterial occlusion.[31]

Abnormal fasting lipid profile, vitamin B_{12}, homocysteine level and if needed, a methionine loading test may also aid in determining the etiology of PAD.

DIFFERENTIAL DIAGNOSIS

Differential diagnosis of PAD includes other disorders that cause similar symptoms of leg pain. The nonvascular conditions that resemble claudication include degenerative joint disease, particularly arthritis of the lumbar spine and the hips; spinal stenosis (pseudoclaudication); prolapsed intervertebral disc; muscle cramps; musculoskeletal pain; peripheral neuropathy; restless legs syndrome; and compartment syndrome. Vascular conditions such as thromboangiitis obliterans (Buerger disease), chronic and acute chronic arterial insufficiency, and deep vein thrombosis may also cause pain resembling intermittent claudication.

The symptoms of spinal stenosis also occur at rest in addition to walking and are often worse while sitting. On the other hand, the pain of PAD is caused by exercise and is relieved by rest. Rather than being localized to the calves as in PAD, the pain usually radiates down the entire extremity. The same can be said about the pain caused by arthritis of the lumbar spine and the hips and prolapsed intervertebral disc. The pain is sharp throbbing or burning in nature, and is associated with numbness and paresthesias. If it is caused by diabetic neuropathy, it is bilateral and extends above the feet. Exercise or rest does not affect the pain of peripheral neuropathy. The pain of restless leg syndrome occurs at night when the legs are still, often awakening the patient and is tingling or crawling. It causes the patient to move the legs restlessly and gets better with walking.[32]

The pain of chronic arterial insufficiency is bilateral, symmetrical, dull aching, or throbbing and usually occurs in the legs because of pooling of blood resulting in edema of feet or legs. In contrast to calf muscle pain of PAD that occurs during walking, the pain occurs after prolonged periods of standing or sitting with legs dangling down and may improve with exercise.

MANAGEMENT

Ironically, patients with PAD are undertreated by physicians from all specialties involved in their care. A recent national physician survey clearly revealed that atherosclerotic risk factor reduction and antiplatelet therapy was prescribed much less frequently in PAD patients compared with CAD patients. It further showed that the physicians perceived antiplatelet therapy and cholesterol-lowering therapy to be more important for the CAD than for the PAD patient. In contrast to vascular surgeons, cardiologists were noted to be prompt in initiating cholesterol-lowering interventions for the patient with PAD.[33]

The patients with PAD are at a much higher risk of death resulting from cardiovascular and cerebrovascular causes than the risk of limb loss,[29] stressing the need to address the overall atherosclerotic disease process involving all vascular beds rather than focusing on individual vascular beds separately.

The management of PAD aims at improvement of functional status and quality of life by providing relief of intermittent claudication, prolongation of survival by prevention of thrombotic events in peripheral, coronary, and cerebrovascular circulation and prevention of complications by aggressive risk factor modification and pharmacological therapy. With aggressive risk factor modification and adequate pharmacotherapy, patients with PAD can have an improved quality of life as well as prolonged survival. Focus should be on smoking cessation, blood pressure reduction to levels below 130/85 mm Hg, low-density lipid levels in the range of 100 mg/dL and effective control of diabetes mellitus (glycosylated hemoglobin levels lower than 7%).

Avoiding tobacco, dieting to reduce cholesterol, and controlling diabetes and blood pressure along with exercise are the cornerstones of nonpharmacological measures for exertional claudication. Exercise, such as walking 30–60 min/day for 5 day/wk at approximately 2 mile/h, will increase walking distances before symptoms occur and provides an overall better functioning status.

Smoking is the most preventable cause and the greatest risk factor of cardiovascular morbidity and mortality in patients with PAD, with the relative risk associated with PAD being 32% with current smoking and 40% with past smoking. Unlike CAD and stroke, previous smoking appears to have a persistent effect on the risk of PAD.[34] All patients with PAD should be educated, encouraged, and assisted in smoking cessation by using both behavioral and adjunctive medical therapies such as nicotine replacement therapy, bupropion, and the newer agent varenicline (Chantix). Patients who quit smoking have an approximately 2–5 year better survival rate compared with those who continue to smoke.[35]

Diabetes mellitus should be intensively controlled to lower glycosylated hemoglobin levels to below 7%, to decrease micro- and macrovascular complications.[36,37]

Hypertension and smoking were found to be the two most important modifiable risk factors for PAD with odd ratio of 2.2 and 2.0, respectively, in the Framingham Offspring Study.[38]

Table 12.2. Management of PAD

Aggressive Risk Factor Modification

Stop smoking

Reduce cholesterol

Increase exercise

Control blood pressure

Control diabetes

Pharmacological Treatment

pentoxifylline

cilostazol

clopidogrel

aspirin

vasodilators

Vascular Interventions

Angioplasty

Stents

Bypass

Reconstruction

Optimal blood pressure control in hypertensive patients leads to significant decrease in stroke, myocardial infarction, congestive heart failure, renal failure, and death. Similar benefits are noted in elderly patients with isolated systolic hypertension[39] and in patients with cardiovascular risk factors.[40] Blood pressure lowering to a mean of 127/75 mm Hg resulted in marked reduction of cardiovascular ischemic events in a recent study of 950 patients with PAD and type 2 diabetes mellitus.[41]

All patients with PAD should exercise regularly. Sedentary lifestyle resulting from claudication in patients with symptomatic PAD leads to a worsening of their cardiovascular risk profile and a higher risk of cardiovascular events, thereby increasing mortality. Patients with intermittent claudication should be taught about foot care and advised to walk as much as possible. As soon as claudication occurs, they should rest and then continue walking. Walking may result in symptom control within the first 3 months. Most patients can adjust to walking long distances with frequent rest stops. Others may benefit from structured vascular rehabilitation programs that have been shown to be superior to home-based exercise programs[42] and may improve peak walking distance and pain free walking distance by over 100%.[43] This improvement can then be maintained using a less frequent exercise maintenance program[44] or a short-course training program.[45]

Lipid lowering in patients with PAD is a clearly indicated goal in the Adult Treatment Panel III guidelines; however, more than 50% of patients with PAD treated by primary care physicians,[4] vascular surgeons,[46] and endovascular specialists[47] have lipid levels above the National Cholesterol

Education Program goals. Patients with PAD and no CAD have higher risk of coronary events if they were not treated with statins than patients with CAD and PAD who received lipid-lowering therapy.[48] In addition to preventing cardiovascular events, statins have been shown to improve pain-free walking distance and other leg functioning parameters, and to improve quality of life in patients with PAD.[49–51]

In addition to controlling of risk factors, walking regularly, foot care and weight loss, patients should be advised to avoid positions that may impair circulation such as crossing the legs while sitting. Supplements such as folic acid, vitamin B_6 (pyridoxine), and vitamin B_{12} (cyanocobalamin) are also beneficial.

The results of drug therapy for claudication are mixed. Pentoxifylline (Trental) and cilostazol (Pletal) have been approved for use in patients with intermittent claudication who have not responded well to conservative measures. The consensus statement in 2003 strongly recommended the use of antiplatelet agents in all patients with PAD, usually aspirin.[52] Pentoxifylline or cilostazol should be tried for 3 months. Other medications that help include coagulation modifiers such as clopidogrel, aspirin, angiotensin-converting enzyme inhibitors, statins, and anticlaudication drugs including vasodilators. If there is no improvement in symptoms, the medicine can be discontinued.

One of the first drugs approved for treating claudication, pentoxifylline (400 mg three times a day), decreases blood viscosity and improves red blood cell flexibility, leading to improved blood flow through arterioles and capillaries and resulting in increased mean walking distance. Although it has few adverse effects, it has not shown increases in muscle blood flow sufficient to prevent claudication.

Cilostazol, a phosphodiesterase inhibitor, with antiplatelet and vasodilatory properties, produces a mild-to-moderate increase in walking distance comparable to that produced by pentoxifylline, at a dose of 100 mg twice a day. A meta-analysis of six trials has shown that treatment with cilostazol was associated with greater improvements in community-based walking ability and health-related quality of life in patients with intermittent claudication than treatment with placebo.[51] It has also been shown to favorably alter plasma lipid profile by elevating high-density lipoprotein cholesterol and lowering triglycerides.[53] Because of its cardiovascular toxicity it is contraindicated in patients with heart failure.

Clopidogrel (75 mg daily) was shown to have a small incremental benefit of 8.7% over aspirin in preventing stroke, myocardial infarction, and vascular death in a prospectively stratified group of patients with PAD in the Clopidogrel Versus Aspirin in Patients at Risk of Ischemic Events study, probably because as many as 40% of PAD patients had an inadequate response to aspirin.[54]

Aspirin 81–325 mg daily, in addition to being cost effective, has been found to be beneficial overall in patients with PAD and atherosclerotic CAD.

Because of their favorable effect on atherosclerotic CAD, β-blockers may help patients with heart disease and claudication.

Other agents that have been shown to benefit intermittent claudication include naftidrofuryl, heparan, and intra-venous glutathione infusion; the results have been variable. Patients with critical limb ischemia who are not good candidates for endovascular or surgical revascularization may benefit from long-term intermittent use of prostanoids including prostaglandin E1, iloprost, and treprostinil.[55,56] These agents reduce rest pain and ulcer size, but have a controversial benefit in intermittent claudication. Hyperbaric oxygen, artificial CO_2 foot bathing, and intermittent pneumatic compression devices have also shown promise in healing of patients with critical limb ischemia with ulceration or gangrene.[57,58]

Patients with refractory rest pain, limb ischemia, nonhealing ulcers, dependent rubor, tissue loss or gangrene, or those with functional disability are candidates for surgical reconstruction. Elderly patients who do not have tissue loss or pain at rest should not undergo surgery, even if they have marked dependent rubor. For patients with severe heart disease, amputation is sometimes preferable to the risk of bypass surgery. Common surgical processes are aortoiliofemoral reconstruction, infrainguinal bypass such as femoropopliteal and femorotibial bypass and extraanatomical bypass such as axillofemoral and femorofemoral bypass. These have a perioperative mortality of approximately 2%–5%.

Potential benefits of surgery must be weighed against risks. If collateral vessels are cut during surgery, the bypass may worsen circulatory impairment. Lower-risk procedures such as a subcutaneous femorofemoral bypass across the lower pelvic area may help save a limb if the disease is unilateral. When a limb is threatened, the presence of stenoses in many areas is not a contraindication to surgery. Patients' general health, lifestyle, age, the presence of heart disease, and location of the lesions must be considered. Increased operative mortality rate in patients with significant CAD is a contraindication to peripheral artery surgery. Angina manifesting after a successful bypass surgery may limit the improvement in walking distance. Angiography is performed before surgery to determine the patency of a major vessel beyond the obstruction and the distal flow beyond the patent vessel.

The most effective treatment for intermittent claudication is arterial bypass surgery or, for less severe cases, percutaneous transluminal angioplasty. Bypass of the most proximal occlusion often increases collateral flow around more distal occlusions sufficiently to salvage the limb. Bypass surgery and angioplasty are generally reserved for patients who have claudication because of isolated aortoiliac disease and severe symptoms. Angioplasty is used on short, discrete stenotic lesions in the iliac or femoropopliteal artery before bypass surgery. Atherectomy, stent placement, and lasers are other techniques. If the lesion is more proximal, the bypass surgery has better clinical results, and the graft remains patent for a longer period. The 5-year patency rate for patients with localized aortoiliac disease is more than 90%, for patients with femoropopliteal disease it is approximately 60%–70% for bypasses above the knee but for bypasses across the knee into the distal popliteal or proximal tibial arteries the patency rate is somewhat lower. The 5-year patency rate for distal femorotibial grafts is less than 50%. Patients with generalized disease have much lower patency rates. A femoropopliteal bypass may uncover claudication in the opposite limb when arterial occlusion is bilateral, leading to only slight clinical improvement and making it necessary to have a second surgery to significantly increase claudication-free walking distance. An autologous saphenous vein is preferable for a femoropopliteal bypass because long-term patency rates are higher, but for aortoiliac and aortofemoral bypass grafts a prosthetic material such as Teflon is used.

Angioplasty is often associated with lower procedural morbidity and mortality rates. Although surgery frequently provides greater long-term patency, the later failure of percutaneous therapies may require reintervention. Most of the newer endovascular technologies are applicable in the treatment of PAD. Subintimal angioplasty is becoming effective in revascularization in patients with lesions of the superficial femoral artery.[59,60] Endovascular brachytherapy has also been found to improve the patency of femoropopliteal arteries undergoing percutaneous angioplasty in nondiabetic patients with long occlusions[61] but may result in thrombotic occlusion in the long term.[62] The drug-eluting stents, which have shown good results in the coronary circulation, have also shown potential in the prevention of restenosis in lesions of superficial femoral artery.[63] The use of tenecteplase–tissue plasminogen activator for catheter-directed thrombolysis in patients with acute limb ischemia was shown to produce marked improvement or complete resolution in more than 87% of patients with a reasonable safety profile.[64]

In patients primarily considered for surgical treatment, antiplatelet and anticoagulant drug therapy can be used to promote graft patency, and β-blockers can be used to reduce the perioperative risks associated with vascular surgery. In patients with gangrene, limb salvage after injection of vascular endothelial growth factor into the calf muscle is being tried as an alternative approach.

Several newer devices, catheters, balloons, and stents are being developed. Other modalities in the process of development include therapeutic angiogenesis to induce angiogenesis by using angiogenic growth factors, bone marrow mononuclear cells, fibroblast growth factor, vascular endothelial growth factor, and hepatocyte growth factor.

COMPLICATIONS

Complications of PAD result from decreased or absent blood flow. Claudication is a marker for generalized atherosclerosis, subjecting PAD patients to a higher risk of death from cardiovascular events than from limb loss. Regardless of whether the PAD is symptomatic, the most significant complications of PAD are stroke and heart attack, with an annual mortality rate of 5%–10%. Strokes are three times more likely in persons with PAD. Critical limb ischemia or acute ischemia of a limb caused by sudden cut off of the blood flow to the limb is also an important complication of PAD, which, if not treated promptly, may result in amputation. Diabetic patients with claudication experiencing acute ischemic event have a much higher risk than the

1% annually among all patients with claudication. Peripheral aneurysms especially of the popliteal artery also result as complications of the PAD. These aneurysms if not surgically resected or bypassed may rupture or thrombose, leading to limb loss. Other complications of PAD include amputation, poor wound healing, restricted mobility due to pain or discomfort with exertion, and severe pain in the affected extremity. Complications of PAD can be prevented by exercise, tobacco abstinence, and following an aggressive treatment plan.

REFERENCES

1. Criqui MH, Langer RD, Fronek A, et al. Mortality over a period of 10 years in patients with peripheral arterial disease. *NEJM.* 1992;326(6):381–386.
2. Fowkes FGR, Housley E, Riemersma RA, et al. Smoking, lipids, glucose intolerance, and blood pressure as risk factors for peripheral atherosclerosis compared with ischemic heart disease. *Am J Epidemiol.* 1992;135:331–340.
3. Belch JJ, Topol EJ, Agnelli G, et al. Critical issues in peripheral arterial disease detection and management: a call to action. *Arch Intern Med.* 2003;163(8):884–892.
4. Hirsch AT, Criqui MH, Treat-Jacobson D, et al. Peripheral arterial disease detection, awareness, and treatment in primary care. *JAMA.* 2001;286(11):1317–1324.
5. Hirsch AT, Hiatt WR. PAD awareness, risk and treatment: new resources for survival – the USA PARTNERS program. *Vasc Med.* 2001;6(3 suppl):9–12.
6. Dormandy JA, Rutherford RB. Management of peripheral arterial disease (PAD). TASC Working Group. TransAtlantic Inter-Society Consensus (TASC). *J Vasc Surg.* 2000;31(1 Pt 2):S1–S296.
7. Meijer WT, Hoes AW, Rutgers D, Bots ML, Hofman A, Grobbee DE. Peripheral arterial disease in the elderly: the Rotterdam Study. *Arterioscler Thromb Vasc Biol.* 1998;18(2):185–192.
8. Collins TC, Petersen NJ, Suarez-Almazor M, Ashton CM. The prevalence of peripheral arterial disease in a racially diverse population. *Arch Intern Med.* 2003;163(12):1469–1474.
9. Higgins JP, Higgins JA. Peripheral arterial disease – Part I: Diagnosis, epidemiology and risk factors. *J Okla State Med Assoc.* 2002;95(12):765–769; quiz 770–771.
10. Pradhan AD, Rifai N, Ridker PM. Soluble intercellular adhesion molecule-1, soluble vascular adhesion molecule-1, and the development of symptomatic peripheral arterial disease in men. *Circulation.* 2002;106(7):820–825.
11. McDermott MM, Greenland P, Green D, et al. D-dimer, inflammatory markers, and lower extremity functioning in patients with and without peripheral arterial disease. *Circulation.* 2003;107(25):3191–3198.
12. Van Den Bosch MA, Kemmeren JM, Tanis BC, et al. The RATIO study: oral contraceptives and the risk of peripheral arterial disease in young women. *J Thromb Haemost.* 2003;1(3):439–444.
13. McDermott MM, Greenland P, Guralnik JM, et al. Depressive symptoms and lower extremity functioning in men and women with peripheral arterial disease. *J Gen Intern Med.* 2003;18(6):461–467.
14. Brevetti G, Piscione F, Silvestro A, et al. Increased inflammatory status and higher prevalence of three-vessel coronary artery disease in patients with concomitant coronary and peripheral atherosclerosis. *Thromb Haemost.* 2003;89(6):1058–1063.
15. Kelly R, Staines A, MacWalter R, Stonebridge P, Tunstall-Pedoe H, Struthers AD. The prevalence of treatable left ventricular

systolic dysfunction in patients who present with noncardiac vascular episodes: a case-control study. *J Am Coll Cardiol.* 2002;39(2):219–224.

16. Kurvers HA, van Der Graaf Y, Blankensteijn JD, Visseren FL, Eikelboom BC. Screening for asymptomatic internal carotid artery stenosis and aneurysm of the abdominal aorta: comparing the yield between patients with manifest atherosclerosis and patients with risk factors for atherosclerosis only. *J Vasc Surg.* 2003;37(6):1226–1233.

17. Cassar K, Bachoo P, Ford I, Greaves M, Brittenden J. Platelet activation is increased in peripheral arterial disease. *J Vasc Surg.* 2003;38(1):99–103.

18. Flex A, Gaetani E, Pola R, et al. The- 174 G/C polymorphism of the interleukin-6 gene promoter is associated with peripheral artery occlusive disease. *Eur J Vasc Endovasc Surg.* 2002;24(3):264–268.

19. Ness J, Aronow WS, Ahn C. Risk factors for peripheral arterial disease in an academic hospital based geriatrics practice. *J Am Geriatr Soc.* 2000;48:312–314.

20. Boushey CJ, Barasford SAA, Omen GS, Motulsky AG. A quantitative assessment of plasma homocysteine as a risk factor for vascular disease. Probable benefits of increasing folic acid intakes. *JAMA.* 1995;274:1049–1057.

21. Mya MM, Aronow WS. Increased prevalence of peripheral artery disease in older men and women with subclinical hypothyroidism. *J Gerontol Med Sci.* 2003;58A:M68–M69.

22. Criqui MH, Fronek A, Barrett-Conner E, Klauber MR, Gabriel S, Goodman D. The prevalence of peripheral arterial disease in a defined population. *Circulation.* 1985;71:516–521.

23. McKenna M, Wolfson S, Kuller L. The ratio of ankle and arm arterial pressure as an independent predictor of mortality. *Atherosclerosis.* 1991;87(2–3):119–128.

24. Gokce N, Keaney JF Jr, Hunter LM, et al. Predictive value of noninvasively determined endothelial dysfunction for long-term cardiovascular events in patients with peripheral vascular disease. *J Am Coll Cardiol.* 2003;41(10):1769–1775.

25. Komarov A, Panchenko E, Dobrovolsky A, et al. D-dimer and platelet aggregability are related to thrombotic events in patients with peripheral arterial occlusive disease. *Eur Heart J.* 2002;23(16):1309–1316.

26. Gerdes VE, ten Cate H, de Groot E, et al. Arterial wall thickness and the risk of recurrent ischemic events in carriers of the prothrombin G20210A mutation with clinical manifestations of atherosclerosis. *Atherosclerosis.* 2002;163(1):135–140.

27. ACC/AHA 2005 Practice Guidelines for the Management of Patients with Peripheral Arterial Disease (Lower Extremity, Renal Mesenteric and Abdominal Aortic). *Circulation.* 2006;113:1474–1547.

28. http://www.ahrq.gov/clinic/uspstf/uspspard.htm.

29. Ouriel K. Peripheral arterial disease. *Lancet.* 2001;358(9289):1257–1264.

30. Padberg FT, Back TL, Thompson PN, Hobson RW, 2nd. Transcutaneous oxygen (TcPO2) estimates probability of healing in the ischemic extremity. *J Surg Res.* 1996;60(2):365–369.

31. Ofer A, Nitecki SS, Linn S, et al. Multidetector CT angiography of peripheral vascular disease: a prospective comparison with intraarterial digital subtraction angiography. *AJR Am J Roentgenol.* 2003;180(3):719–724.

32. Herr KA. Night leg pain. *Geriatr Nurs.* 1992;13:13–16.

33. McDermott MM, Hahn EA, Greenland P, et al. Atherosclerotic risk factor reduction in peripheral arterial disease: results of a national physician survey. *J Gen Intern Med.* 2002;17(12):895–904.

34. Fowler B, Jamrozik K, Norman P, Allen Y. Prevalence of peripheral arterial disease: persistence of excess risk in former smokers. *Aust NZ J Public Health.* 2002;26(3):219–224.

35. Faulkner KW, House AK, Castleden WM. The effect of cessation of smoking on the cumulative survival rates of patients with symptomatic peripheral vascular disease. *Med J Aust.* 1983;1:217–219.

36. UK Prospective Diabetes Study Group. Efficacy of atenolol and captopril in reducing risk of macrovascular and microvascular complications in type 2 diabetes: UKPDS 39. *BMJ.* 1998;317(7160):713–720.

37. UK Prospective Diabetes Study Group. Tight blood pressure control and risk of macrovascular and microvascular complications in type 2 diabetes: UKPDS 38. *BMJ.* 1998;317(7160):703–713.

38. Murabito JM, Evans JC, Nieto K, Larson MG, Levy D, Wilson PW. Prevalence and clinical correlates of peripheral arterial disease in the Framingham Offspring Study. *Am Heart J.* 2002;143(6):961–965.

39. SHEP Cooperative Research Group. Prevention of stroke by antihypertensive drug treatment in older persons with isolated systolic hypertension. Final results of the Systolic Hypertension in the Elderly Program (SHEP). *JAMA.* 1991;265(24):3255–3264.

40. Yusuf S, Sleight P, Pogue J, Bosch J, Davies R, Dagenais G. Effects of an angiotensin-converting-enzyme inhibitor, ramipril, on cardiovascular events in high-risk patients. The Heart Outcomes Prevention Evaluation Study Investigators. *NEJM.* 2000;342(3):145–153.

41. Mehler PS, Coll JR, Estacio R, Esler A, Schrier RW, Hiatt WR. Intensive blood pressure control reduces the risk of cardiovascular events in patients with peripheral arterial disease and type 2 diabetes. *Circulation.* 2003;107(5):753–756.

42. Degischer S, Labs KH, Hochstrasser J, Aschwanden M, Tschoepl M, Jaeger KA. Physical training for intermittent claudication: a comparison of structured rehabilitation versus home-based training. *Vasc Med.* 2002;7(2):109–115.

43. Gardner AW, Poehlman ET. Exercise rehabilitation programs for the treatment of claudication pain. A meta-analysis. *JAMA.* 1995;274(Sep 27):975–980.

44. Gardner AW, Katzel LI, Sorkin JD, Goldberg AP. Effects of long-term exercise rehabilitation on claudication distances in patients with peripheral arterial disease: a randomized controlled trial. *J Cardiopulm Rehabil.* 2002;22(3):192–198.

45. Ambrosetti M, Salerno M, Tramarin R, Pedretti RF. Efficacy of a short-course intensive rehabilitation program in patients with moderate-to-severe intermittent claudication. *Ital Heart J.* 2002;3(8):467–472.

46. Cote MC, Ligeti R, Cutler BS, Nelson PR. Management of hyperlipidemia in patients with vascular disease. *J Vasc Nurs.* 2003;21(2):63–7; quiz 68–9.

47. Mukherjee D, Lingam P, Chetcuti S, et al. Missed opportunities to treat atherosclerosis in patients undergoing peripheral vascular interventions: insights from the University of Michigan Peripheral Vascular Disease Quality Improvement Initiative (PVD-QI2). *Circulation.* 2002;106(15):1909–1912.

48. Aronow WS, Ahn C. Elderly diabetics with peripheral arterial disease and no coronary artery disease have a higher incidence of new coronary events than elderly nondiabetics with peripheral arterial disease and prior myocardial infarction treated with statins and with nonlipid-lowering drug. *J Gerontol A Biol Sci Med Sci.* 2003;58(6):573–575.

49. McDermott MM, Guralnik JM, Greenland P, et al. Statin use and leg functioning in patients with and without lower-extremity peripheral arterial disease. *Circulation.* 2003;107(5):757–761.

50. Mondillo S, Ballo P, Barbati R, et al. Effects of simvastatin on walking performance and symptoms of intermittent claudication in hypercholesterolemic patients with peripheral vascular disease. *Am J Med.* 2003;114(5):359–364.

51. Regensteiner JG, Ware JE Jr, McCarthy WJ, et al. Effect of cilostazol on treadmill walking, community-based walking ability, and health-related quality of life in patients with intermittent claudication due to peripheral arterial disease: metaanalysis of six randomized controlled trials. *J Am Geriatr Soc.* 2002;50(12):1939–1946.

52. Antiplatelet therapy in peripheral arterial disease. Consensus statement. *Eur J Vasc Endovasc Surg.* 2003;26(1):1–16.

53. Grouse JR 3rd, Allan MC, Elam MB. Clinical manifestation of atherosclerotic peripheral arterial disease and the role of cilostazol in treatment of intermittent claudication. *J Clin Pharmacol.* 2002;42(12):1291–1298.

54. Roller RE, Dorr A, Ulrich S, Pilger E. Effect of aspirin treatment in patients with peripheral arterial disease monitored with the platelet function analyzer PFA-100. *Blood Coagul Fibrinolysis.* 2002;13(4):277–281.

55. Chattaraj SC. Treprostinil sodium pharmacia. *Curr Opin Invest Drugs.* 2002;3(4):582–586.

56. Mohler ER 3rd, Hiatt WR, Olin JW, Wade M, Jeffs R, Hirsch AT. Treatment of intermittent claudication with beraprost sodium, an orally active prostaglandin I2 analogue: a double-blinded, randomized, controlled trial. *J Am Coll Cardiol.* 2003;41(10):1679–1686.

57. Toriyama T, Kumada Y, Matsubara T, et al. Effect of artificial carbon dioxide foot bathing on critical limb ischemia (Fontaine IV) in peripheral arterial disease patients. *Int Angiol.* 2002;21(4):367–373.

58. Montori VM, Kavros SJ, Walsh EE, Rooke TW. Intermittent compression pump for nonhealing wounds in patients with limb ischemia. The Mayo Clinic experience (1998–2000). *Int Angiol.* 2002;21(4):360–366.

59. Lipsitz EC, Ohki T, Veith FJ, et al. Does subintimal angioplasty have a role in the treatment of severe lower extremity ischemia? *J Vasc Surg.* 2003;37(2):386–391.

60. Shaw MB, DeNunzio M, Hinwood D, Nash R, Callum KG, Braithwaite BD. The results of subintimal angioplasty in a district general hospital. *Eur J Vasc Endovasc Surg.* 2002;24(6):524–527.

61. Hansrani M, Overbeck K, Smout J, Stansby G. Intravascular brachytherapy for peripheral vascular disease. *Cochrane Database Syst Rev.* 2002;(4):CD003504.

62. Bonvini R, Baumgartner I, Do DD, et al. Late acute thrombotic occlusion after endovascular brachytherapy and stenting of femoropopliteal arteries. *J Am Coll Cardiol.* 2003;41(3):409–412.

63. Duda SH, Pusich B, Richter G, et al. Sirolimus-eluting stents for the treatment of obstructive superficial femoral artery disease: six-month results. *Circulation.* 2002;106(12):1505–1509.

64. Razavi MK, Wong H, Kee ST, Sze DY, Semba CP, Dake MD. Initial clinical results of tenecteplase (TNK) in catheter-directed thrombolytic therapy. *J Endovasc Ther.* 2002;9(5):593–598.

13

STROKE IN THE OLDER ADULT

Kerri S. Remmel, MD, PhD

EPIDEMIOLOGY

Stroke is the leading cause of long-term disability and is the third leading cause of mortality in the United States. Each year, approximately 700,000 people have a stroke, approximately 200,000 of which are recurrent.[1] Of all stroke cases, 87% are ischemic and 12% are hemorrhagic.[2] Approximately 14% of those who have an ischemic stroke or transient ischemic attack (TIA) will have another event within 1 year (see Figures 13.1 and 13.2). Approximately 22% of men and 25% of women with stroke will die within a year and this percentage is higher among people aged 65 years and older. In addition, the prevalence of TIA is estimated to be approximately 240,000 cases annually and the prevalence of silent ischemic stroke between the ages of 55 and 64 years is approximately 11%, 22% between the ages of 65 and 69 years, 28% between the ages of 70 and 74 years, 32% between the ages of 75 and 79 years, 40% between the ages of 80 and 85 years, and 43% by the age of 85 years and older.[2,3] Thus, age is a risk factor for stroke.

STROKE SUBTYPE

Ischemic stroke can be classified based on the presumed mechanism into the modified Trial of Org 10172 in Acute Stroke Treatment or TOAST criteria: 1) large-artery atherosclerosis, 2) cardioembolism, 3) small-vessel occlusion, 4) stroke of other determined etiology (such as arterial dissection or hypercoagulable states), and 5) stroke of undetermined etiology.[6]

In patients in whom the cause of stroke is known , a thorough work up should still be performed to address appropriate risk factor reduction because the patient may have more than one etiology (e.g., severe carotid stenosis and atrial fibrillation).

MANAGEMENT OF STROKE

Over the last few years, improvements have been made in stroke prevention, treatment, and rehabilitation. The approval of the intravenous (IV) thrombolytic (IV tissue plasminogen activator [tPA]) by the Food and Drug Administration in 1996 and advancements in endovascular procedures have been shown to improve outcomes in patients with acute stroke. The availability of scientifically based guidelines and recommendations help to establish consistent treatment protocols, clinical pathways, and standing orders for management of stroke patients. All of which have been shown to improve quality of care during hospitalization and to improve outcomes.

Failure to identify stroke patients immediately on their arrival to the emergency department (ED) may result in expiration of the time window for IV-tPA administration in ischemic stroke patients. A "stroke code" system should be in place to notify rapidly the acute stroke team. In a stroke center, one member of the stroke team should be at patients' bedside within 15 minutes of arrival. Utilization of a "rapid assessment room," usually designated for trauma victims, shortens the time of initial stabilization and assessment (see Table 13.1).

Noncontrast computed tomography (CT) scanning of the brain should be completed within 25 minutes after the patient's arrival in the ED and be read within 45 minutes after arrival in the ED.[9] Noncontrast CT scanning of the brain will identify most cases of hemorrhage and helps discriminate nonvascular causes of stroke such as a brain tumor (Grade B).[10] Based on the result of a noncontrast CT scan, further assessment and management of the acute stroke patient will be performed.

Management of Acute Ischemic Stroke

Patients Who Qualify for IV-tPA

Regardless of age, all acute stroke victims with time of onset less than 3 hours should be assessed for their qualification to receive IV-tPA. It is very important to determine the time of onset or time last known at baseline. Rapid evaluation of the inclusion and exclusion criteria is important to ensure patients

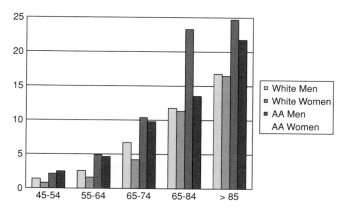

Figure 13.1. Increasing incidence of stroke rate for each 10-year period after the age of 55 years.[4]

will meet all inclusion criteria and that they have no past or present conditions that would exclude them from receiving IV-tPA (see Table 13.2).

In the era of stroke centers, we expect to see an increasing number of stroke patients who will be eligible for acute thrombolytic treatment. Many of these patients will be elderly. The data from The National Institute of Neurological Disorders and Stroke trial showed a favorable outcome in 31%–50% of acute ischemic stroke patients who received IV-tPA (0.9 mg/kg IV, maximum 90 mg) compared with 20%–38% in the untreated group. The benefit is also seen after 1-year follow up. Symptomatic brain hemorrhage was seen in 6.4% of patients who received IV-tPA compared with 0.6% in the placebo group. No difference, however, was found in mortality rate at a 3-month follow up.[11,12]

Many physicians still hesitate to treat older acute stroke patients aggressively. Advanced age should not be a criterion for decision making in older patients with acute stroke. Risks and benefits should be assessed carefully and should be discussed with patients and/or their legal guardian. A patient's baseline

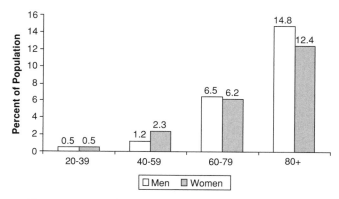

Figure 13.2. Prevalence of stroke by age and sex (NHANES: 1999–2004).[5]

Table 13.1. Assessment of the Acute Stroke Patient in the Rapid Response Room

1. Assess airway, breathing, and circulation and evaluate baseline vital signs.

2. Provide oxygen. Oxygen supplementation via nasal cannula or nonrebreather mask should be used on patients with low oxygen saturation ($\leq$92%) (grade I) or nonhypoxemia (grade IIB).[7]

3. Establish IV access and obtain blood samples including platelet count and coagulation studies.

4. Check blood glucose and promptly treat hypoglycemia. Hyper- or hypoglycemia has an impact on the morbidity and mortality of stroke patients. Therefore, it should be treated promptly although it should not delay the administration of IV-tPA.[8]

5. Perform a neurological screening assessment. Use the National Institutes of Health Stroke Scale or similar tool.

6. Obtain a stat noncontrast CT scan of the brain.

7. Obtain a 12-lead electrocardiogram and portable chest x-ray (do not delay CT scan to obtain these procedure and do not delay CT scan to treat hemodynamically stable patient with arrhythmia.[1]

level of independence and activities of daily living, cognitive function, and wishes should be considered. Prior to excluding the elderly group from standard acute treatments, it is an important consideration that this group will also have a higher complication rate and a worse outcome if untreated. Several studies reported that thrombolysis in the elderly (>80 years old) showed as favorable an outcome after tPA compared with placebo as in younger patients. Increase of symptomatic hemorrhage was still controversial in previous studies. Two European studies reported higher risk of hemorrhage, but results from National Institute of Neurological Disorders Stroke and the tPA Stroke Survey did not find differences in intracranial hemorrhage for stroke patients older than 80 years old compared with the younger group.[11,13,14]

Blood pressure needs to be monitored closely and cautiously in the acute stroke setting. (See Tables 13.4 and 13.5 for management of blood pressure in patients eligible and ineligible for tPA.)

Patients Who Do Not Qualify for IV-tPA, but Who May Benefit from Endovascular Procedures

Intraarterial thrombolysis or other endovascular procedures should be performed within 6 hours after the onset of stroke symptoms. A longer time period has been recommended for the posterior circulation because of its devastating morbidity and mortality and its reversibility.[15–17] Mechanical disruption of clot with the Mechanical Embolus Removal in Cerebral Ischemia clot retrieval device (approved by the Food and Drug Administration in 2004),[18] angioplasty, and cerebrovascular stent placement are used to achieve vascular reperfusion.[19]

Table 13.2. Inclusion and Exclusion Criteria for IV-tPA

Inclusion Criteria

- Age 18 years or older
- Stroke symptom onset ≤3 h
- Clinical diagnosis of ischemic stroke causing a measurable neurological deficit

Exclusion Criteria

- Evidence of intracranial hemorrhage on CT scan
- Symptoms minor or isolated
- Symptoms clearing spontaneously
- Symptoms causing severe deficits
- Symptoms of subarachnoid hemorrhage
- Onset to treatment >3 h or time of onset unknown
- Previous head trauma or stroke in last 3 months
- Myocardial infarction within the last 3 months
- Gastrointestinal or urinary tract hemorrhage within 21 days
- Major surgery within 14 days
- Arterial puncture at a noncompressible site within 7 days
- History of intracranial hemorrhage
- Blood pressure >185/110 mm Hg requiring aggressive treatment
- Evidence of active bleeding or acute trauma
- International normalized ratio >1.7
- Platelet count ≤100,000 mm^3
- Blood glucose ≤50 mg/dL
- Heparin within 24 h, partial thromboplastin time must be within normal range
- Seizure at onset with postictal neurological impairments
- >1/3 hypodensity on CT scan

Table 13.3. Management of Blood Pressure in the Ischemic Stroke Patient Who is Eligible for Thrombolytic Therapy

BP Level (mm Hg)	Treatment
Pretreatment	
SBP >**185** or DBP > **110**	**Labetalol** (may repeat once) or **nitropaste** If BP not reduced and maintained, do **not** administer tPA
During and After tPA	
SBP **180–230** or DBP **105–120**	**Labetalol**
SBP >**230** or DBP **121–140**	**Nicardipine** or **labetalol** If BP not controlled consider nitroprusside
DBP >**140**	**Nitroprusside**

BP, blood pressure; DBP, diastolic blood pressure; SBP, systolic blood pressure.

Table 13.4. The Prevalence (%) of Risk Factors for Stroke in Relation to Advancing Age

	50–59 y	60–69 y	70–79 y	80–89 y
Hypertension	38.2	51.7	63.1	71.6
Atrial fibrillation	0.5	1.8	4.8	8.8
Coronary artery disease	6.6	14.1	20.6	27.7
Chronic heart failure	0.8	2.3	4.9	9.1

Patients Who Do Not Qualify for Acute Thrombolysis or Endovascular Intervention

Ineligibility for acute thrombolysis could result from conditions such as:

1. Ischemic stroke symptoms rapidly improving and resolved;
2. Prior or present conditions in which IV or intraarterial thrombolysis may result in more harm than benefit (see Table 13.2);
3. Hemorrhagic conversion of a large ischemic stroke;
4. Patient refuses thrombolytic therapy;
5. No vascular stenosis was found during evaluation for endovascular procedures.

It is also essential for acute stroke patients to get vascular studies as soon as possible. CT angiography, magnetic resonance (MR) angiography, or conventional angiography can be used to evaluate vasculature in stroke patients. For acute stroke patients who receive IV-tPA, imaging can be done during, or shortly after, thrombolytic therapy is completed. For a stroke patient who may be a candidate for endovascular procedures, the availability of immediate noninvasive imaging may help to identify appropriate candidates for intraarterial thrombolysis and eliminate the need to activate the endovascular intervention team if there is no stenosis found. CT perfusion or MR perfusion can be utilized to assess for hypoperfusion of brain tissue.[1]

Management of Acute Hemorrhagic Stroke

Hemorrhagic stroke is associated with a 30%–50% mortality rate.[20] CT scanning of the head may be used to classify the type and severity of hemorrhage, which includes intraparenchymal hemorrhage, intraventricular hemorrhage, and subarachnoid hemorrhage. The presence of subdural or epidural hematomas must also be identified. Common causes of hemorrhagic stroke are:

1. Hypertension. Hypertension is the most common etiology of hemorrhagic stroke;[20]
2. Cerebral amyloid angiopathy. Amyloid angiopathy results from disposition and infiltration of amyloid β peptide protein into the media and adventitia of the cortical arterioles of the brain. The prevalence of cerebral amyloid angiopathy

Table 13.5. Management of Blood Pressure in the Ischemic Stroke Patients Who Is not Eligible for Thrombolytic Therapy

BP Level (mm Hg)	Treatment
SBP ≤220 or DBP ≤120	No treatment unless end organ involvement
SBP >220 or DBP >121–140	**Nicardipine** or **labetalol** to 10%–15% ↓ in BP
DBP >140	**Nitroprusside** to 10%–15% ↓ in BP

increases with age.[20] Recurrent hemorrhage was reported in 5%–15% of cases;[21]

3. Aneurysms;
4. Vascular malformations;
5. Brain tumors;
6. Anticoagulant associated intracerebral hemorrhage. Gradient-echo MR imaging of the brain has been used to detect petechial hemorrhage, which is typical of the disease.[22] The imaging results are useful in evaluating risks and benefits of anticoagulation.

IDENTIFICATION OF RISK FACTORS AND SECONDARY PREVENTION

Risk factors for stroke can be classified as well or not well documented and based on nonmodifiable, modifiable, and potentially modifiable.

A. Nonmodifiable risk factors
   1. **Age**
      Age is one of the most important nonmodifiable risk factors.
      The risk of stroke doubles for each 10-year period after the age of 55 years.[4]
   2. **Race**
      The incidence of ischemic stroke in the African-American population is two- to threefold higher than that for whites. The incidence of hemorrhagic stroke is also higher in African Americans compared with whites.[23] It is unclear how much uncontrolled modifiable risk factors play a role in this number. Epidemiological studies also showed high incidences of stroke in Hispanic and Asian populations.[24,25]
   3. **Sex**
      The prevalence of stroke is higher in men than women. More women than men die of stroke each year, however. The incidence of stroke in women is higher in the postmenopausal group, raising the question about its relationship with aging and hormonal status.[4,5]
   4. **Family history of stroke or TIA and genetic factors**
      The Framingham study showed that both paternal (n = 1,762; relative risk = 2.4; 95% confidence interval

0.96–6.03) and maternal (n = 2,074; relative risk = 1.4; 95% confidence interval 0.60–3.25) histories were associated with an increased risk for stroke.

Several genetic disorders have been associated with stroke. Cerebral autosomal dominant arteriopathy with subcortical infarcts and leukoencephalopathy, Marfan syndrome, Fabry disease, and neurofibromatosis types I and II are associated with an increased risk of ischemic stroke. Many hypercoagulable states are inherited as autosomal dominant traits, including protein C and S deficiencies, factor V Leiden mutations, which can lead to increased risk of venous thrombosis or may also increase risk of arterial thrombosis.[4] The risk of stroke is also higher in a person with birth weight ≤2,500 g compared to those with birth weight >4000 g.[27]

B. Well-documented modifiable risk factors
   1. **Hypertension**
      Hypertension is a significant risk factor for both ischemic and hemorrhagic stroke. The prevalence of hypertension increases with advancing age. Normal blood pressure is defined as ≤120/80 mm Hg (class IIa, level of evidence B).[28] More than two-thirds of people the age of 65 years and older have hypertension.[28] Antihypertensive treatment is recommended for prevention of recurrent stroke in stroke patients with a history of hypertension (class I, level of evidence A) or with no history of hypertension (class IIa, level of evidence B). An absolute target blood pressure level and reduction are uncertain and should be individualized, but benefit has been associated with reduction of 10/5 mm Hg. The Systolic Hypertension in the Elderly Program Trial found a 36% reduction in the incidence of stroke with treatment using chlorthalidone with or without a ß-blocker.[29]
   2. **Diabetes mellitus**
      Control of blood glucose is recommended among diabetics with ischemic stroke or TIA to reduce microvascular complications (class I, level of evidence A) and macrovascular complications (class IIn, level of evidence B). Normal fasting glucose is defined as glucose ≤100 mg/dl (5.6 mmol/L). The goal of hemoglobin A1C should be ≤7% (class IIa, level of evidence B). More rigorous control of blood pressure and treatment of hyperlipidemia should be considered in patients with diabetes (class IIa, level of evidence B).
   3. **Smoking**
      Cigarette smoking is an independent risk factor for ischemic and hemorrhagic stroke and the risk is present at all ages, and in both sexes and different racial groups.[30,32] The risk of stroke decreases significantly after 2 years of smoking cessation.[30] Every patient with stroke or TIA should quit smoking (class I, level of evidence C).[30] Counseling, nicotine products, and oral smoking cessation medications have been found to be

effective in helping smokers to quit (class IIa, level of evidence B).

4. **Hyperlipidemia**

Patients with ischemic stroke or TIA with elevated cholesterol, comorbid coronary artery disease, or evidence of an atherosclerotic origin should be managed according to National Cholesterol Education Program II guidelines, which include lifestyle modification, dietary guidelines, and medication recommendations (class I, level of evidence A). Statin therapy is recommended and the target goal is low-density lipoprotein cholesterol of $\leq$100 mg/dL and low-density lipoprotein of $\leq$70 mg/dL for very high risk patients with multiple risk factors (class I, level of evidence A).[19]

5. **Atrial fibrillation**

Atrial fibrillation is an independent risk factor for stroke.[33] The attributable risk of stroke from atrial fibrillation increases with age. In the 80 to 89 year-old age group, the attributable risk of stroke is 23.5%. Approximately 18% of patients with stroke have newly diagnosed atrial fibrillation with an additional 4.4% of patients with intermittent atrial fibrillation noted within 14 days after stroke. Up to 92% of these patients continue to have atrial fibrillation in a chronic or paroxysmal form.[34] Strokes from atrial fibrillation are frequently preceded by TIAs and are often devastating large-vessel cortical strokes. Adjusted-dose warfarin reduced stroke in patients with atrial fibrillation by 62%; absolute risk reductions were 2.7% per year for primary prevention and 8.4% per year for secondary prevention. Aspirin reduced stroke in patients with atrial fibrillation by 22%; absolute risk reductions were 1.5% per year for primary prevention and 2.5% per year for secondary prevention.[35] Anticoagulation with warfarin is the standard of care treatment and the only proved treatment for prevention of stroke in patients with atrial fibrillation (class IA).[36] For patients with ischemic stroke or TIAs with persistent or paroxysmal atrial fibrillation, adjusted-dose warfarin (target international normalized ratio 2.0–3.0) is recommended (class I, level of evidence A).

For those with atrial fibrillation and documented contraindication for anticoagulation, aspirin 325 mg/day is recommended (class I, level of evidence A). Severe congestive heart failure has also been associated with increased risk of stroke. Unlike atrial fibrillation, the benefit of anticoagulation for patients with severely reduced systolic function but without atrial fibrillation is still unclear (level IIb recommendation).[37] Falls risk, cognitive impairment, uncontrolled hypertension, and previous gastrointestinal hemorrhage should be taken into consideration when making a decision to start anticoagulation on older patients.

6. **Carotid and other large-artery stenosis**

This invasive management should follow the current guidelines for prevention of stroke in patients with ischemic stroke or TIA.

1. For patients with recent TIA or ischemic stroke within the last 6 months and ipsilateral severe (70%–99%) carotid artery stenosis, carotid endarterectomy (CEA) is recommended (class I, level of evidence A). For ipsilateral moderate (50%–69%) carotid stenosis, CEA is recommended depending on patient-specific factors such as age, sex, and comorbidities and severity of initial symptoms (class I, level of evidence A). When CEA is indicated, surgery within 2 weeks is suggested rather than delaying the surgery (class IIa, level of evidence B). CEA is the most frequently performed surgical procedure to prevent stroke and, in 2004, an estimated 98% of CEA procedures were performed in the United States.[2]

2. For symptomatic stenosis >70% in lesions that are difficult to access or when medical conditions or other conditions increase the risk of surgery, carotid artery stenting is not inferior to CEA (class IIb, level of evidence B).

3. External carotid/internal carotid bypass surgery is not routinely recommended (class III, level of evidence A). Safety and efficacy clinical trials are ongoing to determine whether bypass surgeries are beneficial for patients with complete occlusion of the carotid arteries.

4. Endovascular treatment may be considered for patients with extracranial vertebral stenosis who are still symptomatic despite medical therapies (antithrombotics, statins, and other treatment for risk factors) (Class IIb, level of evidence C)

5. For patients with significant intracranial stenosis who are still symptomatic despite medical therapy, the usefulness of endovascular therapy (angioplasty and/or stent placement) is uncertain and is considered investigational (Class IIb, level of evidence C)

7. **Obesity**

Although the relationship of obesity and stroke is complex, obesity is strongly related to several risk factors for stroke including hypertension, diabetes, and hyperlipidemia.[30] Weight reduction is recommended to control blood pressure (Class I, level of evidence A).[4] The recommended goal is a BMI between 18.5 and 24.9 kg/m^2 and a waist circumference of $\leq$35 in for women and $\leq$40 for men (class IIb, level of evidence C).[30]

8. **Physical inactivity**

Moderate-intensity physical exercise for at least 30 minutes may be considered to reduce the risk of recurrent stroke (class IIb, level of evidence C).[30]

9. **Postmenopausal hormone replacement therapy**

The incidence of stroke is higher in postmenopausal women compared with premenopausal women. It is still uncertain that this increased incidence results from age, hormone status, and/or the role of hormone replacement therapy. The result of The Heart and Estrogen/Progestin Replacement Study did not show any reduction in stroke risk with the use of combined progesterone and estrogen (conjugated equine estrogen 0.625 mg) and medroxyprogesterone acetate (2.5 mg).[38] Some clinical studies showed an increased incidence of stroke in postmenopausal women who use conjugated equine estrogen (Premarin) or a combination of estrogen plus progestin (PremPro).[39,40]

10. **Dietary factors**

Sodium intake $\leq$2.3 g/day (100 mmol/day), and potassium intake $\geq$4.7 g/day (120 mmol/day) is recommended for patients with hypertension (class I, level of evidence A). A diet that is rich in fruits and vegetables may lower the risk of stroke and may be considered (class IIb, level of evidence C).[4]

As in acute stroke treatment, many clinicians avoid aggressive secondary prevention treatments for stroke in the elderly population. This may be from concern for adverse events or drug interactions. Some physicians are also reluctant to institute and maintain aggressive secondary prevention regimens because of the lack of evidence-based studies regarding the cost-effectiveness of such therapies in the elderly population.[41]

Community education to help recognize the signs and symptoms of stroke is the first and most important step toward the improvement of stroke care. This education should also include immediate use of 911 to alert and transport possible stroke patients. For elderly individuals who live alone, the use of alarm systems (such as Lifeline) may be beneficial, especially after falls and with difficulty reaching a phone. A study showed that patients older than the age of 65 years were less likely than those younger than 65 years to know the signs or symptoms of stroke (28% vs. 47%).[42]

Antiplatelet Agents for Secondary Prevention of Stroke

Aspirin (50 mg–325 mg daily), a combination of aspirin and dipyridamole, or clopidogrel is recommended to reduce the risk of stroke in patients with noncardioembolic ischemic stroke or TIA (class I, level of evidence A). The combination of aspirin and extended-release dipyridamole may be more favorable compared with aspirin alone (class IIa, level of evidence A) and clopidogrel may be considered instead of aspirin (class IIb, level of evidence B).[36] There is no proved benefit of stroke risk reduction for the combination of antiplatelets, and the risk of bleeding was higher in the dual antiplatelet group.[43,44]

Prevention of Associated Morbidities: Rehabilitation and Outcome in Stroke

Stroke rehabilitation begins during acute hospitalization as early as possible to optimize the functional outcome. The primary goal of rehabilitation is to prevent complications (such as deep vein thrombosis or pressure ulcers), minimize impairment, and maximize function. A swallowing study should be done prior to oral intake because dysphagia occurs in 45% of all patients with stroke. Monitoring of nutritional intake is also important to prevent malnutrition.[45] Periodic turning in bed and a thorough examination for the presence of pressure ulcers should be done daily (evidence level C). A Foley catheter should be used cautiously because of the risk for infection. Constipation is also common in the acute stroke setting and use of laxatives or stool softeners may be helpful.[45,46] Depression is commonly seen after stroke and can be difficult to diagnose because of other symptoms such as aphasia or neglect. Several studies showed that the treatment of depression can improve rehabilitation outcomes (evidence level A).[45,47] Selective serotonin reuptake inhibitors are the preferred agents, mainly because of the high incidence of anticholinergic effects caused by tricyclic antidepressants in elderly patients.

Age is one important factor in the outcome of stroke. In one study of stroke patients older than 65 years, the disabilities at 6 months poststroke were as follows:[48]

1. 50% with hemiparesis;
2. 30% unable to walk without assistance;
3. 26% were dependent in activities of daily living;
4. 19% with aphasia;
5. 35% with depressive symptoms;
6. 26% live in a nursing home.

Older patients, however, also show comparable improvement during rehabilitation, and intensive rehabilitation should not be withheld in stroke patients simply because of advanced age.[49]

Stroke and Dementia (Vascular Cognitive Impairment)

Several studies report that stroke significantly increases the risk of dementia, especially in patients who have mild cognitive impairment prior to a stroke. Stroke increases the odds of subsequent dementia fivefold compared with individuals without stroke. In 68% of stroke patients with dementia, the diagnosis is made within 1 year after the stroke.[50] In the Framingham study during the 10-year follow-up period, dementia developed in 19.3% of the stroke patients compared with 11.0% of matched controls. This result was independent of age, sex, education, hemispheric location, and type of stroke.[51] The mechanisms by which stroke increases the risk of cognitive decline are not clear.[50–53]

REFERENCES

1. 2005 American Heart Association Guidelines for Cardiopulmonary Resuscitation and Emergency Cardiovascular Care. *Circulation.* 2005; 112(24 Suppl):IV1–203.

2. Howard G, Wagenknecht LE, Cai J, Cooper L, Kraut MA, Toole JF. Cigarette smoking and other risk factors for silent cerebral infarction in the general population. *Stroke.* 1998;29:913–917.

3. Bryan RN, Wells SW, Miller TJ, et al. Infarctlike lesions in the brain: prevalence and anatomic characteristics at MR imaging of the elderly–data from the Cardiovascular Health Study. *Radiology.* 1997;202:47–54.

4. Goldstein LB, Adams R, Alberts MJ et al. Primary prevention of ischemic stroke: a guideline from the American Heart Association/American Stroke Association Stroke Council: cosponsored by the Athero-sclerotic Peripheral Vascular Disease Interdisciplinary Working Group; Cardiovascular Nursing Council; Clinical Cardiology Council; Nutrition, Physical Activity, and Metabolism Council; and the Quality of Care and Outcomes Research Interdisciplinary Working Group. *Circulation.* 2006;113:e873–e923.

5. Rosamund W, Flegal K, Friday G et al. Heart disease and stroke statistics–2007 update: a report from the American Heart Association Statistics Committee and Stroke Statistics Subcommittee. *Circulation.* 2007;115:e69–e171.

6. Adams, HP Jr, Bendixen BH, Kappelle LJ et al. Classification of subtype of acute ischemic stroke. Definitions for use in a multicenter clinical trial. TOAST. Trial of Org 10172 in Acute Stroke Treatment. *Stroke.* 1993;24:35–41.

7. Adams H, Adams R, Del Zappo G, Goldstein LB; Stroke Council of the American Heart Association; American Stroke Association. Guidelines for the early management of patients with ischemic stroke: 2005 guidelines update a scientific statement from the Stroke Council of the American Heart Association/American Stroke Association. *Stroke.* 2005;36:916–923.

8. Fulgham JR, Ingall TJ, Stead LG, Cloft HJ, Wijdicks EF, Flemming KD. Management of acute ischemic stroke. *Mayo Clin Proc.* 2004;79:1459–1469.

9. Alberts MJ, Latchaw RE, Selman WR et al. Recommendations for comprehensive stroke centers: a consensus statement from the Brain Attack Coalition. *Stroke.* 2005;36:1597–1616.

10. Adams HP Jr, Adams RJ, Brott T et al. Guidelines for the early management of patients with ischemic stroke: a scientific statement from the Stroke Council of the American Stroke Association. *Stroke.* 2003;34:1056–83.

11. Tissue plasminogen activator for acute ischemic stroke. The National Institute of Neurological Disorders and Stroke rt-PA Stroke Study Group. *NEJM.* 1995;333:1581–1587.

12. Kwiatkowski TG, Libman RB, Frankel M et al. Effects of tissue plasminogen activator for acute ischemic stroke at one year. National Institute of Neurological Disorders and Stroke Recombinant Tissue Plasminogen Activator Stroke Study Group. *NEJM.* 1999;340:1781–1787.

13. Tanne D, Gorman MJ, Bates VE et al. Intravenous tissue plasminogen activator for acute ischemic stroke in patients aged 80 years and older: the tPA stroke survey experience. *Stroke.* 2000;31:370–375.

14. Hemphill JC 3rd, Lyden P. Stroke thrombolysis in the elderly: risk or benefit? *Neurology.* 2005;65:1690–1691.

15. Wijdicks EF, Nichols DA, Thielen KR et al. Intra-arterial thrombolysis in acute basilar artery thromboembolism: the initial Mayo Clinic experience. *Mayo Clin Proc.* 1997;72:1005–1013.

16. Schonewille WJ, Algra A, Serena J, Molina CA, and Kappelle LJ. Outcome in patients with basilar artery occlusion treated conventionally. *J Neurol Neurosurg Psychiatry.* 2005;76:1238–1241.

17. Smith WS, Intra-arterial thrombolytic therapy for acute basilar occlusion: pro. *Stroke.* 2007;38:701–703.

18. Gobin YP, Starkman S, Duckwiler GR et al. MERCI 1: a phase 1 study of mechanical embolus removal in cerebral ischemia. *Stroke.* 2004;35:2848–2854.

19. Cha JH, Bateman BT, Mangla S et al. Endovascular recanalization therapy in acute ischemic stroke. *Stroke.* 2006;37:419–424.

20. Manno EM, Atkinson JL, Fulgham JR and Wijdicks EF. Emerging medical and surgical management strategies in the evaluation and treatment of intracerebral hemorrhage. *Mayo Clin Proc.* 2005;80:420–433.

21. Mayer SA, Rincon F. Treatment of intracerebral haemorrhage. *Lancet Neurol.* 2005;4:662–672.

22. Smith EE, Eichler F. Cerebral amyloid angiopathy and lobar intracerebral hemorrhage. *Arch Neurol.* 2006;63:148–151.

23. Rosamond WD, Folsom AR, Chambless LE et al. Stroke incidence and survival among middle-aged adults: 9-year follow-up of the Atherosclerosis Risk in Communities (ARIC) cohort. *Stroke.* 1999;30:736–743.

24. Sheinart KF, Tuhrim S, Horowitz DR, Weinberger J, Goldman M, Godbold JH. Stroke recurrence is more frequent in Blacks and Hispanics. *Neuroepidemiology.* 1998;17:188–198.

25. Frey JL, Jahnke HK, Bulfinch EW. Differences in stroke between white, Hispanic, and Native American patients: the Barrow Neurological Institute stroke database. *Stroke.* 1998;29:29–33.

26. Kiely DK, Wolf PA, Cupples LA, Beiser AS and Myers RH. Familial aggregation of stroke. The Framingham Study. *Stroke.* 1993;24:1366–1371.

27. Barker DJ, Lackland DT. Prenatal influences on stroke mortality in England and Wales. *Stroke.* 2003;34:1598–1602.

28. Chobanian AV, Bakris GL, Black HR et al. The seventh report of the Joint National Committee on Prevention, Detection, Evaluation, and Treatment of High Blood Pressure: the JNC 7 report. *JAMA.* 2003;289:2560–2572.

29. SHEP Cooperative Research Group. Prevention of stroke by antihypertensive drug treatment in older persons with isolated systolic hypertension. Final results of the Systolic Hypertension in the Elderly Program (SHEP). *JAMA.* 1991;265:3255–3264.

30. Sacco RL, Adams R, Albers G et al. Guidelines for prevention of stroke in patients with ischemic stroke or transient ischemic attack: a statement for healthcare professionals from the American Heart Association/American Stroke Association Council on Stroke: co-sponsored by the Council on Cardiovascular Radiology and Intervention: the American Academy of Neurology affirms the value of this guideline. *Circulation.* 2006;113:e409–449.

31. Wolf PA, D'Angostino RB, Belanger AJ, Kannel WB. Probability of stroke: a risk profile from the Framingham Study. *Stroke.* 1991;22:312–318.

32. Kurth T, Kase CS, Berger K, Gaziano JM, Cook NR, Buring JE. Smoking and risk of hemorrhagic stroke in women. *Stroke.* 2003;34:2792–2795.

33. Wolf PA, Abbott RD, Kannel WB. Atrial fibrillation as an independent risk factor for stroke: the Framingham Study. *Stroke.* 1991;22:983–988.

34. Lin HJ, Wolf PA, Benjamin EJ, Belanger AJ, D'Agostino RB. Newly diagnosed atrial fibrillation and acute stroke. The Framingham Study. *Stroke.* 1995;26:1527–1530.

35. Hart RG, Benavente O, McBride R, Pearce LA. Antithrombotic therapy to prevent stroke in patients with atrial fibrillation: a meta-analysis. *Ann Intern Med.* 1999;131:492–501.

36. Sacco, RL, Adams R, Albers G et al. Guidelines for prevention of stroke in patients with ischemic stroke or transient ischemic attack: a statement for healthcare professionals from the American Heart Association/American Stroke Association Council on Stroke: co-sponsored by the Council on Cardiovascular Radiology and Intervention: the American Academy of Neurology affirms the value of this guideline. *Stroke.* 2006;37:577–617.

37. Witt BJ, Brown RD Jr, Jacobsen SJ et al. Ischemic stroke after heart failure: a community-based study. *Am Heart J.* 2006;152:102–109.

38. Simon JA, Hsia J, Cauley JA et al. Postmenopausal hormone therapy and risk of stroke: The Heart and Estrogen-progestin Replacement Study (HERS). *Circulation.* 2001;103:638–642.

39. Wassertheil-Smoller S, Hendrix SL, Limacher M et al. Effect of estrogen plus progestin on stroke in postmenopausal women: the Women's Health Initiative: a randomized trial. *JAMA.* 2003;289:2673–2684.

40. Anderson GL, Limacher M, Assaf AR et al. Effects of conjugated equine estrogen in postmenopausal women with hysterectomy: the Women's Health Initiative randomized controlled trial. *JAMA.* 2004;291:1701–1712.

41. Ovbiagele B, Hills NK, Sauer JL, Johnston SC. Secondary-prevention drug prescription in the very elderly after ischemic stroke or TIA. *Neurology.* 2006;66:313–318.

42. Kothari R, Sauerbeck L, Jauch E et al. Patients' awareness of stroke signs, symptoms, and risk factors. *Stroke.* 1997;28:1871–1875.

43. Diener JC, Bogousslavsky J, Brass LM et al. Aspirin and clopidogrel compared with clopidogrel alone after recent ischaemic stroke or transient ischaemic attack in high-risk patients (MATCH): randomised, double-blind, placebo-controlled trial. *Lancet.* 2004;364:331–337.

44. Bhatt DL, Fox KA, Hacke W et al. Clopidogrel and aspirin versus aspirin alone for the prevention of atherothrombotic events. *NEJM.* 2006;354:1706–1717.

45. Bates B, Choi JY, Duncan PW et al. Veterans Affairs/Department of Defense Clinical Practice Guideline for the Management of Adult Stroke Rehabilitation Care: executive summary. *Stroke.* 2005;36:2049–2056.

46. Nakayama H, Jørgensen HS, Pedersen PM, Raaschou Ho, Olsen TS. Prevalence and risk factors of incontinence after stroke. The Copenhagen Stroke Study. *Stroke.* 1997;28:58–62.

47. Cole MG, Elie LM, McCusker J, Bellavance F, Mansour A. Feasibility and effectiveness of treatments for post-stroke depression in elderly inpatients: systematic review. *J Geriatr Psychiatry Neurol.* 2001;14:37–41.

48. Kelley-Hayes M. The impact of poststroke rehabilitation guidelines on functional recovery. *Stroke.* 2002;33:177–178.

49. Luk JK, Chenog RT, Ho SL, Li L. Does age predict outcome in stroke rehabilitation? A study of 878 Chinese subjects. *Cerebrovasc Dis.* 2006;21:229–234.

50. Gamaldo A, Moghekar A, Kilada S, Resnick SM, Zonderman AB, O'Brien R. Effect of a clinical stroke on the risk of dementia in a prospective cohort. *Neurology.* 2006;67:1363–1369.

51. Ivan CS, Seshadri S, Beiser A et al. Dementia after stroke: the Framingham Study. *Stroke.* 2004;35:1264–1268.

52. Pohjasvaara T, Erkinjuntti T, Vataja R, Kaste M. Dementia three months after stroke. Baseline frequency and effect of different definitions of dementia in the Helsinki Stroke Aging Memory Study (SAM) cohort. *Stroke.* 1997;28:785–792.

53. Reitz C, Luchsinger JA, Tang MX, Manly J, Mayeux R. Stroke and memory performance in elderly persons without dementia. *Arch Neurol.* 2006;63:571–576.

14

NEUROLOGICAL PROBLEMS IN THE ELDERLY

Michele Zawora, MD, Tsoa-Wei Liang, MD, Hadijatou Jarra, MD

The elderly are affected by many neurological symptoms as they age, which often have an impact on their health, ability to function, and overall quality of life. This chapter will examine some of the most common complaints and symptoms encountered by the primary care provider. The main goal is to distinguish the cause(s) and to determine the best course of action. Many of these symptoms can be evaluated and treated by the patient's primary care provider, whereas some may require consulting with a neurologist. This chapter will discuss the following topics: gait dysfunction, sensory loss, seizures, headaches, weakness, tremor, and parkinsonism.

GAIT DISORDERS

General Concepts

Gait impairment is a significant cause of morbidity and mortality in the elderly. As many as 15%–20% of patients older than 65 years will suffer from gait impairment, often requiring an assistive device. This percentage increases with age, with an estimated 40%–50% of those older than 85 years, and up to 70% in those older than 90 years.[1]

Gait impairment leading to falls in the elderly represents the most common cause of injury.[2] Some 30% of all elderly will fall at least once annually, with the risk as high as 50% of those older than 80 years. In addition, 50% of long-term care residents will fall at least once annually.[3] One-half of all falls are related to gait impairment and another one-third to balance impairment or postural instability.[4]

Normal locomotion depends on intact motor and sensory systems to maintain equilibrium and balance. The sensory input from vestibular, peripheral nervous, and visual systems is integrated by the cortex, cerebellum, and basal ganglia. The body also uses anticipatory and reactive postural reflexes to maintain equilibrium in response to environmental changes.

Disruptions or lesions in any of these structures may result in gait impairment.

Historically, slowed gait has been considered a natural part of the aging process; however, this is no longer thought to be true. Some of the common changes seen with advancing age include bent posture, slower pace, shortened stride, increased time in double support phase, truncal and limb rigidity, widened base, and en bloc turning.[3] For the majority of elderly patients, gait speed declines by 12%–16% each decade, stride length shortens, and step frequency increases. The time in double support phase increases from 18% in younger patients to 26% by the age of 70 years.[5] The distinction between the so-called senile gait of the elderly and a true pathological gait is often controversial. In general, a disabling gait, one that causes functional impairment, no matter what the age, should be investigated thoroughly for a potentially reversible cause.

Differential Diagnosis

Most gait disorders develop insidiously and may go unnoticed by the patient. Caregiver reports are often necessary for an accurate history. Patients may describe gait impairment in general terms such as "I'm off balance" or "I feel weak." Caregivers may narrow the differential by reporting that the patient appears "drunk" (suggesting cerebellar ataxia) or that the feet appear "frozen to the ground" (suggesting an extrapyramidal gait disorder).

The differential diagnosis of gait impairment is extensive. Please refer to Table 14.1 for a complete list. We will focus on some of the gait disorders most commonly encountered by the primary care provider. Complicating the diagnosis is the fact that gait impairment in the elderly may be multifactorial, so that several causes may be seen in the same patient.

Associated symptoms are often helpful in localizing the lesion and narrowing the differential (refer to Table 14.2).

Table 14.1. Causes of Gait Disorders in the Elderly

Structural disorders
- NPH
- Neoplasms

Vascular
- Multiinfarct state/Binswanger disease
- Stroke
- Subdural/Epidural hematoma
- Subarachnoid hemorrhage (uncommon)
- Spinal cord arteriovenous malformation

Neurodegenerative disorders
- PD
- Huntington's disease
- Anterolateral sclerosis
- Alzheimer's disease
- Frontotemporal dementia

Hereditary disorders
- Spinocerebellar ataxia

Myelopathy

Acquired metabolic/nutritional disorders
- Diabetic neuropathy
- Wernicke–Korsakoff syndrome
- Vitamin B12 deficiency/Subacute combined degeneration

Infectious diseases
- Tertiary syphilis/Tabes dorsalis

Demyelinating diseases
- Multiple sclerosis
- Guillain-Barré Syndrome

Autoimmune/inflammatory disorders

Systemic lupus erythematosus, Sjögren, myasthenia gravis, sarcoid, vasculitis

Trauma

Toxins and drugs
- Neuroleptics
- Sedative-hypnotic agents
- Anticonvulsants

Patients with sensory neuropathy causing ataxia often complain of distal paresthesias and sensory loss. Sensory ataxia is classically associated with more difficulty at night or in the dark, when visual input is limited. Lumbar nerve root compromise generally causes radicular or radiating back or leg pain and would generally not cause gait impairment unless affecting multiple lumbar root levels. Myelopathy or spinal cord com-

Table 14.2. Localization by Associated Signs and Symptoms

Sign	Diagnoses to Consider
Dementia, cognitive impairment	NPH
Nystagmus	Vestibular, cerebellar, or brainstem dysfunction
Dysarthria	Cerebellar, basal ganglia, or corticobulbar dysfunction
Rigidity, tremor, bradykinesia	Parkinsonism
Hyperreflexia, spasticity with Babinski sign	Corticospinal tract disease
Sensory loss, paresthesias, hyporeflexia	Peripheral neuropathy
Dizziness, vertigo	Vestibular disease

pression is often associated with muscle weakness and spasticity unless the pathological entity affects the dorsal columns in which sensory symptoms predominate. Concomitant memory and cognitive issues suggest a cerebral cause such as normal-pressure hydrocephalus (NPH), although dysarthria, depending on its quality, suggests cerebellar, basal ganglia, or hemispheric disease. Vestibular disorders such as labyrinthitis or Ménière's disease are often recognized more by the disequilibrium or vertigo that they cause than the gait impairment. Extrapyramidal disorders may initially lead to a primary gait disorder, but inevitably associated features such as tremor, rigidity, and bradykinesia emerge. Sudden gait failure generally implies a catastrophic medical illness, such as stroke, medication toxicity, infection, meningitis, or myocardial infarction.

Examination

A general gait screen should be incorporated into every encounter with the patient and begins by simply watching a patient enter or exit the examination room. Features of gait that should be observed include stance, base, initiation, velocity, stride length, cadence, fluidity of movements, and deviation. Patients should be observed walking normally, in tandem, and briefly on heels and toes to assess for distal muscle strength. Romberg testing and pull testing should also be performed to assess postural stability. Table 14.3 lists physical findings that may lead to the diagnosis.

A person with a normal gait pattern will hold their body erect, head straight, feet slightly apart, with both arms hanging loosely at the sides and will move forward easily with the opposite leg. Hips and legs flex with each step, whereas the ankle dorsiflexes. The heel strikes the ground first, moving smoothly along the sole and pushing off with the toes. Stride length should be equal with each step. Some abnormalities may only be elicited through gait testing with obstacles or distractions, such as walking through a doorway or over objects on the floor. Examination of footwear for pattern of wear may also be useful.

Table 14.3. Physical Findings and Diagnosis of Gait Disorders

Maneuver/Condition	Finding	Implication
Sitting	Unable to sit upright	Profound imbalance and/or weakness
	Titubation (tremor of the trunk and head)	Cerebellar disease
	Leaning to one side	Hemiparesis or basal ganglia disorder
Rising from chair	Unable to rise without using arms to push-off	Proximal muscle weakness (myopathy), arthritis, or basal ganglia disorder
Standing	Wide-based stance	Cerebellar disease, dorsal column dysfunction
	Stiff neck and head, avoiding motion	Vestibular disease, pain
	Unstable with sternal nudge	Back problems or neurological problems
Walking on toes and heels		Peripheral neuropathy
Gait	Freezing or start hesitation	Parkinsonism
	Reduced arm swing	Parkinsonism
	Involuntary movements	Huntington's disease, basal ganglia disease
Turning	Widened base, extra steps rather than pivoting on one foot	Cerebellar disease, hemiparesis, reduced proprioception
	En bloc turns	Parkinsonism, cautious gait, frontal lobe gait
Romberg sign	Sway/instability with eyes closed	Impaired proprioception

The Get Up and Go Test is a timed test in which the patient is observed rising from a chair, walking 3 m, turning around, and returning to the chair. A score of less than 10 seconds is considered normal, greater than 14 seconds is abnormal, whereas a time greater than 20 seconds indicates severe gait impairment. Although useful as a screen for functional capabilities, this test cannot distinguish between different causes of a gait disorder.

Evaluation

In most cases, careful history-taking and simple observation of the patient in motion will help to narrow the differential diagnosis. The laboratory evaluation will depend on the initial presentation, findings on physical examination, and may include complete blood count, metabolic panel, fasting blood glucose, glycosylated hemoglobin, erythrocyte sedimentation rate (ESR), rapid plasma reagin, thyroid-stimulating hormone, vitamin B12, folic acid levels, and brain imaging with computed tomography (CT). Additional testing if indicated may consist of magnetic resonance imaging (MRI), electromyography (EMG), and nerve conduction study (NCS). Special gait tests exist to define an unusual gait and to clarify its cause.

Gait Patterns and Select Causes

Parkinson's disease (PD) and parkinsonism lead to a slow gait with shortened stride length, and low step height, often described as shuffling. When trying to walk faster, patients with parkinsonism tend to increase step speed out of proportion to stride length or step height. In the earliest stages of PD, gait impairment is very subtle, with patients noting dragging of one leg or difficulty getting in and out of a car or low seat. The typical posture of a patient with PD consists of flexion of the neck, elbows, waist, and knees. Hesitation and freezing may occur on initiating gait, turning, and maneuvering through a doorway. The term festination refers to the short accelerating steps that occur when the center of gravity is moved forward, leading to forward propulsion, and the need for the legs to race to catch-up with the upper body. When making a turn, the upper and lower body move as a unit, with decreased arm swing and hip rotation, so-called en-bloc turning. Loss of postural stability is generally a late manifestation of idiopathic PD. Table 14.4 reviews the most common gait patterns encountered in the geriatric population.

Frontal lesions lead to a gait pattern similar to a parkinsonian gait. In contrast to a parkinsonian gait, the gait is often more clumsy-appearing, ataxic, and unsteady with difficulty initiating gait. Patients with frontal lesions tend to hold their trunk upright, appear stiff, have a wide-based gait, and show prolonged time in double support phase.[6] Patients are prone to falling backward. Frontal lesions often lead to a magnetic gait, referring to the appearance that the feet are stuck to the ground. The lower body is predominantly involved, so that arm swing is preserved and may even be exaggerated when a patient attempts to "release" the legs from the ground. Gait initiation fails, but patients show improvement with continued walking. The term "gait apraxia" is used to describe the fact that gait is impaired despite preserved sensation, muscle strength, and leg movements not related to walking. Associated frontal lobe signs such as primitive reflexes (e.g., snout, grasp, or suck), cognitive impairment, or disinhibited behaviors may be present.

Table 14.4. Gait Patterns

Type of Gait	Description	Associated Signs	Causes
Parkinsonian	Short-stepped, shuffling, with hips, knees, and spine flexed, festination, en bloc turns	Bradykinesia, muscular rigidity, postural instability, rest tremor, reduced arm swing	PD, and atypical or secondary forms of parkinsonism
Frontal gait disorder (Gait apraxia)	Magnetic, start and turn hesitation, freezing, marche petit pas	Frontal lobe signs, dementia, incontinence	NPH, multiinfarct state, frontal lobe degeneration
Sensory ataxia	Unsteady, worse without visual input and at night	Romberg sign present, impaired position and vibratory sensation, distal sensory loss	Sensory neuropathy, neuronopathy, dorsal column dysfunction
Cerebellar ataxia	Wide-based, staggering gait	Dysmetria, dysarthria, dysdiadochokinesia, postural instability, Romberg sign present, nystagmus, titubation, impaired check, rebound, intention tremor	Cerebellar degeneration, stroke, drug or alcohol intoxication, thiamine and B12 deficiency, multiple sclerosis
Vestibular ataxia	Unsteady gait, falling to one side, postural instability	Vertigo, nausea, nystagmus, normal sensation, reflexes, strength	Acute labyrinthitis, Ménière disease
Steppage gait	Resulting from foot-drop, excessive flexion of hips and knees when walking, short strides, slapping quality, tripping	Atrophy of distal leg muscles, loss of ankle jerk, distal sensory loss and weakness foot drop	Motor neuropathy
Waddling gait	Wide based, swaying, toe-walk, lumbar lordosis, symmetrical	Proximal muscle weakness of lower extremities, hip dislocation, use arms to get up from chair	Myopathy, muscular dystrophy
Antalgic gait	Limping, unable to bear full weight, limited range of motion, slow and short steps	Pain worsening with movement and weight-bearing	Degenerative joint disease, trauma
Hemiparetic	Extension and circumduction of weak and spastic limb, flexed arm	Face, arm, and leg weakness, hyperreflexia, extensor plantar response	Hemispheric or brainstem lesion
Paraparetic	Stiffness, extension, adduction, and/or scissoring of both legs	Bilateral leg weakness, hyperreflexia, spasticity, extensor plantar responses	Spinal cord bilateral cerebral lesions
Dystonic	Abnormal posture of foot or leg, distorted gait, foot dragging, hyperflexion of hips	Worse with the action of walking, may improve when walking backward	
Choreic	Irregular, dancelike, slow and wide-based, spontaneous knee flexion and leg rising	Choreoathetotic movements of upper extremities	Huntington's disease, levodopa induced dyskinesia
Cautious gait	Wide-based, careful, slow, like walking on ice, arms and legs abducted, en bloc turns	Associated with anxiety, fear of falling or open spaces	Post-fall syndrome, visual impairment, deconditioning
Psychogenic	Bizarre and nonphysiological gait, rare fall or injury, lurching, "astasia abasia"	Give-way weakness, absence of objective neurological signs	Factitious, somatoform disorders or malingering

Frontal gait impairment is thought to arise because of a disconnection among frontal, basal ganglia, brainstem, and spinal cord gait centers. A wide variety of pathological conditions lead to frontal lobe dysfunction including NPH, diffuse cerebrovascular disease, and frontal degenerative conditions such as frontotemporal dementia, or progressive supranuclear palsy (PSP).

Communicating hydrocephalus or NPH is an often misunderstood and potentially underdiagnosed entity. Early recognition of the condition is imperative, because it may be reversible in the proper clinical setting. Classically, NPH is associated with the triad of gait impairment, urinary incontinence, and dementia; however, the full triad is not usually present. Furthermore, the course may be chronic and progressive, mimicking a neurodegenerative disorder; acute or subacute, mimicking a vascular insult; or static. Gait impairment is usually the first symptom that develops, with memory and urinary symptoms following later. The gait is often wide-based, and unsteady, characterized by small short steps with the feet barely lifting off the floor.

Table 14.5. Cerebellar Signs and Symptoms

Gait ataxia

Titubation

Dysmetria, past-pointing

Nystagmus

Impaired check

Rebound

Dysdiadochokinesia

Scanning dysarthria

Intention tremor

The diagnosis of NPH relies highly on clinical suspicion, and the finding of enlarged ventricles on brain imaging (CT or MRI). It is important to differentiate between ventricular enlargement from hydrocephalus and so-called hydrocephalus ex vacuo that results from cerebral atrophy. This latter entity is characterized by both ventricular enlargement and increased sulcal size, and it occurs as a result of neurodegenerative diseases and aging. In addition, communicating hydrocephalus needs to be differentiated from obstructive hydrocephalus, which is caused by an obstruction along the ventricular system.

Confirmatory testing includes a large volume lumbar puncture (the so-called tap test), which involves removal of 30–40 mL of spinal fluid with careful examination of gait and cognitive function before and after the procedure. A patient with NPH will have a dramatic response to the procedure. Although a positive response to the tap test confirms the diagnosis, in practice, issues that may confound the test include an inability to remove a sufficient volume of spinal fluid, and a clinical examination that is not sensitive enough to detect subtle improvements, delayed improvement, and placebo response.

Patients with an indeterminate response may benefit from observation with a 3-day lumbar drain placed by a neurosurgeon. The procedure increases the ability to detect responders and often helps to confirm the potential benefit of controlled drainage of fluid, before resorting to a permanent shunt. A ventriculoperitoneal shunt is the definitive treatment of choice, although other procedures such as third ventriculostomy may be considered by the surgeon.

Cerebellar lesions cause gait ataxia in combination with a wide variety of signs and symptoms (Table 14.5). The gait is jerky, clumsy, and unsteady. The stance and base are broad. There is often truncal sway when sitting or standing. Patients are aware of the imbalance and take great effort to ambulate. Lurching of the body may occur as the patient overcompensates to maintain balance. Stepping, direction, distance, and timing are irregular. Step height and stride length are reduced. Tandem gait is impaired because of improper response to postural sway.

Patients with cerebellar dysfunction demonstrate dysmetria with past-pointing on finger-to-nose testing. Speech becomes ataxic or scanning with variations in rhythm, volume, and pitch. Rapid alternating movements show impaired rhythm or dysdiadochokinesia, which is demonstrated by rapid tapping of the hand or foot. In the geriatric population, acute cerebellar ataxia is generally from a vascular insult whereas chronic, progressive ataxia is likely from a neurodegenerative process. Subacute ataxia may be related to infection, nutritional deficiency, or autoimmune disorder. Multiple sclerosis is a common cause of acute ataxia in young adults. In the geriatric population, acute or subacute ataxia without a structural cause on MRI is suggestive of paraneoplastic cerebellar degeneration. Hereditary spinocerebellar ataxias are marked by an autosomal dominant pattern of inheritance, onset in the 3rd–5th decades, and progressive loss of function.

Sensory polyneuropathy leads to ataxia when dorsal column or large fiber sensory loss occurs. A Romberg sign is often present. Proper examination for a Romberg sign consists of having the patient stand with feet together and eyes closed. Therefore, testing for a Romberg sign would be impractical, if the patient is unsteady with eyes open. See Sensory loss section for further details.

Spastic Gait

Corticospinal tract lesions anywhere along its course from the cerebrum to spinal cord will cause weakness and spasticity. Spasticity is defined as increased tone to passive range of motion. Bilateral corticospinal tract lesions caused by spinal cord injury or cerebral palsy will lead to a "scissoring" gait. Both legs are spastic, extended, and internally rotated. The hips adduct excessively.

Hemiparetic gait is caused by a unilateral lesion of the corticospinal tract that most commonly occurs after a stroke. The weak leg is spastic, stiff, and extended and circumducts or makes an arc so that the foot can clear the ground. The weak arm is usually flexed at the elbow and pulled toward the chest.

Waddling gait is associated with weakness of hip girdle muscles leading to the dropping of the pelvis toward the swinging leg and compensatory lean toward the standing leg.

Steppage gait occurs as a result of foot drop as the knee and hip flex excessively to compensate for foot drop. Slapping of the feet to the ground may occur as well.

Cautious gait is commonly observed in the elderly who have suffered a fall, usually a severe accidental fall resulting in injury. Acute anxiety develops surrounding the risk of falling again. Physical activity is often decreased and agoraphobia may develop. The appearance of the gait mimics the gait of a normal person walking on ice. The arms are tense, stance is wide based, and the body turns en bloc. Once a patient has found physical support, the gait is improved.

Patients with acute vertigo resulting from vestibular disease may appear ataxic and this condition mimics a cerebellar syndrome. Patients often deviate or veer to the side of the lesion while walking. Nystagmus is present with eyes open. Sensory, strength, and reflexes should be normal.

Treatment

Treatment of gait disorders involves addressing reversible causes and treating chronic medical conditions that exacerbate the gait problems. Physical and occupational therapy can improve strength, balance, and confidence. Medications should always be evaluated with special attention to psychotropic medications and anticholinergic or antihistaminergic agents. Other treatment modalities include assistive devices, adaptive equipment training, drivers training, and nutritional counseling. Although not rigorously studied, exercise programs such as pilates, yoga, and Tai chi are thought to improve balance and gait.

In addition to dopaminergic agents for PD and ventriculoperitoneal shunting for NPH, there are very few specific pharmacological agents for gait disorders. Amantadine, buspirone, and acetazolamide have shown mixed results in patients with cerebellar ataxia.

SEIZURES

General Concepts

Seizures are thought of primarily as a childhood disease or as a chronic disease that continues from an early age. Seizures, however, have a bimodal incidence, with the first peak in the first year of life, and a second peak in the elderly starting at the age of 60 years.[7] In fact, 25%–50% of all new-onset seizures occur in those older than the age of 65 years, and 25% of all epileptics are elderly.[8] Seizure types also differ between the elderly and younger patients. Although the most common type of seizures in children are febrile seizures or tonic–clonic seizures, the most common type in elderly patients are partial seizures with or without secondary generalization. A seizure is classified as partial when the involvement is confined to a specific area of the brain, whereas a generalized seizure involves the entire brain. A symptomatic seizure is defined as a provoked event that is not expected to recur in the absence of the specific trigger.[8]

The incidence of first-time seizures in the elderly increases starting at the age of 60 years, with an estimated annual incidence of 100/100,000 by the age of 65 years.[7] There are 2.3 million Americans living with epilepsy. Approximately one quarter of this number are older than the age of 65 years and 11% are in long-term care facilities. The most common causes of seizure in this age group include poststroke seizure, intracranial tumors, toxic-metabolic disturbances, and head injuries. Thirty percent of first-time seizures are idiopathic, that is, with no known cause identified after workup has been completed.[9] In fact, patients older than 75 years of age have the highest prevalence of unprovoked seizures of any other age group.

Epilepsy is defined as recurrent, unprovoked seizures that are expected to recur in the absence of treatment.[8] The risk of recurrence is 12% in the elderly.[10] Poststroke seizure represents the most common cause of new-onset seizure and epilepsy in the elderly, accounting for one third–one half of all cases. In another one third–one half of all cases of epilepsy the cause is unknown or cryptogenic. These seizures are likely from vascular causes, as most of these patients have vascular comorbidities or risk factors, including cerebrovascular disease, hypertension, hypercholesterolemia, coronary artery disease, or peripheral vascular disease.

Most younger patients who present in status epilepticus have tonic–clonic convulsions. A number of elderly patients will, however, present without visible convulsions. This type of seizure is referred to as nonconvulsive status epilepticus, and it can be a very hard to diagnose. Elderly patients may present with mental status changes, ranging from confusion and lethargy to frank psychosis and coma. The absence of visible convulsions can often lead to misdiagnosis and therefore inadequate management. Electroencephalography (EEG) performed during status episodes will demonstrate focal rhythmic discharges in the frontotemporal regions. The majority of cases are caused by alcohol or benzodiazepine withdrawal, acute organ failure, and drug toxicity.

Clinical Features

Most seizures in the elderly are partial, with or without secondary generalization and the majority are complex partial seizures, with origin in the frontal cortex. Elderly patients may not present with prodromal symptoms such as déjà vu or olfactory hallucinations, which are more common in temporal lobe epilepsy. In addition, geriatric patients are less likely to have facial and motor automatisms and are much more likely to report nonspecific symptoms, such as dizziness, paresthesias, myalgias, confusion, fatigue, and clumsiness.[8] The elderly are likely to have a prolonged postictal period, which may last several days to weeks. Many are misdiagnosed with mental status changes, confusion, blackouts, memory disturbances, syncope, dizziness, dementia, transient ischemic attack (TIA), depression, psychiatric disorder, or metabolic disorder.

Differential Diagnosis

Conditions that may mimic seizure include: cardiac arrhythmias, hypoglycemia, orthostatic hypotension, adverse drug effects, TIA, vasovagal syncope, drop attacks, transient global amnesia, rhythmic movement disorders, migraines, and low-output cardiac syndromes (Table 14.6).[11] Thorough evaluation is imperative in cases in which cardiac disease is suspected, to avoid missing a life-threatening condition.

Etiology

Poststroke seizures account for 30%–50% of all new-onset symptomatic seizures in the elderly population.[7] The incidence of seizures occurs after 4%–9% of all strokes, and usually occurs within the first 2–4 weeks after the event (Table 14.7).[8] Acute poststroke seizure is seen within the first 7 days. A seizure that occurs more than 7 days after event is considered a remote seizure. When compared with the general population, elderly

Table 14.6. Differential Diagnosis of Seizures

Cardiac arrhythmias

Hypoglycemia

Orthostatic hypotension

Adverse drug effects

TIA, CVA

Syncope

Drop attacks

Transient global amnesia

Psychiatric disorder

Sleep disorder

Movement disorders

Migraines

Low-output cardiac syndromes

Table 14.7. Most Common Causes of New-Onset Seizure in the Elderly

Poststroke

Metabolic disturbances

Toxins and drugs

Intracranial tumors

Dementia

Head injury and trauma

Subarachnoid hemorrhage

Intracranial infections

patients who have had a stroke have a 23-fold increased risk of having a seizure and a 17-fold increased risk of developing epilepsy.[12] There are certain qualities of strokes that put a patient at greater risk of having a poststroke seizure. These include large infarct size, the presence of associated hemorrhage, and cortical ischemia. Other risk factors include heavy alcohol use, history of seizure, loss of consciousness, confusional state, persistent paresthesias, stroke recurrence, and cardioembolic cause.[12]

Metabolic disturbances leading to encephalopathy account for 6%–30% of seizures.[8] The most common metabolic disturbances seen in the elderly include hypoglycemia, nonketotic hyperglycemia, hyponatremia, hypocalcemia, uremia, and hepatic encephalopathy. These represent potentially reversible causes of new-onset seizures; the risk of recurrence is greatly reduced if these are addressed and corrected.

Toxins and drugs, both prescribed and illicit, account for 10% of new-onset seizures.[8] Polypharmacy and hypersensitivity place the elderly at higher risk of developing seizures. The physiological changes in drug metabolism and elimination seen with aging make the elderly more susceptible to drug toxicity and more likely to suffer a seizure from alcohol, benzodiazepine, or barbiturate withdrawal.

Intracranial tumors are responsible for 10%–15% of new-onset seizures,[8] although seizures are not likely to be the presenting symptom of a mass lesion. Tumors commonly present with confusion, aphasia, or memory loss. The tumors that are most common in the elderly are meningiomas, gliomas, and metastatic lesions from a distant primary tumor.

Dementia increases the risk of seizure development. Eight percent–10% of the geriatric population is affected by dementia. Patients with Alzheimer dementia have a 5–10-fold increased risk of developing a seizure disorder, with up to one quarter of patients having at least one unprovoked seizure during the course of their disease process. Most seizures do not develop until 6 years after the diagnosis of dementia has

been made. The risk increases as the disease progresses; 11% of patients have had a seizure at 10 years, and 26% by 15 years.[12] Patients who have dementia associated with presenilin I or amyloid precursor protein mutations are at greater risk for seizures. Dementia predisposes patients to seizure development by causing epileptogenic foci in the brain with loss of inhibitory neurons. Changes in neurotransmitters and excitatory ion channels have also been implicated in seizure activity.[13] In addition, preexisting dementia places patients at an increased risk for developing seizures in the poststroke period. The comorbidity of dementia makes patients more resistant to treatment of their seizures and may lead to difficulties in management.

Head injury and trauma account for 4%–17% of new-onset seizures. In addition, 18%–26% of elderly patients with subarachnoid hemorrhage will suffer a seizure, whereas intracranial infections account for less than 3%.[8]

Evaluation

A thorough history-taking is crucial in making the diagnosis of seizure. The history should include associated symptoms, loss of consciousness, time course, medication history, drug use, medical history (including history of seizures and strokes), recent or distant head injury, and recent or current fevers and illnesses. Unfortunately, elderly patients are often alone when these episodes occur, and a detailed history may not be readily available. Unless witnessed, the diagnosis may be difficult in patients with cognitive impairment or dementia. Most patients are amnestic for the event, and postictal confusion may be misinterpreted as worsening of dementia.

A complete physical examination should include an evaluation for any injuries, including oropharyngeal examination for possible tongue or buccal mucosa lacerations. The basic laboratory studies often include complete blood count, electrolytes, blood urea nitrogen, creatinine, liver function tests, glucose, calcium, magnesium, as well as ESR, thyroid function tests, rapid plasma reagin, and lipids. Additional studies should include electrocardiography, EEG, and head CT. Based on history and physical findings, other considerations include urine toxicology screen, serum alcohol, lumbar puncture, and blood and urine cultures.

A normal EEG does not exclude the diagnosis of seizure, as only 26%–38% of elderly patients will have epileptiform abnormalities on a single EEG study.[8] Furthermore, an abnormal EEG study does not make a diagnosis of epilepsy, because focal slowing may be seen in up to one third of all elderly patients who do not experience seizures. The use of video and/or ambulatory EEG improves the sensitivity of diagnosing seizures; however, this is not usually indicated with first-time seizures. Evaluation with EEG can be particularly helpful in diagnosing nonconvulsive status epilepticus. There are several nonspecific EEG findings in acute stroke patients: periodic lateralizing epileptiform discharges, sharp waves, and focal slowing.[12] All elderly patients who present with a new-onset seizure should undergo brain imaging. MRI is useful in detecting acute ischemic lesions, small infarcts, cortical malformations, and neoplasms. Gadolinium-enhanced MRI increases the sensitivity for infection, neoplasm, and inflammatory conditions.

Management

If you are the first responder to a patient who is actively having a seizure or appears to be in a postictal confused state, close attention to basic life support is imperative with the goal of preventing injury. The first step in management is to correct any reversible causes of seizure; for example, toxin exposure, medication overdose or withdrawal, and electrolyte imbalances. Management for first-time seizure in the elderly should include measures to prevent future seizures, as well as safety promotion to prevent injury to self and others. Patients should be counseled about the risks of driving and swimming and should take showers instead of baths, until a cause can be determined or until the disorder is under control. Driving restrictions can pose a significant dilemma for both the patient and physician and decisions should be based on recurrence risk. There are specific state laws regarding driving restrictions, and they can usually be obtained from the state's department of motor vehicles.

Depression and anxiety are underdiagnosed and undertreated in the geriatric population and show a strong association with seizures. Twenty percent–55% of patients with recurrent seizures have signs of depression. Even when epilepsy is controlled, up to 10% of patients suffer from depression.[11] Therefore it is important to screen for these issues in those who have a history of seizures.

Treatment

The decision of when to start a medication is an ongoing dilemma. Currently there are no randomized controlled trials in the geriatric population to define who should be treated and for how long. Current evidence is Level III and below. In general, it is recommended to begin treatment after the second acute seizure, prolonged first seizure, or when the patient presents in status epilepticus. For patients with acute cerebrovascular accident (CVA) or trauma that leads to new-onset seizures, the current recommendations are to treat with antiepileptics for a limited time, in those with high risk for recurrence.[8] For unprovoked seizures, treatment with antiepileptics should be started and continued long term.[8] Antiepileptics have been shown to reduce the risk of acute seizures within the first 7 days after traumatic brain injury, but they do not decrease the risk of remote seizures or mortality. The American Heart Association guidelines state that there is no evidence to start prophylactic agents after *ischemic* stroke and few data to support starting antiepileptics in patients who do suffer a poststroke seizure. There is Level V evidence to consider prophylactic antiepileptics in *hemorrhagic* strokes, treating for 1 month and then tapering medication.[12]

If it is determined that medications are needed to avoid future seizures, the goal of therapy should be to choose the lowest effective dose of a single agent. There are specific age-related physiological changes that occur in the elderly that make choosing an antiepileptic medication a challenge. The elderly have decreased lean body mass and decreased protein-binding capability, which result in altered distribution of medications. Impaired hepatic metabolism and decreased renal clearance, both of which decrease by 10% for each decade after 40 years, lead to slower overall drug metabolism in the elderly.[13] Therefore, lower doses are usually necessary to provide adequate prophylactic treatment. In addition, the elderly will exhibit signs of toxicity at much lower doses than their younger counterparts. It is important to use the antiepileptics carefully in this population and to monitor blood levels closely, with particular attention to any signs of toxicity.

Choosing a medication is complicated by the age-related physiological changes mentioned previously, and there are the risks of polypharmacy and adverse side effects such as confusion, impaired gait, sedation, tremor, dizziness, visual changes, hyponatremia (especially with concurrent diuretics), and vertigo. Osteoporosis is an underappreciated side effect of certain antiepileptic medications. Active bone loss is seen in patients on long-term phenytoin, phenobarbital, and carbamazepine. Health care providers should start patients on calcium and vitamin D supplements for those on long-term antiepileptics and obtain regular screening dual-energy x-ray absorptiometry scans.

In general, the newer anticonvulsants are preferred, as they may have fewer side effects, linear pharmacokinetics, and decreased incidence of interactions with other medications. Table 14.8 reviews common medication choices, along with possible side effects and contraindications that are important in the elderly. The newer drugs include gabapentin, lamotrigine, topiramate, tiagabine, oxcarbazepine, zonisamide, levetiracetam, and pregabalin. When making the choice about which medications to prescribe, consideration must be given to comorbid conditions (especially hepatic or kidney disease), other medications, route of administration, route of metabolism and excretion, dosing schedule, and expense to the individual. There is level A, class I and II evidence that gabapentin and lamotrigine are effective and safe as first-line agents in elderly patients.[14] Carbamazepine has equal effectiveness, but significantly more side effects, which leads to decreased medication compliance.[15] Gabapentin, lamotrigine,

Table 14.8. Seizure Medications

Medication	Considerations in the Elderly	Side Effects	Contraindications	Indications, Recommendations
Phenytoin	Heavily protein bound, requires lower doses, high risk for toxicity, interacts with many medications	Worsened cognitive deficits, osteomalacia, increased falls, liver toxicity, rash, gingival hyperplasia, GI upset	Liver and renal disease, hypoalbuminemia, sinus bradycardia, SA block, second and third degree AV block	Useful in status epilepticus
Carbamazepine*	High protein binding and decreased clearance, use lower and less frequent doses, many drug interactions	SIADH, hypertension, hypotension, rash, GI upset, dizziness, somnolence, nystagmus, diplopia. Black box warning for aplastic anemia and agranulocytosis	Arrhythmias, MAO inhibitors, bone marrow disorders	Epilepsy, bipolar disorder, TN
Valproic acid	High protein binding, use lower doses, longer half-life, increased side effects in elderly, many drug interactions (including lamotrigine)	Weight gain, alopecia, GI upset, tremor, reversible, ataxia, dizziness, mood swings parkinsonism, thrombocytopenia, liver toxicity. Black box warning for hepatotoxicity and pancreatitis	Hepatic disease, urea cycle dysfunction	Partial and complex seizures, mania, migraines
Oxcarbazepine	Fewer drug interactions than carbamazepine	Severe hyponatremia, GI upset, ataxia, tremor, vertigo, diplopia, fatigue	Cardiac arrhythmias, CYP medications	Partial seizures, may increase alertness and attention
Gabapentin*	Well tolerated	Somnolence, dizziness, ataxia, fatigue	Avoid antacids, caution in renal insufficiency	Little effect on cognition, few drug interactions, partial seizures, TN, peripheral neuropathy, migraine, social phobia
Lamotrigine*	Well tolerated	Rash common, GI upset, ataxia, headache, dizziness, blurred vision	Caution in patients with cardiac disease	Partial and tonic–clonic seizure, bipolar disorder. Little cognitive effect, less dosage and elimination issues, may be used in chronic kidney disease
Topiramate		Decreased cognition, anorexia, weight loss, renal calculi, dizziness, motor retardation, fatigue	Behavior or cognitive disorders, renal or hepatic impairment	Partial and tonic–clonic seizure, migraines

* Recommended as first-line agents for elderly patients.

SIADH, syndrome of inappropriate antidiuretic hormone secretion.

and topiramate are effective for monotherapy, although currently not Food and Drug Administration–approved for this use.[15] In general, benzodiazepines and barbiturates should be avoided in the elderly, because of the high risk of adverse side effects, toxicity, and potential for abuse. In patients who present in status epilepticus, quick management of basic life support, followed by cessation of seizure is imperative. It is recommended to start with intravenous diazepam or intravenous lorazepam, followed by intravenous phenytoin or fosphenytoin as second-line agents.

As is the case with when to start a patient on medication, there is also controversy surrounding the decision of if and when to stop treatment. Most neurologists recommend weaning attempts only after a seizure-free interval of 2–3 years. However, some will attempt to discontinue medications after 6–12 months.[12] There are a few nonpharmacological treatment options available, such as vagal nerve stimulation and surgical interventions; however there is currently no adequate evidence to recommend for or against these interventions in this age group.

Prognosis

The overall incidence of seizure recurrence is 3%–12% in the elderly; however, the incidence has been shown to be as high as 34% in some studies.[10] Recurrence risk increases in patients who have associated postical paralysis, abnormal EEG, or abnormal neurological examination. Patients with history of CVA, dementia, intracranial tumors, or alcohol abuse are also at increased risk of recurrence. Eighty percent of patients who have epileptiform foci on EEG will have recurrent seizures. In those patients who have a second seizure, the incidence of a third seizure is 73% at 4 years.[10] Mortality of acute onset of status epilepticus can be as high as 50% in those patients older than 80 years.[8] Up to 70% of patients respond to pharmacological therapy in poststroke epilepsy. This rate is significantly lower in patients with preexisting dementia. The majority of studies do not find that either early or remote seizures increase the risk of dependency or mortality following a stroke event.[12] A seizure itself, however, can be the cause of death, particularly in the case of status epilepticus or recurrent undiagnosed seizures. Usually, the underlying disease process leading to the seizure causes more morbidity and mortality than the seizure itself in the geriatric patient.

SENSORY LOSS

General Concepts

In determining the cause of sensory loss, it is important to define the distribution of the loss and the sensory modalities that are effected. Large, myelinated nerve fibers are responsible for the sensations of proprioception, vibration, pressure, and touch stimuli. Small, relatively unmyelinated fibers respond to pain, temperature, and touch stimuli. Pain and temperature sensations mediated by these fibers reach the dorsal root ganglion, cross the spinal cord, ascend in the contralateral lateral spinothalamic tract, and terminate within the ventral thalamus. In contrast, position and vibration senses ascend in the ipsilateral dorsal column (cuneate and gracilis fasciculi) and cross in the medulla (medial lemniscus), reaching the contralateral thalamus and terminate within the parietal cortex. Because the two modalities cross at different levels, large lesions of one half of the spinal cord will often lead to dissociated sensory signs (so-called Brown-Séquard syndrome).

Specific terms used to describe sensory loss are often used interchangeably but should be distinguished. *Hypesthesia* is defined as a diminished ability to perceive pain, temperature, touch, or vibration. *Anesthesia* is the complete loss of the ability to perceive these sensations. *Hyperesthesia* is an exaggerated sensation to stimuli. *Dysesthesia* is an altered sensation to stimuli. *Hypalgesia* is used to describe decreased sensitivity to painful stimuli, whereas *analgesia* is complete loss of sensitivity to pain. *Allodynia* is a painful response to a normal, usually nonpainful, stimuli.[16]

A mononeuropathy is a disorder of a single peripheral nerve usually caused by compression or trauma. Mononeuritis or mononeuropathy multiplex refers to multiple single peripheral nerve lesions occurring simultaneously or in conjunction with the same pathological process. The condition is thought to be related to microvascular infarction of peripheral nerves either due to diabetes or an immunological disorder such as cryoglobulinemia.

In the primary care setting, peripheral polyneuropathy is the most common cause of sensory loss and will be discussed in more detail in the following section.

History and Localization

A detailed history should include specific symptoms: the time course over which they have occurred; the distribution and severity of symptoms; exacerbating factors; medical history; history of trauma; medication use; over the counter drugs; diet; toxic exposures, including alcohol, tobacco, and other illicit drug use; human immunodeficiency virus (HIV) risk factors; foreign travel; family history; and psychosocial history.

Acute sensory loss may occur after a traumatic neuropathy or with a cerebrovascular lesion. Subacute sensory symptoms may be associated with either a central or peripheral demyelinating lesion. Table 14.9 lists the clinical signs that distinguish central from peripheral lesions. Chronic progressive symptoms may suggest a toxic neuropathy, metabolic derangement, or hereditary neuropathy.

The sensory examination can be time consuming and is often left for last. In general, it is best to use the history to narrow the localization before an exhaustive sensory examination is undertaken. For instance, if a patient complains of distal symmetrical paresthesias and numbness one must consider a peripheral neuropathy first followed by radiculopathy or spinal cord lesions. These complaints are unlikely to be caused by a

Table 14.9. Differentiating Central Versus Peripheral Causes of Sensory Loss

	Peripheral	*Central*
Reflexes	Decreased or absent	Hyperreflexia, clonus, Babinski sign
Tone	Normal or decreased, atrophy, fasciculations	Increased tone
Strength	Symmetrical, proximal, or distal weakness	Incoordination without weakness
Pattern of sensory loss	Confined to a peripheral nerve or nerve root distribution, may be exacerbated by position changes, length dependent stocking-glove distribution	Presence of sensory level
Gait	Antalgic, steppage, waddling	Spastic, paraparetic, hemiparetic

Table 14.10. Patterns of Sensory Loss

Type of Sensory Loss	Site of Lesion	Symptoms	Exam Findings	Examples
Mononeuropathy	Individual peripheral nerve Caused by trauma, entrapment, or vasculopathy	Numbness, paresthesias in specific distribution	Sensory loss along one specific nerve distribution	Carpal tunnel syndrome (median nerve), ulnar neuropathy at elbow, meralgia paresthetica (lateral femoral cutaneous nerve), diabetes, pregnancy
Radiculopathy	Individual nerve root, radiation in dermatome or myotome	Symptoms may be mild because of overlap. Present with severe, intermittent, lancinating pain, toothachelike. May be exacerbated by coughing, sneezing, or straining	Sensory loss, especially pinprick along dermatome, may have tenderness over nerve	S-1 radiculopathy with sciatic nerve distribution. May be caused by diabetes, trauma, tumor, infection, herniated disk
Peripheral neuropathy	Length-dependent axonal neuropathy, because of axonal death and "dying back"	Numbness, paresthesias, pain in feet, legs > hands. Pain may be burning, lancinating, aching, lightening-like. May also have areas of hypesthesia	Stocking-glove distribution. Decreased pinprick, temperature, vibration. Decreased or loss of ankle jerk	Diabetes, alcohol, Vit B12 deficiency, HIV, Lyme, uremia, vasculitis, paraneoplastic neuropathy, amyloidosis, syphilis
Sensory neuronopathies	Degeneration of dorsal root ganglion	Difficulty with walking, balance. Numbness, paresthesias in hands, feet	Asymmetrical, no motor loss, sensory ataxia, decreased vibration, pinprick, position, decreased reflexes, normal strength	Sjögren, Anti-HU paraneoplastic syndrome, Vit B6 toxicity, cisplatin treatment
Cape distribution	Central cervical cord		Loss of pain and temp only in shoulders, arms, torso	Tumor, syrinx, demyelinating disease
Brown-Séquard syndrome	Hemisection of spinal cord	Weakness	Ipsilateral loss of vibration, proprioception, weakness. Contralateral loss of pain and temperature below the level of lesion	
Brainstem lesion	Brainstem		Incomplete hemibody, loss of pain and temperature in ipsilateral face and contralateral trunk and limbs	Wallenberg syndrome (lateral medulla)
Proximal sensory loss (rare)	Axonal neuropathy "bathing suit distribution"	Weakness, acute onset	Proximal motor weakness or paralysis, sensory loss of torso and proximal limbs, loss of proximal deep tendon reflexes, preserved patellar reflex	Porphyria, Tangiers disease, can be seen in diabetes, brachial plexus neuropathy
Thalamic lesions	Thalamus	Severe, intermittent pain in half of body	Complete hemibody, hyperesthesia in contralateral hemibody	Lacunar infarcts, Dejerine–Roussy syndrome
Intracutaneous sensory loss	Dorsal roots	Painless injuries, Charcot joints	Loss of pain and temperature sensation in extensor surfaces of extremities, malar area	Tabes dorsalis, leprosy
Functional sensory loss	Psychogenic, somatic	Complete loss of sensation	Distinct boundaries of pain, temperature, vibration loss that are not anatomically explained	Psychogenic, somatic, malingering, Münchhausen

central cerebral lesion. If a patient complains of sensory symptoms in one hand, mononeuropathy such as median neuropathy at the wrist (carpel tunnel syndrome) or ulnar neuropathy should be considered first. A patient with a lateral femoral cutaneous nerve lesion (meralgia paresthetica) will often be able to map out the distribution of the nerve himself or herself. Refer to Table 14.10 for patterns of sensory loss.

Small-fiber neuropathies may present primarily with neuropathic symptoms of burning, stinging, or cold sensations, whereas large-fiber neuropathies tend to cause tingling, pins and needles, and electrical sensations. Dorsal column dysfunction from tabes dorsalis, B12 deficiency, or demyelination may be marked by mild, vague distal or diffuse sensory symptoms, and the patient may demonstrate significant ataxia and postural instability.

In general, the examination should focus on subjective areas of sensory loss and should begin with application of the stimuli in abnormal areas, progressing to normal areas. Using proportions or analogies such as 50% or 50 cents to describe the degree of sensory loss is often helpful. One may begin by asking the patient to note that the normal body area is 100% or 1 dollar and compare that to the abnormal areas that may be 50 cents or 50%, 25 cents or 25%, and so forth.

Pain sensation should be tested with a safety pin, wooden tongue depressor, or swab that is snapped and splintered. Facial expression and grimacing can be helpful in determining the sensation of pain in patients unable to express pain verbally such as an aphasic or demented individual. Temperature sensation may be assessed using a cool piece of metal, such as the end of a tuning fork or reflex hammer and marching from distal to proximal limbs.

Position sense can be tested by grasping the great toe or index finger, making short excursions up or down and asking the patient to identify the direction of movement. Vibration sense is tested by applying a 128-Hz tuning fork to the bony prominence of the great toe joint, medial malleolus, or knee. Loss of vibration sensation usually occurs in a graded fashion distally to proximally. Complete loss of vibration sense almost never occurs proximally at the knees or elbows without affecting the distal extremities; so again examining the great toe is often the highest yield. Because most neuropathic conditions tend to be length dependent and distally predominant, more useful information may be obtained from examining the feet rather than the hands.

The Romberg test is a test of integration of position sense and proper muscle tone, and postural stability. A positive Romberg test occurs when a patient is able to stand with feet together, arms extended in front, and eyes open, but then the patient loses balance when the eyes are closed. The interruption of visual input leads to complete dependence on the proprioceptive system which when impaired will lead to falls. Patients with poor position sense classically have more difficulty walking in the dark or at night.

Spinal cord lesions may cause vague, diffuse numbness, or paresthesias. A sensory level may be present and is best elicited using a pin to march up and down both sides of the back, asking the patient whether or not they feel a significant change in the sensation at a certain level. The sensory level suggests a lesion of the anterolateral spinal cord. Additional findings such as the presence of hyperreflexia, Babinski sign, clonus at the ankles, or spasticity suggest additional corticospinal tract involvement in either the spinal cord or cerebrum. Hemisensory loss involving the face, arm, and leg localizes to the contralateral cerebrum. Sensory loss or paresthesias are characteristically absent in neuromuscular junction disorders, although muscle pain may be present.

Peripheral Neuropathy

The incidence of peripheral neuropathy increases with age, affecting 26% of adults 65–74 years of age, and up to 54% of those older than 85 years.[17] Elderly patients with peripheral neuropathy will have loss of ankle jerk, followed by loss of fine touch. Predictors of bilateral sensory deficits include increasing age, obesity, vitamin B12 deficiency, lower socioeconomic status, and concurrent rheumatoid arthritis.[17] Peripheral neuropathy may be asymptomatic; however, it is strongly linked with gait and balance dysfunction, falls and injuries, restless legs syndrome, leg cramps and pains, cellulitis, ulcers, and decreased quality of life. The differential diagnosis of peripheral neuropathy is quite extensive (Table 14.11).

Presentation, Signs, and Symptoms

Patients with a length-dependent peripheral polyneuropathy typically present with complaints of distal numbness and tingling beginning in the feet. Over time, the symptoms may slowly progress proximally. Painful or uncomfortable paresthesias, restless legs–like symptoms, imbalance, or gait impairment may be present. Loss of grip strength, tripping over toes, difficulty getting up out of a chair or holding objects may be present in sensorimotor neuropathies.

Examination of a patient with suspected peripheral neuropathy should include orthostatic vital signs to exclude autonomic dysfunction. Neuropathies may also cause trophic skin changes including distal hair loss, edema, and discoloration. A comprehensive neurological examination should be performed with particular attention to fine touch, position and vibration sense at the great toe, deep tendon reflexes at the ankle and patella, and gait testing. Table 14.12 describes physical exam findings in patients with peripheral neuropathy.

Reflexes are often decreased or absent at the ankle in patients with peripheral neuropathy. There is loss of sensitivity to one or more sensory modalities, muscle wasting, weakness of lower extremities, or fasciculations. Other findings include weakness in dorsiflexion of the toes and feet, hammertoes, and pes cavus may also be found. Because of the nerve length dependency of polyneuropathy, the hands are generally not involved until the sensory loss in the legs reaches the knees.

Table 14.11. Differential Diagnosis of Peripheral Neuropathy

Metabolic Disease	Infectious Disease
Diabetes	HIV, acquired immunodeficiency syndrome
Hypothyroidism	Lyme disease
Acromegaly	Leprosy
Hypophosphatemia	
Nutritional deficiencies	*Toxin/Medication*
Vitamin B12 deficiency	Carbon monoxide
Folate deficiency	Organophosphates
Thiamine deficiency	Glue sniffing
Alcoholic disease	Lead
Niacin deficiency	Arsenic
Pyridoxine (B6) deficiency	Cisplatin
Vitamin E deficiency	Ethylene oxide
	Acrylamide
Rheumatological diseases	Vincristine
Rheumatoid arthritis	Mercury
Systemic lupus erythematosus	Gold
Polyarteritis nodosa	Thallium
Amyloidosis	Thalidomide
Sarcoidosis	
Malignancy	
Renal cell carcinoma	
Myeloma	
Lymphoma	
Lung carcinoma	

Table 14.12. Painful Peripheral Neuropathies

Type of Neuropathy	Exam Findings	EMG/NCS
Diabetic peripheral neuropathy	Reduced or absent reflexes, distal sensory loss, +/− orthostatic hypotension	Abnormal
Idiopathic, small-fiber neuropathy	Reduced pinprick in legs, otherwise normal exam	Often normal
Inherited neuropathy	Pes cavus or hammer toes, reduced reflexes and distal sensation	Abnormal
Connective tissue disease	Reduced reflexes and sensation	Abnormal
Vasculitis	Multifocal findings	Abnormal

Evaluation

An initial evaluation for the cause of neuropathy should include urinalysis with attention to protein and glucose levels, complete blood count, ESR, vitamin B12, folate, fasting blood glucose, blood urea nitrogen, creatinine, and thyroid-stimulating hormone.

Referral to a neurologist may be indicated for confirmation and electromyogram (EMG) and nerve conduction studies (NCS). These studies are helpful in distinguishing mononeuropathy, polyneuropathies, and radiculopathies from myopathies and neuromuscular junction disorders. Prognostic information can also be obtained by differentiating between axonal or demyelinating disorders.

Second-tier testing may include serum and urine protein electrophoresis, oral glucose tolerance test, and a rheumatological screen including angiotensin-converting enzyme, antinuclear antibody, antineutrophilic cytoplasmic antibodies, and Sjögren antibodies. Anti-Hu antibody should be ordered to exclude a paraneoplastic neuronopathy from small cell lung cancer. An examination of the cerebrospinal fluid may reveal signs of inflammation (chronic inflammatory demyelinating polyneuropathy [CIDP]), infection, or neoplasm.

Etiology

Diabetes is the most common cause of peripheral neuropathy in the United States. Twenty-eight percent–45% of diabetics older than the age of 40 years suffer from some sort of peripheral neuropathy, defined as at least one area of loss of sensation with monofilament testing.[18] Not all diabetic patients will have neuropathy and not all neuropathy is caused by their diabetic disease. Up to a one third of cases were found to be caused by concurrent vasculitic disease, CIDP, alcoholic neuropathy, and radiculopathy.[19] The most common form of peripheral neuropathy in the United States is symmetrical and distal, caused by diabetes. Up to 10% of nondiabetics have evidence of peripheral neuropathy, and 26% of undiagnosed diabetics, defined as fasting blood glucose over 126 mg/dL, without previous diagnosis, were found to have peripheral neuropathy.[20] Patients do not usually present with neuropathic symptoms until after having the diagnosis of diabetes for 10 years or more. The most common presenting symptoms are pain and paresthesias, gait impairment, limb weakness, and autonomic symptoms.[19]

Chronic alcoholism is the second most common cause of neuropathy in the United States. The specific pathophysiology is unclear, but is thought to be due to thiamine (B1) deficiency. There is no definite evidence that alcohol causes direct damage to peripheral nerves.

Vitamin B12 deficiency can cause any combination of polyneuropathy, cognitive and behavioral impairment, and myelopathy. Deficiency may result from nutritional deficiency from a vegan diet, pernicious anemia, or very rarely brief nitrous oxide exposure. Demyelination of dorsal columns and corticospinal tracts may also occur, with loss of proprioception and fine touch, along with weakness.[21] As with diabetes, the incidence of vitamin B12 deficiency increases with age, with as many as 15% of patients older than 65 years having laboratory proved deficiency.[21] Elderly patients are at higher risk for dietary deficiency, especially those with concurrent alcoholism, poor diets, and those who follow a strict vegan diet. The incidence of malabsorption disorders also increases with age, with decreased acid production in cases of atrophic gastritis and increased rates of pernicious anemia. The chronic use of acid blocking medications, often used in treating gastroesophageal reflux disease, may lead to decreased absorption of vitamin B12 in the gastrointestinal (GI) tract.

Guillain-Barré syndrome (GBS) is an acute demyelinating neuropathy involving both sensory and motor nerves. GBS is caused by an autoimmune response directed against Schwann cells or myelin causing diffuse demyelination of proximal nerve roots and peripheral nerves. Although sometimes idiopathic, the syndrome is often associated with antecedent respiratory or GI illness.

Patients with GBS typically present with distal paresthesias in the hands and feet, evolving over hours to days to flaccid paralysis of the legs with areflexia, and eventually ascending to the arms. Many patients develop respiratory muscle involvement leading to neuromuscular respiratory failure. Autonomic instability including blood pressure lability and arrhythmia are also common. For this reason, early GBS patients with mild symptoms should be hospitalized for observation because critical care and ventilatory support is often required. The diagnosis is confirmed by EMG/NCS, although typical demyelinating neuropathic features may not be present at the time of diagnosis. An examination of cerebrospinal fluid showing an elevated protein and few white cells further confirms the diagnosis. Treatment with intravenous immunoglobulin often improves the prognosis for recovery.[22]

CIDP is a chronic condition marked by relapsing bouts of demyelination affecting predominantly motor nerves and roots. The treatment of choice is periodic pulses of steroids for exacerbations followed by long-term steroid therapy.

Causes of pure small-fiber sensory neuropathies include diabetes, celiac disease, Lyme disease, immunoglobulin G monoclonal gammopathy, vitamin B12 deficiency, connective tissue disease, inflammatory bowel disease, and thyroid disease.

Although uncommon in the geriatric population, functional or psychogenic causes of sensory loss may be encountered. Patients with concurrent depression, anxiety, and personality disorders or who are under a significant amount of social stress will be at higher risk for somatization and factitious disorders. Normal laboratory, imaging, and electrophysiological evaluations should be documented because these conditions are diagnoses of exclusion. Patients with psychogenic disease may show inconsistent findings on examination, such as abrupt demarcation of sensation loss.

Inherited neuropathies such as Charcot-Marie-Tooth disease and acute intermittent porphyria generally do not develop in the elderly and will not be discussed further in this chapter.

Treatment

One of the most common presenting symptoms of peripheral neuropathy is pain that is difficult to treat in many cases. The first-line treatment for peripheral neuropathy includes gabapentin, opioids, lidocaine patch, tramadol, and tricyclic antidepressants (TCAs).[23] Physicians may choose to start with TCAs, especially in those patients with concurrent depression and/or insomnia, moving to carbamazepine, oxcarbazepine, or gabapentin if not effective.[24] Special attention must be given with the use of TCAs because of increased risk of side effects and toxicity in the elderly. Gabapentin should be started with once daily dosing and increased as tolerated to three times daily dosing for pain relief. Opioids have classically been avoided in neuropathic pain treatment; however, there is evidence that these agents can be used as first-line treatment or as adjuvants to other methods. It is recommended to start the patients on short-acting opioids and then switch them to equianalgesic doses of long-acting opioids after 1–2 weeks. Opioids inhibit central ascending pain impulses and have been shown to decrease not only pain but allodynia, sleep disturbances, and overall disability.[25] Lidocaine patches can also be used, especially in cases of specific areas of hyperesthesis, by placing a patch directly over this area of skin. Second-line agents for neuropathic pain include other antispasmodics, such as lamotrigine and carbamazepine, and other antidepressants such as bupropion, citalopram, paroxetine, and venlafaxine.[23] These agents can be used as adjuvants or alone, if other treatment options have failed.

Headache

Headache is one of the most common medical complaints in the primary care setting.

Primary headaches are defined as headache syndromes that occur without underlying anatomical pathological conditions. Most primary headaches begin before middle age and decrease in incidence with age.

General Approach to the Elderly Person with Headaches

The single most important determination to make when evaluating a patient with headache is to determine whether the headache is a new symptom or an exacerbation of a chronic long-standing headache. Furthermore, if a patient describes a new or worsening pattern of headache, it is prudent to err on the side of caution and not presume that the symptom merely represents a change in a previous headache pattern. Although many primary headache syndromes do evolve with age, a change in a headache pattern in the elderly should prompt investigation, particularly brain imaging. Not every patient presenting with headache should undergo imaging. The duration of symptoms is often helpful in determining the need for imaging. A person with 10 years of nonprogressive headache is much less likely to have a malignant or secondary cause for headache such as a hemorrhage or neoplasm.

Primary headaches can begin at any age but usually begin in childhood or between the ages of 20 and 50 years. Migraines

Table 14.13. Headache Types

Headaches	Duration	Characteristics	Associated Symptoms
Migraine	4–72 h	Unilateral, pulsating quality, moderate to severe intensity, aggravated by activity, improved with rest/sleep	Nausea, vomiting, photophobia, and phonophobia
Tension-Type	30 min–7 d	Bilateral, pressing or tightening, no pulsating quality, mild to moderate intensity, not aggravated by activity	No more than one of the following: nausea, vomiting, photophobia, or phonophobia
Cluster	15–180 minutes	Unilateral orbital, supraorbital, or temporal pain	Conjunctival injection, lacrimation, nasal congestion, rhinorrhea, forehead and facial sweating, miosis, ptosis, and eyelid edema

tend to decrease in frequency with age and new-onset migraine headaches later in life are decidedly uncommon, accounting for approximately 2% of all migraines. For this reason, *new-onset headaches after the age of 50 years should be considered secondary until proved otherwise.*

"Worst headache of my life," focal neurological signs or symptoms, meningismus, and altered mental state are clear indications for evaluation including neuroimaging and lumbar puncture.

Associated symptoms before, during, or after episodes of headaches can be helpful in narrowing the differential diagnosis. Photophobia, phonophobia, and presence of aura are characteristics of migraine headaches whereas ipsilateral autonomic features are highly suggestive of cluster headaches. A headache that is worse when the patient is supine and relieved by standing or sitting is suggestive of increased intracranial pressure.

The geriatric population (aged 65 years and older) accounts for one third of all prescriptions written in the United States. This population also has the highest risk of drug–drug interactions and adverse reaction to medications. Discontinuing medications that are not essential is often helpful in eliminating or narrowing down the possible causes of headache.

A thorough medical history can identify uncontrolled hypertension, sinusitis, or meningitis as the cause for headache. Intracranial processes causing headache include primary tumors, metastatic lesions, and intracranial vascular disorders. Inquiring about trauma, falls, and procedures particularly in the elderly can provide valuable information in the history. Head trauma can trigger a primary headache or lead to concussion and intracranial hemorrhages. Procedures such as lumbar puncture may lead to a low-pressure headache characterized by throbbing frontal or occipital headache, dizziness, nausea, and vomiting that are worse when standing and relieved when supine.

A patient with a primary headache syndrome should have a complete neurological examination, including mental status, level of arousal, and an evaluation of cranial nerves, strength, coordination, reflexes, sensation, and gait. Vital signs, fundoscopic examination, and cardiovascular evaluations should also be performed.

Primary Headache Syndromes

Primary headache syndromes such as migraine, tension-type, and cluster headaches account for the majority of headaches in all age groups, including the elderly (Table 14.13).

Migraine

Migraine headache is one of the leading causes of pain-related disability. A migraine may be divided into four phases: premonitory phase, aura, headache, and postdrome. All four phases do not need to be present to diagnose a migraine. The premonitory phase occurs hours to days before the headache onset and consists of psychological symptoms including irritability, depression, fatigue, and systemic symptoms such as anorexia, food cravings, or sluggishness. The aura is a stereotyped focal neurological symptom preceding or accompanying the headache. Visual auras are the most common and are described as hemianoptic flashes or scotomas migrating across the visual field. A typical migraine headache is usually unilateral, throbbing, and aggravated by physical activity. Common associated symptoms contribute to the disability experienced by a migraineur including photophobia, phonophobia, nausea, and vomiting. The postdromal symptoms of migraine may include poor concentration, fatigue, irritability, hypersomnia, and myalgias.

Migraine headaches tend to decrease in frequency with age but when they persist through middle age symptoms may evolve. Auras may be less common. In some cases, auras may occur without headache (acephalgic migraine) mimicking a cerebrovascular event. Acute migraine headache may be aborted with either nonspecific or migraine-specific medications. Several selective serotonin agonists or triptans are available in both oral and parenteral forms. All are recommended for the treatment of acute migraine attacks and show similar efficacy compared with placebo.

Analgesics and nonsteroidal antiinflammatory drugs (NSAIDs) are effective in aborting an attack when administered as early as possible. Ketorolac (Toradol), a parenteral NSAID, is an option for therapy of severe migraines secondary to its relatively rapid onset and long duration of action. Narcotic use should be avoided for chronic daily headaches because it can lead to dependency, rebound headaches, and eventual loss of efficacy. Antiemetics such as metoclopramide (Reglan) and prochlorperazine (Compazine) not only alleviate nausea and emesis associated with migraines, but also provide synergistic analgesia when administered with an NSAID. Special attention should be given prior to starting metoclopramide in an elderly patient, as the risk for side effects and drug interactions is great and can lead to serious injury.

Preventative medications should be used in patients with frequent headaches (more than four per month), prolonged or uncomfortable auras, and aura characterized by focal neurological symptoms (complicated migraine). Beta-blockers, calcium channel blockers, and antidepressants have all been shown to be effective.

Tension-Type Headache

Tension-type headache is a common but less disabling headache syndrome. It is described as a nonpulsating, bilateral headache not often associated with other features such as photophobia, phonophobia, or nausea. Movement does not usually worsen the headache. Analgesics such as acetaminophen, aspirin, and NSAIDs are very effective but their *use should be limited to no more than 2 days per week*. Prophylactic therapy should be considered in patients with chronic headaches requiring daily analgesics. TCAs such as amitriptyline have been shown to reduce headache frequency, the need for analgesics, and headache-related disability. TCAs, however, are generally not well tolerated in the geriatric population because of their anticholinergic and antihistaminic properties. Serotonin reuptake inhibitors may be used, although their usefulness in treating tension-type headache has been unproved. Behavioral techniques such as psychotherapy, stress management, and biofeedback used alone or in combination with antidepressant medications may also reduce headaches and analgesic medication use.

Cluster Headache

Cluster headache is a unilateral headache associated with cranial autonomic features. Compared with migraine and tension-type headache, cluster headache is relatively rare and has a predilection for middle aged men. Attacks are described as excruciating pain over or behind one eye, lasting minutes to hours. Patients may describe the pain as a "hot poker" in the eye. In contrast to migraineurs who often find relief after sleep, patients with cluster headache find it hard to sleep and have a tendency to pace or rock. Cluster headache often occurs in rest or during rapid eye movement (REM) sleep, suggesting a circadian relationship. Because the attacks build up so rapidly, many oral medications are often not effective abortive agents. Subcutaneous sumatriptan (6 mg) given at the onset of an attack has been shown to be effective and safe in aborting the headache. Oxygen is a safe and effective abortive agent. One hundred percent oxygen given at 7–12 L/min via a nonrebreathing facemask over 15–20 minutes should be given. High doses of verapamil (240–960 mg daily in divided doses) has been shown to be effective for preventing attacks but caution

is advised because of the potential induction of arrhythmias. Lithium (600–1200 mg/day) is similarly effective but its use in the elderly is limited by its side effect profile and narrow therapeutic window. Recognizing and avoiding potential triggers including alcohol, volatile fumes, and nitroglycerine is important in the prevention of cluster headache.

SECONDARY HEADACHE SYNDROMES

Three secondary headache syndromes become more common with increasing age: temporal arteritis, trigeminal neuralgia, and postherpetic neuralgia.

Giant cell arteritis (GCA) also known as temporal arteritis is a systemic vasculitis with a predilection for the temporal arteries. The prevalence of GCA increases with advancing age and should be suspected in anyone with *new-onset headache presenting after the age of 50 years*. Headache is the most common presenting symptom occurring in 75% of cases. The headache classically occurs over the temporal artery, and often escalates in severity over days to weeks. Jaw claudication or pain upon chewing is another hallmark feature. Systemic manifestations include malaise, myalgias, and arthralgias mimicking polymyalgia rheumatica.

On physical examination, a prominent, tender, or pulseless temporal artery may be present. The ESR is almost always markedly elevated (over 100). Definitive diagnosis of GCA requires temporal artery biopsy performed by an ophthalmologist or neurosurgeon. Optic neuropathy is the most dreaded complication of GCA. If the diagnosis is missed or delayed, irreversible vision loss may occur. Therefore, if the diagnosis is suspected, waiting for a biopsy is unnecessary and treatment should be instituted immediately with high-dose oral corticosteroids (prednisone 40–60 mg/day). Steroid dosing should be based on symptom relief, whereas the duration of treatment is based on normalization of the ESR.

Trigeminal neuralgia (TN) is a relatively common cause of facial pain in the elderly. The pain is classically described as paroxysms of excruciating sharp, shooting, electrical pains often triggered by minor cutaneous stimuli around the face or jaw. The pain is unilateral, most commonly involving the lower trigeminal divisions (V1 and 2), whereas isolated involvement of the ophthalmic division (V1) is relatively uncommon. The bursts of pain may be interrupted by brief periods of relief or prolonged remissions. The pain is often immobilizing; chewing, eating, talking, or any cutaneous stimulation of the face may be impossible during an attack. Even cold air or the slightest touch may trigger an attack.

Primary TN is almost always unilateral; therefore, *bilateral TN should prompt a search for an underlying lesion*. Primary TN is thought to be related to an underlying pathological condition at the nerve root entry zone in the brainstem or anywhere along the length of the trigeminal nerve. Vascular compression with focal demyelination isa common theory but has never been proven. Secondary or symptomatic TN can result from a number of structural causes including mass lesions, demyelinating plaques, brainstem strokes, dilated or tortuous blood vessels, or basilar artery aneurysms. Signs of jaw weakness, sensory loss, or involvement of other cranial nerves should prompt a workup including dedicated imaging of the brainstem.

Carbamazepine (400–800 mg/day), phenytoin (300–500 mg/day), and baclofen (50–60 mg/day) alone or in combination are effective therapeutic options. Gabapentin and lamotrigine may be better tolerated, but their efficacy has not been proved. Clobazam is effective and easier to use in frail, elderly patients. Several denervation procedures are available for patients in whom medical therapy fails.

Postherpetic Neuralgia

Herpes zoster may affect up to 50% of persons older than the age of 85 years. With increasing age, risk for developing postherpetic neuropathic pain increases. The trigeminal nerve is the most commonly affected dermatome. Postherpetic neuralgia (PHN) is characterized by burning or stabbing with dysesthesia and hyperesthesia over the affected dermatome. Oral or intravenous acyclovir and oral famciclovir are effective for reducing the duration and severity of symptoms. Oral prednisone in addition to acyclovir has been shown to reduce acute zoster symptoms, but there is no evidence that it reduces the risk for developing PHN. TCAs and gabapentin have become the pharmacological agents of choice in PHN, largely because of the lack of other effective agents. More recently, pregabalin and duloxetine have been shown to be beneficial in PHN.

Other Secondary Causes of Headache

Isolated headaches are rarely the presenting symptom of an intracranial mass lesion. Instead the headache is often mild and insidious. More often than not other neurological features such as ataxia, cranial nerve palsies, paresis, nausea, and vomiting are present. Focal or diffuse headaches may be the presenting symptom of subdural hematomas. The diagnosis should be considered in anyone with headache and cognitive impairment, on anticoagulation therapy, or prone to falls whether or not there is a history of head trauma.

Cervical spondylosis and degenerative disc disease may be an underrecognized cause of headache. The head pain is usually a dull, aching pain located over the occipital region, which is aggravated by neck movement. Treatment includes physical therapy and antiinflammatory agents for pain relief.

Carbon dioxide retention in chronic obstructive airway disease causes intracranial vasodilation leading to dull or throbbing headaches that are worse in the morning (because of prolonged recumbent position) and improve with activity. Carbon monoxide poisoning should be suspected in a patient presenting with dull, diffuse headache and confusion, similar symptoms are present in family members, and/or a possible source of the gas is suspected. The headache is also worse on awakening and improves with activity and fresh air. Hypoglycemia or hypoxia can also cause a similar headache. Treatment of headache involves correction of hypoxia and hypercapnia.

Depressed patients may complain of headaches and patients with chronic headaches may become depressed. In the elderly, depression is more likely to generate somatic complaints such as headache rather than emotional problems. Dental caries and abscess, temporomandibular joint dysfunction, and parotiditis may also cause headaches in the elderly, particularly those with xerostomia.

Tremor

Tremors are the most common movement disorder seen in practice and occur as a result of dysfunction of the basal ganglia, cerebellum, or the brainstem connections between these systems. The causes of tremor are myriad but in the geriatric population, tremor may occur as a result of medications, structural lesions, parkinsonism, or essential tremor (ET). Tremors are defined as an involuntary, rhythmic, oscillatory movement that can affect any part of the body. Like most movement disorders, tremors disappear during sleep and rarely awaken one from a deep sleep. Refer to Table 14.14 for diagnostic approach. Tremors are categorized based on the type of activity that maximizes the tremor, that is, rest, posture-holding, or targeted hand movements (Table 14.15).

Rest Tremor

A rest tremor is observed when the affected body part is supported and completely at rest, for example, when the hands are supported in ones lap or hanging at the side. A rest tremor is generally suppressed during voluntary activity, but may reemerge with a sustained posture. Therefore, rest tremors are rest predominant, but not solely present at rest. A rest tremor is often pathognomonic for parkinsonism but may also occur in cerebellar or brainstem lesions (i.e., rubral or Holmes tremor). A typical parkinsonian rest tremor has a low-to-medium frequency and often involves the fingers in a so-called "pill-rolling" motion. There is often a reemergent postural component, and rest tremor worsens with mental distraction such as counting backward with the eyes closed, walking, or contralateral hand movements. A parkinsonian tremor may also involve the chin or tongue, but usually spares the head and neck. Generally, a mild rest tremor causes little disability aside from social embarrassment, but can cause anxiety because of its association with parkinsonism. Dopaminergic agents such as levodopa are generally effective treatments for a rest tremor, as are anticholinergic agents such as trihexyphenidyl.

Postural-Action Tremor

A postural tremor is present with a sustained posture or during movement of the affected body part and disappears when the affected body part is relaxed. ET is the prototypical postural-action tremor and the most common adult-onset movement disorder. An action tremor is noticeable with daily activities such as writing, holding utensils, and drinking. The most commonly affected body part is the arm and may be

Table 14.14. Diagnostic Approach to Tremors

History

- What body parts are affected by tremor?

- How did the tremor begin? Has the tremor progressed? What was the time course from onset to maximal severity or disability?

- Is there a family history of tremor?

- What factors exacerbate or improve tremor?

- Are there preexisting medical conditions, medications, exposures that may explain or exacerbate the tremor?

Examination

- Is the movement disorder a tremor (e.g., a rhythmic oscillatory movement)?

- What body parts are affected?

- In what condition is the tremor most prominent? At rest? With arms in sustention (posture holding)? Or action or targeted hand movements (e.g., writing, finger-to-nose, pouring a cup of water)?

- Is it task specific, such as with writing?

- Does the tremor increase in amplitude as the goal is approached? (Intention tremor) Does it increase with mental distraction? (parkinsonian-rest tremor)

- Are there other associated neurological features to help with localization?

Laboratory and studies

Thyroid function

Blood Glucose

Blood urea nitrogen and creatinine

Brain imaging if other localizing signs are present on examination

Serum ceruloplasmin, copper, and liver function for persons younger than 40 years to screen for Wilson's disease

Table 14.15. Categories of Tremor

Types	Examples
Rest tremor	PD
	Severe ET
Postural-action tremor	ET
	Enhanced physiological tremor
	Most drug-induced tremors
	Primary writing tremor
Intention tremor (Multiple sclerosis, stroke, trauma, degenerative disease)	Midbrain/cerebellar lesions

autosomal dominant with reduced penetrance. The condition has been linked to genes on chromosome 2p (ETM) and 3q (FET).[27,28] ET may remain static or nonprogressive for years to decades. Most people with ET have mild symptoms and do not seek medical attention for years, leading to the label "benign" ET. Generally, the term is avoided because the condition has a tendency to progress with age, generally requires medical therapy, and occasionally requires neurosurgical intervention if refractory to medications.

The main indicators for treatment are social, occupation, or functional disability. Disability arises from difficulty holding utensils or drinks, impaired fine motor activity, speech, or social embarrassment often leading to anxiety that further exacerbates the tremor. In more than 50% of cases, alcohol may dampen the tremor.[29] Effective tremor medications either lower adrenergic tone or increase gamma aminobutyric adrenergic tone. Beta-blockers (e.g., propranolol and atenolol) and primidone are first-line agents for the treatment of ET.[30] Both agents decrease tremor amplitude but generally do not abolish the tremor. Second-line agents such as topiramate, gabapentin, benzodiazepines, and phenobarbital should be tried in individuals who are intolerant of or refractory to first-line agents. Occasionally, the medications are more effective in combination, although polypharmacy should be avoided because of additive central nervous system (CNS) depressant effects. Both stereotactic thalamotomy and high-frequency thalamic stimulation can be dramatically effective for medically refractory ET.[31] The primary advantages of stimulation compared with thalamotomy are the ability to reverse therapy and the lower morbidity associated with stimulation.[32]

Physiological tremor is a normal tremor whose amplitude is too low to be detected by the human eye. Physiological tremor can be accentuated by conditions that produce catecholamine release such as caffeine, anxiety, fear, exercise, hypoglycemia, thyrotoxicosis, pheochromocytoma, and medications/toxins. This accentuated tremor is called enhanced physiological tremor. Treatment when needed is directed at correcting the underlying problem.

Obtaining a thorough medication history in the geriatric population is imperative because polypharmacy is common

unilateral in onset. In ET, by definition, the remainder of the neurological examination in a patient with ET is unremarkable with the exception of "cogwheeling," a ratchety quality found on passive range of motion of the involved limb. The term should not be confused with "cogwheel rigidity," which implies a state of increased tone in extrapyramidal syndromes.

ET generally affects the arms but may involve the head or voice in isolation. Head tremor can result in horizontal or vertical bobbing (as a "no-no" or "yes-yes" movement) and seems to be more common in women. Leg tremor rarely occurs in isolation and is usually found in association with diffuse ET. If bilateral, the tremor may be asymmetrical. Handwriting is often irregular and tremulous.

ET is often considered the most common movement disorder with prevalence estimates ranging from 0.4%–5% and increasing in persons older than 60 years.[26] The prevalence of ET is higher in whites than blacks but is similar between men and women. A family history of similar tremor is often present. In families with the condition, the pattern of inheritance is

Table 14.16. Medications and Toxins that Induce or Exacerbate Tremor

Beta-adrenergic agonists

Epinephrine

Isoproterenol

Albuterol

Theophylline

Amphetamines

Lithium

Phenothiazines, butyrophenones

TCAs

Prednisone

Antiarrhythmics

Amiodarone

Procainamide

Mexiletine

Antimicrobials

Trimethoprim-sulfamethoxazole

Acyclovir

Antiepileptics

Valproic acid

Carbamazepine

Xanthines (in coffee and tea)

Heavy metals

Mercury

Lead

Arsenic

Bismuth

and drug-induced tremors are often reversible, avoidable, or treatable. The diagnosis of drug-induced tremor is made by exclusion of medical causes of tremor, establishing a temporal relation to the start of therapy with the drug, and a dose–response relationship. Table 14.16 lists medications commonly associated with tremor. Many tend to be psychotropic medications, but other drugs commonly associated with tremor include albuterol, amiodarone, prednisone, and theophylline. Chronic treatment with lithium carbonate causes a fine postural or action tremor. In overdose or toxicity, lithium may also be associated with a cerebellar or parkinsonian syndrome.[33,34] Withdrawal from benzodiazepine, alcohol, or other CNS depressants often results in tremor. If the causative medication cannot be discontinued, treatment with a medication such as propranolol may be considered.

Intention Tremor

An intention tremor is a specific type of action tremor in which the amplitude increases as the affected limb approaches a goal. The common test to use at the bedside is finger-to-nose testing. Cerebellar lesions often produce dysmetria or limb ataxia, which is a slow, high-amplitude oscillation that occurs as a limb approaches its target. A true intention tremor results from dysfunction of the tracts exiting the cerebellum, leading to cerebellar outflow tremor. The term rubral tremor may be used and implies dysfunction of the midbrain red (rubral) nucleus, although this tremor may arise from lesions outside the midbrain. Gordon Holmes first described the syndrome in World War I soldiers who suffered cerebellar injuries, hence the eponym Holmes tremor. Multiple sclerosis, trauma, stroke, and degenerative diseases of the brainstem and cerebellum may produce this tremor.[35] A rest component may be present, as well as titubation (head and trunk oscillation when the trunk is unsupported), proximal muscle involvement, and gait ataxia. Wilson's disease may cause such a tremor and has been classically associated with a "wing-beating" tremor when the arms are brought close to the chest and the elbows are lifted. Midline cerebellar dysfunction resulting from a toxin or degenerative condition usually causes a bilateral tremor whereas a focal structural lesion results in a unilateral tremor, ipsilateral to the lesion. These tremors are very disabling as they can severely impair activities of daily living even when nonprogressive or static. They are notoriously difficult to treat, and surgery is often attempted with limited success.

Weakness

Weakness is a common complaint in the primary care setting. The term weakness is sometimes confused by patients with asthenia or fatigue. *Asthenia* is defined as a sense of weariness and exhaustion in the absence of muscle weakness. *Fatigue* is defined as the inability to continue performing a task after multiple repetitions. *Intrinsic or primary muscle weakness* is defined as the inability to perform the first repetition of the task in the presence of muscle weakness.

Asthenia and fatigue can be associated with other disorders such as chronic fatigue syndrome, depression, and chronic heart, lung, and kidney disease. The first step in assessing a patient with the chief complaint of weakness is to distinguish between these terms to guide the physical examination and further workup including appropriate laboratory, radiological, electrodiagnostic, and pathological studies. Patients with asthenia present with the complaint, "I am weak" whereas a patient with true muscle weakness complains of being unable to perform a specific task or feeling heaviness or stuffiness in limbs.

If the patient's symptoms are consistent with asthenia or fatigue, then a thorough medical history, review of systems, and screening (i.e., depression) for diseases associated with these symptoms is warranted. Primary or intrinsic muscle weakness has a myriad of causes, which have been divided into several major categories (Table 14.17). These categories include infectious, inflammatory, neurological, endocrine, rheumatological, genetic, electrolyte-induced, and drug-induced disorders. Neurological, infectious, and drug-induced disorders are the most common causes of myopathy in the adult population.

Table 14.17. Causes of Myopathy

Infectious Causes of Myopathy	Endocrine Disorders
Epstein–Barr virus	Adrenal dysfunction
HIV	Cushing's syndrome
Influenza	Thyroid disorders
Lyme disease	Hyperthyroidism
Meningitis	Hypothyroidism
Polio	Hyperparathyroidism
Rabies	
Syphilis	
Toxoplasmosis	

Neurological disorders that can cause muscle weakness can be subdivided based on an understanding of the neuromuscular system, which is made up of the CNS and the peripheral nervous system (PNS). The CNS is composed of upper motor neurons (motor cortex and corticospinal tracts) and pathology in these regions can result in muscle weakness. Examples of such pathological conditions include acute stroke, CNS space-occupying lesions, spinal cord lesions (related to trauma, infection, tumor,) vascular anomalies (arteriovenous malformations, aneurysms, and amyloid angiopathy), hypertrophic degenerative skeletal changes, demyelinating diseases, and congenital leukodystrophies. The processes usually produce localized nervous system symptoms and signs. The PNS is composed of spinal nerves, dorsal root ganglion, and receptors (neuromuscular junction). Table 14.18 provides examples of some of the disorders of the nervous system and a brief description of each.

Multiple sclerosis is an idiopathic inflammatory disease of the CNS that results in demyelination and subsequent axonal degeneration. It commonly affects the young more than older adults and women more than men. The initial symptoms usually resolve spontaneously with relapses occurring within months or years, but some patients have a primary progressive course from onset.

GBS is an autoimmune syndrome of the PNS resulting in nerve demyelination. It has an overall low incidence but is the most common cause of acute paralysis and requires a high index of suspicion in those patients presenting with acute weakness.

Neoplasms of the nervous system (primary or secondary in origin) can also cause muscle weakness depending on the location of the lesion. Leptomeningeal metastases of non-Hodgkin lymphoma can involve the nerve roots (radiculopathy), resulting in muscle weakness at the level of root affected.

Myasthenia gravis is an autoimmune syndrome characterized by autoantibodies directed at acetylcholine receptors on the postsynaptic membrane of the neuromuscular junction. This disorder can occur at any age, with a peak in women in the second and third decades of life; the peak in men occurs in the fifth and sixth decades.

Radiculopathies caused by disc herniation, degenerative disease, and spinal stenosis can produce muscle weakness by compression or irritation of a nerve root and/or nerve. Paresthesia can often accompany weakness and radiating pain of radiculopathies. Radicular pain is sensitive for the presence of herniation, especially in the lumbar spine.

Spinal cord injuries are a risk factor in our older population because of the increased prevalence of degenerative changes of the spine, cancer, and osteopenia. The elderly are at risk for spinal fracture even with trivial trauma.

Drug-induced myopathies are common especially in our elderly population with polypharmacy. Table 14.19 provides a list of a few medications whose side effect profile includes muscle weakness.

Corticosteroids are often used to treat several inflammatory and rheumatological disorders. They have been found to cause weakness mainly to the proximal muscles of the upper and lower limbs and neck flexors. The chronic or classic form occurs after prolonged use of corticosteroids and has a more insidious course. The acute form is less common, is associated with rhabdomyolysis, and occurs abruptly while the patient is receiving high-dose corticosteroids. Steroid-induced myopathy is more frequent with the use of fluorinated steroids (dexamethasone or triamcinolone) than with nonfluorinated (prednisone or hydrocortisone).

Statins' adverse effects include myositis and rhabdomyolysis, mild serum creatine kinase (CK) elevations, myalgia with and without elevated CK levels, muscle weakness, muscle cramps, and persistent myalgia and CK elevations after statin withdrawal. The mechanism of muscle injury is not clear. Associated symptoms may include fever and malaise. Concomitant medical conditions (hypothyroidism, diabetes), drug–drug interactions, and compromised liver and or kidney function can exacerbate the adverse effects of statins.

Infectious causes of myopathy are numerous, but influenza and Epstein–Barr virus are two of the most common. Table 14.20 provides a brief list of some infections associated with myopathies. Specific infections should be investigated based on patient's risk factors for example, HIV.

Endocrine disorders are less common causes of muscle weakness. Thyroid disease is relatively common in the general population, particularly in the older age groups, but related myopathies are uncommon, except in advanced disease such as myxedema of hypothyroidism.

Inflammatory disease is more common in older adults than in younger adults. Dermatomyositis, polymyositis, and inclusion body myositis (IBM) are common inflammatory disorders associated with muscle weakness. IBM is the most common progressive muscle disease of persons older than age 50 years. IBM muscle contains lymphocytic inflammatory cells.

Rheumatological disorders can cause pain and stiffness, and constitutional symptoms can contribute to muscle weakness. Lupus and rheumatoid arthritis are common rheumatological disorders that are found in both the younger and older populations.

Table 14.18. Cerebrovascular Disease

	Description	*Diagnostic Tests*
Stroke	Weakness of face, arm, and leg on one side of the body without other signs or with ataxia.	Neuroimaging and or lumbar puncture
	Accompanied by aphasia, hemisensory loss, visual deficits.	
	Presence of risk factors for vascular disease.	
	Thromboembolism onset of neurological signs is sudden or rapid.	
	Hemorrhagic: onset gradual	
Subdural/epidural hematoma	Focal neurological signs: gradually over minutes to hours.	CT and MRI
	Accompanied by headache, vomiting, and decrease in level of consciousness (if large intracranial hemorrhage)	
	Usually risk factors for hemorrhage (hypertension, amphetamine or cocaine, intrinsic bleeding diathesis, anticoagulants)	
Demyelinating disorders		
GBS	Subacute onset of bilateral ascending weakness (prominent in the proximal muscles, legs more than arms), decrease or disappearance of deep tendon reflexes, paresthesias spreading proximally, rarely extending past the wrists and ankles	Lumbar puncture: elevated protein (>0.55 g/dL) without pleocytosis
Multiple sclerosis	Insidious or sudden onset.	MRI during or following a first attack
	Symptoms: monocular visual impairment with pain (optic neuritis), numbness, weakness, dizziness, depression.	
	Signs: action tremor, decreased pain, vibration, or position perception; decreased strength, hyperreflexia, spasticity, Babinski; impaired coordination and balance; nystagmus	
Neuromuscular disorders		
Myasthenia gravis	Associated symptoms include fluctuating or fatigable weakness in oculobulbar muscles, followed by limb and respiratory muscles, slurred speech, dysphagia	autoantibody testing
Lambert–Eaton myasthenic syndrome	Insidious onset of proximal hip muscle weakness, a distal limb paresthesia, areflexia, and autonomic instability, and dry mouth	autoantibody testing

Electrolyte-induced myopathy may be primary or secondary in nature. Potassium imbalance is a common cause of muscle weakness and can secondarily be caused by renal disease or angiotensin inhibitor toxicity.

Genetic disorders (muscular and myotonic dystrophies) and metabolic disorders (glycogenoses, lipidoses, and mitochondrial defects) are rare causes for muscle weakness. These disorders usually have a genetic component with a significant family history. The diagnoses of these disorders usually occur in early life and not in the older population.

History

The history assists in narrowing down the cause of the muscle weakness to one of the major categories based on associated symptoms, onset and progression, and pattern of muscle weakness. Family history can also narrow down the differential diagnosis to genetic, metabolic, or rheumatological disorders. Review of pharmaceutical use can identify medications, herbals, and/or narcotics that could cause or contribute to muscle weakness. Clues to finding the cause of muscle weakness may include

risk factors for vascular disease, concurrent medical conditions, risky sexual behaviors, occupational and environmental exposures, and possible exposure to endemic infections.

The onset of disease makes certain etiologies more likely than others. Acute onsets are more suspicious for infectious or cerebrovascular events. Subacute onset can indicate drug-induced disease, electrolyte imbalance, or inflammatory or rheumatological disease. Chronic onset implies genetic or metabolic myopathies.

The pattern or distribution of muscle weakness can also assist in identifying the cause. Focal muscle weakness can be unilateral in nature or involve a specific nerve distribution or intracranial vascular area. Global muscle weakness is bilateral, proximal, distal, or both. The patient's physical activity limitations help determine the pattern of muscle weakness. Proximal muscle weakness is reported by patients as difficulty rising from a chair or combing their hair, representing hip muscle and shoulder girdle weakness, respectively. Many myopathies are associated with proximal muscle weakness. Distal muscle weakness is demonstrated by difficulty standing on toes or

Table 14.19. Medications with Adverse Effects of Myopathy

Amiodarone	Fibric acid derivatives (gemfibrozil)
Antithyroid agents	Interferon
Antiretroviral medications	Leuprolide (Lupron)
Chemotherapeutic agents	NSAIDS
Cimetidine (Tagamet)	Penicillin
Cocaine	Sulfonamides
Corticosteroids	Statins

Table 14.20. Laboratory Findings

Infectious disease	Titers
	Cultures
Electrolyte imbalances	Serum chemistry panel
	Calcium, magnesium
Endocrine disorders	Thyroid-stimulating hormone 24-h cortisol
Rheumatological disorders	ESR
	Antinuclear antibody
	Rheumatoid factor
	Antidouble stranded DNA antibodies
	Antiphospholipid antibodies (Lupus)
	Anticentromere antibodies (scleroderma)

performing fine motor activities such as writing. Distal myopathies are less common and are usually associated with inflammatory or genetic disorders.

Physical Examination

The examination should test the power or strength of the muscles, focusing on severity and pattern. Observations should be made of functional activity to determine if muscle weakness is proximal, distal, or both. A complete neurological examination is paramount in determining if a neurological cause of weakness is a pathological condition of the CNS or PNS. A deficit of a single radicular distribution verses hemiparesis differentiates peripheral radiculopathy from a cerebrovascular event. If the focused neurological examination is unremarkable, then a general physical examination is necessary for extramuscular signs suggestive of a specific disorder.

Further investigation for weakness is guided by the findings on the history and physical examination. When a particular type of myopathy is suspected, laboratory tests specific to that disease or disorder should be performed (Table 14.20). CK is a nonspecific marker of muscle breakdown. CK is an enzyme found predominantly in the heart, brain, and skeletal muscle and when elevated, it usually indicates injury or stress to one or more of these areas. The CK level may be normal in endocrine and electrolyte myopathies, highly elevated in inflammatory myopathies (10–100 times normal range), moderately to highly elevated in muscular dystrophies, and mildly to moderately elevated in metabolic myopathies.

Imaging

If neurological disease, particularly of the CNS, is suspected, early neuroimaging (CT scan or MRI) is indicated. Examples of diseases needing prompt imaging include cerebrovascular disease, intracranial hemorrhages, tumor, meningitis, encephalitis, and multiple sclerosis. Histories and physical examinations for radiculopathies may require plain films and/or MRI to locate the cause. Blood and cerebrospinal fluid testing may also be indicated to distinguish a toxic, metabolic, or infectious process.

Procedures

EMG is indicated when the etiology of the myopathy remains uncertain after history-taking, physical examination,

and laboratory and/or imaging studies. EMG is nonspecific and is helpful only to indicate if a neuropathy or neuromuscular disease is present or to confirm the diagnosis of a primary myopathy. The procedure can cause mild discomfort for patients but is overall well tolerated.

Muscle biopsy is indicated if the diagnosis remains uncertain after EMG. The pathological analysis of the biopsy specimen includes histology, histochemical, electron microscopic, genetic, and biochemical changes. Biopsies of the affected muscle are helpful in identifying genetic, metabolic (glycogen storage diseases), and inflammatory disorders as well as miscellaneous disorders such as sarcoidosis and amyloidosis.

PARKINSONISM

General Concepts

Parkinsonism is a general term used to describe a clinical syndrome characterized by rest tremor, bradykinesia, rigidity, and postural instability. Although most cases of parkinsonism are sporadic, idiopathic, and neurodegenerative, parkinsonism may also occur as a result of a structural lesion, drugs, or toxins affecting basal ganglia function. Common secondary causes of parkinsonism include vascular parkinsonism, drug-induced parkinsonism, and NPH and will be discussed individually in the following sections.

The most common neurodegenerative form of parkinsonism is PD. Currently, the cause of PD is not known, although most studies point to both environmental and genetic factors. Although PD can occur on a familial basis, most cases are sporadic. The hallmark of the condition is the selective degeneration of midbrain dopaminergic neurons, which leads to the cardinal features of the disorder and the characteristic response to levodopa.

Finally, several related degenerative disorders known as Parkinson plus or atypical parkinsonian syndromes are either lumped together or split, often leading to confusion for patients and practitioners. Furthermore, as the pathophysiological bases of these disorders are elucidated, eponyms such as Shy–Drager syndrome have largely been replaced by clinicopathological terms (i.e., multiple system atrophy). Features common to this group of disorders include:

1. Poor response to levodopa;
2. More rapid progression to severe disability than idiopathic PD;
3. Additional neurological features that make them atypical for PD.

Clinical Features of Parkinsonism

Tremor is the most recognizable aspect of a parkinsonian condition, but it is not always present and its absence does not exclude parkinsonism (Table 14.21). Tremor should be observed under three conditions: rest, sustained posture, and during active movements or intention. The typical tremor of PD and other parkinsonian conditions is most prominent at rest. It can affect the hands, legs, jaw, or tongue. Because the tremor is most prominent when the limb is relaxed, patients are generally not as bothered by it as are family members or friends. Frequency and amplitude will vary, but the tremor is classically described as a low-to-medium frequency tremor. The term pill-rolling is used to describe the pronation-supination at the wrist and flexion-extension of the fingers typical of the parkinsonian tremor. The absence of a pill-rolling quality does not, however, exclude a parkinsonian tremor. More importantly, mental concentration (e.g., counting backward) and anxiety enhance a parkinsonian tremor. Lifting the arms to sustain a posture will dampen the tremor temporarily, but the original amplitude and frequency will return after a delay of 2–3 seconds. This so-called reemergent component of the tremor when present is arguably the most specific feature of a parkinsonian tremor.

Tone is tested in a relaxed patient by using passive multidirectional movements of the extremities. The increase in tone associated with basal ganglia or extrapyramidal lesions is constant throughout the range of movement leading to the descriptive term, lead-pipe rigidity. Active movements of the contralateral limb will lead to an increase in tone (Froment sign) and may be used to confirm subtle hypertonicity.

Bradykinesia refers not only to slowing of movements but also hesitancy, arrests, decreased amplitude, or poverty of movements. The presence of bradykinesia is the most diagnostic sign of a parkinsonian disorder. Impaired finger dexterity, loss of facial expression (hypomimia), and small handwriting (micrographia) are some of the earliest signs of bradykinesia resulting from parkinsonism. The voice can be hypophonic and monotone with a loss of diction. The combination of rigidity and bradykinesia leads to difficulty with ordinary tasks such as turning in bed, rising from a chair, or getting in and out of a car.

Table 14.21. Features of PD

Cardinal features
- Rest tremor
- Bradykinesia
- Rigidity
- Postural instability

Secondary features
- Dystonia
- Dysphagia
- Dysarthria, palilalia, hypophonia
- Hypomimia
- Micrographia
- Festination, retropulsion, freezing, start hesitation, en bloc turning
- Stooped posture, kyphosis, scoliosis
- Drooling/sialorrhea
- Constipation
- Overactive bladder
- Erectile dysfunction
- Seborrheic dermatitis
- Pain/paresthesias

Because of the loss of dexterity and range of motion, dressing and routine hygiene can become laborious.

Gait Impairment and Postural Instability

In early disease, examination findings may consist only of decreased arm swing or dragging of one leg. Patients often report that walking feels unnatural. A characteristic stooped posture develops with forward flexion of the trunk, neck, elbows, shoulders, and knees. Stride height and length are reduced, leading to a shuffling gait. The stooped posture and shift in the center of gravity contribute to a tendency to fall forward (propulsion) and an inability to stop (festination). Turning occurs "en bloc," as the head, neck, torso, and extremities no longer rotate independently due to rigidity and bradykinesia. Start hesitation causes difficulty rising from a chair or initiating walking. Patients may describe freezing as though the feet are transiently stuck or "glued" to the ground. The phenomenon typically occurs in doorways, narrow hallways, or near obstacles. Patients often find that visual cues such as floor or sidewalk markings and thresholds will release them from freezing. Freezing is one of the more debilitating symptoms encountered in parkinsonian states and often leads to immobility and falls. Unfortunately, freezing is more often than not refractory to levodopa therapy.

Postural stability is tested using the pull test in which the examiner firmly tugs the patient from behind and assesses the

Table 14.22. Neuropsychiatric Manifestations of Parkinsonism

- Cognitive and intellectual impairment
- Dementia
- Visual hallucinations
- Delusions
- Depression
- Anxiety or akathisia
- Apathy or amotivation
- Sleep disorders such as insomnia, excessive daytime somnolence, REM behavior disorder, periodic leg movements of sleep
- Addictive or compulsive behaviors

Table 14.23. Differential Diagnosis of Parkinsonism

Sporadic neurodegenerative

- Idiopathic PD
- DLB
- PSP
- MSA (formerly, Shy–Drager syndrome, olivopontocerebellar atrophy, and striatonigral degeneration)
- Corticobasal ganglionic degeneration
- Amyotrophic lateral sclerosis–Parkinsonism Dementia (Complex of Guam)
- Alzheimer's disease with extrapyramidal features

Secondary

- Cerebrovascular disease/multiinfarct state
- Drug induced (Neuroleptics, antiemetics such as metoclopramide or prochlorperazine, presynaptic dopamine depleters such as reserpine and tetrabenazine)
- Toxin-induced (MPTP, carbon monoxide, manganese)
- Posttraumatic parkinsonism (Dementia Pugilistica)
- Postencephalitic parkinsonism (Von Economo's disease)
- NPH
- Basal ganglia neoplasm, infarct, hemorrhage, infection

Hereditary neurodegenerative

- Parkin, α-synuclein, UCH-L1 kindreds
- Wilson's disease
- Juvenile Huntington's disease
- Neurodegeneration with brain iron accumulation (Hallervorden–Spatz syndrome)
- Dentatorubral pallidoluysian atrophy
- Spinocerebellar ataxia type 3 (Machado–Joseph's disease)

Psychogenic

ability to maintain an upright stance. Retropulsion or toppling backward occurs when the ability to adjust or maintain the center of gravity is lost. Because of the combination of flexed posture and postural instability, forward falls are typical of moderate-to-advanced stages of PD.

Secondary features of parkinsonism include dysphagia, excess saliva or drooling (sialorrhea), constipation, overactive bladder, erectile dysfunction, seborrheic dermatitis, orthostatic hypotension, pain, paresthesias, and sleep disturbances including REM sleep behavior disorder, periodic limb movements during sleep, restless legs syndrome, insomnia, and obstructive sleep apnea. Numbness, tingling, and aching pains, fatigue, and weakness are common complaints of PD that may be dismissed early in the diagnosis or mistaken for other neurological or medical conditions.

Neuropsychiatric symptoms that may occur in a parkinsonian disorder include subcortical dementia, depression, apathy, anxiety, hallucinations, or delusions (Table 14.22).

Differential Diagnosis

The diagnosis of PD or an atypical parkinsonian disorder is made purely by clinical examination. No radiological or laboratory study can confirm a diagnosis. When all cardinal symptoms are present, the diagnosis is fairly obvious. Diagnostic difficulty usually arises in early stages of the disease when intermittent and subtle symptoms predominate. Nevertheless, even in the hands of movement disorder neurologists experienced in differentiating the conditions, up to 20% of patients have an alternative diagnosis at autopsy, whereas cases with atypical features may prove to have PD (Table 14.23).[36]

Arguably the single most important feature distinguishing idiopathic PD from secondary and atypical forms of parkinsonism is the response to levodopa. Patients with true idiopathic PD display a robust response to levodopa that lasts for many years because PD primarily affects midbrain dopaminergic neurons in the substantia nigra. The lack of response characteristic of other forms of parkinsonism results from degeneration of postsynaptic receptors and nondopaminergic systems.

Red flags suggesting an atypical or secondary form of parkinsonism include: ocular motor palsy, cerebellar signs, early and prominent gait, cognitive, or cranial nerve dysfunction, autonomic failure, or pyramidal signs (Table 14.24). These conditions tend to be more rapidly progressive than PD, in part because of the lack of treatment options. It is unusual for patients with PD to present with postural instability leading to falls and this should alert the physician to alternate forms of parkinsonism.

PSP is so named because of the characteristic eye movement abnormality associated with the condition. The hallmarks of the condition are an akinetic-rigid form of parkinsonism with early balance impairment leading to frequent falls. The characteristic eye movement or gaze abnormality is not always a presenting

Table 14.24. Parkinson Plus Syndromes

	First Description	MRI Findings	Primary Pathology
PD	1817 James Parkinson	Normal	Nigrostriatal degeneration, Lewy bodies
PSP	1964 Steele et al.	Midbrain atrophy, "hummingbird sign"	Midbrain degeneration, frontal lobe degeneration, Tau-positive neurofibrillary tangles
MSA	1900 Dejerine and Thomas, 1960 Shy and Drager, 1960 Adams et al., 1969 Graham and Oppenheimer	Lower brainstem and cerebellar atrophy, "hot-cross bun sign," linear putaminal hyperintensity	Striatonigral, olivopontocerebellar, intermediolateral cell column degeneration, glial cytoplasmic inclusions
DLB	1996 McKeith et al.	Global atrophy	Diffuse cortical and subcortical Lewy bodies and dystrophic neurites
Corticobasal Ganglionic Degeneration	1968 Rebeiz et al.	Asymmetrical frontoparietal atrophy	Ballooned neurons

feature but invariably develops over time. The term supranuclear refers to the fact that although ocular muscles and cranial nerves are intact, brainstem gaze centers and tracts above the level of the nuclei are impaired. Vertical eye movements, which are mediated by midbrain gaze centers, are impaired before horizontal eye movements, whereas reflexive eye movements are preserved. Other characteristic features include a prominent stare with a worried or astonished facial expression and dysarthria. Patients with PSP often develop personality changes and cognitive impairment from the frontal lobe degeneration that occurs. The combination of cognitive impairment and lack of insight often leads to difficulty with medication compliance, social withdrawal, and falls. Microscopically, a microtubule-associated protein called tau accumulates, forming neurofibrillary tangles, so that the pathology of PSP is in fact closer to Alzheimer's disease than it is to PD.

Dementia with Lewy bodies (DLB) is a relatively new diagnostic entity that is the second most common cause of dementia after Alzheimer's disease. Patients with DLB present with a combination of mental symptoms and parkinsonism, with the mental symptoms often overshadowing the movement disorder. Visual hallucinations develop insidiously and, like medication-induced visual hallucinations in PD, are well formed and complex. In contrast to PD, visual hallucinations in DLB develop in the absence of dopaminergic medication exposure or with relatively low doses. Delusions revolving around spousal infidelity or neighbors, friends, or relatives stealing from them are also common. Striking cognitive fluctuations differentiates DLB from other causes of dementia. Patients may be relatively intact at one moment and minutes later become confused, disoriented, psychotic, or obtunded.

When present, several secondary features help to confirm the diagnosis. Repeated falls occur due to postural instability. Syncope and transient loss of consciousness may mimic seizures, stroke, TIA, or a cardiac event and often prompt repeated evaluations or hospitalizations. DLB patients may be very sensitive to dopamine receptor blockers and can develop delirium or akinetic-rigid crises with neuroleptic treatment.

For this reason, only quetiapine or clozapine can be considered safe to use in DLB.

Both PD and DLB have in common characteristic pathological inclusion called the Lewy body (LB). LBs are cytoplasmic inclusions containing the synaptic protein α-synuclein. In DLB, Lewy bodies are present throughout the brainstem and cortex, leading to the pathological term diffuse Lewy Body disease.

Multiple system atrophy (MSA) is a clinical term used to lump three formerly distinct parkinsonian conditions, Shy–Drager syndrome, olivopontocerebellar atrophy, and striatonigral degeneration. The current accepted designations are MSA-A (autonomic form) for Shy–Drager syndrome, MSA-C (cerebellar form) for olivopontocerebellar atrophy, and MSA-P (parkinsonian form) for striatonigral degeneration. Autonomic features include orthostatic hypotension, bowel or bladder incontinence, and sexual dysfunction. Cerebellar features include dysarthria, gait ataxia, and limb incoordination. In practice, overlap of these syndromes is common, so that varying combinations of symptoms are present.

Although the response to levodopa is generally not satisfactory, some patients may experience partial benefit and so should be given levodopa at least once. On the other hand, even if there is a response, side effects such as orthostasis or nausea may limit treatment.

Secondary features suggestive of the diagnosis include REM behavior disorder, which may precede the diagnosis of MSA by many years, stridor, and obstructive sleep apnea due to brainstem respiratory and sleep center dysfunction.

Pathologically, all three syndromes share a common synuclein containing glial cytoplasmic inclusion. The clinical phenotype is largely determined by the location of pathology. In MSA-A, it is the autonomic centers in the brainstem and the upper and sacral spinal cord. In MSA-C, it is the medullary olives, pons, and cerebellum. In MSA-P, it is primarily the substantia nigra and the striatum.

Corticobasal ganglionic degeneration is a condition with both cognitive and movement symptoms and, pathologically, it resembles Alzheimer's disease and frontotemporal dementia. Clinically, it may present primarily as either a parkinsonian or dementia illness. The classic corticobasal syndrome consists of asymmetrical parkinsonism with prominent limb rigidity and dystonic posturing. There may be myoclonic jerking, cognitive impairment involving frontal lobe function, memory systems, or visuospatial systems. Gait impairment is common. One of the most distinctive features of the syndrome is limb apraxia, or inability to perform a voluntary movement that is not from muscle weakness, sensory loss, or ataxia. With time, the so-called alien limb syndrome may develop in which the limb may assume unusual postures, wander in space, or seem out of the control of the person. Over time, rigidity and dementia predominate.

In clinical practice, the most common secondary forms of parkinsonism that one needs to consider are vascular parkinsonism, drug-induced parkinsonism, and NPH. Although the insult may occur once, subsequent lesions or worsening of the underlying lesion may lead to a progressive clinical syndrome that may be mistaken for a neurodegenerative illness. For example, parkinsonism from hydrocephalus will naturally worsen if the hydrocephalus worsens. Drug-induced parkinsonism worsens as the duration of exposure to the dopamine receptor–blocking agent increases.

Cerebrovascular disease is a relatively common cause of parkinsonism, occurring as a result of both strategically placed lacunar infarctions in the basal ganglia or diffuse white matter disease. Patients may present with abrupt onset of a gait disorder or "lower body" parkinsonism. A stepwise pattern of progression is often a clue to recurrent small-vessel ischemic events. Levodopa is not typically effective but should be attempted for both diagnostic and therapeutic purposes. Cerebrovascular risk factors, a history of stroke or transient neurological events, cognitive disturbance, or gait apraxia are often present.[37]

Parkinsonism resulting from chronic antipsychotic treatment is a potentially reversible syndrome that may be identical to idiopathic PD. The risk of parkinsonism from antipsychotic medications is dose dependent and increases in the elderly. With the exception of clozapine, no antipsychotic is free of this risk. Other medications that potentially may induce parkinsonism include antiemetics, such as metoclopramide or prochlorperazine, because of their dopamine blocking capabilities, dopamine depleters such as reserpine or tetrabenazine, and lithium. The compound 1-methyl-4-phenyl-1, 2,3,6-tetrahydropyridine (MPTP) that causes selective nigrostriatal degeneration was discovered after it led to acute parkinsonism in a group of heroin addicts.[38] In addition to MPTP, other toxins associated with parkinsonism include manganese,[39] and carbon monoxide.[40]

Treatment of PD

Possible Neuroprotective Therapy

The ultimate goal in PD research today is to design an agent that will slow or arrest the progression of the disease (neuro-

protection or disease modification). Unfortunately, determining whether or not an agent is neuroprotective is inherently difficult because of the lack of specific clinical endpoints, confounding resulting from a symptomatic benefit, and the lengthy follow-up required.

One of the first agents studied for its potential neuroprotective effects was *Selegiline*, an irreversible monoamine oxidase (MAO) type B inhibitor with antioxidant properties. In the landmark Deprenyl and Tocopherol Antioxidative Therapy of Parkinsonism study, selegiline treatment was found to delay disability and the need for levodopa therapy.[41] The effect, however, was deemed to be at least partly symptomatic, and a clear neuroprotective benefit was never demonstrated.

Coenzyme Q10 is an electron acceptor for complexes I and II of the mitochondrial electron transport chain. A multicenter blinded, randomized trial of 80 patients with early untreated PD demonstrated significantly less decline in Unified Parkinson's Disease Rating Scale scores with high-dose coenzyme Q10 (1200 mg) compared with placebo.[42] Although suggestive of a neuroprotective benefit, a larger-scale study is currently underway to confirm these results.

Dopamine receptor agonists have been proposed to be neuroprotective through various mechanisms, including decreased dopamine metabolism, free radical scavenging, and protection against neurotoxins. Functional imaging with positron emission tomography (PET) and single-photon emission computed tomography has served as surrogate markers of dopaminergic neuron loss. The ReQuip® as Early therapy versus Levodopa PET study followed the [^{18}F] dopa PET scans in newly diagnosed PD patients treated with either levodopa or ropinirole for 2 years.[43] Changes in the single-photon emission computed tomography ligand [$^{123}\beta$]-CIT ([N-(3-fluoropropyl)-2 β-carbomethoxy-3 β-(4-iodophenyl)nortropane]) were studied in a subset of the randomized patients in the Comparison of the Agonist Pramipexole versus Levodopa on Motor complications of PD trial.[44] Both studies revealed decreased loss of dopamine uptake in treated groups; however, it is unclear whether the imaging changes represented an actual neuroprotective effect or pharmacological changes induced by the agonist, unrelated to the degree of neuron loss.

A third-generation MAO-B inhibitor has shown the most promise in recent neuroprotective studies. The Rasagiline Mesylate [TVP-1012] in Early Monotherapy for PD Outpatients study utilized a novel delayed start design.[45] Patients on rasagiline at the beginning of the trial showed significantly more improvement at 1 year compared with patients initiated on placebo and switched to rasagiline at 6 months, even though both groups were on the same treatment for the last 6 months of the study. These results may suggest that rasagiline has a mild effect on the disease course.

Early Symptomatic Therapy

Symptomatic treatment is typically initiated when patients begin to experience social or functional disability. Factors to consider when deciding to initiate treatment include problematic symptoms, age, functional status, comorbid medical

Table 14.25. Medications for the Symptomatic Treatment of PD

Medication	Mechanism of Action	Typical Therapeutic Dosage
Selegiline	MAO-B inhibitor	5–10 mg/day
Rasagiline	MAO-B inhibitor	1–2 mg/day
Benztropine	Anticholinergic	0.5–4 mg/day
Trihexyphenidyl	Anticholinergic	2–8 mg/day
Amantadine	NMDA antagonist	200–400 mg/day
Pergolide	Dopamine agonist	0.75–5 mg/day
Bromocriptine	Dopamine agonist	10–40 mg/day
Pramipexole	Dopamine agonist	1.5–4.5 mg/day
Ropinirole	Dopamine agonist	7.5–24 mg/day
Levodopa		150–600 mg/day
Entacapone	COMT inhibitor	200 mg/day

NMDA, N-methyl-D-aspartate.

conditions, and cognitive status. A wide range of medications with proven symptomatic effects exist for PD, including MAO inhibitors, anticholinergic agents, amantadine, catechol-O-methyltransferase (COMT) inhibitors, dopamine agonists, and levodopa (Table 14.25).

Both selegiline and rasagiline irreversibly inhibit MAO-B, which results in modest enhancement of striatal dopamine levels. In practice, insomnia is the most common reported side effect, making daytime administration more appropriate.

Anticholinergic agents such as benztropine and trihexyphenidyl were among the first treatments for PD. They have moderate effects on tremor, rigidity, and dystonia; however, side effects such as urinary retention, cognitive impairment, dry mouth, and blurred vision limit their use in the elderly.[46]

Amantadine, originally developed for use against influenza, is a tricyclic amine with multiple putative mechanisms including enhancing dopamine release, inhibition of dopamine reuptake, antimuscarinic effects, and N-methyl D-aspartate receptor antagonism. In addition to its use in early PD, antidyskinetic properties make it useful for patients with advanced PD with motor fluctuations. Amantadine is generally well tolerated but lower extremity edema, mental confusion, and hallucinations may complicate treatment. In patients with renal insufficiency, dose adjustments need to be made based on creatinine clearance because amantadine is excreted renally.

Dopamine agonists directly stimulate striatal dopamine receptors and are used both in early PD and as an adjunct in advanced PD with motor fluctuations. Bromocriptine, pergolide, ropinirole, pramipexole, and apomorphine are available in the United States. Subcutaneous apomorphine has been recently Food and Drug Administration–approved for the treatment of refractory "off" periods when medication is not working. Agonists have similar efficacy and side effects common to the class including nausea, lightheadedness, pedal edema, hallucinations, and sedation. Most adverse effects are dose related and can be avoided by slow titration of the drug. The ergot agonists (e.g., bromocriptine and pergolide) carry the additional risk of retroperitoneal fibrosis and Raynaud phenomenon. Furthermore, cardiac valvular abnormalities have been attributed to pergolide and it was recently withdrawn from the U.S. market.[47] Recent reports suggest that agonists, particularly pramipexole, may be associated with compulsive or addictive behaviors such as gambling.

Studies of ropinirole and pramipexole monotherapy compared with levodopa have both demonstrated reduced motor fluctuations and dyskinesiasy.[48,49]

Despite the recent advances in pharmacotherapy, levodopa remains the most time-honored and effective treatment for symptoms of PD. The majority of PD patients will attain significant, long-lasting benefit from levodopa superior to any of the previously mentioned agents. It is well tolerated and effective at a large dose range as long as administered with a peripheral decarboxylase inhibitor (e.g., carbidopa). Without such an inhibitor, levodopa would be intolerable because of peripheral side effects of dopamine such as orthostatic hypotension, nausea, and emesis. In the United States, carbidopa is combined with levodopa in various formulations (10/100, 25/100, 25/250) and marketed as Sinemet® allowing for flexible dosing. The half-life of Sinemet® is approximately 90 minutes, so that multiple daily doses are necessary. We typically start with one half of a 25/100 tablet three times daily, increasing over a few weeks to 1–2 tablets three times daily. CNS side effects such as sedation, insomnia, visual hallucinations, confusion, or psychosis are more likely to occur in the elderly (>80 years) or in later stages of PD.

For convenience, medication dosing may be scheduled around meal times; however, because levodopa absorption occurs in the duodenum through a saturable amino acid transporter, bioavailability may be limited by meals containing large protein content. To maximize bioavailability, patients with fluctuating disease should be instructed to take levodopa on an empty stomach, that is, at least 45 minutes before a meal or 1–2 hours after a meal.

Controlled-release Sinemet (CR)® has a half-life of approximately 3 hours but with a slower onset of action and decreased bioavailability. Sinemet CR comes in 25/100 and 50/200 formulations. In early disease, Sinemet CR can be taken twice a day and is often used at bedtime to prevent wearing-off on awakening. Clinicians should be aware that Sinemet CR translates to less regular Sinemet® during conversion from one to the other (100 mg regular Sinemet is equivalent to 133 mg of Sinemet CR).

Medical Treatment of Advanced Disease

Initially, the dose range and therapeutic window of levodopa is wide and low doses of levodopa have sustained benefits for several years; however, the dosage often needs to be

Table 14.26. Motor Complications

Wearing-off

Delayed-on

Dose failures

On-off phenomenon

Levodopa-induced dyskinesia

Off dystonia

Table 14.27. Management of Psychosis and Hallucinations

■ Exclude infection or other intercurrent illness that may cause delirium

■ Obtain detailed medication history with emphasis on recent additions, dosage changes, withdrawals, or possible ingestions

■ Withdraw medications in this order: anticholinergics, amantadine, selegiline, dopamine agonists, and COMT inhibitors. If troubling hallucinations persist, then consider decreasing levodopa dosage

■ Treatment with quetiapine

■ Clozapine for refractory psychosis

increased (as high as 1,000–1,500 mg) to maintain a stable level of function.

With chronic treatment, at least half of patients receiving dopaminergic therapy develop motor complications or response fluctuations (Table 14.26).[50] As the disease progresses, levodopa's therapeutic window becomes narrowed, leading to clinically apparent fluctuations from "on" (levodopa is working) to "off" (levodopa is not working). In other words, the dose–response curve in advanced disease mirrors the short half-life of levodopa.

Several types of response fluctuations exist. The effect of levodopa may last several hours after a dose and is usually the first type to develop. The duration of the response may progressively shorten (wear off), responses may become unpredictable (on-off phenomenon) and painful limb dystonias or dyskinesias and an overexpression of movement may develop. Dosing intervals may need to be shortened to 1–2 hours to maintain symptom control.

Strategies at this point focus on maximizing on time and minimizing off time, dyskinesias, and side effects. The development of fluctuations may be related to a combination of progressive loss of striatal dopamine storage capacity, pulsatile stimulation of striatal receptors, and receptor hypersensitivity.[51] Therefore, it follows that strategies that minimize pulsatile stimulation may prevent the development of motor complications.

More frequent dosing is the most basic therapeutic maneuver but is limited by the patient's ability to handle frequent round-the-clock dosing and levodopa failures. Use of Sinemet CR may prolong on time, but in our experience, unpredictable responses occur in advanced patients. Furthermore, direct comparison of Sinemet CR with regular Sinemet has shown no major difference in the incidence of dyskinesias and motor complications.[52]

Dopamine agonists are effective in reducing off time, improving function, and reducing levodopa dosages; however, adverse effects such as dyskinesias and hallucinations are more common. Amantadine has been shown to have antidyskinetic properties.

The COMT inhibitors, tolcapone and entacapone, inhibit the breakdown of levodopa in the periphery and CNS and enhance CNS availability of levodopa. Because the action of COMT inhibitors is dependent on the presence of levodopa, COMT inhibitors have no effect on parkinsonian symptoms if levodopa is not administered. Entacapone significantly increases the area under the curve and the half-life of levodopa without increasing maximal plasma concentrations.[53] Specific side effects of entacapone include severe diarrhea and an orange discoloration of urine. Both entacapone and tolcapone have been shown to improve motor fluctuations by reducing wearing off and off time and increasing on time.[19,20] Tolcapone is used infrequently due to cases of fulminant hepatitis.

A Clinical Algorithm

In summary, the medical treatment of PD has advanced dramatically in the last decade but is limited by the relentless progression of the disease. To date, no effective disease-modifying therapies have been discovered. The current state of treatment rests primarily on a symptom-based approach.

Although levodopa remains the most effective therapy for symptoms of PD, we typically begin treatment of mild PD with a dopamine agonist or MAO inhibitor alone. Mild symptoms are often adequately controlled for several months to years on this agent and delaying levodopa treatment may delay the onset of response fluctuations and dyskinesias.

For patients older than 65 years, the incidence of motor complications is low and side effects of agonists are more common. In this population, we advocate starting with levodopa (25/100 three times daily), using the lowest effective dose possible. The dose may be increased by one half to a whole tablet increments as needed. There is no fixed dosage ceiling, although 1,000 mg of levodopa is generally considered more than adequate to control symptoms.

Mild predictable wearing off is easily addressed by increasing the frequency of dosing. Frequent dosing, however, becomes impractical at 2 hours or less. Entacapone (200 mg) can be added to each dose of levodopa to increase the duration of the response, thus increasing daily on time. A concomitant reduction in levodopa dosage by 15%–30% is recommended if the patient is at the high end of the therapeutic window.

The response to levodopa may become more unpredictable with advancing disease. Response failures may occur with absent or delayed onset of action, sudden or unpredictable turning off. The addition of a dopamine agonist is often useful

Table 14.28. Secondary Symptoms of PD and Therapeutic Strategies

Symptom	Nonpharmacological	Pharmacological
Constipation	Increase dietary fiber and fluid intake, regular exercise, discontinue anticholinergics	Stool softeners (docusate), osmotic laxatives (lactulose, milk of magnesia) stimulant laxative (bisacodyl), enemas
Drooling	Speech evaluation and therapy	Botulinum toxin injections, peripheral anticholinergic agent (glycopyrrolate)
Dysarthria/hypophonia	Speech therapy (Lee Silverman technique)	If off symptom, increase dopaminergic therapy
Dysphagia	Dysphagia evaluation, soft-mechanical diet, schedule meals with on time, gastrostomy	If off symptom, increase dopaminergic therapy
Freezing	Physical-occupational therapy for gait training, visual cues	If off symptom, increase dopaminergic therapy
Postural instability/falls	Physical-occupational therapy for gait training or home safety evaluation. Cane, walker, wheelchair, or other form of assistance. Evaluation for orthostasis	If off symptom, increase dopaminergic therapy
Male impotence	Review medications, evaluate for diabetes or underlying endocrine disorder. Urological evaluation	Sildenafil trial, alprostadil (intracavernous injections or intraurethral suppository)
Orthostasis	Elevate head of bed 10–30°, encourage dietary salt intake, compression stockings	Discontinue potential hypotensive drugs, salt-retaining mineralocorticoid (e.g., fludrocortisone) Pressors (e.g., midodrine, ephedrine)
Overactive bladder	Avoid bedtime fluid intake. Exclude infection, prostatism, or other urological problems	Antimuscarinic agents (oxybutynin, tolterodine, imipramine)
Seborrheic dermatitis		Coal tar or selenium-based shampoos, topical steroids

in patients with complex or unpredictable motor complications as long as dyskinesias, visual hallucinations, and other levodopa-related side effects are manageable (Table 14.27).

In a certain subset of patients, the secondary symptoms of PD can become quite disabling. Often increasing dopaminergic therapy is not effective. Table 14.28 outlines some of the most common secondary symptoms of PD and the accepted therapeutic strategies.

Surgical Therapy

In recent years, lesioning surgery, or the selective destruction of basal ganglia targets (e.g., pallidotomy) has fallen out of favor and deep brain stimulation (DBS) has become the surgical treatment of choice. DBS for PD is performed by stereotactically implanting microelectrodes into one of two locations in the basal ganglia, the globus pallidus internus or the subthalamic nucleus. The electrodes are connected to a pulse generator implanted into the chest wall and through a handheld programming device, voltage, frequency, and pulse width may be adjusted to allow for adequate symptom control.

Although the exact mechanism of DBS is not known, it is believed that high-frequency electrical stimulation blocks or inhibits the stimulation target, which rebalances the basal ganglia circuitry. The main advantages of DBS over lesioning therapy include: minimal brain trauma, ability to modify treatment externally, and reversibility of side effects induced by stimulation. Complications unique to DBS include electrical malfunction, lead fracture, battery replacement (every 1–5 years), lengthy initial stimulator programming, infection, skin erosion, and intracerebral hemorrhage or infarct.

The appropriate candidate should have idiopathic PD with disabling symptoms responsive to levodopa, be free of cognitive or neuropsychological illness, have the emotional capabilities and social support to cope with a potentially life-altering surgery, and be able to make the often frequent and involved visits required after surgery. No firm age requirement has been recommended although it is generally believed that patients older than 75 years of age may respond less well to the rigors of surgery and incur greater risk resulting from medical comorbidities and cognitive status.

REFERENCES

1. Verghese J, Le Valley A, Hall, CB, Katz MJ, Ambrose AF, Lipton RB. Epidemiology of gait disorders in community-residing older adults. *J Am Geriatr Soc.* 2006;54:255–261.
2. Sudarsky LR. Gait impairment and falls. In: *Principles of Ambulatory Neurology and the Approach to Clinical Problems.* 25–28.
3. Ruzicka E, Jankovic JJ. Disorders of gait. In: *Parkinson's Disease and Movement Disorders.* 409–429.

4. Mouton CP, Espino DV. Health screening in older women. *Am Fam Physician.* 1999;59:1835–1842.

5. Barak Y, Wagenaar RC, Holt KG. Gait characteristic of elderly people with a history of falls: a dynamic approach. *Phys Ther.* 2006;86:1501–1510.

6. Gilman S. *Merritt's Neurology.* 10th ed. Philadelphia: Lippincott Williams & Wilkins; 2000.

7. Baddour RJ, Wolfson L. Nervous system disease. In: Duthie EH, Katz PR. (eds). Duthie: Practice of Geriatrics. 3rd ed. Philadelphia: WB. Saunders; 1998: 317–327.

8. Stephen LJ, Brodie MJ. Epilepsy in elderly people. *Lancet.* 2000;355(9213):1441–1446.

9. Waterhouse E, Towne A. Seizures in the elderly: Nuances in presentation and treatment. *Cleveland Clin J Med.* 2005;72(Suppl 3): S26–S37.

10. Arroyo S. Treating epilepsy in the elderly. *Drug Safety.* 2001;24: 991–1015.

11. Cloyd J, Hauser W, Towne A, et al. Epidemiological and medical aspects of epilepsy in the elderly. *Epilepsy Res.* 2006;68(Suppl 1):39–48.

12. Ferro JM, Pinto F. Poststroke epilepsy: epidemiology, pathophysiology and management. *Drugs Aging.* 2004;21:639–653.

13. Mendez MF, Lim GTH. Seizures in elderly people with dementia: epidemiology and management. *Drugs Aging.* 2003;20:791–803.

14. Glauser T, Ben-Menchem E. ILAE treatment guidelines: evidence-based analysis of antiepileptic drug efficacy and effectiveness as initial monotherapy for epileptic seizures and syndromes. *Epilepsia.* 2006;47:1094–1120.

15. Bergey GK. Initial treatment of epilepsy. *Neurology.* 2004;63:S40–S48.

16. Morgan GW. Proprioception, touch, and vibratory sensation. In: Goetz CG, Pappert EJ. (ed). Goetz: *Textbook of Clinical Neurology.* 2nd ed. Philadelphia: WB Saunders; 2003:315–332.

17. Mold JW, Vesely SK, Keyl BA. The prevalence, predictors, and consequences of peripheral sensory neuropathy in older patients. *J Am Board Fam Pract.* 2004;17:309–318.

18. Bastyr EJ, Price KL, Bril V. Development and validity testing of the neuropathy total symptom score 6: questionnaire for the study of sensory symptoms of diabetic peripheral neuropathy. *Clin Ther.* 2005;27:1278–1294.

19. Lozeron P. Symptomatic diabetic and non-diabetic neuropathies in a series of 100 diabetic patients. *J Neurol.* 2002;249:569–575.

20. Koopman RJ, Mainous AG, Liszka HA, et al. Evidence of nephropathy and peripheral neuropathy in US adults with undiagnosed diabetes. *Ann Fam Med.* 2006;4:427–432.

21. Oh RC. Vitamin B12 deficiency. *Am Fam Physician.* 2003;(67):979–994.

22. Hughes, RAC. Peripheral neuropathy. *BMJ.* 2002;324:466–469.

23. Dworkin RJ, Backonja M, Rowbotham MC, et al. Advances in neuropathic pain: diagnosis, mechanisms, and treatment recommendations. *Arch Neurol.* 2003;60:1524–1534.

24. Pascuzzi RM. Peripheral neuropathies in clinical practice. *Med Clin N Am.* 2003;87:697–724.

25. Stillman M. Clinical approach to patients with neuropathic pain. *Cleveland Clin J Med.* 2006;73:726–739.

26. Louis ED, Ottman R, Hauser WA. How common is the most common adult movement disorder? Estimates of the prevalence of essential tremor throughout the world. *Mov Disord.* 1998;13:5–10.

27. Higgins JJ, Pho LT, Nee LE. A gene (ETM) for essential tremor maps to chromosome 2p22-p25. *Mov Disord.* 1997;12:859–864.

28. Glucher JR, Jonsson P, Kong A, et al. Mapping of a familial essential tremor gene, FET1, to chromosome 3q13. *Nat Genet.* 1997;17:84–87.

29. Koller WC, Busenbark K, Miner K. The relationship of essential tremor to other movement disorders: report on 678 patients. Essential Tremor Study Group. *Ann Neurol.* 1994;35:717–723.

30. Zesiewicz TA, Elble R, Louis ED, et al. Practice parameter: therapies for essential tremor: report of the Quality Standards Subcommittee of the American Academy of Neurology. *Neurology.* 2005;64:2008–2020.

31. Koller W, Pahwa R, Busenbark K, et al. High-frequency unilateral thalamic stimulation in the treatment of essential and parkinsonian tremor. *Ann Neurol.* 1997;42:292–299.

32. Schuurman PR, Bosch DA, Bossuyt PM, et al. A comparison of continuous thalamic stimulation and thalamotomy for suppression of severe tremor. *NEJM.* 2000;342:461–468.

33. Tyrer P, Alexander MS, Regan A, Lee I. An extrapyramidal syndrome after lithium therapy. *Br J Psychiatry.* 1980;136:191–194.

34. Niethammer M, Ford B. Permanent lithium-induced cerebellar toxicity: Three cases and review of literature. *Mov Disord.* 2007;22:570–573.

35. Deuschl G, Bain P, Brin M. Consensus statement of the Movement Disorder Society on Tremor. Ad Hoc Scientific Committee. *Mov Disord.* 1998;13(Suppl 3):2–23.

36. Hughes AJ, Daniel SE, Blankson S, Lees AJ. A clinicopathologic study of 100 cases of Parkinson's disease. *Arch Neurol.* 1993;50:140–148.

37. Winikates J, Jankovic J. Clinical correlates of vascular Parkinsonism. *Arch Neurol.* 1999;56:98–102.

38. Langston JW, Ballard P. Parkinsonism induced by 1-methyl-4-phenyl-1,2,3,6-tetrahydropyridine (MPTP): implications for treatment and the pathogenesis of Parkinson's disease. *Can J Neurol Sci.* 1984;11:160–165.

39. Olanow CW. Manganese-induced Parkinsonism and Parkinson's disease. *Ann NY Acad Sci.* 2004;1012:209–223.

40. Klawans HL, Stein RW, Tanner CM, Goetz CG. A pure parkinsonian syndrome following acute carbon monoxide intoxication. *Arch Neurol.* 1982;39:302–304.

41. The Parkinson Study Group. Effects of tocopherol and deprenyl on the progression of disability in early Parkinson's disease. *NEJM.* 1993;328:176–183.

42. Shults CW, Oakes D, Kieburtz K, et al. Effects of coenzyme Q10 in early Parkinson disease: evidence of slowing of the functional decline. *Arch Neurol.* 2002;59:1541–1550.

43. Whone AL, Watts RL, Stoessl AJ, et al. Slower progression of Parkinson's disease with ropinirole versus levodopa: the REAL-PET study. *Ann Neurol.* 2003;54:93–101.

44. [Anonymous]. Dopamine transporter brain imaging to assess the effects of pramipexole vs levodopa on Parkinson disease progression. *JAMA.* 2002;287:1653–1661.

45. The Parkinson Study Group. A controlled trial of rasagiline in early Parkinson disease: the TEMPO study. *Arch Neurol.* 2002;59:1937–1943.

46. Calne DB. The role of various forms of treatment in the management of Parkinson's disease. *Clin Neuropharmacol.* 1982;5(Suppl 1):S38–S43.

47. Pritchett AM, Morrison JF, Edwards WD, Schaff HV, Connolly HM, Espinosa RE. Valvular heart disease in patients taking pergolide. *Mayo Clin Proc.* 2002;77:1280–1286.

48. Rascol O, Brooks DJ, Korczyn AD, et al. A five-year study of the incidence of dyskinesia in patients with early Parkinson's disease who were treated with ropinirole or levodopa. O56 study group. *NEJM.* 2000;342:1484–14891.

49. [Anonymous]. Pramipexole vs levodopa as initial treatment for parkinson disease: A randomized controlled trial. Parkinson Study Group. *JAMA.* 2000;284:1931–1938.

50. Rinne UK, Rinne JO, Rinne JK, Laakso K, Laihinen A, Lonnberg P. Brain receptor changes in Parkinson's disease in relation to the disease process and treatment. *J Neural Transm Suppl.* 1983;18:279–286.

51. Mouradian MM, Heuser IJ, Baronti F, Chase TN. Modification of central dopiminergic mechanisms by continuous levodopa therapy for advanced Parkinson's disease. *Ann Neurol.* 1990;27:18–23.

52. Block G, Liss C, Reines S, Irr J, Nibberlink D. Comparison of immediate-release and controlled release carbidopa/levodopa in Parkinson's disease. A multicenter 5-year study. the CR first study group. *Eur Neurol.* 1997;37:23–27.

53. Nutt JG, Woodward WR, Beckner RM, et al. Effect of peripheral catechol-O-methyltransferase inhibition on the pharmacokinetics and pharmacodynamics of levodopa in Parkinsonian patients. *Neurology.* 1994;44:913–919.

15

Recognition and Management of Delirium

James G. O'Brien, MD, Stephanie Garrett, MD

DELIRIUM

Delirium may be the most common and serious psychiatric problem affecting hospitalized older adults. Delirium is an acute fluctuating process of brain failure affecting, especially, attention and cognition. It is associated with many negative sequelae including increased mortality, cost, duration of stay, and risk of nursing home placement, or extended care at home. Despite this fact, delirium is frequently not recognized and if recognized not properly treated.

Delirium can be conceptualized as brain failure similar to heart failure or renal failure in which the cause or precipitating event may be intrinsic to the organ or, more commonly, extrinsic to the organ. Thus infection, electrolyte imbalances, metabolic disturbances, or medications may result in delirium. Delirium is to the older adult what fever is to the infant – a nonspecific manifestation of an underlying problem. In the older adult, the brain may be similar to a circuit breaker, thus the weakest link, in an electrical system, which, when subjected to overload, will be the first to fail. Delirium in the older adult is probably a more common manifestation of illness than fever or pain.

EPIDEMIOLOGY

Delirium is a frequent event in hospitalized elderly patients with 14%–24% being affected at time of admission (prevalence) with an additional 6%–56% developing delirium during the course of hospitalization (incidence).[1] Data from the United Kingdom suggest similar prevalence and incidence with reports of 7%–61% of older patients developing delirium during hospitalization.[2] Delirium adds greatly to the cost of care both in the hospital and postdischarge.

In intensive care units, up to 87% may be affected.[3] Delirium is a common finding in the emergency department, and usually indicates a negative prognosis. Some individuals will not recover and will require prolonged institutional care. Complete recovery has been reported to occur in only 52% of patients who survived hospitalization.[4] Hospital mortality rates range from 6% to 18% and are twice that of matched controls.[5] Other studies indicate mortality may be as high as 76% for hospitalized patients, which is similar to the mortality for myocardial infarction.[6] Delirium is almost always an inevitable feature of the dying process.

DEFINITION

Delirium is an acute confusional state characterized by a disturbance of consciousness and attention interspersed with lucid intervals. Global cognition is impaired, which may be manifested by speech that is incoherent or rambling. Additional features include altered perception with delusions and hallucinations. Patients with delirium may be hypoactive – the most common type – and display lethargy and decreased motor function or may be hyperactive with agitation and aggressive behavior. A combination of both types is also encountered and may pose a greater challenge in terms of management, especially with the use of psychoactive medications. Sleep cycle may also be disturbed with nighttime insomnia and daytime drowsiness. To make this diagnosis one needs to be aware that delirium is common and that careful observation by both physicians and nurses is essential for detection. There is no specific test to verify the presence or absence of the syndrome and many unnecessary imaging studies of the brain are performed to rule out relatively rare causes of this problem.

An essential feature of delirium is reduced awareness and attentiveness to the environment. This results in increased distractibility, loss of ability to remain focused on one topic, and difficulty in maintaining a coherent stream of thought, speech, or action.[7] What is usually manifested to nursing staff and physicians is some abnormal behavior that generally presents as one of three subtypes – hyperactive, hypoactive and mixed. Typically all of the preceding features are interspersed with periods of lucidity, which help separate delirium from dementia.

PATHOPHYSIOLOGY

The pathophysiology of delirium is still poorly understood but it appears that there is a major disruption of neurotransmission. The most common scenario is when a biological stressor occurs in a vulnerable host. This phenomenon can be conceptualized as occurring on a sliding scale. A healthy younger adult with an excess reserve capacity would require a massive insult to develop delirium; conversely, an elderly individual with minimal reserve and multiple comorbid conditions can develop delirium with a minor stressor such as a urinary tract infection. Older individuals are particularly vulnerable as a result of increased cell fallout and a decrease in neurotransmitters, especially acetylcholine.

It is well established that cholinergic deficiency results in delirium and can be induced with anticholinergic medications. Serum anticholinergic activity is increased in delirium and cholinesterase inhibitors have been shown to reverse delirium even in those cases not caused by anticholinergic medications.[8]

Neuropsychological and neuroimaging studies demonstrate disruption of higher cortical function with compromise of many other areas of the brain including the prefrontal cortex, subcortical structures, thalamus, basal ganglia, frontal and temporoparietal cortices, fusiform cortex, and lingual gyri especially on the nondominant side.[9] It also appears that many other neurotransmitters play a causative or contributory role such as dopamine, which influences the release of acetylcholine. Other neurotransmitters such as serotonin, norepinephrine, and gamma aminobutyric acid have been implicated, with the cholinergic system being the final common pathway. Chronic stress and the release of cytokines that alter the permeability of the blood–brain barrier may also contribute.

DIFFERENTIAL DIAGNOSIS

Dementia and delirium are frequently confused and not uncommonly delirium is superimposed on dementia. Acuity of onset typically hours or days, a disturbance in level of consciousness, and the presence of lucid periods are all hallmarks of delirium, but not dementia. Depression can be detected by history-taking and use of a depression screening test such as the Geriatric Depression Scale.

EVALUATION

The causes of delirium are legion and in most instances there is more than one precipitating event. Causal factors can be conceptualized as being extrinsic or intrinsic. Factors extrinsic to the brain, infection, drugs, and alteration in hydration are more common inciters of delirium than intrinsic causes such as stroke or meningitis.

An initial prudent step is to identify all vulnerable adults on admission to the hospital with a previous diagnosis of dementia or mild cognitive impairment by using a mental status screening test such as Mini-mental status clock drawing test on admission. Verifying the presence of delirium can be accomplished via careful observation, history-taking and use of a diagnostic instrument such as the Confusion Assessment Method (CAM) [10]. The CAM Training Manual and Coding Guide is available at elderlifemed.yale.edu/pdf/The_Confusion_Assessment_Method.pdf.

HISTORY

History should include information regarding onset and prior cognitive function such as the ability to live independently, manage finances, telephone, and so forth. A medication history should include all prescribed drugs (multiple physicians), over the counter, herbal, and other medications. Alcohol history, nutrition status, weight loss, and psychiatric history or episodes of confusion should be noted as should the presence of incontinence of bowel or bladder, a history of recent falls particularly with head trauma, sensory deficits such as vision and hearing impairments and whether compensatory aids such as glasses and hearing aids are being used. Comorbid medical conditions such as diabetes mellitus, congestive heart failure, and renal failure need to be documented.

EXAMINATION

The physical examination needs to be comprehensive as the underlying contributing problems may be multiple and usually are remote from the central nervous system such as pneumonia or a urinary tract infection. Essential elements of the examination include determining the of level of consciousness; presence of lucid periods; vital signs for evidence of fever or hypothermia; arrhythmia and brady- or tachyarrhythmia that impairs cerebral blood flow, which is already reduced in older patients; blood pressure, both lying and standing, to detect postural hypotension; and careful examination of lungs to detect pneumonia or congestion. Sites of infection include skin with cellulitis, an acute abdomen, or a distended bladder. A rectal examination is essential to rule out fecal impaction. Deep vein thrombosis may also precipitate delirium.

A neurological examination is needed to detect a central nervous system pathological condition such as cerebral infarction or hemorrhage. Presence of tremors, if new in onset, may be secondary to alcohol withdrawal.

INVESTIGATIONS

Further investigations should be guided by indicators from the history and physical examination.

LABORATORY TESTS

Laboratory tests should include the following: a complete blood count to detect infection or anemia; a metabolic panel that includes blood urea nitrogen/creatinine to identify dehydration and renal failure; blood sugar and electrolytes which are frequent contributors; liver function; and urinalysis, preferably a catheter specimen to check for urinary tract infection.

OTHER INVESTIGATIONS

Chest x-ray films to diagnose pneumonia, congestive heart failure, or other lung pathology and an electrocardiogram to identify an arrhythmia or silent myocardial infarction can be helpful. Blood cultures and pulse oximetry are all simple bedside evaluations that are likely to identify the majority of causes.[11]

NONROUTINE INVESTIGATIONS

In refractory cases or when the previous investigations have failed to reveal a satisfactory explanation, additional tests that are appropriate include thyroid function tests, B-12 and folate levels, arterial blood gas levels, and lumbar puncture in a febrile patient with an unknown source for fever.

Neuroimaging usually has a low yield and should be utilized primarily for those with new focal signs or recent head trauma. This is in contrast with what frequently happens today when an imaging study is performed first.[1]

Electroencephalography is rarely used but may be helpful in detecting occult seizures and separating delirium from other psychiatric diagnoses.

Refractory cases require continued evaluation including repeating various investigations.

MANAGEMENT

It is axiomatic in treating delirium that the underlying cause(s) must be treated before any improvement can be expected.

Frequently, a multipronged approach is indicated. Infections should be treated; dehydration and metabolic abnormalities should be corrected appropriately. Supportive measures such as protecting the airway, assuring oxygen delivery, addressing problems of malnutrition, preventing complications such as falls, pressure ulcers, and deep vein thrombosis and avoiding the use of restraints are essential. Medication management strategies include limiting the number of drugs and withdrawing all nonessential drugs, reducing psychoactive drugs or using safer replacements. In a suspected alcoholic, the use of intravenous thiamine is indicated. Special attention should be paid to bowel and bladder care, avoiding constipation and limiting the use of indwelling catheters.

Providing sleep aids such as warm milk at bedtime and assuring a comfortable temperature can be helpful.

ENVIRONMENT

Creating a safe environment is vital. This can be accomplished most effectively in an Acute Care for the Elderly unit but if not available a room preferably shared closest to the nursing station should be utilized.

A quiet appropriately lit environment with reduced noise levels; use of clocks, calendars, and photos to help with orientation; cueing by staff; and provision of sensory aids for hearing and vision with early and regular mobilization is very helpful. Additional approaches include a consistent staff approach, encouragement of family involvement in care, preferably round the clock or securing the services of a sitter. Use lucid periods to explain to the patient what is happening and reorient them. Special attention should be paid to symptom relief such as adequate treatment of pain or other symptoms such as nausea and vomiting.

PHARMACOLOGICAL MANAGEMENT

The use of psychopharmacological agents should be judicious and should never be utilized to compensate for inadequate staff or family support. Ideally pharmacological agents should only be used when the patient poses a risk to him/herself or others or to preserve a vital treatment such as an intravenous line or an oxygen cannula.

According to American Psychiatric Association guidelines for the agitated, delusional patient, a high potency antipsychotic such as haloperidol is indicated.[12] The exception may be in patients with Parkinson's disease and those experiencing alcohol withdrawal. Haloperidol can be given orally, intramuscularly, and, occasionally, intravenously, but only in true emergency situations as it has the potential to induce life-threatening arrhythmias when given in this form.

Use of atypical antipsychotic medications has not been studied enough to recommend their routine use despite the fact that they are used frequently to manage delirium. Among

Table 15.1. Pharmacological Treatment of Delirium

Class and Drug	Dose	Adverse Effects	Comments
Antipsychotic Haloperidol	0.5–1.0 mg twice daily orally, with additional doses every 4 hrs as needed (peak effect, 4–6 hr)	Extrapyramidal symptoms, especially if dose is >3 mg per day	Usually agent of choice Effectiveness demonstrated in randomized, controlled trials
	0.5–1.0 mg intramuscularly, observe after 30–60 min and repeat if needed (peak effect, 20–40 min)	Prolonged correct QT interval on electrocardiogram Avoid in patients with withdrawal syndrome, hepatic insufficient, neuroleptic malignant syndrome	Avoid intravenous use because of short duration of action
Atypical antipsychotic Risperidone Olanzapine Quetiapine	0.5 mg twice daily 2.5–5.0 mg once daily 2.5–5.0 mg once daily	Extrapyramidal effects equivalent to or slightly less than those with haloperidol Prolonged corrected QT interval on electrocardiogram	Tested only in small, uncontrolled studies Associated with increased mortality rate among older patients with dementia
Benzodiazepine Lorazepam	0.5–1.0 mg orally, with additional doses every 4 hr as needed*	Paradoxical excitation, respiratory depression, oversedation	Second-line agent Associated with prolongation and worsening of delirium symptoms demonstrated in clinical trial Reserve for use in patients undergoing sedative and alcohol withdrawal, those with Parkinson's disease, and those with neuroleptic malignant syndrome
Antidepressant Trazodone	25–150 mg orally at bedtime	Oversedation	Tested only in uncontrolled studies

* Intravenous use of lorazepam should be reserved for emergencies.

existing studies stronger data support the use of risperidone and olanzapine, although well-designed studies do not exist.[13,14] The use of cholinesterase inhibitors such as Aricept, Exelon, and Razadyne intuitively make sense as they may combat a deficiency of acetylcholine. Benzodiazepines are only indicated for alcohol withdrawal and then only short-acting drugs such as lorazepam should be used.[9] Patients should be weaned from these medications when there is evidence of improvement.

Table 15.1 provides a summary of pharmacological agents used in delirium.

PREVENTION

It is thought that perhaps as many as a third of all cases of delirium can be prevented.[14,15] A group at particular risk are nursing home residents, many of whom have cognitive impairment or are demented and are transferred to the hospital with an acute illness and admitted via the emergency room. The stress of illness, transportation, and general chaos in the emergency room and hospital is likely to overwhelm any defense and result in delirium. Perhaps a significant number of these individuals

Table 15.2. Risk Factors for Delirium

Age >65	Functional impairment
Male	Multiple medical problems
Alcohol abuse	Malnutrition
Cognitive Impairment	Polypharmacy
Neurological impairment such as stroke	
Terminal illness	

Table 15.3. Delirium Precipitants

Drugs – especially psychoactive medications			
Severe Illness			
Infection	Intensive Care Placement	Shock	Physical Restraints
Hypoxia	Pain		Bladder Catheter
Iatrogenic Complications		Surgery	Sleep Deprivation

could be treated at their nursing facilities given the portability of diagnostic tools and the ability to administer potent medications such as intravenous antibiotics. This does obligate the physician or nurse practitioner to provide assessment and care on site. Certainly for most pneumonias and urinary tract infections this approach is feasible and preferable and likely to result in significant cost savings. Many authors have identified risk factors for delirium (Table 15.2) that when present on admission increase the probability of delirium developing.

When risk factors that can be considered as patient characteristics are combined with precipitating external factors such as dehydration and sepsis or the use of restraints, delirium is almost certain to develop. Inouye et al. has identified precipitating factors, a summary of which is included in the Table 15.3.

Screening on admission of those who are vulnerable and have risk factors is a strategy that needs to be implemented at all hospitals. The Yale prevention trial addressed the following domains and significantly reduced the incidence of delirium.[14] Actions included orientation and maintaining cognition; early mobilization; minimizing the use of psychoactive drugs; use of nonpharmacological approaches such as normalizing sleep patterns, enhancing communication; and restoring aids such as glasses and hearing devices; preventing and restoring volume depletion; and limiting the use of bladder catheters. Most of these actions fall under the purview of nursing.

SUMMARY

Delirium is a serious life-threatening problem that is very common in hospitalized older adults. It is frequently misdiagnosed and mismanaged. It increases mortality, duration of hospital stay, and both inpatient and posthospital cost. It increases the risk of long-term nursing home placement.

With the use of screening instruments, early detection, and rapid treatment of underlying causes in a safe, appropriate environment, outcomes can be significantly improved.

The management of delirium in a competent manner should be within the purview of any physician responsible for the care of hospitalized older adults.

REFERENCES

1. Inouye SK. Delirium in hospitalized older patients. *Clin Geriatr Med.* 1998;14:745–764.
2. Royal College of Psychiatrists. Who cares wins: improving the outcome for older people admitted to the general hospital. Report of a working group for the Faculty of Old Age Psychiatry. London: Royal College of Psychiatrists. 2005. Available at: www.bgs.org.uk/PDF%20Downloads/WhoCaresWins.pdf.
3. Pisani MA, McNicoll L, Inouye SK. Cognitive impairment in the intensive care unit. *Clin Chest Med.* 2003;24:727–737.
4. Rockwood K. The occurrence and duration of symptoms in elderly patients with delirium. *J Gerontol.* 1993;48(4):M162–M166.
5. Landefeld CS, Palmer RM, Kresevic DM, Fortinsky RH, Kowal J. A randomized trial of care in a hospital medical unit especially designed to improve the functional outcomes of acutely ill older patients. *NEJM.* 1995;332:1338–1344.
6. American Psychiatric Association. Practice guideline for the treatment of patients with delirium. *Am J Psychiatry.* 1999;156(5 Suppl):1–20.
7. American Psychiatric Association. *Diagnostic and Statistical Manual of Mental Disorders.* 4th ed. Washington DC: American Psychiatric Association; 1994.
8. Trzepacz P, van der Mast R. The neuropathophysiology of delirium. In: Lindesay J, Rockwood K, Macdonald A, eds. *Delirium In Old Age.* Oxford: Oxford University Press; 2002:51–90.
9. Inouye SK. Delirium in older persons. *NEJM.* 2006;354:1157–1165.
10. Inouye SK, van Dyck CH, Alessi CA, Balkin S, Siegal AP, Horwitz RI. Clarifying confusion: the confusion assessment method. A new method for detection of delirium. *Ann Intern Med.* 1990;113:941–948.
11. Potter GJ. Guideline Development Group. The prevention, diagnosis and management of delirium in older people: concise guidelines. *Clin Med.* 2006;6:303–308.
12. Cook IA. Guideline watch: practice guideline for the treatment of patients with delirium. Arlington, VA: American Psychiatric Association. 2004. www.guidelines.gov/summary/summary.aspx?ss=15&doc_id=2180&nbr=1406.
13. Boehger S, Breitbart W. Atypical antipsychotics in the management of delirium: A review of the empirical literature. *Pall Care.* 2005;3:227–238.
14. Inouye SK, Bogardus ST Jr, Charpentier PA, et al. A multicomponent intervention to prevent delirium in hospitalized older patients. *NEJM.* 1999;340:669–676.
15. Marcantonio ER, Flacker JM, Michaels M, Resnick NM. Delirium is independently associated with poor functional recovery after hip fracture. *J Am Geriatr Soc.* 2000;48:618–624.

16

EVALUATION AND MANAGEMENT OF DEMENTIA

Lauren G. Collins, MD, Barry N. Rovner, MD, Marjorie M. Marenberg, MD, PhD, MPH

DEFINITION

Dementia is characterized by memory and learning impairment as well as deficits in at least one other cognitive domain. These include: impairment in communication (aphasia); impairment in recognition and manipulation of objects (agnosia and apraxia); impairment in reasoning ability; and impairment in handling complex tasks (executive function). These cognitive symptoms must represent a significant decline from a previous level of functioning and interfere with functional status and social activities. The disturbances must be insidious in onset and progressive and must not be better accounted for by another psychiatric diagnosis, such as delirium, or systemic disease.[1]

Epidemiology

The prevalence of dementia has been estimated to be approximately 6%–10% of individuals aged 65 years or older. The prevalence of dementia increases with age, rising from 2% among those aged 65 to 74 years to more than 30% of those 85 years and older.[2–4] Incidence rates of Alzheimer's disease (AD) demonstrate exponential growth, doubling every 5 years after the age of 65 years, at least until the age of 85 years.[5]

The cost of caring for people with dementia is substantial; dementia has been estimated to increase the mean annual health care cost per older patient by $4,134, primarily as a result of increased hospitalization costs and increased expenditures on skilled nursing facilities.[6] The current annual economic cost of dementia is approximately $100 billion.[7] With the anticipated doubling of the population aged 65 years and older by 2030,[8] the financial impact of dementia on our society will be even more dramatic.

Risk Factors

Determining risk factors for dementia has been an area of intense study (see Table 16.1). Many risk factors for dementia are not modifiable; thus, the search for ways to prevent dementia has garnered much attention. Studies have shown that social, mental, and physical activity appear to be inversely associated with the risk for dementia, but these data come from large observational studies and meta-analyses and require additional validation.[9–11] It is unclear if adopting these lifestyle characteristics will prevent the development of dementia.

Dementia Subtypes

There are several different subtypes of dementia, of which AD is the most common. The definitive diagnosis for the etiology of dementia requires pathological evaluation. However, recent dementia research has demonstrated much overlap between the various dementia syndromes, particularly between AD and vascular dementia (VaD).[12,13] The etiology of certain dementia syndromes may be traced to a common pathophysiology. For example, it appears that the neurodegenerative dementias, such as Alzheimer's dementia, frontotemporal dementia (FTD), dementia with Lewy bodies (DLB), and prion disorders may actually be linked mechanistically to the conversion of normal proteins into insoluble aggregates. These aggregates form cerebral deposits or neuronal inclusions prompting neurotoxic cascades that attempt to remove the misfolded proteins.[14]

Alzheimer's Disease

AD is the most common form of dementia in the elderly, accounting for 60% to 80% of all cases.[15–17] It is estimated that more than 4.5 million adults with AD are currently living in the United States.[18] The cost of caring for one patient with AD is $47,000 per year.[19] The economic burden of this disease is surpassed only by the tremendous social and emotional burden on patients, families, and caregivers.

Epidemiological research has identified the following risk factors for AD: age, presence of the apolipoprotein E epsilon 4

Table 16.1. Risk Factors for Dementia

Identified Risk Factors

Age

Family history

APOE genetic endowment

Down syndrome

Head trauma

MCI

Additional Probable Risk Factors

Vascular risk factors

Hypertension

Diabetes mellitus

Hyperlipidemia

Elevated plasma homocysteine level

High dietary fat intake

Smoking

Adapted from References.[9,10,11]

(APO E4) genotype, family history, Down syndrome, and head trauma. Vascular risk factors, such as diabetes, hypertension, and lipid abnormalities have also been associated with AD. Researchers in AD now concur that what is good for the heart is good for the brain.

Recently, higher education has been found to be a protective risk factor for AD. Individual differences in how tasks are processed may allow for a degree of cognitive reserve from brain pathology. Participation in both leisure and physical activity may also be protective for development of AD.

Brain pathology consistent with AD includes the presence of extracellular amyloid-β protein-42 (Abeta42) deposition and intracellular neurofibrillary tangles (NFTs).[20] AD is characterized by neuronal loss, especially among neurons that release the neurotransmitter acetylcholine.[21]

The etiology of neuronal damage in the brains in AD patients, particularly in the medial temporal lobes and the hippocampus, is still not well understood. To date, the pathophysiology of AD traces back to a family of amyloid precursor proteins that are cleaved by specific secretases. When amyloid precursor protein is cleaved by a γ-secretase on one end and a β-secretase on the other end, a highly amyloidogenic Abeta42 protein is released. This protein appears to aggregate in diffuse plaques, which evolve into dense neuritic plaques.[22] Abeta oligomers, therefore, are probable mediators of neurotoxicity.[23] Once the neuritic plaque has formed, secondary cascades of inflammation, excitotoxicity, and apoptosis may trigger additional damage.

The formation of NFTs and their role in the pathophysiology of AD remains controversial. NFTs consist of a hyperphosphorylated form of the microtubule-associated protein, tau. Severity of cognitive decline correlates with NFT burden more so than with amyloid deposition, suggesting that a mutant tau protein, rather than the NFT, may be the primary neurotoxic mediator.[24,25] Cleavage of tau, a critical step in NFT formation, appears to be triggered by accumulation of Abeta42 protein through activation of caspases.

Clinically, AD is characterized by an insidious onset and early detection is often the result of informant concerns. Early symptoms include loss of short-term memory, repeating statements, and exercising poor judgment. Behavioral symptoms such as personality changes, apathy, delusions, and hallucinations are also common features in patients with moderate AD. In late stages of AD, patients frequently become dependent on others for activities of daily living (ADLs), such as bathing and toileting.

AD is marked by a gradually progressive course and a shortened life expectancy. In one large population-based study, the median survival from time of diagnosis was 4.2 years in men and 5.7 years in women. Mortality predictors include dementia severity at time of diagnosis, abnormal neurological findings, and the presence of comorbidities, such as heart disease and diabetes.[26] Pneumonia is the most common terminal event in patients with progressive dementia.

Vascular Dementia

VaD accounts for 10%–20% of cases of dementias in older adults.[27] The identification of VaD has suffered partly because of a lack of uniform diagnostic criteria.[28,29] Traditionally, VaD was thought to have an abrupt onset of cognitive impairment with stepwise deterioration and focal neurological impairments following a cerebrovascular insult. More recent research has shown that 20% of cases of VaD are actually characterized by a subtle onset and gradual course, making the distinction between VaD and AD on presentation less clear.[30] In fact, diagnostic criteria for VaD have been relatively unsuccessful in predicting pathological findings.[12] Also, autopsy examinations have revealed that coexistence of vascular lesions with AD pathology is common and a "mixed dementia" may be much more common than previously suspected.[31]

Despite suffering from a lack of uniform diagnostic criteria, clinical features that may suggest the diagnosis of VaD include: onset of cognitive decline following a stroke, abrupt onset of symptoms followed by a stepwise deterioration, findings on physical examination that are consistent with a previous stroke, and bilateral and/or lacunar infarcts that involve cortical or subcortical gray matter on cerebral imaging.[12,29] White matter changes in the periventricular regions seen on magnetic resonance imaging (MRI) are thought to be related to microvascular ischemia but are not now part of the diagnostic criteria for VaD. The prognosis of VaD is generally considered to be worse than that of AD, with a median survival of only 3 years following diagnosis.[12]

Frontotemporal Dementia

FTD is a heterogeneous entity that primarily affects the portion of the brain that controls planning, social behavior, and language perception. In contrast to VaD and AD, FTD usually develops at an earlier age, with presentation after the age of 75 years, rare.[32] Recent research suggests that FTD may be more common than was previously believed and that it has a high rate of familial aggregation (20%–40% of cases).[33,34] Prognosis for FTD is variable, with life expectancy after diagnosis ranging from 3 to 10 years.[12]

Pathologically, FTD is characterized by focal atrophy of the frontal and temporal lobes, in the absence of findings consistent with AD.[35] Specific regions of atrophy correlate with the clinical and neuropathological syndrome.[36] These regions often show decreased perfusion on single photon emission computed tomography, positron emission tomography (PET), and perfusion MRI.[37,38] Three neuropathological subtypes of FTD have been described according to the presence or absence of tau and ubiquitin inclusions: tau positive, tau and ubiquitin negative, and ubiquitin negative/tau positive pathology.

Although mutations in the tau gene on chromosome 17 have been implicated in familial FTD, the pathogenesis of nonfamilial FTD remains unclear.[39,40] Autopsy, neuroimaging, and cerebrospinal fluid studies suggest that FTD is characterized by a serotonergic deficit, which likely contributes to the behavioral abnormalities associated with FTD.[41]

There are three distinct clinical subtypes of FTD: behavioral, language, and motor.[32,42] The behavioral subtype is the most common form of FTD, with 90% of patients developing personality changes during the course of their illness. The personality change is often dramatic and is characterized by social inappropriateness, poor judgment, and disinhibition. Impairment of executive function, insight, and memory are also common features in behavioral FTD.[43,44] Findings on perfusion imaging studies often correlate with behavioral symptoms. For example, prominent frontal hypoperfusion is associated with apathy and poor hygiene and self-care, and prominent temporal hypoperfusion is associated with hypomania and compulsive behaviors.[37]

Early progressive language dysfunction is the second most common phenotype in FTD and is characterized by two subtypes: primary progressive nonfluent aphasia (or logopenic aphasia) and progressive fluent aphasia (or semantic dementia).[42] Progressive nonfluent aphasia is characterized pathologically by prominent frontal lobe atrophy and clinically by word-finding difficulty despite preserved understanding of speech. Progressive fluent aphasia is associated with marked temporal lobe involvement.[13] Patients often present with difficulty in naming and in understanding words, secondary to involvement of left temporal lobe, or in face and object recognition, secondary to involvement of right temporal lobe. With progression, patients may develop logorrhea (abundant unfocused speech), echolalia (spontaneous repetition of words), and palilalia (compulsive repetition of phrases).[42]

The third type of FTD involves a prominent motor component in the presentation. Patients often present with extrapyramidal motor symptoms or with signs of bulbar and spinal motor neuron disease. Patients with bulbar or spinal motor neuron disease (FTD–motor neuron disease) often have motor symptoms within 12 months of disease onset and have, generally, a rapidly progressive disease course.[43]

Dementia with Parkinsonism

A number of parkinsonian disorders are associated with dementia. The two most common forms of dementia with Parkinson's are DLB and Parkinson's disease dementia (PDD). Atypical parkinsonian syndromes such as progressive supranuclear palsy (PSP), multisystem atrophy, and corticobasilar ganglionic degeneration also produce dementia syndromes.

Dementia with Lewy Bodies

DLB now appears to be the second most common form of neurodegenerative dementia in older adults, with prevalence estimates ranging from 15% to 20% of all cases.[45,46]

Pathologically, numerous Lewy bodies characterize DLB but plaques and NFTs, often seen in AD, may also be present.[46] New immunocytochemical staining for ubiquitin and α-synuclein has aided greatly in the detection of cortical Lewy bodies and significantly improved the detection of the disorder in postmortem studies.[14]

Despite improved pathological detection, the clinical diagnosis of DLB is still challenging. Patients with DLB can be distinguished from those with AD and VaD by marked cognitive fluctuations, persistent well-formed hallucinations, and coexisting rapid eye movement (REM) sleep behavior disorders.[12,46] DLB should be suspected in patients with signs of parkinsonism such as bradykinesia, muscular rigidity, and tremor. Supportive features for the diagnosis include a history of repeated falls, syncope, sensitivity to neuroleptic medications, delusions, hallucinations in nonvisual modes, and depression.[46] Of note, distinguishing DLB from AD and other dementias may be particularly important because of the risk of adverse events with antipsychotic medications in these patients.[45] Also, patients with DLB may benefit from a trial of levodopa therapy, making early detection even more valuable. Prognosis for DLB appears to be slightly worse than that for AD, with some patients having a rapidly progressive course.[12]

Parkinson's Disease Dementia

Patients PD have a significantly increased risk of developing associated dementia.[47] In one prospective cohort study, 30% of patients developed dementia within 5 years.[48]

Patients with PD have gray matter atrophy in the limbic, paralimbic, and prefrontal regions. On pathological examination, PDD correlates with cortical and limbic Lewy bodies.[49,50]

Although PDD shares features of DLB pathologically, its clinical presentation differs from that of DLB in that it is defined by the onset of dementia in the setting of PD for at least 1 year. The dementia associated with PD is characterized by executive dysfunction, attention impairment, and memory impairment.[50]

Progressive Supranuclear Palsy

PSP mimics PD in its early stages, and patients are often found to have postural instability, bradykinesia, and rigidity. PSP is distinguished from PD by the presence of vertical supranuclear palsy with downward gaze abnormalities. Also, in contrast to PD, the bradykinesia and rigidity is often symmetrical.[51] Patients with PSP generally have a poor response to levodopa.[52] and frequently develop a pseudobulbar palsy with dysarthria and dysphagia.[53]

Pathologically, patients with PSP have globose NTF made up of hyperphosphorylated tau proteins. These lesions are found in the substantia nigra, subthalamic nucleus, globus pallidus, superior colliculus, and midbrain and pons with associated neuronal loss. Cortical involvement generally involves the frontal lobe as well.

Not surprisingly, the dementia associated with PSP is frequently a frontal lobe syndrome; however, it is more rapidly progressive than many other neurodegenerative dementias, with a median time to death following diagnosis of only 6 years.[54]

Creutzfeldt-Jakob Disease

Creutzfeldt-Jakob disease (CJD) is a rare, neurodegenerative disease caused by prions, which presents with a rapid onset of cognitive impairment as well as motor deficits and seizures. CJD should be suspected in any patient presenting with a dementing illness with a subacute onset over weeks to months. There are six recognized subtypes of CJD. Motor manifestations may be cerebellar, extrapyramidal, or extraocular and usually develop shortly after cognitive symptoms. Myoclonus and seizures are less common symptoms and generally occur later in the course of the disease. Electroencephalography and cerebrospinal fluid studies can be helpful in determining the diagnosis and may be supported by gray matter abnormalities on diffusion MRI. CJD is a rapidly progressive dementia and is usually fatal within 1 year after onset.[12]

Reversible Dementia

Although potentially reversible causes of dementia account for less than 10% of cases of dementia, identifying and treating these disorders remains a top priority.[8,55,56] Vitamin deficiencies, thyroid dysfunction, depression, and normal-pressure hydrocephalus (NPH) have all been identified as more common reversible causes of dementia to consider in the initial differential diagnosis (see Table 16.2) of a patient presenting with cognitive impairment, but there are numerous causes of potentially reversible dementias in an expanded differential (see, Table 16.3). Although these syndromes are considered "potentially" reversible, it is important to note that the majority of patients with these syndromes do not improve even when these

Table 16.2. Differential Diagnosis of Cognitive Impairment

AD
VaD
FTD
PD
DLB
CJD
PSP
NPH
Alcohol-related dementia
Medication-induced dementia
AIDS dementia
Delirium
Major depressive disorder with cognitive impairment
MCI
Metabolic disorders

Adapted from Reference.[137]

Table 16.3. Potentially Reversible Dementias

Medication induced
Analgesics
Anticholinergics
Psychotropic medications
Sedative hypnotics
Steroids
Alcohol-related
Intoxication
Withdrawal
Metabolic disorders
Thyroid disease
Vitamin B12 deficiency
Hyponatremia
Hypercalcemia
Hepatic dysfunction
Renal dysfunction
Depression (pseudodementia)
Central nervous system neoplasm
Chronic subdural hematoma
Chronic meningitis
NPH
Human immunodeficiency virus
CJD

Adapted from References.[55,56]

disorders are promptly discovered and treated. Rates of reversal range from only 0.6% to 11% of cases.[56,57]

Normal-Pressure Hydrocephalus

Patients with NPH often present with a triad of gait disturbance ("magnetic gait"), urinary incontinence, and cognitive dysfunction. Although NPH should be considered in patients with these symptoms, it is also important to recognize that many older adults have one or more of these symptoms in the absence of NPH. Nevertheless, NPH is amenable to treatment and, therefore, should still be considered in patients who fit the clinical scenario. Confirmatory studies include imaging studies, radioisotope diffusion studies, and the Fisher test, which involves gait assessment before and after the removal of 30 mL of cerebrospinal fluid. The Fisher test is also useful in predicting response to ventriculoperitoneal shunting, the treatment of choice.[12]

Delirium

Delirium (see Chapter 15), a condition characterized by fluctuating levels of consciousness and inattention, must also be distinguished from dementia. Whereas dementia is characterized by an insidious onset, the onset of delirium is usually abrupt and often precipitated by illness, intoxication, or medication. Delirium is associated with a high morbidity and mortality, but unlike dementia, delirium typically resolves if the underlying cause is addressed.[58] Still, recovery from delirium may be protracted in older adults and may even become chronic in some patients making it difficult to distinguish from dementia.

Mild Cognitive Impairment

Dementia is increasingly recognized as an endpoint on a continuum of cognitive decline.[55] Recent efforts to understand dementia, therefore, have focused on cognitive impairment that precedes dementia. Terms that have been used to describe the range of cognitive and functional conditions between normal and demented include: cognitively impaired not demented, possible dementia prodrome, and age-associated cognitive impairment. What unites all of these terms is the concept that there is some cognitive loss, but not enough to cause significant changes in functioning, which is the hallmark of dementia.

Mild cognitive impairment (MCI) is a recent research construct that attempts to define this period of cognitive impairment before dementia. The definition of MCI is, however, very heterogeneous, and the progression is variable. Many consider that the cognitive impairment associated with short-term memory loss short of dementia (so-called amnestic MCI) is actually "prodromal AD."[14]

DIAGNOSTIC APPROACH

Although a definitive diagnosis of a particular dementia syndrome often requires a postmortem examination, a comprehensive approach with a thorough history-taking, physical examination, tailored laboratory work and imaging studies, and neuropsychiatric testing when appropriate permit a probable diagnosis in the majority of cases. In fact, in studies of AD, a diagnosis of "probable" AD was accurate in 90% of cases based on history from the patient and family members in combination with clinical examination.[59] Clinical pathways to assist in the diagnosis of dementia are available.[14]

History

Most patients with dementia do not present with a subjective complaint of memory loss. Rather, a caregiver or family member often raises the concern of memory loss or behavioral change to the practitioner. For example, informants may report that the patient has had trouble remembering events and preparing finances, has gotten lost in familiar settings, cannot find appropriate words, or has been demonstrating unusual behaviors.

Informants play an integral role in helping practitioners understand the onset, nature, and progression of symptoms.

A thorough history-taking also hinges on a systematic review of prescription medications and over-the-counter medication use. Use of medications that may impair cognition such as anticholinergics, psychotropics, and sedative hypnotics should be determined. Performing a functional assessment is another key step in the evaluation of patients with dementia. Functional impairment is often assessed by asking the patient and family members or informants about instrumental ADLs (i.e., managing finances, household chores, and taking medications) and ADLs (i.e., dressing, grooming, and toileting). The Global Deterioration Scale and Functional Assessment Staging is another standardized tool that can be used to measure dementia-related dependency.[60]

Physical Examination

A comprehensive history-taking and functional assessment should be followed by a complete physical examination. During the physical examination, special attention should be given to the neurological examination to evaluate other possible causes of memory impairment. Focal neurological deficits consistent with previous stroke, signs of parkinsonism, and abnormal gait and eye movements may be particularly revealing.

Cognitive Assessment

Although agreement between history and physical examination is suggestive of a diagnosis of dementia, cognitive assessment is necessary to diagnose and differentiate dementia syndromes. Cognitive performance is, however, influenced by numerous factors, not all of which are indicative of dementia. For example, inefficient learning strategies, slowed processing, decreased attention, and sensory deficits may affect results of cognitive testing. Age, education, and demographic factors may alter performance and must be incorporated into analyses of test results.[61]

The Mini-mental Status Examination (MMSE) is the most commonly used screening test for dementia. The examination tests orientation, registration, attention, and calculation, and it is used to diagnose and stratify patients into mild, moderate, and severe dementia. Traditionally, a perfect score is 30; scores of 25–29 suggest MCI; scores 19–24 indicate mild dementia; scores of 15–19 indicate moderate dementia; and, scores 14 or less are consistent with severe dementia. Using a cutoff of 24, the MMSE has a sensitivity of 87% and a specificity of 82% in a large population-based sample.[62] The MMSE is not sensitive to mild dementia and is influenced by age, education, language, and motor and/or visual impairments. Tools that incorporate age, sex, and educational attainment are now available that help to correct the interpretation of these results.[63,64] For example, in patients with less than 9 years of education, a score of 17 or less is consistent with mild, not moderate, impairment.

MMSE testing can be used not only to diagnose cognitive impairment or dementia, but also to follow its progression. Over time, most patients will display a steady deterioration in their MMSE testing scores. For example, in patients with AD, the average decline in MMSE is 2 to 4 points per year. More recently, the MMSE has also been used to assess decision-making competency. Studies suggest that scores higher than 23 or scores lower than 19 are reliable in distinguishing competency from incompetency. Intermediate scores may require a more complete evaluation.[65,66]

The Clock-Drawing Test (CDT) is a quick screen for cognitive impairment, taking less than 5 minutes to perform. During this test, the patient is asked to draw a clock face with all of the numbers and label the face with a specified time, such as "10 minutes to 2 o'clock." The person is given one point for labeling all 12 numbers, 3 points for placing the 12 at the top, 1 point for drawing two hands, and 1 point for correct identification of the time. A score less than 4 is impaired.[67] The CDT is appealing because of ease of administration, but like the MMSE it is not sensitive to mild impairment.[68]

The Mini-Cog is another brief screening test that combines and the CDT and the three-item recall from the MMSE. Patients who recall none of the three words are classified as demented, those who recall all of the three words are nondemented, and those who recall one or two of the three words are classified as either demented or nondemented based on the results of their CDT.[69] A retrospective analysis suggests that the sensitivity and specificity of the Mini-Cog is similar to that of the MMSE.[69] The advantage of the Mini-Cog is its high sensitivity, ease of administration, and lack of influence by the patient's education level.

Neuropsychological testing encompasses a wide array of tests and involves a more extensive evaluation of multiple cognitive domains. In a practice parameter from 2001, the American Academy of Neurology (AAN) concluded that neuropsychological testing is useful in distinguishing MCI from dementia in patients presenting with memory loss and in distinguishing different dementia syndromes. The five instruments deemed most reliable by the AAN were the Animal Naming test, the Modified Boston Naming test, the MMSE, Constructional Praxis, and Word List Memory.[70] An aggregate total score from these five tests has been shown to differentiate accurately patients undergoing normal aging from patients with AD.[71]

Finally, an assessment of premorbid literacy is crucial to determining the extent of dementia in a patient. The National Adult Reading Test involves the pronunciation of 50 English words and has been validated as an estimator of premorbid ability in a study of 80-year-olds.[72] This test is often administered prior to a full neuropsychiatric evaluation.

Laboratory Evaluation

The only laboratory evaluation recommended for all patients with suspected dementia includes screening for hypothyroidism and B12 deficiency.[12] Tailored laboratory evaluation is otherwise guided by clinical findings and may include assessment of the complete blood count, liver function studies, electrolytes, syphilis and Lyme serology, and human immunodeficiency virus status. The cost effectiveness of obtaining multiple laboratory studies has been called into question because of the low likelihood of detecting a reversible dementia.[73]

Genetic Testing

Genetic testing in patients with dementia is not currently recommended.[74] Although screening for the presence of the APO E4 allele has garnered much research interest because it is a known risk factor for AD, its utility as a diagnostic test is limited because not all persons who are homozygotes for the allele develop AD.[75] The potential for harm based on overdiagnosis of the disease is tremendous. Similarly, measurements of Abeta42 protein levels and tau protein levels appear to provide some research benefit, but their clinical value remains unclear.[76]

Neuroimaging

The role of neuroimaging in patients with suspected dementia is in evolution. Although many clinical prediction rules do not recommend routine screening with neuroimaging, the AAN recommends neuroimaging in the initial evaluation of all patients with dementia.[12] The Alzheimer's Association Position Statement recommends the use of MRI in clinical diagnosis of dementia and cognitive impairment to identify small lacunar infarcts, white matter ischemic changes, hippocampal atrophy, and volumetric changes.[77] MRI findings can lend support to a presumed diagnosis; for example, generalized or focal atrophy may be suggestive of AD and white matter lesions may indicate ischemic disease.[12] Several studies suggest that hippocampal atrophy might allow early detection of AD, may help in following the course of the disease, and may guide future treatment decisions.[78,79] The Alzheimer's Disease Neuroimaging Initiative is a large, multisite study that is now underway and is designed to evaluate the specific role of neuroimaging in the diagnosis of AD and in monitoring of progression of MCI.[80]

The use of functional imaging studies, such as PET and single photon emission computerized tomography, in the diagnosis of dementia is also under study. Preliminary findings suggest that functional studies may detect temporoparietal deficits of AD or diffuse irregular deficits of VaD when the clinical history and examination are equivocal. In one study of 146 patients with cognitive symptoms, PET findings were sensitive predictors of the presence of AD and of neurodegenerative disease, in general.[81] In 2005, the Centers for Medicare and Medicaid (CMS) approved reimbursement for fluorodeoxyglucose-PET as an adjunctive diagnostic tool for dementia. There is no evidence, however, that the additional diagnostic accuracy provided by PET leads to improved patient outcomes or cost-effective medical care. At present, The Alzheimer's Association Imaging Position Statement does not advocate routine use of PET imaging for diagnosis of dementia and cognitive impairment.

In the future, neuroimaging may be improved by the use of amyloid imaging tracers. One agent called the Pittsburgh Compound-B has shown good binding to amyloid B peptide (CAA) amyloid deposition in postmortem studies of the human brain and may improve our diagnostic accuracy of dementia.[82]

Brain Biopsy

The brain biopsy as a diagnostic tool has become nearly obsolete. It is rarely used in younger patients with acute onset of cognitive impairment or those with an atypical clinical presentation suggesting a reversible disorder, brain biopsy is invasive, carries a low diagnostic yield, and rarely leads to specific treatment interventions.

Screening Guidelines

Despite the availability of guidelines for the diagnosis of dementia, routine screening of all older adults is not currently recommended. Rather, the U.S. Preventive Services Task Forces, AAN, and Canadian Task Force on Preventive Health has concluded that there is insufficient evidence (1 recommendation) to support routine screening for dementia in older adults.[83] There are insufficient data to support a beneficial effect of early diagnosis and treatment. Also, the feasibility, cost effectiveness, and potential harms of routine screening of all older adults are largely unknown.

Treatment of Dementia

Advances in the understanding of the pathophysiology of dementia have allowed for development of more targeted pharmacological therapies, however, the cornerstone of the management of dementia is still symptomatic and geared largely toward minimizing functional disability, addressing behavioral disturbances, and preventing injury. Despite a number of setbacks, the search for effective disease-specific and disease-modifying therapies holds promise.

Pharmacological Management

Cholinesterase Inhibitors

Destruction of neurons that release the neurotransmitter acetylcholine appears to play a role in the pathogenesis of AD and other dementias. By blocking the enzyme that breaks down acetylcholine, medications that inhibit cholinesterase raise acetylcholine levels in the brain. There are currently four Food and Drug Administration (FDA)–approved cholinesterase inhibitors (ChIs): tacrine, donepezil, rivastigmine, and galantamine. Tacrine was the first agent used in the treatment of AD but carries a risk of hepatotoxicity and is rarely prescribed. Efficacy and tolerability of the other three medications appear to be similar.[84]

The clinical benefit and cost effectiveness of these ChIs is somewhat controversial. The average benefit of patients taking CHIs is a short-term improvement in cognition and ADLs.[85,86] In a meta-analysis of 29 randomized, controlled trials, patients on ChIs improved only 0.1 standard deviations on ADL scales and 0.9 standard deviations on instrumental ADL scales, a change comparable to preventing a 2-month per year decline in a typical patient with AD.[84] The long-term benefit of these medications, such as a delay in nursing home placement, is still unclear.[87,88] The only nonindustry study, AD2000, showed no effect on timing of nursing home placement or progression of disability.[89] Additional evidence suggests that response to ChIs is variable, with 30%–50% of patients experiencing no benefit and a smaller percentage experiencing a significantly greater than average benefit. CHIs appear to be most effective early in the course of dementia, and, in the absence of other options, many patients and families may opt for a trial of this medication.

The most common side effects of these medications are nausea, diarrhea, sweating, bradycardia, and insomnia occurring in 10%–30% of patients. Generally, the medications are titrated over 2–4 weeks to reach the maximum recommended dose. Benefits may extend to 1–2 years; although no symptomatic improvement may be noted, treated patients may function better than they otherwise would without treatment. If the patient, family, and practitioner do not see a response, however, it is reasonable to discontinue the medication. These medications are also often discontinued when patients progress to advanced dementia and are only reintroduced if there is a deterioration following removal.

Disease-Modifying Agents

The search for disease-modifying agents to help slow the progression of AD has been disappointing. In fact, memantine is the only potentially disease-modifying medication that is approved by the FDA in the treatment of dementia.

Memantine (Namenda®) is an N-methyl-D-aspartate receptor antagonist that blocks pathological stimulation of N-methyl-D-aspartate receptors by glutamate and may protect against excitatory neurotoxicity in patients with dementia. Memantine has been shown to have a small clinical benefit on cognition, ADLs, and behavior in patients with moderate or severe AD. This benefit, however, was not seen in patients with mild to moderate AD or in patients with VaD.[90]

Memantine may also be helpful when used in combination with CHIs. One study suggests that patients taking memantine plus donepezil had better outcomes than those taking donepezil plus placebo on scales measuring cognition, ADLs, global outcome, and behavior.[91] It is still unclear if memantine is neuroprotective. The cost effectiveness of memantine is unknown.

In general, memantine is well tolerated; the most common side effect is dizziness. Confusion, hallucinations, and increased agitation have also been noted rarely in patients with AD and DLB. Withdrawal of the medication should be considered if any patient worsens shortly after starting it.[92]

Researchers have investigated the use of antioxidants, such as vitamin E, vitamin C, and selegiline with mixed results.[93–95] Although vitamin E had some positive results at high doses, a recent meta-analysis revealed an increased risk of all-cause mortality, especially with high doses, leading many to abandon vitamin E supplementation.[96]

Investigation into nonsteroidal antiinflammatory drugs (NSAIDs) and estrogen replacement therapy for the prevention and treatment of dementia has also yielded disappointing outcomes.[97] The side-effect profile of NSAIDs led to significant withdrawal rates from studies.[98,99] New evidence of increased risk of cardiovascular events in individuals receiving celecoxib, rofecoxib, and naproxen sodium led to the suspension of a large prevention trial of NSAIDs.[14] Similarly, studies have shown that estrogen replacement therapy does not improve cognitive or functional outcomes in patients with dementia and that hormone replacement therapy may actually increase the risk of developing dementia.

Despite attracting public interest, ginkgo biloba is also not recommended in the treatment of dementia. Although a Cochrane Review of 33 trials showed some efficacy of ginkgo, the studies lacked intention to treat analyses and suffered from methodological errors.[100] Lack of regulation of the herbal extract, including variability in the dosing and contents, has led many experts to discourage its use at least until better data are available.[101]

More recently, one potential disease-modifying treatment, 3-amino-1-propanselfunoic acid (3APS), has garnered a lot of interest among researchers. This compound binds to amyloid B (AB), a toxic protein known to aggregate, leading to amyloid plaque deposition in the brain. Initial studies have shown that this compound is safe, well tolerated, and reduces amyloid B levels in patients with mild-to-moderate AD.[102]

Nonpharmacological Management

Lifestyle

In several small studies, mental activities, such as reading, playing games or puzzles, and playing a musical instrument have been associated with a decreased risk of cognitive impairment.[103–105] Better cognitive function has been demonstrated in both men and women who pursued high levels of long-term physical activity.[106,107] Physical activity also appears to promote functional autonomy as well as nutritional and cognitive status in those with AD.[108–110]

Nutrition

Inadequate nutrition is common in patients with dementia and is associated with increased morbidity and mortality. Oral nutritional supplements may help to offset this risk by increasing weight and fat-free mass.[111]

Risk Factor Reduction

Aggressive identification and treatment of vascular risk factors may also help to slow cognitive decline. Statin use has been hypothesized as a potential agent in the prevention and treatment of dementia; however, support from randomized clinical trials is not yet available.

OTHER MANAGEMENT ISSUES

Behavioral Disturbances

Psychotic and affective disturbances occur in 50%–90% of patients with dementia and account for much of caregiver stress.[112] Aggression, assault, wandering, and loss of recognition of caregiver are predictive of nursing home placement;[113] therefore, attention to these behaviors is paramount in the care of patients with dementia.

Improving communication and patient perception is one strategy to reduce behavioral disturbances. Reduction of sensory impairment is imperative in communicating with demented patients; glasses and hearing aids should always be available and environmental noise and visual disturbances should be minimized. Caregivers should be encouraged to interact with the patient at eye level, avoid threatening stances or gestures, and speak softly and slowly.

Caregiver training to identify antecedents, response, and consequences of a problematic behavior may also be helpful. Using an "ABC" method, caregivers are asked first to identify the antecedents (A) or triggers for certain behavior such as a change in schedule, interpersonal conflict, or physical stressor; once identified, these antecedents can be avoided or minimized. The caregiver is then asked to describe the behavior (B) elicited by the antecedent and to understand when, where, and how often it occurs. Finally, the caregiver notes the consequences (C) of the behavior, such as how the caregivers reinforce or deter the activity and what happens after the behavioral disturbance.[114]

Another strategy to addressing behavioral disturbance approaches the patient from a social, environmental, and medical perspective. The patient's point of view, environmental triggers, and undiagnosed or underrecognized medical diagnoses are evaluated to design patient-specific interventions.[115]

Tailored behavioral strategies may also help to offset particular types of behavioral disturbances. Psychotic symptoms, such as delusions, hallucinations, and paranoia, are present in up to 30% of patients with dementia.[116] These symptoms may be reduced by minimizing change in routine, correcting sensory deficits and improving lighting. Furthermore, physical activity, distraction, and gentle touch may help to win patient trust.

Affective symptoms, such as apathy, depression, anxiety, and sleep disturbance occur in up to one quarter of all demented patients.[112] Depressive symptoms may be modified by avoidance of sad memories, increased social interaction, and increased activity level. Behavioral interventions to minimize sleep disturbance include improving sleep hygiene as well as addressing nighttime pain and nocturia.

Verbally disruptive behaviors, such as screaming, abusive language, and repetition, may result from cortical disinhibition, but may also signal untreated pain, sensory deprivation, or social isolation. Social interaction and sensory stimulation may improve this behavior. Sundowning, or confusion that increases at nighttime, is common among many elderly demented patients, especially in the acute care setting. Food, brief personal contact, music, and improved hearing and vision have been shown to reduce sundowning.[117]

Aggressive behavior particularly during personal care is also common; this behavior is often a self-protective response and may be secondary to confusion or misunderstanding. Helping caregivers to understand that this behavior is not intended to be harmful may be beneficial. Also, employing assistance during bathing and other personal care efforts has been shown to be successful.[118]

Wandering and pacing pose safety issues for many patients with dementia because of the associated potential for getting lost and for injury. Addressing unmet needs such as hunger, pain, and toileting may minimize pacing. Also, engaging the patient in low-risk exercise or structured physical therapy may help to reduce wandering. Finally, continuous supervision may be necessary to ensure patient safety.

In the absence of other effective therapies, antipsychotic medications may be needed to address certain behavioral disturbances. In the setting of acute agitation or aggression that is not responsive to behavioral interventions, haloperidol is often the drug of choice.[119] It may be given as an intramuscular injection (0.5 mg) or in liquid form. If the initial dose is not effective, a second dose may be given 30 minutes later.

For longer-term treatment of behavioral and psychological disturbances, a trial of atypical antipsychotics may be warranted. These agents include clozapine, olanzapine, risperidone, and quetiapine. Several reviews suggest that these agents have, at most, modest efficacy.[120–122] Also, the Clinical Antipsychotic Trial of Intervention Effectiveness study, released in 2006, suggests that adverse effects leading to intolerability may offset advantages in the efficacy of atypical antipsychotic drugs for the treatment of psychosis, aggression, or agitation in patients with AD.[120]

Despite higher expense, atypical antipsychotic agents do have a lower risk of extrapyramidal side effects than traditional antipsychotic medications. Still, adverse events are common with these medications and include extrapyramidal symptoms, somnolence, and gait dysfunction. To offset some of these adverse events, low doses are recommended. Olanzapine is started at 2.5 mg daily and titrated to a maximum of 5 mg twice a day; olanzapine has been associated with significant weight gain and insulin resistance and requires monitoring of fasting blood glucose. Quetiapine is started at 25 mg at bedtime and titrated to a maximum of 100 or 125 mg daily. Risperidone is started at 0.5 mg a day and titrated to 1 mg a day. At higher doses, significant extrapyramidal side effects may become a problem with risperidone. Clozapine is rarely used now because it carries a risk of agranulocytosis and requires frequent blood monitoring.

Despite frequent clinical use, atypical antipsychotic agents are not FDA approved for management of behavioral disorders, and these medications carry an associated mortality risk. In April 2005, the FDA issued a public health advisory about the use of second-generation atypical antipsychotic agents because of increased mortality found in elderly patients taking these medications.[123] A subsequent meta-analysis confirmed these results and concerns have since been raised about the mortality risk of conventional antipsychotics as well.[124,125]

Given the valid safety concerns associated with antipsychotic medications, they should be reserved for the patient who is at imminent risk of harming himself or others. Practitioners must explain the risks and benefits of these medications and obtain informed consent from the patient and/or family members prior to use. Of note, patients with DLB may be particularly sensitive to the extrapyramidal side effects of antipsychotics and their use in these patients should be avoided.

Depression

Depression, presenting with symptoms of low mood, apathy, social withdrawal, and sleep impairment, is seen in many demented patients. Whether depression and dementia share a neurobiological pathway has not yet been fully elucidated, but older patients with these depressive symptoms do benefit from treatment of depression.[126] As with younger patients, psychotherapy in combination with antidepressant medications appears to have the greatest success in older adults.

Selective serotonin reuptake inhibitors (SSRIs) are first-line agents for treating depression in patients with dementia. Despite a paucity of studies comparing specific agents, longer-acting SSRIs, such as Fluoxetine (Prozac®), are usually avoided in the elderly because of an increased risk of side effects. Paroxetine (Paxil®) is the most anticholinergic of the SSRIs and is also generally avoided. In contrast, Sertraline (Zoloft®) and Citalopram (Celexa®) have been shown to be moderately effective in the elderly and are generally well tolerated. Side effects may include nausea and jitteriness.

Tricyclic antidepressants (TCAs) are second-line agents in this population. Despite moderate efficacy in treating depression, TCAs are associated with confusion and additional anticholinergic side effects, and they carry a significant risk of adverse events in this population.

In certain instances, other classes of antidepressants may be considered to address individual patient characteristics. Bupropion (75–150 mg twice daily) can be used in patients who cannot tolerate side effects of other medications or to augment patients who respond only modestly to SSRIs. Side-effect profiles of some antidepressants may also make them appealing choices in certain cases. For example, mirtazapine (7.5–30 mg) improves both sleep and appetite and may help patients who suffer from insomnia and weight loss.[127] Trazodone (25–200 mg) is also very sedative and, therefore, may be helpful in the agitated or sleep-deprived depressed patient, although evidence of its efficacy is limited. Methylphenidate (5–15 mg after meals) is a rapid-onset stimulant that may be useful in apathetic or somnolent depressed patients. Despite their anxiolytic properties, benzodiazepines are generally avoided in this population because of increased cognitive impairment, sedation, and falls.

Safety

One of the most important safety issues to address in patients with dementia is driving. Patients with AD have been shown to have an increased risk of motor vehicle accidents, a risk that increases each year following diagnosis.[128] Early in the disease, many patients are able to drive safely, but with disease progression, it often becomes unsafe to drive.

Discussions of driving cessation are challenging. Losing a driver's license equates to loss of independence for many patients and may signal progression of disability. Many patients are unaware of their deficits and have difficulty accepting the potential danger associated with their driving.

The majority of states do not mandate physician-reporting of patients with dementia to the Department of Motor Vehicles. Still, the majority of physicians refer patients to driver safety evaluations when family members express concern if an office evaluation indicates significant cognitive impairment. Direct reporting of patients to the Department of Motor Vehicles will also enact a system for evaluating the patient's safety to drive, which includes roadside testing with retesting at regular intervals if the patient passes the test.

The AAN has issued guidelines for driving in patients with AD based on the Clinical Dementia Rating (CDR). Based on this guideline, patients with a rating of 1 or greater should not drive an automobile because of significantly increased risk of accidents and driving performance errors.[129]

In addition to driving, cooking may pose a significant safety hazard to patients with dementia because of distractibility, forgetfulness, and impaired judgment. Early use of microwave ovens may help to maintain independence while minimizing risk for injury or fire.

Advance Care Planning

Comprehensive care for the patient with dementia is not complete without addressing advance care planning. The first step in advance care planning involves education of the family or caregiver as to the natural history of the disease. Many families are not aware that dementia carries an average time to death from time of diagnosis of less than 6 years.[26] Preparing patients, families, and caregivers for the progressive and terminal nature of the disease can help to set expectations and focus discussions around end-of-life wishes and goals of care. Early referral to supportive services may also help to allay the stress on the family and/or caregivers. Opening the discussion of end-of-life issues early in the course of disease can give patients the opportunity to designate a health care power of attorney or complete an advance directive or values history if they have not already done so. Discussion of specific wishes of the patient or the proxy decision maker regarding cardiac resuscitation, future hospitalization, antibiotic use, and artificial nutrition are extremely important, often take place over multiple visits, and need to be readdressed regularly.

Placement of feeding tubes in patients with dementia has been an area of intense controversy and deserves special attention. It is important to recognize that difficulty with feeding is often a sign of severe dementia and a marker for a terminal prognosis. Furthermore, artificial hydration and nutrition in patients with advanced dementia has not been shown to prolong life or reduce patient suffering.[130]

Caregivers

Caregivers play a pivotal role in the well-being of persons with dementia. Caregiver stress, however, is nearly universal; this stress has been associated with increased rates of depressive symptoms and sense of burden. It is estimated that 20%–60% of primary family caregivers develop clinical depression.[131,132] The presence of depression in the caregiver is one of the strongest predictors for nursing home placement.[133]

Providing caregiver support is a critical component of caring for the patient with dementia. Teaching caregivers techniques for handling patients with behavioral disturbance has been shown to lessen depressive symptoms in caregivers.[134] Caregiver support programs, respite care, case management, and adult day services may also relieve caregiver stress and enhance caregiver quality of life.[134–136]

Resources for caregivers (see Table 16.4) include the Alzheimer's Association, which is available online at www.alz.org and provides caregiver support group information as well as information on finding missing individuals with dementia. The

Table 16.4. Community Resources

Alzheimer's Organization

Web site: www.alz.org

Phone: 800–621–0379

Administration on Aging

Web site: www.aoa.gov

Eldercare Locator

Web site: www.eldercare.gov/Eldercare/Public/Home.asp

Phone: 800–677–1116

National Association of Home Care

Web site: www.nahc.org

Phone: 202–547–7424

ABA Commission of Legal Problems of the Elderly

Web site: www.abanet.org

Phone: 202–662–8690

U.S. Administration on Aging, accessible at www.aoa.gov, also provides information on state and local area agencies on aging.

REFERENCES

1. American Psychiatric Association. *Diagnostic and Statistical Manual of Mental Disorders.* 4th ed. Washington, DC: APA Press; 1994.
2. Hendrie HC. Epidemiology of dementia and Alzheimer's disease. *Am J Geriatr Psychiatry.* 1998;6:S3–S18.
3. Ebly EM, Parhad IM, Hogan DB, Fung TS. Prevalence and types of dementia in the very old: results from the Canadian Study of Health and Aging. *Neurology.* 1994;44:1593–1600.
4. Mohs RC, Breitner JCS, Silverman JM, Davis KL. Alzheimer's Disease; morbid risk among first-degree relatives approximates 50% by 90 years of age. *Arch Gen Psychiatry.* 1987;44:405–408.
5. Kukull WA, Higdon R, Bowen JD, et al. Dementia and Alzheimer disease incidence; a prospective cohort study. *Arch Neurol.* 2002;59:1737–1746.
6. Hill JW, Futterman R, Duttagupta S, et al. Alzheimer's disease and related dementias increase costs of comorbidities in managed Medicare. *Neurology.* 2002;58:62–70.
7. Ernst RL, Hay JW. The US economic and social costs of Alzheimer's disease revisited. *Am J Public Health.* 1994;84:1261.
8. Chapman DP, Williams SM, Strine TW, Anda RF, Moore MJ. Dementia and Its Implications for Public Health. Available at: www.cdc.gov/pcd/issues/2006/apr/05_0167.htm. Accessed May 25, 2008.
9. Fratiglioni L, Paillard-Borg S, Winblad B. An active and socially integrated lifestyle in late life might protect against dementia. *Lancet Neurol.* 2004;3:343.
10. Simonsick EM. Fitness and cognition: encouraging findings and methodological considerations for future work. *J Am Geriatr Soc.* 2003;51:570.
11. Coyle JT. Use it or lose it – -do effortful mental activities protect against dementia? *NEJM.* 2003;348:2489.
12. Knopman DS, Boeve BF, Petersen RC. Essential of the proper diagnoses of mild cognitive impairment, dementia, and major subtypes of dementia. *Mayo Clin Proc.* 2003;78:1290–1308.
13. Snowden JS. Semantic dysfunction in frontotemporal lobar degeneration. *Dement Geriatr Cogn Disord.* 1999;10(Suppl 1):33.
14. Morris JC. Dementia update 2005. *Alzheimer Dis Assoc Disord.* 2005;19(2):100–117.
15. Bachman DL, Wolf PA, Linn R, et al. Prevalence of dementia and probably senile dementia of the Alzheimer type in the Framingham study. *Neurology.* 1992;42:115.
16. Evans DA. Estimated prevalence of Alzheimer's disease in the United States. *Milbank Q.* 1990;68:267.
17. Evans DA, Funkenstein HH, Albert MS, et al. Prevalence of Alzheimer's disease in a community population of older persons. Higher than previously reported. *JAMA.* 1989;262:2551.
18. Hebert LE, Scherr PA, Bienias JL, et al. Alzheimer disease in the US population: prevalence estimates using the 2000 census. *Arch Neurol.* 2003;60:1119.
19. Whitehouse PJ. Pharmacoeconomics of dementia. *Alzheimer Dis Assoc Disord.* 1997;11:S22.
20. Cummings JL, Vinters HV, Cole GM, Khachaturian ZS. Alzheimer's disease: etiologies, pathophysiology, cognitive reserve, and treatment opportunities. *Neurology.* 1998;51(Suppl 1):S2–S17.
21. Mash DC, Flynn DD, Potter LT. Loss of M2 muscarine receptors in the cerebral cortex in Alzheimer's disease and experimental cholinergic degeneration. *Science.* 1985;228:1115–1117.
22. Cummings JL. Alzheimer's disease. *NEJM.* 2004;351:56.
23. Gandy S. The role of cerebral amyloid beta accumulation in common forms of Alzheimer disease. *J Clin Invest.* 2005;115(5):1121–1129.
24. Tanzi RE. Tangles and neurodegenerative disease – a surprising twist. *NEJM.* 2005;353:1853.
25. Santacruz K, Lewis J, Spires T, et al. Tau suppression in a neurodegenerative mouse model improves memory function. *Science.* 2005;309:476.
26. Larson EB, Shadlen MF, Wang L, et al. Survival after initial diagnosis of Alzheimer disease. *Ann Intern Med.* 2004;140:501–509.
27. Duthie EH, Glatt SL. Understanding and treating multi-infarct dementia. *Clin Geriatr Med.* 1988;4:749–766.
28. Chui HC, Mack W, Jackson E, et al. Clinical criteria for the diagnosis of vascular dementia. A multicenter study of comparability and interrater reliability. *Arch Neurol.* 2000;57:191.
29. Pohjasvaara T, Mantyla R, Ylikoski R, et al. Comparison of different clinical criteria (DSM-III, ADDTC, ICD-10, NINDS-AIREN, DSM-IV) for the diagnosis of vascular dementia. *Stroke.* 2000;31:2952.
30. Erkinjuntl T, Sulkava R. Diagnosis of multi-infarct dementia. *Alzheimer Dis Assoc Disord.* 1991;5:112–121.
31. Hulette C, Nochlin D, McKeel D, et al. Clinical-neuropathologic findings in multi-infarct dementia: a report of six autopsied cases. *Neurology.* 1997;48:668–672.
32. McKhann GM, Albert MS, Grossman M, et al. Clinical and pathological diagnosis of frontotemporal dementia: report of the Work Group on Frontotemporal Dementia and Pick's Disease. *Arch Neurol.* 2001;58:1803–1809.
33. Gislason TB, Sjogren M, Larsson L, Skoog I. The prevalence of frontal variant frontotemporal dementia and the frontal lobe syndrome in a population based sample of 85 year olds. *J Neurol Neurosurg Psychiatry.* 2003;74:867–871.
34. Ratnavalli E, Brayne C, Dawson K, Hodges JR. The prevalence of frontotemporal dementia. *Neurology.* 2002;58:1615–1621.

35. The Lund and Manchester Groups. Clinical and neuropathological criteria for frontotemporal dementia. *J Neurol Neurosurg Psychiatry*. 1994;57:416.

36. Whitwell JL, Jack CR Jr, Senjem ML, Josephs, KA. Patterns of atrophy in pathologically confirmed FTLD with and without motor neuron degeneration. *Neurology*. 2006;66:102.

37. McMurtray AM, Chen AK, Shapira JS, et al. Variations in regional SPECT hypoperfusion and clinical features in frontotemporal dementia. *Neurology*. 2006;66:517.

38. Mendez MF, McMurtray A, Chen, AK, et al. Functional neuroimaging and presenting psychiatric features in frontotemporal dementia. *J Neurol Neurosurg Psychiatry*. 2006;77:4.

39. Vanderzee J, Rademakers R, Engelborghs S, et al. A Belgian ancestral haplotype harbours a highly prevalent mutation for 17q21-linked tau-negative FTLD. *Brain*. 2006;129:841.

40. Mackenzie IR, Baker M, West G, et al. A family with tau-negative frontotemporal dementia and neuronal intranuclear inclusions linked to chromosome 17. *Brain*. 2006;129:853.

41. Huey ED, Putnam KT, Grafman J. A systematic review of neurotransmitter deficits and treatments in frontotemporal dementia. *Neurology*. 2006;66:17.

42. Neary D, Snowden JS, Northen B, et al. Dementia of frontal lobe type. *J Neurol Neurosurg Psychiatry*. 1988;51:353.

43. Hodges JR, Davies RR, Xuereb JH, et al. Clinicopathological correlates in frontotemporal dementia. *Ann Neurol*. 2004;56:399.

44. Eslinger, PJ, Dennis, K, Moore, P, et al. Metacognitive deficits in frontotemporal dementia. *J Neurol Neurosurg Psychiatry*. 2005;76:1630.

45. Campbell S, Stephens S, Ballard C. Dementia with Lewy bodies: clinical features and treatment. *Drugs Aging*. 2001;18:397–407.

46. McKeith IG. Spectrum of Parkinson's disease, Parkinson's dementia, and Lewy body dementia. *Neurol Clin*. 2000;18:865–902.

47. Aarsland D, Andersen K, Larsen JP, et al. Risk of dementia in Parkinson's disease. A community-based, prospective study. *Neurology*. 2001;56:730.

48. Stern Y, Marder K, Tang MX, Mayeux R. Antecedent clinical features associated with dementia in Parkinson's disease. *Neurology*. 1993;43:1690.

49. Emre M. Dementia in Parkinson's disease: cause and treatment. *Curr Opin Neurol*. 2004;17:399.

50. Aarsland D, Perry R, Brown A, et al. Neuropathology of dementia in Parkinson's disease: a prospective, community-based study. *Ann Neurol*. 2005;58:773.

51. Quinn N. Parkinsonism–recognition and differential diagnosis. *BMJ*. 1995; 310:447.

52. Litvan I, Campbell G, Mangone CA, et al. Which clinical features differentiate progressive supranuclear palsy (Steele-Richardson-Olszewski syndrome) from related disorders? A clinicopathological study. *Brain*. 1997;120(Pt 1):65.

53. Verny M, Jellinger KA, Hauw JJ, et al. Progressive supranuclear palsy: a clinicopathological study of 21 cases. *Acta Neuropathol (Berl)*. 1996;91:427

54. Maher ER, Lees AJ. The clinical features and natural history of the Steele-Richardson-Olszewski syndrome (progressive supranuclear palsy). *Neurology*. 1986;36:1005.

55. Wivel ME. NIMH report. NIH consensus conference stresses need to identify reversible causes of dementia. *Hosp Community Psychiatry*. 1988;39:22–23.

56. Clarfield AM. The decreasing prevalence of reversible dementias: an updated meta-analysis. *Arch Intern Med*. 2003;163:2219–2229.

57. Clarfield, AM. The reversible dementias: do they reverse? *Ann Intern Med*. 1988;109:476.

58. Tueth MJ, Cheong JA. Delirium: diagnosis and treatment in the older patient. *Geriatrics*. 1993;48:75–80.

59. Small GW, Rabins PV, Barry PP, et al. Diagnosis and treatment of Alzheimer's disease and related disorders. *JAMA*. 1997;278:1363–1371.

60. Auer S, Reisberg B. The GDS/FAST system. *Int Psychogeriatr*. 1997;9:167–171.

61. Folstein M, Anthony JC, Parchad I, et al. The meaning of cognitive impairment in the elderly. *J Am Geriatr Soc*. 1985;33:228–235.

62. Freidl W, Schmidt R, Stronegger WJ, et al. Mini-Mental State Examination: influence of sociodemographic, environmental and behavioral factors and vascular risk factors. *J Clin Epidemiol*. 1996;49:73.

63. Grigoletto F, Zappala G, Anderson DW, et al. Norms for the mini-mental state examination in a healthy population. *Neurology*. 1999;53:315.

64. Dufouil C, Clayton D, Brayne C, et al. Population norms for the MMSE in the very old: estimates based on longitudinal data. *Neurology*. 2000;55:1609.

65. Karlawish JH, Casarett DJ, James, BD, et al. The ability of persons with Alzheimer disease (AD) to make a decision about taking an AD treatment. *Neurology*. 2005;64:1514.

66. Pruchno RA, Smyer MA, Rose MS, et al. Competence of long-term care residents to participate in decisions about their medical care: a brief, objective assessment. *Gerontologist*. 1995;35:622.

67. Stahelin HB, Monsch AU, Spiegel R. Early diagnosis of dementia via a two-step screening and diagnostic procedure. *Int Pyschogeriatr*. 1997;9:123–130.

68. Powlishta KK, Von Dras DD, Stanford A, et al. The clock drawing test is a poor screen for very mild dementia. *Neurology*. 2002;59:898.

69. Borson S, Scanlan J, Brush M, et al. The mini-cog: a cognitive 'vital signs' measure for dementia screening in multi-lingual elderly. *Int J Geriatr Psychiatry*. 2000;15:1021.

70. Petersen RC, Smith GE, Ivnik RJ, et al. Apolipoprotein E status as a predictor of the development of Alzheimer's disease in memory-impaired individuals. *JAMA*. 1995;273:1274–1278.

71. Chandler MJ, Lacritz LH, Hynan LS, et al. A total score for the CERAD neuropsychological battery. *Neurology*. 2005;65:102.

72. McGurn B, Starr JM, Topfer JA, et al. Pronunciation of irregular words is preserved in dementia, validating premorbid IQ estimation. *Neurology*. 2004;62:1184.

73. Weyting MD, Bossuyt PM, van Crevel H. Reversible dementia: more than 10% or less than 1%? A quantitative review. *J Neurol*. 1995;242:466.

74. American College of Medical Genetics/American Society of Human Genetics Working Group on ApoE and Alzheimer disease. Statement on use of apolipoprotein E testing for Alzheimer disease *JAMA*. 1995;274:1627.

75. Henderson AS, Easteal S, Jorm AF. Apolipoprotein E allele epsilon 4, dementia, and cognitive decline in a population sample. *Lancet*. 1995;346:1387.

76. Galasko D. Cerebrospinal fluid biomarkers in Alzheimer disease: a fractional improvement? *Arch Neurol*. 2003;60:1195.

77. Albert M, DeCarli C, DeKosky S, et al. *The Use of MRI and PET for the Clinical Diagnosis of Dementia and Investigation of Cognitive Impairment: Consensus Report*. Available at: http://www.alz.org/national/documents/Imaging_consensus_report.pdf. Accessed May 25, 2008.

78. Killiany RJ, Gomez-Isla T, Moss M, et al. Use of structural magnetic resonance imaging to predict who will get Alzheimer's disease. *Ann Neurol*. 2000;47:430.

79. Adak S, Illouz K, Gorman W, et al. Predicting the rate of cognitive decline in aging and early Alzheimer disease. *Neurology.* 2004;63:108.

80. Mueller SG, Weiner MW, Thal LJ, et al. The Alzheimer's disease neuroimaging initiative. *Neuroimag Clin N Am.* 2005;15:869–877.

81. Silverman DH, Small GW, Chang CY, et al. Positron emission tomography in evaluation of dementia: Regional brain metabolism and long-term outcome. *JAMA.* 2001;286:2120.

82. Klunk WE, Engler H, Nordberg A, et al. Imaging brain amyloid in Alzheimer's disease with Pittsburgh Compound-B. *Ann Neurol.* 2004;55:306–319.

83. Boustani M, Peterson B, Hanson L, et al. Screening for dementia in primary care: a summary of the evidence for the U.S. Preventive services task force. *Ann Intern Med.* 2003;138:927.

84. Trinh NH, Hoblyn J, Mohanty, S, et al. Efficacy of cholinesterase inhibitors in the treatment of neuropsychiatric symptoms and functional impairment in Alzheimer disease. A meta-analysis. *JAMA.* 2003;289:210.

85. Kaduszkiewicz H, Zimmermann T, Beck-Bornhold HP, et al. Cholinesterase inhibitors for patients with Alzheimer's disease: systematic review of randomised clinical trials. *BMJ.* 2005;331:321.

86. Doody, RS, Stevens, JC, Beck, C, et al. Practice parameter: management of dementia (an evidence-based review). Report of the Quality Standards Subcommittee of the American Academy of Neurology. *Neurology.* 2001;56:1154.

87. Geldmacher DS, Provenzano G, McRae T, Mastey V, Ieni JR. Donepezil is associated with delayed nursing home placement in patients with Alzheimer's disease. *J Am Geriatr Soc.* 2003;51:937–944.

88. Grossberg GT. The ABC of Alzheimer's disease: behavioral symptoms and their treatment. *Int Psychogeriatr.* 2002;14(Suppl 1):27–49.

89. Courtney C, Farrell D, Gray R, et al. Long-term donepezil treatment in 565 patients with Alzheimer's disease (AD2000): randomized double-blind trial. *Lancet.* 2004;363:2105.

90. McShane R Areosa Sastre A, Miakaran N. Memantine for dementia. *Cochrane Database Syst Rev.* 2006;2. External Accession Number CD003154.

91. Ridha BH, Josephs KA, Rossor MN. Delusions and hallucinations in dementia with Lewy bodies: worsening with memantine. *Neurology.* 2005;65:481.

92. Reisberg B, Doody R, Stoffler A, et al. Memantine in moderate-to-severe Alzheimer's disease. *NEJM.* 2003;348:1333.

93. Laurin D, Foley DJ, Masaki KH, et al. Vitamin E and C supplements and risk of dementia. *JAMA.* 2002;288:2266–2268.

94. Zandi PP, Anthony JC, Khachaturian AS, et al. Reduced risk of Alzheimer disease in users of antioxidant vitamin supplements: the Cache County Study. *Arch Neurol.* 2004;61:82–88.

95. Morris MC, Evans DA, Bienias JL, et al. Dietary intake of antioxidant nutrients and the risk of incident Alzheimer disease in a biracial community study. *JAMA.* 2002;287:3230–3237.

96. Miller ER, Pastor-Barriuso R, Dalal D et al. Meta-analysis: high dosage vitamin E supplementation may increase all-cause mortality. *Ann Intern Med.* 2005;142:37–46.

97. Aisen PS, Saumier D, Briand R, et al. A Phase II study targeting amyloid-B with 3-APS in mild-to-moderate Alzheimer disease. *Neurology.* 2006;67:1757–1763.

98. Scharf S, Mander A, Ugoni A, Vajda F, Christophidis N. A double-blind, placebo-controlled trial of diclofenac/misoprostol in Alzheimer's disease. *Neurology.* 1999;53:197–201.

99. Rich JB, Rasmusson DX, Folstein MF, Carson KA, Kawas C, Brandt J. Nonsteroidal anti-inflammatory drugs in Alzheimer's disease. *Neurology.* 1995;45:51–55.

100. Birks J, Grimley EV, Van Dongen M. Ginkgo biloba for cognitive impairment and dementia. *Cochrane Database Syst Rev.* 2002;CD003120.

101. Angell M, Kassirer JP. Alternative medicine – the risks of untested and unregulated remedies. NEJM. 1998;339:839.

102. Aisen PS, Schafer KA, Grundman M, et al. Effects of rofecoxib or naproxen vs. placebo on Alzheimer disease progression: a randomized controlled trial. *JAMA.* 2003;289:2819–2826.

103. Wilson RS, Mendes De Leon CF, Barnes LL, et al. Participation in cognitively stimulating activities and risk of incident Alzheimer Disease. *JAMA.* 2002;287:742–748.

104. Wilson RS, Bennett DA, Bienias JL, et al. Cognitive activity and incident AD in a population-based sample of older persons. *Neurology.* 2002;59:1910–1914.

105. Verghese J, Lipton RB, Katz MJ, et al. Leisure activities and the risk of dementia in the elderly. *NEJM.* 2003;348:2508–2516.

106. Weuve J, Kang JH, Manson JE, et al. Physical activity, including walking, and cognitive function in older women. *JAMA.* 2004;292:1454–1461.

107. Van Gelder BM, Tijhuis MAR, Kalmijn S, et al. Physical activity in relation to cognitive decline in elderly men; the FINE study. *Neurology.* 2004;63:2316–2321.

108. Teri L, Gibbons LE, McCurry SM, et al. Exercise plus behavioral management in patients with Alzheimer disease: a randomized controlled trial. *JAMA.* 2003;290:2015–2022.

109. Rolland Y, Rival L, Pillard F, et al. Feasibility of regular physical exercise for patients with moderate to severe Alzheimer disease. *J Nutr Health Aging.* 2000;4:109–113.

110. Dvorak RV, Poehlman ET. Appendicular skeletal muscle mass, physical activity, and cognitive status in patients with Alzheimer's disease. *Neurology.* 1998;51:1386–1390.

111. Lauque S, Arnaud-Battandier F, Gillette S, et al. Improvement of weight and fat-free mass with oral nutritional supplementation in patients with Alzheimer's disease at risk of malnutrition: a prospective randomized study. *J Am Geriatr Soc.* 2004;52:1702.

112. Lyketsos CG, Steinberg M, Tschanz JT, et al. Mental and behavioral disturbances in dementia. *Am J Psychiatry.* 2000;157:708–714.

113. Coleridge, PT, George LK. Predictors of institutionalization among caregivers of patients with Alzheimer's disease. *J Am Geriatr Soc.* 1986;34:493–498.

114. Teri L, Rabins P, Whitehourse P, et al. Management of behavior disturbance in Alzheimer disease: current knowledge and future directions. *Alzheimer Dis Assoc Disord.* 1992;6:77–88.

115. Roca RP. Managing the behavioral complications of dementia. In: Cobbs EL, Duthie EH, Murphy JB, eds. *Geriatric Review Syllabus: A Core Curriculum in Geriatric Medicine.* 4th ed., Iowa: Kendall/Hunt; 1999:183–186.

116. Mega MS, Cummings JL, Fiorello T, et al. The spectrum of behavioral changes in Alzheimer's disease. *Neurology.* 1996;46:130.

117. Cohen-Mansfield J, Werner P. Management of verbally disruptive behaviors in nursing home residents. *J Gerontol Med Sci.* 1996;52:M369–M377.

118. Sloane PD, Hoeffer B, Mitchell CM, et al. Effect of person-centered showering and the towel bath on bathing-associated aggression, agitation, and discomfort in nursing home residents with dementia: a randomized, controlled trial. *J Am Geriatr Soc.* 2004;52:1795.

119. Lonergan, E, Luxenberg, J, Colford, J. Haloperidol for agitation in dementia. *Cochrane Database Syst Rev.* 2002. External Accession Number CD0003154.

120. Schneider LS, Tariot PN, Dagerman KS, et al. for the CATIE-AD Study Group. Effectiveness of atypical antipsychotic drugs in patients with Alzheimer's disease. *NEJM.* 2006;355:1525–1538.

121. Sink KM, Holden KF, Yaffe K. Pharmacological treatment of neuropsychiatric symptoms of dementia: a review of the evidence. *JAMA*. 2005;293:596.

122. Lee PE, Gill SS, Freedman M, et al. Atypical antipsychotic drugs in the treatment of behavioural and psychological symptoms of dementia: systematic review. *BMJ*. 2004;329:75.

123. Kuehn, BM. FDA warns antipsychotic drugs may be risky for elderly. *JAMA*. 2005;293:2462.

124. Schneider LS, Dagerman KS, Insel P. Risk of death with atypical antipsychotic drug treatment for dementia: meta-analysis of randomized placebo-controlled trials. *JAMA*. 2005;294:1934.

125. Wang PS, Schneeweiss S, Avorn J, et al. Risk of death in elderly users of conventional vs. atypical antipsychotic medications. *NEJM*. 2005;353:2335

126. Bains, J, Birks, JS, Dening, TR. The efficacy of antidepressants in the treatment of depression in dementia. *Cochrane Database Syst Rev*. 2002;CD003944.

127. Burrows G, Kremer C. Mirtazipine: clinical advantages in the treatment of depression. *Psychopharmacology*. 1997;17(Suppl): 34S–39S.

128. Drachman DA, Swearer JM. Driving and Alzheimer's disease: the risk of crashes [published erratum appears in *Neurology*. 1994;44:4]. *Neurology*. 1993;43:2448.

129. Dubinsky RM, Stein AC, Lyons K. Practice parameter: risk of driving and Alzheimer's disease (an evidence-based review): report of the quality standards subcommittee of the American Academy of Neurology. *Neurology*. 2000;54:2205.

130. Gillick MR. Rethinking the role of tube feeding in patients with advanced dementia. *NEJM*. 2000;342:206–210.

131. Cohen D, Eisdirfer C. Depression in family caring for a relative with Alzheimer's disease. *J Am Geriatr Soc*. 1988;36:885–889.

132. Gallagher D, Rose J, Rivera P, et al. Prevalence of depression in family caregivers. *Gerontologist*. 1989;29:449–456.

133. Arai Y, Sugiura M, Washio M, Miura H, Kudo K. Caregiver depression predicts early discontinuation of care for disabled elderly at home. *Psychiatry Clin Neurosci*. 2001;55:379–382.

134. Belle SH, Burgio L, Burns R, et al. Enhancing the quality of life of dementia caregivers from different ethnic or racial groups. *Ann Intern Med*. 2006;145:727–738.

135. Newcomer R, Yordi C, DuNah R, Fox P, Wilkinson A. Effects of the Medicare Alzheimer's Disease Demonstration on caregiver burden and depression. *Health Serv Res*. 1999;34:669–689.

136. Gaugler JE, Jarrott SE, Zarit SH, Stephens MA, Townsend A, Greene R. Respite for dementia caregivers: the effects of adult day service use on caregiving hours and care demands. *Int Psychogeriatr*. 2003;15:37–58.

137. Kennedy GJ. Dementia. In: Cassel CK, Leipzig R, Cohen HJ, Larson EB, Meier DE. eds. *Geriatric Medicine: An Evidence-Based Approach*. 4th ed. New York: Springer-Verlag; 2003:1074–1093.

17

CLINICAL GEROPSYCHIATRY

John M. Tomkowiak, MD

INTRODUCTION

Unfortunately, the stigma that pervades mental health care in general is exacerbated when discussing mental health issues in the elderly. Statements such as, "If I were that old I would feel tired too" or "If all my friends were dying I would be depressed too" are all too often heard. This demonstration of ageism, which refers to the unfair judging of the elderly adult simply because of their advanced age, is important in medicine because a negative attitude may influence physicians' aggressiveness toward the diagnosis and treatment of the elderly patient.[1–3] Many older adults are already conditioned to accept functional and cognitive decline as an inevitable part of the aging process, and even more troubling is that many health care professionals may perpetuate this concept and mistake the symptoms that can accompany serious illness as part of that inevitable decline.[4]

Nearly 20% of individuals 55 years and older experience a mental disorder that is not a part of normal aging. The most common disorders, in order of prevalence, are anxiety, severe cognitive impairment, and mood disorders. It is estimated, however, that only half of older adults who acknowledge mental health problems receive treatment from any health care provider, and only approximately 3% of those receive specialty mental health services.[5] According to the American Association of Geriatric Psychiatry, over half of older persons who receive mental health care receive it from their primary care physicians. This makes it imperative that primary care services include evaluation for the mental disorders of late life.

There are several considerations when thinking about mental health in the elderly. Many elderly with mental health disorders will have had a long-standing history of mental illness. Chronic mental illness carries a significant physical, mental, and functional burden. When combined with other factors that elderly patients bring to the table, the potential for adverse outcomes is high. The elderly can also experience mental health problems for the first time in late life. Unfortunately, symptoms related to mental illness are all too often overlooked or attributed to old age. Critical diagnoses can be missed secondary to stereotypical beliefs and ageist attitudes, leaving reversible and/or treatable problems untreated.

Diagnosis of mental illness is particularly difficult in the elderly for a number of reasons. The elderly are more likely to have comorbid medical conditions, which may overlap the symptoms of mental illness. The prevalence of other medical problems also makes older patients more likely to be taking multiple prescriptions and over-the-counter medications. These medications, or combinations of medications, can actually be the cause of psychiatric symptoms. It can be an extremely complicated task to sort out the cause of symptoms as they may result from a primary mental illness, secondary to a medical illness, or secondary to medications.

The elderly experience various psychosocial stressors during the normal process of aging, which can lead to the onset of psychiatric symptoms. These include financial difficulties, changes in living situations, the loss of independence, and the loss of family and loved ones.

So what can we do as health professionals to care better for the elderly? There are five concepts that every health provider should understand and practice in taking better care of the mental health in the elderly. 1) If we do not look for mental illness, then we will not find it. 2) Focusing on patient functioning as opposed to complete symptom resolution will likely improve patient outcomes. 3) Inquire about suicidality. 4) A thorough history-taking is vital in determining the appropriate diagnosis and treatment. 5) If the patient is in a caregiving situation, the risk of mental illness is increased.

EVALUATION: IF WE DO NOT LOOK FOR IT, WE MAY NOT SEE IT!

Mr. Aldanado is a 72-year-old man with longstanding well-controlled hypertension who is taking hydrochlorothiazide. He comes to an outpatient office complaining of feeling more tired. He specifically denies feeling sad. "I just feel exhausted," he remarks.

The completion of a thorough mental health assessment is critical to the development of a successful treatment plan. In this case scenario, the first question may be "How many times has this complaint been voiced?" We have already asked the patient if he feels sad. Have we done enough to screen for mental illness in this patient?

Evidence demonstrates that only 50% of elderly patients with moderate-to-severe depressive symptoms will report their symptoms to a physician.[6] Of course, this means that 50% do not! Elderly patients also have chronic medical illnesses that may produce symptoms similar to the ones that are used to diagnose depression. These symptoms include decreased concentration, fatigue, change in appetite, or a change in sleep.[7] The health care provider is faced with the following dilemma: Are the symptoms caused by major depression or are they related to the chronic illness? Obviously this is hard to determine, but we clinicians should have a high level of suspicion for a depressive disorder in these patients.[8]

After further history-taking, Mr. Aldanado states that he has been having trouble with early insomnia and has gained 8 lb over the last 3 months. He has not changed his blood pressure medicine and he denies taking any over-the-counter remedies.

The fact that elderly patients may have a more complicated clinical picture with potentially overlapping symptoms presents us with an opportunity to develop some sound practices when dealing with elderly patients. The first of these is establishing an accurate timeline of symptom development. Health care providers should be reflecting on the answers to questions such as: Are current symptoms attributable to changes in medication dosage or administration, such as hypokalemia caused by hydrochlorothiazide? Are current symptoms attributable to changes in underlying chronic medical conditions? Were current symptoms present before or after a particular psychosocial stressor?

When asked if he has felt this way before Mr. Aldanado says, "no." when specifically asked if he was ever diagnosed with major depression, however, he responds, "Yeah, when I was in my 40s. But that was nothing like this."

It is important to ask specifically about diagnosis of psychiatric disorders early in life. In some cases psychiatric illness may present with a different symptom complex in early episodes. The elderly patient may not connect their current symptoms with their past psychiatric diagnosis.[9] Past medical records can also be extremely helpful with regard to obtaining this information. This is especially true when screening for other medical problems. Evidence suggests that medical records in some organ system areas (e.g., cardiovascular) gave better information regarding specific diagnosis than self-reported interviews whereas interview data from patients provided a

Table 17.1. Keys to Evaluating Mental Health Disorders in the Elderly

- Know symptom specific differences in disease presentation
- Develop an accurate timeline for symptom initiation
- Obtain psychiatric illness history (importance of medical records)
- Gather information from family/friends*
- Take a good substance abuse history

*Always get consent from the patient first.

better assessment of functional impairment and health in general.[9]

We then ask Mr. Aldanado if it would be all right to bring his wife into the room to ask her some questions concerning his symptoms. He readily agrees. When his wife is asked how Mr. Aldanado has been doing, she responds, "I'm really concerned about him. He's mentioned a few times in the last week that he would be better off dead."

Family and friends who accompany patients are potential sources of information. It is often tempting to cut corners on obtaining consent in this population. A provider must always gain consent from the patient to collect this information, and consent should be obtained when the patient is alone and not in the presence of the other informants. Information solicited from family or friends can often be enlightening and even help solidify a diagnosis; however, the same kinds of confidentiality issues that hold true for younger adults need to be observed for this population.

Lastly, alcohol is the drug that is most commonly abused by elderly patients, and a thorough substance abuse history should be obtained. The prevalence of heavy drinking (12–21 drinks per week) among older adults is estimated at 3%–9%.[10] Alcohol intake is definitely an area in which obtaining information from family members can be enlightening. See Table 17.1 for a summary of items necessary for an effective evaluation of mental illness in the elderly. The remainder of this chapter will focus on the most common mental health disorders and issues encountered in the elderly.

EVIDENCE-BASED PRACTICE IN GERIATRIC MENTAL HEALTH CARE

Reports vary on the prevalence of mental disorders in the elderly but conservatively suggest that 20% of the elderly population has at least one mental health disorder;[11] other estimates suggest the prevalence of mental health disorders is as high as 37% when looking at patients who present to primary care settings. It seems, in general, elderly persons report better overall mental health when compared with younger adults.[12] This chapter will break the mental health diagnoses into three major categories: mood disorders, anxiety disorders, and psychotic disorders. We will also look at suicide and other treatment issues related to the elderly. Other important categories such as dementias and substance abuse are being covered in other chapters of this book.

Mood Disorders Overview

The mood disorder group includes the diagnoses of major depression, dysthymia, bipolar disorder, cyclothymia, mood disorders resulting from general medical condition, and substance-induced mood disorders. Other diagnoses in the mood disorder spectrum would include subsyndromal depression (depression that fails to meet the full diagnostic criteria), adjustment disorders, and bereavement.

Major Depression

Major depression and subsyndromal depression are two of the most common psychiatric disorders diagnosed in the elderly. Major depression is associated with significant morbidity and mortality and has also been found to be a significant risk factor in the recovery from other major medical conditions such as heart disease.[13] Researchers have reported that depression in the elderly population is frequently underdiagnosed and undertreated. In one study, the diagnosis was missed in approximately half of all elderly persons who presented with symptoms of a mood disorder.[14]

What can we health practitioners do to diagnose depression more accurately in elderly patients? Mood disorders in the elderly often present with multiple vague somatic complaints, and patients may have medical conditions that account for some of the complaints. If there is a sudden change in the overall number of complaints, in the severity of complaints, or a significant change in functioning, it is important to look closer for the mood diagnosis. A study of elderly inpatients with major depression concluded that three quarters had at least one comorbid medical condition on hospital discharge, and almost half of the patients had two. Comorbid physical illness and cognitive impairment have been negatively associated with depressed elderly patients' functional impairment at discharge.[15]

Accurately identifying the comorbid conditions and referring the patient to the appropriate health care provider is an important step in managing their mental health. Conversely, patients who have medical conditions such as cardiovascular disease, stroke, and hip fracture who are slow to recover, seem to be resistant to treatment, or have extremely poor compliance might also be at risk for suffering from a mood disorder and the mood disorder diagnosis should be thoroughly examined.

DEPRESSION TREATMENT

Ms. Jones is an 88-year-old woman who has a history of major depression previously treated with imipramine. She most recently was diagnosed with a right bundle branch block. She describes a current textbook episode of major depression, and would like to be given another trial of imipramine because it was so successful in the past.

Over the last 10 years, more and more pharmacotherapy treatment options have become available to the health care professional. The serotonin and norepinephrine reuptake inhibitors seem to be as effective as the tricyclic antidepressants (TCAs) with, in some cases, a more favorable side-effect profile.[16] There is some suggestion that older patients respond as well as younger patients to antidepressant medication, but more slowly.[17] Patients who rate their overall health as fair or poor are at greater risk of not responding to a usual treatment regimen.[18] Starting at half the usual dose of younger adults is a standard approach; however, ultimate final doses can vary widely depending on the patient. A common mistake is not to advance the dose of medication to a higher level after a partial response and an appropriate amount of time. Common medication side effects of all antidepressants to consider include drowsiness, agitation, appetite change, and anticholinergic side effects. Anticholinergic side effects such as urinary retention, blurred vision, and constipation are particularly troublesome in the elderly and occur more commonly with TCAs such as imipramine and amitriptyline. In addition, anticholinergic side effects may add to the confusion in patients already suffering from dementia. TCAs also have quinidine-like properties and can cause prolongation of the PR and QRS intervals and make them more dangerous in overdose attempts.

Adverse side effects among the selective serotonin reuptake inhibitors (SSRIs) are very similar, regardless of the medication, with paroxetine and sertraline having a minimally less potential for orthostatic hypotension than the other SSRIs, and paroxetine having a slightly higher potential for weight gain. Although the SSRIs appear to be better tolerated overall, providers must be vigilant for the development of hyponatremia,[19] as well as serotonin syndrome, which causes lethargy, flushing, confusion, tremor and, in extreme cases, renal failure and death. The elimination half-life varies among SSRIs with fluoxetine having a half-life of 2–3 days with a long elimination half-life (7–9 days) of its active metabolite, norfluoxetine. In patients who are on medications with a long half-life, extra consideration should be given when switching medications. In addition, monitoring for drug–drug interactions should occur even after the medication has been stopped. Finally, secondary to the potentially serious interaction between SSRIs in general and monoamine oxidase inhibitors, it is advisable to stop taking one medication from 2 to 5 weeks before starting the other, depending on the specific medications involved.

Another consideration in the elderly is treatment compliance. A recent study that evaluated differences in compliance between adult patients initiating an SSRI found that, overall, more than 50% of patients were deemed to be noncompliant with antidepressant therapy over a 6-month period. The results of the study also highlighted that the SSRI agents were not equivalent in compliance to therapy. After adjusting for baseline covariates in this study, the rate of compliance for the immediate-release SSRI agents was significantly lower than the rate of compliance for controlled-release paroxetine (13.6% lower).[20] Finally, other antidepressants commonly used in the adult population that might be used in appropriate elderly patients include venlafaxine (Effexor®), mirtazapine (Remeron®) bupropion (Wellbutrin®), and duloxetine (Cymbalta®).

Psychotherapy is also an appropriate and effective treatment modality in the elderly. Psychotherapy was found to be more effective than no treatment or placebo in a meta-analysis of 17 studies of psychotherapy interventions in elderly patients with depression.[21] Expert consensus suggests that a combination of medication and psychotherapy, such as cognitive behavioral therapy, might yield the best results in the elderly.[22]

In the elderly, one has to consider further the impact of depression on activities of daily living and physical activity. This is especially important in the cohort of the oldest old (>85 years).[23] In addition, this population may have more recurrences of symptoms during maintenance therapy.[24] For our patient Ms. Jones who was described at the beginning of this section, the best option would *not be* to restart Ms. Jones on imipramine because of the potential for worsening her heart block. Choosing another class such as an SSRI, combining this treatment with supportive psychotherapy, and monitoring frequently during her maintenance stage would be preferred.

Bereavement

Studies suggest that as many as 30% of bereaved individuals will develop major depression during the first year following spousal death. Although bereavement itself is a normal process, it can progress into a full-blown major depression. Caregivers might specifically be at risk after the death of the care recipient.[25] It is common in patients who are experiencing normal grieving to report sadness, appetite disturbance, sleep disturbance, and difficulty concentrating. If, however, excessive guilt, feelings of worthlessness, psychomotor retardation, hallucinations, or persistent suicidal thoughts are present for more than 2 weeks, a diagnosis of major depression should be considered. In general, the clinical literature suggests that less than 25% of bereaved spouses who meet the criteria for major depression are treated with an antidepressant. There are no antidepressants that are specifically indicated, and so the usual treatment considerations for the elderly would apply.

Bipolar Disorder

Ms. Johnson is a 71-year-old woman diagnosed with bipolar disorder who has been successfully treated with lithium 450 mg three times a day. She presents with her husband who complains that over the last 2 days she has become "loopy." Further history-taking reveals they have been working in their yard quite a bit (in the middle of summer), and examination reveals that Ms. Johnson is disorientated to time and place.

Elderly patients with bipolar disorder are a small subset of patients who have affective disorders but account for a disproportionate amount of resources in terms of hospitalizations and cost.[26] Unlike the psychotic disorders, which seem to have a decrease in symptoms with aging, bipolar patients continue to be symptomatic into old age.[27] There is evidence suggesting that with increasing age, bipolar patients are less responsive to treatment.[28] Bipolar patients seem to have more problems with cognitive impairment, and this leads to poorer overall functioning and a greater need for more intensive care.

Bipolar disorder is diagnosed when a patient has had at least one full-blown manic episode. Depressive episodes are also common and many patients diagnosed with bipolar disorder have primarily depressive symptoms. The most common age range in which bipolar disorder first appears is the late teens and early 20s, but it can, in rare cases, occur as a primary illness in the elderly. When a manic episode is diagnosed, care must be taken to rule out medical and drug causes of mania. Substance abuse issues are common in this illness and can make it more difficult to diagnose, as can cognitive impairments that might be present in the elderly. Some patients may be willing to report episodes of depression but will not report episodes of mania because they do not feel they are ill when they are manic.

TREATMENT

There have been very few studies related to the treatment of bipolar disorder in the elderly. The primary treatment of this illness is the use of a mood stabilizer. It is important to realize that patients exhibiting only depressive symptoms may become manic after starting an antidepressant. If a depressed patient has a history of a manic episode at any time in their past, they must be started on a mood stabilizer prior to starting antidepressant therapy. Lithium, which is the gold standard treatment in bipolar disorder, should be used cautiously in the elderly population.[29] Studies have shown that elderly patients need 25%–50% of the usual dose given to younger patients. Because lithium is excreted by the kidneys, elderly patients have an increased susceptibility to toxicity, especially in the summer time when sodium is easily secreted in sweat, and lithium blood levels can rise quickly. Other mainstay treatments in younger adults such as valproic acid have shown some promise, but few controlled studies in geriatric patients have been performed.[30] Recent research suggests that lamotrigine, a newer anticonvulsant, may be helpful.[31] Additionally, preliminary reports on the use of clozapine, risperidone, olanzapine, and quetiapine suggest a role for the use of these agents in late-life bipolar disorder, but more data will need to be collected before definitive recommendations can be made.[32]

Ms. Johnson is probably lithium toxic and may need hospitalization. A lithium blood level should be performed and her lithium should be held until the blood levels fall. Because she has been successfully treated with lithium in the past, it is reasonable to restart her on lithium but with one quarter the dose and frequent monitoring of blood levels, especially during summer, when the patient may be active.

Anxiety Disorders Overview

Ms. Smith is a 65-year-old woman who presents with feelings of anxiety, constant worry, muscle aches and pains, irritability, and difficulty sleeping for 6 months. She states, "I just can't stop worrying."

Anxiety disorders in the elderly, like mood disorders, have been found to be associated with disability, impairment in quality of life, and an increased mortality rate. Anxiety disorders are common in the elderly and often go undiagnosed. Studies have shown that among older adults, anxiety disorders occur anywhere from two to seven times more often than depression problems such as major depressive disorder. This suggests that anxiety disorders are a very real and relatively common problem among older adults experiencing mental health problems.[33] The overall prevalence rates for any anxiety symptoms may be as high as 20%, with the prevalence of anxiety disorders among adults aged 65 years and older being approximately 5.5%.[33] Rates for anxiety disorders may be even higher among elderly adults living in institutional settings such as nursing homes. Older adult women are twice as likely to have an anxiety disorder than older men. Common anxiety disorders include generalized anxiety disorder (GAD), panic disorder (PD), posttraumatic stress disorder (PTSD), obsessive–compulsive disorder, and phobias. Overall phobias and obsessive symptoms seem to be less prominent in the elderly.

GAD and obsessive–compulsive disorder seem to present similarly in later life as in younger adults, but PD and PTSD have slightly different presentations.[34] Late-onset PD appears to be milder with less arousal, less avoidance, and overall higher functioning. Elderly patients with PTSD have less avoidance, dissociation, intrusive symptoms, and survivor guilt, but more estrangement from other people.

The lifetime prevalence of PTSD is 8% in the general population and the incidence in the elderly is thought to be somewhat less frequent. Elderly patients may experience new-onset PTSD or may have developed the disorder previously in life, especially war veterans. A history of a traumatic life event, even if it is not recent, should prompt a thorough review of PTSD symptomatology. Although PTSD presents similarly in younger adults and the elderly, the elderly may experience more intense symptoms of hyperarousal. The symptoms of PTSD may worsen later in life, even in patients who previously had periods of time in which they were symptom free. The loss of social support structure, increased time to think about past experiences, and a decreased ability to control the activities of daily life may lead to increased exposure to traumatic cues or memories.

TREATMENT

There is little evidence related to pharmacotherapy and its effectiveness in the elderly for treatment of anxiety disorders. Traditionally, benzodiazepines have been the treatment of choice for most anxiety disorders. This treatment approach is concerning secondary to the sedating properties and potential longer half-life in the elderly population. For this reason, the use of benzodiazepines that are directly conjugated in the liver (lorazepam, oxazepam, and temazepam) are preferable in older adults.[35] Still benzodiazepines should be used sparingly in this population not only because of the deleterious effects on cognition and the risk of sedation, but also for the addiction potential as well. For GAD, buspirone produces significantly less sedation and has been found to be helpful in anxious older

patients. For PD, SSRIs are the treatment of choice; however, jitteriness in some patients may make symptoms worse. These symptoms may dissipate after a couple of weeks of treatment, but if symptoms continue, or the SSRI makes the patient's symptomatology worse, then alternatives should be found.

Psychotherapy can be helpful when dealing with anxiety disorders. Anxiety management, cognitive therapy, and exposure therapy are the therapies most commonly utilized with the elderly. Anxiety management includes techniques such as relaxation training, thought stopping, positive thinking, and assertiveness training. Psychotherapy alone may be useful for mild cases of acute or chronic PTSD. Severe cases of PTSD may require the addition of pharmacotherapy. When this is the case, antidepressants, particularly SSRIs and venlafaxine are the recommended initial treatment of choice.

Ms. Smith most likely is suffering from GAD. Combination therapy with buspirone and cognitive therapy would be an appropriate initial treatment approach.

Psychotic Conditions

Mr. Delany is a 72-year-old man who has been happily married for 52 years. His wife brings him in for a visit because lately he is getting very angry with her. He paces around the house and yells at her for "cheating" on him. He recently told an appliance repairman that he could not "see" his wife anymore. The patient's wife is exasperated.

Psychotic conditions in the elderly vary widely with prevalence, being fairly low in community samples, but higher in nursing home populations. These disorders are characterized by either auditory or visual hallucinations or delusions. Although patients can carry chronic mental illnesses into old age, acute psychotic disorders or psychosis secondary to other illness are the predominate diagnoses in the elderly.

Psychosis associated with major depression, dementia, Parkinson's disease, substance abuse, and delirium is common in the elderly, diagnoses of schizophrenia and delusional disorder are less common. Many drugs can cause psychosis in susceptible elderly patients, common offenders being anti-Parkinson compounds, anticholinergics, and steroids. Behavioral disturbances are common in the psychotic elderly and these behaviors are often the reason patients are brought to the attention of health care providers. Patients who have psychosis secondary to another primary condition are less likely to have suicidal ideation and behavior than patients with a primary psychotic disorder such as schizophrenia or delusional disorder.

Schizophrenia is thought to have an incidence of approximately 1% in the elderly. Although this number is small, the economic burden of late-life schizophrenia is high. Approximately 75% of the elderly schizophrenia patients are thought to have developed symptoms in adulthood and continue to have symptoms in old age, whereas 25% of these patients have very late onset schizophrenia.[36] In general, it is thought that schizophrenia symptoms are diminished somewhat with advancing age, although sustained remission may be less frequent than previously thought.[37] Women in their 60s are at greater risk to

Table 17.2. Suicide Risk in the Elderly

➤ Significant Risk Factors

■ Elderly white men >85 y in highest risk category

■ Mental disorders (especially major depression)

■ Family discord

➤ Ask: "Do you have thoughts of killing yourself?"

➤ Ask: "Do you ever feel like you would be better off dead?"

➤ Ask: "Do you own a firearm or have access to one?"

---

develop a delusional disorder and may be reluctant to seek treatment secondary to the paranoia that is often present.[38]

Pharmacotherapy directed at psychotic symptoms usually begins at a low dose. Hallucinations and/or delusions may not change in intensity for 3–4 weeks after starting treatment. Initial reduction in symptom intensity is usually attributed to the sedating properties of antipsychotic medications. Newer atypical antipsychotic medications such as olanzapine, quetiapine, and risperidone have been shown to be effective in reducing psychotic symptoms in the elderly, while having somewhat lesser risk for extrapyramidal side effects.[39–41] Frequent concerns with these medications include the risk of orthostasis, sedation, and developing diabetes mellitus type II with prolonged use. There is also some evidence that suggests an increased risk of cerebrovascular events with the use of olanzapine and risperidone in the elderly, especially those older than the age of 80 years, who have a dementing diagnosis. Caution should be used with these drugs in that population.[42] In addition, all of the newer atypical antipsychotics (aripiprazole [Abilify®], clozapine [Clozaril®], olanzapine [Zyprexa®], quetiapine [Seroquel®], risperidone [Risperdal®], ziprasidone [Geodon®], and the olanzapine/fluoxetine combination [Symbyax®]) have a black box warning that there is an increased mortality rate in elderly patients with dementia-related psychoses.[43]

Clozapine is another medication that is effective in younger adults, but because of the potential for increased incidence of agranulocytosis in the older population, it is not considered a first-line drug.[44] Ziprasidone, has had limited study in the elderly and concerns over increasing the QTc interval usually lead to this drug not being used as a first-line agent.[45]

Mr. Delany is paranoid and having delusions of jealousy, a common symptom in elderly patients with psychosis. A thorough investigation of medication changes and other primary illnesses should be made. Starting the patient on a low dose of an atypical antipsychotic such as risperidone would be a good first option.

Suicide in the Elderly

Suicide is a disproportionate cause of death in the elderly population (Table 17.2). It remains a significant cause of mortality, especially in white men older than the age of 85 years. Even

more concerning is the potential that these numbers are probably underreported because there may be "silent suicides" (i.e., medication overdoses and "accidents"). Elderly people who do not comply with life-saving medical treatment (e.g., such as insulin for diabetes) or who stop eating may be indirectly attempting to commit suicide. What should health providers really know and understand about this condition?

Studies have demonstrated that on average 58% of older adults who commit suicide have seen a primary care provider within 1 month of suicide, and 75% within 1 year.[46] Elderly suicide victims are more likely to have an axis I psychiatric diagnosis (91%),[47] with major depression being the most common diagnosis. Elderly patients who appear to be overwhelmed, anxious, sad, or agitated warrant a basic inquiry into their mental health. If any suicide risk factors are present, suicide ideation should be asked about directly. Questions should address both active suicidal ideation, "Have you thought about killing yourself?" and passive suicidal ideation, "Do you ever have thoughts that you would be better off dead?" Additionally, because firearms are a primary means by which suicide is attempted in this population, additional questions about firearm ownership and access to firearms should be asked.[48] Evaluation of suicide risk also includes asking about details of a person's plan (e.g., what would you do? how? and when?). A person with a suicide plan or thoughts of suicide should be referred to a mental health professional for evaluation; if the suicide plan is lethal and immediate (e.g., I will shoot myself with a gun tonight and I have the gun and bullets), they should be taken for evaluation right away.

Suicide in the old elderly (>75 years): There are a number of risk factors that have been identified in this age group. Those factors include: loneliness, family conflict, serious physical illness, and both major and subsyndromal depression.[49] Psychosocial risk factors for suicide in the elderly suggest that a history of mental disorders and family discord are also significant risk factors for suicide in this population.[50] The old-elderly who successfully commit suicide are less likely to have had treatment for depression, thus emphasizing the importance of identifying these disorders in this population. One large multisite trial with elderly patients demonstrated that when patients with suicidal ideation and depressive symptoms were followed by a Master's level depression care manager, there was a significant reduction in suicidal ideation and improvement in symptoms.[51]

Psychotherapy and Other Therapies

Psychotherapy is the treatment, by psychological means, of problems of an emotional nature in which a trained person deliberately establishes a professional relationship with the patient with the object of 1) removing, modifying, or retarding existing symptoms, 2) mediating disturbed patterns of behavior, and 3) promoting positive personality growth and development.[52] The most frequently practiced psychotherapies in the elderly are supportive psychotherapy, brief psychotherapy, interpersonal psychotherapy, cognitive behavioral psychotherapy, problem-solving therapy, and occasionally group therapy.

What are the conditions for which elderly patients are most often referred for psychotherapy? Bereavement and depression are at the top of the list. Psychotherapy is also often used in this population to treat other disorders such as dysthymia, generalized anxiety disorder, PD, PTSD, substance abuse, and early dementia. In addition, psychotherapy can be helpful in addressing stress and behavior problems (e.g., insomnia) that may not be associated with a specific mental illness. Finally, therapy has been shown to reduce pain among nursing home patients.

A meta-analysis of 17 studies of psychotherapy interventions in elderly patients with depression found psychotherapy to be more effective than no treatment or placebo.[21] In addition, psychotherapy in combination with medication often provides optimal treatment for depression in the elderly. It is important to note that issues such as decreased social support, financial difficulties, and hearing and/or vision problems, although not unique to the elderly, can play a significant role in a patient's ability to engage successfully in therapy. Because the literature shows that almost 50% of elderly men have difficulty hearing and 20% have problems with vision, it is important to assess the sensory limitations of a patient prior to beginning therapy. Similarly, memory impairment is common with approximately 10% of people older than 65 years having some problems with memory and more than 33% of those older than the age of 85 years having moderate problems with memory. Psychotherapy can be useful for patients with mild cognitive impairment; however, in patients with moderate cognitive impairment it is usually not helpful. Psychotherapy can play a significant role in the appropriate recovery of elderly patients with depression and other mental health problems. Benefits of psychotherapy include the reduction of stress, decrease in pain, and positive effects on other medical conditions that an individual may have. Finally, finding a therapist who works with elderly patients and knows a variety of therapeutic techniques will more likely produce a good outcome.

Electroconvulsive therapy (ECT): ECT is the treatment of choice for many depressed older persons. It can be a rapid, effective form of treatment for the patient and is safer than antidepressant management in the frail elderly patient.[53] Despite fears and active myths surrounding ECT, it is a life-saving modality that can be used on an inpatient or outpatient basis without risk of major complications. There are no absolute contraindications to ECT but increased intracranial pressure is a relative contraindication.

Regardless of the type of therapy utilized, management plans for older adult patients with mental health issues should be driven by the medical and psychological assessment findings. The symptoms that are present on patient assessment are important because they are predictive of the response to treatment.

Cultural Issues in Maintaining Mental Health in the Elderly: According to the Surgeon General's report little is known about cultural differences and mental health. Some research has suggested that African Americans may have higher rates of cognitive impairment but a lower incidence of mood disorders.[54] Similarly, few differences in rates of depression have been found in older Asian Americans. One area where cultural differences need to be recognized is in the area of psychosis. Cultural acceptance of certain beliefs, for example, sorcery, possession, and witchcraft, may very well be consistent in a specific patient's culture. Not only identification of these differences in patients presenting with current symptoms, but also reevaluation of mental health disorders in relation to their culture is warranted.[55]

Treatment Issues in Patients Who Have Severe Life-long Mental Illness: When contemplating the care of patients who have severe life-long mental illness the health care practitioner needs to consider additional factors. Medication monitoring should always include strategies to place patients on the minimum medication dosages that can successfully control their symptoms. The minimum dose may change over time; occasional dosage reductions after a period of stability should be attempted after discussing with the patient the risks and benefits of doing so. Continued psychoeducation of patients is a common practice that is often overlooked. Patients should be made aware of advances in our understanding of the disorders as well as new treatment options that may have become available over the course of their illness. In addition, a recent study suggested that even though patients may understand their illness is a chronic condition, patients want their care providers to be optimistic and provide hope for their recovery.[56] Finally, new symptomatology should not be assumed to be a part of the patients' previously diagnosed condition. Because comorbidity of psychiatric conditions is common in patients with life-long mental illness, a thorough investigation of other possible causes for the symptoms should be made.

Psychosocial considerations become especially important in aging patients with chronic mental illness. Many times these patients are living with family or friends who themselves are older. When these caregivers die, patients may experience significant stress from the loss itself and also from potential living situation disruptions.[57] Planning for loss and alternative living arrangements can help ease this incredibly stressful time for these patients. Finally, a collaborative model of care that includes all the providers engaged in care of the patient as well as the utilization of available community resources can be the difference between relapse and treatment success.

REFERENCES

1. Dale DC. Poor prognosis in elderly patients with cancer: the role of bias and undertreatment. *J Support Oncol.* 2003;1(4 Suppl 2):11–17.
2. Williams D, Bennett K, Freely J. Evidence for an age and gender bias in the secondary prevention of ischaemic heart disease in primary care. *Br J Clin Pharmacol.* 2003;55:604–608.
3. Uncapher H, Arean PA. Physicians are less willing to treat suicide in older patients. *J Am Geriatr Soc.* 2000;48:188–192.

4. Alliance for Aging Research. Medical Never-Never Land: Ten Reasons Why America is not Ready for the Coming Age Boom. Washington, DC. US Senate Special Committee on Aging, pp. 8–9. URL: www.agingresearch.org/content/article/detail/698/.

5. Lebowitz BD, Pearson JL, Schneider LS, et al. Diagnosis and treatment of depression in late life. Consensus statement update. *JAMA.* 1997;278:1186–1190.

6. O'Connor DW, Rosewarne R, Bruce A. Depression in primary care 1: elderly patients' disclosure of depressive symptoms to their doctors. *Int Psychogeriatr.* 2001;13:359–365.

7. American Psychiatric Association: *Diagnostic and Statistical Manual of Mental Disorders.* 4th ed. Washington, DC: American Psychiatric Association, 2000.

8. Drayer RA, Mulsant BH, Lenze EJ, et al. Somatic symptoms of depression in elderly patients with medical comorbidities. *Int J Geriatr Psychiatry.* 2005;20:973–982.

9. Wilhelmson K, Rubenowitz LE, Andersson C, Sundh V, Waern M. Interviews or medical records, which type of data yields the best information on elderly peoples' health status? *Aging Clin Exp Res.* 2006;18:25–33.

10. Liberto JG, Oslin DW, Ruskin PE. Alcoholism in older persons: a review of the literature. *Hosp Community Psychiatry.* 1992;43:975–984.

11. Jeste DV, Alexopoulos GS, Bartels SJ, et al. Consensus statement on the upcoming crisis in geriatric mental health: research agenda for the next two decades. *Arch Gen Psychiatry.* 1999;56:848–853.

12. Centers for Disease Control and Prevention. *The State of Aging and Health in America 2004.* Available at: http://www.cdc.gov/aging/pdf/State_of_Aging_and_Health_in_America_2004.pdf. Accessed May 28, 2008.

13. Mallik S, Krumholz HM, Lin ZQ, et al. Patients with depressive symptoms have lower health status benefits after coronary artery bypass surgery. *Circulation.* 2005;111:271–277.

14. Mulsant BH, Ganguli M. Epidemiology and diagnosis of depression in late life. *J Clin Psychiatry.* 1999;60 (Suppl 20):9–15.

15. Proctor EK, Morrow-Howell NL, Dore P, et al. Comorbid medical conditions among depressed elderly patients discharged home after acute psychiatric care. *Am J Geriatr Psychiatry.* 2003;11:329–338.

16. Bartles SJ, Dums AR, Oxman TE, et al. Evidence-based practices in geriatric mental health care: an overview of systematic reviews and meta-analyses. *Psychiatry Clin North Am.* 2003;26:971–990.

17. Reynolds CF, Frank E, Kupfer DJ, et al. Treatment outcome in recurrent major depression: a post hoc comparison of elderly ("young old") and midlife patients. *Am J Psychiatry.* 1996;153:1288–1292.

18. Miller MD, Schultz R, Paradis C, et al. Changes in perceived health status of depressed elderly patients treated until remission. *Am J Psychiatry.* 1996;153:1350–1352.

19. Strachan J, Shepard J. Hyponatraemia associated with use of selective serotonin re-uptake inhibitors. *Aust NZ J Psychiatry.* 1998;32:295–298.

20. Keene MS, Eaddy MT, Mauch RP, et al. Differences in compliance patterns across the selective serotonin reuptake inhibitors (SSRIs). *Curr Med Res Opin.* 2005;21:1651–1659.

21. Scogin F, McElreath L. Efficacy of psychosocial treatments for geriatric depression: a quantitative review. *J Consult Clin Psychol.* 1994;62:69–74.

22. Alexopoulos GS, Katz IR, Reynolds CF, Carpenter D, Docherty JP. Pharmacotherapy of depressive disorders in older patients. *Expert Consensus Guideline Series.* Oct. 2001:1–86.

23. Blazer DG. Psychiatry and the oldest old. *Am J Psychiatry.* 2000;157:1915–1924.

24. Reynolds CF, Frank E, Dew MA, et al. Treatment of 70+-year-olds with recurrent major depression. *Am J Geriatr Psychiatry.* 1999;7:64–69.

25. Rebollo P, Alonso J, Ramon I, et al. For the 'Dying Elderly in Catalonia' Study Group. Health-related quality of life during the bereavement period of caregivers of a deceased elderly person. *Qual Life Res.* 2005;14:501–509.

26. Bartels SJ, Forester B, Miles KM, Joyce T. Mental health service use by elderly patients with bipolar disorder and unipolar major depression. *Am J Geriatr Psychiatry.* 2000;8:160–166.

27. Angst J. Clinical typology of bipolar illness, in Mania: an Evolving Concept. Ed: Belmaker RH, van Praag HM. Lancaster MTP Press. SP Medical & Scientific Books, NYC, 1980.

28. Young RC, Falk NR. Age, manic psychopathology, and treatment response. *Int J Geriatr Psychiatry.* 1989;4:73–78.

29. Eastham JH, Jeste DV, Young RC. Assessment and treatment of bipolar disorder in the elderly. *Drugs Aging.* 1998;12:205–224.

30. Young RC, Gyulai L, Mulsant BH, et al. Pharmacotherapy of bipolar disorder in old age. *Am J Geriatr Psychiatry.* 2004;12:342–357.

31. Sajatovic M, Gyulai L, Calabrese JR, et al. Maintenance treatment outcomes in older patients with bipolar I disorder. *Am J Geriatr Psychiatry.* 2005;13:305–311.

32. Sajatovic M, Madhusoodanan S, Coconcea N. Managing bipolar disorder in the elderly: defining the role of the newer agents. *Drugs Aging.* 2005;22:39–54.

33. Stanley MA, Beck JG. Anxiety Disorders. *Clin Psychol Rev.* 2000;20:731–754.

34. Wetherall JL, Maser JD, van Balkom A. Anxiety disorders in the elderly: outdated beliefs and a research agenda. *Acta Psychiatr Scand.* 2005;111:401–402.

35. Sheikh JI, Cassidy EL. Treatment of anxiety disorders in the elderly: issues and strategies. *J Anxiety Disord.* 2000;14:173–190.

36. Jeste DV, Twamley EW. Understanding and managing psychosis in late life. *Psychiatric Times.* XX (3). 2003;20:19–22.

37. Auslander LA, Jeste DV. Sustained remission of schizophrenia among community-dwelling older outpatients. *Am J Psychiatry.* 2004;161:1490–1493.

38. Targum SD. Treating psychotic symptoms in elderly patients. *Primary Care Companion J Clin Psychiatry.* 2001;3:156–163.

39. Mintzer J, Targun S. Psychosis in elderly patients: classification and pharmacotherapy. *J Geriatr Psychiatry Neurol.* 2003;16:199–206.

40. Barak Y, Shamir E, Zemishlani H, Mirecki I, Toren P, Weizman R. Olanzapine vs. haloperidol in the treatment of elderly chronic schizophrenia patients. *Prog Neuropsychopharmacol Biol Psychiatry.* 2002;26:1199–1202.

41. Madhusoodanan S, Sinha S, Brenner R, Gupta S, Bogunovic O. Use of olanzapine for elderly patients with psychotic disorders: a review. *Ann Clin Psychiatry.* 2002;13:201–213.

42. Royal College of Psychiatrists, Royal College of General Practitioners, British Geriatric Society, et al. (2004). *Guidance for the Management of behavioural and psychiatric symptoms in dementia and the treatment of psychosis in people with history of stroke/TIA following CSM restriction on Respiridone and Olanzapine.* Faculty of the Psychiatry of Old Age, Royal College of Psychiatrists.

43. Howard R. Late-onset schizophrenia and very late-onset schizophrenia-like psychosis. In: Jacoby R, Oppenheimer C, eds. Psychiatry in the Elderly. Oxford: Oxford University Press; 2002:744–761.

44. U.S. Food and Drug Administration. Atypical antipsychotic drugs information. Available at: http://www.fda.gov/cder/drug/infopage/antipsychotics/default.htm. Accessed May 28, 2008.

45. Greco KE, Tune LE, Brown FW, van Horn WA. A retrospective study of the safety of intramuscular ziprasidone in agitated elderly patients. *J Clin Psychiatry.* 2005;66:928–929.

46. Luoma JB, Martin CE, Pearson JL. Contact with mental health and primary care providers before suicide: a review of the evidence. *Am J Psychiatry.* 2002;159:909–916.

47. Henriksson MM, Marttunen MJ, Isometsa ET, et al. Mental disorders in elderly suicide. *Int Psychogeriatr.* 1995;7:275–286.

48. Gorina Y, Hoyert D, Lentzner H, Goulding M. Trends in causes of death among older persons in the United States. U.S. Department of Health and Human Services, Center for Disease Control and Prevention, National Center for Health Statistics. www.cdc.gov/nchs/data/ahcd/agingtrends/06olderpersons.pdf.

49. Waern M, Rubenowitz E, Wilhelmson K. Predictors of suicide in the old elderly. *Gerontology* 2003;49:328–334.

50. Rubenowitz E, Waern M, Wilhelmson K, Allebeck P. Life events and psychosocial factors in elderly suicides – a case-control study. *Psychol Med.* 2001;31:1193–1202.

51. Bruce ML, Ten Have TR, Reynolds CF, et al. Reducing suicidal ideation and depressive symptoms in depressed older primary care patients. *JAMA.* 2004;291:1081–1091.

52. Wolberg LR. *The Technique of Psychotherapy.* New York: Grune & Stratton; 1977.

53. Cole SA. Mood misorders. In: Noble J, ed. Primary Care Medicine. St. Louis: Mosby-Year Book; 1996:1738–1747.

54. Kales HC, Blow FC, Bingham CR, Copeland LA, Mellow AM. Race and inpatient psychiatric diagnoses among elderly veterans. *Psychiatric Serv.* 2000;51:795–800.

55. Faison WE, Armstrong D. Cultural aspects of psychosis in the elderly. *J Geriatr Psychiatry Neurol.* 2003;16:225–231.

56. Lester QT, Sorohan H. Patients' and health professionals' views on primary care for people with serious mental illness: focus group study. *BMJ.* 2005;330:1122.

57. Lefley HP, Agnes BH. Helping parental caregivers and mental health consumers cope with parental aging and loss. *Psychiatric Serv.* 1999;50:369–375.

18

Alcohol and Other Drug Abuse in Older Patients

Richard D. Blondell, MD, Lynne M. Frydrych, MS, Rita M. Sawyer, MSN

Acknowledgments: This work was supported, in part, by grant K23-AA015616 from the National Institute on Alcohol Abuse and Alcoholism (RDB and LMF).

INTRODUCTION

Alcohol and drug use disorders are significant problems among older patients. These problems may be underappreciated by health care professionals because of limited clinical evidence and research data to form practice guidelines, insufficient training, and rushed office visits that tend to focus on acute and chronic physical problems, which can easily consume all the clinician's attention leaving little time to screen, diagnose, and perform an intervention for a substance use disorder.

Diagnosis of a substance use disorder can be difficult in the older patient. Embarrassment, shame, and fear of disapproval by family members may lead older individuals to conceal their drinking or drug use. Family members, who would be unlikely to ignore alcohol or drug abuse in a young person, may tolerate alcohol or drug abuse in an older person because they may think that after a long life the person "deserves it," or that "it makes no difference anyway." Family members may also believe that an oversedated elderly patient is "more manageable." Furthermore, the signs and symptoms of substance abuse often mimic the clinical presentation of other common medical or psychiatric disorders and health care providers may perceive their diagnostic role as being directed mainly toward the chief complaint.[1]

Definitions

There is a confusing array of terms used to describe individuals who use and misuse alcohol and other drugs: "alcohol abuse," "alcoholism," "chemical dependency," "drug addiction," and "substance abuse." These descriptions depend on biological, psychological, and social consequences of repeated self-administration of alcohol and/or drugs. These terms vary with the context of their use and may mean different things to the lay public, law enforcement officials, and nonmedical or medical professionals.

A dichotomous diagnostic approach is taken by the International Classification of Diseases and in the *Diagnostic and Statistical Manual of Mental Disorders*, 4th ed.[2] These disease-oriented approaches are useful for coding medical records, research data, and medical billing, and therapeutic interventions focus on disease-oriented control or cures. *Substance abuse* is defined as a maladaptive pattern of substance use leading to a pattern of clinically significant impairment over a 12-month period. It is associated with repeated use in hazardous situations resulting in recurrent social, interpersonal, or legal problems and failure to fulfill major life obligations. *Substance dependence* is characterized by a maladaptive pattern of substance use over a 12-month period plus at least three of the following: tolerance; evidence of withdrawal; use of larger amounts or use over a longer period than intended; persistent desire or unsuccessful efforts to cut down; a great deal of time spent in drinking or drug-related activity; a loss of important social, occupational, or recreational activities as a result of use; or substance use despite knowledge of having a persistent or recurrent physical or psychological problem resulting from the use of substances. It should be noted that this definition does not include amounts/quantities used.

A health risk approach is taken by the National Institutes of Health (NIH) and the World Health Organization (WHO), which assert that substance use is a continuum ranging from limited use to highly excessive abuse and therapeutic interventions focus on "harm reduction." The NIH uses the terms, "at-risk," "alcohol-related problems," and "alcohol dependent,"[3] but WHO also includes the term "hazardous use."[4] In the United States, the threshold for "at-risk" use, as defined by the NIH, for all persons aged 65 years or older and for younger women is more than seven drinks per week or more than three drinks on any given day. "One drink" is considered to be 12 oz of regular beer, 5 oz of table wine, or 1.5 oz of distilled spirits, which all contain approximately 12 g of ethanol. There is some evidence to suggest that these drinking levels for older men are too restrictive and that the levels could be closer to those for younger men (14 drinks per week with a maximum or 4 in any given day).[5]

Basic Pharmacology

Psychoactive substances exhibit the objective pharmacological phenomenon of behavioral reinforcement, tolerance, and physical dependence.[6] *Behavioral reinforcement* is produced by a mood-altering substance that creates an artificial state of reward leading to compulsive substance use mediated by neural mechanisms, which are now only beginning to be understood. *Tolerance* refers to the progressive decrease in the sensitivity to the effects of a substance with repeated use such that a greater quantity of a substance is required to achieve the same effect or that the same quantity produces a lesser effect. *Physical dependence* may develop over time as the central nervous system's adaptation to frequent/heavy use of many, but not all mood-altering substances. This adaptation is revealed as a withdrawal syndrome when the intake stops. The nature of the withdrawal syndrome varies with the substance. Agitation, seizures, and hallucinations may occur with alcohol withdrawal; mydriasis, vomiting, diarrhea, and piloerection may occur with opioid withdrawal; and hypersomnolence is frequently seen with stimulant withdrawal. Alcohol pharmacokinetics (i.e., absorption, metabolism, and excretion) are not appreciably altered with increasing age;[7] however, changes in body composition may influence the effects of alcohol in the elderly. Compared with younger people, the elderly have a larger proportion of body fat, and this may explain the finding that older men achieved a 20% higher peak in blood alcohol concentration following an intravenous administration of a similar amount of alcohol than did younger men.[8] Age-related decreases in hepatic or renal function may affect the pharmacokinetics of drugs. For example, decreased liver function may prolong the half-live of a benzodiazepine, especially those with active metabolites (e.g., diazepam).

Prevalence

It is difficult to quantify objectively alcohol use and determine exactly when abuse occurs. The prevalence of alcohol problems depends on the study population selected and the definitions used. In a national household survey of 87,915 participants, 55% of those aged 50 years or older consumed alcohol, but the prevalence of alcohol dependence was 1.6%.[9] In another study of over 12,000 elderly primary care patients, 15% were found to engage in excessive alcohol consumption.[10] In a similar study of 3,954 primary care patients, the prevalence was 10.6%.[11] Among 865 community-dwelling elderly individuals living in

public housing 4% were current problem drinkers, but the lifetime prevalence was 22%.[12]

Illicit drug use is not common among older patients; however, they are often prescribed controlled substances, and it is difficult to determine precisely when appropriate prescription drug use evolves from frequent use to misuse, to abuse, to dependence and finally to addiction. For example, one study found that the life-time prevalence of illicit drug dependence was less than 1% for those aged 60 years or older.[13] The misuse of prescription drugs, however, can pose as much of a health problem among older patients as it does in young patients. For example, in 2005, the rate of visits to hospital emergency departments for the nonmedical use of opioids was approximately 30/100,000 for those aged 55 or older; a rate similar to the 12–22 year age group.[14] Furthermore, there may be a cohort effect. As members of the "baby boom" generation age, those who abused illicit drugs when they were young may be likely to abuse prescription drugs when they are elderly. Therefore, overall rates of drug abuse may be expected to increase. It has been estimated that the demand for substance abuse treatment services in older persons will increase by 70% from 1.7 million in 2001 to 4.4 million by the year 2020.[15] Typically, however, older patients are less likely than younger adults to view their substance misuse as problematic, indicating the need for clinicians to consider routinely substance abuse among one of the possible diagnoses for the older patient.[16]

Etiology

The etiology of substance use disorders is not known. Estimates of heritability from twin studies suggest that up to a third of the variance observed for alcohol use disorders is under genetic control.[17] Learned behaviors also appear to be important in the maintenance of substance use problems.[18]

SCREENING, DIAGNOSIS, AND INITIAL TREATMENT

Recommendation: "The U.S. Preventive Services Task Force (USPSTF) recommends screening and behavioral counseling interventions to reduce alcohol misuse by adults, including pregnant women, in primary care settings." (Level B, Systematic review) [19]

The basic clinical approach of older patients with drug or alcohol problems is similar to that of any other chronic preventable disease; it can be summarized by the "5 A's: Ask, Assess, Advise, Assist, and Arrange."

Ask: Screening for Alcohol and Drug Problems

There are many screening questionnaires available for clinical use. The 25-question Michigan Alcohol Screening Test has been available for more than three decades.[20] Although useful

Table 18.1. ASK: Screening for Alcohol Problems among Older Patients

Question	Positive Response
1. Have you ever had a problem with alcohol?	Yes
2. When was the last time you had any drink containing alcohol?	Within past month
3. On average, how many days per week do you drink alcohol?	*
4. On a typical day when you drink, how many drinks do you have?	*
5. What is the maximum number of drinks you have had on any given occasion during the last month?	More than 4
6. Have you ever felt that you should *Cut* down on your drinking?	Yes
7. Have people *Annoyed* you by criticizing your drinking?	Yes
8. Have you ever felt bad or *Guilty* about your drinking?	Yes
9. Have you ever had a drink first thing in the morning to steady your nerves or get rid of a hangover? *(Eye-opener)*	Yes

Either question 1 or 2 can be used as an opening question. Questions 3 through 5 relate to the quantity and frequency of drinking, whereas questions 6 through 9, the "CAGE questions," relate to the patterns and consequences of drinking. Drinking in excess of low-risk levels or a positive response to any of the CAGE questions suggests the possibility of an alcohol problem.

* An at-risk drinking level for older adults is more than seven drinks per week or more than three drinks in a given day. One "standard drink" is equal to 12 oz of regular beer, 5 oz of wine, or 1.5 oz of distilled spirits.

Adapted from: *Helping Patients with Alcohol Problems: A Health Practitioner's Guide.* Rockville, MD: National Institute of Alcohol Abuse and Alcoholism, US Dept of Health and Human Services; 2003. NIH Publication No. 03–3769.

in research settings, it is somewhat cumbersome to use in clinical settings. This led to the development of a 13-item questionnaire, the Short Michigan Alcohol Screening Test.[21] A 24-question version has also been designed for use with a geriatric population.[22] An international group associated with the WHO developed the Alcohol Use Disorders Identification Test, a 10-item questionnaire that can be used throughout a multitude of cultures across different age groups.[23] A series of short questions, however, may have more use in clinical situations than formal screening questionnaires.[3] These are summarized in Table 18.1. Either of the first two questions (i.e., "Have you ever had a problem with alcohol?" or "When was the last time you had any drink containing alcohol?") can be asked of older patients; additional questions are only pertinent if there is a positive response to one of the first two.

There is no current evidence to either support or oppose routine screening for drug abuse.[24] In routine clinical encounters, however, certain "clues" noted during the medical history or physical examination may suggest problematic substance use (see Table 18.2) and should trigger further assessment. Screening instruments for drug use disorders have been developed including the CAGE-Adapted to Include Drugs (CAGE-AID), which contains alcohol screening questions that were modified to assess drug problems as well.[25] For example, the question "Have you ever felt bad or guilty about your drinking?" was changed to "Have you ever felt bad or guilty about your drinking or drug use?" One study reported that the CAGE-AID was able to discriminate both alcohol and drug users from

controls in individuals older than the age of 50 years and that it was "well-suited" in screening for alcohol as well as drug abuse in geriatric patients.[26] Pharmacy records can be obtained to quantify the number and dosages of tablets dispensed, or in jurisdictions where they are available, governmental electronic pharmacy dispensing datasets can be queried, which often yield useful information.[27]

Assess: Clinical Assessment and Diagnosis

A clinical assessment can be performed for diagnostic purposes if screening or clinical suspicion suggests a drug or alcohol use disorder. The recent patient history, medical history, family and social history, the physical examination, routine laboratory tests, or diagnostic images can provide clues about the severity of a substance use disorder. These are summarized in Table 18.2.

It may be difficult for health care professionals, family members, and even patients themselves to recognize a substance use disorder until the consequences have become catastrophic, particularly among older women.[28] Death rates of women with drinking problems are twice those for men.[29] Benzodiazepines have been associated with health problems among older individuals including: femur fractures,[30] hip fractures,[31] falls,[32] and motor vehicle accidents.[33] In North America, there has been a dramatic rise in the legitimate use of opioids for pain control over the past decade, but there has also been a parallel increase in deaths from opioid poisoning.[34] The problem is

Table 18.2. ASSESS: Findings Suggesting Substance Abuse on Clinical Assessment

Recent history

General malaise, vague pains, gastrointestinal complaints, hypertension, sexual dysfunction

Memory problems, behavioral changes, new-onset depression, sleep problems

Self-neglect, recurrent falls, decline in health status, malnutrition, geriatric squalor syndrome

History

Medical: liver problems, pancreatitis, peptic ulcers, seizures, vague chronic pains

Surgical: multiple surgical procedures for pain problems, recurrent traumatic injuries, burns

Psychiatric: recurrent depression, anxiety disorders, prior treatment for alcohol or drug problems

Family and Social History

Family history of alcohol or drug problems

History of heavy drinking or preoccupation with drinking

Employment problems, frequent work absenteeism, early retirement

Marital or family problems, domestic violence

Arrests for driving while intoxicated or public intoxication

Any history of illicit drug use or drug-related arrests

Physical Examination

Malnutrition, cachexia, alcohol odor on breath

Multiple facial scars, nasal irritation, parotid hypertrophy, poor oral hygiene

Gynecomastia, cardiomegaly, hepatomegaly, testicular atrophy

Peripheral neuropathy, spider angioma, old (or new) needle marks

Laboratory

Elevated mean corpuscular volume, thrombocytopenia

Elevated liver or pancreatic enzymes, hyperglycemia, hyperlipidemia

Blood alcohol level of intoxication, urine toxicology positive for unprescribed drugs

Imaging

Old rib fractures on chest radiogram

Cortical atrophy on CT scan

expected to worsen as the population ages, with increased rates of painful conditions such as arthritis, back pain, cancer, and neuropathic disorders.[35] Requests for an increase in prescribed benzodiazepines or opioids should prompt a clinical assessment or reassessment.

Patients can also be assessed for their "readiness to change."[36] Some patients have not even considered making a change in their alcohol or drug use and are said to be in a "precontemplative" stage. Others have considered making a change ("contemplative"), want to change ("determinative"), or are completely ready to change and are in an ("action") stage. The type of advice that the clinician gives the patient will depend on the patient's willingness to change. If the patient is willing to change, the clinician can offer direct advice. A referral to a treatment agency for a formal evaluation can also be useful. If the patient is not willing to change or accept a referral, the clinician may perform an intervention designed to motivate the patient to change substance abuse–related behaviors or accept a referral to a treatment program.

Advise: Interventions

If a substance use disorder is identified, the primary care clinician has several options for an initial intervention: brief advice, bibliotherapy, or brief interventions. Brief advice from a trusted health care professional can motivate some older patients who drink excessively to quit or cut-down. The advice may be simple because some patients may respond to straightforward advice such as "I do not want you to drink any alcohol at all until you return to the office when I will recheck your liver tests."

Bibliotherapy is a useful alternative. Some older patients may be given printed information and encouraged to read it and "just think about it" before returning to the office for a reevaluation. Literature from self-help groups (e.g., Alcoholics Anonymous [AA]) may be particularly useful for this purpose, and several excellent books are available in the "self-help" section of many large bookstores.

Brief interventions have been used to address problem drinking among a wide variety of patients. One group of authors reviewed 32 controlled studies from 14 countries that involved more than 6,000 drinkers and found encouraging evidence that the course of harmful alcohol use can be effectively altered by well-designed brief intervention strategies in primary care settings.[37] Similar positive findings have been demonstrated specifically in older adults.[38] The essentials of one model for a brief intervention are summarized in Table 18.3. Brief interventions appear to be most effective if patients are approached in a concerned, nonjudgmental manner.

Assist and Arrange

A referral could also be made to a self-help group or to a professional treatment program for a planned intervention or an evaluation before initiating behavioral therapy. Medications may be needed to manage a withdrawal syndrome.

Self-help groups such as AA or Narcotics Anonymous (NA) can be important allies of the health care provider. Local, national, and international meeting schedules can be accessed from the Internet. When a call is made to a local AA office, the receptionist who answers the telephone is often willing to speak immediately with a patient waiting in an ambulatory clinic or physician office. This receptionist is usually "in recovery" and can provide encouragement to attend AA meetings or can even

Table 18.3. ADVISE: Sample FRAMES "Brief Intervention" for Problem Drinking

Feedback	Express a specific concern about the patient's drinking: "I'm concerned that your drinking is causing you to fall."
Responsibility	Emphasize that change is the patient's responsibility: "Only you can make a decision to change and prevent future problems."
Advice	Advise action by suggesting a specific goal or action to do: "I would like you to see a counselor for an evaluation."
Menu	Provide the patient with alternatives (menu of options): "You could go to an AA meeting or just think about what I have said."
Empathy	Express empathy and provide comfortable context for dialogue: "I know this may be hard for you to talk about."
Self-efficacy	Support self-efficacy and instill optimism: "You can do this and if you reach out for help, you'll get better."

Information from: Miller WR, Rollnick S. *Motivational Interviewing: Preparing People to Change Addictive Behavior.* 2nd ed. New York: The Guildford Press; 2002.

arrange for an AA member to visit the patient for a face-to-face meeting (known as a "12th Step Call"). Arrangements can also be made to have AA literature mailed to the patient's home.

"Planned interventions" usually coming at the request of a family member, spouse, or partner may be useful for alcohol-dependent patients who do not respond to brief interventions, who do not accept referrals, or who are not motivated to change. The families of these patients can be referred to a treatment center that will help orchestrate a planned intervention, originally developed at the Johnson Institute.[39] An "intervention" involves convening a meeting with a number of the patient's friends and family members to discuss their concerns, write letters to the patient, and rehearse their parts for the actual intervention. Subsequently, they all meet with the patient, read their letters out-loud that express their concerns, and voice a specific recommendation such as, "I love you, but please get help at the rehabilitation center." These interventions are designed to create an artificial crisis that prompts the patient to follow the clinical recommendations and accept treatment.

Often, older patients need assistance accepting and implementing the recommended treatment plan (see Table 18.4). They often need the clinician to make arrangements to be admitted for detoxification, to schedule an appointment with a treatment agency, to deal with the preauthorization requirements of health insurance companies, or to arrange appropriate follow-up for coexisting mental health or physical problems.

Table 18.4. ASSIST and ARRANGE: Linking Patients to Treatment Services

Assist

Patient in accepting treatment plan

Family in making arrangements for care

Arrange

Admission for detoxification, if indicated

Appointments to treatment agencies

Health insurance preauthorization, if required

Contact with self-help groups

Appropriate follow-up

PHARMACOTHERAPY

Recommendation: Patients with serious psychiatric involvement (e.g., suicidal ideation), concurrent acute illness, or severe Alcohol Withdrawal Syndrome symptoms, or those who are at high risk for developing seizures or delirium tremens, are best detoxified in inpatient settings. (Level C, Expert opinion).[40]

Management of Alcohol Withdrawal (Detoxification)

Medical management of the alcohol withdrawal syndrome (i.e., detoxification) may be indicated for those patients who have the signs and symptoms of withdrawal on cessation of drinking. Patients with advanced age (especially those without a reliable caregiver) or those who have concurrent medical problems (e.g., neurological disorders, heart disease, hepatic dysfunction, coagulopathies, malnutrition, or diabetes) may be best managed in a hospital setting. Because of the risk for recurrent seizures, hospitalization for the management of benzodiazepine withdrawal should also be considered. Withdrawal from opiates can be safely performed in outpatient settings, but it is extremely difficult to coordinate unless there is a reliable caregiver who is able to access medical backup promptly.

Recommendation: Benzodiazepines are the drugs of choice for monotherapy in patients with the Alcohol Withdrawal Syndrome. (Level B, Systematic review).[41,42]

Long-acting agents such as chlordiazepoxide or diazepam are the preferred agents as they appear to be more effective at preventing alcohol withdrawal seizures and delirium than short-acting agents;[41,42] however, these agents have several active metabolites and long half-lives (several days). Therefore, among elderly patients, particularly those with cognitive disorders or liver dysfunction, short-acting benzodiazepines such as oxazepam or lorazepam should be considered. Of these, only oxazepam is approved by the Food and Drug Administration (FDA) for the management of alcohol withdrawal. Lorazepam has similar actions and has the convenience of being available

Table 18.5. FDA-Approved Treatment Regimens for Alcohol Withdrawal

Chlordiazepoxide (Librium®)	Initial dose is 50–100 mg, to be followed by repeated doses as needed until agitation is controlled – up to 300 mg/day.
Diazepam (Valium®)	10 mg, 3 or 4 times during the first 24 hours, then 3 or 4 times daily as needed.
Oxazepam (Serax®)	15–30 mg, 3 or 4 times daily.

* Adapted from product information package inserts approved by theFDA.

not only in oral forms but also parenteral preparations. These medications are summarized in Table 18.5.

Elderly patients with alcohol problems often neglect their nutrition; therefore, thiamine should *always* be given to prevent Wernicke–Korsakoff syndrome. Because of delayed absorption with oral administration, the first dose should be given parenterally. Hyperadrenergic signs (e.g., tachycardia and hypertension) can be managed with β-adrenergic antagonists with good central nervous system penetration (e.g., propranolol) or centrally acting α-adrenergic agonists (e.g., clonidine). Neuroleptics can be used to calm agitated patients with psychotic symptoms once they have been adequately sedated with a benzodiazepine. Haloperidol is preferred to the phenothiazines because it is believed that it poses a lower seizure risk. Carbamazepine has been widely used in Europe for alcohol withdrawal.

Recommendation: A validated scale such as the CIWA-Ar should be used to monitor patient response to alcohol withdrawal pharmacotherapy. (Level C, Expert opinion).[43]

Patients hospitalized for detoxification should be monitored with an objective rating scale of alcohol withdrawal such as the Clinical Institute Withdrawal Assessment for Alcohol, revised (CIWA-Ar).[44] The items on this assessment scale are summarized in Figure 18.1.

Medications are provided if patients score at least 6 points on this scale; a score of 15 points or more suggests that the alcohol withdrawal is significant and requires immediate attention. The goal is to prevent alcohol withdrawal delirium and seizures.

Pharmacotherapy for Drug Withdrawal (Detoxification)

The medical management of sedative withdrawal can be performed in outpatient settings by gradually decreasing the dose of the prescribed sedative, usually over several weeks to a few months. Withdrawal from hypnotic benzodiazepines is associated with improved cognitive function.[45] Sedative withdrawal seizures can be life threatening. Patients who are receiving multiple prescriptions from multiple physicians are unreliable, do not have a dependable caregiver, or have serious medical conditions are best managed as inpatients. Detoxification can be accomplished by gradually reducing doses of benzodiazepines or phenobarbital over 7–10 days. Withdrawal from opiates can be accomplished by gradually reducing the dose of the prescribed opiate over several weeks or with tapering doses of either buprenorphine or methadone over a few days. In the United States, however, elective methadone or buprenorphine detoxification (i.e., outside of acute medical care settings) is regulated and requires special permits. The management of cocaine withdrawal is largely supportive because there is no specific pharmacotherapy. Although basic treatment for alcohol and drug withdrawal is not complicated, clinical experience is often essential when dealing with these patients, who often have psychosocial and personality issues that can be a challenge to manage (Table 18.6). There are additional issues of liability that lead to most medically managed detoxifications being accomplished in specialized programs and facilities.

BEHAVIORAL THERAPY

Not all experts in the addiction field share the same treatment goals for substance use disorders. Traditionally, abstinence is the goal of most programs in the Untied States; however, there are some who argue that reduction of substance use to low-risk levels is more appropriate. Still others find benefit in adding methadone or buprenorphine maintenance to behavioral therapy for the management of opiate dependence. At the present time, the clinician might pick the strategy that would benefit the patient most.

The goals of most behavioral treatment programs are to promote abstinence, decrease health risks associated with substance abuse, and improve social functioning. There is no shortage of behavioral treatment program options for patients with drug and alcohol problems. Common approaches include: motivational enhancement therapy (MET),[46] cognitive behavioral therapy (CBT),[47] group therapy, and Twelve-step facilitation.[48] MET seeks to increase patient motivation to maintain abstinence from drugs and alcohol. CBT seeks to reframe the patient's thinking about his/her drug or alcohol use and is often based on the premise that patients are "self-medicating" some underlying psychiatric or behavioral problem. Once these problems are reframed and patients are given "the appropriate tools" to deal with their psychological issues, their need to drink or use drugs will diminish over time as they gain insight into the nature of their problem and learn to recognize the benefits of abstaining from drugs or alcohol. Group therapy relies on the support and confrontation of peers, under the guidance of a professional therapist, to encourage behavioral change and/or abstinence. Twelve-step facilitation is designed to encourage patient participation with self-help groups, such as AA or NA. Most treatment programs are not pure entities of any of these approaches and combine elements of MET with CBT during one-on-one sessions with a

Table 18.6. Pharmacotherapy of Drug Problems

Problem	Medication	Comments
Sedative withdrawal	Benzodiazepines Phenobarbital	Withdrawal from sedatives may be severe and complicated by seizures (see text for details).
Opioid withdrawal	Buprenorphine Methadone	The use of buprenorphine or methadone for detoxification is regulated in the United States.
Cocaine withdrawal	None	The care of patients with cocaine withdrawal is largely supportive.
Opioid maintenance	Buprenorphine/naloxone (Suboxone®) Methadone	In the United States, physicians who prescribe buprenorphine with or without naloxone for maintenance must be registered with government agencies, and the use of methadone for maintenance is limited to organizations with special government-issued permits. It is also forbidden to prescribe any other opioid to patients for the maintenance of opioid dependency.

NAUSEA AND VOMITING – **"Do you feel sick to your stomach? Have you vomited?" Observation:**	
0 = no nausea and no vomiting 1 = mild nausea with no vomiting	4 = intermittent nausea with dry heaves 7 = constant nausea, frequent dry heaves, and vomiting
TREMOR – **Arms extended and fingers spread apart. Observation:**	
0 = no tremor 1 = not visible, but can be felt fingertip to fingertip	4 = moderate, with patient's arms extended 7 = severe, even with arms not extended
PAROXYSMAL SWEATS – **Observation:**	
0 = no sweats visible 1 = barely perceptible sweating, palms moist	4 = beads of sweat obvious on forehead 7 = drenching sweats
ANXIETY – **"Do you feel nervous?" Observation:**	
0 = no anxiety, at ease 1 = mildly anxious	4 = moderately anxious or guarded 7 = equivalent to acute panic states as seen in severe delirium or acute schizophrenic reactions
AGITATION – **Observation:**	
0 = normal activity 1 = somewhat more than normal activity	4 = moderately fidgety and restless 7 = paces back and forth during most of the interview, or constantly thrashes about
TACTILE DISTURBANCES – **"Have you any itching, pins and needles sensations, any numbness or do you feel bug scrawling on or under your skin?" Observation:**	
0 = none 1 = very mild itching, pins/needles, burning/numbness 2 = mild itching, pins/needles, burning/numbness 3 = moderate itching, pins/needles, burning/numbness	4 = moderately severe hallucinations 5 = severe hallucinations 6 = extremely severe hallucinations 7 = continuous hallucinations
AUDITORY HALLUCINATIONS – **"Are you more aware of sounds around you? Are they harsh? Do they frighten you? Are you hearing anything that is disturbing to you? Are you hearing things that you know are not there?" Observation:**	
0 = not present 1 = very mild harshness or ability to frighten 2 = mild harshness or ability to frighten 3 = moderate harshness or ability to frighten	4 = moderately severe hallucinations 5 = severe hallucinations 6 = extremely severe hallucinations 7 = continuous hallucinations
VISUAL HALLUCINATIONS – **"Does the light appear to be too bright? Is its color different? Does it hurt your eyes? Are you seeing anything that is disturbing to you? Are you seeing things that you know are not there?" Observation:**	
0 = not present 1 = very mild sensitivity 2 = mild sensitivity 3 = moderate sensitivity	4 = moderately severe hallucinations 5 = severe hallucinations 6 = extremely severe hallucinations 7 = continuous hallucinations
HEADACHE, FULLNESS IN HEAD – **"Does your head feel different? Does it feel like there's a band around your head?" Observation:** (Do not rate for dizziness or lightheadedness. Otherwise, rate severity.)	
0 = not present 1 = very mild 2 = mild 3 = moderate	4 = moderately severe 5 = severe 6 = very severe 7 = extremely severe
ORIENTATION AND CLOUDING OF SENSORIUM – **"What day is this? Where are you? Who am I?" Observation:**	
0 = oriented and can do serial additions 1 = cannot do serial additions or is uncertain about date 2 = disoriented for date, no more than 2 calendar days	3 = disoriented for date, no more than 2 calendar days 4 = disoriented for place and/or person
TOTAL	
Total score is a simple sum of each item score (maximum score = 67).	

Figure 18.1. Clinical Institute Withdrawal Assessment Scale for Alcohol, Revised (CIWA-Ar).

Table 18.7. FDA-Approved Medications for Maintenance of Abstinence from Alcohol

Medication	Dosage*	Comments
Disulfiram (Antabuse®)	*Initial dose*: *Maximum* 500 mg/day for 1–2 wk *Average dose*: 250 mg/day (range, 125–500 mg/day)	Contraindicated in patients with coronary artery disease. Use with caution during concomitant phenytoin administration. May cause optic neuritis or peripheral neuropathy.
Acamprosate (Campral®)	Two 333 mg tablets, 3 times daily	Contraindicated in patients with impaired renal function (creatinine clearance <30 mL/min). Adverse effect profile is similar to placebo.
Naltrexone, oral tablets (ReVia®)	50 mg/day	Contraindicated in patients with a hypersensitivity to naltrexone or with acute hepatitis. May need to follow liver enzymes in healthy patients.
Naltrexone, extended release for intramuscular injection (Vivitrol®)†	380 mg/mo	Similar to oral form. Also contraindicated in patients who are receiving or currently dependent on opioids, or who have a positive urine screen for opioids, as use may cause acute opioid withdrawal. Use may pose a problem for patients who subsequently require opioids for pain control.

* Adapted from product information package inserts approved by the FDA.

† In the United States, intramuscular naltrexone must be ordered from company that markets the product (Cephalon, Inc.) via telephone (1–800-848–4876), FAX (1–877-329–8484) or on-line at www.vivtrol.com.

professional and include group therapy sessions while encouraging patients to participate in self-help groups.

Outpatient treatment settings may be appropriate for individuals who have good social support and have few medical or psychosocial problems; inpatient treatment may be best for those who do not. Older patients are often placed in treatment programs along with younger people and treated in a similar manner; however, the elderly have special needs. They frequently do not mix comfortably with younger, "street-wise" people and special treatment programs have been developed to address issues more germane to the elderly. Whether these special programs produce better outcomes than generic approaches is unknown. Although participation in self-help groups such as AA or NA seems to benefit many older adults, the effectiveness of these self-help programs has not been subjected to scientific scrutiny.

PHARMACOTHERAPY TO PROMOTE ABSTINENCE

Although psychosocial support is an essential component of the treatment of drug and alcohol dependence, relapse rates remain high when it is used alone. Psychosocial support or counseling targets the cortex where decision making takes place, but it may not fully address the addictive disease because addictive drives are not primarily conscious. Therefore, there is an interest in using pharmacotherapy as a way to promote recovery from addiction. There are a number of pharmacological agents that can be used to promote abstinence from alcohol or opiates. Pharmacotherapy targets portions of the brain that are associated with reward pathways and subconscious generation of drives.

Three medications are approved for the maintenance of abstinence from alcohol in the United States: disulfiram, naltrexone, acamprosate. These are summarized in Table 18.7. Disulfiram has been available in the United States for more than half a century and is used as an aversive agent that causes the inhibition of aldehyde dehydrogenase, which is responsible for the breakdown of acetaldehyde, the primary metabolite of ethanol. If a patient consumes ethanol after taking disulfiram for at least 3 consecutive days, subsequent high levels of acetaldehyde will cause nausea, vomiting, diarrhea, tachycardia, dyspnea, and facial flushing. Severe reactions include respiratory depression, shock, acute congestive heart failure, myocardial infarction, convulsions, and sudden death. Therefore, its use among older patients is limited. Moreover, disulfiram appeared to have little or no measurable benefit in many clinical trials.

The oral opioid agonist naltrexone is thought to reduce drinking by decreasing the pleasurable, positively reinforcing effects of alcohol. In the COMBINE study of 1,383 recently alcohol abstinent volunteers, it was found that those receiving routine medical management in primary care settings with encouragement to attend AA combined with either oral naltrexone *or* psychotherapy faired better on drinking outcomes than those receiving medical management alone.[49] Patients who are taking or may require opiates for analgesic purposes may not be able to take naltrexone. A once monthly injectable depot form of naltrexone is also available in the United States.

Acamprosate is structurally similar to several endogenous amino acids present in the brain. Its mechanism of action is not entirely clear, but it appears to modulate the glutamatergic neurotransmission and thus reduce cravings for alcohol. Although the COMBINE study did not observe a benefit for

Table 18.8. Guidelines for the Use of Controlled Substances for the Treatment of Pain

Guideline	Comments
Patient evaluation	There must be documentation of a medical history and physical examination. The record should include information about the nature of the pain, prior treatment, and the medical indication for the use of controlled substances.
Treatment plan	There must be a written treatment plan that includes other modalities if necessary. The physical and psychosocial goals of treatment need to be clear.
Informed consent	The risk and benefit of treatment need to be discussed with the patient. Only one pharmacy should be used by the patient. A written agreement or a signed consent should be considered outlining patient responsibilities, including: toxicology testing, frequency of prescription refills, and reasons for discontinuation of drug therapy.
Periodic review	The clinical course related to treatment response (e.g., pain control, level of function, quality of life) should be documented periodically. Information from family or caregivers may be important.
Consultation	Patients whose progress is less than satisfactory or who show signs of medication misuse may require referral to an expert in the management of such patients.
Medical records	The physician should keep accurate and complete records.
Legal compliance	The physician must be familiar with and comply with all federal, state, and local regulations.

Adapted from: Federation of State Medical Boards of the United States, Inc. *Model policy for the use of controlled substances for the treatment of pain*. Available at: www.fsmb.org/pdf/2004_grpol_Controlled_Substances.pdf. Accessed January 29, 2007.

this medication, many European studies have demonstrated modest effectiveness.[50]

In the United States, methadone and buprenorphine are used for maintenance in opioid dependence. The combination of buprenorphine and naloxone (Suboxone®) can be prescribed by physicians who have completed a brief training program and have received a special authorization. Methadone maintenance must occur in a federally approved methadone maintenance treatment program. Although elderly patients are not common in buprenorphine or methadone maintenance programs, these programs do have older patients among their rosters who benefit from long-term opiate maintenance, but tend to have more medical problems than younger patients.[51]

Long-Term Monitoring

Primary care clinicians have skills that can be instrumental for the long-term treatment of patients with substance use disorders. Patient progress in recovery can be monitored through regularly scheduled office visits for routine medical care and for renewal of medications to promote abstinence.[52] Clinicians can ask about progress in substance abuse rehabilitation programs, involvement with self-help groups, the use alcohol and or other drugs, and functioning at home or in interpersonal relationships. Patients in solid recovery from a drug or alcohol use disorder do not drink or take drugs and regularly attend counseling sessions or self-help meetings. They take care of their physical health and rarely forget or cancel appointments. They get along socially with friends and family, function well

at activities of daily living, and obey the law, especially the laws related to diversion of prescription controlled substances. Failure to do these things may precede a relapse, which may be prevented by reinitiating or intensifying involvement in self-help groups or professional treatment. Controlled substances should be used with great caution, if at all. The use of sedatives (e.g., benzodiazepines) should generally be avoided.

Pain Management

Occasionally, some patients, who are in recovery from a substance use disorder, may require opioids for the treatment of pain. For short-term use, limited supplies should be given, and the patient seen frequently for reevaluation. Medications should be discontinued when no longer indicated. Some patients will required medically managed detoxification if they are unable to discontinue use without great physical or psychological discomfort. Patients who require long-term opioids should be managed according to recent medical licensure policies as outlined in Table 18.8. Before prescribing opioids, especially propoxyphene, meperidine or tramadol, it may be prudent to review the patient's list of medications for potential drug–drug interactions. In one study of 27,617 Medicare enrollees, more than 20% of them were prescribed opioid analgesics and in this patient sample, opioids were involved in approximately 5% of all adverse drug events.[53] Some older patients may divert their medications to others. Some of these diverted medications end up being resold in the illicit drug trade, and these older patients may even come to rely on this to supplement their retirement income. Physicians who prescribe controlled substances need to be vigilant, least they unwittingly contribute to a growing societal problem of prescription drug diversion.

Team Concept

Drawing on the therapeutic relationship and their existing skills, the members of the primary care team (e.g., physicians, nurse practitioners, nurses, psychologists, physical therapists, and social workers) all have an important role in the long-term management of the patient recovering from a substance use disorder. The challenge to caregivers of older patients with alcohol and drug use disorders is immense and concerns issues of trust, compliance with treatment, and appropriate use of health care resources. Treatment must be age-specific and sensitive, tailored to the psychological and medical needs of older patients. It involves direct patient care as well as teaching and reinforcing accurate information about addiction treatment and treatment follow-up.

A physician or specialty-trained nurse practitioner initiates treatment after a careful assessment that includes a thorough drug and alcohol history-taking. Detoxification is performed under their close medical supervision with management of medical comorbidities and continual reassessment of symptoms and signs.

Clinical nurses, who have the skills to interact effectively with older patients, have an important role to play in hospitals, ambulatory clinics, and substance abuse treatment centers. They observe the effects of all medications given to patients and record the effects on standardized scales (e.g., CIWA-Ar). Nurses can coordinate the nonpharmacological management of anxiety, pain, insomnia, and other distressing symptoms. They can also offer brief educational interventions that may be effective, as older patients have many misconceptions about alcohol and drug use. Important educational topics include metabolism of alcohol and drugs in the aging body, the potential for alcohol–drug or drug–drug interactions and discussions of healthy lifestyles.

Addiction counselors are a necessary part of the team, especially those who possess skills in various psychosocial treatment approaches. These approaches may include individual behavioral therapy, the use of group and individual psychotherapy, and brief intervention techniques. Behavioral counseling educates patients about how to initiate abstinence, function without alcohol or other drugs, handle cravings, and recognize situations that may lead to relapse. Effective counselors provide emotional support that allows the patient to explore fears, express concerns, and discuss practical issues. Counselors offer support by setting limits and realistic goals as well as providing adequate referral sources for treatment follow-up.

SUMMARY

Alcohol and drug use problems may frequently go undetected among older patients. All older patients should be screened for alcohol problems and those who screen positive or those suspected of a drug problem should undergo further assessment and receive an appropriate intervention to address substance abuse problems. Some patients will require medical management for alcohol or drug withdrawal. Hospitalization is indicated for those at-risk for complications of withdrawal, where the treatment can be monitored by specifically trained nurses using objective rating scales. A multidisciplinary team is usually necessary to manage the long-term needs of the older patient who is recovering from an alcohol or drug use disorder.

REFERENCES

1. McInnees E, Powell J. Drug and alcohol referrals: are elderly substance abuse diagnoses and referrals being missed? *BMJ.* 1994;308:444–446.
2. American Psychiatric Association. *Diagnostic and Statistical Manual of Mental Disorders.* 4th ed. Washington, DC: American Psychiatric Association; 1994.
3. National Institute on Alcohol Abuse and Alcoholism, US Department of Health and Human Services. *Helping Patients Who Drink Too Much: A Clinician's Guide.* Rockville, MD: National Institutes of Health; 2007. NIH publication 07–3769.
4. Saunders JB, Aasland OG, Amundsen A, Grant M. Alcohol consumption and related problems among primary care patients: WHO collaborative project on early detection of persons with harmful alcohol consumption. *Addiction.* 1993;88:349–362.
5. Lang I, Guralnik J, Wallace RB, Melzer D. What level of alcohol consumption is hazardous for older people? Functioning and mortality in U.S. and English national cohorts. *J Am Geriatr Soc.* 2007;55:49–57.
6. Carr LA. The pharmacology of mood-altering drugs of abuse. *Primary Care.* 1993;20:19–31.
7. Scott RB. Alcohol effects in the elderly. *Compr Ther.* 1989;15:8–12.
8. Vestal R, McGuire E, Tobin JD, Andres R, Norris M, Mezey E. Aging and alcohol metabolism. *Clin Pharmacol Ther.* 1977;21:343–354.
9. Kandel D, Chen K, Warner LA, Kessler RC, Grant B. Prevalence and demographic correlates of symptoms of last-year dependence on alcohol, nicotine, marijuana, and cocaine in the U. S. population. *Drug Alcohol Depend.* 1997;44:11–29.
10. Barry KL, Blow FC, Walton MA, et al. Elder-specific brief intervention: 3-month outcomes. *Alcohol Clin Exp Res.* 1998;22:30A.
11. Callaghan CM. Health services use and mortality among older primary care patients with alcoholism. *J Am Geriatr Soc.* 1995;43:1378–1383.
12. Black BS, Rabins PV, McGuire MH. Alcohol use disorder is a risk factor for mortality among older public-housing residents. *Int Psychogeriatr.* 1998;10:309–327.
13. Hinkin CH, Castellon SA, Dickinson-Fuhrman E, Daum G, Jaffe J, Jarvik L. Screening for drug and alcohol abuse among older adults using modified version of CAGE. *Am J Addict.* 2001;10:319–326.
14. Substance Abuse and Mental Health Services, Office of Applied Studies. Drug Abuse Warning Network: emergency department visits involving nonmedical use of selected pharmaceuticals. *The New Dawn Report-Special Topics.* 2006;(23):1–4.
15. Gfroerer J, Penne M, Pemberton M, Folsom R. Substance abuse treatment need among older adults in 2020: the impact of the

aging baby-boom cohort. *Drug Alcohol Depend.* 2003;69:127–135.

16. Nemes S, Rao PA, Zeiler C, Munly K, Holtz KD, Hoffman J. Computerized screening of substance abuse problems in a primary care setting: older vs. younger adults. *Am J Drug Alcohol Abuse.* 2004;30:627–642.

17. Devor EJ, Cloninger CR. Genetics of alcoholism. *Annu Rev Genet.* 1989;23:19–36.

18. Wilson GT. Cognitive studies in alcoholism. *J Consult Clin Psychol.* 1987;55:325–331.

19. US Preventive Services Task Force. *Screening for Alcohol Misuse.* Available at: http://www.ahrq.gov/clinic/uspstf/uspsdrin.htm. Accessed May 28, 2008.

20. Selzer ML. The Michigan Alcoholism Screening Test: the quest for a new diagnostic instrument. *Am J Psychiatry.* 1971;127:1653–1658.

21. Selzer ML Vinokur A, Rooijen LV. A self-administered Short Michigan Alcoholism Screening Test (SMAST). *J Stud Alcohol.* 1975;36:117–126.

22. Blow FC, Brower KJ, Schulenberg JE, Demo-Dananberg LM, Young JP, Beresford TP. The Michigan Alcoholism Screening Test-Geriatric Version (MAST-G): a new elderly-specific screening instrument. *Alcohol Clin Exp Res.* 1992;16:372.

23. Babor TF. From clinical research to secondary prevention: international collaboration in the development of the Alcohol Use Disorders Identification Test (AUDIT). *Alcohol Health Res World.* 1989;13:371–374.

24. McPherson TL, Hersch R. Brief substance use screening instruments for primary care settings: a review. *J Subst Abuse Treat.* 2000;18:193–202.

25. Brown RL, Leonard T, Saunders LA, Papasouliotis O. The prevalence and detection of substance use disorders among inpatients ages 18–49: an opportunity for prevention. *Prev Med.* 1998;27:101–110.

26. Hinkin CH, Castellon SA, Dickson-Fuhrman E, Daum G, Jaffe J, Jarvik L. Screening for drug and alcohol abuse among older adults using a modified version of the CAGE. *Am J Addict.* 2001;10:319–326.

27. Blondell RD, Dodds HN, Blondell MN, Droz DC. Is the Kentucky prescription reporting system useful in the care of hospitalized patients? *J Ky Med Assoc.* 2004;102:15–19.

28. Finfgeld-Connett DL. Treatment of substance misuse in older women: using a brief intervention model. *J Gerontol Nurs.* 2004;30:30–37.

29. Smith WB, Weisner C. Women and alcohol problems: a critical analysis of the literature and unanswered questions. *Alcohol Clin Exp Res.* 2000;24:1320–1321.

30. Herings RM, Stricker BH, de Boer A, Bakker A, Sturmans F. Benzodiazepines and the risk of falling leading to femur fractures: dosage more important than elimination half-life. *Arch Intern Med.* 1995;155:1801–1807.

31. Wagner AK, Zhang F, Soumerai SB, et al. Benzodiazepine use and hip fractures in the elderly: who is at greatest risk? *Arch Intern Med.* 2004;164:1567–1572.

32. Kurtzthaler I, Wambacher M, Golser K, et al. Alcohol and benzodiazepines in falls; an epidemiological view. *Drug Alcohol Depend.* 2005;79:225–230.

33. Hemmelgarn B, Suissa S, Huang A, Boivin JF, Pinard G. Benzodiazepine use and the risk of motor vehicle crash in the elderly. *JAMA.* 1997;278:27–31.

34. Paulozzi LJ, Budnitz DS. Increasing deaths from opioid analgesics in the United States. *Pharmacoepidemiol Drug Saf.* 2006;15:618–627.

35. Kuehn BM. Opioid prescriptions soar. *JAMA.* 2007;297:249–251.

36. Prochaska JO, DiClemente CC, Norcross JC. In search of how people change: applications to addictive behaviors. *Am Psychol.* 1992;47:1102–1114.

37. Bien TH, Miller WR, Tonigan JS. Brief interventions for alcohol problems: a review. *Addiction.* 1993;88:315–335.

38. Fleming MF, Manwell LB, Barry KL, Adams W, Stauffacher EA. Brief physician advice for alcohol problems in older adults: a randomized community-based trial. *J Fam Pract.* 1999;48:378–384.

39. Johnson VE. *I'll Quit Tomorrow.* San Francisco: Harper & Rowe; 1980.

40. Saitz R, O'Malley SS. Pharmacotherapies for alcohol abuse. Withdrawal and treatment. *Med Clin North Am.* 1997;81:881–907.

41. Mayo-Smith MF. Pharmacological management of alcohol withdrawal. A meta-analysis and evidence-based practice guideline. American Society of Addiction Medicine Working Group on Pharmacological Management of Alcohol Withdrawal. *JAMA.* 1997;278:144–151.

42. Williams D, McBride AJ. The drug treatment of alcohol withdrawal symptoms: a systematic review. *Alcohol Alcohol.* 1998;33:103–115.

43. Mayo-Smith MF. Management of alcohol intoxication and withdrawal. In: Graham AV, Schultz TK, eds. *Principles of Addiction Medicine.* 2nd ed. Chevy Chase, MD: American Society of Addiction Medicine, Inc.; 1998:431–440.

44. Sullivan JT, Sykora K, Schneiderman J, Naranjo CA, Sellers EM. Assessment of alcohol withdrawal: the revised clinical institute withdrawal assessment for alcohol scale (CIWA-Ar). *Br J Addict.* 1989;84:1353–1357.

45. Curran HV, Collins R, Fletcher S, Kee SCY, Woods B, Iliffe S. Older adults and withdrawal from benzodiazepines hypnotics in general practice: effects on cognitive function, sleep, mood, and quality of life. *Psychol Med.* 2003;33:1223–1237.

46. National Institute on Alcohol Abuse and Alcoholism, US Department of Health and Human Services. *Motivational Enhancement Therapy Manual.* Rockville, MD: National Institutes of Health; 1994. NIH publication 94–3723.

47. National Institute on Alcohol Abuse and Alcoholism, US Department of Health and Human Services. *Cognitive-Behavioral Coping Skills Therapy Manual.* Rockville, MD: National Institutes of Health; 1994. NIH publication 94–3724.

48. National Institute on Alcohol Abuse and Alcoholism, US Department of Health and Human Services. *Twelve Step Facilitation Therapy Manual.* Rockville, MD: National Institutes of Health; 1994. NIH publication 94–3722.

49. Anton RF, O'Malley SS, Ciraulo DA, et al. Combined pharmacotherapies and behavioral interventions for alcohol dependence: the COMBINE study: a randomized controlled trial. *JAMA.* 2006;295:2003–2017.

50. Acamprosate (Campral) for alcoholism. *Med Lett Drugs Ther.* 2005;47:1–3.

51. Lofwall MR, Brooner RK, Bigelow GE, Kindbom K, Strain EC. Characteristics of older opioid maintenance patients. *J Subst Abuse Treat.* 2005;28:265–272.

52. Friedmann PD, Saitz R, Samet JH. Management of adults recovering from alcohol or other drug problems: relapse prevention in primary care. *JAMA.* 1998;279:1227–1231.

53. Gurwitz JH, Field TS, Harrold LR, et al. Incidence and preventability of adverse effects among older persons in the ambulatory setting. *JAMA.* 2003;289:1107–1116.

19

AGING IN ADULTS WITH DEVELOPMENTAL DISABILITIES

Paula M. Minihan, MPH, PhD

The present generation of older persons with developmental disabilities are survivors. They are also often referred to as pioneers. In effect though, they are persons who have no role models as they and others close to them anticipate the challenges of their later years of life.[1] (p. 137)

INTRODUCTION

For the first time in our nation's history, a significant number of older adults with developmental disabilities (DD) are living in community settings and turning to community-based physicians for care, but information to guide physicians is limited. According to the U.S. Centers for Disease Control and Prevention (CDC):

Developmental disabilities are a diverse group of severe chronic conditions that are due to mental and/or physical impairments. People with developmental disabilities have problems with major life activities such as language, mobility, learning, self-help, and independent living. Developmental disabilities begin anytime during development up to 22 years of age and usually last throughout a person's lifetime.[2]

The CDC statement reflects the federal statutory definition of DD as codified in Public Law 106–402, The Developmental Disabilities Assistance and Bill of Rights Act of 2000.[3] The federal definition notes that most individuals with DD will require special services, supports, and other forms of assistance throughout their lives. Mental retardation, now generally referred to as intellectual disability (ID), autism spectrum disorders, cerebral palsy, hearing loss, and vision impairment are among the most common DD.

In previous generations, only a small proportion of individuals with DD survived into older adulthood and they generally lived in large state institutions where physicians who were removed from mainstream health care systems managed their care.[4] The contemporary network of services and supports for people with DD, in contrast, is community-based, and individuals with DD are now expected to seek care from physicians in the communities where they live. These revolutionary changes in the support system for people with DD have been accompanied by marked gains in life expectancy, particularly for individuals with nonorganic forms of DD.[4–7] Older adults with DD have benefited from the gains in life expectancy enjoyed by the general population; they have also benefited from remarkable improvements in their access to quality health care services and to greatly expanded societal opportunities. Many adults with DD residing in the community, at present, live in supervised residences that are publicly financed and administered by state government (specifically, state agencies for people with DD). Other adults with DD live with their families where they may receive services and supports through the state DD agency. This significant demographic change presents challenges, particularly for primary care physicians, who may have limited experience managing the care of older adults with DD and who have few places to turn for information about best practices with respect to this emerging population.

This chapter is intended to provide health care providers with information about the health needs of older adults with DD who are living in community settings, with an emphasis on characteristics that may differ from those of older adults without DD. The chapter begins with background information about DD. This is followed by a profile of older adults with DD, including information about the size of this population and where these individuals reside. The main body of this chapter is devoted to issues related to life expectancy and causes and predictors of mortality for older adults with DD; the clinical management of adult patients with DD; and age-related health concerns common to older adults with DD, including those with particular syndromes.

DEVELOPMENTAL DISABILITIES

The most prevalent DD is mental retardation, more recently called ID. This change in terminology is relatively new, and both terms are in use in the DD literature at present. The American Association on Intellectual and Developmental Disabilities (AAIDD), the new name adopted by the American Association on Mental Retardation (AAMR) in 2007, defines mental retardation as a disability characterized by significant limitations both in intellectual functioning and in adaptive behavior as expressed in conceptual, social, and practical adaptive skills. This disability originates before the age of 18 years.[8] In many instances, the cognitive limitations seen in individuals with ID are accompanied by physical, sensory, or psychiatric impairments of varying levels of severity that may influence the course of the aging process.[9] The AAIDD definition is predicated on several assumptions, including the importance of determining functional limitations within the context of community environments typical of the individual's age peers and culture, recognition that limitations and strengths often coexist within an individual, and the expectation that supports tailored to the person's limitations will lead to functional gains. Historically, the AAIDD definition of mental retardation took into account levels of impairment, determined largely by IQ scores and ranging from mild to profound; in the current AAIDD definition, intensity of support needs are rated from intermittent to persuasive, and add a new dimension to level of disability discussions.[10]

There are many causes of ID including "biomedical, social, behavioral, and educational risk factors that interact during the life of an individual and/or across generations from parent to child."[8] Some of the more common known causes include Down syndrome, fetal alcohol syndrome, fragile X syndrome, and congenital conditions that affect the brain, such as hydrocephalus. In many situations, however, the cause of an ID is not known.[11] Studies indicate that both cause and level of ID are related to morbidity and mortality across all age groups.[4,6,7,12–14] Individuals with lower IQ scores often have associated medical conditions and functional limitations, such as nonmobility and lack of basic self-help skills, that are associated with morbidity and mortality.

Autism spectrum disorders refer to a group of DD defined by significant impairments in social interaction and communication and the presence of unusual behaviors and interests.[15] Although the incidence of autism spectrum disorders is rising and there is concern about the implications of aging for individuals with diagnoses on the autism spectrum, this diagnostic category is relatively new compared with other DD diagnoses, and there are few older adults in this population. A search of the biomedical literature for research findings with respect to older adults with autism yielded no results.

With the exception of older adults with cerebral palsy, a group for whom there is limited information, information about older adults with other DD is almost nonexistent. Almost all of the information currently available about older adults with DD refers to people with intellectual disabilities, particularly Down syndrome, and this emphasis is reflected in this chapter.

PROFILE OF OLDER ADULTS WITH DEVELOPMENTAL DISABILITIES

Prevalence

There is limited information about the nationwide number of older adults with DD. The national surveillance systems created to monitor the health status of Americans by using probability samples have just recently begun to identify people with disabilities as a subpopulation. The service networks administered by states for people with DD maintain management information systems, but these networks do not serve every individual with DD; no one knows how many adults with DD do not receive services from state DD agencies. In addition, state DD agencies use different eligibility criteria – all serve people with mental retardation but some do not serve individuals with other DD diagnoses, such as, autism.[16] Furthermore, societal definitions of when one is "old," based on chronological age, may not be appropriate for some individuals with DD, particularly those who appear to age earlier than members of the general population.[17–19] Persons with Down syndrome, for example, have a known predisposition to premature aging.[16,20]

This lack of consensus about when a person with DD should be considered "old" has implications for health care providers and for service organizations requiring some determination of when an individual becomes eligible for services. Janicki and Breitenbach identified the sixth decade of life, when people with DD are in their 50s, as the chronological time period most associated with age-related changes in this population. Age of 50 years has been identified as the age when mortality risks begin to increase markedly for persons with severe intellectual disabilities.[4] Age of 50 years has also been identified as the age when adults with Down syndrome are at increased risk for losses in adaptive behavior;[20] adaptive behavior refers generally to common activities of daily living.

From the perspective of making determinations about eligibility for "elder" services, public agencies are increasingly using age 60 years, particularly for planning purposes.[18] The 1987 reauthorization of the Older Americans Act of 1965 (P.L. 89–73, as amended), which included specific provisions for older persons with disabilities for the first time, specifies age 60 years as the age of eligibility for services.[18] This legislation requires equal access to services by older adults with disabilities, including adults with intellectual disabilities.

The AAIDD estimates that nationwide there are currently between 600,000 and 1.6 million older adults with DD.[21] Heller et al.[22] estimate that 641,161 adults with intellectual disabilities older than the age of 60 years live in the United States. These numbers are expected to double by 2030 when the youngest members of the postwar baby boom generation reach the age of 60 years.

Place of Residence

Community-based living is now the norm for adults with DD, although there are no data about where older adults with DD currently reside. Nationwide, families are the major providers of care for adults with intellectual disabilities; estimates of the percentage of adults of all ages who live with their families range as high as 76%.[22] Of concern, many family caregivers of adults with DD are older than the age of 60 years and facing their own age-related challenges.[23–25] State systems for people with DD offer a range of formal, supervised residential options. In 2004, these systems served approximately 492,000 individuals: 37% lived in settings such as group homes, apartments, and foster homes serving up to 6 residents; 31% lived in small "supported living settings" that they themselves selected; 11% lived in larger group homes serving up to 15 residents; 14% lived in large public or private institutions; and 6% lived in large nursing homes or facilities.[26] Historically, nursing homes provided the primary placement for adults with DD older than the age of 65 years, but this is no longer the case. The determination that many individuals with DD were inappropriately placed in nursing homes, made following the mandatory review of nursing home placements for people with DD under the Omnibus Budget Reconciliation Act of 1987, has reduced nursing home placements considerably.[5]

LIFE EXPECTANCY FOR ADULTS WITH DEVELOPMENTAL DISABILITIES

Introduction

The life expectancy for persons with DD increased dramatically during the 20th century. According to reports, the mean age at death for persons with intellectual and developmental disabilities increased from 19 years in the 1930s, to 59 years in the 1970s, to 66 years (the latter excludes individuals with Down syndrome) in 1993.[7,22] Similar dramatic gains in life expectancy have been reported for adults with intellectual disabilities in Australia.[6] In a study investigating mortality among a large number of adults with ID, aged 40 years and older, over a 10-year period, Janicki and colleagues [7] found:

> Although individuals in the current generation of older adults with ID still generally die at an earlier age than do adults in the general population (average age at death: 66.1 years), many adults with ID live as long as their age peers in the general population. (p. 284)

Janicki and Breitenbach[9] note "most adults with intellectual disabilities who live past their third decade are likely to survive into old age and experience the normal aging process" (p. 6).

The life expectancy for individuals with Down syndrome has also increased markedly, although these individuals still have shorter life expectancies on average than other individuals with ID but without Down syndrome and the general

population. In the Janicki et al. study,[7] the average age at death for adults with Down syndrome was 55.8 years compared with 66.1 years for adults with ID but without Down syndrome and 70.4 years for adults in the state's general population.

Causes of Mortality

The leading causes of death among adults older than age 40 years in Janicki et al's cohort were similar to those in the state's general older population, with some exceptions. The causes of death among adults with ID in rank order were: cardiovascular diseases (33%); respiratory diseases (20%), cancers (16%), digestive system diseases (6%), septicemia (2%), renal diseases (2%), and injuries (1%), respectively.[7] In contrast, proportionately more deaths in the general population were attributed to cardiovascular disease, cancer, and injuries and fewer to respiratory diseases and digestive system diseases than in the ID population. When deaths in the ID cohort were examined by International Classification of Diseases codes, acute myocardial infarction was the most prevalent single cause of death (26.5%). Among deaths from respiratory disease, pneumonia was the most prevalent cause, particularly among the oldest persons in the cohort.

Predictors of Mortality

Level of ID has long been reported to be a strong predictor of mortality, but this association is now more fully understood to reflect confounding by the life-threatening medical conditions and/or functional limitations that often accompany severe ID.[4,7] Eyman and Borthwick-Duffy[4] report that functional deficits, such as immobility and lack of eating skills, remain strong predictors of mortality regardless of etiology, including Down syndrome. Among individuals with Down syndrome overall, age remains an important predictor of mortality.[4,7,9,27]

Although data with respect to sex and mortality are limited in the ID literature, two studies [6,7] reported that males were dying at earlier ages and at higher rates than females, paralleling the experiences of the general population.

The issue of racial and ethnic health disparities is just emerging in the ID literature and appears to warrant further attention. A California-based study of people with Down syndrome of all ages[27] found higher mortality rates among Blacks than among those in the "White/Hispanic/Asian" category, whereas an Australian study[6] found that people with ID from "indigenous Australian parentage" had a significantly reduced life expectancy compared with those from the majority population.

ISSUES IN THE CLINICAL MANAGEMENT OF PATIENTS WITH DEVELOPMENTAL DISABILITIES

In 1987, Garrard[28] voiced concern that community-based physicians were not adequately prepared to manage the care of people with mental retardation who were moving into communities from institutions. He worried that physicians lacked clinical experience with patients with mental retardation, particularly adults; were uncertain about the adequacy of their skills for examining and communicating with such patients and unsure about how to proceed in the face of resistance to preventive, diagnostic, or therapeutic procedures; could find it difficult to recognize health problems when patients were unable to communicate directly concerning their needs; and could be discouraged because of extraordinary time requirements and inadequate financial reimbursement.

Over the intervening 20 years, physicians have gained considerable experience with respect to patients with DD, particularly adults, and some have shared experiences from their practices.[14,29–31] Nonetheless, information about the issues the nation's physicians face when managing the care of adults with DD remains in short supply.

The greatest obstacle that physicians in Maine reported they faced with respect to the clinical management of patients with mental retardation was the inadequacy of medical information.[32] According to physicians, some patients with cognitive or communication limitations were unable to report what was troubling them or provide a sufficient verbal history and they were not always accompanied to the visit by someone who could speak knowledgeably on their behalf. Others have reported that comprehensive medical records may not be available.[29] Some individuals may not know how to monitor their own health or interpret or report symptoms, which further complicates the problem.[33,34]

Under these circumstances, a major challenge for health care professionals, according to Adlin,[33] "can be in properly diagnosing and treating some of these common conditions" (p. 50). Martin[29] notes that it is generally more difficult to distinguish biological from psychological problems in the DD population. He observes, "A change of behavior may be due to an infection, a social stressor, a medication side effect, new seizure activity or a mental disorder" (p. 5). This makes health care professionals highly dependent on the observations and assistance of caregivers to recognize health problems and follow through with treatment regimens.[1,9,29,31,33] Caregivers may be either direct support staff or family members.

Other issues with respect to the clinical management of adults with DD have been noted in the literature, and they are listed below. Many have particular relevance to the care of older adults.

- **Some adults with DD have multiple complex conditions that require the involvement of specialty physicians and other health care professionals, including behavioral specialists.** When individuals with DD and complex medical and behavioral needs receive care from several different specialists, their care may be fragmented or even at cross-purposes.[35] A primary care physician can do much to enhance overall quality of care by coordinating the efforts of multiple health care providers.[1] Although seeking specialty

consultations is a routine aspect of primary care, many physicians in the Maine survey reported they lacked knowledge about specialists who were experienced in treating patients with DD to whom they could refer patients for consultations and/or management of complex conditions.[32] Interdisciplinary geriatric assessment teams have much to offer older adults with multiple and complex conditions, including older adults with DD.[1,36]

- **Adults with DD may be at increased risk for a number of health problems, referred to as secondary conditions or disabilities, which are largely preventable at the primary, secondary, or tertiary levels.**[14,37,38] The 2005 Surgeon General's Report[38] defines secondary conditions as "medical, social, emotional, family, or community problems for which a person with a primary disabling conditions is at increased risk" (p. 13). Physicians who are knowledgeable about risk factors and potential interventions can do much to prevent these conditions and/or limit their impact.[14] People with cerebral palsy or other mobility impairments, for example, face increased risks for osteoporosis and bone fractures as they age; adequate calcium and vitamin D intake, screening, and medication, if warranted, can reduce these risks.[39]

- **Medication-related problems, including polypharmacy, adverse drug effects, drug interactions, and risks associated with long-term use, may be a particular concern for many adults with DD.** According to Adlin,[33] "Older adults with developmental disabilities are at very high risk for complications associated with polypharmacy due to the nature of the types of medication they are frequently prescribed" (p. 50). She recommends frequent review of medication use in this group, readjustment of dosages when indicated, and elimination of medications "in the absence of proven need and efficacy" (p. 51), and others concur with her recommendations.[14,36,40] One of the few studies to examine medication use in older persons with DD found that 27% were using psychotropic medications, excluding seizure medications, and 19% were using antipsychotic medications.[1] Zigman and colleagues[20] (1994) warned "The questionable use of psychoactive medications, particularly antipsychotic medications, is an issue of particular concern. These medications, which have the potential to produce significant adverse reactions, especially among older persons, are often prescribed for control of maladaptive behaviors, with or without determination of an appropriate psychiatric diagnosis" (p. 81).

  Long-term use of some medications, for example, psychotropic or anticonvulsant medications, increases the risk for developing secondary conditions (e.g., tardive dyskinesia, conditions associated with obesity, or osteoporosis).[1]

- **There is a danger of "diagnostic overshadowing" when evaluating behavioral problems and/or other symptoms of mental illness in adults with DD.** Reiss and coworkers[41] were the first to use this term to describe the tendency of clinicians to attribute symptoms of mental illness in persons with mental retardation to the underlying mental retardation. Diagnostic overshadowing can lead clinicians to diagnose mental illness less accurately in persons with mental retardation than in persons without mental retardation, decreasing the likelihood that these individuals will receive appropriate treatment.[20,42] A variation of diagnostic overshadowing may also apply to situations involving physical health. In a survey in which more than half of the adults with DD who were studied were obese, based on body mass index calculations,[43] nurse respondents rarely reported obesity as a health problem. The authors expressed concern that some health care professionals "may be accepting obesity as normal among adults with intellectual disabilities and are not aggressively addressing the health consequences" (p. 295).

- **Special care must be taken with respect to medical procedures requiring informed consent.** Adults with DD are assumed to be legally competent to give informed consent unless they have been deemed incompetent by a formal court decision, and a legal guardian or some other surrogate decision maker has been appointed to make decisions on their behalf. Legal issues involving consent may be complex and have the potential to delay or prevent the timely delivery of diagnostic testing and other procedures.[30,31,36] For this reason, Martin[29] recommends that physicians determine the legal status of patients with mental retardation when they first enroll in a medical practice. The ARC,[44] the world's largest grassroots organization of and for people with ID and DD, advises that adults with DD who are unable to make their own medical decisions should have surrogate decision makers appointed to make these decisions, in advance of a possible medical emergency. It is important to note that consent issues may vary from state to state. Regardless of the patient's legal status, patients with DD should be involved in decisions about their own care as much as possible.[29,30,34]

- **Some individuals with DD are unable to cooperate with standard screening, diagnostic, or treatment procedures without special supports.** These supports may include extended appointment times to explain procedures to patients in a way that they are able to comprehend; extra appointments to desensitize patients to the upcoming procedure (e.g., gynecological examinations); previsit medication, and, on occasion, general anesthesia.[7,29,30,32] Under some circumstances (e.g., a colonoscopy or complex dental procedures for a patient with severe DD), health care professionals must consider the benefit to the patient, weighing his or her personal risk factors and disease status, against the potential risks to a patient who may not have the ability to understand what is occurring or why.[29,30]

- **Almost all older adults with DD are dependent on Medicaid and/or Medicare to pay for their health care.** Medicaid and Medicare reimbursement rates, particularly rates for primary care services, are generally deemed inadequate to compensate physicians for the cost of providing care to most patients, including patients with DD.[1,29,32,34] This may create barriers to physician services for older adults with DD.

AGE-RELATED HEALTH ISSUES

Introduction

Older adults with DD constitute a subgroup of the older U.S. population who are linked both by the presence of a lifelong disability and the potential need for services and supports that differ by type and/or intensity from those required by older adults without lifelong disabilities. A growing body of research is helping to elucidate the age-related health issues experienced by persons with Down syndrome, which are unique to that diagnosis, and these will be discussed later. It is likely that individuals with other DD with organic etiologies are also at risk for syndrome-specific health issues when they age, although these have yet to receive the attention that has been devoted to Down syndrome.

Other factors that are known to influence the health status of individuals who are aging include receipt of health care services, health behaviors, and attitudes, but how these factors influence aging among people with DD is not well understood.[45] Many of today's older adults with DD were denied access to quality health care services when they were younger and this may have compromised their health in ways in which future generations of older people with DD will not be affected. Also, the importance of health behaviors such as healthy eating and regular physical activity was neither well understood nor addressed by DD service systems when this cohort was younger,[34] and it is doubtful these individuals have benefited from health gains associated with healthy lifestyles.

Nonetheless, Janicki and Breitenbach[9] suggest this generation of older adults with DD may be healthier in many respects than younger cohorts of persons with DD because of the phenomenon of "differential mortality" – the tendency for healthier people to live longer. Still, information remains limited about the medical conditions and other health problems experienced by older adults with DD that are not syndrome specific. Most information is derived from cross-sectional studies based on small convenience samples, including some from medical practices, and it is not known if this information is generalizable. The lack of information from prospective cohort studies makes it especially difficult to identify the risk factors associated with particular conditions seen among older adults with DD.

Common Health Issues

Current information suggests that most older people with DD have health care needs that are similar to those of older people without lifelong disabilities; many also have multiple chronic conditions, and these are often accompanied by functional losses in the areas of mobility, vision, and hearing.[1,7,18,21,33,40,43,46] In a review of the extant literature about the age-associated health problems of older adults with

DD, Seltzer and Luchterhand[1] listed sensory losses (e.g., vision and hearing), musculoskeletal changes (e.g., arthritis, osteoporosis, loss of muscle), cardiovascular problems (e.g., high cholesterol, hypertension, heart disease), and gastrointestinal problems (e.g., constipation). Older adults with DD are said to experience type 2 diabetes, some forms of cancer, and dementia at rates similar to the general population.[21,36,40] Zigman et al.[46] reported an increased prevalence of thyroid disease and cardiac arrhythmias among a cohort of elderly adults with mental retardation without Down syndrome compared with the general population. Hearing loss and vision loss are thought to be significantly underdiagnosed among older people with DD.[1,36,46] Significant untreated dental disease is also a concern. Many older adults with DD take medications that are associated with periodontal disease (e.g., anticonvulsants). They may also have lacked access to regular dental care for most of their lives and have histories of poor oral hygiene at home.[1,29,36]

It is as important to work with caregivers to maximize the functioning of older adults with DD, as it is with any older adult. It is particularly important that health care providers not automatically attribute functional losses seen in older adults with DD to aging; some may be associated with medical conditions, such as hypothyroidism, adverse medication reactions, or hearing deficits, that are treatable and reversible.[1,9,33] Preserving and even maximizing functioning can enable the older person with DD to continue to perform activities of daily living; maintain their level of independence, whatever that level is; and preserve important social relationships.

Most older adults with DD are thought to face the same risk factors for age-related chronic conditions as older adults without lifelong disabilities, with the possible exception of behavioral risks such as smoking, alcohol abuse and illicit drug use, options not readily available to this cohort when they were younger.[7,21] In one of the few empirical reports of behavioral risk factors among a large cohort of adults with DD living in the community,[43] over half were obese, based on their body mass index, and more than half were reported not to engage in exercise and another 43% were reported to exercise lightly. Only 8% were reported to use tobacco and less than 1% to use alcohol. Promising results from a controlled study of an exercise training program for adults with Down syndrome[47] – specifically, improvements in cardiovascular fitness and muscle strength and some weight loss – suggest that adults with DD can benefit from structured efforts to reduce chronic disease risk through behavioral changes. Such efforts have been very limited to date.

Extant research concerning mental illness among older adults with DD is focused mainly on changes in cognitive functioning, particularly Alzheimer[1] and other forms of dementia. Age is the strongest risk factor for developing dementia in this group as it is in the general population. Most estimates of the prevalence of dementia among adults with DD are problematic because they were derived from samples with different age ranges and/or included people with Down syndrome who are known to experience a higher incidence of dementia at earlier

ages than other individuals with DD. In a large, statewide, cross-sectional study of adults aged 40 years and older, excluding persons with Down syndrome,[48] the prevalence of dementia was 3% among adults aged 40 years and older; 6% among those aged 60 years and older, and 12% among those aged 80 years and older. The age-specific prevalence rates of dementia in a more recent prospective cohort study involving elderly adults with mental retardation without Down syndrome[46] were found to be equivalent to or lower than in the general population.

Assessing dementia in people with IDs is particularly difficult because, by definition, these individuals have cognitive impairments *prior* to "age-related cognitive decline, making the detection of decline in cognitive abilities very challenging."[49] Furthermore, diagnosis may be heavily dependent on direct behavioral observations.[1,49] Because clinical presentation is often atypical, some recommend that diagnostic criteria be modified in this group. Martin,[29] for example, notes that the signs and symptoms of dementia may be subtle, including "a loss of social, verbal or job skills, a decreased ability to perform the activities of daily living, changes in behavior and sleep patterns and/or forgetfulness." Careful interviews with caregivers can help inform the clinician's understanding of the patient's putative cognitive and functional changes in the context of their daily routines; they can also enable the clinician to compare and contrast the patient's current level of cognitive functioning with the past.[49] To address concerns related to diagnosing dementia in persons with lifelong cognitive limitations, the AAMR-International Association for the Scientific Study of Intellectual Disability (AAMR-IASSID) Task Force[50] issued "Practice Guidelines for the Clinical Assessment and Care Management of Alzheimer's Disease and Other Dementias Among Adults with Intellectual Disability." This report can be accessed online.[51]

Little is known about the prevalence of other emotional and mental health problems among older adults with DD.[20] Many people, including people with DD, experience losses as they age, but it is unclear how older people with DD experience these losses given the lifelong nature of their disabilities, particularly cognitive limitations.[18] It is also unclear how often these losses are associated with behavioral and emotional problems. According to Seltzer and Luchterhand,[1] depression is the most frequently occurring psychiatric disorder in a specialty clinic for older adults with DD; they and others note depression is a particularly difficult condition to diagnose in this population, a problem that may deprive patients of access to beneficial treatments.[20] The issue of grief and bereavement also warrants attention. Because it is unclear how people with DD conceptualize or interpret their emotions about death, "normal" grief processes could be construed as pathological.[1] Health care providers also need to be cognizant that older adults with DD, like other vulnerable populations, face elevated risks for abuse and neglect; such problems could present as emotional or behavioral issues.[31,52]

An issue of increasing concern and interest with respect to older adults with DD is end-of-life care.[53] It is hoped that the expanded services and supports, and increased sensitivity to the needs of people at the end of life, which has transformed care for many in the general population in recent years, can be extended to adults with DD.

PREVENTIVE HEALTH RECOMMENDATIONS FOR OLDER ADULTS WITH DEVELOPMENTAL DISABILITIES

To guide health care providers, the Massachusetts Department of Mental Retardation, in partnership with the University of Massachusetts Medical School, has issued detailed health recommendations for adults with mental retardation.[54] The recommendations supplement evidence-based preventive health recommendations for the general population with information about special health considerations and vulnerabilities associated with DD. The recommendations are presented by age, including categories for the ages 50–64 years and 65 years and older, and note the appropriate periodicity and nature of screening for older adults. The recommendations may be accessed online.[54]

The Down Syndrome Medical Interest Group, William Cohen, editor,[55] has also issued preventive health recommendations – *Health Care Guidelines for Individuals with Down Syndrome: 1999 Revision* – which list additional tests and evaluations recommended for children and adults with Down syndrome. Health recommendations for adults are intended for all individuals older than the age of 18 years, but do include several references to older adults. This document may be accessed online.[55]

SPECIAL POPULATIONS

Down Syndrome

Despite remarkable recent gains, persons with Down syndrome have shorter life expectancies and also exhibit signs and symptoms of aging earlier than either other adults with DD or members of the general population.[1,4,7,9,20,21,27,48,50,56] Research has shown that almost all older adults with Down syndrome, at autopsy, have the neuropathological changes that are indicative of Alzheimer's disease, yet not all exhibit clinical signs of dementia.[20,49,56] Zigman et al.[20] reviewed the extant literature on age-related behavioral changes among adults with Down syndrome and reported the majority of studies consistently found that fewer than 50% exhibited significant signs and symptoms of dementia. They concluded:

> There is a substantial body of research supporting the hypothesis that adults with Down syndrome older than 50 years of age are at increased risk for losses in adaptive skills ... One issue in need of further clarification is whether observed age-related declines in adaptive skills are manifested in similar ways among adults with Down syndrome at different levels of mental retardation. It also remains to be determined whether these losses are

due to precocious but otherwise "normal" aging or to an increased age-specific susceptibility to Alzheimer's disease. (p. 72)

Answering these questions will require the conduct of cohort studies that assess the cognitive and behavioral functioning of people with Down syndrome and then follow them over time to assess cognitive and functional changes.

Older adults with Down syndrome are also at increased risk for early development of age-related hearing and vision losses, particularly cataracts, thyroid disease, seizures, musculoskeletal problems that interfere with mobility, obstructive sleep apnea, and earlier onset of menopause.[1,9,33,43,57] A number of these conditions could be mistaken for signs and symptoms of Alzheimer's disease and other forms of dementia; accuracy of diagnosis and effectiveness of treatment will do much to maintain functioning. Congenital heart disease is common among children with Down syndrome and it is typically repaired surgically early in life; these individuals may have an increased susceptibility to heart conditions as they age.[33] A large study investigating mortality in persons with Down syndrome,[27] found that mortality associated with circulatory system diseases (congenital and noncongenital) exceeded that in the general population; rates of mortality from leukemia and respiratory diseases was similarly elevated. A high prevalence of obesity has also been reported among adults with Down syndrome, although there are no data with respect to older adults.[58]

Cerebral Palsy

Cerebral palsy refers to a group of disorders that affect a person's ability to move and to maintain balance and posture.[59] Information about the effect of aging on the health care needs of people with cerebral palsy is sparse, largely anecdotal, and complicated by the heterogeneity seen among individuals with cerebral palsy, particularly with respect to cognitive functioning and associated medical conditions.[1,39] In a large, population-based survey of children with DD conducted by the CDC, 75% of children with a diagnosis of cerebral palsy had one or more other disabilities, including epilepsy, mental retardation, hearing loss, or vision impairment.[59] Although cerebral palsy is considered nonprogressive, many individuals experience functional losses, affecting ambulation and balance, at earlier ages than individuals without cerebral palsy.[1,39] Adults with cerebral palsy are also particularly susceptible to secondary conditions and disabilities, including chronic pain, musculoskeletal deformities and arthritis, overuse syndromes, poor oral health, and fatigue.[39] Some older adults with CP are also at increased risk for osteoporosis because of their lifelong immobility, inadequate calcium intake, low levels of vitamin D associated with limited sun exposure, and also medication use, which increases their risk for bone fractures.[1,33] Data concerning the life expectancy of adults with cerebral palsy are very limited but suggest that the most important predictor of life expectancy is functional level. In a large study in California,[13] adults with cerebral palsy who were high functioning (i.e., had full motor and feeding abilities) had life expectancies close to that of the general population whereas adults with cerebral palsy who lacked basic functional skills, including mobility and feeding, had much shorter life spans.

DISCUSSION

In a prescient 1988 paper, Pincus and Massad[60] cautioned that traditional care patterns for people with DD, which relied heavily on subspecialists, particularly pediatric subspecialists, could promote fragmented care within community-based health care systems, and they advocated that family physicians assume a larger responsibility for the care of this group. In their words:

> Family physicians are uniquely suited to both understand the health problems of developmentally disabled persons as they age and to serve as the "case managers" for their frequently complex health care needs. (p. 322)

This chapter shows that primary care physicians have an important role to play with respect to the clinical management of older adults with DD and that family physicians, by virtue of their training and their "culture," appear particularly well suited to assume this role. This is the first generation of older adults with DD who are living in the community and turning to community-based primary care physicians for their care, and, although information to guide physicians remains limited, more and more data are emerging about the health needs and experiences of this very heterogenous group. Their presence in communities around the country is a testimony not only to the dramatic improvements in life expectancy this group has experienced over the past 50 years, but also to their expanded access to quality health care services and to vastly enhanced societal opportunities over that same time period.

Most research about the health needs of this group is based on cross-sectional surveys that provide "snapshots" of the health care needs of disparate, often small, samples of older adults with DD at particular points in time. By virtue of these designs, it is unclear if findings from these studies can be generalized to the larger population of older adults with DD; it is also impossible to identify risk factors and other antecedents and influences on aging in this group using cross-sectional designs. The "evidence" so central to the practice of evidence-based medicine simply does not exist right now to guide physicians with respect to DD. Longitudinal studies that follow large cohorts of adults with DD as well as randomized control trials designed to evaluate the efficacy of various preventive and therapeutic interventions are needed to elucidate fully the health needs of this group. Building on preventive health recommendations for the general population, two expert physician panels have issued preventive health recommendations for adults with mental retardation and also for people with Down syndrome to guide health care providers.[54,55]

Considerable research attention has been focused on older adults with Down syndrome because these individuals are known to exhibit signs and symptoms of aging at earlier ages than both other adults with DD and members of the general population; they also appear to have a special susceptibility to dementia of the Alzheimer type. Among adults with Down syndrome and other types of DD with organic etiologies, it is unclear how the "normal" aging process interacts with characteristics related to the underlying medical condition.

Cross-sectional studies of older adults with DD who do not have Down syndrome or other types of DD with organic etiologies – a group that comprises "most" older adults with DD – suggest that these individuals generally face the same age-related health problems as individuals without lifelong disabilities. Concerns that older adults with DD, but without Down syndrome, faced increased risks for dementia and other conditions associated with cognitive and behavioral losses appear to be ungrounded; most recent research suggests the incidence of these conditions among older people with DD without Down syndrome is similar to that of older people without lifelong disabilities. Information about mental health problems, such as depression and anxiety disorders, among older adults with DD is especially limited and this area of inquiry deserves special attention.

Data about behavioral risk factors for this group are in especially short supply but emerging information suggests these individuals are not immune from national trends associated with the obesity epidemic; elevated rates of overweight and obesity have been reported in several studies, along with information about high rates of unhealthy diets and sedentary behavior. Risks associated with alcohol abuse, illegal drug use, and smoking, on the other hand, appear lower, perhaps because of historical considerations – most of the nation's older adults with DD lived in protected environments like institutions or their family's home when they were younger and may have had less access to these substances than the general population.

If, in fact, most older adults with DD face many of the same age-related health risks as older adults without lifelong disabilities, this still presents primary care physicians with challenges. Tyler and Bourguet[14] advise physicians to "think of geriatric syndromes" when providing primary care to adult patients with mental retardation and this advice applies even more directly to older adults. According to Tyler and Bourguet:[14]

> Evaluation and management strategies developed for geriatric medicine can be applied to adults with mental retardation, regardless of age. The "geriatric syndromes," including incontinence, falls, immobility, functional impairment, cognitive decline, osteoporosis, and polypharmacy, may emerge before the 6th decade and require recognition and careful evaluation.

Many older adults with DD come to the physician's office with inadequate medical information, which presents special challenges. Under these circumstances, diagnosing common medical conditions can be difficult, and diagnosing complex medical and behavioral conditions may feel next to impossible. Physicians are highly dependent on the observations and assistance of caregivers – both family members and direct support staff – to diagnose and treat older adults with DD. Physicians may find it helpful to consult with interdisciplinary geriatric assessment teams around the needs of older adults with DD and complex medical and behavioral conditions.

The concept of "healthy aging" is beginning to be heard within service systems for older adults with DD and these discussions have great promise.[61] The notion that aging persons with DD can be helped to avoid disease and disability, maintain high cognitive and physical function, and continue engaging in rewarding activities should be a goal for families, service and support systems, and physicians, although what will be required to help the majority of older people with DD achieve this goal has yet to be defined. Janicki and Breitenbach[9] believe that the next frontier with respect to improving the health status and quality of life for aging persons with DD lies in the area of lifestyle or health behavior changes, for example, promoting regular physical activity, although the literature on this topic at present is sparse.

Physicians could play an important role in promoting healthy lifestyles among their older patients with DD; at a minimum, they should follow the same guidelines for routine screening and other dimensions of clinical prevention as with other patients of the same sex and age, but without life-long disabilities. Counseling patients and caregivers about the importance of healthy eating, regular physical activity, and limited sedentary behavior will help to emphasize the importance of day-to-day behaviors on health status.

Finally, physicians should be aware that under the aegis of state government, there are formal community-based service and support networks for people with DD and a parallel network of community-based services and supports for people who are aging. The robustness of these systems varies from state to state. Unfortunately, older adults with DD sometimes "fall between the cracks" and do not receive the appropriate level and type of services they require from either service network. Across the country, however, there are encouraging signs that DD service networks are beginning to respond to the special needs of older adults and the aging service network is becoming more welcoming to individuals with DD. This is a cohort whose numbers will only increase, and it is heartening to see that the publicly funded systems that are responsible for their supervision are beginning to put in place services and supports to safeguard health and functioning and, optimally, to promote healthy aging among members of this group.

REFERENCES

1. Seltzer GB, Luchterhand C. Health and well-being of older persons with developmental disabilities: a clinical review. In: Seltzer MM, Krauss MW, Janicki MP, eds. *Life Course Perspectives on Adulthood and Old Age*. Washington DC: American Association on Mental Retardation; 1994:109–142.

2. US Centers for Disease Control and Prevention. Developmental Disabilities Topic Home. Available at: http://www.cdc.gov/ncbddd/dd/default.htm. Accessed May 28, 2008.

3. US Department of Health and Human Services, Administration on Developmental Disabilities. The Developmental Disabilities Assistance and Bill of Rights Act of 2000. Available at: http://www.acf.hhs.gov/programs/add/ddact/DDACT2.html. Accessed May 28, 2008.

4. Eyman RK, Borthwick-Duffy SA. Trends in mortality rates and predictors of mortality. In: Seltzer MM, Krauss MW, Janicki MP, eds. *Life Course Perspectives on Adulthood and Old Age*. Washington DC: American Association on Mental Retardation; 1994:93–105.

5. Anderson DJ. Health issues. In: Sutton E, Factor AR, Hawkins BA, Heller T, Seltzer GB, eds. *Older Adults with Developmental Disabilities*. Baltimore: Brookes Publishing Co.; 1993:29–48.

6. Bittles AH, Petterson BA, Sullivan SG, Hussain R, Glasson EJ, Montgomery PD. The influence of intellectual disability on life expectancy. *J Gerontol A Biol Sci Med Sci*. 2002;57:M470–M472.

7. Janicki MP, Dalton AJ, Henderson CM, Davidson PW. Mortality and morbidity among older adults with intellectual disability: health services considerations. *Disabil Rehabil*. 1999;21(5/6):284–294.

8. American Association on Intellectual and Developmental Disabilities. Definition of mental retardation. Available at: http://www.aamr.org/Policies/faq_mental_retardation.shtml. Accessed May 28, 2008.

9. Janicki MP, Breitenbach N. *Aging and Intellectual Disabilities – Improving Longevity and Promoting Healthy Aging: Summative Report*. Geneva: World Health Organization; 2000.

10. Luckasson RA, Borthwick-Duffy S, Buntinx WHE, Coulter DL, Craig EM, Reeve A. *Mental Retardation: Definition, Classification, and Systems of Supports*, 10th ed. Washington, DC: American Association on Mental Retardation; 2002.

11. US Centers for Disease Control and Prevention. Developmental Disability – Intellectual Disability. Available at: http://www.cdc.gov/ncbddd/dd/mr3.htm. Accessed May 28, 2008.

12. Shavelle RM, Strauss, DJ, Pickett J. Causes of death in autism. *J Autism Dev Disord*. 2001;31(6):569–576.

13. Strauss D, Shavelle R. Life expectancy of adults with cerebral palsy. *Dev Med Child Neurol*. 1998;40:369–375.

14. Tyler CV, Bourguet C. Primary care of adults with mental retardation. *J Fam Pract*. 1997:44(5):487–494.

15. US Centers for Disease Control and Prevention. Autism Information Center. Available at: http://www.cdc.gov/ncbddd/autism/index.htm. Accessed May 28, 2008.

16. Krauss MW, Greenberg JS, Seltzer MM. Aging in adults with developmental disabilities and severe and persistent mental illness. In: Gallo JJ, Busby-Whitehead J, Rabins PV, Silliman RA, Murphy JB, Reichel W, eds. *Reichel's Care of the Elderly*. Philadelphia: Lippincott Williams & Wilkins; 1999:241–251.

17. Adlin M. Older adults with developmental disabilities and chronic mental illness. In: Reichel W, Gallo JJ, Busby-Whitehead J, Delfs JR, Murphy JB, eds. *Care of the Elderly: Clinical Aspects of Aging*. 4th ed. Baltimore: Williams & Wilkins; 1995:161–167.

18. Janicki MP. Policies and supports for older persons with mental retardation. In: Seltzer MM, Krauss MW, Janicki MP, eds. *Life Course Perspectives on Adulthood and Old Age*. Washington, DC: American Association on Mental Retardation; 1994:143–165.

19. McNellis CA. Mental retardation and aging: Mental health issues. *Gerontol Geriatr Educ*. 1997;17(3):75–86.

20. Zigman WB, Seltzer GB, Silverman WP. Behavioral and mental health changes associated with aging in adults with mental retardation. In: Seltzer MM, Krauss MW, Janicki MP, eds. *Life Course Perspectives on Adulthood and Old Age.* Washington, DC: American Association on Mental Retardation; 1994:67–91.

21. American Association on Intellectual and Developmental Disabilities. Fact Sheet: AGING – Older adults and their aging caregivers. Available at: http://www.aamr.org/Policies/faq_aging.shtml. Accessed May 28, 2008.

22. Heller T, Janicki M, Hawkins B. Healthy aging and community participation. In: Lakin KC, Turnbull A, eds. *National Goals & Research for People with Intellectual & Developmental Disabilities.* Washington, DC: American Association on Mental Retardation; 2005:311–332.

23. Braddock D. Aging and developmental disabilities: demographic and policy issues affecting American families. *Ment Retard.* 1999;37(2):155–161.

24. Heller T, Factor A. Facilitating future planning and transitions out of the home. In: Seltzer MM, Krauss MW, Janicki MP, eds. *Life Course Perspectives on Adulthood and Old Age.* Washington, DC: American Association on Mental Retardation; 1994:39–50.

25. Seltzer MM, Krauss MW. Aging parents with coresident adult children: the impact of lifelong caregiving. In: Seltzer MM, Krauss MW, Janicki MP, eds. *Life Course Perspectives on Adulthood and Old Age.* Washington, DC: American Association on Mental Retardation; 1994:3–18.

26. Braddock D, Hemp R, Rizzolo MC, Coulter D, Haffer L, Thompson M. *The State of the States in Developmental Disabilities – 2005 (Preliminary Report).* Washington, DC: American Association on Mental Retardation; 2005.

27. Day SM, Strauss DJ, Shavelle RM, Reynolds RJ. Mortality and causes of death in persons with Down syndrome in California. *Dev Med Child Neurol.* 2005;47:171–176.

28. Garrard SD. Community health issues. In: Matson JL, Mulick JA, eds. *Handbook of Mental Retardation.* New York: Pergamon Press; 1983:289–305.

29. Martin BA. Primary care of adults with mental retardation living in the community. *Am Fam Physician.* 1997;56(2):485–494.

30. Smith DS. Health care management of adults with Down syndrome. *Am Fam Physician.* 2001;64(6):1031–1038, 1039–1040.

31. Prater CD, Zylstra RG. Medical care of adults with mental retardation. *Am Fam Physician.* 2006;73(12):2175–2184.

32. Minihan PM, Dean DH, Lyons CM. Managing the care of patients with mental retardation: a survey of physicians. *Ment Retard.* 1993;31(4):239–246.

33. Adlin M. Health care issues. In: Sutton E, Factor AR, Hawkins BA, Heller T, Seltzer GB, eds. *Older Adults with Developmental Disabilities.* Baltimore: Brookes Publishing Co.; 1993:49–60.

34. Edgerton RB, Gaston MA, Kelly H, Ward TW. Health care for aging people with mental retardation. *Ment Retard.* 1994;32(2):146–150.

35. Seltzer MM. Continuity of health services throughout life – Scientific presentation. Paper presented at the Surgeon General's Conference on Health Disparities and Mental Retardation. October 10, 2001, Washington, DC.

36. Carlsen WR, Galluzzi KE, Forman LF, Cavalieri TA. Comprehensive geriatric assessment: applications for community-residing, elderly people with mental retardation/development disabilities. *Ment Retard.* 1994;32(5):334–340.

37. Traci MA, Seekins T, Szalda-Petree A, Ravesloot C. Assessing secondary conditions among adults with developmental disabilities: a preliminary study. *Ment Retard.* 2002;40(2):119–131.

38. US Department of Health and Human Services. *The Surgeon General's Call To Action To Improve the Health and Wellness of Persons with Disabilities.* Available at: http://www.surgeongeneral.gov/library/disabilities/calltoaction/calltoaction.pdf. Accessed May 28, 2008.

39. Zaffuto-Sforza CD. Aging with cerebral palsy. *Phys Med Rehabil Clin N Am.* 2005;16:235–249.

40. Cooper SA. Clinical study of the effects of age on the physical health of adults with mental retardation. *AJMR.* 1998;102(6):582–589.

41. Reiss S, Levitan G, Szyszko J. Emotional disturbance and mental retardation: diagnostic overshadowing. *AJMD.* 1982;86:567–574.

42. Jopp DA, Keys CB. Diagnostic overshadowing reviewed and reconsidered. *AJMR.* 2001;106(5):416–433.

43. Janicki MP, Davidson PW, Henderson CM, et al. Health characteristics and health services utilization in older adults with intellectual disability living in community residences. *JIDR.* 2002;46(4):287–298.

44. TheARC. Position statements – Health care. Available at: http://www.thearc.org/NetCommunity/Page.aspx?&pid=1372&srcid=405. Accessed May 28, 2008.

45. Seltzer MM, Krauss MW, Janicki MP. Preface. In: Seltzer MM, Krauss MW, Janicki MP, eds. *Life Course Perspectives on Adulthood and Old Age.* Washington, DC: American Association on Mental Retardation; 1994:vii–viii.

46. Zigman WB, Schupf N, Devenny DA, et al. Incidence and prevalence of dementia in elderly adults with mental retardation without Down syndrome. *AJMR.* 2004;109:126–141.

47. Rimmer JF, Heller T, Wang E, Valerio I. Improvements in physical fitness in adults with Down syndrome. *AJMR.* 2004;109(2):165–174.

48. Janicki MP, Dalton AJ. Prevalence of dementia and impact on intellectual disability services. *Ment Retard.* 2000;38(3):276–288.

49. Shultz J, Aman M, Kelbley T, et al. Evaluation of screening tools for dementia in older adults with mental retardation. *AJMR.* 2004;109(2):98–110.

50. Janicki MP, Heller T, Seltzer GB, Hogg J. Practice guidelines for the clinical assessment and care management of Alzheimer's disease and other dementias among adults with intellectual disability. *JIDR.* 1996;40(4):374–382.

51. American Association on Mental Retardation–International Association for the Scientific Study of Intellectual Disability Task Force. *Practice Guidelines for the Clinical Assessment and Care Management of Alzheimer and Other Dementias Among Adults with Mental Retardation.* Available at: http://www.aamr.org/Reading_Room/Practical/practical_guidelines.pdf. Accessed May 28, 2008.

52. Strickler HL. Interaction between family violence and mental retardation. *Ment Retard.* 2001;39(6):461–471.

53. Botsford AL. Status of end of life care in organizations providing services for older persons with a developmental disability. *AJMR.* 2004;109(5):421–428.

54. Massachusetts Department of Mental Retardation, University of Massachusetts Medical School's Center for Developmental Disabilities Evaluation and Research. Preventive health recommendations for adults with mental retardation. Available at: http://www.guideline.gov/summary/summary.aspx?doc_id=4201. Accessed May 28, 2008.

55. Cohen WI, Patterson B, eds. Down Syndrome Medical Interest Group. Health Care Guidelines for Individuals with

Down syndrome – 1999 Revision. Available at: http://www.ndsccenter.org/resources/healthcare.pdf. Accessed May 28, 2008.

56. Bush A, Beail N. Risk factors for dementia in people with Down syndrome: issues in assessment and diagnosis. *AJMR.* 2004;109(2):83–97.

57. Gill CJ, Brown AA. Overview of health issues of older women with intellectual disabilities. In: Hammel J, Nochajski SM, eds. *Aging and Developmental Disability: Current Research, Programming, and Practice Implications.* New York: The Haworth Press, Inc.; 2000:23–36.

58. Braunschweig CL, Gomez S, Sheean P, Tomey KM, Rimmer J, Heller T. Nutritional status and risk factors for chronic disease in urban-dwelling adults with Down syndrome. *AJMR.* 2004;109(2):186–193.

59. US Centers for Disease Control and Prevention. Developmental Disabilities – Cerebral Palsy. Available at: http://www.cdc.gov/ncbddd/dd/ddcp.htm. Accessed May 28, 2008.

60. Pincus S, Massad R. Family medicine and the developmentally disabled: a relationship worth building. *Fam Med.* 1988;20(5):322–323.

61. Davidson PW, Heller T, Janicki MP, Hyer K. *The Tampa Scientific Conference on Intellectual Disability, Aging, and Health. Final Report.* Chicago: Rehabilitation and Training Center on Aging with Developmental Disabilities, University of Illinois at Chicago; 2003.

20

PULMONARY ISSUES IN THE ELDERLY

David DeFeo, MD, Shannon S. Carson, MD

Most of the pulmonary diseases present in the elderly also exist in younger patients; however, the incidence and presentation of these diseases can differ greatly between these two age groups. Elderly patients tend to have other comorbidities that can increase the difficulty with which diagnoses are made and interfere with recovery. This is particularly true when disease processes advance to cause respiratory failure.

PHYSIOLOGICAL CHANGE WITH AGING

Changes to the respiratory system occur with aging that have an impact on pulmonary reserve and decrease the respiratory system's ability to respond to physiological stress and disease. These "normal aging" changes are mild and usually not clinically relevant in the healthy state. The changes discussed later should never limit a patient's usual activity or cause significant dyspnea at rest in the absence of lung disease.

As a patient ages, elastic tissue in the lung is replaced by collagen. This change results in smaller airway size.[1] Airway diameter decreases significantly after the fourth decade, resulting in increased air trapping as small airways collapse at end expiration. The alveolar–arterial oxygen gradient increases with advancing age because of a number of factors including increased collagen deposition in the walls of alveoli, changes in alveolar structure, and decreased alveolar surface area. The thoracic cage and respiratory muscles also change with age. Arthritis of the costovertebral joints, kyphoscoliosis, and calcification of intercostal cartilage result in decreased chest wall compliance and increased stiffness.[2] Diaphragmatic strength diminishes with age because of an unknown mechanism.[3]

A number of changes can occur that affect mechanical defenses of the lung. Elderly patients can be susceptible to mechanical dysfunction of the swallowing mechanism from central nervous disorders, primary swallowing dysfunction, and sedating medications. Neurological dysfunction can also

lead to a decreased cough reflex. Finally, mucociliary clearance decreases with age.[4]

OBSTRUCTIVE LUNG DISEASES

Dyspnea, wheezing, and cough are clinical symptoms often reported by patients. In the elderly, the differential diagnosis of the symptoms is broad and includes chronic obstructive pulmonary disease (COPD), asthma, congestive heart failure, anemia, pneumonia, and pulmonary embolus to name a few. Asthma and COPD are commonly grouped together under the term obstructive lung diseases. They represent a continuum of obstructive lung diseases from COPD, which is characteristically irreversible, to asthma, which represents reversible lung disease. It can be difficult to truly differentiate between the two disease processes. It is common for elderly patients with asthma not to have fully reversible disease. This is related to the diminishing function of the sympathetic nervous system that occurs with aging, leading to a diminished response to β-agonists.[5]

Asthma

The National Institutes of Health defines asthma as "A chronic inflammatory disease of the airways in which many cells play a role, in particular, mast cells, eosinophils, and T-lymphocytes. In susceptible individuals, this inflammation causes recurrent episodes of wheezing, breathlessness, chest tightness, and cough, particularly at night or in the early morning. These symptoms are usually associated with widespread but variable airflow limitation that is at least partially reversible either spontaneously or with treatment. This inflammation also causes an associated increase in airway hyperresponsiveness to a variety of stimuli."[6] Asthma is a disease that may occur at any age. Approximately 10% of children suffer from asthma. The prevalence declines to 5% in patients in their third and fourth

Table 20.1. Asthma Classification and Treatment

| Asthma Severity | Symptoms | | Peak Flow Rate | Treatment |
	Day	Night		
Mild intermittent	<2/wk	<2/mo	>80% predicted	As needed therapy with a short-acting β-agonist
Mild persistent	>2/wk	>2/mo	>80% predicted	Low-dose inhaled corticosteroid or leukotriene antagonist or cromolyn
Moderate persistent	Daily	>1/wk	60%–80% predicted	Low-to-medium dose inhaled corticosteroid with long-acting β-agonist
				Consider theophylline
Severe persistent	Continuous		<60% predicted	Oral corticosteroid w/ high-dose inhaled corticosteroid and long-acting β-agonist

decades of life. After the age of 65 years, the prevalence rises to approximately 8%. This prevalence may be underestimated given that elderly patients are less likely to complain of dyspnea. The symptoms may also overlap with other diseases, leading clinicians to attribute them falsely to these other diseases. This, in turn, may result in less use of pulmonary function testing, which is vital in diagnosing asthma.

Although the incidence of asthma in developed countries is increasing, mortality rates for asthma have declined overall since the 1980s. Most of these deaths occur in patients older than 45 years of age, underscoring the importance of diagnosing asthma in the elderly. A study using the Nationwide Inpatient Sample examined all of the hospitalizations for asthma recorded in the database in the year 2000. Patients who were older than 55 years accounted for 30.2% of the more than 65,000 hospital admissions resulting from asthma exacerbations. Multivariate analysis identified age, having more comorbid conditions, and male sex as being associated with an increased risk of mortality.[7]

The diagnosis of asthma hinges on the ability to demonstrate reversible airway obstruction. Spirometry provides measurements of forced expiratory volume in 1 second (FEV1), forced vital capacity (FVC), and peak expiratory flow, which are useful in demonstrating the presence of obstructive lung disease. A greater than 15% and 200 mL improvement in FEV1 spontaneously or after administration of a β-agonist supports the diagnosis of asthma. With normal spirometry, a broncho-provocation study such as a methacholine challenge, may be used to diagnose asthma. This test is safe to perform and well tolerated. A decrease of 20% in FEV1 is considered a positive study at a concentration of methacholine of less than 4 mg/mL. Although a positive methacholine challenge test is not specific for asthma, a negative test in the absence of asthma treatment virtually rules out asthma. Patients can also measure peak expiratory flows over several days. If there is evidence of diurnal variation greater than 20% and at least 60 L/min, this lends credence to the diagnosis of asthma.

The treatment of asthma involves first characterizing the frequency of the patient's asthma symptoms and the variability in peak expiratory flows (Table 20.1). Mild intermittent asthma is characterized by daytime symptoms occurring less than two times per week and nighttime symptoms less than two times

per month. Also FEV1 and peak expiratory flow rates generally are greater than 80% of those predicted with less than 20% variability in these measurements. These patients can be treated simply with as needed β2-agonists.

Patients with mild, persistent asthma have daytime symptoms more than two times per week, with nighttime symptoms occurring more than two times per month. FEV1 and peak expiratory flow rates remain greater than 80% of those predicted, but there is typically 20%–30% variability in these measurements. The foundation of therapy for these patients is antiinflammatory agents such as inhaled corticosteroids, leukotriene antagonists, or less commonly, cromolyn. β2-agonists are used for quick relief of symptoms.

Patients with moderate, persistent asthma have daily symptoms requiring daily use of their β2-agonist rescue inhaler, more than two exacerbations per week, and one nighttime exacerbation per week. FEV1 and peak expiratory flow rates can be 60%–80% of those predicted, with variability greater than 30% in peak expiratory flows. For these patients, antiinflammatory agents remain the cornerstone of therapy, along with the addition of a long-acting β-agonist. Patients should be educated to avoid doses of long-acting β-agonists beyond daily recommendations, especially during exacerbations, as overuse may increase the risk of complications such as arrhythmias or possibly death. Consideration should be made to increasing the dose of the inhaled corticosteroid and possibly adding theophylline.

Severe, persistent asthma is characterized by continuous symptoms of asthma, frequent exacerbations, and nighttime symptoms. FEV1 and peak expiratory flow rates can be below 60% of those predicted with variability greater than 30%. Treatment involves maximizing all of the above classes of therapies in addition to limited courses of oral corticosteroids.

Once control of symptoms has been achieved, as evidenced by a minimal use of rescue β-agonists, therapy can be deescalated in a stepwise manner. This is a strategy supported by the British Thoracic Society guidelines for the management of asthma. For example, in a patient with moderate, persistent asthma with well-controlled symptoms who is being treated with a combination corticosteroid and long-acting β-agonist inhaler, one could consider "stepping down" the patient's therapy to a corticosteroid inhaler only.

Many of the inhaled therapies described previously come in the form of metered-dose inhalers (MDIs). Drug delivery is dependent on the correct use of MDIs. This, in turn, is dependent on the correct timing of the triggered drug release and inspiratory effort. The elderly patient may have difficulty with MDIs as a drug delivery system because of a number of reasons such as cognitive impairment, arthritic disease of the hands, or difficulty with near vision.[8] The failure to use the MDI correctly results in inadequate deposition of drug into the lungs of the patient, and thus less bronchodilatory or antiinflammatory effect of the medication.[9] Use of a spacer device makes correct timing of the actuation of the inhaler with the inhalation effort unnecessary. In one study, 97% of patients were able to use an MDI correctly with a spacer compared with only 87% of patients not using a spacer.[10] Lung deposition of drug has been shown to be improved with spacers.[11] This is a result of reduced oral deposition of drug, which in the case of inhaled corticosteroids also results in less throat irritation and oral candidiasis. Dry powder inhalers may also be a solution to the incorrect timing issue of MDIs. Although these devices do not require the coordination needed for the correct use of MDIs, repeated patient education on use of the device is necessary.

Chronic Obstructive Pulmonary Disease

The Global Initiative for Chronic Obstructive Lung Disease (GOLD) report defines COPD as a disease state characterized by airflow limitation that is not fully reversible. The airflow limitation is usually both progressive and associated with an abnormal inflammatory response of the lungs to noxious particles or gases.[12] Airflow limitation is confirmed by spirometry revealing an FEV1/FVC ratio <70%. The GOLD criteria further classify COPD severity according to FEV1 as follows: stage 1 is an FEV1 ≥80% of predicted; stage 2 is an FEV1 50%–<80% predicted; stage 3 is an FEV1 30%–<50% predicted; and stage 4 is an FEV1 < 30%.

Two disorders are included under the heading of COPD. These include chronic bronchitis and emphysema. Chronic bronchitis is a clinically defined entity and is characterized by the presence of a productive cough for 3 months in each of 2 successive years, with other causes of chronic cough ruled out. Emphysema is defined anatomically as the destruction of alveolar walls and permanent enlargement of the air spaces distal to the terminal bronchioles. This destruction of the elastic tissue of the lung results in premature closing of airways on exhalation, leading to airflow limitation. The majority of patients have features of both disorders.

COPD continues to be one of the leading diseases responsible for morbidity and mortality in the United States. It currently is the fourth leading cause of death in the United States. It is one of only a few diseases in which the death rate has been increasing over the past several years. It is estimated that, in the next few years, COPD will become the third ranked cause of death in the United States. COPD resulted in 8 million physician office outpatient visits, 1.5 million emergency room visits,

Table 20.2. COPD Classification and Treatment

COPD Stage	FEV1 (% Predicted)	Treatment
Stage 1	>80%	Ipratropium or albuterol as needed
Stage 2	>50% but <80%	Long-acting bronchodilator such as tiotropium
Stage 3	>30% but <50%	Inhaled corticosteroids and long-acting bronchodilator
Stage 4	<30%	As above with the addition of oxygen if necessary for hypoxia or cor pulmonale

726,000 hospitalizations, and 119,000 deaths in the year 2000.[13] In 2004, the direct cost of COPD in the United States was $20.9 billion dollars.[14]

The GOLD guidelines prescribe treatment for COPD based on the severity of illness (Table 20.2). A short-acting bronchodilator such as ipratropium or albuterol is usually all that is required for stage I disease. Stage II disease may require the addition of a long-acting bronchodilator or a switch to a long-acting anticholinergic such as tiotropium. By stage III, inhaled corticosteroids should be considered. Although the benefit of inhaled corticosteroids for survival is controversial, they have been shown to decrease exacerbation rates.[15] Stage IV disease usually requires treatment with oxygen for chronic respiratory failure. Supplemental oxygen is indicated when the hemoglobin oxygen saturation is below 88% or the PaO_2 is <55 mm Hg. If the PaO_2 is 56–59 mm Hg, then oxygen is indicated only when there are signs of cor pulmonale or secondary erythrocytosis. The Nocturnal Oxygen Therapy Trial demonstrated that continuous oxygen in these patients results in improved survival when compared with patients who only use nocturnal oxygen.[16]

Other options exist for the treatment of COPD. The usefulness of theophylline is limited by its narrow therapeutic index. It may cause a small improvement in FEV1 as well as improvement in exercise capacity and symptoms; however, even at therapeutic levels, side effects such as nausea, diarrhea, headaches, and irritability may occur, especially in the elderly. At toxic blood levels, seizures and cardiac arrhythmias may occur. Mucolytic agents have not been shown to improve outcomes in acute exacerbations in any randomized, controlled trial. Antibiotics have demonstrated favorable results when used during an exacerbation of COPD. Systemic corticosteroids are also useful for acute exacerbations of COPD, but should be rapidly tapered. Rarely do prolonged courses of steroids benefit COPD patients. As the duration of oral steroid treatment increases, the side effects of osteoporosis, cataracts, diabetes, and skin thinning become more common. A randomized, placebo-controlled trial demonstrated that a 2-week course of corticosteroid therapy is as effective as an 8-week course.[17]

Pulmonary rehabilitation can be used to improve functional capacity. Lower extremity exercise training improves exercise tolerance. Upper extremity exercise training is also advised, as many patients experience dyspnea while sedentary and performing activities of daily living. These regimens, along with breathing technique training have been shown to improve symptoms in patients with COPD.[18]

Lung volume reduction surgery represents another possible treatment for severe COPD. Its benefit is based on the assumption that the removal of overdistended, hyperinflated lung allows less diseased lung to expand, thereby improving lung function. The National Emphysema Treatment Trial examined the efficacy of this procedure in COPD. Patients with primarily upper lobe emphysema and very poor exercise tolerance had the greatest benefit. In this group, mortality rates were lower, exercise capacity higher, and overall quality of life improved compared with medically managed patients.[19]

Among all interventions for COPD patients, smoking cessation remains one of the most important as it will reduce the rate of loss of pulmonary function over time. Long-term quit rates of 5%–10% have been demonstrated when physicians make a recommendation to quit smoking, Emphasizing the benefits of smoking cessation with patients may provide the motivation needed to quit. These benefits include reduced cough from reduced sputum production, improved exercise tolerance, improved ability to taste, and lower risk for cardiac events and cerebrovascular accidents. It should be emphasized to patients that even when they quit smoking late in life, exsmokers have a slower rate of decline in lung function when compared with smokers.[20] Pharmacological intervention improves quit rates significantly when compared with counseling alone, and the combination of the two have proved to be the best. Nicotine replacement with or without the antidepressant bupropion remains the standard regimen for smoking cessation. A new medication, varenicline, is a partial nicotine receptor agonist that has shown promise in early trials. There have been no specific trials in the elderly for the above pharmacological agents.

Yearly vaccination against influenza A and B is another important aspect in the management of COPD and appears to be well tolerated by most patients. These recommendations are based on a number of randomized trials that show patients who have received the influenza vaccine have fewer exacerbations.[21] It is also recommended that COPD patients be vaccinated with the pneumococcal vaccine, and then again in 5 years if the first dose was given prior to the age of 65 years.

PULMONARY EMBOLISM

Pulmonary embolism (PE), a condition with a 30% mortality rate if untreated,[22] remains a challenging diagnosis for clinicians to make. This results from the variability in clinical presentation. Symptoms in the elderly can be nonspecific and attributable to other underlying cardiovascular diseases. The incidence of venous thromboembolism (VTE) increases with age, beginning at the age of 45 years, and then undergoes a significant increase after the age of 65 years.[23] In patients aged 60–75 years, the incidence of VTE is approximately 3.5 per 1000,

Table 20.3. Diagnostic Options for PE

Diagnostic Modality	Advantages	Disadvantages
D-dimer	Minimally invasive; high sensitivity	Usually elevated nonspecifically in elderly; low specificity
Doppler ultrasound	Minimally invasive; high specificity	Misses pelvic vein thrombosis; low sensitivity
V/Q scan	Minimally invasive	High percentage of inconclusive scans in the elderly
hCT	Minimally invasive	IV contrast; misses peripheral pulmonary emboli
Pulmonary angiogram	Gold standard	Invasive; IV contrast

increasing to 9 per 1000 in patients aged 75 years and older.[24] Pulmonary embolism is associated with a higher short-term mortality rate in the elderly compared with younger patients.[25]

The major risk factors for VTE include hypercoagulability states, venous stasis, and endothelial injury. Immobility in the elderly is a common cause for venous stasis, as demonstrated in one study in which 65% of patients older than 65 years diagnosed with a PE had been confined to bedrest for more than 4 days.[26] Other causes of venous stasis include congestive heart failure, prior thrombosis, and hyperviscosity syndromes. Endothelial injury can be a result of knee or hip surgery, trauma, and other surgical procedures. Surgical procedures can also result in immobility leading to venous stasis, giving elderly postoperative patients two risk factors for VTE. Hypercoagulable states can result from malignancy, trauma, burns, inherited deficiencies of anticoagulant proteins, or acquired conditions such as the lupus anticoagulant.

A review of the Prospective Investigation of Pulmonary Embolism Diagnosis study revealed that patients older than 70 years had similar symptoms of PE compared with younger patients. The more common symptoms and signs included dyspnea, pleuritic chest pain, cough, anxiety, tachypnea, and tachycardia.[27] In one series comparing patients younger than 64 years to an older group of patients, the older group was more likely to have cardiac arrest and/or falling to the floor.[28] This may result from the lack of cardiopulmonary reserve observed in the elderly as part of the aging process. Thus, the elderly patient may be more prone to right ventricular dysfunction for a given degree of pulmonary vascular obstruction than a younger patient.

Diagnostic tests used for PE tend to have lower specificities in the elderly than in younger patients (Table 20.3). D-dimer is the degradation product formed from the fibrinolysis of venous thrombosis. The D-dimer enzyme-linked immunosorbent assay test has a sensitivity of between 87% and 100%; however, the specificity is usually much lower. In a cohort of over 1,000 patients grouped by decade of age, the sensitivity of the enzyme-linked immunosorbent assay D-dimer test remained high in all groups, but the specificity dropped dramatically in the elderly age groups.[29] In this cohort, only 5% of patients had a negative assay (defined as <500 μg/L) in the older than 80 years age group, limiting the diagnostic utility of this test. Thus, in a patient with a low probability of deep vein thrombosis(DVT)/PE, a negative D-dimer essentially rules out PE. Unfortunately, this is an uncommon occurrence in the elderly patient, which leads to further investigation for PE.

Lower limb venous compression ultrasonography is a useful tool when attempting to diagnose VTE. In patients with confirmed PE, DVT is found via ultrasonography in 50%–80% of patients.[30] The specificity of ultrasonography for proximal lower extremity DVT is greater than 97%.[31] There is no evidence that ultrasonography of the lower extremities is limited in any way in elderly patients when compared with younger patients.

The Prospective Investigation of Pulmonary Embolism Diagnosis study demonstrated the usefulness of ventilation-perfusion lung scanning as a diagnostic test for suspected PE. The test has a high sensitivity to exclude PE with a normal perfusion scan. Conversely, the test has a high specificity to confirm PE with a high-probability scan.[32] The major limitation in ventilation-perfusion scanning occurs with intermediate probability results, which are considered inconclusive. When a large cohort of patients underwent perfusion scanning for suspected PE, the number of inconclusive scans increased from 32% in patients younger than 40 years to 58% in patients aged 80 years or older.[31] This is likely related to changes to the lung parenchyma that occur with aging, which are more likely to affect the results of a functional test such as ventilation-perfusion scanning.

Helical computed tomography's (hCT) role in diagnosing VTE has grown significantly over the past several years. Early single-detector units were adequate for imaging central vessels, but not more peripheral vessels, thus limiting the sensitivity to approximately 70%. Because of the low sensitivity, hCT had to be combined with another diagnostic test, usually lower extremity ultrasound, to reduce the false-negative rate. In a study using these two modalities, the 3-month thromboembolic risk was 0.5% among patients with negative hCT and ultrasound, a number similar to that seen with pulmonary angiography.[33] Multidetector hCT allows for better definition of the vasculature and thus has improved sensitivity. Studies of patients with elevated D-dimer levels who underwent hCT without lower extremity ultrasound demonstrated a 3-month thromboembolic risk of 0.6%–1.3% in patients with negative studies.[34,35] Given the lower usefulness of the D-dimer assay in the elderly, it is unclear how these data apply to this subset of patients.

Anticoagulation prevents the extension of existing clots and recurrence of VTE, and it reduces the incidence of fatal PE by 70%.[36] Anticoagulation should be withheld in patients who have a contraindication such as active gastrointestinal bleeding or an intracranial process such as hemorrhage or neoplasm. The elderly appear to be especially susceptible to bleeding while receiving anticoagulation therapy but this should not be withheld unless one of the aforementioned contraindications exists.[37] Intravenous unfractionated heparin is typically the initial agent used for anticoagulation. Low-molecular-weight heparins (LMWHs) have also been shown to be effective as initial treatment in VTE. LMWHs have the benefit of not requiring laboratory monitoring, as opposed to unfractionated heparin.[38] Their use is limited in patients with renal insufficiency. Once therapeutic anticoagulation is achieved, patients are typically started an oral anticoagulation regimen with warfarin. The duration of anticoagulation is dependent on risk factors for recurrent VTE and whether or not these factors are reversible. The risk of bleeding is increased in patients older than 80 years or in patients with neurological impairment who are prone to falls.[39]

Thrombolytic therapy involves the intravenous administration of agents that directly dissolve the thrombus. Currently available agents include urokinase, streptokinase, and recombinant tissue plasminogen activator. Thrombolytic therapy is reserved only for patients with hemodynamic instability as these agents are associated with a greater than threefold increase in the risk of major bleeding compared with heparin.[40]

Inferior vena cava filters are indicated in patients with known lower extremity DVT and a contraindication to anticoagulation therapy.[41] Whether or not inferior vena cava filters have any role in long-term management of VTE is questionable, as they do not prevent thrombus formation or extension. One retrospective study did not show a significant reduction in readmission for PE after 1 year.[42] Additional studies are needed to evaluate the safety and efficacy of inferior vena cava filters in the elderly, especially with the availability of retrievable filters that can be removed once anticoagulation is no longer contraindicated.

TUBERCULOSIS

For information on other infectious processes in the lung, please refer to Chapter 22 on infections in the elderly.

The elderly account for more than 20% of tuberculosis (TB) cases in the United States. In 1999, the elderly case rate was almost double that for the overall population at 11.7 per 100,000.[43] This likely reflects the higher frequency of exposure and infection in the early 1900s. Also, people who had positive tuberculin skin tests but were older than the age of 35 years were not treated because of concerns about hepatotoxicity prior to the most recent TB treatment guidelines. This places them at risk for reactivation of prior infection. Elderly patients have also been shown to be at risk for reinfection in close-living situations such as nursing homes.[44] Clinical manifestations of TB infection in the elderly are nonspecific and include fever, weight loss, weakness, and cough to name a few. The diagnosis is aided by clinical suspicion, the tuberculin skin test radiological findings, and results of sputum culture testing. Even with this testing strategy, the diagnosis can remain elusive. Between 1985 and 1988, 5.1% of TB cases reported in the United States were found at autopsy, with 60.3% of these cases in patients older than 65 years.[45]

Currently, treatment of latent TB should be undertaken in all patients regardless of age. Nine months of isoniazid therapy is recommended. Other treatment options include 2 months of rifampin and pyrazinamide or 4 months of rifampin. Treatment of active TB should be initiated with four-drug therapy, unless the patient is in an area with less than a 4% incidence in isoniazid resistance. Elderly patients are at increased risk for isoniazid-induced hepatitis and should have liver function studies monitored every 1–2 months while receiving therapy.[46] The current guidelines also recommend directly observed therapy for all active cases of TB to ensure compliance with the drug regimen.[47]

SLEEP-DISORDERED BREATHING

Both the young and old can be afflicted with sleep-disordered breathing (SDB); however, the prevalence of SDB is much higher in patients older than 60 years compared with those younger. SDB occurs in between 45% and 62% of the elderly versus 4% and 9% of middle aged patients.[48] Symptoms of SDB include snoring, nonrestorative sleep resulting in excessive daytime sleepiness, and witnessed apneas if a bed partner is present. Patients may report falling asleep during the daytime at inappropriate times. Risk factors for SDB include obesity and cigarette smoking.[49] Patients with congestive heart failure or cerebrovascular accidents are at risk for central apneas. SDB has been shown to be a risk factor for the development of hypertension, along with other cardiac problems including arrythmias.[50]

Diagnosis of SDB is made via overnight polysomnography. If the study demonstrates an apnea–hypopnea index (the average number of times a patient has apneas or hypopneas per hour) to be greater than 10–15, the diagnosis of SDB is supported. The treatment of choice for SDB is positive airway pressure, utilizing CPAP or BiPAP.[51] The air pressure acts as a splint to keep the upper airway open and prevent obstruction of the airway. The pressure is titrated to the required setting during polysomnography either in a split-night fashion or with a second visit to the sleep laboratory.

Other options exist for treatment. Weight loss in obese patients can reduce or eliminate SDB.[52] Frequently, with mild to moderate SDB, body position can be adjusted to prevent apneas. Avoidance of the supine position, where the tongue falls back into the oropharynx, can reduce the number and severity of apneas.[53] Avoidance of sedating medications and alcohol can help resolve apneas.[54] Uvulopalatopharyngoplasty involves pharyngeal reconstruction of excess tissue in the soft palate, tonsils, and enlarged uvula. This procedure is effective in only approximately 50% of cases.[55] Oral appliances exist that either advance the mandible or tongue forward to maintain airway patency; however, these only have a success rate of 50% in reducing the apnea–hypopnea index.[56]

INTERSTITIAL LUNG DISEASE

The interstitial lung diseases are a group of diseases that ultimately cause damage to the lung with resultant scarring. These diseases affect people of varying ages, some with a known cause, others without an identifiable agent causing the disease. Most are uncommon in the elderly, with the exception of idiopathic pulmonary fibrosis (IPF). The prevalence of IPF in adults older than 75 years is 175 per 100,000 compared with only 2.7 per 100,000 in adults between 35 and 44 years old.[57] Many exposures have been associated with an increased risk for the development of IPF, but no specific etiology has been proved.

Patients with IPF typically present with progressive dyspnea on exertion over several years. This is usually associated with a cough. Physical examination reveals fine, end-inspiratory crackles in more than 85% of patients with IPF. Digital clubbing can be noted in more than half of patients.[58] Pulmonary function studies reveal a restrictive defect, the severity of which is dependent on the degree of fibrosis. Radiological studies are the key to diagnosis. Chest radiographs demonstrate bibasilar shadowing early in the disease. High-resolution chest CT has allowed for confident diagnosis of IPF, often saving the patient from an invasive diagnostic biopsy procedure.[59] The scans typically reveal a patchy, heterogeneous distribution of fibrosis, with a proclivity for the subpleural and bibasilar regions of the lung. Bronchiectasis can also be seen. The extent of disease demonstrated on the high-resolution CT typically correlates with the severity of the functional impairment.[60]

The course of IPF can be relentless, leading to a mean survival of 3 to 5 years.[61] Some patients stabilize after an initial period of decline.[62] Treatment for IPF remains controversial, with corticosteroids having been the cornerstone of therapy for decades; however, no randomized, placebo-controlled studies have been performed to evaluate efficacy. Retrospective studies have failed to demonstrate survival benefit with corticosteroids.[61,63] Other immunosuppressants such as azathioprine or cyclophosphamide have been used in patients who cannot tolerate the side effects of corticosteroids. These agents, also, have not been demonstrated to have a survival benefit. Current consensus statements advise treatment with immunosuppressive agents only in those patients with a deteriorating course or evidence of alveolitis on high-resolution CT.[64] Follow up studies in this subgroup are underway. Another trial evaluated N-acetylcysteine, an antioxidant, added on to the usual immunosuppressive therapy for IPF. Patients in the treatment group had slower deterioration in pulmonary function than the control group, but there was no mortality difference between the two groups.[65]

CRITICAL CARE

Elderly patients account for approximately half of the patients in acute hospital Intensive Care Units (ICUs).[66] The incidence of respiratory failure in the 65–84 years age group is twice that of the 55–64 years age group, so critical care utilization for this portion of the population will increase dramatically over the next several years as the baby boom generation ages.[67]

Despite the high utilization of ICU beds by elderly patients, age is a factor in decisions to withhold aggressive therapies.[68] Physicians, however, may often be unaware of desires of elderly patients to undergo invasive care and may withhold care inappropriately. Many health care providers assume that the elderly have poor outcomes from critical care relative to younger patients but chronological age accounts for only 3% of explanatory power for risk of death. Acute physiological abnormalities and severity of underlying comorbidities are much more important factors.[66] Although elderly patients receive fewer invasive therapies when faced with critical illness, this has little impact on survival when accounting for other variables.[69] This suggests that the higher amount of resources utilized in younger patients provides limited benefit over the amount of resources typically used for elderly critically ill patients. Elderly survivors of critical illness are often left with significant functional limitations but measures of emotional health are usually good, and almost all survivors would opt to undergo ICU care again if the need arose.[70]

As stated previously, respiratory failure is more common in the elderly than younger age groups. This is likely because of changes that occur with aging not only with the respiratory system, as described previously, but also with the aging of other organ systems. These changes serve to decrease the reserve available to deal with the stresses of critical illness. There are many causes of respiratory failure including pulmonary causes such as COPD, interstitial lung diseases, and pneumonia, along with nonpulmonary causes such as cardiac or neurological dysfunction and severe sepsis. In a cohort of 300 mechanically ventilated patients admitted to ICUs, 49% had pulmonary diagnoses responsible for the respiratory failure.[71]

Acute lung injury, including the acute respiratory distress syndrome, is one of the more common causes of respiratory failure seen in the ICU. It represents a form of noncardiogenic pulmonary edema, characterized by a $PaO_2:FiO_2$ ratio less than 300, no evidence of left heart failure, and bilateral infiltrates. In the year 2000, the acute respiratory distress syndrome network low tidal volume (6 cc/kg) versus high tidal volume (12 cc/kg) trial was published, demonstrating an 8.8% absolute reduction in mortality associated with lower tidal volumes.[72] In that study cohort, elderly patients had higher adjusted mortality risk than younger patients. Elderly patients also required more time for liberation from mechanical ventilation after passing trials of spontaneous breathing.

Liberation from mechanical ventilation is an important concern when placing an elderly patient on ventilatory support. Weaning protocols using daily spontaneous breathing trials have been shown to be superior to more gradual withdrawal of ventilator support (Table 20.4).[73–75] One reason why elderly patients have more difficulty with extubation after passing spontaneous breathing trials may be delirium. Delirium is more common in elderly critically ill patients, and its presence

Table 20.4. Approach to Liberation from Mechanical Ventilation

Screen patients daily for appropriateness of discontinuation of mechanical ventilation by assessing the following:

- Is the underlying process that led to intubation reversed?
- Is the patient hemodynamically stable?
- Does the patient have the ability to cough and gag (mental status)?
- Is the FiO_2 less than or equal to 0.5 with a peep less than 8?
- Frequency to tidal volume ratio <100 while breathing spontaneously for 1 min?

If patient meets the above criteria, then a spontaneous breathing trial (SBT) should be undertaken by one of the following for 30 min:

- PSV 5 cm H_2O w/ 0 peep
- T-piece trial

Assess patient's tolerance of the SBT by evaluating the following:

- Adequacy of oxygenation and ventilation
- Hemodynamic stability
- Stable ventilatory pattern and work of breathing
- Adequate cough

If the patient appears to have tolerated the SBT, proceed to extubation.

is associated with longer duration of hospital stay and higher hospital mortality.[71] Prevention of delirium by limiting use of long-acting sedatives such as lorazepam can decrease duration ventilation.[76]

Elderly patients are at higher risk for prolonged mechanical ventilation after acute illness.[77] Prolonged mechanical ventilation in elderly patients is associated with high 1-year mortality and very poor functional status in survivors. Although aggressive and systematic approaches to liberation from ventilation described previously can limit the incidence of prolonged mechanical ventilation, the most effective approach is to avoid intubation when possible. Judicious use of noninvasive positive pressure ventilation in patients presenting with respiratory failure due to COPD reduces the incidence of mechanical ventilation and improves the risk of mortality.[78]

Elderly patients are also at higher risk for severe sepsis. The incidence for patients older than 80 years is 26.2 per 1,000 population compared with 3 per 1,000 overall.[79] Considering the high incidence of diastolic dysfunction in the elderly and underlying renal dysfunction, they may be more likely to benefit from early aggressive resuscitation than younger patients. Elderly patients also gain more benefit from use of activated protein C in severe sepsis than younger patients, despite having a slightly higher bleeding risk.[80]

REFERENCES

1. Bode FR, Dosman J, Martin RR, Ghezzo H, Macklem, PT. Age and sex differences in lung elasticity and in closing capacity of nonsmokers. *J Appl Phys.* 1976;41:129–135.

2. Chan ED Welsh CH. Geriatric respiratory medicine. *Chest.* 1998;114:1704–1733.

3. Tolep K, Higgins N, Muza S, et al. Comparison of diaphragm strength between healthy adult elderly and young men. *Am J Respir Crit Care Med.* 1995;152:677–682.

4. Puchelle E, Zahm JM, Bertrand A. Influences of age on bronchial mucociliary transport. *Scand J Respir Dis.* 1979;60:307–313.

5. Pfeifer MA, Weinberg CR, Cook D, et al. Differential changes in the autonomic nervous system function with age in man. *Am J Med.* 1983;75:249–258.

6. National Heart, Lung, and Blood Institute. Guidelines for the Diagnosis and Management of Asthma.Expert Panel Report 3; 2007. Available at: http://www.nhlbi.nih.gov/guidelines/asthma/asthgdln.pdf. Accessed May 28, 2008.

7. Krishnan V, Diette GB, Rand CS, et al. Mortality in patients hospitalized for asthma exacerbations in the United States. *Am J Respir Crit Care Med.* 2006;174:633–638.

8. Armitage JM, William SJ. Inhaler technique in the elderly. *Age Ageing.* 1988;17:275–278.

9. Lindgren S, Bake B, Larsson S. Clinical consequences of inadequate inhalation technique in asthma therapy. *Eur J Respir Dis.* 1987;70:93–98.

10. Connolly MJ. Inhaler technique of elderly patients: comparison of metered dose inhalers and large volume spacer devices. *Age Ageing.* 1995;24:190–192.

11. Newman SP, Newhouse, MT. Effect of add-on devices for aerosol drug delivery: deposition studies and clinical aspects. *J Aerosol Med.* 1996;9:55–70.

12. Executive Summary: Global Strategy for the Diagnosis, Management, and Prevention of COPD 2008. Available at: http://www.goldcopd.org/Guidelineitem.asp?l1=2&l2=1&intId=996. Accessed May 28, 2008.

13. Mannino DM, Homa DM, Akinbami L, Ford ES, Redd SC. Chronic obstructive pulmonary disease surveillance – United States,1971–2000. *MMWR.* 2002;51:1–6.

14. National Heart, Lung and Blood Institute. Morbidity and mortality chartbook on cardiovascular, lung, and blood diseases 2007. Available at: http://www.nhlbi.nih.gov/resources/docs/cht-book.htm. Accessed May 28, 2008.

15. Alseedi A, Sin DD, McAlister FA. The effects of inhaled corticosteroid in chronic obstructive pulmonary disease: a systematic review of randomized placebo-controlled trials. *Am J Med.* 2002;113:59–65.

16. Nocturnal Oxygen Therapy Group. Continuous or nocturnal oxygen therapy in hypoxemic chronic obstructive lung disease: a clinical trial. *Ann Intern Med.* 1980;93:391–398.

17. Niewoehner DE, Erbland ML, Deupree RH, et al. Effect of systemic glucocorticoids on exacerbations of chronic obstructive pulmonary disease. *NEJM.* 1999;340:1941–1947.

18. ACCP/AACVPR Pulmonary Rehabilitation Guidelines Panel. Pulmonary rehabilitation: joint ACCP/AACVPR evidence-based guidelines. *Chest.* 1997;112:1363–1396.

19. Fishman A, Martinez F, Naunheim K, et al. A randomized trial comparing lung-volume-reduction surgery with medical therapy for severe emphysema. *NEJM.* 2003;348:2059–2073.

20. Scanlon PD, Cannett JE, Waller LA, et al. Smoking cessation and lung function in mild-to-moderate chronic obstructive pulmonary disease. *Am J Respir Crit Care Med.* 2000;161:381–390.

21. Poole PJ, Chacko E, Wood-Baker RW, Cates CJ. Influenza vaccine for patients with chronic obstructive pulmonary disease. *Cochrane Database Syst Rev.* 2006;25:CD002733.

22. Lilienfeld DE, Chan E, Ehland J, et al. Mortality from pulmonary embolism in the United States: 1962–84. *Chest.* 1990;98:1067–1072.

23. Anderson Jr FA, Wheeler HB, Goldberg RJ, et al. A population based perspective of the hospital incidence and case fatality rates of deep vein thrombosis and pulmonary embolism. The Worcester DVT Study. *Arch Intern Med.* 1991;151:933–938.

24. Oger E. Incidence of venous thromboembolism: a community-based study in Western France. EPI-GETBP Study Group. *Thromb Haemost.* 2000;83:657–660.

25. Kniffin WD, Baron JA, Barrett J, et al. The epidemiology of diagnosed pulmonary embolism and deep venous thrombosis in the elderly. *Arch Intern Med.* 1994;154:861–866.

26. Masotti L, Ceccarelli E, Cappelli R, et al. Pulmonary embolism in the elderly: clinical, instrumental and laboratory aspects. *Gerontology.* 2000;46:205–211.

27. Stein P, Gottshalk A, Saltzman H, et al. Diagnosis of acute pulmonary embolism in the elderly. *J Am Coll Cardiol.* 1991; 18:1452–1457.

28. Timmons S, Kingston M, Hussain M, Kelly H, Liston R. Pulmonary embolism: differences in presentation between older and younger patients. *Age Ageing.* 2003;32:601–605.

29. Righini M, Goehring C, Bounameaux H, et al. Effects of age on the performance of common diagnostic tests for pulmonary embolism. *Am J Med.* 2000;109:357–361.

30. Elias A, Colombier D, Victor G, et al. Diagnostic performance of complete lower limb venous ultrasound in patients with clinically suspected acute pulmonary embolism. *Thromb Haemost.* 2004;91:187–195.

31. Kearon C, Julian JA, Newman TE, et al. Noninvasive diagnosis of deep venous thrombosis. McMaster Diagnostic Imaging Practice Guidelines Initiative. *Ann Intern Med.* 1998;128:663–677.

32. The PIOPED Investigators. Value of the ventilation/perfusion scan in acute pulmonary embolism. Results of the prospective investigation of pulmonary embolism diagnosis (PIOPED). *JAMA.* 1990;263:2753–2759.

33. Anderson DR, Kovacs MJ, Dennie C, et al. Use of spiral computed tomography contrast angiography and ultrasonography to exclude the diagnosis of pulmonary embolism in the emergency department. *J Emerg Med.* 2005;29:399–404.

34. Writing Group for the Christopher Study Investigators. Effectiveness of managing suspected pulmonary embolism using an algorithm combining clinical probability, D-dimer testing, and computed tomography. *JAMA.* 2006;295:172–179.

35. Ghanima W, Almaas V, Aballi S, et al. Management of suspected pulmonary embolism (PE) by D-dimer and multislice computed tomography in outpatients: an outcome study. *J Thromb Haemost.* 2005;3:1926–1932.

36. Hull R, Hirsh J, Carter C, et al. Diagnostic value of ventilation-perfusion lung scanning in patients with suspected pulmonary embolism. *Chest.* 1985;88:819–828.

37. Kuijer P, Hutten B, Prins M, et al. Prediction of the risk of bleeding during anticoagulant treatment for venous thromboembolism. *Arch Intern Med.* 1999;159:457–460.

38. Columbus Investigators. Low-molecular-weight heparin in the treatment of patients with venous thromboembolism. *NEJM.* 1997;337:657–662.

39. Fihn S, Callahan C, Martin D, et al. The risk for and severity of bleeding complications in elderly patients treated with warfarin. The National Consortium of Anticoagulation Clinics. *Ann Intern Med.* 1996;124:959–962.

40. Arcasoy S, Kreit J. Thrombolytic therapy of pulmonary embolism. *Chest.* 1999;115:1695–1707.

41. Athanasoulis C, Kaufman J, Halpern E, et al. Inferior vena cava filters: review of a 26-year single center clinical experience. *Radiology.* 2000;216:54–66.

42. White R, Zhou H, Kim J, et al. A population-based study of the effectiveness of inferior vena cava filter use among patients with venous thromboembolism. *Arch Intern Med.* 2000;160:2033–2041.

43. Centers for Disease Control and Prevention, Division of Tuberculosis Elimination. National Surveillance System highlights from 2000. Atlanta: Center for Disease Control and Prevention; 2001.

44. Steed WW, Lofgren JP, Warren E, et al. Tuberculosis as an endemic and nosocomial infection among the elderly in nursing homes. *NEJM.* 1985;312:1483–1487.

45. Rieder HL, Kelly GD, Bloch AB, et al. Tuberculosis diagnosed at death in the United States. *Chest.* 2001;100:678–681.

46. Rajagopalan S, Yoshikawa TT. TB in long-term care facilities. *Infect Control Hosp Epidemiol.* 2000;21:611–615.

47. Centers for Disease Control and Prevention. Treatment of Tuberculosis, American Thoracic Society, CDC, and Infectious Diseases Society of America. *MMWR.* 2003;52:1–77.

48. Ancoli-Israel S, Kripke DF, Klauber MR, et al. Sleep-disordered breathing in community-dwelling elderly. *Sleep.* 1991;14:486–495.

49. Wetter DW, Young TB, Bidwell TR, Badr MS, Palta M. Smoking as a risk factor for sleep-disordered breathing. *Arch Intern Med.* 1994;154:2219–2224.

50. Lavie P, Herer P, Hoffstein V. Obstructive sleep apnea syndrome as a risk factor for hypertension: population study. *Br Med J.* 2000;320:479–482.

51. Grunstein RR. Nasal continuous positive pressure treatment for obstructive sleep apnea. *Thorax.* 1995:1106–1113.

52. Loube DI, Loube AA, Mitler MM. Weight loss for obstructive sleep apnea: the optimal therapy for obese patients. *J Am Diet Assoc.* 1994;94:1291–1295.

53. Ancoli-Israel S. Sleep problems in older adults: putting myths to bed. *Geriatrics.* 1997;52:20–30.

54. Guilleminault C, Silvestri R, Mondini S, Coburn S. Aging and sleep apnea: action of benzodiazepine, acetazolamide, alcohol, and sleep deprivation in a healthy elderly group. *J Gerontol.* 1984;39:655–661.

55. Walker RP, Grigg-Damberger M, Gopalsami C. Uvulopalato-pharyngoplasty versus laser-assisted uvulopalatoplasty for the treatment of obstructive sleep apnea. *Laryngoscope.* 1997;107:76–82.

56. Schmidt-Nowara WW, Lowe A, Wiegand L, Cartwright R, Perez-Guerra F, Menn S. Oral appliances for the treatment of snoring and obstructive sleep apnea: a review. *Sleep.* 1995;18:501–510.

57. Coultas D, Zumwalt R, Black W, et al. The epidemiology of interstitial lung disease. *Am J Respir Crit Care Med.* 1994;150:967–972.

58. Johnston I, Prescott R, Chalmers J, et al. British Thoracic Society study of cryptogenic fibrosing alveolitis: current presentation and initial management. *Thorax.* 1997;52:38–44.

59. Grenier P, Chevret S, Biegelman C, et al. Chronic diffuse infiltrative lung disease: determination of the diagnostic value of clinical data, chest radiography, and CT with Bayesian anaylsis. *Radiology.* 1994;191:383–390.

60. Xaubert A, Agusti C, Lubrich P, et al. Pulmonary function tests and CT scan in the management of idiopathic pulmonary fibrosis. *Am J Respir Crit Care Med.* 1998;158:431–436.

61. Hubbard R, Johnston I, Britton J. Survival in patients with cryptogenic fibrosing alveolitis: a population-based cohort study. *Chest.* 1998;113:396–400.

62. Lynch JP III, Wurfel M, Flaherty K, et al. Usual interstitial pneumonia. *Semin Respir Crit Care Med.* 2001;22:357–385.

63. Douglas WW, Ryu JH, Schroeder DR. Idiopathic pulmonary fibrosis: impact of oxygen and colchicine, prednisone, or no therapy on survival. *Am J Respir Crit Care Med.* 2000;161:1172–1178.

64. The American Thoracic Society. Idiopathic pulmonary fibrosis: diagnosis and treatment. *Am J Respir Crit Care Med.* 2000;161:646–664.

65. Demedts, M, Behr J, Buhl R, et al. High-dose acetylcysteine in idiopathic pulmonary fibrosis. *NEJM.* 2005;353:2229–2242.

66. Knaus WA, Wagner DP, Draper EA, et al. The APACHE III prognosis system: Risk prediction of hospital mortality for critically ill hospitalized adults. *Chest.* 1991;100:1619–1636.

67. Behrendt CE. Acute respiratory failure in the United States: incidence and 31-day survival. *Chest.* 2000;118:1100–1105.

68. Hamel MB, Teno JM, Goldman L, et al. Patient age and decisions to withhold life-sustaining treatments from seriously ill, hospitalized adults. SUPPORT Investigators. Study to Understand Prognoses and Preferences for Outcomes and Risks of Treatment. *Ann Intern Med.* 1999;130:116–125.

69. Hamel MB, Davis RB, Teno JM, et al. Older age, aggressiveness of care, and survival for seriously ill hospitalized adults. SUPPORT Investigators. Study to Understand Prognoses and Preferences for Outcomes and Risks of Treatment. *Ann Intern Med.* 1999;131:721–728.

70. Danis M, Patrick DL, Southerland LI, Green ML. Patients' and families' preferences for medical intensive care. *JAMA.* 1988;260:797–802.

71. Ely EW, Evans GW, Haponik EF. Mechanical ventilation in a cohort of elderly patients admitted to an intensive care unit. *Ann Intern Med.* 1999;131:96–104.

72. The Acute Respiratory Distress Syndrome Network. Ventilation with lower tidal volumes as compared with traditional tidal volumes for acute lung injury and the acute respiratory distress syndrome. *NEJM.* 2000;342:1301–1308.

73. Ely EW, Baker AM, Dunagan DP, et al. Effect of the duration on mechanical ventilation of identifying patients capable of breathing spontaneously. *NEJM.* 1996;335:1864–1869.

74. Esteban A, Alia I, Gordo F, et al. Extubation outcome after spontaneous breathing trials with T-tube or pressure support ventilation: the Spanish Lung Failure Collaborative Group. *Am J Respir Crit Care Med.* 1997;156:459–465.

75. Brochard L, Raauss A, Benito S, et al. Comparison of three methods of gradual withdrawal from ventilatory support during weaning from mechanical ventilation. *Am J Respir Crit Care Med.* 1994;150:896–903.

76. Carson SS, Kress JP, Rodgers JE, et al. A randomized trial of intermittent lorazepam versus propofol with daily interruption in mechanically ventilated patients. *Crit Care Med.* 2006;34:1326–1332.

77. Carson SS. Outcomes of prolonged mechanical ventilation. *Curr Opin Crit Care.* 2006;12:405–411.

78. Keenan SP, Sinuff T, Cook DJ, Hill NS. Which patients with acute exacerbation of chronic obstructive pulmonary disease benefit from noninvasive positive-pressure ventilation? A systematic review of the literature. *Ann Intern Med.* 2003;138:861–870.

79. Angus DC, Linde-Zwirble WT, Lidicker J, et al. Epidemiology of severe sepsis in the United States: analysis of incidence, outcome, and associated costs of care. *Crit Care Med.* 2001;29:1303–1310.

80. Ely EW, Angus DC, Williams MD, et al. Drotrecogin alfa (activated) treatment of older patients with severe sepsis. *Clin Infect Dis.* 2003;37:187–195.

21

GASTROENTEROLOGICAL DISEASE IN THE OLDER ADULT

Christine Hsieh, MD, Cuckoo Choudhary, MD

The gastrointestinal (GI) tract is affected by physiological changes of aging as well as by comorbid disease processes such as atherosclerosis and diabetes mellitus (DM). Multiple medication use in the elderly often has direct effects on intestinal mucosa and motility. GI problems may be the cause of common problems seen in the elderly such as dysphagia, weight loss, and constipation. GI disease in the elderly may also present atypically, have higher complication rates, and more complex treatment issues.

ESOPHAGUS

Dysphagia

Dysphagia is a common problem among older adults. In the nursing home the prevalence of dysphagia is as high as 50%–60%.[1] Dysphagia is defined as the inability to initiate a swallow or a sensation that solids or liquids do not pass easily from the mouth into the stomach. In older patients, difficulty with eating may not only be associated with pharyngoesophageal disease or the GI tract, but also with cognitive and psychiatric problems, neurological deficits, and dental disease.[2] In oropharyngeal dysphagia, the main complaint is food getting stuck in the throat, nasal regurgitation, and coughing. Swallow-related coughing occurs because of the misdirection of the food bolus into the airway. Oropharyngeal dysphagia is usually caused by local, neurological, or muscular disease such as esophageal cancer, cerebrovascular accident, and muscular dystrophy. Patients with esophageal dysphagia complain of food getting stuck in the sternum region. Dysphagia for both solids and liquids from the onset usually implies a motility disorder of the esophagus such as achalasia, whereas mechanical obstructing lesions such as Zenker diverticulum initially cause dysphagia for solids only, but may progress to involve liquids.

The treatment of dysphagia depends on finding the underlying cause. A careful history may help localize the etiology to oropharyngeal or esophageal dysphagia. A detailed review of medications is important because certain drugs such as anticholinergics and antihistamines can reduce salivary flow and produce a dry mouth making swallowing difficult. The initial diagnostic study in the evaluation of dysphagia in most cases is a barium videofluoroscopy of the oropharynx and esophagus.[3] Videofluoroscopy is aimed at analyzing functional impairment of the swallowing mechanism.[4] At the level of the esophagus, barium studies may identify the level and nature of obstruction such as a stricture, achalasia, or malignancy, but it is not usually diagnostic. For patients with symptoms of esophageal dysphagia, diagnostic testing may also include manometry and endoscopy. Esophageal manometry is considered the "gold standard" in the diagnosis of esophageal motility disorder. Upper endoscopy has the advantage of allowing direct visualization of the mucosa, biopsy of any suspicious lesions, and therapeutic intervention, such as esophageal dilation.[3]

Gastroesophageal Reflux Disease

Gastroesophageal reflux (GERD) is one of the most common complaints in older patients. The prevalence of GERD in older adults is approximately 20%.[5] The most common clinical symptom of GERD is heartburn, described as a retrosternal burning sensation or discomfort.[6] Other symptoms of GERD include regurgitation, hypersalivation, dysphagia, dyspepsia, and odynophagia. Less common symptoms include coughing, sore throat, and wheezing.[6] GERD is caused by transient inappropriate lower esophageal sphincter relaxations that lead to acid reflux into the esophagus.[7] Sliding hiatal hernia may contribute to acid reflux and a higher frequency of esophagitis.[8] Studies have shown that elderly patients have milder symptoms compared with younger patients, but they have a higher prevalence of esophagitis and Barrett's esophagus.[5]

Patients with mild or uncomplicated heartburn or acid regurgitation can begin empiric treatment with an acid-suppressing medication such as hydrogen receptor antagonists or proton pump inhibitors.[9] Symptomatic improvement may be considered diagnostic of GERD; however, patients with severe or long-standing heartburn, dysphagia, odynophagia, GI bleeding, and atypical symptoms such as chest pain or weight loss require diagnostic testing to determine the extent and severity of disease. A barium swallow can characterize the anatomy as well as identify structural lesions such as hiatal hernia, diverticulum, strictures, ulcerations, and mass lesions such as cancer.[6] The barium swallow is not specific or sensitive for the diagnosis of GERD.[6] Upper endoscopy with biopsy is the gold standard used to directly visualize the esophagus and evaluate mucosal integrity.[6] Esophageal manometry can be used to document the presence of effective esophageal peristalsis. The 24-hour ambulatory esophageal pH testing is a noninvasive test to monitor esophageal acid exposure; it can quantify the degree of reflux and correlate symptoms to reflux episodes.[6]

Treatment for GERD begins with lifestyle modifications for reducing symptoms of reflux. Patients are advised to elevate the head of the bed, lose weight, eat small meals, avoid eating at bedtime, and avoid foods that lower the lower esophageal sphincter pressure such as alcohol, caffeine, smoking, tomato and citrus juices and sauces, and peppermint. Medications that may lower lower esophageal sphincter pressure and cause mucosal damage to the esophagus such as nonsteroidal antiinflammatory drugs (NSAIDs) should also be avoided.

The medical treatments for GERD include hydrogen receptor antagonists, proton pump inhibitors, and prokinetic agents. Hydrogen receptor antagonists may improve symptoms in nonerosive GERD; however, hydrogen receptor antagonists have a lower healing rate for severe esophagitis.[6] The treatment of choice for patients with severe GERD or reflux esophagitis is proton pump inhibitors for eight weeks.[10] They have been shown to be superior to hydrogen receptor antagonists in healing reflux esophagitis and relieving symptoms.[6] There is no significant difference in efficacy among the various proton pump inhibitors. Prokinetic agents, such as metoclopramide, have been used for the treatment of GERD. Metoclopramide, however, is not used often in the elderly because of a high rate of central nervous system side effects. In addition, prokinetic agents have not been shown to be more effective compared with hydrogen receptor antagonists.[6] Recurrence of symptoms is common after therapy is discontinued, and maintenance therapy may be needed because of the chronic nature of GERD.[11] Patients with severe, persistent regurgitation despite proton pump therapy may be considered for antireflux surgery.

Patients with long-standing GERD are at greatest risk for developing Barrett's esophagus. The annual incidence of adenocarcinoma in patients with Barrett's esophagus has been estimated at 0.5%.[12] The risk of esophageal cancer increases with age, with a mean age at diagnosis of 67 years.[13] Esophageal adenocarcinoma is more prevalent in Caucasian men (Caucasian/African American ratio, 5:1; male/female ratio, 8:1).[14] Squamous cell carcinoma (SCC) of the esophagus is more common than adenocarcinoma in the United States, although the incidence of the latter is on the rise. The incidence of SCC is higher in men than in women and higher in African Americans than in Caucasians. Predisposing conditions for SCC include factors that cause chronic irritation and inflammation of the esophageal mucosa such as smoking and excessive alcohol consumption.[15] Other sources of chronic irritation include achalasia and esophageal diverticula. Patients with esophageal cancer complain of dysphagia, odynophagia, and weight loss.[12] A barium radiography or endoscopy is usually the initial diagnostic study, and endoscopic biopsy is performed to confirm the diagnosis.[12] Computed tomography (CT) scans of the chest, abdomen, and pelvis are usually obtained to evaluate for metastatic disease.[12] Localized esophageal cancer may be treated with resection alone, with median survival ranging from 13 to 19 months. The 5-year survival rates ranged from 15% to 24%.[12] Currently, strategies combining surgery, radiotherapy, and chemotherapy are being investigated to improve survival in patients with localized esophageal cancer. In advanced disease, both SCC and adenocarcinoma of the esophagus are responsive to chemotherapy; however, the response typically lasts a few months and survival is usually less than a year.[12]

Medication-Induced Esophageal Injury

Pill-induced esophagitis occurs more frequently in older adults probably because of the increased use of medications such as potassium chloride, alendronate, aspirin, NSAIDs, and doxycycline. In addition, disordered motility, decreased salivary flow, pills taken while supine or with little liquid increase this risk.[3] Anatomically aortic or left atrial enlargement may create a pseudostricture in the esophagus leading to dysphagia. Another common site of injury is at the level of the esophagogastric junction. Patients usually present with odynophagia, chest pain, vomiting, and dysphagia.[16] Upper endoscopy is the most sensitive diagnostic test and may reveal a discrete ulcer. Endoscopy may exclude reflux and infectious esophagitis and malignancy. Barium radiography is not as sensitive but may exclude malignancy and extrinsic compression on the esophagus. Pill-induced ulcers usually heal spontaneously within a few days.[3] Sucralfate may provide a protective coating on the mucosa and promote healing.[17] There is currently no evidence that proton pump inhibitors, hydrogen receptor blockers, or antacids are effective in healing these lesions. Patients should be advised to take oral medications with liquid and maintain an upright posture for at least 30 minutes after taking medications.[3]

Infectious Esophagitis

Older patients are at higher risk for infectious esophagitis because they are more likely to be immunocompromised because of comorbid medical conditions such as malignancies and diabetes mellitus and the use of immunosuppressant medications.[18] Infections may be fungal, viral, or bacterial. *Candida albicans* is the most common cause of fungal esophagitis. Patients with infectious esophagitis generally present with acute onset of dysphagia and odynophagia. Diagnosis is usually made by endoscopy and biopsy for histological sampling and culture. Therapy is guided by identification of the infectious organism.[3]

Achalasia

Achalasia is an idiopathic esophageal motor disorder characterized by incomplete lower esophageal sphincter relaxation and absent peristalsis because of loss of myenteric neurons controlling esophageal smooth muscle function.[18,19] It is more prevalent with advancing age.[3] Patients generally present with dysphagia to both solid and liquids. Other symptoms include regurgitation of food, chest pain, and even recurrent aspiration pneumonia. The diagnosis is usually made by a barium esophagram, which demonstrates dysmotility and delayed emptying of the esophagus. Esophageal manometry reveals a normal to high resting lower esophageal sphincter pressure with incomplete relaxation and abnormal peristalsis of the esophagus. Endoscopy is indicated in older patients to exclude esophageal cancer, which may give the appearance of pseudoachalasia.[3] Injection of botulinum toxin into the lower esophageal sphincter, pneumatic balloon dilation, and surgery including laparoscopic surgery have been used for the treatment of achalasia.[3]

STOMACH

Peptic Ulcer Disease

Peptic ulcer disease should always be considered in older patients complaining of dyspepsia, nausea, abdominal discomfort, marked weight loss, or GI bleeding. Peptic ulcer disease is considered to be more serious in the elderly because they have more ulcer-related complications, resulting in higher mortality rates.[20] The mortality rate is 30%–50% in elderly patients with perforated ulcers.[21] Older patients are more likely to be hospitalized with peptic ulcer disease for GI bleeding, or their complications such as obstruction or perforation.[22] The incidence of peptic ulcer disease increases with age.[23] The two most common risk factors for peptic ulcer disease are NSAID use and *Helicobacter pylori* infections. Peptic ulcer disease is seen in the elderly in part because of comorbid medical conditions and medications used to treat them. For example, older patients often use aspirin or anticoagulation therapy for cardiopulmonary diseases. NSAIDs are used more frequently in the elderly to treat chronic conditions such as arthritis. In one study, the concurrent use of oral anticoagulation and NSAIDS in the elderly increased the risk 13-fold of developing GI bleeding.[24] Gastric mucosal injuries have been reported in 70%–80% of patients taking NSAIDS, and gastric or duodenal ulcers have been shown to occur in 10%–30% of patients taking NSAIDS regardless of age.[25] Misoprostol[26]

and proton pump inhibitors[27] have been shown to reduce NSAID-induced mucosal injury.

The prevalence of *H. pylori* increases with age, approximately 60% by the age of 70 years.[28] *H. pylori* infection is associated with 60% of gastric ulcers and 80% of duodenal ulcers. Serum enzyme-linked immunosorbent assay serology is an initial, noninvasive approach to diagnosing *H. pylori* infection in symptomatic patients or asymptomatic patients with a history of peptic ulcer disease. The average sensitivity for the enzyme-linked immunosorbent assay test is 86%–94%, and the specificity is 78%–95%.[29] Serology cannot distinguish between past or active infections. The test may be less accurate in elderly patients.[30] Alternative noninvasive tests include histological examination, rapid urease tests, polymerase chain reaction assays, urea breath testing, and stool antigen assay.[6] The gold standard diagnosis of peptic ulcer disease is made by endoscopy. Endoscopy allows direct visualization and biopsy of abnormal tissue, which is useful to reveal gastritis and differentiate benign gastric ulcers from gastric cancer. Barium radiography can be used to diagnose peptic ulcer; however, it is not as sensitive or specific as endoscopy.[6]

The treatment for peptic ulcer disease begins with suppression of gastric acid to heal the ulcer. The healing rates for duodenal and gastric ulcers are more rapid with proton pump inhibitors compared with hydrogen receptor antagonists. The healing rate for duodenal ulcers when using omeprazole was 93% in 2 weeks and 100% at 4 weeks.[31] In comparison, the healing rate with hydrogen receptor antagonist was 70%–80% at 4 weeks and 80%–95% after 8 weeks.[32] Treatment of patients with *H. pylori* infection has been shown to decrease the risk of recurrence of peptic ulcers.[33] Treatment for patients with peptic ulcer disease with *H. pylori* includes a combination regimen, generally a proton pump inhibitor to suppress acid production and clarithromycin, and either metronidazole or amoxicillin to eradicate the organism.[6] NSAIDs and *H. pylori* may work synergistically to cause ulcers, thus NSAIDs should be avoided in patients with an ulcer history. If an NSAID is required then a proton pump inhibitor or misoprostol should be used concomitantly; however, proton pump inhibitors have been shown to be more effective and have fewer side effects.[34] Maintenance therapy with a proton pump inhibitor may be required beyond 4 weeks in patients with complicated peptic ulcer disease.

Gastric Cancer

The incidence of gastric cancer increases with advancing age, peaking after 60 years of age.[35] Almost 95% of gastric cancers are adenocarcinomas. Lymphomas account for 4%, and the remaining 1% consists of SCC, carcinoid tumors, and leiomyosarcomas. *Helicobacter pylori*, chronic atrophic gastritis, and intestinal metaplasia have been associated with the development of gastric adenocarcinoma.[36] Environmental risk factors include a diet high in smoked or salted foods, cigarette smoking, low socioeconomic status, and low intake of fruits and vegetables.[26] Patients with gastric cancer usually complain of early satiety, anorexia, nausea, vomiting, and weight loss.[37] Upper endoscopy with tissue biopsy is the mainstay for diagnosis. Whereas a CT scan is obtained to exclude distant metastasis, an endoscopic ultrasound is used to stage the tumor locally.[38] The only cure is resection; however, recurrence usually develops within 5 years and the 5-year survival rate ranges from 20% to 42% after resection.[39] Chemotherapy and radiation have not been found to improve survival in patients with gastric cancer.[40]

PANCREAS

Pancreatitis

The most common cause of acute pancreatitis in the elderly is gallstone pancreatitis, accounting for 65%–75% of cases.[41] Alcohol accounts for only 20% of cases of acute pancreatitis.[42] Other causes include drugs and malignancy. The most commonly associated medications include azathioprine, 6-mercaptoprine, mesalamine, angiotensin-converting enzyme inhibitors, and methyldopa.[43] The incidence of medication-induced pancreatitis may be rising in the elderly because of the use of multiple medications. Pancreatic ductal obstruction resulting from malignancy or other causes may also lead to acute pancreatitis.[44] Another category of pancreatitis seen in the elderly is a form of chronic pancreatitis known as late-onset or senile idiopathic pancreatitis. The cause is not entirely clear but may be result from atherosclerosis of the blood vessels supplying the pancreas.[44] Older patients may complain of the classic abdominal pain, nausea, and vomiting; however, they can also present atypically with hyperglycemia, shock, and multiorgan failure. The evaluation for acute pancreatitis begins with serum amylase and lipase levels. Serum amylase levels have been found to be higher in older adults, but lipase appears to be less variable in older adults and may be more specific for the diagnosis of acute pancreatitis.[45] Ultrasound and CT scanning of the abdomen are the most commonly used imaging tests for the diagnosis of acute pancreatitis and its complications such as abscesses and pseudocysts. Endoscopic retrograde cholangiopancreatography (ERCP) is used to visualize and extract gallstones and drain the pancreatic duct or look for obstructive causes such as adenomas and carcinomas. Usually patients will require ERCP in the presence of concomitant cholangitis, persistent common bile duct stones, jaundice, and in patients with severe gallstone pancreatitis.[44] In the elderly, ERCP may be indicated in unexplained pancreatitis to evaluate for malignancy.[44] Treatment for mild pancreatitis includes bowel rest, intravenous fluids, and pain management. Severe pancreatitis may lead to pulmonary, cardiac, and renal complications. In gallstone pancreatitis, ERCP and biliary sphincterotomy have been shown to be effective treatment in the elderly, particularly for elderly patients with high surgical risks.[44] Broad-spectrum antibiotics may be required for developing necrotizing pancreatitis. If there is no response to antibiotics, a percutaneous CT-guided aspiration is recommended for culture of the organism.[46] Surgical debridement is usually reserved for patients with pancreatic necrosis and abscesses in multiorgan failure.

Pancreatic Cancer

The incidence of pancreatic cancer increases with age and is almost 20 times higher in people older than 65 years.[47] Sixty percent of patients at the time of diagnosis have liver metastasis, malignant ascites, or other signs of tumor dissemination. Most patients die within 1 year of diagnosis of pancreatic cancer.[38] The overall 5-year survival rate is less than 5%.[47] Risk factors for developing pancreatic cancer include cigarette smoking, high fat or meat intake, gallstones, diabetes mellitus, and chronic pancreatitis.[38] Patients may present with abdominal pain caused by tumor invasion and jaundice from extrahepatic biliary obstruction. Other nonspecific presenting symptoms include weight loss, anorexia, fatigue, nausea, and pruritus.[38] There are no specific serum tumor markers for pancreatic cancer. Serum CA 19–9 seems to be elevated in some patients with pancreatic cancer, but also elevated in patients with gallbladder and bile duct cancers.[48] Laboratory tests may show elevated liver enzymes, serum alkaline phosphatase, and bilirubin. Ultrasound or CT scanning is usually the initial imaging study. ERCP is also very sensitive and specific (>90%) for the diagnosis of pancreatic cancer.[38] Endoscopic ultrasound-guided fine-needle aspiration of regional lymph nodes is used to diagnose and stage pancreatic cancer.[38] Chemotherapy and radiation have not been shown to be effective in treating pancreatic cancer. Radical pancreaticoduodenectomy surgery (Whipple procedure) is the only curative treatment for pancreatic cancer.[38] Elderly patients who underwent the surgery and were otherwise healthy had mean survival times ranging from 28 to 42 months.[49] Many elderly patients, however, present with advanced disease when curative resection is not an option. Palliative treatment for nonresectable pancreatic cancer includes biliary stents to relieve obstruction, radiation therapy, and pain control.[38]

LIVER DISEASE

Chronic liver disease was the ninth most common cause of death in the United States in 1998.[50] The rate of mortality from chronic liver disease was highest among patients aged 65–74 years.[51] Age-related changes in the liver include decline in liver volume and a decrease in hepatic blood flow. Many studies show age-related decline in the clearance of drugs undergoing liver metabolism.[52] The liver in older persons also has decreased regenerative capacity, which may be the reason the elderly have more difficulty recovering from hepatic injury.[52] Aging does not seem to affect liver blood tests such as serum bilirubin, serum aminotransferases, and hepatic alkaline phosphatase.[53] Hepatic dysfunction in the elderly may present with anorexia, jaundice, and elevated liver transaminases, alanine aminotransferase (ALT), and aspartate aminotransferase (AST). One of the most important causes of hepatic dysfunction to consider in older patients is medication. Older patients with multiple chronic medical problems often take multiple medications. Many prescription and over-the-counter medications may cause liver function abnormalities in older patients because of alterations in drug metabolism. For example, Isoniazid-induced hepatitis occurs in greater than 2% of persons older than 50 years of age but is uncommon in younger patients.[54] Systemic diseases such as congestive heart failure may affect the liver. Older patients with obesity, hyperlipidemia, and DM may have a steatohepatitis. The differential diagnosis for an elderly patient with elevated liver transaminases should also include viral and alcoholic hepatitis. In most cases, alcoholic hepatitis can be differentiated from viral hepatitis by the pattern of serum aminotransferases. Patients with alcoholic hepatitis have an AST:ALT ratio of at least 2:1, whereas in acute viral hepatitis the ALT is equal or greater than the AST. Alcohol-induced hepatitis is associated with a twofold elevation of the gamma glutamyltransferase. Patients with signs of acute viral hepatitis should be tested to differentiate the viral etiology. Hepatitis A virus (HAV) occurs rarely in patients older than 65 years; however, older patients tend to develop more severe HAV infections and have a higher incidence of acute liver failure and a higher rate of mortality compared with younger patients.[52] Acute Hepatitis B virus (HBV) is not common in the elderly population because of the decrease risk of transmission through high-risk sexual behavior and intravenous drug use. The rate of progression to become a chronic HBV carrier seems to be higher in elderly adults who develop an acute HBV infection.[55] Similarly, older patients who acquire the Hepatitis C virus (HCV) have a more rapid progression of disease. In addition to male sex, daily alcohol use, older age of infection was a major risk factor for more rapid progression of liver fibrosis.[56] The most common source of HCV transmission in infected elderly persons is prior transfusions with blood and blood products or injection drug use.[52] The treatment of HCV in the elderly is not entirely clear. Studies are controversial on whether older patients can achieve a sustained viral response to interferon-α therapy alone, and there is the concern about the side effects of the medication.[52] In younger patients, the combination of interferon-α and Ribavirin increased the rate of sustained response; however, the efficacy and tolerability of this combination is not well studied in the elderly population.[52]

Hepatocellular Cancer

Hepatocellular carcinoma usually develops in older patients with chronic liver disease. The risk factors for hepatocellular carcinoma include cirrhosis, HBV infection, chronic HCV, and hemochromatosis.[57,58] Metastasis to the liver from other GI malignancies is also seen in the elderly. Patients usually present late in the course of the disease with symptoms of abdominal pain, weight loss, jaundice, anorexia, hepatomegaly, and ascites. One commonly used laboratory marker for hepatocellular carcinoma is serum α-fetoprotein.[59] Diagnosis can usually be made with a rising serum α-fetoprotein in conjunction with a classic appearance on imaging studies such as ultrasound,

CT, magnetic resonance imaging, or angiography.[60] Focal liver lesions with an uncertain diagnosis may require a liver biopsy. The risks of liver biopsy include bleeding and seeding of the tumor along the needle track.[61] The treatment for hepatocellular carcinoma may include resection, cryoablation, and chemotherapy. One study showed that fewer older patients underwent hepatic resection, but among those patients who did there were no significant differences in morbidity, hospital mortality, or long-term survival rates.[62] Because most patients present with advanced disease, the median survival following diagnosis is 20 months.[63]

CHOLELITHIASIS

Elderly patients are predisposed to gallstone formation because of the physiological changes with aging including decreased bile acid production, increased cholesterol saturation of bile, reduced gallbladder contractions, and decreased response to cholecystokinin.[44] The prevalence of gallstone disease in the elderly is estimated to be between 14% and 27%.[44] Clinical presentation of biliary colic is acute, severe right upper quadrant or epigastric pain. The pain may radiate to the back or scapula and is often associated with nausea and vomiting; however, many patients are asymptomatic with gallstones and do not require treatment. Elderly patients have more complications from gallstones such as acute cholecystitis, pancreatitis, ascending cholangitis, or obstructive jaundice.[44] In patients with symptoms of biliary colic, liver function studies should be obtained. Ultrasound is usually the initial imaging modality. CT scanning of the abdomen or magnetic resonance cholangiography may be used if common bile duct stones or ductal obstruction are suspected. In patients with obstructive jaundice, cholangitis, or suspected biliary pancreatitis, ERCP is both diagnostic and therapeutic.[44] The treatment for symptomatic cholelithiasis for patients who are able to undergo surgery is laparoscopic cholecystectomy.[44] Elderly patients have more complications resulting in higher conversion from laparoscopic to open cholecystectomy.[64] Compared with open cholecystectomy, the laparoscopic technique has a lower rate of complications, including bleeding, infection, or injury to bile duct or bowel and faster recovery with less pain. Noninvasive treatments for symptomatic gallstones including extracorporal shock-wave lithotripsy and oral dissolution therapy are not commonly used.[44] Patients with gallstones in the common bile duct or gallstone pancreatitis require ERCP with sphincterotomy. Compared with surgery for acute cholangitis, ERCP and sphincterotomy showed lower rates of morbidity and mortality.[65]

Gallbladder Cancer

Gallbladder cancer is relatively uncommon, but the incidence does increase with age, peaking at 60 years.[38] Risk factors include gallstone, female sex, and a history of smoking.[44] In one study, gallbladder cancer was found to be associated with

Table 21.1. Manning Criteria for the Diagnosis of IBS

IBS is defined by the presence of three or more of the following:

1) Pain relieved with defecation

2) More frequent stools at the onset of pain

3) Looser stools at the onset of pain

4) Abdominal distension

5) Passage of mucus through the rectum

6) Sensation of incomplete evacuation

Information from reference.[68]

Table 21.2. Rome II Criteria for IBS

Recurrent abdominal pain or discomfort for at least 3 days per month in the last 3 months associated with 2 or more of the following:

1) Improvement with defecation

2) Onset associated with change in frequency of stool

3) Onset associated with change in form (appearance of stool)

Criteria fulfilled for symptoms present at least 3 months over 1 year with symptom onset at least 6 months prior to diagnosis.

Information from Reference.[67]

gallstones in 50%–88% of patients.[66] Most gallbladder cancer presents in an advanced stage, and the resectability rates range from 15% to 30%.[38]

SMALL AND LARGE INTESTINE

Irritable Bowel Syndrome

Irritable bowel syndrome (IBS) is a functional bowel disorder characterized by abdominal pain and altered bowel habits without any identifiable organic cause.[67] The abdominal pain is generally located in the lower abdomen, often on the left side with variable intensity. Patients may also complain of abdominal bloating and increased gas production. Pain may be exacerbated by stress or eating, and it is often relieved with defecation. Patients with IBS also complain of diarrhea, constipation, or alternating diarrhea and constipation. A diagnosis is based on the presence of symptoms as defined by the Manning criteria (Table 21.1)[68] or the more updated diagnostic Rome II Criteria (Table 21.2).[67] IBS is considered a diagnosis of exclusion. Especially in older patients, the possibility of an organic disease must first be excluded. The American College of Gastroenterology recommends a careful assessment of the patient's symptoms and identifying dietary factors or medications that may contribute to the symptoms.[69] Laboratory evaluation may include stool hemocult, complete blood count, chemistry panel, and thyroid function testing. A colonoscopy is usually recommended for older patients, especially because of the higher risk of colon cancer, but it should also be considered with any "red flag" symptoms, such as hematochezia, weight loss, family history of colon cancer, fever, anemia, and chronic severe diarrhea.[69] Symptomatic treatment for IBS begins with dietary changes. Patients should be encouraged to keep a diary to monitor symptoms and identify triggers. Fiber supplementation may improve constipation-predominant symptoms, although patients may experience increased bloating with high-fiber diets. Anticholinergics are antispasmodic agents that may decrease fecal urgency and abdominal pain. Antidiarrheals, such as loperamide, inhibit excessive GI motility but may exacerbate constipation. Alosetron, a serotonin receptor antagonist, blocks receptors in the GI tract that cause hypersensitivity and hyperactivity of the intestines. Alosetron has been approved only for women with severe chronic diarrhea-predominant IBS; however, the medication has restrictions limiting its use because of serious and unpredictable GI adverse events. Tegaserod, which had been on the market for the past few years, was approved for constipation-predominant symptoms. It was recently taken off the market for presumably causing increased risk of coronary events and strokes. Patients started on empiric treatment should be reevaluated in 3 to 6 weeks and if symptoms do not improve additional testing may be necessary based on the patient's symptoms.[69] Psychological factors need to be considered in patients who do not respond to treatment. Stress relaxation and counseling to reduce anxiety and other psychological symptoms may help to decrease symptoms of irritable bowel. Antidepressants, such as tricyclic antidepressants, may be recommended for abdominal pain because of their analgesic properties in addition to their psychotropic effects. Selective serotonin reuptake inhibitors may treat the psychological symptoms and have a low side-effect profile.[69] Along the spectrum of IBS, chronic constipation is another common problem of the elderly discussed in another chapter.

Inflammatory Bowel Disease

Inflammatory bowel disease, such as Crohn's disease and ulcerative colitis, may occur in older patients, although initial presentation is usually between the ages of 15 and 40 years. Patients may complain of diarrhea, rectal bleeding, abdominal pain, weight loss, and fever. Crohn's disease may involve the entire GI tract. Ulcerative colitis may involve the entire colon or be confined to the rectum or rectosigmoid. More severe disease may involve the distal colon and typically present with severe cramps, low-grade fevers, frequent loose stools, and rectal bleeding. Colonoscopy with biopsy sampling is useful in determining the extent and severity of the disease. The goal of treatment is to control the inflammation.[70] Mild-to-moderate disease can be managed with 5-aminosalicylic acid compounds.[71] In addition, symptomatic treatment with loperamide and cholestyramine is recommended.[70] Corticosteroids and immunosuppressants may be beneficial in severe and refractory disease.[72] Resection is indicated for severe, intractable ulcerative colitis and is curative. Surgery may have an impact on bowel function or necessitate an ileostomy pouch.[73] Resection is not curative for Crohn's disease, but is indicated for complications such as abscess, bleeding, and obstruction.[74] Periodic colonoscopy is recommended in patients with long-standing ulcerative colitis and Crohn colitis because of the increased risk of colon cancer.[70]

Diarrhea and Fecal Incontinence

Diarrhea occurs commonly in older people. Diarrhea is defined as the passage of loose stools with greater water content than normal.[75] Acute diarrhea lasts for less than 2 weeks and is often caused by intestinal infections.[76] The most common organisms found in patients with acute diarrhea include *Shigella*, *Salmonella*, and *Campylobacter jejuni*.[76] Most causes of acute gastroenteritis are believed to be viral.[77] A common cause of infectious diarrhea in hospitalized patients or patients in nursing homes is *Clostridium difficile*. *Clostridium difficile* is a more prevalent cause of diarrhea seen after antibiotic therapy.[77] The diagnosis is made by detecting cytotoxins in the stool. The treatment is a 7- to 14-day course of metronidazole or vancomycin; however, relapse occurs in many patients, who require retreatment.[78]

Chronic diarrhea is defined as diarrhea that lasts for more than 2 weeks. Causes of chronic diarrhea include IBS, inflammatory bowel disease, and intestinal malabsorption.[77] Medication side effects may also be a possible cause of diarrhea, particularly antibiotics, colchicine, and laxatives.[77] Overflow diarrhea may also occur because of impaction, which is often seen in institutionalized patients.[77] Alterations in bowel habits, including diarrhea, is an indication for colonoscopy to exclude colon cancer in older patients.

The prevalence of fecal incontinence seems to increase with age. It is unclear whether the increased prevalence in the elderly results from age-related changes in the anal sphincter function or increased prevalence of diseases such as DM neurological disorders, and cognitive impairment that may affect the anal sphincter. The history and physical examination may distinguish loss of anal sphincter function from overflow incontinence secondary to fecal impaction. Loss of anal sphincter function may be evaluated by anorectal manometry to measure anal canal pressure, rectal sensation, and rectal compliance.

Diverticular Disease of the Colon

The prevalence of diverticulosis of the colon increases with age. Fifty percent of persons older than the age of 70 years and more than 66% older than 85 years have colonic diverticulosis.[79] It is thought to occur because of high intraluminal pressures that form diverticula in the colonic wall, commonly because of prolonged colonic transit time and decreased stool volume. It is a more significant problem in developed countries and the established risk factor is low dietary fiber diet. Vegetarians who include more dietary fiber in their diet have a lower incidence of diverticular disease.[80] The majority of patients with diverticulosis are asymptomatic. Clinical manifestations include painful diverticular disease, diverticular hemorrhage, diverticulitis, and

complications of diverticulitis. Diverticular bleeding is one of the most common causes of lower GI bleeding in older adults, followed by bleeding from angiodysplasia.[79] Approximately 10%–25% with diverticular disease have bleeding per rectum.[79] Diverticula are found more commonly on the left colon; however, bleeding diverticula often originate from the right colon. Diverticular bleeding is usually abrupt and painless, often associated with mild abdominal cramping and passage of blood clots or melena.[79] The majority (70%–80%) of diverticular bleeding stops spontaneously but one-quarter of patients will have a recurrent episode.[81] Patients with lower GI bleeding require colonoscopic evaluation to diagnosis diverticulosis and to exclude other causes of bleeding such as angiodysplasia, infectious colitis, colonic polyps, and colon cancer. The treatment for diverticular bleeding is usually conservative because most bleeding spontaneously resolves.[79] Approximately 3%–5% of patients experience a massive bleed requiring blood transfusion.[79] In patients with active bleeding, a radionuclide scan may localize the approximate site of bleeding. Arteriography is more invasive but more specific in localizing the site of bleeding. After localizing the bleeding, interventional radiology techniques such as intraarterial infusion of vasopressin or transcatheter embolization may achieve hemostasis. Surgery is indicated in patients in whom conservative management fails and who have recurrent or persistent bleeding.[79]

Diverticulitis occurs in 10%–20% of patients with diverticular disease.[82] Diverticulitis occurs most commonly in the sigmoid colon and patients usually present with left lower quadrant abdominal pain often associated with peritoneal signs. In patients with suspected diverticulitis, a CT scan of the abdomen is highly sensitive and specific in acute diverticulitis.[82] Double-contrast studies and endoscopy with air insufflation are not recommended because of the risk of perforation.[79] The treatment in mild cases is bowel rest, oral hydration, and oral broad-spectrum antibiotics with amoxicillin and clavulanic acid or trimethoprim-sulfamethoxazole with metronidazole for anaerobic coverage.[82] Ciprofloxacin may be a substitute for trimethoprim-sulfamethoxazole, and clindamycin is a substitute for anaerobic coverage.[82] Severe cases or lack of improvement with outpatient treatment may require hospital admission for intravenous antibiotics, bowel rest, and intravenous hydration. Patients who respond to conservative management should have a colonic evaluation 8 weeks following the resolution of symptoms to exclude other conditions such as colon cancer.[79] Approximately 15%–30% of hospitalized patients do not respond to conservative management and require surgery.[82] Complications of diverticulitis that may require surgical intervention are diverticular abscess, fistula, intestinal obstruction, and free colonic perforation.[79]

Ischemic Bowel Disease

Ischemic bowel diseases occur when blood flow is diminished to the mesenteric circulation. Intestinal ischemia is classified into acute mesenteric ischemia, chronic mesenteric ischemia, and colonic ischemia.[83] Colonic ischemia is the most common vascular disorder in the elderly. Risk factors include atherosclerosis, hypotension, embolism, and aortic surgery.[83] The most common sites of colonic ischemia are the splenic flexure, descending colon, and sigmoid. Patients usually present with sudden onset of mild left lower quadrant abdominal pain and bloody diarrhea.[83] Colonoscopy is the procedure of choice to diagnosis ischemic colitis and exclude other causes such as inflammatory bowel disease, infectious colitis, diverticulitis, and colon cancer. The initial treatment of colonic ischemia is supportive management including monitoring, bowel rest, hydration, and administration of systemic antibiotics. In mild cases, colonic ischemia is reversible and clinical symptoms subside in 24–48 hours followed by mucosal healing within 1–2 weeks.[83] Only 5% of patients have recurrent episodes that may result in chronic ischemic colitis, gangrene, perforation, or strictures.[83] Resection is usually indicated in these patients with irreversible mucosal damage. Colonic infarction is a surgical emergency and patients may present with fever, leukocytosis, abdominal rebound, or guarding.[83]

Acute mesenteric ischemia occurs when there is decreased blood flow to the superior mesenteric artery, which affects the small intestines and possibly the right half of the colon. Approximately 50% of cases results from superior mesenteric artery embolus. It is most commonly seen in elderly patients with cardiovascular disease such as congestive heart failure, cardiac arrhythmia, myocardial infarction, and hypotension. The hallmark of acute mesenteric ischemia is that patients usually complain of severe abdominal pain but have a relatively benign abdominal examination.[83] The development of an acute abdomen (rebound and guarding) usually indicates that ischemia has progressed to infarction. Clinicians need to have a high degree of suspicion to make the diagnosis before infarction occurs. Other signs of ischemia may include abdominal distension and GI bleeding.[83] Laboratory studies may show leukocytosis and metabolic acidosis. Initial plain radiographs of the abdomen may be normal, radiological signs such as thumbprinting, ileus, and intramural air suggests that infarction may have occurred.[83] Angiography can be used to assess the circulation and detect the presence and site of emboli and thromboses. An angiographic catheter may then be used to administer intraarterial vasodilators or thrombolytics to improve blood flow.[83] The treatment for superior mesenteric artery embolus is surgical embolectomy.[83] Exploratory laparotomy is performed in patients with an acute abdomen to remove necrotic bowel and restore blood flow.[83] The prognosis is poor for acute mesenteric ischemia, with an average mortality rate of 71%.[84]

REFERENCES

1. Shaker R. Oropharyngeal dysphagia: practical approach to diagnosis and management. *Semin Gastrointest Dis.* 1992;3:115–128.
2. Steele CM, Greenwood C, Ens I, et al. Mealtime difficulties in a home for the age: not just dysphagia. *Dysphagia.* 1997;12:43–50.
3. Shaker R, Staff D. Esophageal disorders in the elderly. *Gastroenterol Clin N Am.* 2001;30:335–359.
4. Achem, SR, DeVault KR. Dysphagia in Aging. *J Clin Gastroenterol.* 2005;39(5):357–371.
5. Mold JW, Reed LE, Davis AB, et al. Prevalence of gastroesophageal reflux in elderly patients in a primary care setting. *Am J Gastroenterol.* 1991;86:965–970.
6. Linder JD, Wilcox CM. Acid peptic disease in the elderly. *Gastroenterol Clin N Am.* 2001;30:363–376.
7. Dent J, Dodds WJ, Friedman RH, et al. Mechanism of gastroesophageal reflux in recumbent asymptomatic human subjects. *J Clin Invest.* 1980;65:256–267.
8. Patti MG, Godbert HI, Arcerito M, et al. Hiatal hernia size affects lower esophageal sphincter function, esophageal acid expose, and degree of mucosal injury. *Am J Surg.* 1996;171:182–186.
9. DeVault KR, Castell DO. Updated guidelines for the diagnosis and treatment of gastroesophageal reflux disease: the Practice Parameters Committee of the American College of Gastroenterology. *Am J Gastroenterol.* 1999;94:1434–1442.
10. DeVault KR, Castell DO. Updated guidelines for the diagnosis and treatment of gastroesophageal reflux disease. *Am J Gastroenterol.* 2005;100:190.
11. Hetzel DJ, Dent J, Reed WD, et al. Healing and relapse of severe peptic esophagitis after treatment with omeprazole. *Gastroenterology.* 1988;95:903.
12. Enzinger PC, Mayer RJ. Medical progress: esophageal cancer. *NEJM.* 2003;349(23):2241–2252.
13. Ries LAG, Eisner MP, Kosary C, et al., eds. *SEER Cancer Statistics Review, 1973–1999.* Bethesda, Md.: National Cancer Institute, 2002.
14. Devesa SS, Blot WJ, Fraumeni JF Jr. Changing patterns in the incidence of esophageal and gastric carcinoma in the United States. *Cancer.* 1998;83:2049–2053.
15. Terry P, Lagergren J, Ye W, Nyren O, Wolk A. Antioxidants and cancers of the esophagus and gastric cardia. *Int J Cancer.* 2000;87:750–754.
16. Abid S, Mumtaz K, Jafri W, et al. Pill-induced esophageal injury: endoscopic features and clinical outcomes. *Endoscopy.* 2005;37(8):740–744
17. Pinos T, Figueras C, Mas R. Doxycycline-induced esophagitis: treatment with liquid sucralfate. *Am J Gastroenterol.* 1990; 85:902.
18. Baehr PH, McDonald GB. Esophageal infections: risk factors, presentation, diagnosis, and treatment. *Gastroenterology.* 1994;106:509.
19. Massey BT, Hogan WJ, Dodds WJ, et al. Alteration of the upper esophageal sphincter belch reflex in patients with achalasia. *Gastroenterology.* 1992;103:1574–1579.
20. McCarthy D. Acid peptic disease in the elderly. *Clin Geriatr Med.* 1991;7:231–254.
21. Coleman JA, Denham MJ. Perforation of peptic ulcer in the elderly. *Age Ageing.* 1980;9:257.
22. Gabriel SE, Jaakkimainen L, Bombardier C. Risk for serious gastrointestinal complications related to use of nonsteroidal anti-inflammatory drugs. A meta-analysis. *Ann Intern Med.* 1991; 115:787–796.
23. Sonnenberg A. Temporal trends and geographical variations of peptic ulcer disease. *Aliment Pharmacol Ther.* 1995;9 (Suppl 2):3–12.
24. Shorr RI, Ray WA, Daugherty JR, Griffin MR. Concurrent use of nonsteroidal anti-inflammatory drugs and oral anticoagulants places elderly persons at high risk for hemorrhagic peptic ulcer disease. *Arch Intern Med.* 1993;153:1665–1670.
25. McCarthy D. Nonsteroidal anti-inflammatory drug-related gastrointestinal toxicity: definitions and epidemiology. *Am J Med.* 1998;105:3S–5S.

26. Koch M, Dezi A, Ferrario F, Capurso I. Prevention of nonsteroidal anti-inflammatory drug-induced gastrointestinal mucosal injury. A meta-analysis of randomized controlled clinical trials. *Arch Intern Med.* 1996;156(20):2321–2332.

27. Hooper L, Brown TJ, Elliott R, et al. The effectiveness of five strategies for the prevention of gastrointestinal toxicity induced by non-steroidal anti-inflammatory drugs: systematic review. *BMJ.* 2004;329:948.

28. Banatvala N, Mayo K, Megraud F, Jennings R, Deeks JJ, Reldman RA. The cohort effect and Helicobacter pylori. *J Infect Dis.* 1993;168:219–221.

29. Smoot DT, Cutler AF. Helicobacter pylori: diagnostic tests. *Gastroenterol Endoscopy News.* 1997;48:28.

30. Liston R, Pitt MA, Banerjee AK. IgG ELISA antibodies and detection of Helicobacter pylori in elderly patients. *Lancet.* 1996;347:269.

31. Maton PN. Omeprazole. *NEJM.* 1991;324:965.

32. Feldman M, Burton ME. Histamine 2-receptor antagonists: standard therapy for acid peptic diseases (part 2). *NEJM.* 1990;323:1749.

33. Hopkins RJ, Girardi LS, Turney EA. Relationship between H. pylori eradication and reduced duodenal and gastric ulcer recurrence: a review. *Gastroenterology.* 1996;110:1244.

34. Hawkey CJ, Karrasch JA, Szczepanski L, et al. Omeprazole compared with misoprostol for ulcers associated with nonsteroidal anti-inflammatory drugs: Omeprazole versus misoprostol for NSAID-Induced Ulcer Management (OMNIUM) study group. *NEJM.* 1998;338:727–734.

35. Mettlin C. Epidemiologic studies in gastric adenocarcinoma. In: Douglass HO Jr. (ed). Gastric Cancer. New York: Churchill Livingstone; 1988.

36. Fuchs CS, Mayer RJ. Gastric carcinoma. *NEJM.* 1195;353:32–42.

37. Wanebo HJ, Kennedy BJ, Chmiel J, et al. Cancer of the stomach. A patient care study by the American College of Surgeons. *Ann Surg.* 1993;218:583–592.

38. Sial SH, Catalano MF. Gastrointestinal tract cancer in the elderly. *Gastroenterol Clin N Am.* 2001;30:565–590.

39. Boland R, Scheiman J. Tumors of the stomach. In: Yamada T, Alpers D, Owyang C, et al. (eds). Textbook of Gastroenterology. ed 2. Philadelphia: JB Lippincott; 1995:1494–1523.

40. Luk G. Tumors of the stomach. In: Feldman M, Scharschmidt BF, Sleisenger MH (eds). *Gastrointestinal and Liver Disease.* ed 6. Philadelphia: WB Saunders; 1998:772.

41. Lankish PG, Burchard-Reckert S, Petersen M, et al. Etiology and age have only a limited influence on the course of acute pancreatitis. *Pancreas.* 1996;13:344–349.

42. Browder W, Patterson MD, Thompson JL, et al. Acute pancreatitis of unknown etiology in the elderly. *Ann Surg.* 1993;217:469–475.

43. Eland IA, van Puijennbroek EP, Sturkenboom MJ, et al. Drug-associated acute pancreatitis: twenty-one years of spontaneous reporting in The Netherlands. *Am J Gastroenterol.* 1999;94:2417–2422.

44. Ross SO, Forsmark CE. Pancreatic and biliary disorders in the elderly. *Gastroenterol Clin N Am.* 2001;30:531–544.

45. Kohn HD, Wider G, Bayer PM, et al. Immunoreactive trypsin, alpha-amylase and lipase in serum – is there an age-dependence? *Clin Biochem.* 1982;15:49–51.

46. Freeny PC, Hauptmann E, Althaus AJ, et al. Percutaneous CT-guided catheter drainage of infected acute necrotizing pancreatitis: techniques and results. *AJR.* 1998;170:969.

47. Ries LAG, Eisner MP, Kasary CL, et al. SEER Cancer statistics review: National Cancer Institute 1973–1992, Bethesda; 2000.

48. Ritts RE, Nagorney DM, Jacobsen DJ, et al. Comparison of preoperative serum CA 19–9 levels with results of diagnostic imaging modalities in patients undergoing laparotomy for suspected pancreatic and gallbladder disease. *Pancreas.* 1994;9:707.

49. Sohn TA, Yeo CJ, Cameron JL, et al. Should pancreaticoduodenectomy be performed in octogenarians? *J Gastrointest Surg.* 1998;2:207–216.

50. National Vital Statistics Report 2000;48:1–105.

51. Deaths and hospitalization from chronic liver disease and cirrhosis – United States, 1980–1989. *MMWR.* 1993;41:969.

52. Regev A, Schiff ER. Liver disease in the elderly. *Gastroenterol Clin N Am.* 2001;30:547–563.

53. MacMahon M, James OFW. Liver disease in the elderly. *J Clin Gastroenterol.* 1994;18:330.

54. Kopanoff DE, Snider DE Jr, Caras GJ. Isoniazid related hepatitis. *Am Rev Respir Dis.* 1978;117:991.

55. Kondo Y, Tsukada K, Takeuchi T, et al. Higher carrier rate after hepatitis B virus infection in the elderly. *Hepatology.* 1993;18:768.

56. Poynard T, Bedossa P, Opolon P. Natural history of liver fibrosis progression in patients with chronic hepatitis C. *Lancet.* 1997;349:825–832.

57. Davila JA, Morgan RO, Shaib Y, McGlynn KA, El-Serag HB. Hepatitis C infection and the increasing incidence of hepatocellular carcinoma: a population-based study. *Gastroenterology.* 2004;127:1372–1380.

58. Elmberg M, Hultcrantz R, Ekbom A, et al. Cancer risk in patients with hereditary hemochromatosis and in their first-degree relatives. *Gastroenterology.* 2003;12:1733–1744.

59. Collier J, Sherman M. Screening for hepatocellular carcinoma. *Hepatology.* 1998;27(1):273–278.

60. Bruix J, Sherman M. Management of hepatocellular carcinoma. *Hepatology.* 2005;42:1208–1236.

61. Ohlsson B, Nilsson J, Stenram U, Akerman M, Tranberg KG. Percutaneous fine-needle aspiration cytology in the diagnosis and management of liver tumours. *Br J Surg.* 2002;89:757–762.

62. Poon RT, Fan ST, Lo CM, et al. Hepatocellular carcinoma in the elderly: results of surgical and non surgical management. *Am J Gastroenterol.* 1999;94:2460.

63. The Cancer of the Liver Italian Program (CLIP) investigators. A new prognostic system for hepatocellular carcinoma: a retrospective study of 435 patients. *Hepatology.* 1998;28(3):751–755.

64. Magnuson TH, Ratner LE, Zenilman ME, et al. Laparoscopic cholecystectomy: applicability in the geriatric population. *Am Surg.* 1997;63:91–96.

65. Lai ECS, Mok FPT, Tan ESY, et al. Endoscopic biliary drainage for severe acute cholangitis. *NEJM.* 1992;326:1582–1586.

66. Kimura W, Shimada H, Kuroda A, et al. Carcinoma of the gallbladder and extrahepatic bile duct in autopsy cases of the aged, with special reference to its relationship to gallstones. *Am J Gastroenterol.* 1989;84:386–390.

67. Thompson WG, Longstreth GF, Drossman DA, et al. Function bowel disorders and D. Functional abdominal pain. In: Drossman DA, Talley NJ, Thompson WG, Whitehead WE, Corazziari E, (eds). *Rome II: Functional Gastrointestinal Disorders: Diagnosis, Pathophysiology, and Treatment.* 2nd ed. McLean, VA: Degnon Associates; 2000;351–432.

68. Talley NJ, Zinsmeister AR, Van Dyke C, Melton LJ III. Epidemiology of colonic symptoms and the irritable bowel syndrome. *Gastroenterology.* 1991;101:927–934.

69. American Gastroenterological Association. AGA guideline: irritable bowel syndrome. *Gastroenterology.* 2002;123:2105–2107.

70. Botoman VA, Bonner GF, Botoman DA. Management of inflammatory bowel disease. *Am Fam Physician.* 1998;57:27(2):166–168.

71. Brzezinski A, Rankin GB, Seidner DL, Lashner BA. Use of old and new oral 5-aminosalicylic acid formulations in inflammatory bowel disease. *Cleve Clin J Med.* 1995;62:317–323.

72. American Gastroenterological Association Institute. American Gastroenterological Association Institute Medical position statement on corticosteroids, immunomodulators, and Infliximab in inflammatory bowel disease. *Gastroenterology.* 2002;130:935–939.

73. Weiss E, Wexner S. Surgical therapy for ulcerative colitis. *Gastroenterol Clin N Am.* 1995;24:559.

74. Glotzar D. Surgical therapy for Crohn's disease. *Gastroenterol Clin N Am.* 1995;24:527.

75. Fine KD, Schiller LR. AGA technical review on the evaluation and management of chronic diarrhea. *Gastroenterology.* 1999;116:1464.

76. Jewkes J, Larson HE, Price AB, et al. Aetiology of acute diarrhea in adults. *Gut.* 1981;22(5):388–392.

77. Holt PR. Diarrhea and malabsorption in the elderly. *Gastroenterol Clin N Am.* 2001;30:427–444.

78. McFarland LV, Mulligan ME, Kwok RYY, et al. Nosocomial acquisition of *Clostridium difficile* infection. *NEJM.* 1989;320:204.

79. Farrell RJ, Farrell JJ, Morrin MM. Diverticular disease in the elderly. *Gastroenterol Clin N Am.* 2001;30:475–496.

80. Gear JSS, Fursdon P, Nolan DJ, et al. Symptomless diverticular disease and intake of dietary fibre. *Lancet.* 1979;11:511–514.

81. McGuire HH. Bleeding colonic diverticula: a reappraisal of natural history and management. *Ann Surg.* 1994;220:653–656.

82. Ferzoco LB, Raptopoulos V, Silen W. Acute diverticulitis. *NEJM.* 1998;338:1521–1526.

83. Greenwald DA, Brandt LJ, Reinus JF. Ischemic bowel disease in the elderly. *Gastroenterol Clin N Am.* 2001;30:445–473.

84. Brandt LJ, Boley SJ. AGA technical review on intestinal ischemia. *Gastroenterology.* 2000;118:954.

22

Serious Infections in the Elderly

David Alain Wohl, MD

INTRODUCTION

Diseases caused by infectious pathogens are a major cause of illness and death among the elderly.[1] Many of the most serious infectious diseases have a predilection for those at the extremes of age – individuals with relatively deficient immune function. In addition, infections common to persons of all ages can be devastating when they occur in those of more advanced age. Elderly individuals also are frequently found in environments, such as hospitals and nursing facilities, where antibiotic-resistant organisms are prevalent and indwelling catheters breech the protection offered by an intact integument. On the other end of the functionality spectrum, many older individuals are active and may spend their postretirement years traveling to locales where they are exposed to exotic organisms. Similarly, many elders are sexually active and remain at risk for sexually transmitted infections, especially when establishing new intimate partnerships.

Compounding their increase in risk of infection, older individuals may suffer from delays in diagnosis as their infections often present atypically. Infectious diseases in older persons frequently present without fever or leukocytosis and can be challenging to detect and localize – especially in those who suffer from cognitive impairments. Therefore, the diagnostic approach must be modified when the patient is elderly, and the clinician must appreciate the unique characteristics of this growing population.

THE ELDER HOST

Immune function changes with age and during advanced age can begin to falter. Both humeral and cellular immunity can wane during senescence.[2,3] Memory T-cells, primed by prior antigen exposure, proportionally increase whereas the pool of naïve T-cells, responsible for responses to new antigens, declines

coincident with the progressive involution of the thymus that occurs during aging.[4,5] CD8+ cells also diminish, as do immunoglobulin M memory B cells, further reducing the ability to contain infections.[4–7] Vaccine responses become muted along with delayed hypersensitivity in older persons.[8,9] The important barriers to infection such as skin and mucosal surfaces also weaken. Skin thins and glandular secretions decrease, and along with age-related immune deficits, raise the risk for soft tissue infection and/or systemic spread. Concomitant illnesses can also enhance risk of infectious diseases. Conditions common in the elderly including diabetes mellitus, malignancies, chronic obstructive pulmonary disease, prosthetic joints, and bladder emptying disorders are associated with a higher incidence of infections. Immunosuppressive drugs used in the treatment of connective tissue diseases and other conditions common in the aged further raise the risk of infection. Malnutrition secondary to comorbid disease, poverty, poor dentition, or other causes of inadequate caloric intake further reduces host defenses against infection.

THE ENVIRONMENT

Approximately 5% of persons older than 65 years of age reside in a nursing facility but the rate increases to almost 20% by age 85 years.[2] Hospitalization rates for individuals aged 65 years and older are three times that of the general population.[10] In addition, many elderly individuals regularly attend clinics or require hospitalization at some point. These encounters increase the risk colonization with infectious pathogens, including those resistant to antimicrobials such as methicillin-resistant staphylococci, exposure to outbreaks of endemic infections such as tuberculosis (TB) and nosocomial infectious diseases like *Clostridium difficile*. The illnesses that attend advancing age often lead to instrumentation, catheterization, and surgery – each of which carries a risk of infection.

Table 22.1. Factors Increasing Vulnerability to Infectious Diseases during Aging

Host	Environment
Immunological	Nursing home residence
↓ Naïve T cells	Hospitalization
↓ CD8 + cells	Instrumentation
↓ IgM memory B cells	Exposure to drug-resistant organisms
Skin thinning and breakdown	Exposure to endemic infectious diseases during travel
↓ Glandular secretions	
↓ bCough reflex	
Cognitive impairment	
Malnutrition	
Poor dentition	
Tobacco use	
Poverty	

Few hospital admissions of elderly patients do not include a urinary catheter and intravenous line and many also entail even more invasive diagnostic and therapeutic procedures – further contributing to infection risk. Table 22.1 summarizes factors related to increased vulnerability to infection during aging.

APPROACH TO THE ELDERLY PATIENT WITH SUSPECTED INFECTIOUS DISEASE

The diagnosis of infectious diseases in elderly patients can be challenging. Classic features of some infections such as fever and leukocytosis may be absent in older individuals even during fulminant infection, dangerously delaying diagnosis.[11] Approximately 40% of older adults may not mount a febrile response to serious infection.[12] Therefore, small elevations in temperature above individual baseline should be concerning and fevers of 38.3°C should be considered alarming.[13] Localizing symptoms of infection may be subtle, and impaired cognition because of dementia or as a manifestation of the infection may render the patient unable to describe symptoms accurately. Delirium, in particular, is common during infection in the elderly.[14] In addition, infections among older patients can present atypically with vague aches, anorexia, or confusion as the only indication that an acute illness is present. A high degree of suspicion for underlying infectious processes is necessary when older individuals present with such subtle changes. Failure to consider adequately the possibility of infection in the elderly patient and overreliance on indicators of infection that are more common among younger patients can lead to tragic misdiagnosis of potentially treatable conditions.

Among more functional older patients, a complete travel and sexual risk behavior history-taking is mandatory. Elderly individuals are increasingly traveling to areas where endemic infectious diseases may be encountered. This includes domestic as well as international travel. Many elderly individuals remain sexually active into their 80s and 90s and assumptions regarding sexual orientation and monogamy can be dangerous and interfere with disease prevention and treatment efforts. The Centers for Disease Control and Prevention recommends that human immunodeficiency virus (HIV) testing should be ordered at least once for all persons seeking health care who are aged 13–65 years.[15] Many experts believe that testing should continue to be offered to those older than 65 years of age if they remain sexually active and at risk of acquiring HIV infection. Repeated testing is always warranted in persons with continued higher-risk behaviors.

MAJOR INFECTIOUS DISEASES

Urinary Tract Infections

Bacterial infection of the urinary tract is the most common bacterial infection in older adults and is the major source of bacteremia in this population.[16] Urinary catheters – both urethral and condom types – greatly increase urinary tract infection (UTI) risk.[11] Furthermore, host factors including neurogenic bladder, prostate enlargement in men, and vaginal atrophy and increase in vaginal pH in women can foster bacterial colonization that predisposes to UTI.[11] Frequent bladder emptying is protective against urinary infection; however, with aging the volume of urine required to sense a need to void increases and many elderly patients have reduced urinary flow because of poor fluid intake, obstruction and/or decreased bladder contractility, which further fosters bacterial colonization of the urine.[17]

Clinical Manifestations/Diagnosis

Classic symptoms of UTI such as dysuria, urinary frequency and urgency, suprapubic tenderness, and fever are telltale when present. As mentioned previously, however, some or all of these symptoms may be absent despite serious UTI. Atypical presentation of UTI with nausea, vomiting, dehydration, and confusion are common.[18,19] Urinalysis of a clean catch urine specimen demonstrating pyuria, increased leukocyte esterase, and nitrite is highly suggestive in the setting of the aforementioned clinical presentations. Confirmation of infection with urine culture also permits guidance of antibiotic therapy. Blood culture should be obtained in patients with more concerning acute illness to assess for urosepsis.

Quantitative clean catch urine culture revealing 100,000 CFU/mL or greater (for women, confirmed on repeated testing) in persons without symptoms of UTI is considered evidence of asymptomatic bacteriuria. Asymptomatic bacteriuria is common in elderly patients, especially women and has been linked to institutionalization, bladder-emptying disorders, diabetes, and prior UTI.[20]

Management

Gram-negative organisms are the most commonly cultured UTI pathogens and empiric therapy should broadly be directed toward these organisms until culture results return.[18,21] Patients with indwelling urinary catheters are also at increased risk for *Enterococcus* and, in such patients, coverage of this Gram-positive organism may be prudent. Detection of *Staphylococcus aureus* in the urine raises concern for endovascular infection such as endocarditis because this organism is often spread to the urine hematogenously. Echocardiography and blood cultures are indicated when *S. aureus* is retrieved from clean catch urine.

Treatment of asymptomatic bacteriuria has not been demonstrated to have an impact on morbidity or mortality and is generally not recommended.[16] Removal of urinary catheters should be considered and the need for such catheters regularly assessed. Following antibacterial treatment, typically for 7–14 days, repeated urine analysis and culture can be obtained to demonstrate clearing of the organism and resolution of pyuria.

Candida is not infrequently encountered in the urine of elderly hospitalized patients, especially those treated with broad-spectrum antibacterials. In most cases, treatment is unnecessary; however, in patients who are immunocompromised, exhibit symptoms of UTI, or are in need of urological instrumentation, treatment of candiduria should be strongly considered.

Bacterial Pneumonia

Respiratory infections are a leading cause of infectious disease–associated deaths among older individuals and can be acquired in the community or at nursing/medical facilities.[1] A number of factors conspire to raise the risk of pneumonia in the elderly, including a decline in pulmonary function, diminished cough reflex, reduced mucociliary transport, and decreased lung elasticity.[2,22,23] These mechanical factors lead to trapping of air, diminished ability to clear oral secretions, and colonization of pharynx with pathogenic bacteria.[23] Aspiration of such secretions is a major cause of pneumonia among elderly patients with impaired swallowing and/or cognition and is exacerbated by poor dentition. Prior or current smoking and its sequelae, including chronic obstructive pulmonary disease, further enhance the risk of respiratory infections among older patients.

Clinical Manifestations/Diagnosis

As with other infections in the elderly, pneumonia may not be heralded by the usual signs and symptoms. Cough may not be prominent, fever can be absent or mild, and shortness of breath subtle. Nonspecific symptoms of confusion or other mental status change, lethargy, and falling may be the only indications that something is amiss.[24,25] A high index of suspicion is required and a chest radiograph should be obtained when the physician is confronted with such changes. X-rays often reveals an infiltrative process; however, absence of an infiltrate on the film does not preclude pneumonia because dehydration may minimize radiographic evidence of infection.[26] The presence of a cavity suggests anaerobic abscess, TB, or mycotic infection. Sputum analysis, although potentially valuable in

the identification of causative organisms, is rarely available as older individuals may be unable to cooperate with specimen collection or expectorate. When respiratory secretions can be obtained, Gram stain and routine bacterial culture should be performed. Blood cultures may also yield an organism associated with pneumonia. Pulse oximetry and, in some cases, arterial blood gas level should be measured to assess oxygenation status. Viral and other atypical pneumonias, malignancy, and pulmonary embolus need to also be considered in the differential diagnosis of the older patient in whom pneumonia is suspected.

Management

Treatment of bacterial pneumonia should be guided by sputum Gram stain and culture. Given the difficulty of establishing a specific bacterial cause of pneumonia via sputum analysis and the seriousness of such infections in elderly patients, empiric therapy directed at the likely culprits is prudent and recommended.[27] Delays in the initiation of therapy risks progression of disease and, therefore, treatment should begin within hours of presentation.[28] For community-acquired pneumonia, *Streptococcus pneumoniae*, *Hemophilus influenza*, enteric Gram-negative bacilli, influenza, and other respiratory viruses are most common; however, *S. aureus* and atypical organisms such as *Mycoplasma*, *Legionella*, and *Chlamydia* also occur.[29] *Legionella* can be acquired in the community or nosocomially and urine testing for *Legionella* antigen can assist in the diagnosis of this infection. Patients residing in nursing homes more commonly experience pneumonia caused by the enteric Gram-negative organisms, oral aerobes and anaerobes, and *S. aureus*.[2] These organisms (see Table 22.2) are responsible for the lion's share of pneumonia in the hospitalized patient but more unusual organisms including *Acinetobacter* and *Pseudomonas* may also cause disease. Obviously, those patients who are more ill and those unable to tolerate oral intake require inpatient care and intravenous administration of antibiotics. Treatment of most bacterial pneumonia lasts for 7–14 days.

Antibiotic choice must be guided by host and environmental factors such as concomitant illnesses, risk of aspiration, and setting in which the patient resides.[27] Broader coverage – taking into account drug-resistant organisms and anaerobes – is typically indicated in institutionalized patients compared with those who live at home who may be able to be treated initially with an antipneumococcal fluoroquinolone, third generation cephalosporin, or macrolide, depending on local drug susceptibility patterns. Detection of a specific organism can lead to the narrowing of antibiotic therapy. Failure to detect improvement during therapy may indicate that the selected therapy is suboptimal and that a change in antibiotics is required. In such cases, the presence of underlying immunodeficiency, such as that from HIV infection, and atypical infections caused by fungi or *P. jiroveci* (formerly *carinii*), should be considered.

Patients with pneumonia who are moderately-to-severely ill should be hospitalized. Findings associated with poor prognosis in elderly patients with community-acquired pneumonia

Table 22.2. Causes of Pneumonia in the Elderly [2]

Community Acquired	Nursing Facility Associated	Hospital Associated
S. pneumonia	Enteric Gram-negative bacilli	Enteric Gram-negative bacilli
H. influenzae	Oral aerobes and anaerobes	Oral aerobes and anaerobes
Enteric Gram-negative bacilli	*S. aureus*	*S. aureus*
S. aureus	*S. pneumonia*	*S. pneumonia*
Legionella pneumophila	*H. influenzae*	*Legionella pneumophila*
Mycoplasma pneumoniae	*Moraxella catarrhalis*	*Moraxella catarrhalis*
Chlamydia pneumoniae	Influenza	*Pseudomonas* spp.
Influenza	Other respiratory viruses	*Acinetobacter* spp.
Respiratory syncytial virus		*Stenotrophomonas* spp.
Other respiratory viruses		Influenza
Pneumocystis jiroveci		Other respiratory viruses

include PaO_2 <60 mm Hg, O_2 saturation <90%, altered mental status, heart rate higher than 125 beats/minute, respiratory rate higher than 30/min, hypo- or hyperthermia, leukocytosis or leukopenia, anemia, hyponatremia, hyperglycemia, multilobar infiltrates, and pleural effusion.[11] In addition, older patients with pneumonia and significant comorbid diseases such as malignancy, immunodeficiency, renal or hepatic insufficiency, or cardiovascular disease may also require inpatient monitoring.

INFLUENZA

Influenza is a cause of viral pneumonia, occurring generally in the winter months in the United States. Recent data suggest that the virus thrives in cool temperatures with limited humidity – accounting for its seasonality.[30] Community and institutional acquisition occur under these conditions because this is a highly infectious virus with an incubation period of only 2–3 days. The infection and its complications can be lethal in elderly individuals.

Clinical Manifestations/Diagnosis

As in bacterial pneumonia, elderly patients with influenza may present atypically with the triad of cough, fever, and acute onset less evident than mental status alteration, generalized malaise, and other nonspecific complaints.[31] Among patients living in confined settings, the report of a similar illness or actual influenza among other residents or staff is an important epidemiological clue. Secondary bacterial infection with streptococci or staphylococci occurs and typically manifests as a period of worsening of disease after an initial improvement. The chest radiograph may demonstrate bilateral infiltrates – suggestive of a viral pneumonia. In addition, the diagnosis can be facilitated by viral culture of respiratory secretions and rapid antigen testing of a nasopharyngeal swab.

In travelers returning from Asia, it is important to assess for infection with more virulent strains of influenza or severe adult respiratory syndrome.

Management

Antiviral drugs active against influenza include amantadine and rimantadine – both of which cover only influenza A – and oseltamivir and zanamivir, which cover both influenza A and B.[32,33] The effectiveness of these agents depends on their timely administration, and there is little evidence that they are beneficial when administered beyond 48 hours after the start of symptoms. Selection of antiviral therapy, when appropriate, should be determined by epidemiological and toxicity factors. Cost may also be a consideration given the wide disparities in expense between the older and newer agents. Both oseltamivir and zanamivir can be used as prophylaxis in elderly unvaccinated patients who are exposed to influenza.

Influenza vaccination is effective at reducing the morbidity and mortality rates associated with influenza and is recommended annually for those 65 years and older and younger individuals with chronic medical conditions or who reside in confined settings.[34,35] The vaccine contains killed virus and cannot cause influenza.

Pulmonary Tuberculosis

More than half the cases of TB in the United States are diagnosed in individuals 65 years of age or older.[36] Age-related waning of cellular immunity, comorbid conditions, immunosuppressant medications, and malnutrition increase the risk of reactivation of latent TB in the elderly. In addition, failure to administer isoniazid to older individuals with a positive tuberculin skin test because of fears of hepatotoxicity may also increase the risk of future reactivation of TB. Primary acquisition of TB also occurs among the elderly and transmission of TB within nursing facilities is well documented.[37]

Clinical Manifestations/Diagnosis

Pulmonary TB presents generally as a nonacute illness characterized by weight loss, fever, night sweats, and cough. Some patients may have hemoptysis. Nonspecific constitutional complaints may mask the more classic symptoms, and the diagnosis of TB should be considered in elderly persons with "failure to thrive." Chest radiographs, tuberculin skin testing and sputum stain, and culture are the foundations of the diagnostic workup for pulmonary TB. Chest films may reveal an area of infiltration – often in the upper lobes – or a cavitary lesion but patterns similar to bacterial pneumonia can also be seen.[38] The diagnosis is made microbiologically with the culture of sputum for *Mycobacterium tuberculosis*. The specimen should undergo an acid-fast stain and be plated on specialized media. Unfortunately, sputum may be difficult to collect and it may take 6 weeks for the culture to grow sufficiently. In some cases, bronchoscopy may be required to obtain specimens for stain and culture. Given the difficulty of establishing a quick diagnosis, empiric therapy is a consideration when suspicion of TB is high, such as in a patient with a classic chest film and a positive tuberculin skin test. Rapid tests for TB are now available and these molecular assays may be of use in some patients.[39] They are generally used to confirm the presence of TB in respiratory specimens that reveal AFB. The use of these assays in acid-fast bacilli–negative smears, although not approved for such use by the U.S. Food and Drug Administration (FDA) is tempting in cases in which TB is suspected despite the smear result and a positive result would be considered strong evidence of the infection.

Tuberculin skin testing is useful for determining prior exposure to TB. As the test relies on cellular immune responses, the false-negative rate of the test increases during advanced age. In some individuals, skin testing itself can boost immune responses to tuberculin such that repeated testing will become positive – giving the appearance of a conversion in the test from initially negative to positive.[40] In settings where skin testing for TB is performed on a regular basis, a two-step procedure at initial intake is advisable. If the initial reaction is negative, a repeated skin test is done 2–3 weeks later and the second result is considered final. Bacillus-Calmette-Guérin vaccination may produce skin reactions to tuberculin. For those who received the vaccine as a child, the cross-reactivity to the skin testing should wane by adulthood and not be a significant factor in elderly individuals. Those who receive Bacillus-Calmette-Guérin vaccination as adults should have skin testing done several months after vaccination to establish a baseline test reaction size. Subsequent skin testing can be compared with this baseline result and increases of greater than 15 mm should be considered positive in persons older than 35 years of age.

Gamma-interferon assays of blood are also used to detect latent TB and are now available through commercial laboratories.[41,42] There are limited data on the accuracy of this assay in the elderly but a positive result indicates prior exposure. The Centers of Disease Control and Prevention have published recommendations regarding the use of the interferon-γ assay QuantiFeron-TB Gold and these state that the test can be used in all circumstances in which tuberculin skin testing is performed.[43]

All patients with either latent or active TB, regardless of age, should be tested for HIV infection.

Management

The therapeutic management of pulmonary TB in the elderly patient is not different from that in younger patients.[44] As discussed previously, empiric therapy for TB may be considered in patients with an illness consistent with pulmonary TB, especially when the sputum reveals acid-fast bacilli. Drug therapy typically consists of four drugs (isoniazid, rifampin, pyrazinamide, and ethambutol) administered for 2 months. Provided drug susceptibility testing indicates sensitivity to isoniazid and rifampin, treatment can be whittled to these two agents for the remainder of the course. As polypharmacy is common in many elderly patients, care must be taken to avoid drug–drug interactions between TB and other medications. Monitoring for drug toxicity, especially changes in hepatic transaminases (alanine aminotransferase and aspartate aminotransferase), is prudent. In general, aspartate aminotransferase or alanine aminotransferase elevations up to five times normal can be tolerated if the patient is free of hepatitis symptoms and up to three times normal if there are signs or symptoms of liver toxicity.[45] When treatment-limiting hepatic toxicity occurs, expert consultation should be sought so that reintroduction of therapy can be considered. Patients receiving ethambutol should have a baseline ophthalmology evaluation and be questioned monthly regarding visual disturbances because this drug can cause optic neuritis. Monthly ocular evaluations are recommended for patients taking doses greater than 15–25 mg/kg, patients receiving the drug for longer than 2 months, and any patient with renal insufficiency.

Latent TB should be treated in elderly individuals.[45,46] In one study, the risk of isoniazid-associated hepatotoxicity increased with age and was 2.3% among those aged 50 years or older.[47] More recent data indicate the risk of isoniazid-related hepatitis was generally rare with only 1 case per 1,000 persons; however, the incidence was not analyzed according to age.[48] Current guidelines recommend that age not be considered when deciding to treat latent TB.[46] Importantly, alcohol raises the risk of the isoniazid-related hepatitis and all patients on this drug need to be warned to abstain. Peripheral neuropathy occurs in up to 2% of patients taking isoniazid and this can be prevented by pyridoxine supplementation.[49,50]

Herpes Zoster

Herpes zoster, or shingles, is a common condition associated with advancing age. It is also a commonly misunderstood disease by both patients and clinicians. The causative organism is the varicella zoster virus (VZV). This virus is the same one that causes chickenpox in younger persons and, like all herpes viruses, remains latent within the body following initial infection. In the case of VZV, the virus resides in the dorsal root ganglion where it can remain without causing illness. With diminished immune function subsequent to aging, drugs or illness, the virus can be activated and lead to the clinical syndrome known as shingles.[51]

Clinical Manifestations/Diagnosis

As opposed to the indistinct, if not misleading, presentation of other infectious diseases in the elderly, herpes zoster almost always announces itself with a constellation of classic symptoms. The illness starts with a 2–7 day prodrome of tingling and pain at the site where soon thereafter an erythematous rash emerges in an area restricted to 1–2 adjacent dermatomal regions and does not usually cross the midline.[51] The rash matures quickly, first becoming papular and then vesicular coincident with an increased intensity of pain and burning. Within 2 weeks, the lesions crust and begin to fade, although they may leave permanent scars. Serious systemic illness is rare although fever, weakness, and anorexia can occur. Involvement of multiple dermatomes, crossing of the midline by lesions, and continued emergence of new lesions suggest more profound immunodeficiency.[51–53]

Although the clinical presentation is usually sufficient to establish the diagnosis of herpes zoster, laboratory confirmation can be achieved by testing of the vesicle fluid for the presence of VZV – either via viral culture, polymerase chain reaction, or Tzanck smear.

Unusually herpes zoster can involve the eye, either externally or at the retina. Zoster lesions at the tip of the nose is an indication of involvement of cranial nerve V. Myelitis and encephalitis are rare, but serious, complications. The most common complication of shingles is postherpetic neuralgia (PHN). Continued pain and hypersensitivity at the area of the rash continues during PHN and can last up to a year.[54]

Management

A number of oral antivirals including acyclovir, valacyclovir, and famciclovir are active against VZV and can be used to reduce the duration of illness.[51] These are most effective in reducing the time to lesion crusting and acute pain resolution when initiated within 72 hours of the onset of the rash. Prompt valacyclovir and famciclovir treatment may also shorten the duration of PHN. Treatment with antivirals should continue until crusting of all the lesions occurs – generally 7–10 days.

Persons with active lesions are infectious and can transmit VZV to those who have not previously been exposed to or vaccinated against the virus. Person with a clear history of chickenpox are at no risk of infection (even if pregnant) and need not take any special precautions regarding VZV. Crusting of the lesions is associated with a marked reduction in infectiousness.

The management of PHN is often difficult. Topical therapies including anesthetics, and capsaicin can be used; however, systemic therapy with narcotics, anticonvulsant drugs (e.g., gabapentin) or antidepressants (e.g., nortriptyline, amitriptyline, desipramine, and sertraline) may be required.[55] Intransi-

gent cases of PHN should be referred to a pain management specialist.

As described in chapter 33, prevention of herpes zoster is possible with a newly FDA-approved zoster vaccine. This vaccine is manyfold more potent than that used for immunizing previously uninfected individuals and is approved for use in immunocompetent persons without a history of shingles who are older than 60 years.[55,56,56a] Use of the vaccine has been found to reduce the risk of herpes zoster by more than 50%.[56] A mild varicella rash can occur as an adverse effect of the vaccine.

Methicillin-Resistant *Staphylococcus aureus*

Methicillin-resistant *S. aureus* (MRSA) is a major cause of nosocomial infections including skin and soft tissue infections, septicemia, endovascular infections, and infections of indwelling catheters or implanted prosthetic devices.[57] The spread of MRSA in health care settings has had a significant impact on both clinical outcomes and health costs.[58] Hospital stays are prolonged, and mortality is higher among those with this infection. Risk factors associated with hospital-acquired MRSA include prolonged hospitalization (often more than 14 days), preceding antimicrobial therapy (especially with cephalosporins or fluoroquinolones), presence in an intensive care unit or burn unit, hemodialysis, surgical site infection, and proximity to a patient colonized or infected with MRSA.[58] As many, if not most, hospital inpatients are elderly, MRSA can be considered a major infection in this population. Furthermore, there is a great potential for the spread of MRSA within nursing facilities given the high rates of colonization with the organism among residents of such facilities.

Recently, community-acquired (CA) MRSA infections are becoming more common. Studies performed between 1997 and 2001 demonstrate that 12%–22% of all staphylococcal isolates in patients presenting from community settings were methicillin resistant.[59] In a study performed in 2004, 59% of staphylococcal isolates obtained strictly from skin and soft tissue infections were characterized as CA-MRSA.[60] Risk factors that have been associated with CA-MRSA infection include African-American race, HIV infection, antibiotic therapy within the past 6 months, and skin trauma.[61]

Clinical Presentation/Diagnosis

MRSA colonizes the nasal mucosa and oropharynx but may also be found on the skin. Colonization itself does not cause illness, but it does increase the risk of subsequent disease from the organism. The clinical manifestations of MRSA infection are protean and include skin and soft tissue infections, pneumonia, endovascular infections, and joint infections.[57,58] CA-MRSA frequently presents as a boil or skin abscess that is painful and erythematous. Clinically, it is impossible to distinguish between MRSA and other bacterial causes of these infections. Culture of the organism from infected tissue or blood is the basis of diagnosis. Given the aggressive nature of many staphylococcal infections, however, a high level of suspicion

Table 22.3. Antibiotic Options for MRSA

Antibiotic	Route	Indications	Routine Dose	Major Side Effects
Trimethoprim-Sulfamethoxazole (Septra, Bactrim)	PO, IV	Skin and soft tissue infections. Not specifically FDA approved for infections resulting from MRSA.	1 double-strength tablet (160 mg TMP/800 mg SMX) po bid	Anemia, neutropenia, rash, pruritus, Stevens–Johnson syndrome. Not recommended during the third trimester of pregnancy.
Minocycline (Minocin) and Doxycycline (Doryx)	PO	Skin and soft tissue infections. Not specifically FDA approved for infections resulting from MRSA.	100 mg po bid	Photosensitivity, rash. Not recommended for use during pregnancy.
Clindamycin (Cleocin)	PO, IV	Skin and soft tissue infections, bone infections. Not specifically FDA approved for infections resulting from MRSA.	300–600 mg po tid-qid	Rash, *Clostridium difficile* colitis
Rifampin (Rifampicin)	PO	Should not be used as a single agent. May be used in combination for treatment and eradication of MRSA.	600 mg po qd	Rash, liver inflammation. High frequency of drug–drug interactions.
Vancomycin (Vancocin)	IV	Endocarditis, bacteremia, bone/joint infections.	1000 mg q 12 h	Hypersensitivity reactions, red man syndrome.
Quinupristin – Dalfopristin (Synercid)	IV	Skin and soft tissue infections.	7.5 mg/kg q 8–12 h	Arthralgias, myalgias.
Linezolid (Zyvox)	IV, PO	Skin and soft tissue infections, pneumonia.	600 mg q 12 h	Bone marrow suppression. Note: not recommended for routine oral use because of potential for inducing resistance, toxicity, and high cost.
Daptomycin (Cubicin)	IV	Skin and soft tissue infections.	4–6 mg/kg q day	Myopathy.

should be maintained in the presence of predisposing conditions such as defects in phagocytic function and diabetes mellitus.

As mentioned previously, a common error in the management of endovascular infections caused by *S. aureus* is the assumption that detection of this organism in the urine indicates only a UTI. Isolation of this organism in the urine should prompt evaluation for the presence of endocarditis or other endovascular infection as this organism commonly enters the genitourinary system hematogenously.

Management

Drainage of infected material and antibiotics are the mainstays of therapy. Skin and soft tissue abscesses require surgical drainage and adjunctive antibiotic therapy. Nonsurgically managed MRSA infections require appropriate antibiotic therapy. There are different drug susceptibility profiles for MRSA seen in hospital- compared with community-acquired isolates.[62] There is also a difference in patterns of drug resistance depending on geography. It is, therefore, important to tailor treatment according to regional antibiotic susceptibility patterns (see Table 22.3). In some cases, drugs such as trimethoprim-sulfamethoxazole and doxycycline can be used to treat a drained abscess. Other infections, resulting from MRSA, may require more active agents against the organism.

In general, vancomycin is active against MRSA. There are reports of some strains of *S. aureus* with reduced susceptibility to vancomycin but these are rare, show only intermediate resistance to this drug, and retain susceptibility to the newer classes of antistaphylococcal antibiotics: the oxazolidinones, quinupristin/dalfopristin, the cyclic lipopeptide daptomycin, and the glycylcycline tigecycline.[63] These alternatives are typically used when vancomycin is not tolerated.

Newer approaches to therapy involve decolonization to prevent person-to-person transmission and to break the cycle of recurrent outbreaks of MRSA skin and soft tissue infections in a single individual. Currently no clear consensus guidelines exist and evidence from controlled trials is limited; however, general measures include intranasal mupirocin, topical antiseptic washes (i.e., chlorhexidine gluconate) during daily showers and weekly Clorox baths (approximately 0.25 cups per bath with a 10 minute soak). One recent encouraging study utilized a triple approach with an oral regimen of rifampin and doxycycline, intranasal 2% mupirocin ointment, and 2% chlorhexidine gluconate for washing.[64] In this study, 112 hospitalized patients who were colonized with MRSA were randomized to receive this decolonization therapy for 7 days or no treatment. Of those treated, 74% had negative MRSA cultures at 3 months, whereas only 32% of those who were not treated were culture negative at follow-up. Eight months later, 54% of those who were treated remained culture negative. This same study found that in patients who were colonized with mupirocin-resistant *S. aureus* at baseline treatment was nine times more likely to fail.

Personal hygiene measures include keeping nails trimmed short and scrubbed daily with soap, single-use only of bath towels and garments, and washing clothes in hot water. If a single patient has recurrent MRSA outbreaks then often oral antibiotics are used in conjunction. Also, all members of the household should be treated with the general decolonization measures. Handwashing and other infection control measures are essential to prevent the spread of MRSA, especially in institutionalized settings.

SUMMARY

The diagnosis and management of infectious diseases in older persons can be challenging. Clinicians must be familiar with the differences in clinical presentation among older and younger patients. In addition, it is important that subtle indicators of serious infection and impending clinical decompensation such as hypothermia or leukopenia not be missed. Timely therapeutic intervention when infection is suspected is essential as a delay in appropriate treatment, even for a few hours, can have devastating consequences. As the population in the United States continues to age, familiarity with the clinical presentation, diagnosis, and management of the major serious infections of elderly individuals becomes an increasingly critical component of general medicine and primary care.

REFERENCES

1. Heron MP, Smith BL. Deaths: leading causes for 2003. *National Vital Statistics Reports.* 2007;55:March 15. Available at: http://www.cdc.gov/nchs/data/nvsr/nvsr55/nvsr55_10.pdf. Accessed May 30, 2008.
2. Htwe TH, Mushtaq A, Robinson Sb, et al. Infections in the elderly. *Infect Clin N Am.* 2007;21(3):711–743.
3. Listi F, Candore G, Modica MA, et al. A study of serum immunoglobulin levels in elderly persons that provides new insight into B cell immunosenescence. *Ann NY Acad Sci.* 2006;1089:487–495.
4. Pster G, Weiskopf D, Lazuardi L, et al. Naive T cells in the elderly: are they still there? *Ann NY Acad Sci.* 2006;1067:152–157.
5. Pawelec G, Koch S, Franceschi C, et al. Human immunosenescence: does it have an infectious component? *Ann NY Acad Sci.* 2006;1067:56–65.
6. Shi Y, Yamazaki T, Okubo Y, et al. Regulation of aged humoral immune defense against pneumococcal bacteria by IgM memory B cell. *J Immunol.* 2005;175:3262–3267.
7. Colonna-Romano G, Aquino A, Bulati M, et al. Memory B cell subpopulations in the aged. *Rejuv Res.* 2006;9(1):149–152.
8. Howells CHL, Vesselinova-Jenkins CK, Evans AD, et al: Influenza vaccination and mortality from bronchopneumonia in the elderly. *Lancet.* 1975;1:381–383.
9. Ammann AJ, Schiffman G, Austrian R: The antibody responses to pneumococcal capsular polysaccharides in the aged. *Proc Soc Exp Biol Med.* 1980;164:312–316.
10. Greenberg S. Administration on Aging. A profile of older Americans: 2005. Available at: http://www.aoa.gov/PROF/Statistics/profile/2005/profiles2005.asp. Accessed May 30, 2008.
11. Mouton CP, Bazaldua OV. Common infections in older adults. *Am Fam Physician.* 2001;63:257–268.
12. Yoshikawa TT, Norman DC. Fever in the elderly. *Infect Med.* 1998;15:704–706.
13. Norman DC. Special infectious disease problems in geriatrics. *Clin Geriatr.* 1999;(Suppl 1):3–5.
14. Fraser D. Assessing the elderly for infections. *J Gerontol Nurs.* 1997;23:5–10.
15. Branson BM, Handsfield HH, Lampe MA, et al. Revised recommendations for HIV testing of adults, adolescents, and pregnant women in health-care settings. *MMWR.* 2006;55(RR-14):1–17.
16. Yoshikawa TT. Ambulatory management of common infections in elderly patients. *Infect Med.* 1991;20:37–43.
17. Pfisterer MH, Griffiths DJ, Schaefer W, et al. The effect of age on lower urinary tract function: a study in women. *J Am Geriatr Soc.* 2006;54:405–412.
18. McCue JD. Treatment of urinary tract infections in long-term care facilities: advice, guidelines and algorithms. *Clin Geriatr.* 1999;(Suppl):11–17.
19. Nicolle LE. Urinary tract infection in long-term-care facility residents. *Clin Infect Dis.* 2000;31:757–761.
20. Zhanel GG, Harding GK, Guay DR. Asymptomatic bacteriuria. Which patients should be treated? *Arch Intern Med.* 1990;150:1389–1396.
21. Lienderrozos HJ. Urinary tract infections: management rationale for uncomplicated cystitis. *Clin Fam Pract.* 2004;6:157–173.
22. Meyer KC. Lung infections and aging. *Ageing Res Rev.* 2004;3:55–67.
23. Meyer KC. Aging. *Proc Am Thorac Soc.* 2005;2:433–439.
24. Venkatesan P, Gladman J, MacFarlane J, et al. A hospital study of community acquired pneumonia in the elderly. *Thorax.* 1990;17:254–258.
25. Riquelme R, Torres A, WI-Ebiary M, et al. Community-acquired pneumonia in the elderly. *Am J Respir Crit Care Med.* 1997;156:1908–1914.
26. Hash R, Stephens J, Laurens M, et al. The relationship between volume status, hydration, and radiographic findings in the diagnosis of community-acquired pneumonia. *J Fam Pract.* 2000;49:833–837.
27. Loeb M. Pneumonia in older persons. *Clin Infect Dis.* 2003; 37:1335–1339.
28. Meehan T, Fine M, Krumholz H, et al. Quality of care, process, and outcomes in elderly patients with pneumonia. *JAMA.* 1997;278:2080–2084.
29. Ruiz M, Ewing S, Marcos M, et al. Etiology of community-acquired pneumonia: impact of age, comorbidity, and severity. *Am J Respir Crit Care Med.* 1999;160:397–405.
30. Lowen AC, Mubareka S, Steel J, Palese P. Influenza virus transmission is dependent on relative humidity and temperature. *PLoS Pathogens.* 2007;3:e151.
31. Govaert TME, Dinant GJ, Aretz K, et al. The predictive value of influenza symptomatology in elderly people. *Fam Pract.* 1998;15:16–22.
32. Winquist AG, Fukuda K, Bridges CB, Cox NJ. Neuraminidase inhibitors for treatment of influenza A and B infections. *MMWR.* 1999;48(RR-14):1–9.
33. Kuhle C, Evans JM. Prevention and treatment of influenza infections in the elderly. *Clin Geriatr.* 1999;7(2):27–35.

34. Centers for Disease Control and Prevention. Recommendations of the Advisory Committee on Immunization Practices (ACIP), 2007–2008. Available at: http://www.cdc.gov/flu/professionals/acip/. Accessed June 1, 2008.

35. Gross PA, Hermogenes AW, Sacks HS, et al. The efficacy of influenza vaccine in elderly persons: a meta-analysis and review of the literature. *Ann Intern Med.* 1995;123:518–527.

36. Dutt AK, Stead WW. Tuberculosis in elderly. *Med Clin North Am.* 1993;77:1353–1368.

37. Zevallos M, Justman JE. Tuberculosis in the elderly. *Clin Geriatr Med.* 2003;19: 121–138.

38. Imperato J, Sanchez LD. Pulmonary emergencies in the elderly. *Emerg Med Clin N Am.* 2006;24:317–338.

39. American Thoracic Society Workshop. Rapid diagnostic tests for tuberculosis: what is the appropriate use? *Am J Respir Crit Care Med.* 1997;155:1804.

40. Menzies D. Interpretation of repeated tuberculin tests. Boosting, conversion, and reversion. *Am J Respir Crit Care Med.* 1999;159:15.

41. Pai M, Riley LW, Colford JM Jr. Interferon-gamma assays in the immunodiagnosis of tuberculosis: a systematic review. *Lancet Infect Dis.* 2004;4:761.

42. Menzies D, Pai M, Comstock G. Meta-analysis: new tests for the diagnosis of latent tuberculosis infection: areas of uncertainty and recommendations for research. *Ann Intern Med.* 2007;146:340.

43. Mazurek GH, Jereb J, Lobue P, et al. Guidelines for using the QuantiFERON-TB Gold test for detecting Mycobacterium tuberculosis infection, United States. *MMWR.* 2005;54:49.

44. Bass J, Farer L, Hopewell P, et al. Treatment of tuberculosis and tuberculosis infection in adults and children. American Thoracic Society and The Centers for Disease Control and Prevention. *Am J Respir Crit Care Med.* 1994;149:1359–1374.

45. Blumberg HM, Burman WJ, Chaisson RE, et al. American Thoracic Society/Centers for Disease Control and Prevention/Infectious Diseases Society of America. Treatment of tuberculosis. *Am J Respir Crit Care Med.* 2003;167:603.

46. Jasmer RM, Nahid P, Hopewell PC. Clinical practice. Latent tuberculosis infection. *NEJM.* 2002;347:1860.

47. Kopanoff DE, Snider DE Jr, Caras GJ. Isoniazid-related hepatitis: a U.S. Public Health Service Cooperative Surveillance Study. *Am Rev Respir Dis.* 1978;117:991–1000.

48. Nolan CM, Goldberg SV, Buskin SE. Hepatotoxicity associated with isoniazid preventive therapy: a 7-year survey from a public health tuberculosis clinic. *JAMA.* 1999;281:1014–1018.

49. Oestreicher R, Dressler SH, Middlebrook G. Peripheral neuritis in tuberculous patients treated with isoniazid. *Am Rev Tuberc.* 1954;70:504–508.

50. Snider DE Jr. Pyridoxine supplementation during isoniazid therapy. *Tubercle.* 1980;61:191–196.

51. Dworkin RH, Johnson RW, Breuer J, et al. Recommendations for the management of herpes zoster. *Clin Infect Dis.* 2007;44:S1–44.

52. Weinberg JM, Vafaie J, Scheinfeld NS. Skin infections in the elderly. *Dermatol Clin.* 2004;22:51–61.

53. Heininger U, Seward J. Varicella. *Lancet.* 2006;368:1365–1376.

54. Schmader KE, Studenski S. Are current therapies useful for the prevention of postherpetic neuralgia? A critical analysis of the literature. *J Gen Intern Med.* 1989; 4(2):83–89.

55. Kost RG, Straus SE. Postherpetic neuralgia – pathogenesis, treatment and prevention. *NEJM.* 1996;335:32–42.

56. Kimberlin D, Whitley RJ. Varicella-zoster vaccine for the prevention of herpes zoster. *NEJM.* 2007;356:1338–1343.

56a. Oxman MN, Levin MJ, Johnson GR, et al. A vaccine to prevent herpes zoster and post-herpetic neuralgia in older adults. *NEJM.* 2005;352(22):2271–2284.

57. Crossley KB, Archer GL. The staphylococci in human disease. New York: Churchill Livingstone; 1997.

58. Kaplan AH. *Staphylococci Infections. Netter's Internal Medicine.* Teterboro, NJ: Icon Learning Systems; 2003.

59. Chambers HF. The changing epidemiology of *Staphylococcus aureus? Emerg Infect Dis.* 2001;7:178–182.

60. Moran GJ, Krishnadasan A, Gorwitz RJ, et al. Methicillin-resistant *S. aureus* infections among patients in the emergency department. *NEJM.* 2006;355:666–674.

61. Centers for Disease Control and Prevention. Outbreaks of Community-associated methicillin-resistant Staphylococcus aureus skin infections-Los Angeles County, California, 2002–2003. *MMWR.* 2003;52:88.

62. Foster TJ. The *Staphylococcus aureus* "superbug." *J Clin Invest.* 2004;114:1693–1696.

63. Liu C, Chambers HF. Staphylococcus aureus with heterogeneous resistance to vancomycin: epidemiology, clinical significance, and critical assessment of diagnostic methods. *Antimicrob Agents Chemother.* 2003;47:3040–3045.

64. Simor A, Phillips E, McGeer A, et al. Randomized controlled trial of chlorhexidine gluconate for washing, intranasal mupirocin, and rifampin and doxycycline versus no treatment for the eradication of methicillin-resistant Staphylococcus aureus colonization. *Clin Infect Dis.* 2007;44:178–185.

23

Human Immunodeficiency Virus in the Elderly

Karen Krigger, MD, MEd, Molly Rose, RN, PhD

Human immunodeficiency virus (HIV) affects the immune system by the destruction of human T-helper cells, or CD4 cells. A significant loss of CD4 cells depletes the body's ability to protect itself from "opportunistic infections," creating the condition of acquired immune deficiency syndrome (AIDS), usually when the CD4 count falls below 200 cells/mm. The time from HIV infection to death without the benefit of antiretroviral therapy is currently 10–11 years in the average patient.[1] Age as a host factor influences the rate of HIV disease progression.[2] Aging is associated with a higher viral load following seroconversion, more aggressive disease progression, shorter survival rates, and increased intolerance of antiretroviral agents. Physiological changes of aging such as involution of the thymus gland may inhibit function of CD4 cells, and CD4 cell regeneration generally slows with age. There are other common changes with aging that can affect disease progression. There is an increased risk of autoimmune disorders, a decrease in renal and lung function, neurological and psychological changes (such as depression and dementia), and postmenopausal vaginal changes. Additionally, comorbidity and poor nutrition could affect disease progression.

Although the term "elderly" is usually applied to patients in the sixth decade, the Centers for Disease Control and Prevention (CDC) defines elderly AIDS patients as those 50 years and older. AIDS cases in persons older than 50 years, originating before 1989, were a result of contaminated blood transfusions from 1978–1985, representing 6%, 28%, and 64% of AIDS among persons aged 50–59 years; 60–69 years; and older than 70 years, respectively.[3] Subsequent voluntary donor deferral and routine screening of blood donations since 1985 significantly reduced cases associated with blood transfusions. Unfortunately, the risk factors of men who have sex with men, intravenous drug use, and heterosexual transmission began to increase. The CDC data reports from 1991–1996 revealed 11% of the total adult AIDS cases from that period were older than 50 years of age.[3] Heterosexual contact was reported as the risk factor responsible for a 94% rise in AIDS cases presenting with opportunistic infections among men older than 50 years from 1991 to 1996. The number of AIDS cases in the United States increased fivefold in the 50 year and older population from 1990 to 2001: 16,288–90,513, representing 19% of the AIDS cases at the end of 2000. Current AIDS cases reported cumulatively through 2005 in the United States are as follows: 45–54 years: 1–576,643 or 16%; 55–64 years: 46,588 or 5%; older than 65 years: 14,647 or 2% for a cumulative total of 23% of all AIDS patients.[4] Data indicated patients older than 50 years were more likely to have wasting syndrome, HIV encephalopathy, and severe immunosuppression at the time of their diagnosis, with death more likely within 30 days.[3,5]

The epidemiology of HIV/AIDS because of highly active antiretroviral therapy (HAART) has evolved into a decrease in AIDS death rates and an increasing number of years of survival. This translates to an increase in the number of people older than the age of 50 years who are living with HIV/AIDS. Individuals diagnosed at a younger age and living to an older age, in addition to the number of adults older than age 50 years with newly diagnosed HIV/AIDS, will have an impact on prevention and clinical practice. Other age-related sociological issues of aging can affect prevention, diagnosis, and treatment issues related to HIV/AIDS. For example, reduced socialization, isolation, stigma, and grandparent caregiving issues can affect stress, time management, and priorities related to one's own health maintenance. Studies have shown that the highest proportion of respondents indicating stigma issues were older adults[6] and that older adults were less likely to disclose their HIV status to relatives, partners, church members, and neighbors.[7] The phenomenon today of grandparents raising grandchildren often becomes a higher priority for the grandparent than personal health.[8,9] Health care providers need to be aware of high-risk behaviors among older adults, become skilled at identifying symptoms of HIV/AIDS, and stay vigilant about screening for HIV/AIDS and the risk factors.[10]

Risk factors for the elderly population are similar to those of the younger population. The greatest risk is unprotected sexual behavior, dispelling the myth that older people are not sexually active. Findings show that 71% of men and 51% of women older than 60 years report that they are sexually active.[11] Male-to-male unprotected sex with an infected partner is the chief risk behavior with this age group. Older men engaging in sex with other men may have less self-identification as gay ("down low" experience) and may be in denial about the risk of HIV. Heterosexual transmission of HIV/AIDS among older adults through unsafe sexual behavior has dramatically increased and accounts for the largest percentage of AIDS cases among heterosexual groups. The popularity of medications such as Viagra may contribute to these numbers. In addition, older adults are less likely to practice safer sex with condoms, perhaps because they do not need to practice birth control and they have a lower perceived susceptibility to sexually transmitted diseases. Studies have shown that approximately 20% of sexually active older adults use condoms.[12,13] Postmenopausal older women are at a greater risk of HIV infection during intercourse than younger women because of age-related physiological changes of decreased vaginal lubrication and thinning of vaginal mucosa resulting from estrogen loss and a decline in the immune system.

Primary HIV prevention interventions and health education materials targeted to the elderly is lacking.[14,15] There has been little public acknowledgement of HIV/AIDS as a concern for older adults. Older adults do not see other older adults in the media with HIV/AIDS.[16] Although older adults engage in risky behaviors, lack of perceived risk leads to failure to adapt safer behaviors.[17] A literature review of transmission risks in older adults categorized findings into individual and system-failure-related risks with factors of inadequate HIV transmission education, poor awareness and risk perception, and insufficient patient/provider communication.[18] One study found that older people had questions and were willing to discuss these issues with their health care providers, but no one asked them and they were uncomfortable broaching the subject.[19] Studies related to interest in HIV education for older adults found that older adults would prefer HIV education at senior centers and from their physicians and other health care providers.[15,16] A prospective clinical trial comparing the impact of clinician-driven health education regarding HIV during medical appointments versus standard of care control group demonstrated a significant decrease in unprotected sex among the intervention group for those older than 18 years of age.[20] Thus, despite the paucity of available HIV prevention programs, health care providers can provide much needed awareness and education to their older adult patients. Older adults need to know that they are at risk for sexually transmitted diseases (including HIV) and strategies to prevent the disease.

In the 1997 Skiest and Keiser survey study, 333 primary care physicians in a large metropolitan U.S. city were more likely to rarely or never ask their older than 50 years patients about HIV risk factors or discuss risk reduction strategies with them.[21] As early as 1998, data suggested persons older than 50 years of age were not receiving prompt testing for HIV infection following the onset of HIV-related illnesses. Physicians were less likely to consider HIV infection among this population, resulting in missed opportunities for preventing disease progression, opportunistic infections, death, and secondary HIV to uninfected individuals.[3] Frank and open conversations regarding sexuality and sexual practices and drug use among the elderly are essential to encouraging prevention and HIV screening.

HIV presents in all age groups during acute infection, 1–2 weeks after exposure, mimicking flu-like syndromes with fever, muscle aches, myalgias, arthralgias, anorexia, nausea, vomiting, diarrhea, and weight loss. Rashes and posterior cervical adenopathy may be present. In the elderly, symptoms of chronic HIV infection or AIDS may be hard to distinguish from common comorbid conditions including constitutional signs of fatigue, weight loss, and anorexia. HIV infection should be included in the differential diagnosis of neurological presentations of neuropathy, atherosclerotic dementia, Alzheimer's, and Parkinson's disease. AIDS dementia presents with early behavioral changes, possibly focal neurological signs (i.e., weakness in the extremities), and, rarely, with aphasia. Cerebrospinal fluid studies are positive for elevated proteins and monocytic pleocytosis compared with Alzheimer's patients who lack behavioral changes and focal neurological signs early in the disease; are aphasic, and have normal cerebrospinal fluid. As AIDS dementia progresses, seizures, neuromuscular tremors, peripheral neuropathy, and ataxia may occur. Alternate presentations include pneumonia, varicella zoster virus, tuberculosis, pneumocystis, candidias, cytomegalovirus, anemia, thrombocytopenia, non-Hodgkin lymphoma, psoriasis, and seborrheic dermatitis.[22–27] Szerlip et al.[28] proposed an albumin/globulin ratio of less than 1.0 combined with a history of alcohol abuse or sexually transmitted disease should prompt HIV screening for patients older than 55. Current screening recommendations by the CDC advocate routine voluntary HIV screening as a normal part of medical practice, similar to screening for other treatable conditions.[29] Pneumocystis presents with progressive dyspnea, fever, cough, and bilateral chest x-ray infiltrates in all ages. Unfortunately, too often this late-stage finding is the triggering event for HIV testing in the elderly despite physician contact for other comorbid conditions.[30]

As of this writing, there are no treatment guidelines for the elderly.[31] Because older patients are usually excluded from clinical trials, controlled data are lacking in this group. Older adults appear to have worse immune suppression at diagnosis, more opportunistic infections, and shorter AIDS-free intervals than their younger counterparts.[4] Yung and Mo[32] reported that aging creates increased gene expression of CCR 1–5 (chemokine receptors). CCR4 and CCR5 are the required coreceptors of HIV-1 and HIV-2 isolates entry into T–cells and monocytes. Chemokine receptor expression level closely relates to HIV viral load (the number of copies of HIV viral particles per milliliter of blood) and disease progression. Involution of the thymus at approximately the age of 50 years has been found to inhibit CD4 cell function, possibly blunting CD4 response to antiretroviral therapy. This would explain higher absolute CD4 gains and shorter response time to antiretroviral therapy in younger patients.[8]

Although few HIV drug studies have included older patients, Dailly et al.[33] published evidence of decreased clearance with a standard dose of Nevirapine, a nonnucleoside reverse transcriptase inhibitor used in HIV treatment in elderly patients, suggesting therapeutic drug monitoring might be advantageous in preventing drug toxicity in this population.[33] Elderly patients with their lower creatinine clearance are at increased risk of renal disease with certain antiretroviral drugs such as Tenovir, a nucleoside reverse transcriptase inhibitor, and Indinavir, a protease inhibitor. Additionally, comorbid illness in the elderly increases the risk of polypharmacy and pharmacological interaction between antiretroviral drugs and drugs used for the treatment of heart disease, hyperlipidemia, psychiatric illness, erectile dysfunction, and so forth.[34,35] Currently, there are no Beers criteria assisting practitioners with HIV medications.[36] HAART has long been associated with increased levels of serum lipids, impaired glucose metabolism, and increased cardiovascular events. Orlando et al.[34] reported more cardiovascular, endocrine-metabolic and neurological disorders in older patients on HAART than their younger cohorts.

Older HIV patients appear to be at increased risk of cognitive impairment compared with younger patients. Elderly patients with detectable viral loads appear to be twice as likely to have impairment as similarly aged patients with nondetectable virus hindering the patient adherence to treatment regimens.[37] In addition to antiretroviral therapies, recommendations are to treat anemia, vitamin B12 deficiency, and testosterone deficiencies that may occur while providing good nutrition, exercise, and mental/social stimulation.

In summary, medical providers should universally screen adolescents, adults, and pregnant women for HIV. The symptom of infected elderly patients, defined by age older than 50 years, may mimic common comorbidities of aging. Although responsive to therapy, these patients need closer surveillance than their youthful counterparts for liver, renal, metabolic, endocrine, and hematological abnormalities while on HAART. It is important to remember the appearance of the aforementioned abnormalities may have a higher incidence in the HIV elderly than their noninfective cohorts because of the disease itself. Finally, provider recognition of HIV infected seniors' decreased socialization and increased isolation, and stigma of the disease can affect their clinical outcomes.

REFERENCES

1. Bartlett J, Gallant JE. *2005–2006 Medical Management of HIV Infection.* Baltimore: Johns Hopkins Medicine Health Publishing Business Group; 2005:18–19.
2. Department of Health and Human Services. HRSA Information Center. *Guide to the Clinical Care of Women with HIV.* Washington, DC: U.S. Government Printing Office; 2005:19–20.
3. Centers for Disease Control and Prevention. *MMWR.* 1998; 47(2):21–27. AIDS among persons aged greater than or equal to 50 years – United States, 1991–1996.
4. Centers for Disease Control and Prevention. HIV/AIDS Surveillance – General Epidemiology through 2006. Available at: http://www.cdc.gov/hiv/topics/surveillance/resources/slides/general/. Accessed June 2, 2008.
5. Gebo KA, Moore RD. Treatment of HIV infection in the older patient. *Expert Rev Anti Infect Ther.* 2004;2:733–743.
6. Centers for Disease Control and Prevention. HIV-related knowledge and stigma: United States, 2000. *MMWR.* 2000;49:1062–1064.
7. Rose MA, Kennedy M, Watson MR. HIV prevention for older adults. *Florida J Public Health.* 1998;10:5–9.
8. Kataoka-Yahiro M, Ceria C, Caulfield R. Grandparent caregiving role in ethnically diverse families. *J Pediatr Nurs.* 2004;19:315–328.
9. Minkler M, Fuller-Thomson E. African American grandparents raising grandchildren: a national study using census 2000 American community survey. *J Gerontol Psychol Sci Soc Sci.* 2005;60:S82–S92.
10. Wilson MMG. Sexually transmitted disease. *Clin Geriatr Med.* 2003;19:637–655.
11. Dunn ME, Cutler N. Sexual issues in older adults. *AIDS Patient Care STDs.* 2000;14:67–69.
12. Rose MA. Knowledge of HIV/AIDS, perception of risk and behaviors among older adults. *Hol Nurs Pract.* 1995;10:10–17.
13. Stall R, Catania J. AIDS risk behaviors among late middle-aged and elderly Americans. *Arch Intern Med.* 1998;154:19–20.
14. Orel NA, Wright JM, Wagner J. Scarcity of HIV/AIDS risk-reduction materials targeting the needs of older adults among state departments of public health. *Gerontologist.* 2004;44:693–696.
15. Altschuler J, Katz AD, Tynan M. Developing and implementing an HIV/AIDS education curriculum for older adults. *Gerontologist.* 2004;44:121–126.
16. Rose MA. Planning HIV education programs: cultural implications. *J Gerontolog Nurs.* 2004;30:34–39.
17. Goodroad BK. HIV and AIDS in people older than 50: a continuing concern. *J Gerontolog Nurs.* 2003;29:18–24.
18. Savasta AM. HIV: associated transmission risks in older adults: an integrative review of the literature. *J Assoc Nurse AIDS Care.* 2004;15:50–59.
19. Linsk NL. HIV among older adults: age-specific issues in prevention and treatment. *AIDS Reader.* 2000;10:430–440.
20. Fisher JD, Fisher WA, Cornman DH, Amico R, Bryan S, Friedland GH. Clinician delivered intervention during routine clinical care reduces unprotected sexual behavior among HIV infected patients. *J Acquir Immune Defic Syndr.* 2006;41:44–52.
21. Skiest DJ, Keiser P. Human immunodeficiency virus infection in patients older than 50 years: a survey of primary care physicians' beliefs, practices, and knowledge. *Arch Fam Med.* 1997;6:289–294.
22. Zelenetz PD, Epstein ME. HIV in the elderly. *AIDS Patient Care and STDs.* 1998;12:255–262.
23. Manfredi R. HIV disease and advanced age: an increasing therapeutic challenge. *Drugs Aging.* 2002;19:647–669.
24. Wooten-Bielski K. HIV and AIDS in older adults. *Geriatr Nurs.* 1999;20:268–272.
25. El-Sadr W, Gettler J. Unrecognized human immunodeficiency virus infection in the elderly. *Arch Intern Med.* 1995;155:184–186.
26. Inelman EM, Gasparini G, Enzi G. HIV/AIDS in older adults: a case report and literature review. *Geriatrics.* 2005;60:26–30.

27. Shavit L, Grenader T. Delayed diagnosis of HIV-associated thrombocytopenia in a man of 70. *J R Soc Med.* 2005;98: 515.

28. Szerlip MA, DeSalvo KB, Szerlip HM. Predictors of HIV infection in older adults. *J Aging Health.* 2005;17:293–304.

29. Centers for Disease Control and Prevention. Revised recommendation for HIV testing of adults, adolescents, and pregnant women in health-care settings. *MMWR.* 2006;55(RR14):1–17.

30. Jedlovsky MD, Fleischman JK. Carinii pneumonia as the first presentation in patients older than fifty. *AIDS Patient Care and STDs.* 2000;14:247–249.

31. DHHS Panel on Antiretroviral Guidelines for Adults and Adolescents Guidelines for the Use of Antiretroviral Agents in HIV-1 Infected Adults and Adolescents. Oct. 10, 2006.

32. Yung RL, Mo R. Aging is associated with increased human T Cell CC chemokine receptor gene expression. *J Interferon Cytokine Res.* 2003;23:575–582.

33. Dailly E, Billaud E, Reliquet V, et al. No relationship between high nevirapine plasma concentration and hepatotoxicity in HIV-1 infected patients naïve of antiretroviral treatment or switched from protease inhibitors. *Eur J Clin Pharmacol.* 2004;60:343–348.

34. Orlando G, Meraviglia P, Cordier L, et al. Antiretroviral treatment and age-related co-morbidities in a cohort of older HIV infected patients. *HIV Med.* 2006;7:549–557.

35. Manfredi R. HIV infection and advanced age: emerging epidemiological, clinical, and management issues. *Ageing Res Rev.* 2004;3:31–54.

36. Fick DM, Cooper JW, Wade WE, Waller JL, Maclean JR, Beers MH. Updating the Beers criteria for potentially inappropriate medication use in older adults: results of a US consensus panel of experts. *Arch Intern Med.* 2003;164:2716–2724.

37. Vance DE, Burrage JW. Promoting successful cognitive aging in adults with HIV: strategies for intervention. *J Gerontolog Nurs.* 2006;32:34–41.

24

Principles of Fluid and Electrolyte Balance and Renal Disorders in the Older Patient

Matthew Russell, MD, MSc, Rebecca A. Silliman, MD, PhD, MPH, James Burke, MD

THE AGING KIDNEY

An age-associated decrease in renal mass is common, although most studies done to explore this issue did not exclude individuals with comorbid conditions. Population selection and design type have limited the assessment of renal changes in the elderly, as many have used hospitalized or otherwise institutionalized elders in a cross-sectional design.[1] Interestingly, in elderly patients who suffered traumatic death and in whom renal disease and/or important comorbid conditions were excluded, there was no significant decrease in renal mass.[2,3] In patients with decreased renal mass, the number of functioning glomeruli decreases with a greater proportion lost in the cortex and relative sparing of medullary glomeruli.[4] Although the number of glomeruli decline, the remaining glomeruli increase in size.[5] Consequently, any injury to remaining nephrons is more consequential. There is an increase in glomerular hyalinization or sclerosis in apparently healthy elderly individuals.[6] Once again, the change in the number of glomeruli varies greatly in elders, although the presence of glomerulosclerosis is indicative of subclinical renal injury from comorbid conditions affecting renal structure.[1]

RENOVASCULAR CHANGES

There is a decrease in glomerular filtration rate (GFR) in elderly patients, although this may occur to a lesser extent in the aging of healthy individuals.[7,8] Nevertheless, an age-related decline in GFR is an independent predictor of adverse outcomes such as death and cardiovascular disease.[9-11] Blood flow decreases more than the GFR, leading to an increased filtration fraction and subsequent increase risk of nephron damage.[12] There are several factors responsible for this change, including renal vasoconstriction, thickening of the glomerular base-

ment membrane, expansion of the glomerular mesangium and extracellular matrix leading to glomerulosclerosis.[13] Additional factors include glomerular ischemia, tubulointerstitial injury, arteriolar hyalinization, and atherosclerosis, which can lead to loss of functioning nephrons.[14] Although these age-related changes may not have a readily demonstrable impact in the absence of underlying diseases, the absence of renal reserve renders the kidney susceptible in the setting of acute insults.[13]

ASSESSING GFR IN ELDERLY PATIENTS

The GFR is the sum of the filtration rates in all of the functioning nephrons. Thus, it gives a rough measure of the number of functioning nephrons. It is used clinically to address the degree of renal impairment and to follow the course of the disease. Additionally, estimation of renal function is key for dosing medications that are cleared by renal excretory pathways. There are several methods to assess GFR,[15] all of which have significant limitations. These include direct measurement via markers, calculation of creatinine clearance by 24-hour urine collection, and estimation equations.

There are direct measures such as inulin or iothalamate clearance but these tests are not readily available to the clinician. Next, there is the creatinine clearance method from 24-hour urine collection. This test estimates GFR by measuring plasma and urine creatinine, and urine volume. This test tends to overestimate the GFR in that it does not take into account the contribution of creatinine secreted by the proximal tubules. In addition, it is a test that relies on urinary collection and either under- or overcollection can lead to an over- or underestimation of preserved renal function, respectively.

There are several estimation equations that are commonly used to determine GFR. The most common are the

Cockcroft–Gault[16] (CG) and Modification of Diet in Renal Disease (MDRD[17]) equations. These equations can be accessed on the Internet at www.kidney.org/professionals/kdoqi/gfr_calculator.cfm.

The CG equation has been criticized in measuring GFR in elders. Goldberg and Finkelstein demonstrated only a moderate correlation (r = 0.74) between creatinine clearance and that calculated using the CG estimation equation in a subset of hospitalized elderly patients.[18] In general, the CG equation has been demonstrated to show lower estimates of GFR at older ages, especially in community-dwelling elders.[19] Newer estimation equations such as the MDRD and the abbreviated MDRD have been found to be accurate in African-Americans and those with diabetic renal disease.[20] Both the MDRD and CG have additional limitations in individuals with variations in dietary intake, malnutrition, extreme obesity or loss of limb (amputees), and renal transplant.[21]

The importance of calculating creatinine clearance in elders cannot be overstated because a change in plasma creatinine that falls within a laboratory range of normal may, in fact, represent a much larger insult. For example, a creatinine of 1.2 mg/dL in a muscular young adult may represent normal renal function, but in an elder with less muscle mass, a change from a serum creatinine of 0.6 mg/dL to 1.2 mg/dL represents loss of over half of all functioning nephrons.

CHANGES IN FLUID AND ELECTROLYTE

Under normal circumstances, age has no effect on basal plasma sodium or potassium levels or the ability to maintain fluid homeostasis.[1] Some studies, however, have found that there is a significant increase in the steady-state blood hydrogen ion and reduction in steady-state plasma bicarbonate.[22] Nevertheless, derangements of fluid and electrolyte balance often accompany acute medical illnesses, suggesting once again a more limited renal reserve.

SODIUM AND WATER HOMEOSTASIS

Because "dehydration" and volume depletion are often used incorrectly interchangeably, and because both problems are common in elderly patients, a clear definition of terms and understanding of sodium and water balance is needed to direct therapy correctly.

Dehydration can be functionally defined as a loss of solute-free water. Consequently, there exists with dehydration, a hyperosmolar state that triggers a series of humoral responses to stimulate increased free water intake and absorption. Common examples of dehydrated states include osmotic diarrheas, and diabetes insipidus. In elders, dehydration is most commonly from an inability to access free water.

Volume depletion, on the other hand, reflects loss of extracellular fluid that is both solute and water. This can be seen in overdiuresis or gastrointestinal losses. The body's response to a volume load or deficit is much more sluggish than the response to a change in plasma tonicity.

Sodium is the main determinant of extracellular fluid volume. Sodium balance is effected by exogenous sodium intake, changes in renin and aldosterone levels, hemodynamics, and minimally by changes in GFR. There appears to be a blunted response to several hormones in the aged kidney. The secretion rate and concentration of aldosterone decline with age.[23] This is partially attributable to a decrease in renin, the secretion of which also decreases by decade both in terms of basal and stimulated plasma levels.[24] Recall that renin activates the angiotensin pathway, which leads to an increase in aldosterone levels. Decrease in aldosterone can lead to urinary sodium wasting and hyperkalemia in elderly patients with renal insufficiency.[25]

Atrial natriuretic peptide is released in response to volume overload. It exerts powerful natriuretic, diuretic, and vascular smooth muscle relaxing effects.[26] It is a natural antagonist to the renin-angiotensin system.[27,28] With aging, the level of atrial natriuretic peptide increases[29] but does not appear to contribute substantially to the alterations in renal mechanisms of sodium homeostasis.[1]

Sodium homeostasis operates with a slower rate of endocrine response in the aged. There is slower renin-aldosterone responsiveness to acute stimuli with advancing age.[24,30] In several experimental models, elderly patients demonstrated significant deficits in response to sodium loads and deprivation. In a study of potential kidney donors, all free of cardiovascular or renal disease, individuals were subjected to dietary sodium and potassium restriction. Patients younger than the age of 25 years were able to decrease urinary sodium excretion more rapidly than those older than 60.[31] Sodium losses have been demonstrated to have a more profound impact on the blood pressure of elders compared to younger individuals. In elderly patients who underwent a 2-kg diuresis, there was a 24-mm Hg decrease in orthostatic systolic pressure, an effect not seen on younger patients who underwent the same diuresis.[32]

Similarly, the ability to handle a high sodium load may also be impaired in the aging kidney. In patients given a 2-L intravenous normal saline infusion over 3–4 hours, those older than 40 excreted less sodium than those younger than age 40 years over the course of the next day.[33] This has a subsequent impact on blood pressure. Indeed, most studies demonstrated that elders are more likely than younger patients to have elevations in blood pressure as a response to increased sodium intake.[34,35] With increased sodium comes increased weight and potential peripheral edema. This effect can be heightened with the use of nonsteroidal antiinflammatory drugs (NSAIDs) by elderly patients. NSAIDs inhibit the synthesis of prostaglandin E2 leading to sodium retention.[36]

There is widespread atherosclerotic vascular disease in many older individuals. The subsequent stiffening of the vasculature contributes to isolated systolic hypertension, which could potentially be worsened by impaired ability of the kidneys to excrete a sodium load. The stiff vasculature also contributes to wide differential pressures, noted to correlate with mortality.

WATER BALANCE

In general, the diluting and concentrating capabilities of the kidney have been shown to be impaired with aging.[37,38] Water homeostasis is maintained in part by means of antidiuretic hormone (ADH), a hormone manufactured in the hypothalamus and released from the posterior pituitary gland. ADH is released in response to osmotic and/or baroreceptor stimuli and stimulates absorption of water in the collecting tubules. Once again, the body's response to osmotic stimuli is much more rapid than to baroreceptor stimuli. Thus ADH's main function is to absorb free water to restore normal plasma tonicity. The secretion of ADH in response to an increase in plasma osmolality was thought to increase in older patients;[39] however, recent studies fail to confirm this.[40,41] There is a decrease in thirst sensitivity in response to osmotic stimulation, leading to an increased risk of dehydration.[42] The study by Philips et al. found that older male patients drank less water and reported less thirst than younger control individuals in response to a 24-hour fluid deprivation. Add to this the observation that renal responsiveness to ADH has been shown to decrease with aging.[37] Indeed in a cross-sectional study of National Health and Nutrition Examination Survey III data, age was positively associated with mild and overt plasma hypertonicity.[43] With regards to the response to volume depletion, several studies have shown that elders have an increased secretion of ADH compared to younger patients.[44,45]

Conversely, the ability to excrete a water load is reduced in elders.[38] One study demonstrated that after a water load, minimal urine osmolality was higher in patients aged 77–88 years than in healthy patients aged 17–40 years.[46] Peak urine flow was also lower in older patients, but when decreased GFR factored in, there was no difference in urine flow rate among the different age groups. Nevertheless, there did appear to be a persistent diluting defect in the older ages.

HYPONATREMIA

Hyponatremia is defined as a serum sodium concentration of less than 137 mEq/L. Nearly 7% of healthy elderly persons have serum concentrations of 137 mEq/L or less.[47] Hyponatremia is a common problem in elders and increases with age.[48,49] A longitudinal study of elders in a nursing home demonstrated that more than half of the residents had at least one episode of hyponatremia over the course of 1 year.[50] The symptoms of hyponatremia are mainly neurological and include nausea and malaise at milder levels, headache, lethargy, obtundation and eventually seizure, and coma and respiratory depression at more extreme levels.[51] Cerebral edema resulting from severe, rapid-onset hyponatremia can lead to encephalopathy.[52]

Hyponatremia can be associated with low, normal, or high plasma tonicity. Dilutional hyponatremia occurs when water intake exceeds the capacity of the kidney to excrete it and there is a subsequent hypoosmolar state. Hyperosmolar hyponatremia occurs when there is an increase in osmotically active solute that is not electrically charged. This can be seen in hyperglycemic states and mannitol infusions. Isosmolar hyponatremia can occur when isosmotic nonsodium-containing fluids, such as glycine or sorbitol, are used for irrigation during urological or gynecological procedures and subsequently gain access to the extracellular space.[53,54] Another entity associated with normal plasma osmolality is pseudohyponatremia. This is a laboratory anachronism, which is no longer of clinical importance.[55,56]

For the most part in elders, hyponatremia represents a disorder in which water excretion is impaired and, thus, there is a low plasma tonicity.[57] The most common causes of hyposmolar hyponatremia in elders are states of decreased effective plasma circulation and the syndrome of inappropriate antidiuretic hormone (SIADH) secretion. Hypoosmolar hyponatremia resulting from true volume depletion occurs when there is a decrease in total body sodium. In the volume-expanded states, when hyponatremia is present, there is total body sodium excess, but decreased effective circulating volume. When there is decreased effective circulation volume, as in congestive heart failure (CHF) and cirrhosis, the decreased perfusion triggers baroreceptors and subsequent secretion of ADH. In the effective circulating volume contracted states achieved via gastrointestinal or renal losses, a similar pathway ensues with electrolyte-free water retention. Gastrointestinal mechanisms of loss include vomiting and diarrhea, and renal mechanisms of loss include commonly used diuretics and salt-wasting kidney diseases. Thiazide diuretics, particularly in small-framed older women, are a common cause of hyponatremia, and electrolytes should be rechecked within a week after starting this class of diuretics in high-risk patients.

Another major category is SIADH secretion. This is commonly attributed to adverse medication effects, pulmonary disease, and ectopic production of ADH by tumor cells, but it can also be observed in advanced renal failure and with hormonal disorders such as hypothyroidism and cortisol deficiency. When SIADH secretion occurs, the urine is inappropriately concentrated in the setting of hypotonic plasma. The body is also in a euvolemic state as opposed to the volume expanded, but with ineffective circulatory states of CHF and cirrhosis and the volume-depleted states mentioned previously. The most common causes of SIADH secretion include malignancy, medications, pulmonary disease, and neurological disorders.

The evaluation of the elder with low serum sodium focuses on the history and physical examination including a thorough review of medications. Laboratory tests that are relevant include serum and urine osmolality and urine sodium. In addition, a basic metabolic profile and thyroid function testing are also useful. Prior laboratory studies are helpful to establish a baseline and to determine the rapidity of onset. It is important to make a valid estimation of the individual's volume status.

Physical examination findings such as reduced skin turgor and dry oral mucous membranes may suggest volume depletion. Peripheral edema or anasarca may suggest a volume-expanded individual with diminished effective circulating volume. Ancillary findings of orthostasis and laboratory evidence of volume depletion are helpful in this matter as well.

The etiology and rate of correction of hyponatremia are key elements in the management of low sodium concentration. It is often difficult to establish the acuity of the electrolyte imbalance and, if the date of onset is unknown, it is advisable to treat the problem as chronic. Fluid repletion in the volume-contracted patient is managed with normal saline solution. Hyponatremia resulting from SIADH secretion can often be treated with fluid restriction alone, although in some cases adjunctive therapy with agents that induce diabetes insipidus may also be used. Demeclocycline and lithium have been used for patients unable to comply with fluid restriction, although these medications require close monitoring for adverse effects such as diabetes insipidus, liver abnormalities, and renal injury.[58] New ADH antagonists are currently being evaluated and may end up as treatment for acute SIADH secretion.

Rapid rate of correction of sodium levels has been associated with osmotic demyelinization in patients with hyponatremia.[59,60] Correcting the levels too slowly can allow for the progression of cerebral edema. Because this is a difficult problem to navigate, it is perhaps best to correct sodium deficits in asymptomatic individuals at a less than maximal rate, specifically, one less than 0.5 mEq/L/h.[51] The sodium deficit is calculated by subtracting the current level from the goal level in millimoles per/liter and multiplying it by the total body water, which is approximately 0.5 times the lean body weight in kilograms for men and 0.45 times the lean body weight in women. Most experts recommend a correction rate of between 8 and 10 mmol/L per day.[61,62]

HYPERNATREMIA

Hypernatremia is defined as a plasma sodium level of 145 mmol/L or greater. It always represents a hyperosmotic state.[63] Although there are several mechanisms by which this may develop, most commonly in elders, the presence of hypernatremia reflects an inability to maintain adequate fluid intake to keep up with free water losses.[64] Insensible free water losses from skin and respiratory system can increase with acute illness, hyperthermia, or exercise.[65,66] Loss of free water can also occur in the setting of gastrointestinal illness and osmotic diuresis because of hyperglycemia or mannitol.[67–69] Additionally, in elders who already have a decreased thirst response, there may be concurrent problems that have an impact on the ability to have access to or ingest free water. This can especially include neurological processes such as cognitive impairment, and functional deficits from cerebrovascular disease or neuromuscular disorders. In rare cases, hypernatremia can result from ingestion or infusion of hypertonic solutions. Hypernatremia can also be caused by impairments in thirst mechanisms because of

hypothalamic impairment, and inadequate secretion or effect of ADH leading to diabetes insipidus.

Diabetes insipidus is a defect in the secretion or effect of ADH on the free water channels of the distal collecting tubules. It can be thought of as having a central etiology if there is a deficiency state of ADH secretion, or a nephrogenic etiology if there is a resistance to or blockade of the effects of ADH. The net effect is that the kidney excretes an inappropriately dilute urine in the setting of a hyperosmolar state.

In elders, the most common causes of central diabetes insipidus are head trauma, neurosurgery, hypoxic or ischemic encephalopathy, tumors, and idiopathic conditions such as infiltrative disease.[63,70] Nephrogenic diabetes insipidus is defined as an inability to appropriately respond to ADH at the renal tubular level. The common causes for elders include chronic lithium ingestion, hypokalemia, and hypercalcemia.[71] Amphotericin B, ofloxacin, demeclocycline, and foscarnet are additional medications associated with nephrogenic diabetes insipidus and multiple myeloma, amyloidosis, and analgesic nephropathy, and obstructive uropathy are additional causes.[72]

Symptoms of hypernatremia include lethargy, irritability, and weakness in mild to moderate stages and can progress to twitching, seizures, and coma.[73] Severe symptoms tend to occur at levels over 158 mm/L.[74,75] In a retrospective study of elderly patients admitted to an acute care geriatric wards, mortality rates were 33.3% and 71.4%, respectively, in patients with serum sodium levels from 151 to 153 mEq/L and in those with values over 154 mEq/L.[76] Age and sodium level were independent risk factors for mortality. Evaluation of elderly patients presenting with hypernatremia includes taking a complete history eliciting recent intake and elimination patterns.

Correction of the hyperosmolar state involves determining the fluid status of the patient. As was previously stated, the etiology of hypernatremia in elders is most commonly from free water losses that exceed fluid intake. In addition to obtaining serum osmolality, urine osmolality and sodium concentrations should also be measured. A maximally concentrated urine with osmolality above 800 mOsm/kg suggests a problem of inadequate fluid intake, whereas a less concentrated urine less than 200 mOsm/kg may represent a form of diabetes insipidus.[63] Calculation of the free water deficit is essential to determine the amount of fluid that is to be administered:

$$\text{Water deficit} = (\text{plasma sodium} - 140)/140 \times \text{TBW}$$

Total body water (TBW) is estimated by multiplying the body weight in kilograms by 0.5 and 0.45 for elderly men and women, respectively.[77] As with hyponatremia, the rate of correction must be slow to prevent complications of rapid solute shifting. In hypovolemic hypernatremic patients, the general rule is to correct the volume loss first with normal saline. Once volume losses have been corrected, the fluid content used should be more dilute. Again, rates of correction should not exceed a change in sodium concentration of more than 0.5 mmol/L in 1 hour or 12 mmol/L over a 24-hour period. Additionally, it is not recommended to correct more than half of the free water deficit in the first 24 hours. It is also important to take into account the continued insensible losses and ongoing illnesses that may contribute to fluid losses when calculating fluid administration schedules.

POTASSIUM HOMEOSTASIS

Potassium is the main electrolyte of intracellular fluid with approximately 98% of total body potassium stores located within cells.[78] Potassium homeostasis is maintained by both extrarenal and renal mechanisms. Extrarenal mechanisms include shifts between the intra- and extracellular spaces mediated by insulin, sympathetic adrenergic agents, hyperosmolar states, acid base changes, and possibly aldosterone.[79] In the kidney, potassium secretion depends on the electrochemical gradient across the distal tubule, which is affected mainly by sodium and water delivery to the distal nephron as well as acid base perturbations. Potassium is secreted by principal cells located in the distal convoluted tubule and collecting ducts in response to hyperkalemia, acid base considerations, and aldosterone.[80] The healthy renal tubular mechanism can typically adapt to wide variations in daily amounts of dietary intake of potassium.

HYPERKALEMIA

Decreased delivery to the distal tubule is a frequent cause of hyperkalemia. Thus, a volume-depleted state and renal failure via any number of mechanisms may be associated with hyperkalemia. As was mentioned previously, there is also a decrease in aldosterone secretion with aging, which also predisposes the elderly kidney to hyperkalemia. In patients with hyporenin and hypoaldosterone states, hyperkalemia can develop. This is commonly seen in patients with diabetic nephropathy.[81] Several commonly prescribed medications may lead to hyperkalemia. Potassium supplements, in the setting of impaired potassium secretion capability, have been associated with hyperkalemia.[82] Angiotensin-converting enzyme (ACE) inhibitors act to prevent the conversion of angiotensin I to angiotensin II, thus decreasing the secretion of aldosterone, leading to the potential for decreased excretion of potassium. This is also seen with angiotensin receptor blockers (ARBs), but to a lesser extent.[83] Patients on potassium-sparing diuretics such as spironolactone, an aldosterone antagonist, may also develop elevated serum potassium concentrations. NSAIDs have been associated with hyperkalemia via the inhibition of prostaglandin synthesis and resultant decreased renal renin secretion.[84] Additional agents associated with hyperkalemia include trimethoprim-sulfamethoxazole, heparin,[85] or low molecular weight heparin, β-adrenergic blocking drugs, and severe digoxin toxicity.

The main complication and risk of mortality in hyperkalemia is cardiac arrhythmia.[86] Symptoms are typically nonspecific and include muscle weakness and paralysis.[87] Gener-

ally speaking, concerning symptoms do not become evident until the serum concentration exceeds 7.0 mEq/L.[88] The detection and treatment of hyperkalemia is focused around stabilizing cell membranes, increasing potassium excretion, shifting potassium from the extracellular space to the intracellular space, and eliminating or preventing underlying causes of hyperkalemia. With critically high levels of potassium, or in clinically symptomatic situations, stabilization of the cardiac cell membrane is key. Infusions of calcium will antagonize the effects of hyperkalemia.[89] Calcium, either as gluconate or chloride, is the first treatment of choice in the emergency setting and has a rapid onset of action.[85] Insulin and β-2 agonists, as well as sodium bicarbonate infusions, aid in shifting potassium into the intracellular space. Volume expansion is also essential and when sufficiently volume replete, intravenous furosemide can be given to aid kaliuresis. Eliminating any of the aforementioned medications that lead to hyperkalemia is essential to reduce recurrence of this electrolyte abnormality. In situations of mild or chronic hyperkalemia, patients may be given a potassium binding resin such as sodium polystyrene sulfonate at set intervals. This resin should be used with caution in elders, given the risk of colonic gangrene related to sorbitol, when repeated doses are used in the setting of reduced bowel perfusion.

HYPOKALEMIA

Hypokalemia can result for many reasons. Increased excretion can be affected by both renal and extrarenal mechanisms. Loss via the gastrointestinal tract because of vomiting, diarrhea, or iatrogenic drainage are potential causes. Renal losses can result from a state of increased aldosterone secretion, metabolic or respiratory alkaloses, renal tubular acidosis (RTA), and various medications. Hypomagnesemia has also been associated with hypokalemia and more difficult potassium deficit repair.[90]

The potassium wasting of type 1 or distal RTA occurs because distal acidification is impaired. Type 2 or proximal RTA can also result in loss of potassium. In this disorder, bicarbonate is not absorbed proximally, and if alkali therapy is given to correct for loss of bicarbonate, it can result in increased sodium delivery and accompanying nonreabsorbable anion to the distal tubule resulting in increased kaliuresis.[91]

In elders who are often medicated for fluid overloaded states, diuretics are common causes of hypokalemia. This is particularly true of thiazide diuretics.[92] Additional medications that can cause hypokalemia include amphotericin B, β-adrenergic agonists, and rarely, chemotherapeutic agents.[93]

RENAL FAILURE

Acute

Acute renal failure (ARF) occurs when the kidney is not able to maintain typical homeostatic processes. In elders, the incidence of ARF is greater than in the general population.[94] Typically, renal failure can be divided into prerenal, renal, and postrenal etiologies. Volume depletion is the most common cause of ARF in elders.[95]

Impairment of blood flow delivery to the kidney can lead to ARF. Decreased effective circulation via intravascular volume depletion, or decreased cardiac output is the common pathway to renal failure. Profound medical illnesses such as sepsis, myocardial infarction, cirrhosis, and pancreatitis are common disease states associated with ARF. Alterations in intrarenal hemodynamics with the use of agents that act on renal arterioles and subsequently reduce effective renal plasma flow can also contribute to prerenal ARF. These agents include ACE inhibitors and NSAIDs. Vascular processes such as bilateral renal artery stenosis are less common causes of renal failure. The patient with ARF resulting from prerenal causes is oliguric. Diagnosis is typically made by analysis of urinary sediment, measurement of serum electrolytes and creatinine, as well as urinary osmolality, creatinine, and sodium. Many sources also recommend calculation of the fractional excretion of sodium, although this may not be helpful because concurrent use of diuretics makes this an unreliable parameter. A urine osmolality greater than 500 mOsm/kg and a fractional excretion of sodium of less than 1 suggests a prerenal state.[96] Again, concurrent use of diuretics will confound this analysis. Treatment is centered on restoring effective renal plasma flow by correcting any ongoing fluid losses and withholding any offending medications.

TUBULOINTERSTITIAL DISEASES

Acute tubular necrosis (ATN) and interstitial nephritis are occasional consequences of drug toxicity and frequent causes of ARF. Acute interstitial nephritis (AIN) is a hypersensitivity response in the kidney and is characterized by ARF, sterile pyuria, eosinophilia,[97] and a urinary sediment with white blood cells and renal epithelial cells, and casts containing those elements. ATN is a major cause of ARF resulting from damage to the tubular epithelium. This can be achieved via states of transient renal hypoperfusion or by direct toxicity of an agent to the tubular epithelium. Most cases of tubulointerstitial disease present with elements of both AIN and ATN, and, in fact, there is a continuum of presentation depending on the nature of the renal insult.

ATN can result from episodes of renal hypoperfusion, which can occur in the settings of sepsis, ischemia, hypotension, and CHF. Direct tubular damage by toxic insult can also result in sloughing of renal tubular epithelial cells and resultant ATN. Agents that are associated with risk of ATN include antibiotics such as aminoglycosides and amphotericin B and cisplatin and radiocontrast media. Elders undergoing angiography or imaging with intravenous radiocontrast agents are at risk for developing ARF via ATN. Cast nephropathy from light chain proteins seen in multiple myeloma can lead to ARF via direct tubular toxicity and tubular obstruction.

In ATN, the urinalysis typically reveals a urinary sediment notable for muddy brown casts or epithelial cells that represent sloughing of the tubular epithelium. Urine electrolyte analysis in the absence of concurrent diuretic use demonstrates an elevated sodium concentration reflecting impaired absorptive capacity of the damaged tubular epithelium.[98] In one study, mortality from ATN in hospitalized and ICU patients was 38% and 79%, respectively.[99] A small percentage of patients do not recover from ATN and thus, approximately 5%–10% of patients will proceed to long-term dialysis.[100] This percentage is higher in ICU patients. Treatment and reduction in mortality centers around rapid recognition and reversal of ATN and supply of hemodynamic and nutritional support as well as timely initiation of hemodialysis.[98] For the older patient with other conditions that lead to ICU levels of care, the concurrent development of ATN suggests a very poor prognosis.

AIN can be induced in response to medications, infections, and has also been demonstrated in cases of patients with autoimmune and neoplastic processes. AIN has been demonstrated in the setting of acute bacterial pyelonephritis, renal tuberculosis, and fungal nephritis.[101] Common medications associated with AIN include β-lactam and other antibiotics (ciprofloxacin, macrolides, vancomycin), NSAIDs, diuretics (furosemide, thiazides), antivirals, antihypertensive agents (amlodipine, captopril, diltiazem), and antiepileptics (phenytoin, carbamazepine).[101] Drug-induced AIN from medication is typically a hypersensitivity-type reaction and, if present, typically appears within several days of starting the medication, although prior exposure can accelerate onset.[102] Although renal biopsy is the gold standard to demonstrate AIN, the diagnosis is typically made based on history of recent addition of medication combined with results from urinalysis (as stated previously), serum chemistry (demonstrating renal insufficiency), and complete blood count with differential (demonstrating eosinophilia). Renal failure resolves within several weeks of withdrawing the offending agent. Although no solid evidence supports the routine use of corticosteroids, many practitioners use them with the hope of accelerating healing.

POSTOBSTRUCTIVE UROPATHY

Partial obstruction of the postrenal urinary system can lead to hydronephrosis and renal failure. Typically, in older patients the causes of obstructive uropathy include prostatic hypertrophy or carcinoma, pelvic or retroperitoneal neoplasms, and calculi.[103] Treatment centers on eliminating or reducing the degree of obstruction.

Glomerular Disease

There are a myriad of mechanisms that induce glomerular damage. There may be autoimmune processes that can cause deposition disease or damage to the basement membrane, mesangial matrix, glomerular vasculature, podocytes, or other components. Glomerular disease can also occur in the setting of systemic diseases such as diabetes, vasculitis, amyloidosis, human immunodeficiency virus, and hepatitis C. Glomerular disease can be a cause of acute or chronic renal failure and is classically divided into two general patterns: nephritic and nephrotic. Many patient presentations do not fall within this strict categorization and have combined elements. Classically, hematuria and a highly active urine sediment notable for red cells and red blood cell casts characterize the nephritic syndrome. With nephritic syndrome, there is an associated drop in GFR because of the inflammation of the glomerular apparatus and subsequent decreased surface area available for filtration. The nephrotic syndrome is defined as proteinuria of greater than 3.5 g/day, edema, and hyperlipidemia. Urine sediment often demonstrates oval fat bodies and fatty casts. Diabetic nephropathy is the most common glomerular disease seen in elders. In comparison to younger age groups, diabetes, amyloidosis, vasculitis, and membranous nephropathy were more common.[104] The most common type of glomerular disease in elderly patients in a study of 334 patients aged 65 years and older who underwent renal biopsy for renal failure demonstrated that the most common causes of proteinuria were membranous glomerulopathy (34.3%), minimal change disease (14.6%), focal segmental sclerosis (11.7%), and amyloidosis (8.8%).[105]

RENOVASCULAR DISEASE

Stenosis of one main renal artery or one of its major branches can lead to renal ischemia, renal failure, and hypertension. With bilateral disease, renal failure can occur. Although impaired blood flow can result from multiple processes including arteritis and renal artery dissection, the majority of renal arterial lesions in elders are attributable to atherosclerosis.[106] Atherosclerotic disease is the predominant lesion detected in patients older than 50 years and in population-based studies; hemodynamically significant stenosis (>60% lumen occlusion) is common (6.8% of individuals >65 years).[107] In one study, renovascular disease was responsible for 3% of all recognized secondary hypertension, and in older patients who had evidence of generalized atherosclerosis, 10% of secondary hypertension was attributable to renovascular disease.[108]

Although a stenotic lesion may be present, this does not necessarily translate into a clinically significant progression to end-stage renal disease. To significantly affect renal function on a vascular basis alone, the entire renal mass must be affected or another parenchymal disease must be present in the contralateral kidney when there is unilateral renovascular disease.[106] Patients with atherosclerotic renovascular disease are more likely to be at accelerated risk for stroke, CHF, and myocardial infarction.

Clinically significant atherosclerotic renovascular disease (ARVD) may present in the elder with a history of chronic hypertension that suddenly becomes difficult to manage or for whom there has been a sentinel event such as cerebrovascular accident. Similarly, ARVD should be considered when renal function declines with the initiation of an ACE inhibitor or any new blood pressure agent, because lowering systemic blood pressure may lead to an increased risk of underperfusion of the poststenotic kidney and subsequent reduction of GFR. The responses to underperfusion of the renal parenchyma include upregulation of the renin–angiotensin system, adrenergic stimuli, oxidative stress pathways, and vasoconstrictor prostaglandins. These responses have been associated with significant clinical consequences including sodium and fluid retention and flash pulmonary edema.[106]

Evaluation and treatment of renovascular disease in elders is controversial and most sources suggest an individualized process. In terms of diagnostic workup, there has been no evidence to support widespread screening for early detection of renal artery stenosis (RAS).[109] Rather, patients with presentations suggestive of RAS, including refractory hypertension, progressive renal failure, and pulmonary edema are more likely to benefit from screening. Screening is most useful to determine who will benefit from revascularization procedures. Patients with renal impairment and kidneys less than 8 cm long are unlikely to benefit from revascularization procedures.[110] Ultrasound is useful to rule out obstruction, and identify the patient with chronic kidney disease (CKD) for whom recovery is unlikely. Computed tomography angiography and magnetic resonance angiography are the accepted standard tests for imaging renal arteries. Treatment via balloon angioplasty revascularization may modestly improve blood pressure control and decreases the number of antihypertensive medications required.[111,112] Patients with recurrent CHF or flash pulmonary edema with severe RAS may have considerable improvement after renal angioplasty and stenting.[113] Outcomes for patients with RAS and concurrent chronic renal impairment do not support revascularization, although the data are not completely clear in this matter.[114]

CHRONIC KIDNEY DISEASE

The prevalence of chronic renal failure in patients older than the age of 65 years is increasing. The National Health and Nutrition Examination Survey III study data found that approximately 25% of all Americans aged 70 years or older had moderately or severely decreased kidney function.[115] Hypertensive disease and diabetes are the main causes for CKD. The number of dialysis patients older than 65 years has more than doubled within 10 years in the United States.[116] CKD is 100 times more prevalent than end-stage renal failure and the incidence is increasing more rapidly.[117] Often times, renal insufficiency is not detected even when patients have access to primary care.[118] In light of these statistics, timely primary care screening for CKD and any effective interventions are key in reducing the progression to end-stage renal failure and renal replacement therapy.

CKD is defined as either kidney damage (e.g., proteinuria) or decreased kidney function, manifested by decreased GFR, for 3 months or more.[11] Patients with risk factors for

CKD should be screened. Risk factors include patients with a family history of kidney disease, patients with diabetes, hypertension, recurrent urinary tract infections or obstruction, and patients with systemic diseases that are known to affect the kidneys.[117] Additionally, a recent study has demonstrated that it is cost effective to screen patients older than the age of 60 years, even when other kidney disease risk factors are absent.[119] Screening markers for kidney damage include persistent proteinuria, an albumin/creatinine ratio greater than 30 mg/g in a random urine "spot" sample, and abnormal urine sediment. GFR is the best measure of overall kidney function and can be determined using an estimation equation (see previously).[120] Patients with risk factors suggestive of obstructive uropathy should undergo imaging of the urinary tract with ultrasonography. Ultrasonography can also help to establish the cause of the renal disease as well as the prognosis. Small, atrophic kidneys seen on ultrasound may herald a worse prognosis and asymmetrical kidney size may suggest renovascular disease.[117]

Once CKD has been identified, the stage of the disease must be determined. The National Kidney Foundation Kidney Disease Outcomes Quality Initiative Classification, Prevalence, and Action Plan for stages of CKD has staged this disease process based on GFR and, at each stage, makes recommendation for action. Patients who possess risk factors and have a GFR of 60 mL/min per 1.73 m^2 or greater are to be screened and should undergo assessment for CKD risk reduction. Patients with kidney damage but normal GFR should undergo diagnosis and treatment of comorbid conditions and cardiovascular disease risk reduction. Patients with an unclear etiology of renal disease or patients with a GFR between 60 and 89 mL/min per 1.73 m^2 should be considered for evaluation by a nephrologist to estimate disease progression. Patients with moderately decreased GFR (between 30 and 60 mL/min per 1.73 m^2) are cared for in partnership with subspecialist nephrology and the goal is to treat the complications and comorbidities that contribute to disease progression and to prepare the patient for eventual renal replacement therapy.[11]

There are several areas of concern for nephrologists and anyone caring for people with CKD. These are blood pressure control,[121] glycemic control in diabetics, calcium and phosphorus metabolism, reduction of proteinuria with an ACE inhibitor or ARB,[122–124] and acidosis. Decreasing or eliminating microalbuminuria may slow the progression to overt nephropathy in patients with type II diabetes.[125] Additional interventions that show promise for delaying progression of renal disease include dietary protein intake reduction,[126,127] management of lipid disorders,[128] and improvement of anemia related to renal failure by erythropoietin administration.[129]

Blood pressure control is clearly the most important medical issue that preserves kidneys. Although ACE inhibitors and ARBs are important, blood pressure control with any drug is crucial. A blood pressure of 125/75 mm Hg is considered optimal for preserving renal function. Regarding calcium and phosphorus, all patients with CKD should be screened for vitamin D3 production. People with levels below 30 should be treated with 1,000 U of vitamin D3 daily. Sun exposure is limited in many people, accounting for much of the deficiency. In patients with GFRs less than 45, levels of parathormone begin to rise. Because the kidney makes the active form of vitamin D (1,25 [COH]2 D3), it should be supplemented on a daily or thrice weekly basis. Phosphorus levels do not begin to rise until late CKD. Because this also stimulates parathormone levels, the phosphorus needs to be controlled. This can be done by decreasing intake (i.e., no dairy products) and the use of calcium acetate. Because the calcium/phosphorus product should not be allowed to rise over 55, calcium acetate should be limited to two to three tablets per meal. Sevelamer hydrochloride and lanthanum-based binders can also be used. Anemia correction is handled with erythropoietin, which can be given subcutaneously or intravenously for patients undergoing dialysis. Doses vary, but should be limited to treating only anemia of less than 10 g/dL of hemoglobin and should be titrated to a hemoglobin no greater than 12 g/dL. Finally, acidosis should be corrected to a venous bicarbonate of 22–24.

RENAL REPLACEMENT

The number of dialysis patients older than 65 years has more than doubled within 10 years in the United States.[116] With the increasing elderly population comes an increased disease burden of end-stage renal disease in this group in the form of dialysis as well as issues surrounding allocation of renal resources. Historically, transplant centers have been resistant to accept patients older than the age of 65 years for consideration for renal transplantation because of concerns about patient life expectancy overall and the perceived superior survival rates on dialysis versus transplantation.[130] In elders, however, there appears to be a superior life expectancy with renal transplantation over dialysis at 5 years.[131,132] Living donor transplants are definitely preferred, and this is particularly true in elderly patients because they may not be able to wait sufficient time for a cadaver kidney, up to 3–6 years depending on blood type. Also, living kidneys work better than cadaver kidneys and generally last twice as long and with better function. Several studies have suggested that, although graft loss from death is higher in elderly patients, death-censored analysis of graft survival rate in elder allograft recipients is comparable or even superior to younger recipients.[133,134] A study of 8-year death-censored graft survival shows significant decrease in older age groups. Sixty-seven percent of patients aged 18–49 years had a death-censored survival rate of 67%, 40–54 of 62%, and for ages older than 65 years, the survival rate was 51%.[135] A more recent study looking at graft survival rates in elders compared with younger patients showed worse outcomes in patients older than 60 years compared with those between 18 and 59 years. When patients with age-related high-risk factors such as nonskin malignancy, vascular disease, and a current history of smoking were eliminated, the patient and graft survival rates were equivalent between the younger and older allograft recipient groups.[136] This suggests that rather than age as a relative contraindication, screening out patients with high-risk factors associated with risk of poor graft survival is the more prudent course.

In the steroid-sparing age of cyclosporine monotherapy, elderly patients appear to do well after transplantation. This has been attributed to superior medical compliance in the older age groups compared with younger.[137] and a decreased inflammatory and blunted immune response in the elderly[138] Additionally, steroid-free immunosuppressive regimens appear to reduce the posttransplant morbidity and mortality seen in elders in older studies by lowering risk of infection and cardiovascular complications such as hypertension and hyperlipidemia. Finally, the issue of calcineurin inhibitor (CNI) toxicity needs to be raised. CNI is now best used until there is an increase in creatinine. If the biopsy reveals CNI toxicity and the patients is at least 6 months posttransplantation, one can consider stopping CNIs because the critical rejection period is over. Also of note is that elderly patients have an immune system that is less robust, making CNI sparing more relevant.

The decision to proceed with renal transplantation versus renal replacement therapy with dialysis requires a patient-centered approach, which focuses on the impact on lifestyle and the ability to comply with complex medical regimens.

ACKNOWLEDGMENTS

Edward Alexander, MD, Section of Nephrology, Boston University School of Medicine; Elizabeth Abernethy, MD, Section of Nephrology, Boston University School of Medicine.

REFERENCES

1. Epstein M. Aging and the kidney. *J Am Soc Nephrol.* 1996;7:1106–1122.
2. Fliser D. Ren Sanus in corpore sano: the myth of the inexorable decline of renal function with senescence. *Nephrol Dial Transplant.* 2005;20:482–485.
3. Kasiske BL, Umen AJ. The influence of age, sex, race and body habitus on kidney weight in humans. *Arch Pathol Lab Med.* 1986;110:55–60.
4. Tauchi H, Tsuboi K, Okutomi J. Age changes in the human kidney of the different races. *Gerontologia.* 1971;17:87–97.
5. McLachlan MSF. The aging kidney. *Lancet.* 1978;2:143–145.
6. McLahan MSF, Guthrie JC, Anderson CK. Vascular and glomerular changes in the aging kidney. *J Pathol.* 1977;121:65–77.
7. Lindeman RD, Tobin JD, Shock NW. Association between blood pressure and the rate of decline in renal function with age. *Kidney Int.* 1984;26:861–868.
8. Fliser D, Franek E, Joest M, Block S, Mutschler E, Ritz E. Renal function in the elderly: impact of hypertension and cardiac function. *Kidney Int.* 1997;51:1196–1204.
9. Fried LP, Kronmal RA, Newman AB, Bild DE, Mittelmark MB, Polak JF, et al. Risk factors for 5-year mortality in older adults: the Cardiovascular Health Study. *JAMA.* 1998;279:585–592.
10. Manjunath G, Tighiouart H, Coresh J, et al. Level of kidney function as a risk factor for cardiovascular outcomes in the elderly. *Kidney Int.* 2003;63:1121–1129.
11. Levey AS, Coresh J, Balk E, et al. National Kidney Foundation practice guidelines for chronic kidney disease: evaluation, classification, and stratification. *Ann Int Medicine.* 2003;139(2):137–149.
12. Kielstein JT, Bode-Boger SM, Haller H and Fliser D. Functional changes in the ageing kidney: is there a role for asymmetric dimethylarginine. *Nephrol Dial Transplant.* 2003;18(7):1245–1248.
13. Baylis C. Changes in renal hemodynamics and structure in the aging kidney;sexual dimorphism and the nitric oxide system. *Exp Gerontol.* 2005;40,4:271–278.
14. Levi, Rowe JW. Renal function and dysfunction in aging. In: D.W. Seldin and G. Giebisch, Editors, The Kidney: Physiology and Pathophysiology 101, Raven Press, New York (1992), pp. 3433–3456.
15. Stevens L, Perrone RD. Assessment of kidney function: serum creatinine; BUN; and GFR. Up to Date Online version 14.3. accessed November 29, 2006.
16. Cockcroft DW, Gault MH. Prediction of creatinine clearance from serum creatinine. *Nephron.* 1976;16:31–41.
17. Levey AS, Bosch JP, Lewis JB, et al. A more accurate method to estimate glomerular filtration rate from serum creatinine: a new prediction equation. Modification of Diet in Renal Disease Study Group. *Ann Intern Med.* 1999;130:461–470.
18. Goldberg TH, Finkelstein MS. Difficulties in estimating glomerular filtration rate in the elderly. *Arch Intern Med.* 1987;147:1430–1433.
19. Malmorse LC, Gray SL, Peiper CF, et al. Measured versus estimated creatinine clearance in a high-functioning elderly sample: MacArthur Foundation study of successful aging. *J Am Geriatr Soc.* 1993;41:715–721.
20. Lewis J, Agodoa L, Cheek D, et al. Comparison of cross-sectional renal function measurements in African Americans with hypertensive nephrosclerosis and of primary formulas to estimate glomerular filtration rate. *Am J Kidney Dis.* 2001;38:744–753.
21. Gaspari F, Ferrari S, Stucchi N, et al. Performance of different prediction equations for estimating renal function in kidney transplantation. *Am J Transplant.* 2004;4:1826–1835.
22. Frassetto LA. Morris RC Jr. Sebastian A. Effect of age on blood acid-base composition in adult humans: role of age-related renal functional decline. *A J Physiol.* 1996;271(6 Pt 2):F1114–F1122.
23. Flood C, Gherondache C, Pincus G, et al. The metabolism and secretion of aldosterone in elderly subjects. *J Clin Invest.* 1967;l46:960–966.
24. Crane MG, Harris JJ. Effect of aging on renin activity and aldosterone excretion. *J Lab Clin Med.* 1976;87:947–959.
25. Bauer JH. Age-related changes in the renin-aldosterone system. Physiological effects and clinical implications. *Drugs Aging* 1993;3:238–245.
26. Silver MA, Maisel A, Yancy CW, et al. BNP Consensus Panel 2004: a clinical approach for the diagnostic, prognostic, screening, treatment monitoring, and therapeutic roles of natriuretic peptides in cardiovascular diseases. *Congest Heart Fail.* 2004 Sep-Oct;10(5 Suppl 3):1–30.
27. Boomama F, Van der Meiracker AH. Plasma A- and B-type natriuretic peptides. Physiology, methodology, and clinical use. *Cardiovasc Res.* 2001;51:442–459.
28. Johnston CI, Hodsman PG, Kohzuki M, et al. Interaction between atrial natriuretic peptide and the renin angiotensin aldosterone system. Endogenous antagonists. *Am J Med.* 1989 Dec 26;87(6B):24S–28S.
29. Ohashi M, Fujio M, Nawata H. High Plasma concentration of human natriuretic polypeptide in man. *Kidney Int.* 1975;8:325–333.

30. Weidmann P, Demyttenaere-Burzstein S, Maxwell MH, DeLima J. Effect of aging on plasma renin and aldosterone in normal man. *Kidney Int.* 1975;8:325–333.

31. Epstein M, Hollenberg NK. Age as a determinant of renal sodium conservation in normal man. *J Lab Clin Med.* 1976;87:411–417.

32. Shannon RP, Wei JY, Rosa RM, Epstein FH,Rowe JH. The effect of age and sodium depletion on cardiovascular response to orthostasis. *Hypertension* 1986;8:438–443.

33. Luft FC, Grim CE, Fineberg N, Weinberger MC. Effects of volume expansion and contraction in normotensive whites, blacks and subjects of different ages. *Circulation.* 1979;59:644–650.

34. Elliot P, Stamler J, Nichols R, et al. Intersalt revisited: further analysis of 24 hour sodium excretion and blood pressure within and across populations. *BMJ.* 1996;312:1248–1253.

35. Mulkerrin EC, Clark BA, Epstein FH. Increased salt retention and hypertension from non-steroidal agents in the elderly.

36. Sanghi S, MacLaughlin EJ, Jewell CW, et al. Cyclooxygenase-2 inhibitors: a painful lesson. *Cardiovasc Hematol Disord Drug Targets.* 2006 Jun;6(2):85–100.

37. Rowe JW, Shock NW, DeFronzo RA. The influence of age on the renal response to water deprivation in man. *Nephron.* 1976;17:270–278.

38. Shannon RP, Minaker KL, Rowe JW. Aging and water balance in humans. *Semin Nephrol.* 1984;4:346–353.

39. Helderman JH, Vestal RE, Rowe JW, et al. The response of arginine vasopressin to intravenous ethanol and hypertonic saline in man: the impact of aging. *J Gerontol.* 1978;33:39–47.

40. Stachenfeld NS, Mack GW, Takamata A, et al. Thirst and fluid regulatory responses to hypertonicity in older adults. *Am J Physiol.* 1996;271:R757–R765.

41. Duggan J, Kilfeather S, Lightman SL. The association of age with plasma arginine vasopressin and plasma osmolality. *Age Ageing* 1993;22:332–336.

42. Weinberg AD, Minaker KL, et al. Dehydration. Evaluation and management in older adults. *JAMA.* 1995;274:1552–1556.

43. Stookey JD. High prevalence of plasma hypertonicity among community-dwelling older adults: results from NHANES III. *J Am Diet Assoc.* 2005 Aug;105(8):1231–1239.

44. Phillips PA, Rolls BJ, Ledingham JG, et al. Reduced thirst after water deprivation in healthy elderly men. *NEJM.* 1984;311:753–759.

45. Bevilacqua M, Norbiato G, Chebat E, et al. Osmotic and nonosmotic control of vasopressin release in the elderly:Effect of metoclopramide. *J Clin Endocrinol Metab.* 1987;65:1243–1247.

46. Lindeman RD, Lee TD, Yiengst MJ, Shock NW: Influence of age, renal disease, hypertension, diuretics and calcium on the antidiuretic responses to suboptimal infusions of vasopressin. *J Lab Clin Med.* 1966;68:206–223.

47. Caird FI, Andrews GR, Kennedy RD. Effect of posture on blood pressure in the elderly. *Br Heart J* 1973;35:527–530.

48. Lye M. Electrolyte disorders in the elderly. *Clin Endocrinol Metab.* 1984;13:377.

49. Kugler JP, Hustead T. Hyponatremia and Hypernatremia in the elderly. *Am Fam Physician.* 2000 Jun 15;61(12):3623–3630.

50. Miller M, Morley JF, Rubinstein LZ. Hyponatremia in a nursing home population. *J Am Geriatr Soc.* 1995;43:1410–1413.

51. Al-Salman J, Hyponatremia. *West J Med.* 2002;176:173–176.

52. Laureno R, Karp BI. Myelinolysis after correction of hyponatremia. *Ann Intern Med.* 1997;126:57–62.

53. Konarzewski WH. Disorders of sodium balance: hyponatraemia can occur during transurethral resection of prostate. *BMJ.* 2006 Apr 8;332(7545):853–854.

54. Estes CM, Maye JP. Severe intraoperative hyponatremia in a patient scheduled for elective hysteroscopy: a case report. *AANA J.* 2003 Jun;71(3):203–205.

55. Oster JR, Singer I. Hyponatremia, hyposmolality, and hypotonicity:tables and fables. *Arch Inter Med.* 1999;159:333–336.

56. Fried LF, Palevsky PM. Hyponatremia and hypernatremia. *Med Clin North Am* 1997;81:585–609.

57. Rennke HG, Denker BM. Renal Pathophysiology: the essentials. 2nd Edition. Lippincott Williams and Wilkins. 2006, pp. 78–82.

58. Cherrill DA, Stote RM, Birge JR, Singer I. Demeclocycline treatment in the syndrome of inappropriate antidiuretic hormone secretion. *Ann Intern Med.* 1975;83:654–656.

59. Adams RA, Victor M, Mancall EL. Central pontine myelinolysis: a hitherto undescribed disease occurring in alcoholics and malnourished patients. *Arch Neurol Psychiatry.* 1959;81:154–172.

60. Martin RJ. Central pontine and extrapontine myelinolysis: the osmotic demyelination syndromes. *J Neurol Neurosurg Psychiatry.* 2004 Sep;75 Suppl 3:iii22–28.

61. Androgue HJ, Madias NE. Hyponatremia. *NEJM.* 2000 May 25;342(21):1581–1589.

62. Karp BI, Laureno R. Central pontine and extrapontine myelinolysis after correction of hyponatraemia. *The Neurologist* 2000;6:255–266.

63. Fall PJ. Hyponatremia and Hypernatremia: a systematic approach to causes and their correction. *Postgrad Med.* 107(5):75–82.

64. Rose BD, Post, TW. Clinical Physiology of Acid-Base and Electrolyte Disorders, 5th ed, McGraw-Hill, New York, 2001, pp. 749–761.

65. Bossingham MJ, Carnel NS, Campbell WW. Water balance, hydration status, and fat-free mass hydration in younger and older adult. *Am J Clin Nutrition.* 2005;81(6):1342–1350.

66. Stout NR, Kenny RA, Baylis PH. A review of water balance in ageing in health and disease. *Gerontology* 1999;45:61–66.

67. Loeb JN. The hyperosmolar state. *NEJM.* 1974 May 23; 290(21):1184–1187.

68. Gault MH, Dixon ME, Doyle M, Cohen WM. Hypernatremia, azotemia, and dehydration due to high-protein tube feeding. *Ann Intern Med.* 1968;68:778.

69. Gipstein RM, Boyle JD. Hypernatremia complicating prolonged mannitol diuresis. *NEJM.* 1965;272:1116–1117.

70. Rose BD, Post TW. Clinical Physiology of Acid-Base and Electrolyte Disorders, 5th ed, McGraw-Hill, New York, 2001, pp. 751–754.

71. Rose BD, Post, TW. Clinical Physiology of Acid-Base and Electrolyte Disorders, 5th ed, McGraw-Hill, New York, 2001, pp. 754–758.

72. Garofeanu CG, Weir M, Rosas-Arellano MP, Henson G, Garg AX, Clark WF. Causes of reversible nephrogenic diabetes insipidus: a systematic review. *Am J Kidney Dis.* 2005 Apr;45(4):626–637.

73. Rose BD, Post TW. Clinical Physiology of Acid-Base and Electrolyte Disorders, 5th ed, McGraw-Hill, New York, 2001, pp. 761–764.

74. Martins D, Adegbenga A, Norris KC. Geriatric emergency: the management of salt and water disturbances in the elderly. *Clinical Geriatrics.* 2001;9(7).

75. Moder KG, Hurley DL. Fatal hypernatremia from exogenous salt intake: report of a case and review of the literature. *Mayo Clin Proc.* 1990 Dec;65(12):1587–1594.

76. Molaschi M, Ponzetto M, Massaia M, Villa L, Scarafiotti C, Ferrario E. Hypernatremic dehydration in the elderly on admission to hospital. *J Nutr Health Aging.* 1997;1(3):156–160.

77. Androgue HJ, Madias NE. *Hypernatremia NEJM.* 2000 May 18;342(20):1493–1499.

78. Rennke HG, Denker BM. Renal Pathophysiology: the essentials. 2nd Edition. Lippincott Williams and Wilkins, 2006, pp. 176–178.

79. Biswas K, Mulkerrin EC. Potassium homeostasis in the elderly. *Quarterly Journal of Medicine.* July 1997;90(7):487–492.

80. Rennke HG, Denker BM. Renal Pathophysiology: the essentials. 2nd Edition. Lippincott Williams and Wilkins, 2006, pp. 180–182.

81. Lush DJ, King JA, Fray JC. Pathophysiology of low renin syndromes: Sites of renal secretory impairment and prorenin overexpression. *Kidney Int.* 1993;43.

82. Lawson DH. Adverse reactions to potassium chloride. *QJM.* 1974;433–440.

83. Hollander-Rodriguez JC, Calvert JF Jr. Hyperkalemia. *American Family Physician.* 2006;73(2):283–290.

84. Schlondorff D. Renal complications of nonsteroidal anti-inflammatory drugs. *Kidney Int.* 1993;44:643–653.

85. Perazella MA, Mahnensmith RL. Hyperkalemia in the elderly:drugs exacerbate impaired potassium homeostasis. *JGIM.* Oct 1997;12(10):646–656.

86. Bashour T, Hsu I, Gorfinkel HJ, Wickramesekaran R, Rios JC. Atrioventricular and intraventricular conduction in hyperkalemia. *Am J Cardiol* 1975 Feb;35(2):199–203.

87. Muensterer OJ. Hyperkalaemic paralysis. *Age Ageing* 2003 Jan;32(1):114–115.

88. Rose BD, Post, TW. Clinical Physiology of Acid-Base and Electrolyte Disorders, 5th ed, McGraw-Hill, New York, 2001, pp. 913–919.

89. Rennke HG, Denker BM. Renal Pathophysiology: the essentials. 2nd Edition. Lippincott Williams and Wilkins. 2006, pp. 190.

90. Whang R, Whang DD, Ryan MP. Refractory potassium repletion. A consequence of magnesium deficiency. *Arch Intern Med.* 1992 Jan;152(1):40–45.

91. Rennke HG, Denker BM. Renal Pathophysiology: the essentials. 2nd Edition. Lippincott Williams and Wilkins, 2006, pp. 194.

92. Isaac G, Holland OB. Drug-induced hypokalaemia. A cause for concern. *Drugs Aging.* 1992 JanFeb;2(1):35–41.

93. Panichpisal K, Angulo-Pernett F, Selhi S, Nugent KM. Gitelman-like syndrome after cisplatin therapy: a case report and literature review. *BMC Nephrol.* 2006 May 24;7:10.

94. Pascual J, Orofino L, Liano F, et al. Incidence and prognosis of acute renal failure in older patients. *J Am Geriatr Soc.* 1990;38:25–30.

95. Kumar R, Hill CM, McGeown MG: Acute renal failure in the elderly. *Lancet.* 1973;1:90–91.

96. Pascual J, Liano F, and Ortuno J. The Elderly Patient with Acute Renal Failure. *J Am Soc Nephrol.* 1995;6(2):144–153.

97. Markowitz GS, Perazella MA. Drug-induced renal failure: a focus on tubulointerstitial disease. *Clinica chimica Acta.* Jan 2005;351(1–2):31–47.

98. Esson ML, Schrier RW. Diagnosis and treatment of acute tubular necrosis. *Ann Int. Med.* 2002;137(9):744–752.

99. Liano F, Junco E, Pascual J, et al. The spectrum of acute renal failure in the intensive care unit compared with that seen in other settings. The Madrid Acute Renal Failure Study Group. *Kidney Int.* 1998;53(suppl 66):S16–S24.

100. Kjellstrand CM, Ebben J, Davin T. Time of death, recovery of renal function, development of chronic renal failure and need for chronic hemodialysis in patients with acute tubular necrosis. *Trans Am Soc Artif Intern Organs.* 1981;27:45–50.

101. Kodner CM, Kudrimoti A. Diagnosis and management of acute interstitial nephritis. *Am Fam Physician.* 2003;67(12):2527–2534.

102. Rennke HG, Denker BM. Renal Pathophysiology: the essentials. 2nd Edition. Lippincott Williams and Wilkins, 2006, pp. 348–350.

103. Rennke HG, Denker BM. Renal Pathophysiology: the essentials. 2nd Edition. Lippincott Williams and Wilkins. 2006 pp. 295.

104. Modesto-Segonds A, Ah-Soune MF, Durand D, Suc JM. Renal biopsy in the elderly. *Am J Nephrol.* 1993;13(1):27–34.

105. Preston RA, Stemmer CL, Materson BJ, et al. Renal biopsy in patients 65 years of age or older. An analysis of the results of 334 biopsies. *Journal of the American Geriatrics Society.* 1990;38(6):669–674.

106. Garovic VD, Textor SC. Renovascular hypertension and ischemic nephropathy. *Circulation.* 2005;112:1362–1374.

107. Hansen KL, Edwards MS, Craven TE, et al. Prevalence of renovascular disease in the elderly: a population based study. *J Vasc. Surg.* 2002;36:443–451.

108. Anderson GH, Blakeman N, and Streeten DH. The effect of age on prevalence of secondary forms of hypertension in 4429 consecutively referred patients. *J Hypertens.* 1994;12:609–615.

109. Shepherd S, Cadwallader K. Does early detection of suspected atherosclerotic renovascular hypertension change outcomes?. *Journal Fam Pract.* 2005;54(9).813–816.

110. Connolly JO, Woolfson RG. Renovascular Hypertension: diagnosis and management. *Brit. J Urol.* 2005;96:715–720.

111. Nordmann AJ, Woo K, Parkes R, et al. Balloon angioplasty or medical therapy for hypertensive patients with atherosclerotic renal artery stenosis? A meta-analysis of randomized controlled trials. *Am J Med.* 2003;114:44–50.

112. van Jaarsveld BC, Krijnen P, Pieterman H, et al. The effect of balloon angioplasty on hypertension in atherosclerotic renal-artery stenosis. *NEJM.* 2001;342:1007–1014.

113. Gray BH, Olin JW, Childs MB, et al. Clinical benefit of renal artery angioplasty with stenting for the control of recurrent and refractory congestive heart failure. *Vasc Med.* 2002;7:275–279.

114. Kennedy DJ, Colyer WR, Brewster PS, et al. Renal insufficiency as a predictor of adverse events and mortality after renal artery stent placement. *Am J Kidney Dis.* 2003;42:926–935.

115. Coresh J, Astor BC, Greene T, et al. Prevalence of chronic kidney disease and decreased kidney function in the adult US population. Third National Health and Nutrition Examination Survey. *Am J Kidney Dis.* 2003;41:1–12.

116. Braun WE. Allocation of cadaveric kidneys: new pressures, new solutions. *Am J Kidney Dis.* 1994;24: 526–530.

117. Snyder S, Pendergraph B. Detection and Evaluation of Chronic Kidney Disease. *Am Fam Physician.* 2005;72(9):1723–1732.

118. McClellan WM, Ramirez SP, Jurkovitz C. Screening for chronic kidney disease: unresolved issues. *J Am Soc Nephrol.* 2003;14(7supp 2):S81–S87.

119. Boulware LE, Jaar BG, Tarver-Carr ME, et al. Screening for proteinuria in US adults: a cost-effectiveness analysis. *JAMA.* 2003;290:3101–3114.

120. Rennke HG, Denker BM. Renal Pathophysiology: the essentials. 2nd Edition. Lippincott Williams and Wilkins, 2006, pp. 17–22.

121. Peterson JC, Adler S, Burkart JM, et al. Blood pressure control, proteinuria, and the progression of renal disease. The Modification of Diet in Renal Disease Study. *Ann Intern Med.* 1995;123:754–762.

122. Jafar TH, Stark PC, Schmid CH, et al. Progression of chronic kidney disease: the role of blood pressure control, proteinuria,

and angiotensin-converting enzyme inhibition; a patient level meta-analysis. *Ann Intern Med.* 2003;139:244–252.

123. Brenner BM, cooper ME, de Zeeuw D, et al. Effects of losartan on renal and cardiovascular outcomes in patients with type 2 diabetes and nephropathy. *NEJM.* 2001;345:861–869.

124. Jafar TH, Schmid CH, Giatras LM, et al. Angiotensin-converting enzyme inhibitors and progression of nondiabetic renal disease: a meta-analysis of patient level data. *Ann Intern Med.* 2001;135:73–87.

125. Parving HH, Lehnert H, Brochner-Mortensen J, et al. Irbesartan in Patients with Type 2 Diabetes and Microalbuminuria Study Group.The effect of irbesartan on the development of diabetic nephropathy in patients with Type 2 diabetes. *NEJM.* 2001;345:870–878.

126. Kasiske BL, Lakatua JD, Ma JZ, Louis TA. A meta-analysis of the effects of dietary protein restriction on the rate of decline in renal function. *Am J Kidney Dis.* 1998;31:954–961.

127. Levey AS, Green T, Beck GJ, et al. Dietary protein restriction and the progression of chronic renal disease: what have all of the results of the MDRD study shown? Modification of Diet in Renal Disease Study group. *J Am Soc Nephrol.* 1999 Nov;10(11):2426–2439.

128. Weiner DE, Sarnak MJ. Managing dyslipidemia in chronic kidney disease. *J Gen Intern Med.* 2004 October; 19(10):1045–1052.

129. Jungers P, Choukroun G, Oualim Z, et al. Beneficial influence of recombinant human erythropoietin therapy on the rate of progression of chronic renal failure in predialysis patients. *Nephrol Dial Transplant.* 2001;16:307–312.

130. Ponticelli C. Should renal transplantation be offered to older patients? *Nephrol Dial transplant.* 2000;15:315–317.

131. Schaubel D, Desmeules M, Mao Y, et al. Survival experience among elderly end-stage renal disease patients. *Transplantation.* 1995;1389–1394.

132. Bonal J, Cleries M, Vela E and the Renal Registry Committee. Transplantation versus hemodialysis in elderly patients. *Nephrol Dial Transplant.* 1997;12:261–264.

133. Gjertson DW. A multi-factor analysis of kidney graft outcomes at one and five years posttransplantation:1996 UNOS Update. *Clin Transplant.* 1996:343–360.

134. Tesi RJ, Elkhammas EA, Davies EA, et al. Renal transplantation in older people. *Lancet.* 994;343:461–464.

135. Meier-Kriesche HU, Ojo AO, Cibrik DM, et al. Relationship of recipient age and development of chromic renal allograft failure. *Transplantation.* 000;70:306–310.

136. Doyle SE, Matas AJ, Gillingham K, Rosenberg ME. Predicting clinical outcome in the elderly renal transplant recipient. *Kidney Int.* 2000;57:2144–2150.

137. Greenstein S, Siegal B. Compliance and non compliance in patients with a functioning renal transplant: a multicenter study. *Transplantation* 1999;66:1718–1726.

138. Becker BN, Ismail N, Becker YT, et al. Renal transplantation in the older stage renal disease patient. *Am J Kidney Dis.* 1996;16:353–362.

25

UROLOGICAL ISSUES IN OLDER ADULTS

Tomas L. Griebling, MD, FACS, FGSA

INTRODUCTION

Urological problems are extremely common in older adults. The prevalence of many urological disorders increases with advancing age in both men and women. Estimates indicate that approximately 20% of all primary care visits include some type of urological complaint. In fact, data from the National Ambulatory Medical Care Survey indicate the specialty of urology ranks third, behind only ophthalmology and cardiology, in the total annual number of outpatient clinical visits by older Medicare recipients in the United States.[1] These trends hold steady even when stratifying for ages older than either 75 or 85 years. This chapter addresses the evaluation and management of many of the common urological conditions seen in older adults. Several topics relevant to urology are also covered in more detail in other chapters including urinary incontinence (Chapter 26), sexuality and sexual health (Chapter 55), and prostate cancer (Chapter 36).

HEMATURIA

Hematuria is a common urological condition seen in people of all ages. The condition may be gross or microscopic, and it may be episodic or persistent. Any episode of gross hematuria should be considered abnormal. On microscopic urinalysis, the generally accepted upper limit of normal is zero to three red blood cells per high-powered field.[2] Because it is a common presenting sign for many types of genitourinary pathology, elderly patients with gross or persistent microhematuria should undergo a thorough evaluation including upper urinary tract imaging and cystourethroscopy. The common sources of hematuria in older adults are summarized in Table 25.1. Intravenous pyelography has been the traditional form of imaging used in the evaluation of hematuria; however, recent stud-

ies have suggested that computed tomography imaging may be equivalent or superior to intravenous pyelography for detection of urological abnormalities.[3] If possible, the study should be done both without and with intravenous contrast. The noncontrast images are particularly useful to evaluate for stones. After contrast administration, immediate and delayed images are obtained. These help to delineate renal function and anatomy, the course and caliber of the ureters, and the general anatomy of the bladder. Delayed images are useful to identify hydronephrosis and potential ureteral obstruction.

Although larger lesions in the bladder may be identifiable on computed tomography imaging or ultrasound, smaller mucosal lesions may not be evident on these studies. Therefore, cystourethroscopy must be considered an essential part of the complete urological evaluation for hematuria. Bladder cancers, particularly transitional cell carcinomas, usually start in the urothelium and are often visible as papillary lesions on cystoscopy. Carcinoma in situ is a particularly aggressive form of bladder cancer that may initially present with either microscopic or gross hematuria. On cystoscopy, this usually appears as a red, velvety patch in the urothelium. Histological examination of bladder biopsies and cytological examination of either voided urine or bladder washing specimens may be useful to help diagnose bladder malignancies. In the United States, transitional cell carcinoma is the most common form of bladder cancer in older adults, and cigarette smoking is one of the most common risk factors.

Although an episode of gross hematuria can be quite distressing for the patient, emergency evaluation is not usually necessary. The exceptions are patients experiencing clot retention with difficulty passing urine or patients requiring blood transfusions for anemia secondary to the hematuria. Cystourethroscopy with clot evacuation may be required in these cases. If a specific bleeding site is identified, electrocoagulation may be useful. In many cases, a specific source cannot

Table 25.1. Causes of Hematuria in Older Adults

Benign Conditions

  Stones

  UTI

  Pyelonephritis

  Glomerular diseases of the kidney

Inflammatory conditions

  Prostatitis

  Cystitis

  Urethritis

Malignant Conditions

  Bladder cancer

  Transitional cell carcinoma

  Squamous cell carcinoma

  Carcinoma in situ

  Ureteral cancer

  Renal cancer

  Renal cell carcinoma

  Prostate cancer

  Urethral cancer

be identified. In cases of persistent gross hematuria, chemical coagulation with bladder infusions of dilute alum or formalin may be required.

In older patients with renal insufficiency, a plain x-ray of the kidneys, ureters, and bladder and renal ultrasound can be performed as the initial imaging evaluation. This should be supplemented with cystourethroscopy and retrograde ureteropyelography to look for abnormalities in the ureters or renal collecting systems. Filling defects may indicate some type of space-occupying lesion such as a stone, tumor, polyp, fungus ball, blood clot, or stricture.

Acute conditions such as urinary tract infection (UTI), prostatitis, or stone passage may be associated with hematuria. Urinalysis should be repeated after these conditions have been treated, and, if hematuria persists, then urological consultation for further evaluation should be obtained. Hematuria is also frequently seen in elderly patients receiving chronic anticoagulation therapy; however, these individuals still require a complete urological evaluation because 15%–20% will be found to have significant underlying genitourinary pathology.

If an older adult patient has persistent microhematuria despite a negative urological evaluation with upper tract imaging, cystourethroscopy, and cytology, then referral to a nephrologist to evaluate for possible glomerular bleeding would be warranted. This is particularly true in patients with a history of either proteinuria or hypertension.[2]

HEMATOSPERMIA

Hematospermia, blood in the ejaculate, is occasionally seen in older men. Although it is most commonly idiopathic and benign, it may be an indication of other underlying genitourinary pathological conditions such as prostatitis or prostate cancer.[4] Bleeding from dilated capillary vessels in the prostate may also cause hematospermia. In some cases, this may be triggered by excessive physical exertion or vigorous sexual activity. Evaluation, including a thorough history-taking and physical examination, may help to identify the cause of the condition. Additional tests that may be useful include cystourethroscopy, transrectal ultrasound, prostate biopsy, and determination of prostate-specific antigen (PSA) levels.

URINARY TRACT INFECTIONS

Bacteriuria and UTI are among the most common urological diagnoses in older adults. The estimated lifetime risk for development of a UTI in women is greater than 50%, and the associated costs are staggering. In the year 2000, the estimated overall annual expenditures for UTI care in the United States were $2.47 billion for women, and $1.03 billion for men.[5,6] Epidemiological studies indicate that the incidence and prevalence of UTIs increases with advancing age.[7] Although seen in both sexes, a higher proportion of women are affected, with a ratio of 3:1. Various age-related physiological changes may predispose older adults to UTIs. These include hormonal and vaginal changes associated with menopause, alterations in cognitive function, prostate disease, and changes in bladder physiology.

Asymptomatic bacteriuria should be differentiated from symptomatic UTI. Symptomatic UTIs should be treated in patients of any age. Diagnosis should be confirmed with urinalysis and urine cultures. Determination of drug sensitivity on urine culture is important to ensure that appropriate antibiotic therapy has been administered. This is particularly important given the increased rates of drug resistance seen with many common bacteria. Typical symptoms of acute UTI include fever, dysuria, urinary urgency and frequency, burning with urination, and suprapubic discomfort. Elderly patients may not develop these symptoms because of normal alterations in overall immune status associated with aging. Older adults may exhibit other symptoms resulting from UTI including lethargy, anorexia, or confusion. In elderly patients with new onset of delirium, a urinalysis and urine culture should be checked to determine if a UTI is present.

Antibiotic therapy for acute UTI is usually administered as an oral preparation. Uncomplicated UTI may be treated with simple, low-cost antibiotics such as amoxicillin or ampicillin, nitrofurantoin, or trimethoprim-sulfamethoxazole. In patients who are allergic to these compounds, cephalosporins and tetracycline may be used as second-line therapy. Fluoroquinolones are usually reserved for complicated UTIs including those associated with concomitant stone disease, pyelonephritis, or sepsis. The choice of appropriate antibiotic therapy should of course be guided by the patient's overall medical condition, renal function status, and the results of the antibiotic sensitivity profile for the specific organism. The duration of therapy generally ranges from 3 to 7 days, and is dependent on a variety of factors including overall complexity of the infection and response to therapy. Intravenous antibiotic therapy may be required in cases of severe infection, pyelonephritis, or urosepsis.

The most common organisms seen in elderly patients with UTI include Gram-negative bacteria such as *Escherichia coli*, *Pseudomonas*, *Klebsiella*, and *Proteus*. The most common Gram-positive organisms seen in older adults with UTI include *Staphylococcus aureus*, and *Enterococcus*.[8] In patients with recurrent, culture-documented UTI, a clinical investigation to search for a nidus of infection is warranted. Common causes of recurrent infection include urolithiasis or other foreign body, chronic urinary retention, and vesicoureteral reflux. Treatment of the underlying condition may lead to resolution or a decrease in the frequency of UTIs.

Asymptomatic bacteriuria is quite common, particularly in elderly women. This is seen both in community-dwelling and institutionalized elders. In a community-based, cross-sectional analysis of 432 people aged 80 years or older, 19.0% of the women and 5.8% of the men were found to have asymptomatic bacteriuria.[9] In this study, urinary incontinence, reduced mobility, and systemic estrogen replacement therapy were identified as independent risk factors for asymptomatic bacteriuria in women. There is general consensus that asymptomatic bacteriuria need not be treated with antibiotic therapy.

UTIs associated with systemic bacteremia in elderly patients carry a high risk of morbidity and mortality. In a retrospective study of 191 patients aged 75–105 years with concomitant positive urine and blood cultures, the in-hospital mortality rate was 33%.[8] A variety of factors associated with impaired physical and cognitive function were associated with increased mortality; however, advanced age itself was not identified as a significant risk factor in this particular study. Other studies have confirmed that mental status changes and a history of frequent UTIs may be associated with increased mortality in elderly patients with UTI.[10]

The role of impaired bladder emptying in development of UTI in older adults has been somewhat controversial. Intuitively, it makes sense that increased postvoid residual urine volume may be associated with UTI. The data, however, have been somewhat conflicting on this topic. A recent retrospective analysis of 101 stroke patients admitted for inpatient rehabilitation demonstrated that a finding of two or more postvoid residual urine volumes of 150 mL or more was independently associated with an increased risk of UTI.[11]

Impaired nutritional status may also be associated with an increased propensity for elderly patients to develop UTIs. In a recent study of 185 hospitalized older adults (mean age 81.6 +/−0.6 years), malnutrition was associated with an increased rate of nosocomial infections, including UTIs.[12]

Indwelling catheterization is clearly associated with an increased risk of UTI in older adults. Intermittent catheteriza-

tion is preferred, if possible, in patients who have problems with urinary retention. Indwelling catheters should be used only if absolutely necessary. A recently published study examined the rates of UTI observed in a group of 277 elderly patients who had an indwelling urinary catheter placed in the emergency room at the time of hospital admission.[13] Overall, 28% of these patients were diagnosed with a UTI during their hospitalization; however, 69% of these individuals either had a UTI diagnosed in the emergency room or had clinically significant bacteriuria ($\geq 10^5$ organisms/mL) prior to the catheter placement. Therefore, 9% of the patients who had an indwelling catheter placed developed a new UTI during hospitalization.

Several treatments may be helpful to prevent development of UTIs in susceptible older adults. Increased hydration may be helpful to decrease bacterial adherence to the urothelium of the bladder and urethra. Vaginal estrogen replacement may help to prevent development of UTI in postmenopausal women with atrophic vaginitis. Estrogen helps to acidify the vaginal fluid that facilitates growth of *Lactobacillus* sp., the natural vaginal flora. *Lactobacillus* is an important component of the natural host-defense mechanism, which helps prevent overgrowth of pathogenic bacteria associated with UTI. The estrogen is administered vaginally to enhance absorption in the vaginal and periurethral tissues. Even in patients already on systemic estrogen therapy, additional vaginal administration may be required to reach appropriate local tissue levels. Administration approximately three times weekly is usually sufficient. Exogenous estrogen administration is typically contraindicated in women with a history of uterine or breast cancer.

Cranberries (*Vaccinium macrocarpon*) have long been considered a preventive agent for UTIs, and consumption of cranberry juice has been associated with decreased rates of UTI in elderly patients.[14] This is most likely because of acidification of the urine and the azo ring chemistry found in the cranberries that prevents bacterial adherence to the urothelium. If patients are going to use cranberry to help prevent UTI, they should be counseled to look for products containing a high percentage of real juice rather than water. Cranberry tablets may be substituted for juice in diabetic patients or those on a reduced calorie diet.

URINARY CATHETERS

In general, the use of indwelling urinary catheters should be avoided if at all possible.[15] Indwelling catheters can be associated with significant potential complications including UTIs, urosepsis, and stone formation. Care should be taken to remove the catheter as soon as feasible, and to monitor the patient for signs and symptoms of UTI. With extended time, chronic catheter irritation may lead to squamous metaplasia of the bladder epithelium and squamous cell carcinoma of the bladder.

If chronic indwelling catheter use is required, suprapubic catheter drainage is usually preferred over urethral catheterization. The suprapubic catheter may be easier for caregivers to change and is often more comfortable for patients. In patients

Table 25.2. Anticholinergic Medications

Medications	Typical Dosages
Oxybutynin	5 mg BI day – QI day
Oxybutynin (time released)	5, 10, or 15 mg once daily
Oxybutynin (transdermal)	3.9 mg/day, patch changed twice weekly
Tolterodine	1 or 2 mg BID
Tolterodine (time released)	4 mg once daily
Darifenacin	7.5 or 15 mg once daily
Solifenacin	5 or 10 mg once daily
Potential side effects of anticholinergic medications	
Dry mouth	
Constipation	
Confusion	
Blurry vision	
Headache	
Tachycardia	
Prolongation of QT interval on electrocardiogram	

who are sexually active, a suprapubic catheter is helpful because it moves the catheter away from the genitals. Chronic urethral catheterization may also lead to urethral or bladder neck erosion and subsequent urinary incontinence. Urinary leakage around an indwelling catheter is usually caused by either catheter blockage or bladder spasms. Gentle irrigation of the catheter with sterile saline can be used to relieve obstruction from urinary sediment. Anticholinergic or antispasmodic agents may be useful to diminish bladder spasms. The most common anticholinergic agents including dosages and potential side effects are listed in Table 25.2. Care should be taken when prescribing these agents in older adults, and the patient and family or caregivers should be instructed to watch closely for any signs of side effects. Placement of larger catheters should be avoided because this will only serve to dilate the urethra or suprapubic tract and will not correct the underlying problem. With time, the use of larger catheters may lead to urethral or bladder neck erosion and worsening urinary incontinence. Treatment of urinary incontinence in patients with this type of urethral erosion may be quite difficult and often involves major surgery such as a cystectomy with urinary diversion or augmentation enterocystoplasty with closure of the bladder neck.

STONE DISEASE

Approximately 20% of all adults will develop urinary stone disease at some point in their lives. In general, rates of stone formation and passage do not differ in elderly patients compared with the general population. Patients with a history of stone disease are at significantly increased risk for development of recurrent stone episodes. One of the primary risk factors for stone disease is inadequate hydration, which is often seen in older adults. A recent epidemiological and health care utilization analysis revealed that Medicare beneficiaries with a diagnosis of stone disease had a 2.5 to 3-fold higher rate of inpatient hospitalization for the condition compared with younger patients.[16] This study also demonstrated that rates of outpatient hospital and office visits for evaluation and treatment of stone disease increased by 29% and 41%, respectively, among Medicare beneficiaries between 1992 and 1998.

Small stones (<5 mm) can often be treated effectively with increased hydration and oral analgesics. In many cases, the stones will pass spontaneously. Patients are encouraged to collect and strain their urine to capture the stones for chemical analysis. Larger stones often require surgical intervention for treatment. Cystoscopy and ureteral stent placement may be required to bypass an obstructing stone and help relieve renal colic. Indications for stent insertion include upper tract obstruction, particularly with significant urinary infection or bacteriuria, a solitary kidney, underlying renal insufficiency, or intractable nausea, vomiting, or pain. Subsequent surgical treatment may include ureteroscopy with stone fragmentation and removal or extracorporeal shock wave lithotripsy. Percutaneous nephrostolithotomy may be required for large stones in the renal pelvis or calyces.

Stone composition may also change with advancing age. Alterations in stone chemistry in older adults may be related to associated changes in vitamin D and calcium metabolism, which can be affected by age-related physiological changes. The overall proportion of uric acid stones also appears to increase with advancing age.[17] This may be related to a progressive defect in urine ammoniagenesis, which is observed with aging, and which leads to a low urinary pH observed in patients who form uric acid stones. In addition, there is evidence that diabetic patients tend to have a higher incidence of uric acid stone production compared with nondiabetics.[18] This may help explain the higher rates of uric acid stone production observed in older adults, who also have a greater tendency to have diabetes mellitus or a history of gout.

Rates of stone recurrence appear to be similar in older adults compared with younger individuals.[19] In a review of 209 stone patients older than 65 years, calcium oxalate and calcium phosphate were the most common types of stones observed. The elderly patients accounted for 9.6% of the total population in this study; however, the older patients demonstrated a significantly higher rate of uric acid stone formation compared with the younger patients. Hyperuricosuria and hypercalcuria appear to be common in older patients with recurrent stone disease.

UROLOGICAL MALIGNANCIES

The incidence and prevalence of most of the urological malignancies increase with advancing age. In some cases, there may be differences in the type or progression of cancer compared with younger patients. For a more detailed discussion regarding evaluation and management of cancers in older adults, please refer to Chapter 36.

Prostate Cancer

Prostate cancer is the most common nonskin cancer diagnosed in men, and the second leading cause of cancer deaths behind lung cancer. It is estimated that approximately 186,320 new cases of prostate cancer will be diagnosed in the United States in 2008, and approximately 28,660 men will die of the disease.[20] The incidence and prevalence of prostate cancer increase with age. In general, prostate cancer is a slow-growing disease, and many men will die of other comorbid conditions rather than of prostate cancer itself. In patients with clinically organ-confined disease, treatment with curative intent by using either radical prostatectomy or radiation therapy may be utilized. Although there is no specific age limitation, curative treatment is most often considered for those men with a predicted life expectancy of at least 10 additional years. In men with metastatic disease or in those who are not deemed to be surgical candidates, hormonal therapy with androgen deprivation may be used to slow the progression of the disease. For additional information on the evaluation and treatment of prostate cancer in elderly men, please refer to Chapter 36.

Routine screening for prostate cancer in elderly men is somewhat controversial. In younger men, the American Urological Association recommends screening with an annual serum PSA level and a digital rectal examination.[21] Guidelines suggest starting routine screening at the age of 50 years, and at 40 years for men considered to be at high risk for prostate cancer. These would include African-American men and those with a family history of prostate cancer. Specific age cutoffs at which to discontinue screening have not been definitively established. In general, routine prostate cancer screening in elderly men with a predicted life expectancy of less than 10 years is not indicated.[22] Decisions to screen for prostate cancer in elderly men should be tailored to each patient's specific clinical situation with consideration of overall health and other comorbid disease.

Bladder Cancer

Bladder cancer often presents initially with either gross painless hematuria or persistent microhematuria. In the United States, the most common type of bladder cancer is transitional cell carcinoma. On cystoscopic examination, this usually appears as either a papillary or sessile tumor of the bladder mucosa. Carcinoma in situ is a particularly aggressive form of bladder cancer. Cystoscopically, this typically appears as a velvety red patch in the bladder mucosa. Bladder wash cytology and biopsies are needed to help establish the diagnosis.

Treatment of bladder cancer is dependent on the grade and stage of the tumor. Low-grade tumors that do not invade into the muscular layer of the bladder are usually treated with endoscopic resection. Tumor recurrence occurs in up to 70% of patients, and careful postoperative follow-up is essential for proper treatment. Follow-up consists of repeated cystoscopy and cytology every 3 months for 2 years, every 4 months for 2 years, every 6 months for 2 years, and then annually. Adjuvant therapy with intravesical administration of Bacillus-Calmette-Guérin or chemotherapeutic agents may be used to help decrease tumor recurrence. High-grade noninvasive tumors may also be treated with a combination of resection and intravesical chemotherapy.

Invasion of tumor into the muscularis propria is an ominous finding and is associated with a high risk of disease progression. The mainstay of therapy is radical cystectomy in women or cystoprostatectomy in men. This is a major surgical procedure that is associated with significant risk of morbidity and mortality. Recent studies indicate that elderly patients can safely undergo this type of surgery, although the risks and potential benefits need to be carefully considered for each individual patient.[23] Options for urinary diversion include both continent and noncontinent options.[24] The traditional diversion is an ileal conduit, which is brought to the skin as a urinary stoma. The urine drains continuously into an ostomy bag that is secured directly to the skin. Methods for continent urinary diversion include a catheterizable pouch, which the patient drains several times daily using intermittent catheterization, or an orthotopic neobladder. The neobladder is a pouch made of detubularized bowel that is anastomosed to the urethra. The patient voids per urethra to empty the pouch, although some patients do need to do periodic intermittent catheterization to completely drain the reservoir. Because the orthotopic diversion relies on the external urinary sphincter for continence, many patients experience some urinary leakage during their sleep.

Urethral Cancer

Primary malignant tumors of the urethra are rare and occur more commonly in women than men. Patients usually present with hematuria or difficulty with urination. The tumor is often palpable on bimanual pelvic examination. Cystoscopy and biopsy are used to help confirm the diagnosis. Treatment consists of excision, and possible adjuvant chemotherapy or radiation.

Kidney Cancer

Cancers of the kidney account for approximately 3%–4% of all diagnosed malignancies in both men and women.[20] The most common types of kidney cancer include renal cell carcinomas, which originate in the renal parenchyma, and transitional cell carcinomas, which originate in the transitional epithelium of the renal collecting system. Early treatment is essential to prevent development of metastatic disease beyond the kidney. For renal cell carcinomas, partial nephrectomy may be considered if the tumor is amenable to resection to spare as many functional nephrons as possible to preserve renal function.

Recent advances in therapeutic methodology have made techniques such as cryotherapy and radio-frequency ablation of renal tumors minimally invasive options for some patients. These types of therapies may be particularly useful in elderly patients who may not be candidates for more invasive surgery. Radical nephrectomy may be required if the tumor is large or not amenable to a nephron-sparing approach. The overall health and potential longevity of the patient must be carefully considered in each case.

Nephroureterectomy has been the traditional treatment for transitional cell carcinomas of the renal collecting system. The ureter is removed because the tumor usually involves a field change within the tissue, and subsequent recurrences in the ureter are extremely common (>70%). Nephron-sparing options including endoscopic tumor resection with administration of chemotherapeutic or immunotherapeutic agents into the renal collecting system. These may be viable options in patients who are not candidates to undergo more involved surgery.

Testis Cancer

Testis cancer is a relatively uncommon malignancy, accounting for approximately 1% of all cancers diagnosed in males.[20,25] Testis cancers can present at any point in a man's life, although the types of cancer differ significantly by patient age. In infants and children, yolk sac tumors and embryonal cell carcinomas are the most common. In young men between the ages of 15 and 35 years, testis cancer is actually the most common solid malignancy, and ranks behind only the leukemias and lymphomas in overall incidence. The most common forms of testis cancer in young men include seminomas and nonseminomatous germ cell tumors. In contrast, the most common testicular tumors in elderly men are lymphomas. These tend to be aggressive tumors and are generally managed with systemic chemotherapy or a combination of chemotherapy and radiation. Recurrence is common, occurring in up to 80% of patients.[26] Extranodal recurrence is not uncommon and may involve the central nervous system. Chemotherapy can be useful in some cases of testicular lymphoma.

BENIGN DISORDERS OF THE PROSTATE

Prostate diseases are among the most common urological conditions that affect older men. The primary nonmalignant conditions affecting the prostate gland in older men include benign prostatic hyperplasia (BPH) and prostatitis.

Benign Prostatic Hyperplasia

The prostate gland secretes fluid that helps form the ejaculate and provides nutrient factors required for the function and survival of sperm. Benign enlargement of the prostate gland typically begins at approximately 40–50 years of age.[27] This enlargement is driven by the presence of serum testosterone.

Proliferation of both the stromal and the epithelial components of the prostate gland can occur in cases of BPH. The effect of prostatic enlargement is variable. Some men experience few symptoms; however, many men develop obstructive voiding symptoms including urinary frequency, hesitancy, nocturia, and a slow urinary stream. Nocturia can be particularly bothersome for some men.[28] Other men experience chronic difficulty emptying the bladder or acute urinary retention. In some cases, men may also experience irritative voiding symptoms with urinary urgency or urge incontinence. Pain is uncommon unless men have acute urinary retention or need to strain to urinate. Prostate size does not always correlate with symptoms. In fact, some men with relatively small prostate glands have severe symptoms, particularly if the median lobe of the prostate gland is involved. Voiding symptoms associated with BPH can have a significantly negative impact on both overall and health-related quality of life.[29,30] Fortunately, there are a wide variety of both surgical and nonsurgical therapies for BPH that can be quite effective in relieving these bothersome symptoms. These are outlined in Table 25.3. In addition, quality indicators for evaluation and management of BPH in vulnerable elderly men have recently been established.[31]

Medical Therapies

Currently, there are three main categories of drugs used for the pharmacological treatment of BPH. These include the α-adrenergic antagonists, the 5-α-reductase inhibitors, and nutritional supplements and phytotherapies. The α-adrenergic antagonists include terazosin (Hytrin), doxazosin (Cardura), tamsulosin (Flomax), and alfuzosin (Uroxatral). These drugs act by blocking α-adrenergic receptors in the tissue of the prostatic urethra and bladder neck. This leads to a relaxation of smooth muscle in these tissues, which causes a decrease in outlet resistance. These drugs have been shown to work well, particularly in men with smaller prostate glands.[32] The medications are usually prescribed once daily at bedtime. This helps to reduce some of the potential side effects of the medication including orthostatic hypotension. Men should be warned to rise slowly and make sure they have their balance before getting up from bed. This is particularly true for men who have nocturia and get up to go to the toilet in the night. There have been associations reported between α-blocker therapy and erectile dysfunction in older men.[33,34] Another potential side effect of this class of drugs is the floppy-iris syndrome.[35] The medications may cause relaxation of the smooth muscle in the iris of the eyes. This can become a problem if the medication is not discontinued prior to cataract surgery. The condition causes intraoperative billowing of the iris musculature with risk of prolapse and progressive miosis. Men taking these medications must advise their ophthalmologist prior to any surgical interventions.

The 5-α-reductase inhibitors act by blocking the enzyme that helps catalyze the conversion of testosterone into dihydrotestosterone. Limiting the amount of circulating dihydrotestosterone leads to a shrinking of the prostate gland,

Table 25.3. Treatment Options for BPH

Medical Therapies	
Alpha-adrenergic antagonists	
Nonselective	
Terazosin (Hytrin)	1–10 mg PO at bedtime (must titrate dose)
Doxazosin (Cardura)	1–8 mg PO at bedtime (must titrate dose)
Selective	
Tamsulosin (Flomax)	0.4–0.8 mg PO at bedtime
Alfuzosin (Uroxatral)	10 mg PO once daily
5-Alpha-reductase inhibitors	
Finasteride (Proscar)	5 mg PO once daily
Dutasteride (Avodart)	0.5 mg PO once daily
Surgical Therapies	
TURP	
Transurethral incision	
Open suprapubic prostatectomy	
Open retropubic (non-radical) prostatectomy	
Minimally Invasive Therapies	
Transurethral electrovaporization	
Transurethral needle ablation	
High-intensity focused ultrasound	
Transurethral microwave thermotherapy	
Lasers (various)	
Prostatic stents	

although the full effect may not be seen for several months after starting the medication.[36] The two main drugs in this category include finasteride (Proscar) and dutasteride (Avodart). These medications generally work better in men with larger prostate glands. The potential side effects include decrease in libido and development of gynecomastia or breast discomfort. The drugs will also cause an approximate 50% reduction in circulating serum PSA. It is recommended that a PSA level be checked prior to initiating these medications. After starting a 5-α-reductase inhibitor, observed PSA levels should be doubled to determine the actual PSA for a given patient.

Several recent studies have suggested that using a combination of an α-adrenergic antagonist and a 5-α-reductase inhibitor may have better overall efficacy compared with monotherapy, particularly for men with larger prostates or more severe voiding symptoms.[37,38] Whereas this dual therapy may be beneficial for some patients, the potential side effects and additive costs of these medications must also be considered.

A number of natural remedies and plant extracts have gained popularity for the treatment of the symptoms of BPH. The most widely used preparation is saw palmetto (*Serenoa repens*). The exact mechanism of action is unknown, but theories suggest it may be similar to either 5-α-reductase inhibitors or other hormonally active agents. To date, there have been relatively few studies examining the efficacy of these types of preparations, particularly in elderly men. These agents are available in health food stores without a prescription. It is difficult to counsel patients about the safety and efficacy of these types of treatments because of the overall paucity of data. These phytotherapeutic agents are also not subject to regulation by the Federal Food and Drug Administration (FDA) and there may be significant variations between products and even between batches of the same product.

The roles of micronutrients and other nutritional components have recently attracted attention as a potential option for treatment and perhaps prevention of BPH.[39,40] Research data are limited, particularly for elderly men; however, this is a rapidly growing area of both basic science and clinical research. Zinc has long been advocated as a mineral important for prostate health. Other agents being examined for their potential influence on prostate physiology include lycopenes, bioflavonoids including soy, and selenium. If these types of nutritional agents show a clinically significant effect in either treating BPH or preventing clinically significant symptoms, it may alter the ways in which this disorder is managed.

Surgery

Surgical treatment may be required in some patients, particularly if medical therapy has not been clinically successful. The traditional options for surgery include open surgical removal of the prostate through either a suprapubic or retropubic approach or transurethral resection. Open surgery is still used in men with very large prostate glands (>100 g). For most men, transurethral surgery has replaced open surgery as the technique of choice, because of lower overall morbidity and mortality and improved recovery. Transurethral resection of the prostate (TURP) remains the gold standard to which all other forms of therapy are compared. The main risks of TURP include bleeding and infection and development of hyponatremia from absorption of hypotonic irrigation solution during surgery. Recent technical advances have led to development of surgical systems that can utilize isotonic saline for intraoperative irrigation. This has reduced the incidence of the post-TURP hyponatremia syndrome and the associated morbidity of the procedure. Another potential side effect is the development of retrograde ejaculation after TURP. In men with a smaller prostate or with an elevated bladder neck, a transurethral incision of the prostate may help to avoid this potential complication.

Minimally Invasive Therapies

A number of minimally invasive surgical therapies have been developed to treat symptomatic BPH.[41,42] Examples include transurethral electrovaporization of the prostate, transurethral needle ablation of the prostate, which utilizes radio-frequency energy, high-intensity focused ultrasound, or transurethral microwave thermotherapy, which heats the prostate leading to sloughing of the treated tissue. Several different techniques using various laser energy methods have also been developed. Intraurethral prostatic stents have been developed for treatment of mild-to-moderate BPH.[43] These devices are placed across the prostatic urethra and function to push open the urethral lumen with a radial springlike configuration. The overall popularity of urethral stents for routine management of BPH has declined because of associated complications including erosion, migration, or stricture. Removal can be difficult as the components of the stent become incorporated in the epithelium of the urethra. Nonetheless, these devices could be useful in highly select patients, such as frail elderly men with diminished life expectancy who may be too ill to undergo a more involved procedure.[44]

Many of these current minimally invasive options do offer potential advantages in elderly patients. Some can be performed with the patient receiving a local anesthetic in the outpatient office setting. This obviates the need for general or regional anesthesia, which may be advantageous for older adults with multiple comorbidities. Some offer a significant reduction in the potential for perioperative bleeding, which is associated with the traditional TURP. This can be beneficial for elderly patients who may have undergone anticoagulation therapy for treatment of cardiovascular disease. Although each of the minimally invasive treatments show promise in clinical trials and with short-term follow-up, the long-term efficacy of each has yet to be fully determined.

Prostatitis

Several different forms of infection and inflammation can affect the prostate. These include acute prostatitis, chronic prostatitis, and prostatodynia. Although the precise prevalence of prostatitis is unclear and varies among studies, recent epidemiological data suggest an overall prevalence of 2%–10% in adult men.[45,46] This study suggested there are preliminary data that may indicate causal associations between a history of prostatitis and subsequent development of either BPH or prostate cancer. The clinical impact of prostatitis in elderly men is significant, and inpatient hospitalization rates to treat prostatitis in Medicare beneficiaries range from 2 to 2.5 times higher compared with younger men.[6,47]

Acute bacterial prostatitis is most often associated with a rapid onset of symptoms including fever, chills, irritative voiding symptoms with frequency and urgency, dysuria, and pelvic or perineal pain. Because of a generalized decrease in immune function, elderly men may not mount a full symptomatic response and the clinical findings may be more subtle. The cause is usually from an ascending infection with bacteria from the distal urethra. This may be exacerbated by sexual activity or urethral instrumentation such as cystoscopy or catheter insertion. Rectal examination will usually reveal a swollen and tender prostate. Prostate massage should *not* be performed if acute bacterial prostatitis is suspected, because this can lead to systemic dissemination of bacteria and subsequent urosepsis. Urine cultures should be obtained to identify the organism involved in the infection and to help guide antibiotic therapy. If the patient is acutely ill, hospitalization with intravenous antibiotic administration may be necessary. Acute urinary retention may need to be treated with suprapubic tube insertion. Urethral catheterization should be avoided to prevent development of urosepsis. Oral antibiotic therapy is usually continued for 4 weeks. The most common antibiotics used for this are doxycycline or the fluoroquinolones because they can achieve adequate tissue concentrations in the prostate. Computed tomography examination may be useful to identify prostatic abscesses that would require surgical drainage.

Chronic prostatitis occurs more commonly than acute prostatitis in elderly men.[48] Typical symptoms include urinary urgency and frequency, dysuria, nocturia, low back pain, scrotal or perineal discomfort, or suprapubic pain. Findings on rectal examination can be variable. Some men will have significant tenderness or swelling of the prostate gland but others will not. Secretions obtained from prostatic massage may be helpful to establish the diagnosis. Microscopic examination may reveal bacteria or white blood cells. A urine culture should be obtained to help guide antibiotic selection. Initial therapy with approximately 2 weeks of antibiotic agents is indicated, although longer courses of antibiotics may be necessary. Avoiding dietary irritants such as caffeine, alcohol, or carbonated beverages may also be helpful.

Prostatodynia refers to a syndrome in which patients have symptoms suggestive of acute or chronic prostatitis without objective clinical findings. Pain is one of the hallmarks of this condition. Antibiotics often do not help to alleviate symptoms in these patients. Other causes of chronic pelvic pain should be considered such as interstitial cystitis, a chronic inflammatory condition of the urinary bladder that can cause similar symptoms. Treatment may be difficult and needs to be individualized for each patient. Antiinflammatory agents, antihistamines, α-adrenergic antagonists, and pain medications may be useful. Conservative therapies with pelvic floor relaxation techniques or biofeedback therapy may also be of some benefit.

PENILE DISORDERS

In addition to penile cancers, a wide variety of benign conditions may affect the male genitalia. Many of these are inflammatory conditions, and these may be influenced by both anatomical factors and other comorbid conditions such as diabetes mellitus.

Phimosis

Phimosis is a condition characterized by narrowing of the foreskin, which makes retraction of the foreskin difficult or impossible. This may lead to pain and inflammation and may be associated with difficult voiding for some patients. Some dermatological conditions such as lichen sclerosis and balanitis xerotica obliterans (BXO) may increase the incidence of development of phimosis.[49,50] Surgical treatment with either a dorsal slit or circumcision may be needed to treat the condition.

Paraphimosis

In paraphimosis, the foreskin is retracted and becomes trapped behind the coronal sulcus. Tissue edema and swelling occurs that prevents the foreskin from reducing back over the glans penis. This can be quite painful, and, if left untreated, may lead to tissue necrosis or significant infection.[51] One of the most common causes of paraphimosis is retraction of the foreskin for placement of a urinary catheter or other manipulation of the penis, with failure to properly reduce the foreskin back to anatomical position after the procedure. Manual reduction of a paraphimosis should be attempted and may require the use of a penile block with injectable local anesthetic. Once an adequate anesthetic level is obtained, gentle pressure can be applied circumferentially to the penis to help reduce tissue edema. The thumbs are then placed on the sides of the glans penis, and the first two forefingers of each hand are used to pull the foreskin back down past the coronal sulcus and over the glans. If this is unsuccessful, surgical reduction with a dorsal slit or

circumcision may be required. Treatment should be considered a urological emergency.

Balanoposthitis

Balanoposthitis or balanitis is an inflammatory condition of the glans penis that may also involve the adjacent foreskin. The condition is frequently associated with diabetes mellitus and may be more common in men whose blood glucose levels are poorly controlled. An evaluation for diabetes should be performed in previously undiagnosed men with an episode of balanitis. Treatment of the condition includes cleansing of the glans penis with mild soap and water, and subsequent application of topical antifungal ointment. Limited administration of topical steroids may also be helpful to reduce inflammation. Oral antifungal agents may be necessary to help completely resolve any infection. If the condition does not improve with topical treatments or oral medication, then surgical intervention with circumcision may be required.

BXO is a specific type of balanitis that may be chronic and difficult to eradicate. In this condition, the tissue becomes firm and sclerotic in response to inflammation. Some studies have identified an association between BXO and an increased risk of developing penile cancers such as squamous cell carcinoma.[50]

Peyronie Disease

One of the more common benign conditions of the penis is Peyronie disease.[52] This condition is characterized by development of a painful lump within the tissue of the penis associated with curvature of the penile shaft toward the lesion with erection. The condition is caused by a fibrous plaque in the tunica albuginea, the dense connective tissue that forms the outer layers of the corpus cavernosum of the penis. The fibrous plaque prevents stretching of this tissue with erection, which causes the penile curvature toward the side of the lesion. The condition may cause painful erections and may lead to significant erectile dysfunction.[53] Originally described more than a century ago, the exact etiology of the condition is still unknown, although research suggests that prior tissue trauma from vigorous sexual activity and systemic vascular disease may be risk factors.[54]

Treatment of Peyronie disease can be difficult, and a variety of different therapies have been tried with variable success.[55] Oral antiinflammatory agents, including vitamin E, colchicine, and p-aminobenzoate (Potaba), have been useful in some men and may reduce the pain associated with both erection and the plaques themselves. Plaque injection has been used with variable success. Agents often used for this include verapamil, interferon, collagenase, and steroids. Excision of the plaques can also be performed, although this may require tissue grafting to replace the tunica albuginea, which is removed. Depending on the technique used, this may also result in foreshortening of the penile shaft length. Placement of a penile prosthesis at the time of plaque excision may be necessary to help treat the associated erectile dysfunction.

SCROTAL DISORDERS

In addition to testis cancer, several benign conditions of the scrotum can occur in elderly men. These can be quite bothersome for patients and often require additional evaluation and treatment.

Epididymitis

Acute epididymitis is one of the most common scrotal problems seen in older men.[46] This is usually caused by a bacterial infection and may be associated with recent urinary tract instrumentation or chronic urethral catheter use. The condition often occurs in conjunction with other genitourinary infections including acute cystitis or prostatitis. Symptoms include swelling of the affected hemiscrotum with pain and swelling of the effected epididymis. Patients may also experience systemic symptoms of fever, chills, and malaise. If the cause of the patient's symptoms is unclear, a scrotal ultrasound can be helpful to establish the diagnosis. Epididymitis is typically associated with increased arterial blood flow to the epididymis in response to the acute inflammation. A urine culture should be obtained to help guide choice of antibiotic therapy, although empiric treatment should be administered prior to obtaining the final culture results. Scrotal support, bed rest, and topical application of ice packs can provide symptomatic relief.

Hydrocele

A hydrocele is caused by collection of fluid surrounding the testicle. It is usually associated with an anatomical defect of the layers of the tunica vaginalis. Diffuse scrotal enlargement is the most common presenting symptom, and this usually occurs gradually. Hydroceles are typically not painful unless there is an associated infection. In many cases, symptoms have been present for months or years before the patient seeks medical attention. Rapid development of hydrocele may be an indication of an underlying scrotal malignancy and appropriate clinical evaluation should be performed. With larger hydroceles, the volume of fluid surrounding the testicle may prevent palpation of the gonad. Positive transillumination of the scrotum is a clinical hallmark of the condition. Scrotal ultrasound may also be useful to establish the diagnosis.

Treatment is usually based on symptoms. Smaller asymptomatic hydroceles may be watched conservatively and often do not need additional therapy. Larger hydroceles can be bothersome for the patient and frequently interfere with walking or dressing. Although aspiration of the hydrocele fluid has been described, this is usually temporary and is associated with an increased risk of scrotal infection. Excision of the hydrocele is often effective and can be done with the patient receiving local or regional anesthetic on an outpatient basis.[56,57] Hydroceles are sometimes associated with an inguinal hernia, which may also require surgical repair.

Spermatocele

Another common cystic enlargement in the scrotum is a spermatocele. These can vary in size and are located adjacent to the testicle, which is usually palpably normal. Spermatoceles typically transilluminate, but differ from hydroceles by the lack of excess fluid surrounding the testis. Spermatoceles are more common in men who have undergone prior vasectomy for control of fertility. In most cases, spermatoceles are asymptomatic and require no additional therapy beyond education and reassurance. Excision is often performed for enlarging or painful spermatoceles.[55]

Varicocele

A varicocele is caused by dilation of the veins of the pampiniform plexus. Patients experience a swelling of the veins in the spermatic cord and may feel a sense of heaviness or fullness in the hemiscrotum. Varicoceles are often unilateral and are most common on the left. Approximately 15% of all adult males have some degree of varicocele. In younger men, varicoceles may be associated with infertility and impaired sperm quality. Many varicoceles are asymptomatic and they often develop over months or years. Rapid development of a varicocele or presence of an isolated right-sided varicocele should prompt clinical and radiographic evaluation for a possible retroperitoneal mass or renal tumor. Tumor thrombus into the vena cava from a renal cell carcinoma or venous obstruction from extrinsic compression by a pelvic mass may cause rapid development of a varicocele. Asymptomatic varicoceles in older adults do not require treatment. If the varicocele is large or painful, excision or radiographic embolization may be performed; however, the patient must be counseled that treatment might not improve symptoms of scrotal pain.

Testicular Torsion

Testicular torsion occurs when the testis rotates on its vascular axis, leading to arterial compromise. The onset of symptoms is usually sudden and includes pain and swelling of the associated hemiscrotum. Scrotal ultrasound with vascular Doppler imaging is useful to help establish the correct diagnosis. This condition is considered a urological emergency, and surgical intervention is indicated if the torsion cannot be manually reduced. Detorsion and fixation of the testis in the scrotum should be performed within 4 hours of the onset of symptoms to help improve clinical outcomes. If treatment is significantly delayed, the decreased arterial flow may result in tissue necrosis and loss of the testicle. Torsion of the testicle is rare in elderly men, and more often occurs in infants, children, and adolescents.

Scrotal Edema

Benign scrotal edema is a very common condition seen in older men, particularly in the acute hospital setting. Patients with vascular disease, hypertension, ascites, congestive heart failure, and pulmonary edema are at increased risk for developing scrotal edema. Excess fluid accumulates in the most dependent areas including the legs and feet, the presacral tissues, and the scrotum. The condition is usually painless. In some cases of severe scrotal swelling, urination may be difficult because of compression of the urethra and penis. This may require placement of a urinary catheter. Treatment typically involves conservative therapy with scrotal elevation and support, and ice packs if the patient has pain. Diuretics may be indicated to treat underlying conditions such as congestive heart failure or pulmonary edema. The scrotal swelling will typically resolve with time once the underlying cause has been adequately treated.

URETHRAL STRICTURES

Urethral strictures are scars that develop in the urethra that may lead to narrowing or even obliteration of the urethral lumen. Historically, sexually transmitted diseases (STDs) such as gonorrhea were a major cause of urethral stricture disease. They are now most often associated with a history of urethral or pelvic trauma. Traumatic urethral instrumentation increases the risk for development of a urethral stricture. In men who have undergone radical prostatectomy for prostate cancer or TURP) for BPH, scarring may develop at the junction between the urethra and bladder, leading to a bladder neck contracture. Urethral strictures are most often treated surgically; however, in some cases of mild strictures, urethral dilation may be adequate.[58] Urethral strictures are uncommon in women, and urethral dilation is not typically indicated unless an instrument cannot be passed easily during surgery. There are no data to support the routine use of urethral dilation in women for the treatment of voiding dysfunction.

BENIGN DISORDERS OF THE LOWER FEMALE URINARY TRACT

Urethral Caruncle

Urethral caruncles typically present as benign, polypoid lesions of the distal urethra and are most often seen in postmenopausal women. These are usually small lesions, although in some cases they can reach up to 1–2 cm in diameter. The etiology is unknown but may be related to urethral prolapse and chronic irritation associated with estrogen deficiency. In some patients the lesion may be painful or may bleed to the touch. Care must be taken to differentiate urethral caruncles, which are typically soft and mobile, from urethral carcinomas, which are typically firm or hard and more fixed in position. Excisional biopsy may be performed if there is a question about the histological composition. In most cases, urethral caruncles can be treated nonsurgically with warm Sitz baths and antiinflammatory medications. Topical estrogen can be quite useful and helps to shrink the lesions. Complete resolution may be observed with continued estrogen application. Excision is indicated if more conservative therapy is ineffective.[59]

Urethral Diverticulum

A urethral diverticulum is an outpouching of the anterior urethra in women that may be associated with significant lower urinary tract symptoms. The classic clinical triad includes dysuria, dyspareunia, and postvoid dribbling. Although the exact etiology is unknown, theories include obstruction of paraurethral ducts with development of an inclusion cyst in the wall of the urethra. Subsequent spontaneous drainage of the cyst cavity into the urethral lumen leads to development of an epithelialized tract between the diverticulum and the urethra. Congenital abnormalities can also lead to a thinning of the anterior urethral wall, which in turn could cause development of an opening between the diverticular space and the urethra. Physical examination usually reveals a soft tissue bulge in the suburethral area in the vagina. These are often tender to palpation because of the trapping of infected urine or sediment in the diverticular sac. Radiographic examination with voiding cystourethrography or pelvic magnetic resonance imaging may be helpful to establish the correct diagnosis. Excision including removal of the entire diverticular sac is indicated for symptomatic diverticula.[59] In some cases, the diverticular sac may be quite close to the external urethral sphincter, and care must be taken not to injure this structure during surgery because this could lead to urinary incontinence. If the opening to the diverticulum is small, the urethra may be repaired primarily; however, a vascularized pedicle flap may be necessary to repair larger defects in the anterior urethra.

Genitourinary Fistulae

A fistula is defined as a connection between two hollow organs or between a hollow organ and the skin. Fistulae can occur in the genitourinary tract in older adults, often resulting from other underlying conditions or after treatment for these conditions. The most common types of fistulae involving the urinary system in older women include vesicovaginal fistulae between the bladder and vagina and vesicoenteric fistulae between the bladder and bowel. In developed countries, most vesicovaginal fistulae are iatrogenic and related to prior pelvic surgery such as hysterectomy. Colonic diverticular disease leads to an increased risk of vesicocolonic fistulae. Inflammatory bowel disorders such as Crohn's disease increase the risk of fistulae between the bladder and small intestine. Other risk factors for development of fistula include prior pelvic surgery or radiation or a history of pelvic malignancy. With a vesicovaginal fistula, women typically experience continuous urinary leakage from the vaginal vault. Chronic UTI with enteric bacteria is the most common problem associated with vesicoenteric or vesicocolonic fistulae. These associated symptoms may have a strong negative influence on quality of life. Evaluation includes identification of the type and location of the fistula tract by using physical examination, endoscopy, and imaging. Treatment is most often surgical with excision of the fistula tract and repair of the effected organs.[61]

Atrophic Vaginitis

In postmenopausal women, the decrease in vaginal estrogen levels may be associated with tissue changes in the vaginal mucosa. The most common condition is atrophic vaginitis, which may involve variable degrees of tissue inflammation. On clinical examination, the tissue appears pale and thin with loss of natural rogations. Patients may experience pelvic pain or dryness. Women who are sexually active may complain of dyspareunia. Unless contraindicated by a history of breast or uterine cancer, topical estrogen replacement is indicated to help reduce symptoms.

Pelvic Organ Prolapse

Various forms of pelvic organ prolapse are common in elderly women. Loss of anterior pelvic floor support results in a protrusion of the bladder into the vaginal vault, which is referred to as a cystocele. A rectocele occurs if the posterior aspect of the vaginal wall is involved. In an enterocele, the apex of the vaginal vault is prolapsed. These entities may occur alone or in combination. Pessaries can be used to reduce the prolapse and provide a nonsurgical form of therapy for some patients. In some cases, surgical repair may be indicated. Additional information on pelvic organ prolapse is provided in Chapter 27 on gynecological disorders in elderly women.

SEXUAL HEALTH

Assessment and treatment of sexual disorders is an important part of health care for many older adults. Several comorbid conditions that are common in older adults can have significant negative influence on sexual health including diabetes, hypertension, heart disease, and vascular insufficiency. Urinary incontinence can negatively influence sexual activity in both men and women.[62,63]

STDs can occur in older adults, and patients with clinical symptoms or those who are at risk should be screened for STDs as indicated.[64] Older adults have generally not been targeted in public health campaigns for prevention of STDs including human immunodeficiency virus (HIV). This is changing, however, and there is an increased awareness that older adults may need education for prevention and treatment of STDs. Some clinical trials are also now focusing on therapy for STDs and HIV in older adults.[65] Issues related to sexual health are discussed in more detail in Chapter 55.

CONCLUSION

A wide variety of urological conditions occur in older adults. Because of associated symptoms such as urinary incontinence, infection, or pain, these may have a significant negative influence on activities and health-related quality of life. Appropriate evaluation and treatment are important for effective management. Successful treatment may lead to reduction or elimination of symptoms and significant improvements in quality of life for elderly patients.[66]

REFERENCES

1. Ambulatory Visits to Physicians By Specialty, Patients 65 years or Older (as a percent of all visits to each specialty) 1999–2004. Status of Geriatrics Workforce Study: Documenting the Development of Geriatric Medicine, Tables 1.16–1.16b, 2006. Cincinnati, OH: Association of Directors of Geriatric Academic Programs. Available at: http://www.adgapstudy.uc.edu/Figures.cfm. Accessed June 3, 2008.
2. Grossfeld DG, Wolf JS Jr., Litwin MS, et al. Asymptomatic microscopic hematuria in adults: summary of the AUA Best Practice Policy recommendations. *Am Fam Physician.* 2001;63:1145–1154.
3. Lang EK, Macchia RJ, Thomas R, et al. Improved detection of renal pathologic features on multiphasic helical CT compared with IVU in patients presenting with microscopic hematuria. *Urology.* 2003;61:528–532.
4. Polito M, Giannubilo W, a'Anzeo G, et al. Hematospermia: diagnosis and treatment. *Arch Ital Urol Androl.* 2006;78:82–85.
5. Griebling TL. Urologic Diseases in America Project: trends in resource use for urinary tract infections in women. *J Urol.* 2005;173:1281–1287.
6. Griebling TL. Urologic Diseases in America Project: trends in resource use for urinary tract infections in men. *J Urol.* 2005;173:1288–1294.
7. Richards CL. Urinary tract infections in the frail elderly: issues for diagnosis, treatment and prevention. *Int Urol Nephrol.* 2004;36:457–463.
8. Tal S, Guller V, Levi S, et al. Profile and prognosis of febrile elderly patients with bacteremic urinary tract infection. *J Infect.* 2005;50:296–305.
9. Rodhe N, Mölstad S, Englund L, et al. Asymptomatic bacteriuria in a population of elderly residents living in a community setting: prevalence, characteristics and associated factors. *Fam Pract.* 2006;23:303–307.
10. Ginde AA, Rhee SH, Katz ED. Predictors of outcome in geriatric patients with urinary tract infections. *J Emerg Med.* 2004;27:101–108.
11. Dromerick AW, Edwards DF. Relation of postvoid residual to urinary tract infection during stroke rehabilitation. *Arch Phys Med Rehabil.* 2003;84:1369–1372.
12. Paillaud E, Herbaud S, Caillet P, et al. Relations between undernutrition and nosocomial infections in elderly patients. *Age Ageing.* 2005;34:619–625.
13. Hazelett SE, Tsai M, Gareri M, Allen K. The association between indwelling urinary catheter use in the elderly and urinary tract infection in acute care. *BMC Geriatr.* 2006;6:15.
14. Henig YS, Leahy MM. Cranberry juice and urinary-tract health: science supports folklore. *Nutrition.* 2000;16:684–687.

15. Pilloni S, Krhut J, Mair D, Madersbacher H, Kessler TM. Intermittent catheterization in older people: a valuable alternative to an indwelling catheter? *Age Ageing.* 2005;34:57–60.

16. Pearle MS, Calhoun EA, Curhan GC, et al. Urologic Diseases in America Project: urolithiasis. *J Urol.* 2005;173:848–857.

17. Daudon M, Doré JC, Jungers P, et al. Changes in stone composition according to age and gender of patients: a multivariate epidemiological approach. *Urol Res.* 2004;32:241–247.

18. Pak CY, Sakhaee K, Moe O, et al. Biochemical profile of stone-forming patients with diabetes mellitus. *Urology.* 2003;61:523–527.

19. Usui Y, Matsuzaki S, Matsushita K, et al. Urolithiasis in geriatric patients. *Tokai J Exp Clin Med.* 2003;28:81–87.

20. Ahmedin J, Siegel R, Ward E, et al. Cancer statistics, 2008. *CA Cancer J Clin.* 2008;58:71–96.

21. Thompson I, Thrasher JB, et al. eds. Guideline for the Management of Clinically Localized Prostate Cancer: 2007 Update. Baltimore: American Urological Association, Education and Research Inc.; 2007. www.usrf.org/CaP%20Guidelines,%20AUA,%202007.pdf.

22. Walter LC, Bertenthal D, Lindquist K, Konety BR. PSA screening among elderly men with limited life expectancies. *JAMA.* 2006;296:2336–2342.

23. Chang SS, Alberts G, Cookson MS, Smith JA Jr. Radical cystectomy is safe in elderly patients at high risk. *J Urol.* 2001;166:938–941.

24. Deliveliotis C, Papatsoris A, Chrisofos M, Dellis A, Liakouras C, Skolarikos A. Urinary diversion in high-risk elderly patients: modified cutaneous ureterostomy or ileal conduit? *Urology.* 2005;66:299–304.

25. Purdue MP, Devesa SS, Sigurdson AJ, et al. International patterns and trends in testis cancer incidence. *Int J Cancer.* 2005;115:822–827.

26. Fonseca R, Habermann TM, Colgan JP, et al. Testicular lymphoma is associated with a high incidence of extranodal recurrence. *Cancer.* 2000;88:154–161.

27. Fitzpatrick JM. The natural history of benign prostatic hyperplasia. *BJU Int.* 2006;97(Suppl 2):3–6.

28. Weiss JP. Nocturia: 'Do the math.' *J Urol.* 2006;175:S16–S18.

29. Bruskewitz RC. Quality of life and sexual function in patients with benign prostatic hyperplasia. *Rev Urol.* 2003;5:72–80.

30. DuBeau CE. The aging lower urinary tract. *J Urol.* 2006;175:S11–S15.

31. Saigal CS. Quality indicators for benign prostatic hyperplasia in vulnerable elders. *J Amer Geriatr Soc.* 2007;55:S253–S257.

32. Resnick MI, Roehrborn CG. Rapid onset of action with alfuzosin 10 mg once daily in men with benign prostatic hyperplasia: a randomized, placebo-controlled trial. *Prostate Cancer Prostatic Dis.* 2007;10:155–159.

33. Giuliano F. Impact of medical treatments for benign prostatic hyperplasia on sexual function. *BJU Int.* 2006;97(Suppl 2):34–38.

34. van Dijk MM, de la Rosette JJ, Michel MC. Effects of alpha(1)-adrenoceptor antagonists on male sexual function. *Drugs.* 2006;66:287–301.

35. Srinivasan S, Radomski S, Chung J, Plazker T, Singer S, Slomovic AR. Intraoperative floppy-iris syndrome during cataract surgery in men using alpha-blockers for benign prostatic hyperplasia. *J Cataract Refract Surg.* 2007;33:1826–1827.

36. Roehrborn CG, Bruskewitz R, Nickel JC, et al. Sustained decrease in incidence of acute urinary retention and surgery with finasteride for 6 years in men with benign prostatic hyperplasia. *J Urol.* 2004;171:1194–1198.

37. Roehrborn CG, Siami P, Barkin J, et al. The effects of dutasteride, tamsulosin and combination therapy in lower urinary tract symptoms in men with benign prostatic hyperplasia and prostatic enlargement: 2-year results from the CombAT Study. *J Urol.* 2008;616–621.

38. Logan YT, Belgeri MT. Monotherapy versus combination drug therapy for the treatment of benign prostatic hyperplasia. *Am J Geriatr Pharm.* 2005;3:103–114.

39. Tamler R, Mechanick JI. Dietary supplements and nutraceuticals in the management of andrologic disorders. *Endocrinol Metabol Clin N Am.* 2007;36(2):533–552.

40. Marks LS, Roehrborn CG, Andriole GL. Prevention of benign prostatic hyperplasia disease. *J Urol.* 2006;176:1299–1306.

41. Hoffman RM, Monga M, Elliot SP, MacDonald R, Wilt TJ. Microwave thermotherapy for benign prostatic hyperplasia. *Cochrane Database Syst Rev.* 2007;17:CD004135.

42. Hoffman RM, MacDonald R, Monga M, Wilt TJ. Transurethral microwave thermotherapy vs. transurethral resection for treating benign prostatic hyperplasia: a systematic review. *BJU Int.* 2004;94:1031–1036.

43. Masood S, Djaladat H, Kouriefs C, Keen M, Palmer JH. The 12-year outcome analysis of an endourethral wallstent for treating benign prostatic hyperplasia. *BJU Int.* 2004;94:1271–1274.

44. Ogiste JS, Cooper K, Kaplan SA. Are stents still a useful therapy for benign prostatic hyperplasia? *Curr Opin Urol.* 2003;13:51–57.

45. Krieger JN, Riley DE, Cheah PY, Liong ML, Yuen KH. Epidemiology of prostatitis: new evidence for a world-wide problem. *World J Urol.* 2003;21:70–74.

46. Nickel JC, Teichman JMH, Gregore M, Clark J, Downey J. Prevalence, diagnosis, characterization, and treatment of prostatitis, interstitial cystitis, and epididymitis in outpatient urologic practice: the Canadian PIE Study. *Urology.* 2005;66:935–940.

47. Pontari MA. Chronic prostatitis/chronic pelvic pain syndrome in elderly men: toward better understanding and treatment. *Drugs Aging.* 2003;20:1111–1125.

48. Pontari MA, Joyce GF, Wise M, et al. Prostatitis. *J Urol.* 2007;177:2050–2057.

49. Aynaud O, Piron D, Casanova JM. Incidence of preputial lichen sclerosus in adults: histologic study of circumcision specimens. *J Am Acad Dermatol.* 1999;41:923–296.

50. Pietrzak P, Hadway P, Corbishley CM, Watkin NA. Is the association between balanitis xerotica obliterans and penile carcinoma underestimated? *BJU Int.* 2006;98:74–76.

51. Williams JC, Morrison PM, Richardson JR. Paraphimosis in elderly men. *Am J Emerg Med.* 1995;13:351–353.

52. Mulhall JP, Creech SE, Boorjian SA, et al. Subjective and objective analysis of the prevalence of Peyronie's disease in a population of men presenting for prostate cancer screening. *J Urol.* 2004;171:2350–2353.

53. El-Sakka AI. Prevalence of Peyronie's disease among patients with erectile dysfunction. *Eur Urol.* 2006;49:564–569.

54. Bjekic MD, Vlajinac HD, Sipetic SB, Marinkovic JM. Risk factors for Peyronie's disease: a case-control study. *BJU Int.* 2006;97:570–574.

55. Cavallini G. Towards an evidence-based understanding of Peyronie's disease. *Int J STD AIDS.* 2005;16:187–195.

56. Kiddoo DA, Wollin TA, Mador DR. A population based assessment of complications following outpatient hydrocelectomy and spermatocelectomy. *J Urol.* 2004;171:746–748.

57. Menon VS, Sheridan WG. Benign scrotal pathology: should all patients undergo surgery? *BJU Int.* 2001;88:251–254.

58. Barbagli G, Palminteri E, Lazzeri M, Guazzoni G, Turini D. Long-term outcomes of urethroplasty after failed urethrotomy versus primary repair. *J Urol.* 2001;165:1918–1919.

59. Park DS, Cho TW. Simple solution for urethral caruncle. *J Urol.* 2004;172:1884–1885.

60. Ljungqvist L, Peeker R, Fall M. Female urethral diverticulum: 26-year followup of a large series. *J Urol.* 2007;177:219–224.

61. Flores-Carreras O, Cabrera JR, Galeano PA, Torres FE. Fistulas of the urinary tract in gynecologic and obstetric surgery. *Int Urogynecol J.* 2001;12:203–214.

62. Tannenbaum C, Corcos J, Assalian P. The relationship between sexual activity and urinary incontinence in older women. *J Am Geriatr Soc.* 2006;54:1220–1224.

63. Griebling TL. The impact of urinary incontinence on sexual health in older adults. *J Am Geriatr Soc.* 2006;54:1290–1292.

64. Wilson MM. Sexually transmitted diseases. *Clin Geriatr Med.* 2003;19:637–655.

65. Nogueras M, Navarro G, Antón E, et al. Epidemiological and clinical features, response to HAART, and survival in HIV-infected patients diagnosed at the age of 50 or more. *BMC Infect Dis.* 2006;6:159.

66. Gerharz EW, Emberton M. Quality of life research in urology. *World J Urol.* 1999;17:191–192.

26

URINARY INCONTINENCE

Jan Busby-Whitehead, MD, Mary H. Palmer, PhD, RN-C, FAAN,
Theodore N. Johnson, MD, MPH

Urinary incontinence (UI), the involuntary loss of urine, has a prevalence of 25%–45% in women.[1] Only approximately 34% of incontinent women have UI to such a degree that they viewed it as a significant bother.[2] Frequent or severe UI can have a devastating impact on people's lives, leading to social withdrawal and depression and contributing to the decision to go into a nursing home.[3] Leaking small amounts can often be managed by wearing pads and has only a modest impact on quality of life. UI is approximately half as common in men compared with women.[1]

UI prevalence increases with age as shown in Figure 26.1. At the age of 60 years approximately 14.8% of women have moderate-to-severe incontinence, but this increases to 20.2% by 70 years and to 27.5% by 85 years.[2] The loss of continence will not always occur with aging. Many specific age-related changes, such as functional impairments in mobility, dexterity, cognition, and reduction in bladder capacity, contribute to UI. Other established risk factors that are not age-related include obesity and parity. The strongest single risk factor in men other than age is prostatectomy or transurethral resection.[2]

An estimated 60% of people with UI who are identified through surveys have not reported their UI to a health care provider,[4] perhaps because they are embarrassed or believe nothing can be done to help.[5] This is unfortunate, because UI is curable in many and can be managed in most cases.[6] Health care providers, therefore, should specifically ask about incontinence.

PHYSIOLOGICAL MECHANISM FOR CONTINENCE AND MICTURITION

Innervation of the lower urinary system is under cholinergic, adrenergic, and somatic control. The early phase of bladder accommodation is mediated by β-adrenergic receptors in the bladder dome. Bladder contraction is mediated by cholinergic (parasympathetic) activity, whereas relaxation of the internal and external sphincters is mediated by adrenergic (sympathetic) pathways in the pudendal nerve via a spinal reflex mediated by the S2–S4 sacral nerve roots. Normal bladder capacity is 300–600 mL.

Central nervous system control of bladder and sphincter function is mostly inhibitory, that is, reflex bladder contractions are actively inhibited until a socially appropriate time and place to urinate is found. This inhibition occurs through neural linkages from the sensorimotor cortex of the frontal lobes to the brainstem, cerebellum, thalamus, and spinal cord. Micturition normally involves a conscious disinhibition of bladder contractions. Thus, stroke and other neurological processes can result in UI because of loss of central cortical inhibition. Excessive bladder filling may overcome higher cortical inhibitory inputs, resulting in the involuntary contraction of the bladder via the reflex arc (referred to as uninhibited bladder contractions).

The urethra is composed of internal (smooth muscle) and external (striated muscle) sphincters. Somatic innervation through the pudendal nerve allows voluntary contraction of the external sphincter and pelvic floor musculature that protects against urine loss from sudden increases in abdominal pressure. Voluntary contraction of the external urethral muscle also reflexly inhibits bladder contraction and can interrupt voiding.

Continence depends on voluntary inhibition of reflex bladder contraction and intermittent, as needed, voluntary contraction of the striated pelvic floor muscles to counter increases in intraabdominal pressure or escape contractions of the bladder. Micturition requires voluntary disinhibition of bladder contractions, which reflexly leads to relaxation of both the internal and external urethral sphincters.

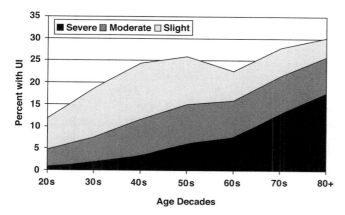

Figure 26.1. Prevalence and severity of UI by age (adapted from EPINCOT).

CLASSIFICATION

Transient incontinence is defined as new leaking of sudden onset that is generally associated with an acute medical or surgical illness or drug therapy, and it is usually reversible with resolution of the underlying problem. Functional incontinence is another term that has been used for this condition. Causes of transient incontinence are diverse (Table 26.1). Drug side effects contribute greatly to this problem, therefore, a review of prescription and over-the-counter medications is extremely important.

Established incontinence is usually chronic, requires investigation, and is amenable to treatment in many cases. There are four types of established incontinence: stress, urge, mixed incontinence, and overflow (also termed chronic urinary retention and incontinence with a high postvoid residual).

URGE INCONTINENCE

Urge incontinence results from unsuppressed bladder contractions (detrusor instability). These uninhibited contractions are associated with an irresistible urge to void and usually result in loss of a large volume (>100 mL). Patients with urge incontinence may also have symptoms of urgency, frequent urination, and nocturia, which is called overactive bladder (OAB). By definition, to have OAB, one must have urinary urgency without a urinary tract infection (UTI).

Reversible causes of urge incontinence include UTI, radiotherapy or chemotherapy, fecal impaction, and bladder outlet obstruction from an enlarged prostate. Special categories of urge incontinence merit comment. Detrusor hyperreflexia is a term describing unsuppressed bladder contractions associated with a neurological disorder. Any damage to the structural integrity of the cholinergic inhibitory center of the central nervous system, or the afferent innervation from the lower spinal cord where the reflex arc is located, can cause detrusor hyperreflexia. Processes such as Alzheimer's disease, cerebro-

Table 26.1. Identification of Reversible Conditions that may Cause or Contribute to Urinary Incontinence

- Conditions affecting the lower urinary tract
  - Urinary tract infection (symptomatic with frequency, urgency, dysuria)
  - Atrophic vaginitis or urethritis
  - Prostatectomy
  - Stool impaction
- Drug side effects
  - Diuretics: polyuria, frequency, urgency
  - Caffeine: aggravation or precipitation of UI
  - Anticholinergic agents: urinary retention, overflow incontinence
  - Stool impaction
  - Psychotropic medications
    - Antidepressants: anticholinergic actions, sedation
    - Antipsychotics: anticholinergic actions, sedation, immobility, rigidity
    - Sedatives, hypnotics, CNS depressants: sedation, delirium, immobility, muscle relaxation
  - Opioid analgesics: urinary retention, fecal impaction, sedation, delirium
  - α-Adrenergic blockers: urethral relaxation
  - α-Adrenergic agonists: urinary retention (found in many cold and diet over-the-counter preparations)
  - β3-Adrenergic agonists: urinary retention
  - Calcium channel blockers: urinary retention
  - Alcohol: polyuria, frequency, urgency, sedation, delirium, immobility
- Increased urine production
  - Metabolic disorders (hyperglycemia, hypercalcemia)
  - Excess fluid intake
  - Volume overload
  - Venous insufficiency with edema
  - Congestive heart failure
- Impaired ability or willingness to reach the toilet
  - Delirium
  - Chronic illness, injury; restraint that interferes with mobility
  - Psychological disorders

Modified from Fantl et al.[6] CNS, central nervous system.

vascular atherosclerosis, multiple sclerosis, Parkinson's disease, spinal cord tumors or transection, and cervical spondylosis (among others) may result in incontinence by this mechanism.[6]

OVERFLOW INCONTINENCE (BLADDER OUTLET OBSTRUCTION AND ATONIC BLADDER)

Bladder outlet obstruction is more common in men than women and it occurs primarily because of benign prostatic hypertrophy (BPH), prostatic neoplasm, or urethral stricture. BPH may result in lower urinary tract symptoms such as frequency, urgency, nocturia, hesitancy, or weak urinary stream. In women, urethral stricture or severe bladder prolapse may also impede urine flow. In both men and women, partial obstruction may become complete obstruction with the use of anticholinergic or α agonist pharmacological agents, or with severe constipation. Atonic and neurogenic bladder are terms describing impaired bladder contractions resulting from low spinal cord lesions, diabetic or alcoholic neuropathy, and/or intake of muscle relaxants, opioids, or antidepressants. The usual clinical presentation of bladder outlet obstruction or atonic bladder is constant dribbling or leaking associated with an enlarged, palpable bladder. The physical examination finding of a grossly enlarged bladder is very specific, but poorly sensitive for establishing the diagnosis of outlet obstruction. Patients generally strain to urinate, and voluntarily and involuntarily voided urine volumes are frequently small.

STRESS INCONTINENCE

Stress incontinence occurs in women more than men and results from a hypermobile urethra, internal sphincter insufficiency, or reduced support by the pelvic floor musculature in the bladder outlet. Multiple childbirths, gynecological surgery, and decreased effects of estrogen on pelvic tissues, vasculature, and urethral mucosa are possible causes. Sphincter weakness may also be the result of urethral inflammation, neurological disease, radiation therapy, or α-blocker drugs such as prazosin or methyldopa. In men, stress incontinence may occur following prostatectomy. Patients are likely to complain of losing small amounts of urine with coughing, straining, lifting, or changing posture. Although this history is highly sensitive, it is only moderately specific, and many patients with these symptoms do not have stress incontinence.[8] Some men following prostatectomy will have constant urinary dribbling.

EVALUATION

Evaluation should begin with a detailed history of the nature, severity, and burden of UI and identifying the most easily remedied contributing causes. An incontinence diary filled out before the patient's visit is helpful. A history of leakage occurring immediately following coughing, laughing, or posture change suggests stress incontinence.[9] An inability to stop urine flow voluntarily suggests the inability to identify properly and use these muscles or pelvic floor muscle weakness. A low mental status screening examination suggests dementia, which may be associated with detrusor instability, indifference to the symptoms, or both.

Classic symptoms of urge incontinence are urine loss with hand washing, hearing running water, or while rushing to the bathroom; these are insensitive and nonspecific.[9] Dysuria and frequency may indicate infection. A decrease in force of the urine stream and straining with urination suggest obstruction or impaired bladder contractility. Important items of the medical history include data about childbirth, pelvic surgery, cancer, neurological disease, diabetes mellitus, congestive heart failure, and previous treatment of UI. Specific questions should be asked about prescription and over-the-counter medication use, alcohol use, and fluid intake. Inquiries should be made about the physical layout of the patient's residence and whether impaired mobility limits access to toilet facilities. The patient should bring a bag containing all prescription and nonprescription drugs to the clinic so that medications that may contribute to incontinence can be identified.

The physical examination should focus on the abdomen and urogenital area and the central and peripheral nervous systems. The abdominal examination is insensitive for a high postvoid residual (PVR) or in chronic urinary retention, but gross bladder distention (for example, >500 mL) can usually be detected. In acute urinary retention, the distended bladder is a firm, midline mass that originates from the pelvis and is dull to percussion. The rectal examination may reveal fecal impaction, a pelvic mass, or an enlarged prostate gland. The size of the prostate does not correlate well with obstruction.[10] It is very important to assess perianal sensation and the patient's ability to contract and relax the anal sphincter voluntarily. An abnormal clinical sign can suggest serious lumbosacral disease, possibly requiring emergency treatment. In women, a pelvic examination is indicated to assess urethral, uterine, or bladder prolapse and to evaluate the patient for any pelvic mass. A gray, dry vaginal mucosa is suggestive of atrophic vaginitis.

The most important diagnostic distinction is between overflow incontinence and the other types of UI. Most studies show a poor correlation between the underlying cause and the patient's symptoms. Incontinence from several causes (mixed incontinence) in many older people limits the usefulness of evaluation algorithms based on symptoms and signs alone.[11]

DIAGNOSTIC TESTS

Selected tests are recommended for the evaluation of incontinent patients. On initial evaluation, a urinalysis and/or a urine culture, if indicated, should be done. Properly collected clean catch urine is adequate for culture even for nursing home residents,[12] although some persons will require an in-and-out catheterization to obtain an appropriate specimen. Although an unlikely, yet serious, cause of new incontinence is bladder carcinoma, urine cytology is not recommended in the routine evaluation of the incontinent patient as a screening test.[13] A workup is indicated for older patients with even transient hematuria, as the risk of malignancy is appreciable if there is no indication of glomerular bleeding. Older patients should generally undergo ultrasonography or helical computed tomography scanning of the lower and upper urinary tract, and urine cytology should be obtained. If these tests are negative, cystoscopy is recommended for those at risk for bladder cancer.[14]

Tests for blood urea nitrogen, creatinine, glucose, and calcium are recommended if compromised renal function or polyuria is suspected in patients not taking diuretics.[6] The PVR urine volume should be measured in all patients with symptoms of incontinence. This can be done by inserting, in sterile fashion, a No.14 French straight catheter into the bladder. Caution is indicated for patients with outflow obstruction, as a single catheterization may cause infection. Alternatively, a bladder ultrasound scan may be obtained 5–10 minutes after the patient has voided. The portable ultrasound scan has been shown to be highly reliable, especially at low and very high bladder volumes. Although the definition of a high PVR is controversial, a volume of 200 mL or more suggests either outlet obstruction or atonic bladder, and is an indication for further urological evaluation.[15]

Clinical tests for stress incontinence in women are useful and highly specific.[16] With a full bladder and, optimally, wearing a preweighed pad, the patient should cough, laugh, or strain to induce urine leakage. The patient then removes the pad, voids, the urine volume is measured, and the pad is weighed. This test should be repeated if the urine volume in the pad and pan is less than 200 mL.

FORMAL URODYNAMIC TESTING

After the basic evaluation, treatment for the presumed type of incontinence should be initiated, unless there is need for further evaluation.[6] Further evaluation is indicated for the following: failure of initial treatment, a history of surgery or radiotherapy, frequent UTIs, marked prolapse on physical examination, severe hesitancy, PVR greater than 200 mL, inability to pass a catheter, or persistent hematuria.[17] Common urodynamic tests that provide more detailed diagnostic information include urine flowmetry, voiding cystourethrography, multichannel cystometrogram, pressure-flow study, urethral pressure profile measurement, and sphincter electromyography.[6] A urologist, gynecologist, or less commonly, a geriatrician trained in pelvic floor disorders generally performs these tests.

TREATMENT

Accurate diagnosis of UI is essential for appropriate treatment. Any cause of transient incontinence identified during evaluation should be addressed specifically. Behavioral, pharmacological, and surgical therapies are all effective in older people. It is generally advisable to begin a treatment regimen with the least risk and burden to the patient and caregiver. In all types of incontinence, except those characterized by obstruction or poor

bladder contractility, behavioral techniques should be considered as first-line therapy unless the patient has a specific preference for another type of therapy.[6]

Management of UI in long-term care settings differs from management in the ambulatory care setting for two principal reasons. First, comorbidities such as dementia and mobility impairment are more frequent and more severe in the long-term care setting and these complicate the management of UI. Second, in the outpatient setting, behavioral interventions can be implemented by the patients themselves or by highly motivated caregivers who are usually family members. In long-term care, these interventions are implemented by nursing assistants whose motivation may be compromised by high patient-to-staff ratios. For these reasons, treatment of UI in the long-term care setting is discussed separately.

AMBULATORY CARE TREATMENT OF UI

Successful treatment of functional incontinence relies on the recognition that physical, pharmacological, psychological, and environmental problems coexist that can cause or worsen UI. Providing the patient with assistive devices such as a urinal or bedside commode; reassessing drug indications, doses, and schedules; treating depression; addressing hostility; eliminating barriers in the path to the toilet; and removing restraints may improve incontinence dramatically. A visit to the patient's home by a visiting nurse and discussion with family members can be very helpful in identifying barriers to continence and implementing simple changes that improve continence. Treatments that are specific to each type of UI are discussed as follows.

URGE INCONTINENCE

The treatment of urge incontinence entails designing interventions to decrease or block uninhibited bladder contractions, improve bladder capacity, and prolong the time from symptoms of urgency to voiding. Effective strategies include 1) dietary and lifestyle changes, 2) behavioral training (timed-voiding), and 3) drugs to reduce bladder contractions.

Dietary Management

Self-monitoring techniques such as reducing caffeine and alcohol intake, management of constipation, and drinking an adequate intake of fluids throughout the day, but decreasing fluid intake close to bedtime, have been shown to be helpful in reducing UI in women.[18]

Behavioral Treatment

The primary behavioral treatment for urge incontinence or OAB is timed voiding. The rationale for this treatment is that patients with urge incontinence may void too frequently and may gradually develop an intolerance for bladder filling. The treatment is to instruct the patient to void at fixed, short intervals such as every 30 minutes and to increase gradually the duration of the interval to 2–3 hours. Patients are encouraged to resist the urge to void between these intervals. Timed voiding may be combined with pelvic floor muscle exercises to strengthen the pelvic floor muscles, and patients may be taught "the knack," which consists of contracting the pelvic floor muscles when they experience an urge to void to reflexly inhibit bladder contractions.[19] A typical regimen for pelvic muscle exercises is described later under treatments for stress incontinence.

Another behavioral technique for urge UI is biofeedback, in which pressure sensors are placed in the bladder, rectum, and urethra to record contractions. The goals of biofeedback training are 1) to teach appropriate pelvic floor muscle contractions and 2) to teach the patient to inhibit bladder contractions voluntarily. Many patients are not able to learn appropriate pelvic floor exercise techniques without biofeedback, or they require repeated verbal guidance to obtain any improvement in continence. In one study, only 50% of patients who had a single, simple verbal instruction in pelvic floor muscle exercises were able to perform the technique properly.[20] Bladder–sphincter biofeedback methods in which vaginal, rectal, and urethral pressures and myoelectrical activity are displayed to assist the patient in learning to relax the bladder and contract pelvic floor muscles, enable patients to learn these techniques more quickly. Biofeedback requires insertion of sensors and the services of a specially trained therapist. Biofeedback in conjunction with bladder retraining has been shown to be effective in teaching voluntary inhibition of bladder contractions to selected patients, achieving 50% or greater improvement in continence.[19] This approach is most useful for patients who are mobile and who have minimal cognitive impairment.

Pharmacological Therapy

Anticholinergic agents are the mainstay of therapy for patients with urge and mixed incontinence. Oxybutynin is a first-line agent that has both anticholinergic and smooth muscle relaxant properties. Studies with the immediate release (IR) formulation have shown a 15%–58% greater reduction in urge UI compared with placebo. The extended release (ER) and transdermal (TD) formulations have similar efficacy. The initial dosage for IR demonstrated to be effective in clinical trials is 2.5–5 mg three times a day, although some elderly patients benefit from only 2.5 mg daily. The initial dosage for the ER formulation is 5 mg daily and can be titrated up to 30 mg daily. The 3.8-mg TD patch is applied twice weekly. Up to 50% of patients in clinical trials of the IR medication had side effects such as dry mouth and constipation that limited therapy. The ER and TD formulations are associated with a lower rate of dry mouth. Narrow-angle glaucoma and urinary retention are contraindications for treatment with oxybutynin.

Tolterodine, a muscarinic receptor antagonist, was found to be as effective as oxybutynin in double-blind studies, but it had a lower incidence and decreased severity of the side effect of dry mouth. As with oxybutynin, tolterodine should not be used in patients with narrow-angle glaucoma or urinary retention. Several case reports note cognitive side effects similar to dementia with tolterodine use.[21]

Trospium is a nonselective muscarinic receptor antagonist metabolized in the kidneys that was approved by the FDA in 2004 for treatment of the OAB symptom complex of urgency, frequency, and incontinence. The dose for older persons and those with renal impairment is 20 mg daily. Trospium must be taken on an empty stomach.

Solifenacin and darifenacin are more selective muscarinic receptor (M3) antagonists. These drugs were also approved by the FDA in 2004 for treatment of OAB symptoms. Initial dosage of solifenacin is 5 mg, which may be titrated to 10 mg, and the dose of darifenacin is 7.5–15 mg daily. Studies have not shown these drugs to be associated with a clear increase in efficacy or decrease in side effects compared with other anticholinergic drugs such as tolterodine.

For all older patients taking anticholinergic drugs, PVRs should be monitored to identify urinary retention that causes worsening of incontinence. In these cases, the drug dose should be reduced, and in severe cases, discontinued.

Other drugs observed in clinical trials to be beneficial include dicyclomine hydrochloride, propantheline, and tricyclic antidepressants, such as imipramine, doxepin, desipramine, and nortriptyline. Use of these medications is generally limited by side effects, and they are not recommended as first-line therapy.

Recently, new surgical approaches have been developed for urge incontinence that remains unresponsive to medical and behavioral treatment. Discussion of these treatments is beyond the scope of this chapter.

STRESS INCONTINENCE (SPHINCTER INSUFFICIENCY/PELVIC FLOOR MUSCLE WEAKNESS)

Behavioral Treatment

The rationale behind behavioral treatments for stress incontinence is that this type of incontinence results from transient increases of bladder pressure above urethral pressure, which can be corrected by strengthening the external urethral sphincter muscle so that urethral sphincter pressure is higher or by elevating the bladder neck. The simplest and least costly behavioral technique is referred to as pelvic floor muscle exercises or Kegel exercises. These are often taught verbally by instructing patients to squeeze the pelvic floor muscles as if they are holding back urine or holding back a bowel movement but to keep their abdominal wall muscles relaxed (i.e., to avoid inappropriate increases in intraabdominal pressure that may increase the likelihood of stress incontinence). These instructions may include the suggestion that patients place a hand on the abdomen to detect abdominal wall contraction or that they continue to breathe while squeezing pelvic floor muscles. Patients are instructed to squeeze pelvic floor muscles and hold a maximum squeeze for 3–10 seconds, with l0-second rest periods in between squeezes. They are told to perform 20–30 squeezes, three–five times a day for at least 8 weeks.[6] One study reported improvement in incontinence symptoms in 54% and cure in 16% of elderly women.[22]

The initial instruction in pelvic floor muscle exercises should be done during a digital rectal or pelvic examination: With the examining finger in the anal canal or vagina, the therapist instructs the patient to squeeze the pelvic floor muscles and provides verbal feedback on whether she is squeezing correctly. The examiner can also hold a hand on the abdominus rectus muscles to detect inappropriate contractions. Biofeedback may also be used to teach pelvic floor muscle exercises in the treatment of stress UI. Although this may be helpful to many patients, studies have generally shown no significant difference in efficacy between biofeedback and Kegel exercise training alone.

Two other techniques for strengthening pelvic floor muscles in patients with stress UI should be noted. First, conical vaginal weights can be placed in the vagina, with the patient being instructed to hold these weights in; this was reported to improve the effectiveness of pelvic floor muscle exercises in selected patients.[23] Second, electrical stimulators placed in the anal canal or vagina have been used to elicit contractions of the pelvic floor to 1) passively exercise the muscles and/or 2) help patients locate these muscles and learn how to contract them voluntarily. To date, there is no strong evidence for increased efficacy compared with behavioral training in stress UI.

An alternative treatment for stress UI in women is to wear pessaries in the vagina to elevate the bladder neck. In theory, this accomplishes the same thing as a bladder suspension continence surgery; elevating the bladder neck makes the angle between the bladder and the urethra more acute so that bladder filling mechanically pinches off the urethral opening. Pessaries come in various sizes and shapes and should be selected based on effectiveness and patient preference/comfort following a therapeutic trial. Referral to a nurse clinical specialist experienced in the use of pessaries or to a urogynecologist should be considered.

Drug Treatment

Because sphincter contraction is mediated by α-adrenergic neurotransmitters, drugs that stimulate α-receptors were previously used for treatment for stress incontinence. The most widely used α-adrenergic agonist, phenylpropanolamine, has been withdrawn from the market.

Estrogen has direct effects on urethral mucosa and periurethral tissues and increases the number and responsiveness of α-receptors in women. Vaginally applied estrogen cream, ring, or tablets may improve stress and mixed UI.[24] The duration of topical estrogen application has not yet been established; however, several large studies have shown that oral estrogen or estrogen plus progesterone worsens stress, urge, or mixed UI. In the Women's Health Initiative study, 23,296 women, aged 50–79 years, received 0.625 mg conjugated estrogen, conjugated

estrogen plus medroxyprogesterone acetate (progesterone) 2.5 mg, or placebo.[25] Those patients who were continent at baseline and were treated with estrogen or estrogen plus progesterone had an increased risk for all types of UI at the 1-year evaluation. The largest increase in risk was for stress UI. Treatment with oral conjugated estrogen 0.625 mg plus progesterone 2.5 mg was associated with worsening of stress, urge, or mixed incontinence in the Heart and Estrogen/Progestin Replacement Study.[26] Based on these data, oral estrogen is not recommended as treatment for UI.

Surgical Management

When conservative therapy has failed, surgery may be appropriate. In women with urethral hypermobility of the bladder neck, retropubic or needle suspension of the urethrovesical junction is the procedure of choice, and cure rates of 78%–84% have been reported.[6] A recent innovation in bladder neck suspension surgery is the use of vaginal tape,[27] which simplifies the surgery and reduces morbidity.

For intrinsic sphincter deficiency, periurethral bulking injections with collagen (less frequently with Teflon) that cause an increase in outlet resistance are recommended as first-line surgical treatment for women with stress incontinence who do not have coexisting urethral hypermobility.

Urethral insufficiency occurs in men following transurethral resection of the prostate but is otherwise rare in men. Biofeedback combined with pelvic floor muscle exercises has been shown to improve stress and mixed UI in this population and is the first-line treatment. In patients with severe cases in whom biofeedback has failed or who have no access to it, periurethral bulking injections or artificial sphincter implantation, which allows the patient to use a pump in the scrotal sac to inflate and deflate a balloon around the urethra, may be appropriate.[6]

OVERFLOW INCONTINENCE (ATONIC BLADDER)

Atonic bladder is a potentially life-threatening condition because it increases the risk of reflux of bacteria to the kidneys. In patients with severe neurological deficits, intermittent clean catheterization every 2–4 hours by the patient or caregiver is often the best management. If this is not possible or practical, an indwelling catheter may be necessary. The use of chronic indwelling catheters is generally not encouraged because of the frequency of complications, including urolithiasis, symptomatic bacteriuria, periurethral abscess, and acute pyelonephritis. Appropriate management of an indwelling catheter depends on proper insertion using sterile technique and maintaining a closed sterile system. Urethral cleansing, routine bladder irrigation, and prophylactic antibiotic therapy should be avoided,[28] as these procedures do not prevent bladder colonization and are likely to result in the selection of resistant organisms.

For patients with mild overflow incontinence, a prompted voiding schedule (reminding the patient to void every

2–3 hours) may be beneficial. Also for mild symptoms, cholinergic agonists such as bethanechol may increase smooth muscle contractions in patients with atonic bladder. Patients respond to doses of 10–30 mg three or four times a day, although side effects have limited their use. The literature does not support the use of bethanechol longer than a month.[29] Overflow incontinence resulting from a hyporeflexic bladder is generally poorly responsive to behavioral or pharmacological therapy. Surgery is not indicated.

OUTFLOW OBSTRUCTION

Use of a questionnaire, such as the American Urological Association Symptom Inventory,[30] is useful in deciding on initial treatment for men with BPH. Men with milder symptoms can be managed by watchful waiting. For men with moderate-to-severe urethral obstruction and severe symptoms, surgery is often the treatment of choice. Current medication approaches for BPH include α-antagonists (such as doxazosin, terazosin, and tamsulosin) that reduce the dynamic component of prostatic obstruction, 5-α reductase inhibitors (such as finasteride and dutasteride), which shrink the prostate gland and antimuscarinic anticholinergic agents (such as tolterodine).Transurethral prostatectomy has a high cure rate for patients with properly functioning bladders, although development of stress UI is a known complication. There is a growing use of minimally invasive surgical techniques that have proved efficacious. These may be attractive because of their shorter recovery time and that they do not require general anesthesia. Women may present with bladder outlet obstruction secondary to pelvic organ prolapse, specifically cystocele. This may require surgical repair. In these patients, full evaluation including urodynamic testing prior to surgery is essential to rule out coexisting causes of incontinence.

MANAGING UI WITH ABSORBENT PADS AND CONTINENCE PRODUCTS

Absorbent pads and other continence products are designed for management rather than treatment of UI. Although evaluation and treatment are recommended, many patients will either depend on continence products exclusively or will use absorbent pads for security in circumstances where they are fearful of incontinence.

Disposable absorbent pads typically consist of a superabsorbent layer surrounded by an outer barrier and an inner membrane that conducts moisture away from the skin. They are supplied both as small pads to be worn in undergarments by patients who typically experience small-volume leakage or as briefs worn in place of undergarments by patients who at least occasionally have large-volume leakage of urine. For men with light incontinence, pads may be constructed as pouches or in the shape of a shield or leaf that surrounds the penis.

For men, sheaths made of latex or plastic that can be attached around the penis and that connect via tubing to a collection bag are more commonly used than absorbent pads. Sheaths are associated with a higher incidence of UTIs than pads, although this risk can be minimized by ensuring that the connection between the sheath and collection device does not kink or become obstructed. Other risks associated with sheaths are allergic reactions to latex, irritation, and compression from sheath binding straps.

Body-worn urinals have also been designed for women, and occlusive devices have been developed for men and women. These are not commonly used and are not reviewed here.[31]

TREATMENT OF UI IN LONG-TERM CARE FACILITIES

Prevalence estimates of UI in both men and women aged 65 years and older residing in long-term care facilities range from 30% to 77%. The prevalence of UI reported in a recent population-based study involving 95,911 older nursing home residents from eight southeastern states was 65% on admission, suggesting that the majority of nursing home residents are incontinent.[32] It is possible to decrease the frequency and severity of UI in at least half of incontinent long-term care patients through prompted voiding, but this approach is rarely used in long-term care facilities because the financial and staff resources needed to implement this program are seen as prohibitive. For the most part, in nursing homes UI is managed rather than treated or prevented: It is usually managed by placing absorbent pads on beds or chairs or by keeping residents in absorbent undergarments, and changing these two–three times per day.

Behavioral Treatment

Prompted voiding is the behavioral program that has been most thoroughly evaluated:[33] A staff member approaches each incontinent resident every 2 hours (or at intervals individualized to each patient) and asks them if they would like assistance to get to the toilet. Assistance is provided if needed, and staff is instructed to encourage patients to void and to praise them for success at remaining continent between prompts. Increasing fluid intake and exercise may also be included. In a large number of studies, this approach reduced the severity of UI (the proportion of times checked that the patient was found to be wet) by approximately 50% overall, although relatively few patients become fully continent. When prompts were no longer provided, the rate of UI quickly returned to its former level. Moreover, approximately half of nursing home residents do not benefit because of the severity of cognitive impairment or other functional limitations.

Management studies have shown that the average time required to assist a patient to the toilet to urinate greatly exceeds the time required to change absorbent undergarments or bed pads and linens. The additional cost is approximately $4.31 compared with regular care.[34]

Table 26.2. Therapeutic Modalities in Urinary Incontinence

Type of Incontinence	Strongly Recommended Therapies	Potentially Useful Therapies
Urge	Diet and fluid management	Pelvic floor electrical stimulation
Behavioral therapy	Timed voiding	Dicyclomine (10 mg qd, titrate up to 20 mg tid)
Drug therapy	Pelvic muscle exercises with or without biofeedback	Propantheline (7.5 mg qd titrated up to 30 mg qd to tid)
	Anticholinergic agents	Imipramine (10–25 mg qd to qid): avoid if potential for orthostatic hypotension
	Oxybutynin (IR 2.5–5 mg qd to tid; ER 5–30 mg qd; 3.8-mg TD patch changed 2×/wk)	
	Tolterodine (IR 1–2 mg bid; 2–4 mg qd ER)	
	Trospium (20 mg qd to bid)	
	Solifenacin (5–10 mg qd)	
	Darifenacin (7.5–15 mg qd)	
Stress	Pelvic muscle exercises with or without biofeedback	Conjugated estrogens:
Behavioral therapy	Timed voiding	Intravaginal only (0.5 gm qd, up to 1 g qd)
Surgery	Hypermobility	Hypermobility
	Retropubic suspension	Anterior vaginal repair
	Intrinsic sphincter deficiency	Needle bladder neck suspension
	Sling procedure (vaginal tape)	Intrinsic sphincter deficiency
	Periurethral bulking agents	Artificial sphincter
Management	Intermittent catheterization	Indwelling catheterization (only if necessary)
Functional	Correct underlying cause	

Modified from Fantl et al.[6]

Treatments recommended for management of urinary continence are adapted from the Agency for Health Care Policy and Research (AHCPR) 1996 clinical practice guideline Urinary Incontinence in Adults with updated drug recommendations.

SUMMARY

UI remains a common, underreported, and vexing problem in elderly patients. New therapeutic options using behavioral, pharmacological, and surgical approaches can lead to symptomatic improvements or cure for this important clinical problem and increased comfort for the patient.

REFERENCES

1. Burgio K, Clark A, Lapitan MC, Nelson R, Sillen U, Thom D. Epidemiology of urinary (UI) and faecal (FI) incontinence and pelvic organ prolapse (POP). In: Abrams P, Cardozo L, Khoury S, Wein A, eds. *Incontinence.* 2005 ed. Paris: Health Publication Ltd; 2005:255–312.

2. Hannestad YS, Rortveit G, Sandvik H, Hunskaar S. A community-based epidemiological survey of female urinary incontinence: the Norwegian EPINCONT study. Epidemiology of Incontinence in the County of Nord-Trondelag. *J Clin Epidemiol.* 2000;53:1150–1157.

3. Thom DH, Haan MN, Van Den Eeden SK. Medically recognized urinary incontinence and risks of hospitalization, nursing home admission and mortality. *Age Ageing.* 1997;26:367–374.

4. Burgio KL, Ives DG, Locher JL, Arena VC, Kuller LH. Treatment seeking for urinary incontinence in older adults. *J Am Geriatr Soc.* 1994;42:208–212.

5. Umlauf MG, Goode S, Burgio KL. Psychosocial issues in geriatric urology: problems in treatment and treatment seeking. *Urol Clin N Am.* 1996;23:127–136.

6. Fantl JA, Newman DK, Colling J, et al. Urinary incontinence in adults: Acute and chronic management. *Clinical practice guideline* 2 (1996 Update). AHCPR 96–0682. 3-1-1996. Rockville, MD: US Department of Health and Human Services, Public Health Service, Agency for Health Care Policy and Research.

7. Brocklehurst JC, Dillane JB. Studies of the female bladder in old age. II. Cystometrograms in 100 incontinent women. *Gerontol Clin (Basel).* 1966;8:306–319.

8. Summitt RL Jr, Stovall TG, Bent AE, Ostergard DR. Urinary incontinence: correlation of history and brief office evaluation with multichannel urodynamic testing. *Am J Obstet Gynecol.* 1992;166:1835–1840.

9. Bergman A, Bader K. Reliability of the patient's history in the diagnosis of urinary incontinence. *Int J Gynaecol Obstet.* 1990;32:255–259.

10. Frimodt-Moller PC, Jensen KM, Iversen P, Madsen PO, Bruskewitz RC. Analysis of presenting symptoms in prostatism. *J Urol.* 1984;132:272–276.

11. DuBeau CE, Resnick NM. Evaluation of the causes and severity of geriatric incontinence. A critical appraisal. *Urol Clin N Am.* 1991;18:243–256.

12. Ouslander JG, Schapira M, Schnelle JF. Urine specimen collection from incontinent female nursing home residents. *J Am Geriatr Soc.* 1995;43:279–281.

13. Khadra MH, Pickard RS, Charlton M, Powell PH, Neal DE. A prospective analysis of 1,930 patients with hematuria to evaluate current diagnostic practice. *J Urol.* 2000;163:524–527.

14. Schroder FH. Microscopic haematuria. *BMJ.* 1994;309:70–72.

15. Ouslander JG, Simmons S, Tuico E, et al. Use of a portable ultrasound device to measure post-void residual volume among incontinent nursing home residents. *J Am Geriatr Soc.* 1994;42:1189–1192.

16. Diokno AC, Normolle DP, Brown MB, Herzog AR. Urodynamic tests for female geriatric urinary incontinence. *Urology.* 1990;36:431–439.

17. Kane RL, Ouslander JG, Abrass IB. *Essentials of Clinical Geriatrics.* New York: McGraw-Hill; 1989.

18. Kincade JE, Dougherty MC, Carlson JR, Hunter GS, Busby-Whitehead J. Randomized clinical trial of efficacy of self-monitoring techniques to treat urinary incontinence in women. *Neurourol Urodyn.* 2007;26:507–511.

19. Nygaard IE, Kreder KJ, Lepic MM, Fountain KA, Rhomberg AT. Efficacy of pelvic floor muscle exercises in women with stress, urge, and mixed urinary incontinence. *Am J Obstet Gynecol.* 1996;174:120–125.

20. Bump RC, Hurt WG, Fantl JA, Wyman JF. Assessment of Kegel pelvic muscle exercise performance after brief verbal instruction. *Am J Obstet Gynecol.* 1991;165:322–327.

21. Tsao JW, Heilman KM. Transient memory impairment and hallucinations associated with tolterodine use. *NEJM.* 2003;349:2274–2275.

22. Burns PA, Pranikoff K, Nochajski T, Desotelle P, Harwood MK. Treatment of stress incontinence with pelvic floor exercises and biofeedback. *J Am Geriatr Soc.* 1990;38:341–344.

23. Olah KS, Bridges N, Denning J, Farrar DJ. The conservative management of patients with symptoms of stress incontinence: a randomized, prospective study comparing weighted vaginal cones and interferential therapy. *Am J Obstet Gynecol.* 1990;162:87–92.

24. DuBeau CE. Estrogen treatment for urinary incontinence: never, now, or in the future? *JAMA.* 2005;293:998–1001.

25. Hendrix SL, Cochrane BB, Nygaard IE, et al. Effects of estrogen with and without progestin on urinary incontinence. *JAMA.* 2005;293:935–948.

26. Grady D, Brown JS, Vittinghoff E, Applegate W, Varner E, Snyder T. Postmenopausal hormones and incontinence: the Heart and Estrogen/Progestin Replacement Study. *Obstet Gynecol.* 2001;97:116–120.

27. Maher C, Baessler K, Glazener CM, Adams EJ, Hagen S. Surgical management of pelvic organ prolapse in women: a short version Cochrane review. *Neurourol Urodyn.* 2008;27:3–12.

28. Wong E. *Guidelines for Prevention of Catheter Associated Urinary Tract Infections.* Philadelphia: Saunders; 1974.

29. Ouslander J. Urinary incontinence. In: Hazzard w, Andres R, Bierman E, Blass J, eds. *Principles of Geriatric Medicine and Gerontology.* 3rd ed. New York: McGraw-Hill; 1990:1123–1142.

30. Svatek R, Roche V, Thornberg J, Zimmern P. Normative values for the American Urological Association Symptom Index (AUA-7) and short form Urogenital Distress Inventory (UDI-6) in patients 65 and older presenting for non-urological care. *Neurourol Urodyn.* 2005;24:606–610.

31. Newman DK, Fader M, Bliss DZ. Managing incontinence using technology, devices, and products: directions for research. *Nurs Res.* 2004;53:S42–S48.

32. Boyington JE, Howard DL, Carter-Edwards L, et al. Differences in resident characteristics and prevalence of urinary incontinence in nursing homes in the southeastern United States. *Nurs Res.* 2007;56:97–107.

33. Schnelle JF. Treatment of urinary incontinence in nursing home patients by prompted voiding. *J Am Geriatr Soc.* 1990;38:356–360.

34. Schnelle JF, Keeler E, Hays RD, Simmons S, Ouslander JG, Siu AL. A cost and value analysis of two interventions with incontinent nursing home residents. *J Am Geriatr Soc.* 1995;43:1112–1117.

27

GERIATRIC GYNECOLOGY

Carmen Sultana, MD

In the 2000 census, 16.3% of the population was older than the age of 60 years.[1] As the numbers of women older than 65 years in the United States increases, projections for the year 2050 note that they will join 100 million elderly or 22.9% of the population.[2] The clinician caring for elderly women should be familiar with the general approach to screening and management of common gynecological problems in this group.[3] It may not be practical for women to be referred immediately for all gynecological complaints and examinations. The primary care physician can triage and manage basic issues and refer as appropriate to their training and skill level. This chapter will discuss the approach to evaluating the patient in the office and nursing home setting, review screening guidelines for gynecological malignancies and osteoporosis, and then present approaches to common presenting complaints that often lead to referral to a gynecologist, including issues concerning hormone replacement therapy (HRT).

APPROACH TO THE PATIENT

The older patient should have regular gynecological care and screening for malignancies of the female genital tract as part of routine primary care evaluations. This includes asking patients about symptoms and problems that they might not volunteer. This area might be overlooked when focusing on a patient's more pressing chronic disease states. Breast and pelvic examination may not be viewed as part of a "routine" examination. If the primary physician is not performing these examinations, they should ensure that the patient is seeing a gynecologist for this part of the examination. Changes in recommendations for the frequency of cervical cytology screening may lead to neglect of the other components of the pelvic examination. Attitudes toward sexuality, incontinence, and genital examination on the part of care providers and patients may also lead to discomfort with this part of the history-taking and physical examination.

The nursing home patient may pose additional challenges in access and availability of resources and facilities for gynecological examinations.

HISTORY AND PHYSICAL EXAMINATION AND ROUTINE SCREENING GUIDELINES

The physical examination of elderly women should not omit breast, pelvic, and rectal examination. Breast and pelvic examination for cancer screening are coded as a procedure under Medicare guidelines using the G0101 CPT codes. The code for a Pap smear is Q0019. A breast examination should be done in the standard fashion, with the examiner first inspecting the breasts visually with the patient's arms extended above the head and then placed on her hips to tense the underlying pectoral muscles. Palpation of the cervical, supraclavicular, and axillary areas should be done to look for lymph node enlargement. If the patient is able to lie flat, the breasts should be examined in that position. The nipples should be squeezed to check for sanguinous discharge. The examiner should be sensitive to the overall physical condition of the woman when considering pelvic examination as well. Patients may need assistance getting on and off examination tables, and care should be taken to avoid leaving them unattended to do so because of the risk of falling. They may not be able to tolerate lying flat with the head of the bed completely down because of cardiac disease or back pain. If the lithotomy position with stirrups is uncomfortable, the frog leg position in which the patient lies supine with heels together is an alternative, in which case the speculum should be inserted with the handle up instead of down. Another alternative is the left lateral decubitus position with knees bent; an assistant can hold up the top leg while the examiner inserts the speculum. For bedbound nursing home patients, examination in bed can be easier if an inverted bedpan covered by a towel is inserted under the patient's sacrum.

The pelvic examination should begin with inspection of the external genitalia, looking for ulcerations, skin lesions, and leukoplakia. Loss of hair and architecture of the labia are part of generalized atrophic conditions, as is the urethral caruncle or ectasia in which urethral tissue everts and may even bleed. This condition also is treated with estrogen creams. The patient should perform the Valsalva maneuver so that a general assessment of prolapse in the supine position can be obtained. A more detailed examination involves the Pelvic Organ Prolapse Quantification system, or POP-Q, in which the genital hiatus, perineal body, position of the cervix and vaginal apex, the length of the vagina, and the lowest points on the anterior and posterior vaginal walls are measured with a ruler using a Graves or Pederson and a Sims' speculum.

The selection of a smaller or larger speculum should be individualized depending on whether atrophy and stenosis or relaxation and a wide introitus predominate. The vagina should be inspected for bleeding and discharge, as well as for degree of prolapse, as described previously. Leaking of urine with cough on Valsalva can also be assessed, especially if the patient has not yet emptied her bladder. Voiding is recommended before the bimanual rectovaginal examination. The size and position as well as any tenderness of the uterus and adnexa are assessed. Any pelvic or rectal masses should be evaluated. Unprepped tests for fecal occult blood are no longer recommended and should be replaced by full colonoscopy or three-prepped test for fecal blood by the patient and a sigmoidoscopy. The full discussion of screening for colon cancer is beyond the scope of this chapter.

Laboratory testing for this age group includes cervical cytology as detailed later; urinalysis, annual mammography, lipid profile, and thyroid-stimulating hormone every 5 years, fasting glucose testing every 3 years, and screening for colon cancer and osteoporosis.

SCREENING AND DIAGNOSIS OF GYNECOLOGICAL CANCERS

Vulvovaginal Cancer

Malignancies of the vulva may present with bleeding or itching, or they may be noted on a routine examination. Vulvar squamous cell carcinoma is variable in appearance: It can be exophytic, ulcerated, or a hyperkeratotic plaque. The color is variable as well, ranging from hypopigmented to hyperpigmented or a similar color as the surrounding skin. Other conditions such as vulvar intraepithelial neoplasia, which is precancerous, and Paget disease (atypical glandular cell intraepithelial neoplasia) have a similar appearance and presentation and should be considered as well. Melanoma of the vulvar area is also not uncommon. Suspicious lesions should undergo biopsy sampling after preparing the skin with povidone iodine solution and injecting the skin with 1% lidocaine, using a Keyes dermatological punch, scissors, and forceps to remove a specimen that should be on the border of the lesion and include some normal dermis. Silver nitrate usually suffices to control oozing.

It is important to inspect carefully the vaginal mucosa for lesions in any patient having vaginal bleeding, especially when there is a history of an abnormal Pap smear. That being said, vaginal cancer is very rare at 0.2–0.4 per 100,000 women, and guidelines no longer recommend routine cytology screening of the vagina in patients whose cervices have been removed as part of a vaginal or total abdominal hysterectomy.

CERVICAL CANCER AND CYTOLOGY SCREENING

The American Cancer Society, the U.S. Preventive Services Task Force (USPSTF), and the American College of Obstetricians and Gynecologists reevaluated their screening recommendations in 2002–2003.[4] Recognizing that human papillomavirus (HPV) is the oncogenic pathogen that causes cervical cancer and that women in their 30s and older are less likely than younger women to acquire new HPV infections, they recommended that patients younger than 30 years be screened annually and those previously well screened women older than 30 years be screened every 2–3 years. When is it appropriate to discontinue screening altogether in older women? Screening can be discontinued in women who have had total hysterectomies (with removal of the cervix) unless they have a recent history of high-grade cervical dysplasia, diethystilbestrol exposure, or are immunocompromised. The American Cancer Society recommends that women may elect to discontinue screening at the age of 70 years if they have had three documented normal cytology tests in the last 10 years without any abnormal ones.[5] USPSTF recommended cessation of screening in women older than 65 years if they have had adequate recent screening with negative Pap tests.[6] The American College of Obstetricians and Gynecologists notes that evidence to set an upper age at which to stop screening is lacking and that individual patient risk factors should be assessed.[7] Practitioners should keep in mind that 25% of new cases of cervical cancer are diagnosed in women older than 65 years,[8] most likely in underscreened women.

If a patient complains of postmenopausal bleeding or postcoital bleeding, and a lesion is visualized on the cervix, a biopsy should be obtained immediately by using a Kevorkian cervical biopsy instrument without waiting for the results of cervical cytology. Monsel solution or silver nitrate can be applied to the site to control bleeding.

OVARIAN CANCER

The median age for the incidence of ovarian cancer is approximately the age of 60 years. The best way to detect early ovarian cancer appears to be a high index of suspicion on the part of patients and physicians. The American College of Obstetricians and Gynecologists recommends annual pelvic examination for screening.[9] Cancer antigen-125 (CA-125) is helpful in guiding referral to a gynecological oncologist for postmenopausal women with pelvic masses, but is not sensitive or specific enough to use for screening in asymptomatic women without palpable masses. Women with high-risk family histories for breast and ovarian cancer, including those carrying BRCA1 and 2 genes, should be counseled about their screening and prevention options.[9]

Uterine cancers are, like most of the other gynecological cancers, most prevalent in older patients. Endometrial cancers are fortunately frequently diagnosed at early stages because they present with postmenopausal bleeding. A low threshold for evaluating bleeding is adequate screening for endometrial cancer (see evaluation of postmenopausal bleeding, later). Sarcomas and other uncommon malignant tumors of the uterine wall may present with bleeding and/or a rapidly enlarging uterus. Diagnosis requires hysterectomy and pathological examination of the uterus.

COMMON PROBLEMS IN THE ELDERLY

Hormone Replacement Therapy

The use and indications for HRT for menopausal symptoms, genital atrophy, osteoporosis, and cardiac disease have undergone dramatic changes in the last 5 years. The history of estrogen use in the United States began in 1942 with the approval of conjugated equine estrogens for the treatment of menopausal symptoms.[10] Sales declined in the 1970s with reports of endometrial cancer in users, but the addition of progestins and reports of the prevention of bone loss by the drug increased use again. There were reports of favorable lipoprotein profiles in women using HRT and many reports of reduced cardiovascular risk in users as well. The 2002 Women's Health Initiative report of increased breast cancer and coronary heart disease events in estrogen–progestin users resulted in a reevaluation of the management of menopausal symptoms and prevention of coronary artery disease.[11] No benefit was found for cardiovascular disease prevention; indeed, there was an excess risk of stroke and cardiac death in the users of combination pills. Hip fractures and colon cancer were decreased. Other studies including meta-analyses, also found no protective effect of HRT for adverse cardiovascular outcomes,[12] or for dementia.[13] The major indication for usage of hormone replacement is for treatment of vasomotor and/or vulvovaginal atrophy, and the FDA recommends that they be used for "the shortest duration possible." The geriatrician may encounter patients who have been on systemic HRT for many years and may be reluctant to discontinue it for various reasons. It is best to have a discussion with the patient and make her aware of the issues so that she can make an informed decision. There is no evidence that HRT needs to be tapered except for the patient's comfort. Unfortunately, hot flashes and other symptoms may recur with attempts to stop the medication. It may be best to try to decrease to the lowest dose that still relieves symptoms if the patient is unable to stop taking it entirely. Other medications that may relieve hot flashes are serotonin uptake inhibitors such as venlafaxine and soy products. Herbal remedies containing black cohosh, such

as remifemin, in general are not found to be more effective than placebo. Older treatments include clonidine, which may cause hypotension in the normotensive patient, and belladonna or other sedatives.

Various formulations of estrogen and progestin combinations are available for these indications, in oral form or as patches, gels, creams, and vaginal rings. Only certain oral and transdermal preparations are indicated for osteoporosis prevention, and none at this time for treatment.

SEXUAL DYSFUNCTION

Older women may suffer from sexual dysfunction or dyspareunia, which they may not tell their physicians about unless they are asked or screened. A recent survey of women older and younger than the age of 65 years revealed that the older women had a similar number of sexual concerns as younger women.[14] Interestingly, older women were less likely to report dyspareunia than their younger counterparts, but those who did had more lubrication difficulties and their levels of desire were more disparate from their partners. For 68%, the topic had never arisen during an office visit; for those who had discussed it, the patient was twice as likely as the physician to have raised it.[14] The categories of sexual dysfunction according to the *Diagnostic and Statistical Manual of Mental Disorders–IV* include hypoactive sexual desire disorder (HSDD), female sexual arousal disorder, and female orgasmic disorder.[15] The diagnosis of HSDD is based on lack of the genital lubrication swelling response, yet women's complaints are usually about lack of subjective sexual arousal.[16] Evidence exists that life stressors, contextual factors, past sexuality, and mental health problems are more significant predictors of sexual interest than menopause status itself.[17] Large population studies have not found positive correlations between sexual function and serum testosterone levels.[18,19] No medications are currently approved by the FDA for the treatment of sexual dysfunction in women other than estrogen therapy for dyspareunia related to atrophy. Nevertheless, the uses of testosterone as a treatment for women with HSDD, especially for women who experience surgical menopause, is of interest to researchers, but hampered by lack of good studies on the appropriate dosage.[20] The lack of instruments or questionnaires that are unbiased makes measurement of outcomes difficult. Serum androgen levels do not correlate with symptoms. The risks of hirsutism, androgenization, and dyslipidemia must be balanced against the benefits. Oral methyltestosterone with estradiol has been demonstrated to improve HSDD but is only FDA approved for vasomotor symptoms.[21] More recent studies have shown that transdermal testosterone is also helpful for women after surgical menopause.[22] Naturally postmenopausal women are more complex; serum total and free testosterone levels do not decrease with age although androstenedione and dehydroepiandrosterone sulfate levels do.[23] A meta-analysis of randomized trials of testosterone plus HRT compared with HRT alone suggested that the addition of testosterone improved sexual function scores for postmenopausal women, with an adverse effect on high-density lipoprotein levels.[24]

As far as dyspareunia is concerned, it is commonly assumed that falling estrogen levels are responsible for vaginal atrophy and that the discomfort during intercourse that some menopausal women experience results from this. Some studies, however, suggest that women who continued coital activity had less atrophy than abstinent women and that continued sexual activity in the elderly was predicted by premenopausal sexual satisfaction.[17]

VULVOVAGINAL PROBLEMS (PRURITUS, DISCHARGE, BLEEDING, LESIONS)

Itching with or without discharge may indicate a vaginal infection such as candidiasis, trichomoniasis, or bacterial vaginosis. Just as in younger patients, physical examination should be augmented by measurement of vaginal pH and a wet prep slide or saline prep. Budding spores or branching hyphae are seen in only 50% of patients with yeast infections. The pH of the vaginal discharge is normally acidic, just as during a candidal infection. The other two infections as well as atrophic vaginitis lead to alkaline pH. The differential diagnosis should also include desquamative inflammatory vaginitis, a condition of unknown etiology characterized by a thin yellow discharge that can be bloody, a high vaginal pH, and superficial dyspareunia. On microscopic wet prep, white cells, increased parabasal cells, and Gram-positive cocci may be seen.[25] It responds to clindamycin cream.

Of course, itching can also result from vulvar irritation or dermatitis, vulvar intraepithelial neoplasia, cancer, lichen sclerosis, squamous cell hyperplasia, and other conditions.

The vulva is embryologically derived from ectoderm, endoderm (the vestibule), and mesoderm (hymenal membrane),[26] which is estrogen responsive. Pruritus can result from the infections discussed previously; from hypoestrogenic atrophic vaginitis; from mechanical irritation and wetness from urinary incontinence, for example; from dermatoses such as lichen sclerosis, lichen planus, psoriasis, and contact and seborrheic dermatitis; as well as itching from premalignant and malignant conditions. These are exclusive of a host of sexually transmitted infections and infestations, which are beyond the scope of this discussion. Likewise, there are systemic causes of itching such as uremia, hepatic disease, diabetes, and thyroid disease and lymphomas, leukemias, and other cancers in other parts of the body, and graft-versus-host disease and so forth.

A general approach to this problem is to take a full history, including any lotions or bath products the patient may have been using. Sexual history-taking should be done as well. Evaluate for vaginitis and atrophy first and other treatable causes. Any ulcerations or lesions should generally be investigated with biopsy to rule out vulvar intraepithelial neoplasia or squamous cell carcinoma, which can both vary in appearance but which frequently itch. Lichen sclerosis peaks in incidence in postmenopausal women.[27] It is characterized by a white "cigarette paper" appearance to the skin and by loss of architecture of the labia minora. It is treated with steroids such as clobetasol. Lichen planus presents as papular plaques with the characteristic white reticular pattern also seen in the buccal mucosa. Topical steroids are the usual treatment.

Vulvodynia has been defined by the International Society for the Study of Vulvovaginal Disease as vulvar discomfort in the absence of gross anatomical or neurological findings.[28] Common causes of discomfort and dyspareunia such as vaginal infection, dermatological conditions, and vaginal atrophy should be ruled out or treated. In the absence of these findings, topical lidocaine, low-dose antidepressants, and low oxalate diet have been used for treatment of pain that localizes to the vestibule on Q-tip testing. Vestibulitis has been linked to HPV. Treatments for this include α-interferon injections and resection of the vestibule.

POSTMENOPAUSAL BLEEDING

Postmenopausal bleeding is defined as bleeding that occurs after 1 year of amenorrhea in a woman not receiving HRT. Bleeding that occurs after cyclic withdrawal of progestins as part of HRT is normal. Some women on continuous combined HRT regimens will also bleed irregularly, especially when starting therapy – 60% in one study had spotting or bleeding in the first 6 months of therapy.[29]

Fortunately, 95% of uterine bleeding in postmenopausal women results from benign, causes, and only 5% is from endometrial carcinoma or complex endometrial hyperplasia with atypia.[29] The most common cause for uterine bleeding after menopause is atrophy of the endometrium, but endometritis, polyps, simple endometrial hyperplasia as well as uterine myomas or sarcomas are possible. Women who are receiving tamoxifen therapy for breast cancer are at risk for polyps and carcinoma. It should be remembered that not all bleeding from the genital tract is uterine and not all bleeding is from the genital tract. Hematuria and rectal bleeding that are mistaken for vaginal bleeding are also part of the differential diagnosis. The entire genital tract should be carefully examined to look for other sources of bleeding such as vaginal or cervical lesions or polyps.

Endometrial cancer has a lifetime incidence of approximately 1 in 100 women. Risk factors include obesity, nulliparity, family history such as hereditary nonpolyposis colorectal cancer syndrome, and unopposed estrogen therapy. Stage 1, grade 1 cancer has a better than 95% cure rate and is easily detected because of bleeding early in presentation. Performing office endometrial biopsy, measurement of endometrial stripe thickness on ultrasound, or hysteroscopy with dilation and curettage can be used to diagnose malignancy in the early stages. Endometrial sampling can be performed without anesthetic in the office or bedside setting by using a disposable plastic instrument such as the Pipelle provided the cervix has not become stenotic; use of a tenaculum on the cervix and dilators such as the Os-finder can help with small degrees of stenosis.

These procedures are 88%–97% sensitive in detecting disease. Alternatively, transvaginal ultrasound may be performed. The sensitivity compares favorably to sampling procedures, with a mean sensitivity of 91%.[29] Sonohysterography, ultrasound performed with saline instilled into the uterus, allows lesions like polyps and myomas to be more clearly defined. An endometrial thickness of 5 mm or greater should lead to a procedure to obtain a tissue sample. It is important to note that this lining appears abnormal in women taking tamoxifen becuase of its estrogen-like effects, but because they are at increased risk for pathological malignancy, any woman taking tamoxifen who is bleeding needs endometrial biopsy and/or dilation and curettage. Endometrial hyperplasia is treated with progestins unless it is complex hyperplasia with atypia. In that case, total hysterectomy with removal of the ovaries is recommended because the progression to cancer or chance of simultaneous cancer is more than 15%. Endometrial cancer is staged with total abdominal hysterectomy–bilateral salpingo oophorectomy and node sampling in most cases.

ADNEXAL MASSES

The adnexal mass or ovarian cyst found on physical examination or imaging studies in a postmenopausal woman raises the possibility of ovarian or fallopian tube cancer. Fortunately, approximately half of tumors in women older than 60 years are benign.[30] Older women can develop benign cysts such as germinal inclusion cysts, despite not ovulating. Screening studies suggest that 3%–5% of asymptomatic postmenopausal women will have an adnexal mass confirmed sonographically.[31] Traditionally, surgical exploration was thought to be necessary in all cases; however, the increasing availability of high-resolution pelvic imaging and CA-125 antigen testing has made it possible to triage these masses. This has been a two-edged sword as well, because the diagnosis of nonmalignant masses in asymptomatic patients undergoing pelvic ultrasound or other imaging techniques for unrelated problems leaves patients at risk for unindicated surgery and other interventions. The assessment of pelvic masses in older women is discussed later; it should also include evaluation of the breast and bowel because of the rates of metastatic colon and breast cancer in this age group.

Criteria developed in the 1980s[32] noted that ovarian masses could be evaluated for high or low risk of malignancy based on size, echogenicity or cystic characteristics, and presence or absence of ascites and matted bowel. Ultrasound findings of solid or papillary areas greater than 3 mm and septations greater than 3 mm in cysts have been associated with three–six times higher rates of malignancy. Parker and Berek[33] found that 25 masses with benign ultrasound characteristics and CA-125 levels less than 35 μ/mL were all benign. If the mass is less than 6 cm, the risk of cancer also decreases. One study found that only 1 of 32 masses less than 5 cm in size was malignant.[34] A study of 2,763 women aged 50 years and older with unilocular cysts up to 10 cm in size found 69% resolved spontaneously and none of the remainder were found to be malignant.[35]

In general, ultrasonography has a negative predictive value for malignancy of 90% or above, whereas the positive predictive value ranges from 30%–73%.[31] Therefore, it is reasonable to follow postmenopausal patients with simple cysts smaller than 5 cm and normal CA-125 levels (<35 μ/mL) or to perform laparoscopic removal of the ovaries with frozen section evaluation and staging laparotomy if cancer is found.[36] If increasing size or complexity of the mass is found or CA-125 levels increase, staging surgery should be done.

PELVIC PROLAPSE

The causes of pelvic prolapse and its frequent companion, urinary and fecal incontinence, are complex and may involve as yet poorly understood risk factors such as collagen changes or deficiencies; childbirth; and weight bearing or straining at stool exacerbated by aging and decreased estrogen levels. It can take the form of uterine prolapse, anterior vaginal wall prolapse or cystocele, posterior vaginal wall prolapse or rectocele, and posthysterectomy vaginal vault prolapse. A quantitative system of measuring and grading prolapse was developed in 1996. The POP-Q grid and staging system attempts to allow comparison between studies of treatment outcomes.[37] Pelvic organ prolapse may be asymptomatic or may cause sensations of heaviness, pressure, and other discomfort. Ureteral obstruction as a result of prolapse is rare, but anterior segment prolapse may cause difficulty emptying the bladder and urinary retention. Rectoceles can be associated with constipation but may not be the cause. The patient's bowel regimen should be optimized before assuming that surgical correction will help. Any accompanying urinary incontinence should be addressed, usually with urodynamic testing. Prolapse can mask underlying stress incontinence and should not be repaired without consideration as to whether a urethropexy or sling should be included as part of the surgical approach. The approach to urinary incontinence is discussed in further detail elsewhere in this book.

Treatment options can include observation, pelvic muscle exercises, pessary, or surgical repair depending on the severity of the symptoms, sexual activity and wish to maintain a functioning vagina, and state of health in terms of tolerating and recovering from a surgical procedure. Elderly patients, who are healthy, have low death rates from benign gynecological surgery and surgery for incontinence.[38] In general, vaginal procedures are less risky than abdominal repairs, but may differ in cure rates depending on the nature of the patient's problem.

Pessaries are often underutilized for pelvic prolapse. Fitting involves making sure the device is not so large that the patient can feel it but not small enough that it falls out during a Valsalva maneuver. If the genital hiatus is large or the levator muscle tone poor, it may not be possible to fit a patient with a pessary that will be retained. Parity and posthysterectomy status are associated with failure to retain a pessary.[39] The patient being fitted with a pessary must be able to void with it in place before leaving the office. Pessaries come in a variety of shapes and sizes, including ring, Gellhorn, Gehrung,

Hodge, cube, and doughnut. Ring pessaries lend themselves to easy removal and reinsertion for patients who wish to remove and clean them themselves, and they can even be left in place during sexual activity. Otherwise, the patient should see her practitioner every 3 months for cleaning and inspection of the vagina to look for ulcerations or bleeding. Estrogen and antibacterial creams can prevent ulceration and malodorous discharge. A trial of pessary use should be considered in most patients before recommending surgery. A recent study noted that 73% of patients with symptomatic prolapse could be successfully fitted with a pessary, and 92% of these patients were satisfied with its use after 2 months.[40] Pessaries may unmask stress incontinence or make it worse because they relieve urethral kinking and allow easier flow of urine. Surgery may be required in these circumstances to address adequately both prolapse and urinary incontinence.

REFERENCES

1. Department of Health and Human Services Administration on Aging. Census 2000 Data on the Aging. Summary Table of Age Characteristics of the Older Population for the United States and for States: 2000. Available at: http://www.aoa.gov/prof/Statistics/Census2000/stateprofiles/ageprofile-states.asp. Accessed June 5, 2008.
2. U.S. Senate Subcommittee on Aging, American Association of Retired Persons, Federal Council on Aging, and U.S. Administration on Aging. Trends and Projections. DHHS Publication No. (FCOA) 91–98001. U.S. Department of Health and Human Services; 1991.
3. American College of Obstetricians and Gynecologists. ACOG Committee Opinion No. 292. Primary and preventive care: periodic assessments. *Obstet Gynecol.* 2003;102:1117–1124.
4. Waxman AG. Guidelines for cervical cancer screening: history and scientific rationale. *Clin Obstet Gynecol.* 2005;48:77–97.
5. Saslow D, Runowicz CD, Solomon D, et al. American Cancer Society guidelines for the early detection of cervical neoplasia and cancer. *CA Cancer J Clin.* 2002;52:342–362.
6. U.S. Preventive Services Task Force. Screening for cervical cancer. Agency for Healthcare Research and Quality 2003. Available at: http://www.ahrq.gov/Clinic/uspstf/uspscerv.htm. Accessed June 5, 2008.
7. American College of Obstetricians and Gynecologists. ACOG Practice Bulletin No.45. Cervical cytology screening. *Obstet Gynecol.* 2003;102:417–427.
8. Cervical cancer. NIH Consensus Statement. 1996;14:1–38. Available at consensus.nih.gov/1996/1996CervicalCancer102PDF.pdf.
9. ACOG Committee Opinion 2002; No.280. The role of the generalist obstetrician-gynecologist in the early detection of ovarian cancer. *Obstet Gynecol.* 2002;100:1413–1416.
10. Stefanick ML. Estrogens and progestins: background and history, trends in use, and guidelines and regimens approved by the US Food and Drug Administration. *Am J Med.* 2005;118:64S–73S.
11. Writing Group for the Women's Health Initiative Investigators. Risks and benefits of estrogen plus progestin in healthy postmenopausal women: principal results from the Women's Health Initiative randomized controlled trial. *JAMA.* 2002;288:321–333.
12. Gabriel SR, Carmona L, Roque M, Sanchez GL, Bonfill X. Hormone replacement therapy for preventing cardiovascular disease in post-menopausal women. *Cochrane Database Syst Rev.* 2005;2:CD002229.
13. Hogervorst E, Yaffe K, Richards M, Huppert F. Hormone replacement therapy to maintain cognitive function in women with dementia. *Cochrane Database Syst Rev.* 2002;3:CD003799.
14. Nusbaum MRH, Singh AR, Pyles AA. Sexual healthcare needs of women aged 65 and older. *J Am Geriatr Soc.* 2004;52:117–122.
15. American Psychiatric Association. *Diagnostic and Statistical Manual of Mental Disorders.* 4th ed. Washington, DC: American Psychiatric Association; 1994.
16. van Lunsen RHW, Laan E. Genital vascular responsiveness and sexual feelings in midlife women: psychophysiologic, brain, and genital imaging studies. *Menopause.* 2004;11:741–748.
17. Hartmann U, Philippsohn S, Heiser K, Ruffer-Hesse C. Low sexual desire in midlife and older women: personality factors, psychosocial development, present sexuality. *Menopause.* 2004;11:726–740.
18. Santoro A, Torrens J, Crawford S, et al. Correlates of circulating androgens in mid-life women: the Study of Women's Health Across the Nation. *J Clin Endocrinol Metab.* 2005;90:4836–4845.
19. Davis SR, Davison SL, Donath S, Bell RJ. Circulating androgen levels in self-reported sexual function in women. *JAMA.* 2005:294:91–96.
20. Vigersky RA. Goldilocks and menopause. *Arch Intern Med.* 2005;165:1571–1572.
21. Lobo RA, Rosen RC, Yang HM, et al. Comparative effects of oral esterified estrogens with and without methyltestosterone on endocrine profiles and dimensions of sexual function in postmenopausal women with hypoactive sexual desire. *Fertil Steril.* 2003;79:1341–1352.
22. Braunstein GD, Sundwall DA, Katz M, et al. Safety and efficacy of a testosterone patch for the treatment of hypoactive sexual desire disorder in surgically menopausal women. *Arch Intern Med.* 2005;165:1582–1589.
23. Laughlin G, Barrett-Connor E, Kritz-Silverstein D, von Muhlen D. Hysterectomy, oophorectomy and endogenous sex hormone levels in older women: the Rancho Bernardo study. *J Clin Endocrinol Metab.* 2000;200;85:645–651.
24. Somboonporn W, Davis S, Seif MW, Bell R. Testosterone for peri- and postmenopausal women. *Cochrane Database Syst Rev.* 2005;4:CD004509.
25. Say PJ, Jacyntho C. Difficult to manage vaginitis. *Clin Obstet Gynecol.* 2005;48:753–768.
26. Bohl TG. Overview of vulvar pruritis through the life cycle. *Clin Obstet Gynecol.* 2005;48:786–807.
27. Lewis FM, Velangi SS. Vulvar ulceration. *Clin Obstet Gynecol.* 2005;48:824–837.
28. Haefner HK, Collins ME, Davis GD, et al. The vulvodynia guideline. *J Lower Genital Tract Dis.* 2005;9:40–51.
29. Good AE. Diagnostic options for assessment of postmenopausal bleeding. *Mayo Clin Proc.* 1997;72:345–349.
30. Katsube Y, Berg JW, Silverberg SG. Epidemiologic pathology of ovarian tumors: a histopathologic review of primary ovarian neoplasms diagnosed in the Denver Standard Metropolitan Statistical Area, 1 July–31 December 1969 and 1 July–31 December 1979. *Int J Gynecol Pathol.* 1982;1:3–16.
31. van Nagell FR, DePriest PD, Reedy MB, et al. The efficacy of transvaginal sonographic screening in asymptomatic women at risk for ovarian cancer. *Gynecol Oncol.* 2000;77:350–356.

32. Hermann UJ, Gottfried LW, Goldhirsch A. Sonographic patterns of ovarian tumors: prediction of malignancy. *Obstet Gynecol.* 1987;69:777–781.

33. Parker WH, Berek JS. Management of selected cystic adnexal masses in postmenopausal women by operative laparoscopy: a pilot study. *Am J Obstet Gynecol.* 1990;163:1574–1577.

34. Rulin MC, Preston AL. Adnexal masses in postmenopausal women. *Obstet Gynecol.* 1987;70:578–581.

35. Modesitt SC, Pavlik EJ, Ueland FR, De Priest PD, Kryscio RJ, van Nagell JR. Risk of malignancy in unilocular ovarian cystic tumors less than 10 cm in diameter. *Obstet Gynecol.* 2003;102:594–599.

36. van Nagell JR, DePriest PD. Management of adnexal masses in postmenopausal women. *Am J Obstet Gynecol.* 2005;193:30–35.

37. Bump RC, Mattiasson A, Bo K, et al. The standardization of terminology of female pelvic organ prolapse and pelvic floor dysfunction. *Obstet Gynecol.* 1996;175:10–17.

38. Sultana CJ, Campbell JW, Pisanelli WS, Sivinski L, Rimm AA. Morbidity and mortality of incontinence surgery in elderly women: an analysis of Medicare data.[see comment]. *Am J Obstet Gynecol.* 1997;176:344–348.

39. Fernando RJ, Thakar R, Sultan AH, Shah SM, Jones PW. Effect of vaginal pessaries on symptoms associated with pelvic organ prolapse. *Obstet Gynecol.* 2006;108:93–99.

40. Clemons JL, Aguilar VC, Tillinghast TA, Jackson ND, Myers DL. Patient satisfaction and changes in prolapse and urinary symptoms in women who were fitted successfully with a pessary for pelvic organ prolapse. *Am J Obstet Gynecol.* 2004;190:1025–1029.

28

Disorders of the Endocrine Glands

Matthew C. Leinung, MD, Paul J. Davis, MD, Faith B. Davis, MD

INTRODUCTION

Although the majority of endocrine diseases present in the elderly patient population with classic symptoms and signs, a substantial minority of patients come to medical attention with subtle or atypical findings. Such presentations require a low threshold in the physician for consideration of endocrine diagnoses. The pituitary–adrenal cortex and pituitary–thyroid endocrine axes remain very much intact over the life span and, therefore, the diagnostics of endocrine disorders in these topical areas remain much as they are in young individuals. Virtually all of the endocrinopathies may have their presentations obscured in the elderly patient population by concomitant nonendocrine disorders that are severe and that distract attention from the possibility of endocrinopathy. Finally, treatment of endocrine diseases in the elderly is often more complex than in younger patients. This results from concomitant nonendocrine illness. Polypharmacy for such conditions complicates dosing of endocrine drugs and increases risks of complications of drug therapy in the older endocrine patient. For example, hypoglycemia in the management of the older diabetic patient occurs in the contexts of metabolic bone disease with attendant increased risk of fractures with falls and of coronary artery disease. Extreme care is required in the development of therapeutic regimens for older endocrine patients so that treatment achieves a satisfactory, albeit compromised, balance between benefit and risk.

PARATHYROID DISEASE AND OTHER DISEASES OF CALCIUM METABOLISM

Primary Hyperparathyroidism

Clinical Features

Primary hyperparathyroidism is a common and subtle endocrinopathy over the life span. Whether by design or

as part of laboratory test templates, the measurement of serum total calcium concentration occurs frequently and has increased practitioners' recognition of asymptomatic parathyroid disease.[1] It is rare to encounter hyperparathyroidism in older patients in whom the serum calcium level is sufficiently elevated to cause polyuria or clouded sensorium. When such findings do occur as a result of hypercalcemia, they are usually because of the presence of nonendocrine tissue cancers that secrete parathyroid hormone–related peptide (PTHrp).

The particular importance of primary hyperparathyroidism in the elderly is its contribution to bone mass loss in this population that is already subject to metabolic bone disease, namely, osteoporosis and osteomalacia. Primary hyperparathyroidism also increases bone turnover in patients with Paget's disease and measurement of circulating PTH is recommended when the elevated serum alkaline phosphatase activity in such a patient does not respond satisfactorily to bisphosphonate administration or other accepted modalities.[2] Hyperparathyroidism should also be suspected in the elderly patient with Paget's disease when hypercalcemia develops in the setting of patient immobilization.

Urinary tract calculi occur with appreciable frequency in men over the lifespan and are found with a frequency in postmenopausal women that begins to approach that of men. Primary hyperparathyroidism is a well-recognized cause of the development of calcium phosphate stones when mild-to-moderate elevations in the filtered load of calcium in the kidney exceed the tubular reabsorption threshold for calcium. The development of more than one urinary tract calculus over time or concurrently should encourage the physician to assess the possibility of primary hyperparathyroidism as a cause; in elderly women, the finding of a single stone warrants a workup for primary hyperparathyroidism.

Significant elevation of serum total calcium concentration may induce blood pressure elevation, but this cause is very rarely the case in elderly patients whose hypertension is difficult to control. Renovascular disease, early congestive heart failure, and pheochromocytoma – which are surprisingly frequent in the older patient – are issues to consider in the setting of blood pressure elevations that require complex medical treatment regimens.

Diagnosis

The hallmark laboratory findings of primary hyperparathyroidism are elevated serum total calcium concentration and depressed serum phosphate level. When present, hypophosphatemia in PTH excess reflects the phosphaturic effect of PTH; hypercalcemia results from the reabsorptive action of PTH on bone, increased renal tubular reabsorption of calcium from the glomerular filtrate of plasma, and enhanced activation of vitamin D that leads to increased gastrointestinal tract absorption of dietary calcium.

There is clinical "noise" in these measurements that can limit their usefulness. For example, depression of serum albumin concentration because of liver disease or inadequate nutrition, particularly common in the elderly, will lower the total calcium concentration because almost 50% of serum calcium is protein bound and albumin accounts for 75% of this bound fraction. Thus, normal serum calcium in the setting of hypoalbuminemia may prevent recognition of mild hypercalcemia due to hyperparathyroidism or other causes. A standard correction for the impact of decreased serum albumin content on serum total calcium concentration is a 0.8–1.0 mg/dL decrease in calcium for each 1.0 g/dL decline in albumin. Decrease in dietary meat content lowers phosphate intake. Hyperglycemia is associated with decrease in serum phosphate concentration, presumably reflecting a concomitant shift of glucose with phosphate into cells from the plasma. Therefore, the isolated finding of hypophosphatemia is not a useful discriminant in making the diagnosis of hyperparathyroidism.

The finding of elevated circulating intact PTH (iPTH) in the presence of normal kidney function is the hallmark of primary hyperparathyroidism. Because of the modest decline in renal function (glomerular filtration rate [GFR]) that occurs with normal aging, there is a small upward trend with age of serum iPTH, but within the normal range; this change does not confuse the diagnostic evaluation of elderly patients for parathyroid disease.

Serum alkaline phosphatase activity will rise in patients with primary hyperparathyroidism who have metabolic bone disease. There are many clinical factors unrelated to PTH that will confound interpretation of elevated circulating alkaline phosphate activity, but fractionation of this measurement into liver- and bone-source fractions in the elderly and in young people at least eliminates a contribution from hepatic disease.

Therapeutic Decision Making

Although serum calcium levels can be lowered pharmacologically, the definitive treatment of primary hyperparathyroidism is surgery. Preoperative radioisotopic scanning of the thyroid bed with gadolinium may allow the localization of the

source of excess iPTH production to one parathyroid gland, when the disease reflects a parathyroid adenoma. Hyperplasia of all four parathyroid glands may occur, however, as the cause of primary hyperparathyroidism. Neck explorations are conducted by endocrine or head-and-neck surgeons. Today, neck exploration as management of primary hyperparathyroidism is 1-day surgery and the morbidity is low, except for very transient immediately postoperative hypocalcemia, which is mild. Such surgery is usually well tolerated by even very elderly patients;[3] however, parathyroid hyperplasia that requires removal of three-and-a-half parathyroid glands can result in permanent hypoparathyroidism.

The critical decision in management of elderly patients with primary hyperparathyroidism is when or whether to endorse parathyroid gland surgery. The usually low-grade short-to-intermediate term morbidity of primary hyperparathyroidism must be viewed in the context in older patients of multiple nonendocrine disorders that may have significant morbidity and mortality and that, like chronic lung disease, pose significant anesthetic risk. If the patient's bone mass is stable on or in the absence of bisphosphonate or calcitonin treatment for osteopenia and in the presence of mild elevation of serum total calcium, surgery is not mandated. Appreciable decrease in bone mass over 6 to 12 months in the setting of primary hyperparathyroidism and/or serum calcium levels of 11 mg/dL or higher is cause to recommend neck exploration in the otherwise healthy elderly patient. A National Institutes of Health (NIH) Consensus Conference, in 2002, recommended parathyroidectomy for a bone mineral density t score below −2.5, but this advisory must be tempered in the elderly patient population by the presence of concomitant illnesses that make such surgery of unacceptable risk. Although control of urinary tract calculus formation can be achieved medically with thiazide administration to decrease urinary calcium excretion, the thiazides exacerbate already elevated serum calcium levels by increasing tubular reabsorption of calcium. Alternative medical management of stone disease is available or parathyroidectomy can be considered in the setting of a 24-hour urinary calcium greater than 400 mg or recurrent urolithiasis in the elderly, just as it is in younger patients.

Secondary Hyperparathyroidism

The most common cause of secondary hyperparathyroidism is vitamin D deficiency (with resultant calcium insufficiency as the driving force for PTH elevation). This is recognized with increasing frequency in the elderly, resulting in part from the fact that the level of 25-hydroxy vitamin D considered to be normal in this age group has recently been increased. Some studies have found vitamin D insufficiency in upward of 40% of the elderly, even in southern latitudes,[4] and a low threshold for screening and treatment should be maintained. Sufficient calcium intake and vitamin D supplementation should normalize circulating PTH levels.

Elevated blood iPTH is a concomitant of chronic renal insufficiency, reflecting the decrease in serum calcium concentration that is a hallmark of the condition and that is multifactorial in origin. Medical management of secondary hyperparathyroidism is beyond the scope of this chapter. Improved management strategies for chronic renal failure and availability of dialysis to the elderly mean that older patients with advanced kidney disease are being encountered with increasing frequency by nephrologists and geriatricians.

Management of metabolic bone disease in older patients with secondary hyperparathyroidism can be complex. Patients are preferably treated with calcitriol (1,25-dihydroxy-vitamin D3), even in the presence of limited renal function,[5] with careful attention to measurements of serum calcium and phosphate levels. Oral bisphosphonate can be used in this setting to treat bone disease, but the manufacturers of the agent do recommend avoiding use of the drug in patients with renal insufficiency (creatinine clearance <35 mL/min). Published experience shows that administration of bisphosphonate in the elderly with varying degrees of kidney disease can be safe,[6,7] but it is appropriate to manage these patients who are receiving bisphosphonate – as well as oral calcium supplementation and vitamin D – very cautiously, and in conjunction with a nephrologist.

Hypercalcemia Resulting from Tumoral Secretion of Parathyroid Hormone–Related Peptide

Clinical Features

Hypercalcemia from cancer is frequent in the elderly, with this patient population's accruing risk of cancer. The most common cause of malignant tumor-related hypercalcemia is the secretion by squamous tumor cells of PTHrp. The organ affected is primarily the lung. Hypercalcemia can be striking in this setting (12–15 mg/dL or higher) and, in contrast to the clinical presentation of primary hyperparathyroidism, may cause the patient to present with altered sensorium and volume depletion because of polyuria induced by profound elevation of serum calcium. Regardless of patient age, patients with lung cancer largely represent the cigarette-smoking population. Hypercalcemia in this setting may be exacerbated by thiazide use and by excessive dietary calcium intake and ingestion of vitamin D initiated by patients as prophylaxis for bone mass loss before the diagnosis of cancer with hypercalcemia is made.

Diagnosis

These hypercalcemic patients will have low or suppressed authentic iPTH in serum and elevated circulating PTH-reactive protein. PTH-reactive protein, in contrast to iPTH, is phosphaturic.[8] The serum phosphate may, therefore, be low or normal if the serum calcium is severely elevated because volume depletion will have decreased GFR, resulting in a decreased filtered load of phosphate. In the acute presentation of hypercalcemic patients with cancer, the chest x-ray may be the first indication of the cause of the elevation in serum calcium, because results of PTH assays are not rapidly available. In some patients,

serum amylase and lipase activities may be increased, reflecting soft tissue calcium deposition in the pancreas.

Therapeutic Decision Making

When tumoral hypercalcemia is not severe (serum calcium concentration <12 mg/dL), loop diuretic treatment is effective via the calciuric action of this family of agents. In severe hypercalcemia, however, that is managed in the intensive care unit by intensivists and endocrinologists, the management includes at least partial restoration of intravascular and extravascular volume with saline prior to, or in conjunction with, furosemide or another loop diuretic. Volume expansion increases GFR and the sodium administered has a specific role in fostering renal tubular calcium excretion (sodium diuresis with calcium diuresis). Concern that excessive saline administration in elderly hypercalcemic patients with histories of congestive heart failure will induce congestive heart failure is real, and monitoring of central venous pressure is endorsed in the acute management of severe hypercalcemia in older patients. The simple estimation of neck vein distention and auscultation of lung fields may be helpful when central line placement is impractical.

The successful treatment of severe hypercalcemia is much improved today by the use of parenteral bisphosphonates. It is important to monitor kidney function during the use of these agents, particularly in the elderly, and although patients with already established decrease in creatinine clearance can in many cases be safely treated with bisphosphonates, as noted in the section on secondary hyperparathyroidism, it is appropriate to manage these individuals in conjunction with the nephrologist and endocrinologist.[9] An association between bisphosphonate therapy and osteonecrosis of the jaw has been reported.[10] A history of invasive dental procedures, age older than 60 years, or female sex may be more important contributing factors to jaw osteonecrosis than bisphosphonate treatment when this bone disease is observed in the setting of bisphosphonate therapy.

Other Forms of Tumoral Hypercalcemia

Hypercalcemia resulting from breast cancer in women and multiple myeloma in men and women are relatively frequently encountered in the geriatric patient population. In the cases of both malignant syndromes, the hypercalcemia may be severe. In women, replacement estrogen administration that antedated clinical appearance of breast cancer may contribute to the level of hypercalcemia. It is worthwhile noting that tamoxifen use in breast cancer patients may also precipitate severe hypercalcemia.[10] Hypercalcemia from B-cell lymphoma in association with elevated calcitriol and suppressed PTH and PTHrP has also been reported,[11] as has hypercalcemia in association with renal cell carcinoma and increased levels of PTHrP.[12]

Other Forms of Nontumoral Hypercalcemia

The differential diagnosis of hypercalcemia is extensive beyond hyperparathyroidism and cancer-related hypercalcemia, but in the aging patient the list of likely causes is manageable. These causes include excessive calcium intake as with over-the-counter antacids (milk-alkali syndrome[13]) and vitamin D intoxication that occurs via dietary supplements.

Hypoparathyroidism

Clinical Features

Decreased parathyroid function is uncommon in older patients. It may be autoimmune in origin or secondary to thyroid gland surgery and surgery for parathyroid gland hyperplasia or irradiation of the neck for cancer of the upper airway. The principal biochemical finding of hypoparathyroidism is decreased serum calcium concentration, which is usually found with increased serum phosphate; this finding is of lower specificity than one would like in the elderly. The reason for this is, as pointed out previously, that serum albumin concentration tends to fall over the lifespan as a consequence of several diseases and because of inadequate nutrition. Fifty percent of serum calcium is bound to circulating albumin and thus hypocalcemia is relatively common in older patients. Mild renal disease in the elderly, resulting principally from hypertension and diabetes mellitus (DM), may result in phosphate retention and an increase in serum phosphate concentration.

What is essential in recognizing the syndrome clinically is discerning neuromuscular irritability. The patient will recount periods of distracting muscle twitching and simple palpation or gentle squeezing of large muscles by the physician may provoke brief episodes of twitching. A clinical test of neuromuscular irritability that has been used in the past is a blood pressure cuff test that involves occluding venous return from the forearm, but not preventing arterial inflow. Flexor muscle contracture in the forearm/wrist and extensor muscle contraction of the fingers may be obtained with this test in the patient who has a low ionized calcium level. This test is *not* recommended, particularly in elderly patients. It is painful and, in the elderly patient with fragile skin and blood vessels, may produce ecchymoses.

Diagnosis

The approach to diagnosis in this syndrome is measurement of ionized calcium concentration in patients who exhibit such neuromuscular irritability, attempting to document whether magnesium depletion is present, as well as measurement of the circulating iPTH level. Secure documentation of total body magnesium depletion by measurement of serum magnesium is difficult because 80% of body magnesium is intracellular and a normal serum Mg^{2+} level does not accurately reflect the abundance of the intracellular ion.

Therapeutic Decision Making

Management of this condition is with dietary calcium supplementation, usually in conjunction with vitamin D. The goal of treatment is a serum calcium level in the lower half of the normal range.

DISORDERS OF THE ADRENAL CORTEX AND ADRENAL MEDULLA

Hypercortisolism

Clinical Features

The pituitary–adrenocortical endocrine axis is intact over the life span and no decline in performance of this axis is expected as a concomitant of normal aging. Pituitary gland-driven hypercortisolism (Cushing's syndrome) is quite uncommon in the older patient population. The reason for the infrequency of this endogenous syndrome is not clear. Hypercortisolism from a nodule in an adrenal cortex also is uncommon in older patients. The findings of excess circulating cortisol on physical examination are well described in standard textbooks of medicine and endocrinology. In brief they involve hypertension, loss of subcutaneous fat in the extremities and accumulation of adipose tissue in the trunk, facial telangiectasias, rounding of the face ("moon facies"), and muscle atrophy. Bone mass loss will accompany hypercortisolism that is well established.

The syndrome of excessive circulating cortisol that is encountered more frequently in geriatric patients is "iatrogenic Cushing's syndrome," resulting from prescription of antiinflammatory steroids for several conditions, including temporal arteritis and the asthmatic component of chronic obstructive pulmonary disease.

Diagnosis

Traditional confirmation of the presence of endogenous Cushing's syndrome in any patient consists of establishing a) an elevated level of 24-hour urinary free cortisol, b) nonsuppressibility of endogenous cortisol secretion, and c) lack of suppression of circulating endogenous adrenocorticotropic hormone (ACTH). Nonsuppressibility is shown with an overnight or 2-day dexamethasone suppression test with measurement of the patient's serum cortisol level in response to this maneuver. The overnight test consists of evening administration of a single 1-mg dose of dexamethasone and measurement of circulating cortisol the following morning. If the cortisol level has fallen to less than 5 μg/dL, normal suppressibility has been demonstrated. Recently, documentation of loss of diurnal variation of cortisol secretion with morning and bedtime salivary cortisol determination has become popular among endocrinologists as a method of diagnosing Cushing's syndrome[14] and appears to be valid in the elderly.[15] Interpretation of other results should be performed with an endocrinologist. Nodular adrenocortical disease with hypercortisolism is not pituitary gland-driven, and it results in suppression of endogenous (pituitary) ACTH. Inferior petrosal sinus sampling of blood for ACTH (after corticotropin-releasing hormone administration) may be used to confirm a pituitary rather than ectopic source of ACTH.

Other laboratory findings that may accompany excess circulating levels of cortisol include hyperglycemia, namely, unmasking of latent DM or worsening of glycemic control in patients with existing diabetes.

Radiological studies that are useful in the consideration of the diagnosis of pituitary–adrenal cortex hyperfunction are pituitary magnetic resonance imaging (pituitary-driven disease, Cushing's disease) and imaging of the adrenal glands for nodularity. In Cushing's disease, there will be bilateral adrenal gland hyperplasia.

Therapeutic Decision Making

The management of endogenous Cushing's syndrome or hyperfunctioning nodular adrenocortical disease in any age group is with endocrine consultation. Iatrogenic hypercortisolism, particularly when antiinflammatory steroid administration has resulted in worsened control of diabetes mellitus or bone mass loss sufficient to have provided a context in which fracture has occurred, calls for alternative antiinflammatory drug interventions in conjunction with rheumatological consultation (temporal arteritis) or with a pulmonologist (chronic obstructive pulmonary disease). Where it is feasible, withdrawal of chronic antiinflammatory corticosteroid treatment is best accomplished with subspecialty consultation to reduce the risk of exacerbation of the underlying condition for which steroid therapy was initiated and to minimize clinical hypoadrenocorticism that can complicate reduction in steroid dosage below 10 mg of prednisone daily or its equivalent. Indeed, steroid treatment of years' duration may occasionally result in a state of apparently permanent adrenal gland atrophy that is incapable of returning to a state of normal function with return of pituitary gland secretion of ACTH when therapeutic steroids are removed.

Ectopic ACTH Production by Nonendocrine Tumors

Lung carcinomas, particularly bronchial carcinoid tumors and other neuroendocrine cancers, are widely recognized to be capable of secreting ACTH and may produce Cushing's syndrome in patients of any age. Most of the affected patients are cigarette smokers. The ectopic ACTH syndrome in the elderly is a marker of very aggressive cancer and patients with the disease may not fully express the cutaneous and adipose tissue hallmarks of the syndrome. What is encountered clinically is profound muscle atrophy and severe hypokalemia, as well as acute DM. The hypokalemia reflects the very high levels of ACTH that induce corticosteroid as well as variable mineralocorticoid overproduction. The levels of circulating glucocorticoids may be sufficiently high to induce hypokalemia as well as immunosuppression. This syndrome is difficult to treat and should be managed jointly by the oncologist and endocrinologist.

Mineralocorticoid Excess

Primary Hyperaldosteronism

Excessive production of mineralocorticoid (aldosterone) by the adrenal cortex causes hypertension that is frequently difficult to treat and that is associated with wasting of urinary potassium. The hypertension that is refractory to conventional pharmaceutical management responds to varying doses of spironolactone. The hypokalemia that results is refractory to conventional doses of oral potassium replacement. This syndrome is not common in the elderly patient and its diagnosis and treatment are the same in young and elderly age groups.

Incidental Adrenal Gland Nodules

Adrenal incidentaloma is an adrenal mass, generally 1 cm or more in diameter, discovered serendipitously during a radiological examination performed for indications other than an evaluation for adrenal disease. Such lesions are a common finding in this era of computed imaging. Autopsy studies have discovered that adrenal cortical nodularity is a consequence of aging. It is estimated that 7% of patients older than 70 years will have an unsuspected adrenal adenoma on computerized abdominal imaging.[16] Despite this association with advanced age, the mean age at diagnosis in a recent review of more than 2,000 cases was only 57 years.[17]

The majority of adrenal incidentalomas are hormonally inactive, benign adrenal adenomas; however, they may represent metastatic lesions, hormonally active adenomas, pheochromocytomas, or adrenocortical carcinoma. The characteristics of the lesion on computed imaging may be useful: hypointensity on computed tomography (10 HU or less) or liver isodensity on T2-weighted magnetic resonance imaging is indicative of benign adenomas. Hyperintensity on T2-weighted images is characteristic of pheochromocytoma. Large size (>6 cm) is suggestive (but not diagnostic) of adrenocortical carcinoma, and generally warrants consideration for removal. Although the incidence of adrenocortical carcinoma peaks in the 4th and 5th decades, it can be found with advanced age.

Although it has been recognized that Cushing's syndrome resulting from adrenal adenomas is uncommon (and especially so in advanced age), appreciation has developed for the existence of "preclinical" or "subclinical" Cushing's syndrome. This occurs when autonomous production of cortisol by an adenoma is insufficient to cause overt, or "clinical," Cushing's syndrome. It has been recognized in up to 10% of adrenal incidentalomas and may be associated with hypertension and diabetes, which can improve after surgical removal of the incidentaloma.[18]

It is now recommended that patients with adrenal incidentalomas undergo hormonal evaluation consisting of an overnight low-dose (1 mg) dexamethasone test to rule out autonomous cortisol secretion. In addition, urine collection for evaluation of metanephrine and catecholamines should be performed. If the patient is hypertensive, screening for hyperaldosteronism with a plasma renin and aldosterone should be performed as well.

The natural history of these lesions has not been adequately defined. There are reports of cortisol secretory autonomy developing over extended periods of time; however, data are insufficient to provide clear recommendations regarding extended follow-up.

Hypocortisolism

Clinical Features

Spontaneous hypoadrenocorticism (Addison's disease) reflects bilateral adrenal gland destruction resulting from autoimmune disease, adrenal hemorrhage, or, occasionally, lung cancer metastatic to both adrenal glands. Iatrogenic adrenal atrophy is due to long-term use of antiinflammatory corticosteroids, as noted previously, and may be irreversible. Hypoadrenocorticism in this setting may be temporary as steroids are withdrawn, or permanent, despite the tapering or total withdrawal of steroid treatment. Spontaneous Addison's disease from autoimmune destruction of the adrenal glands is quite uncommon in the elderly. Bilateral adrenal hemorrhage certainly can occur in the older patient population and requires two contributory features: a hypocoagulable state because of therapeutic anticoagulation or spontaneous bleeding/clotting disorders and some degree of stimulation of the adrenal cortex. Here, stimulation means clinically significant medical stress, that is, a major cardiovascular event, such as a stroke or myocardial infarction with hypotension, or during and after a major surgical procedure. Involvement of the adrenals in metastatic lung cancer occurs in up to 10% of this particular patient population, but relatively few of these patients have sufficient tumor burden in the adrenals to result in hypoadrenocorticism.

The clinical clues to hypoadrenocorticism in the elderly include easy fatigability or weakness and unexplained decline in blood pressure. The latter may occur in patients who were previously hypertensive and may be attributed to antihypertensive drug treatment that was previously only marginally effective. Hyperpigmentation of the creases of the skin of the hands or pigmentary incontinence of the mucous membranes is helpful when present in supporting the suspicion of reduced function of the adrenal cortex in fair-skinned patients, but may be absent in recent onset disease – for example, in the case of bilateral adrenal hemorrhage – or unimpressive or absent in the elderly.

As in younger patients, the elderly may develop adrenocortical hypofunction that results from hypopituitarism (secondary adrenocortical insufficiency), rather than the result of primary failure of the adrenal cortex. In the older patient population, these are more commonly in women than men. In such women, the disease reflects a very much delayed onset of pituitary failure several decades after a difficult delivery at the end of pregnancy resulted in pituitary hemorrhage that only partially infarcted the pituitary gland. Thus, the medical history in older women who are suspected to have secondary adrenal gland failure must include a review of pregnancies and deliveries.

Diagnosis

Mild hyponatremia and mild or substantial hyperkalemia are classic findings of Addison's disease but are sometimes difficult to interpret in older patients because of aging-related decline in renal function. Electrolyte abnormalities are relatively common in older patients, regardless of the state of the adrenal cortex, and these abnormalities are usually due to diuretic therapy. Diuretic treatment may induce primary sodium depletion and, in the case of thiazides, free water clearance impairment that further accentuates any underlying predisposition to hyponatremia. Thiazide and loop diuretics cause hypokalemia, rather than elevation of the serum K^+ concentration that is expected in hypoadrenocorticism. Thus, loop or thiazide diuretic use in patients with hypoadrenocorticism may accentuate hyponatremia and mask hyperkalemia.

Serum cortisol levels are expected to be low in patients with decreased function of the adrenal cortex, but it is important to examine morning values that should peak in the patient with normal adrenocortical function and normal diurnal variation in cortisol. Relative adrenocortical insufficiency (decreased adrenocortical reserve) also occurs in the elderly and here the serum cortisol may be within the normal range in a stressed patient when the hormone should in fact be frankly elevated. Plasma ACTH levels are high in the patient with decreased adrenal gland function and normal pituitary gland function. ACTH is of course low in secondary adrenocortical insufficiency, usually in conjunction with reduced circulating levels of one or more other trophic hormones of the pituitary gland.

Hypoglycemia may occur in Addison's disease in patients of any age group, but it will be difficult to recognize in patients with established DM and baseline hyperglycemia.

Therapeutic Decision Making

Treatment of adrenocortical insufficiency requires replacement glucocorticoid, that is, hydrocortisone, 10 mg by mouth up to three times a day or an equivalent glucocorticoid. We recommend close attention to the need for mineralocorticoid in the elderly. In younger patients, mineralocorticoid replacement is routinely prescribed with glucocorticoids. In the older patient with an established tendency to form edema, very low dosage mineralocorticoid may result in salt and attendant water retention that is sufficient to exacerbate edema formation and/or elevation in blood pressure. Congestive heart failure may be exacerbated by low-dose mineralocorticoid administration. Therefore, institution of glucocorticoid therapy should be followed with monitoring of blood pressure, body weight, and serum K^+ concentration to look for indications for adding an aldosterone equivalent. The indications are borderline low or frankly low blood pressure, loss of even small amounts (1–2 lb) of weight, and a tendency toward or persisting hyperkalemia. When one or more of these measures is documented, Florinef at 0.05 mg by mouth daily or its equivalent may be introduced with continuation of careful monitoring of physical findings, including those of heart failure and serum electrolyte levels.

Pheochromocytoma

Clinical Features

Pheochromocytoma is a surprisingly frequent, unanticipated finding at autopsy in patients older than the age of 65 years. Although most of these tumors must be nonfunctional because of the absence of an antecedent history of hypertension or other symptoms of pheochromocytoma, it seems likely that functional adrenal medullary tumors are underrecognized in the older patient. The internist and geriatrician should not insist on finding the hallmarks of pheochromocytoma in the elderly hypertensive patient before considering a diagnostic workup for the condition. Such hallmarks include paroxysmal elevations of blood pressure, sustained very high levels of blood pressure, excessive sweating, and postural decreases in blood pressure. Excessive sweating in the elderly is not common, regardless of possible cause, such as fever or anxiety. Even when it is demonstrated, the finding of postural hypotension is not easy to interpret in older patients. In the uncomplicated young or elderly pheochromocytoma patient, a decrease in blood pressure with assumption of the upright posture represents the decreased plasma volume that is conditioned by catecholamines. Older hypertensive patients without pheochromocytoma who have been subjected to excessive diuresis will exhibit postural hypotension. Older patients with pheochromocytoma but who are receiving a thiazide diuretic or have mild expansion of blood volume due to early cardiac decompensation may not demonstrate postural hypotension.

Diagnosis

The diagnostic evaluation of the older patient for pheochromocytoma is identical to that of younger patients and is dependent on measurement of plasma fractionated catecholamines or 24-hour urinary catecholamine derivatives, that is, metanephrines. If paroxysmal hypertension *is* encountered in the elderly patient, then the drawing of plasma catecholamines at the time of a paroxysm is desirable, albeit often difficult to accomplish.

There are two important problems in interpreting the results of catecholamine measurements in the older patient population. First, incomplete 24-hour urine collections are common in older patients and if the physician uses this diagnostic approach, it is essential that creatinine in the sample be quantitated to assure completeness of the collection. Most clinical laboratories automatically include this measurement. Second, fractionated plasma catecholamine measurements include norepinephrine, and this catecholamine is readily elevated by unremarkable stress in the elderly. Here, unremarkable stress includes simple arithmetic calculations or questioning. The source of the norepinephrine that is stress generated is the autonomic nervous system, not the adrenal medulla. Free metanephrine levels are available, very sensitive and specific, although results yield a high false-positive rate, particularly in the elderly.

Therapeutic Decision Making

The management of pheochromocytoma is excision. Medical management with α-adrenergic and β-adrenergic receptor blocking agents is possible in the older patient if nonendocrine medical conditions impose unacceptably high anesthetic and surgical risks on the individual. Such management is conducted by the endocrinologist or other hypertension specialist.

DISORDERS OF THE THYROID GLAND

Hypothyroidism

Clinical Features

Primary failure of the thyroid gland is a very common endocrinopathy. The risk of hypothyroidism is approximately 10% over the life span in the U.S. population and the risk of the disease, as is the case for many endocrine diseases, is higher in women than men. The disease is usually from progressive autoimmune destruction of the thyroid gland but may follow head-and-neck irradiation for carcinoma of the upper airway or for lymphoma. Failure to recognize subtle findings of hypothyroidism in the elderly is also common and results from the fact that some of the features common in aging – decreased energy and initiative, cold temperature intolerance, constipation, excessively dry skin, low back muscle aching – are important symptoms of hypothyroidism. Indeed, a series of patients has been reported with low back syndrome as the presenting complaint of hypothyroidism. Slowed, but otherwise unimpaired, cognition is recognized by family members. That is, lapses in the responses to questions are seen. Although angina pectoris and myocardial infarction can occur in hypothyroidism, they are unusual, despite the elevated serum total cholesterol concentration that is common in the disease.

Hypertension may occur in hypothyroidism and sometimes responds to thyroid hormone replacement alone. Tachyarrhythmias occasionally interrupt the bradycardia that is typical of thyroid hypofunction. Body temperature may be 95°F to 97°F. Pallor is common but sometimes the hypercarotenemia of hypothyroidism imparts a slightly tanned to slightly orange color to the skin. Accumulation of myxedema in the skin of the face creates the impression of facial fullness and may minimize facial wrinkling in primary hypothyroidism. Myxedema is the accumulation of fibroblast-source glycosaminoglycans in a variety of tissues, including the skin and striated and cardiac muscle. Myxedema in the vocal cords conditions the hoarseness of voice that is expected in the syndrome. The timber of the voice in thyroid hypofunction, however, is reproduced in euthyroid elderly patients with histories of cigarette smoking. Muffled heart sounds represent accumulation of myxedema in the heart muscle and slowed kinetics of contraction or, commonly, myxedema and obligated water in the pericardial sac around the heart. When it occurs, the accumulation of pericardial fluid is slow and only rarely predisposes to tamponade.

A sometimes striking finding on physical examination in hypothyroid patients is the slowness with which certain precision movements of daily living are accomplished, such as buttoning and unbuttoning of blouses and shirts. Delayed relaxation phase of deep tendon reflexes is a classic finding. Occasionally, one encounters cerebellar signs in hypothyroidism that, in some patients, are reversible with several months' thyroid hormone replacement.

Severe hypothyroidism or myxedema precoma is marked by hypothermia (body temperature, 90°F–94°F), hypotension, bradycardia, and impaired sensorium. This is a medical emergency that is to be managed in the intensive care unit. A history of hypothyroidism may be elicited from family members or associates, together with an account of lapsed replacement therapy. Myxedema precoma can be triggered by coincident, severe nonthyroidal illness, such as sepsis, in which available thyroid hormone is turned over at an accelerated rate, leading to an appreciable, rapid decrease in circulating L-thyroxine (T_4). Conversion of T_4 to 3,5,3′-triiodo-L-thyronine (T_3) in peripheral tissues is ordinarily titrated against tissue need for T_3, the more metabolically active form of thyroid hormone; in severe nonthyroidal illness, this tissue deiodinase–regulated conversion is inhibited and serum T_3 levels are very low. In contrast, patients with advanced hypothyroidism who are not systemically ill with the nonthyroidal illness syndrome may have normal circulating levels of T_3, but low levels of T_4 (see later).

Secondary hypothyroidism is from hypopituitarism. Occasionally, only the pituitary cells that secrete thyroid-stimulating hormone (TSH) are affected in the damaged pituitary gland, but usually the gonadotrophin-ovary or -testicular axis is also affected. Symptoms of this form of hypothyroidism are not as severe in pituitary hypothyroidism as they are in primary thyroid gland failure and accumulation of tissue glycosaminoglycans is unimpressive.

Diagnosis

The diagnostic standard for primary hypothyroidism is increased pituitary gland release of thyrotropin (TSH) and resultant elevated serum TSH concentration. Serum T_4 and free T_4 will be low. Serum T_3 levels may be normal or low, depending on the duration of the hypothyroid state and freedom from systemic nonthyroidal illness. That is, the serum T_3 is the last of the traditional serum thyroid function tests to fall into the low range in hypothyroidism. The reason for this is that the hormone output of the thyroid gland under TSH stimulation features more T_3.

Other laboratory findings include leak of striated muscle creatine kinase (CK) into the circulation. Infrequently, cardiac muscle CK isoenzyme will be found in excess in blood from patients with primary hypothyroidism. Hyponatremia results from impaired renal tubular free water clearance that in encountered in the hypothyroid individual. The decrease in serum sodium concentration is occasionally profound. This is more likely the case in older patients who are at risk for multiple causes for hyponatremia, including thiazide diuretic use and substantial hyperglycemia. A low-grade macrocytic anemia that responds to thyroid hormone replacement therapy may also be seen. The association of autoimmune thyroid gland destruction due to Hashimoto thyroiditis and pernicious anemia places patients with primary hypothyroidism at risk for this hematological syndrome. This specific anemia does not respond to thyroid hormone replacement.

In the setting of secondary hypothyroidism, the serum TSH concentration will be low rather than elevated but serum total and free T_4 and total T_3 will be decreased. Thus, the finding of a low serum TSH in an occasional patient in whom mild hypothyroidism is suspected because of symptoms must be considered a candidate for secondary hypothyroidism. As noted previously in the discussion of hypopituitary hypoadrenocorticism, the clue in the medical history to secondary hypothyroidism may be a difficult delivery of a child several decades earlier that was associated with intrapituitary hemorrhage that was insufficient at the time to cause acute hypopituitarism.

Therapeutic Decision Making

The principal decision for the physician in treating newly recognized primary hypothyroidism is the choice of the initial dose of thyroid hormone replacement. In the elderly hypothyroid patient, this should almost invariably be a conservatively low dose, such as 25 μg L-thyroxine (T_4) by mouth daily. The reason for this conservative dose is to avoid an accelerated increase in myocardial oxygen demand in patients with a high likelihood of some degree of coronary artery disease. This slow titration is particularly important in older patients who have a documented history of heart disease. Thus, although angina pectoris and acute myocardial infarction are infrequent spontaneous events in untreated older hypothyroid patients, these events may occur in the setting of aggressive initial replacement therapy of primary hypothyroidism. The daily dose of T_4 may be increased at 2-week intervals by 12.5–25 μg until the serum TSH has fallen into the normal range. If angina supervenes, apparently as a consequence of replacement thyroid hormone dose adjustment, then slower upward adjustments in dose are required.

T_3 is not recommended as replacement therapy for the hypothyroid patient. The reason for this position is that the half-life of T_3 is short (1 day) and thus replacement may be more importantly influenced by noncompliance than is T_4 therapy. T_4 has a half-life of 7 days. Furthermore, T_3 replacement is associated with a state of several hours of elevated circulating T_3 levels after each ingestion of the hormone. There is no evidence that combination therapy with T_4 and T_3 offers benefits to patients of any age.

When clinical euthyroidism is achieved in the T_4-treated patient, it is expected that ancillary laboratory test results that were abnormal – such as the serum sodium concentration, total cholesterol and CK – will have returned to their normal ranges. Persistence of abnormalities of these measures requires additional diagnostic tests or, in the case of hyperlipidemia, specific therapy. The macrocytic anemia of pernicious anemia will not normalize with thyroid hormone replacement and requires parenteral vitamin B_{12} administration.

Although replacement thyroid hormone therapy is guided by the objective measure of the serum TSH concentration, the critical endpoint in thyroid hormone replacement is freedom of the treated patient from symptoms and signs of hypothyroidism. The latter usually is concordant with the return of TSH to the normal range. Unless symptoms clearly from hypothyroidism persist, there is no therapeutic advantage to titration of the serum TSH downward within the normal range, once the latter has been achieved. There may be therapeutic disadvantages to such pressure on the serum TSH. These disadvantages include the exacerbation of symptoms or signs of preexisting heart disease or the possibility of fostering cell proliferation in stable cancer syndromes if these are present. For example, published clinical evidence suggests that certain cancers, including those of breast, brain, and head-and-neck, may be partially thyroid hormone dependent.[18,19] These tumors of course are encountered with some frequency in the older patient population.

Acute hypoadrenocorticism may be precipitated by rapid thyroid hormone replacement in the patient with primary hypothyroidism. This complicating syndrome is heralded by a significant decrease in blood pressure and other signs of decreased intravascular volume. Short-term glucocorticoid replacement may be required in this situation and management of this more complex clinical picture is best conducted in conjunction with endocrine consultation.

Management of secondary hypothyroidism also involves conservative dose escalation of thyroid hormone replacement, but serum TSH is not a chemical guideline. Relief of symptoms is the endpoint. Serum free T_4 and total serum T_3 concentrations usually return to their normal ranges when clinical relief is obtained.

Subclinical Hypothyroidism

Elevation of the serum TSH concentration in the absence of clinical findings suggestive of primary hypothyroidism is termed subclinical hypothyroidism. It may occur in any age group. It is not clear that any morbidity accompanies this isolated laboratory abnormality and we usually do not proceed to treatment of these patients until clinical symptoms or signs consistent with hypothyroidism emerge or the serum TSH level exceeds 10 μU/mL in the absence of symptoms.[20]

Hyperthyroidism

Clinical Features

The majority of the hyperthyroid elderly patient population presents clinically with clusters of the classic symptoms and signs of thyrotoxicosis encountered in younger patients.[20] These findings include sinus tachycardia, systolic hypertension, hyperkinetic behavior, increased appetite, weight loss and frequent stools. However, thyroid gland enlargement (goiter) occurs in more than 90% of younger patients with hyperthyroidism and is absent in about 40% of older hyperthyroid patients. Endocrine ophthalmopathy (proptosis, conjunctival injection, limitation of extraocular muscle function) is rare in the elderly with diffuse toxic goiter (Graves' disease). Compared with younger individuals, older patients with hyperthyroidism have an increased incidence of toxic nodules but diffuse goiter remains more common than nodular thyroid gland enlargement in older thyrotoxic patients.

There are three other important differences between old and young individuals with hyperthyroidism. First, "monosystemic hyperthyroidism" is thyrotoxicosis that predominantly affects one organ system, such as the heart, and it is substantially more common in the elderly. Second, the symptom triad

of decreased appetite, constipation, and weight loss that is commonly associated with colon cancer occurs in approximately 15% of older hyperthyroid patients and indicates the difficulty that is sometimes encountered in recognizing thyrotoxicosis in the elderly. Third, atrial fibrillation occurs with high frequency (40%) in the elderly with thyroid hyperfunction, but this cardiac arrhythmia is encountered in only 5% of young patients with the disease. Further, atrial fibrillation remits spontaneously in the younger patient during successful treatment of thyrotoxicosis, whereas remission of atrial fibrillation during treatment is uncommon in the elderly.[20]

Pharmacological β-adrenergic blocker treatment is effective management for certain symptoms and the tachycardia of established thyrotoxicosis in patients of all ages. The widespread, appropriate use of pharmacological β-blockade in patients with heart disease means that many elderly patients with cardiovascular disease, who then develop hyperthyroidism, may have the cardiovascular and neurological symptoms of thyroid disease blunted. The practitioner must be prepared to recognize very subtle hyperthyroidism in the elderly who present with monosystemic thyroid disease that is somewhat muted by β-adrenergic blockade therapy. The clues may be unexplained weight loss, shortened attention span, or, paradoxically, apathy.

"Thyroid storm" is a state of exaggeration of symptoms of hyperthyroidism, usually cardiovascular or neurological, which is accompanied by fever that reflects severe hypermetabolism. It can be triggered by systemic infection. It is a medical emergency and is occasionally encountered in the older patient population, particularly after treatment of hyperthyroid patients with an ablative dose of radioactive iodine (see later).

Diagnosis

Suppression of serum TSH is the hallmark of spontaneous hyperthyroidism. The serum total T_4 concentration, free T_4 and total T_3 levels are elevated. In fewer than 5% of patients, only the serum T_3 concentration is abnormally high and TSH may be low or fully suppressed. This syndrome is "T_3-toxicosis." In elderly patients with concomitant nonthyroidal illness such as cancer or active heart disease with heart failure, the T_3-toxicosis state may be marked by borderline high T_3 rather than a frankly elevated value. Elevated thyroidal radioactive iodine uptake (RAIU) is useful in confirming the diagnosis of conventional hyperthyroidism or T_3-toxicosis, but the RAIU may be borderline high and not definitively increased in elderly patients with classic or atypical thyroid hyperfunction. Human B lymphocyte-source thyroid-stimulating immunoglobulin mediates Graves' disease but measurement of circulating human B lymphocyte-source thyroid-stimulating immunoglobulin levels is very expensive and its utility has not been standardized in elderly patients with Graves' disease (diffuse toxic goiter).

Factitious hyperthyroidism resulting from patient self-administration of excessive amounts of thyroid hormone is encountered across the life span. When L-thyroxine is being ingested by the patient, the laboratory test findings are elevated serum total T_4 and free T_4, suppressed circulating TSH, and, diagnostically, low or suppressed RAIU and low thyroglobulin levels. If T_3 is the form of thyroid hormone that has been used to induce factitious hyperthyroidism, then serum T_3 concentration will be elevated, total T_4 will be reduced, and TSH and thyroidal RAIU will be very low.

A handful of patients of various ages have been reported who have pituitary tumors that secrete excess amounts of TSH that causes hyperthyroidism. This very rare state has a unique serum thyroid function test profile, in that the serum TSH concentration rather than being suppressed is elevated.

Therapeutic Decision Making

The standard treatment of hyperthyroidism in the older patient population is ablation of the thyroid gland with radioactive iodine (^{131}I). Radioablation of the thyroid will frequently result in permanent hypothyroidism, a result the patient must be warned to anticipate. The release of preformed hormone from the thyroid gland 1–2 weeks following administration of ablative ^{131}I may exacerbate symptoms of hyperthyroidism in older and in young patients and rarely will provoke life-threatening thyroid storm. Even in low doses, β-adrenergic blockade therapy is effective preventive management against the possibility of thyroid storm at the time of radioablation of the thyroid gland.

Some elderly thyrotoxic patients may reject radioablation treatment and are then treated with a thioamide drug: propylthiouracil or methimazole. The choice and dose of thioamide are best made in conjunction with an endocrinologist, particularly if the patient has a hematological disorder, such as a low peripheral white blood cell count, or a history of liver disease.

Subclinical Hyperthyroidism

The finding in an asymptomatic patient of a low or suppressed serum TSH level with an otherwise normal serum thyroid function test profile defines "subclinical hyperthyroidism." Whether this syndrome is a mandate for treatment in all cases remains a point of discussion in endocrinology, but this patient population with a suppressed serum TSH level and no symptoms of thyroid disease has an increased risk of developing atrial fibrillation and osteoporosis and has a worsened all-cause mortality rate. This patient population should be managed by an endocrinologist.

Goiter

Clinical Features

Asymptomatic thyroid enlargement, particularly multinodular goiter that is accompanied by normal serum thyroid function test results, is common in the older patient population. As is the case with nodules of the adrenal cortex, nodularity of the thyroid is a concomitant of normal aging. Goiter is of course detected by inspection and palpation of the neck and is frequently brought to the attention of the physician by the patient.

Diagnosis

It is important to consider the possibility of thyroid cancer in the enlarged thyroid gland. This is rarely a consideration in diffuse thyromegaly detected on physical examination. Ultrasonography-guided aspiration of nodules at risk for harboring thyroid cancer is conducted by the endocrinologist. Such nodules are >1.0–1.5 cm in diameter or larger and are solid on sonography. Radioactive iodine scanning of the nodular thyroid gland continues to be used in some centers for the evaluation of nodules at risk for cancer. That is, nodules that do not take up the isotope have approximately a 25% risk of containing cancer. Cystic, nonmalignant nodules also fail to take up isotope.

Therapeutic Decision Making

The chemically euthyroid nodular goiter, that is, thyroid gland enlargement associated with normal serum thyroid function test results, requires endocrinological evaluation.

Thyroid Cancer

Thyroid cancer is common and, when found histologically to be papillary, can be indolent. Thyroid cancers, for a given histological type and grade, are more aggressive in the elderly than in younger patients. Metastatic papillary tumors spread locally in the neck. Follicular thyroid cancer tends to metastasize regionally, notably to the lung, and anaplastic carcinoma is highly aggressive, widely metastatic, and resistant to treatment. Papillary and follicular lesions are managed with extirpation and postoperative, large-dose radioactive iodine to destroy remaining primary or metastatic tissue that has retained the cellular iodine trap to take up iodine. Thyroid cancer is managed by the endocrinologist, nuclear medicine specialist, and oncologist.

The critical issue in thyroid cancer for the internist and geriatrician is recognizing early disease. This means 1) recording of a medical history relevant to thyroid cancer, and 2) careful evaluation of thyroid nodules and isolated cervical lymph node enlargement. The pertinent medical history in the elderly patient population involves questions about low-dose head-and-neck irradiation exposure for tonsillar or adenoidal enlargement and for acne that was practiced in the U.S. in the 1950s and into the 1960s. Such low-dose radiation exposure is a risk factor for thyroid cancer that is usually papillary. The other thyroid cancer risk is environmental hazardous exposure. The radiation accident at Chernobyl is the prime example of such exposure. Again, the form of thyroid cancer that has emerged years in the wake of the incident is papillary. Other environmental exposures may have occurred early in the development and testing of nuclear devices by research teams and military personnel in various countries.

PITUITARY DISEASES

Clinical Features

Pituitary-driven adrenocortical disease (Cushing's disease) has been discussed previously in the section on the adrenal glands and is rare in the elderly. Extremely rarely, the TSH-producing cells (thyrotropes) of the pituitary gland autonomously produce excess TSH and hyperthyroidism, as noted.

Pituitary tumors are appreciated to occur with some frequency in the older patient population. These are largely (75%) nonsecretory lesions and thus present as hypopituitarism and/or visual field losses. The prolactin-producing cells of the pituitary may become tumoral, but are very rarely secretory. When the lesions are secretory, the primary product is growth hormone (GH) that leads to subtle or occasionally pronounced acromegaly. Some "nonsecretory" pituitary adenomas in the elderly may derive from gonadotropic cell lines and may secrete nonfunctional β-LH subunit.

Hypopituitarism in the older patient population is clinically marked by loss of gonadotropin secretion, which is more readily appreciated in male patients as loss of libido. Also evident in older patients are secondary hypothyroidism and secondary hypoadrenocorticism.

Diagnosis

Visual field examination and evaluation of patients for secondary hypogonadism and pituitary hypothyroidism as well as secondary adrenocortical hypofunction are required. End-organ secretory products, such as testosterone, thyroid hormones, cortisol, are low, but there is no corresponding increase in luteinizing hormone, TSH, or ACTH, and the circulating levels of these polypeptide hormones may be very low. Radiological evaluation of the sella turcica and pituitary gland is essential and is usually done by magnetic resonance imaging.

Therapeutic Decision Making

The treatment regimens for hypopituitary patients and for those with excessive growth hormone production are developed in conjunction with an endocrinologist and neurosurgeon. Radiotherapy is utilized when there is a need for reduction in adenoma size.

REFERENCES

1. Scholz DA, Purnell DC. Asymptomatic primary hyperparathyroidism: 10-year prospective study. *Mayo Clin Proc.* 1981;56:473–478.
2. Gutteridge DH, Gruber HE, Kermode DG, Worth, GK. Thirty cases of concurrent Paget's disease and primary hyperparathyroidism: sex distribution, histomorphometry, and prediction of the skeletal response to parathyroidectomy. *Calcif Tissue Int.* 1999;65:427–435.
3. Politz D, Norman J. Hyperparathyroidism in patients over age 70: clinical characteristics and their ability to undergo outpatient parathyroidectomy. *Thyroid.* 2007;17:133–139.
4. Holick MF. Vitamin D deficiency. *NEJM.* 2007;357:266–281.
5. Quarles LD, Yohay DA, Carroll BA, et al. Prospective trial of pulse oral versus intravenous calcitriol treatment of hyperparathyroidism in ESRD. *Kidney Int.* 1994;45:1710–1721.
6. Indridason OS, Quarles LD. Comparison of treatments for mild secondary hyperparathyroidism in hemodialysis patients. *Kidney Int.* 2000;57:282–292.
7. Linnebur SA, Milchak JL. Assessment of oral bisphosphonate use in elderly patients with varying degrees of kidney function. *Am J Geriatr Pharmacother.* 2004;2:213–218.
8. Stewart AF. Clinical practice. Hypercalcemia associated with cancer. *NEJM.* 2005;352:373–379.
9. Machado CE, Flombaum CD. Safety of pamidronate in patients with renal failure and hypercalcemia. *Clin Nephrol.* 1996;45:175–179.
10. Pazanias M, Miller P, Blumentals WA, Bernal M, Kothawala P. A review of the literature on osteonecrosis of the jaw in patients with osteoporosis treated with oral bisphosphonates: prevalence, risk factors, and clinical characteristics. *Clin Ther.* 2007;29:1548–1558.
11. Arumugam CP, Sundravel S, Shanthi P, Sachdanandam P. Tamoxifen flare hypercalcemia: an additional support for gallium nitrate usage. *J Bone Miner Metab.* 2006;24:243–247.
12. Klatte T, Said JW, Belidegrun AS, Pantuck AJ. Differential diagnosis of hypercalcemia in renal malignancy. *Urology.* 2007;70:179e7–179e8.
13. Sourbier C, Massfelder T. Parathyroid hormone-related protein in human renal cell carcinoma. *Cancer Lett.* 2006;240:170–182.
14. Picolos MK, Lavis VR, Orlander PR. Milk-alkali syndrome is a major cause of hypercalcemia among non-end-stage renal disease (non-ESRD) inpatients. *Clin Endocrinol (Oxf).* 2005;63:566–557.
15. Findling JW, Raff H. Cushing's syndrome: important issues in diagnosis and management. *J Clin Endocrinol Metab.* 2006;91:3746–3753.
16. Raff H. Personal communication, 2007.
17. Young WF. The incidentally discovered adrenal mass. *NEJM.* 2007;356:601–610.
18. Thompson RG, Young WF. Adrenal incidentaloma. *Curr Opinion Oncol.* 2003;15:84–90.
19. Hercbergs AA, Goyal LK, Suh JH, et al. Propylthiouracil-induced chemical hypothyroidism with high-dose tamoxifen prolongs survival in recurrent high grade glioma: a Phase I/II study. *Anticancer Res.* 2003;23:617–626.
20. Cristofanilli M, Yamamura Y, Kau SW, et al. Thyroid hormone and breast carcinoma: primary hypothyroidism is associated with a reduced incidence of primary breast carcinoma. *Cancer.* 2005;103:1122–1128.

29

OSTEOPOROSIS AND OTHER METABOLIC DISORDERS OF THE SKELETON IN AGING

Karen D. Novielli, MD

BACKGROUND

Osteoporosis is a disorder of the skeletal system in which low bone mass and a deterioration of skeletal microarchitecture result in reduced bone strength and increased risk of fracture. Peak bone mass typically occurs in the third decade of life and is a result of genetic factors, nutrition, physical activity, and hormonal status. Age-related bone loss begins in the fourth or fifth decade of life and is accelerated in women during the early years of menopause. Factors that impair peak bone mass or accelerate bone loss can lead to osteoporosis. Medical conditions such as malabsorption and endocrine disorders that can impact peak bone mass and/or the rate of bone loss can increase the likelihood of osteoporosis.

The World Health Organization operationally defines osteoporosis as a bone mineral density (BMD) that falls 2.5 standard deviations or more below the mean for healthy young adults of the same race and sex. The T-score is the term given to express the number of standard deviations that an individual's BMD differs from the mean for healthy young adults of the same race and sex. A T-score lower than −2.5 is classified as osteoporosis and a T-score between −1.0 and −2.5 is considered to indicate osteopenia.

The primary clinical manifestations of this disorder are fractures of the spine and hip, although fractures may occur at any skeletal site. Osteoporosis exerts a significant toll on the quality of life and life expectancy of the elderly. One in two women and one in five men older than the age of 50 years can expect to experience an osteoporosis-related fracture in their lifetime.[1] Fractures of the hip are associated with a loss of independence. For example, only one third of women who experience a hip fracture return to their previous living arrangements and functional abilities.[2] Vertebral fractures are associated with loss of height, chronic pain, and difficulty with daily activities. There is also a higher age-adjusted relative risk of dying following a hip fracture and following a clinical vertebral fracture of 6.68 and 8.64, respectively.[3]

SCREENING FOR OSTEOPOROSIS

In clinical practice, decisions surrounding screening for osteoporosis – who to screen, when to screen, how often to screen and by what modality to screen – are far from settled. In reviewing the available evidence for the U.S. Preventive Services Task Force (USPSTF) in establishing their 2002 recommendations on screening for osteoporosis, Nelson and colleagues[4] noted that there were no trials in which the effectiveness of screening was evaluated and therefore no direct evidence that screening improves outcomes. It is not surprising then that there is a lack of consensus in clinical guidelines on screening for osteoporosis.

The best available, although tenuous, evidence for screening comes from a 2005 study by Kern et al.[5] These authors studied a population-based cohort from four states enrolled in a cardiovascular health study. Participants in two states underwent hip dual-energy x-ray absorptiometry (DXA) scanning, whereas participants in the other two states received usual care. Although the use of hip DXA was associated with 36% fewer incident hip fractures over the 6 years of study compared with usual care, differences in osteoporosis treatments between the screened and unscreened groups did not seem to account for the differences in hip fracture rates. Thus, although there appears to be a positive effect of screening, the mechanism remains unclear and the effect could be a result of confounding variables.

Despite a lack of clear evidence for benefit, the USPSTF[6] and the National Osteoporosis Foundation [7] both recommend routine screening for osteoporosis for all women aged 65 years and older regardless of risk factors. The USPSTF gives this recommendation with a rating of B, finding at least fair evidence that the service improves important health outcomes and that benefits outweigh harms. In making this recommendation, the USPSTF determined that there was good evidence that the risk for osteoporosis and fracture increases with age and other factors, that BMD measurements accurately predict short-term risk for fractures, and that treating asymptomatic women with osteoporosis reduces their risk for fracture. A National Institutes of Health Consensus Statement,[8] on the other hand, notes that although the value of bone density in predicting fracture risk is established, the value of universal screening, especially in perimenopausal women has not been established. They recommend that until there is good evidence to support the cost effectiveness of routine screening or the efficacy of early initiation of preventive drugs, an individualized approach is recommended and that a bone density measurement be considered when it will help the patient decide whether to institute treatment to prevent osteoporotic fractures.

In a meta-analysis of the ability of bone density measurement to predict fracture, Cumming[9] noted that "measuring bone density is at least as good for predicting fractures as high blood pressure is for predicting stroke and high serum cholesterol is for predicting coronary heart disease." In a separate meta-analysis by Marshall et al.,[10] the authors concluded that when all measurement sites and all measurement methods were combined, the overall relative risk for fracture was 1.5 (95% confidence interval [CI] 1.4–1.7) for 1 standard deviation decrease in bone density. They also concluded that BMD measurement at the hip was better for predicting hip fracture (RR 2.6, 95% CI 2.0–3.5) and that measurement at the lumbar spine was a better predictor for fracture at that site (RR 2.4, 95% CI 1.8–3.2).

Using estimates of age-specific prevalence rates, treatment effects, and adherence rates, Nelson et al.[4] estimated that in the 65–69 age group, 731 women would need to be screened to prevent one hip fracture in 5 years and that 88 women with low bone density would need to be treated to benefit 1 woman. Two hundred and forty-eight women would need to be screened to prevent one vertebral fracture and 30 women would need to be treated to benefit 1 woman. The authors noted that these numbers become more favorable with advancing age because of rising prevalence of osteoporosis with age. Relative to women aged 50–54 years, the risk of having osteoporosis is 5.9 times higher in women aged 65–69 years, and 14.3 times higher in women aged 75–79 years.[11]

With respect to women younger than the age of 65 years, the USPSTF recommends that routine screening begin at age 60 years for women at increased risk of fractures from osteoporosis and makes no recommendation for or against screening in postmenopausal women who are younger than 60 years or in women aged 60–64 years who are not at increased risk for osteoporotic fractures.[6] The National Osteoporosis Foundation recommends screening for younger postmenopausal women with one or more risk factors (other than being white, postmenopausal and female)[7] and the National Institutes of Health Consensus Statement recommends that bone density measurement

should be considered in patients receiving glucocorticoid therapy for 2 months or more and in patients with other conditions placing them at high risk for osteoporotic fractures.[8]

A subject of debate is determining which risk factors other than age place a postmenopausal woman at higher risk for osteoporotic fractures and when a discussion about earlier screening should be initiated. In postmenopausal women aged 60–64 years, lower body weight (<70 kg) is the single best predictor of low BMD.[6] There is less evidence to support the use of other risk factors such as smoking, weight loss, family history, decreased physical activity, alcohol use, caffeine use, low calcium intake, low vitamin D intake, and the use of certain medications, in guiding decision making about whether to begin screening at an earlier age.[6]

Specific instruments to aid the clinician in the assessment of risk for osteoporosis and fracture generally have moderate-to-high sensitivity and low specificity. The best validated instruments include the 3-item Osteoporosis Risk Assessment Instrument and the 6-item Simple Calculated Osteoporosis Risk Estimation tool.[12,13] The Osteoporosis Risk Assessment Instrument uses age, weight, and current use of hormone replacement therapy to identify women at risk for osteoporosis and has a 94% sensitivity and 41% specificity. The Simple Calculated Osteoporosis Risk Estimation instrument has a 91% sensitivity and a 40% specificity.[12,13]

No studies have evaluated the optimal interval for repeated screening for osteoporosis. Screening should not be more frequent than every 2 years as this amount of time is be needed to measure reliably a change in BMD; however, longer intervals may prove adequate.[14] Repeated screening is likely to prove more beneficial in women at higher risk, namely older women, women with lower BMD at baseline, and those with other risk factors for fracture.

As to which test is best to screen for osteoporosis, bone density measurement at the femoral neck by DXA is the best predictor of hip fracture and is comparable to forearm measurements for predicting fracture at other sites.[14] Other methods of testing, such as peripheral bone testing in the primary care setting, can help to identify postmenopausal women at high risk of fracture in the short-term; however, further research is needed to compare the accuracy of peripheral bone density with DXA. In general, the likelihood of being diagnosed with osteoporosis varies with the location and the number of sites tested and the type of bone density test used.[14]

EVALUATION OF THE PATIENT WITH OSTEOPOROSIS

Routine evaluation of the patient with osteoporosis should be performed to exclude secondary causes of osteoporosis such as thyroid disorder, hyperparathyroidism, or chronic liver or kidney disease and should include thyroid function tests, calcium, phosphate, alkaline phosphatase, kidney and liver function tests, a complete blood count, and an erythrocyte sedimentation rate. Consideration should also be given to obtaining serum immunoglobulins and paraproteins and urinary Bence-Jones proteins to exclude multiple myeloma.

PREVENTION AND TREATMENT OF OSTEOPOROSIS

A number of studies have documented that DXA testing alone is a poor predictor of who will sustain a fracture. Approximately half of the fractures experienced by community-dwelling individuals occur in those with a T-score greater than –2.5.[15] Silverman[16] recommends considering risk factors other than BMD, particularly age and prior fracture, in treatment decisions and using a 10-year probability of fracture rather than relative risk of fracture to guide treatment decision making. Most guidelines recommend treating older patients with osteoporosis (T-score < –2.5) and not treating those with a T score greater than –1.5. Patients who have already sustained a fragility fracture are at increased risk of sustaining a further fracture and should be treated. For those with a T-score between –1.5 and –2.5, other clinical risk factors such as older age and weight can help to decide which patients are most likely to benefit from treatment.

Nonpharmacological Modalities

Patients with osteoporosis and those at risk for developing osteoporosis should be counseled about risk factor reduction and lifestyle modifications where appropriate. Medications associated with increased risk of osteoporosis such as glucocorticoids, thyroid hormone replacement, and certain anticonvulsants (for example, phenytoin) should be reviewed and reduced or eliminated if possible. Patients should be counseled to stop smoking and to avoid alcohol and caffeine.

Optimal intake of calcium and vitamin D is thought to be important for reducing bone loss and suppressing bone turnover, and may, particularly in institutionalized older individuals, be associated with fewer fractures.[17] The majority of clinical trials evaluating pharmacological agents for treatment of osteoporosis have included adequate calcium and vitamin D supplementation. Generally, adequate amounts of daily calcium and vitamin D are considered important adjuncts to the prevention and treatment of osteoporosis but insufficient as lone therapy for treatment.

Although the optimal source of calcium is dietary, most patients do not obtain enough calcium or vitamin D through dietary sources and require supplementation. The Institute of Medicine recommends that men and women older than the age of 50 years consume at least 1,200 mg of calcium per day and those 50–70 years or older from 400 IU to 600 IU of vitamin D daily. There appears to be no advantage to the use of vitamin D analogs such as calcitriol over vitamin D in the treatment of osteoporosis and the use of analogs may lead to an increased incidence of adverse events.[17]

Weight-bearing exercise is critical for development and maintenance of bone mass. To the degree that exercise pro-

motes coordination, balance, and muscle strength, it may also be important for fall prevention. For many individuals, a regular walking program is the simplest way to achieve the benefits of exercise. Progressive resistance strength training may improve muscle strength, however, if not supervised appropriately, can result in musculoskeletal injury. This is of particular concern in patients with osteoporosis, in whom resistance training with loads to the spine for instance could result in a fragility fracture.

For patients at high risk of falling, additional measures to reduce the likelihood of falling and the impact of falling should be considered. Occupational therapists evaluate the home environment and provide suggestions that can reduce the likelihood of falling. Physical therapists can assist with a program to improve muscle strength, gait, and balance. They will also evaluate the patient for appropriate use of assistive devices. Other measures that can reduce the impact of falling, such as hip protectors, should also be considered.

Natural Health Products

A review article by Whelan et al.,[18] identified 45 natural health products that were noted in the literature as having value in the management of osteoporosis in women. Of the 45 health products, only 3 health products (dehydroepiandrosterone [DHEA], Vit K2, and phytoestrogens) met criteria for their evidence-based review. The other agents either did not have randomized controlled trials available to support their use or the randomized controlled trials were of combination products and not the individual product alone.

Two trials for DHEA were evaluated. One showed improvement in BMD of older women who took DHEA in a dose of 50 mg/day. The other trial showed no benefit to BMD in healthy women who took DHEA for 6 months at a dose of 100 mg/day.

Five trials of vitamin K2 were evaluated. Two studies using 45 mg/day of vitamin K2 for 24 months in postmenopausal women with osteoporosis found fewer vertebral fractures among the vitamin K2 group than among the controls. In the trials evaluated, vitamin K2 also appeared to preserve bone density. Further studies of natural health products should be obtained before they can be recommended for either prevention or treatment of osteoporosis.

Eleven trials of phytoestrogens were evaluated. The authors concluded that data from the trials were equivocal, with some studies showing benefit and others not showing a benefit.

Pharmacological Modalities

Currently, the bisphosphonates alendronate, ibandronate, and risedronate, as well as calcitonin, estrogen, parathyroid hormone (PTH), and raloxifene are all approved by the U.S. Food and Drug Administration (FDA) for the prevention and/or treatment of osteoporosis. The bisphosphonates, calcitonin, estrogen, and raloxifene are classified as antiresorptive medications as they slow or stop the bone resorption portion of the bone remodeling cycle. PTH is the only approved medication that increases bone formation.

Bisphosphonates

The bisphosphonates etidronate, alendronate, and risedronate have been shown to increase the BMD at the hip and spine in a dose-dependent manner. In postmenopausal women with osteoporosis, etidronate and alendronate reduced the incidence of vertebral fractures.[19,20] In postmenopausal women with osteoporosis and preexisting vertebral fractures at baseline, both alendronate and risedronate were effective at reducing the number of new vertebral and nonvertebral fractures.[21,22] In a meta-analysis of data from randomized trials of bisphosphonates,[23] the relative risk reduction for vertebral fractures was 48% for alendronate and 36% for risedronate, and for nonvertebral fractures 49% for alendronate and 27% for risedronate. Both alendronate and risedronate are approved for treatment of glucocorticoid-induced osteoporosis, and alendronate is approved for the treatment of osteoporosis in men. Once weekly doses of bisphosphonates are considered to be therapeutically equivalent to daily doses and have a safety and tolerability profile at least as good as daily doses and comparable to placebo.[24] Ibandronate is approved for the treatment of postmenopausal osteoporosis and is administered once a month.

The bisphosphonates inhibit osteoclastic bone resorption and accumulate in the skeleton.[25] The effect of long-term use of bisphosphonates on bone turnover and strength is unknown. Ten-year follow-up data from phase III studies of alendronate have shown that spine BMD increases progressively for at least 10 years during continued treatment and the initial increases in BMD seen with alendronate treatment at other skeletal sites are maintained during this time period. It appears that reductions in vertebral and nonvertebral fracture risk are also maintained during 10 years of treatment.[26] Although many of the bisphosphonates are approved for the prevention of osteoporosis, because they accumulate in the skeleton and may have an impact on bone turnover and bone strength, very long-term data are needed to evaluate appropriately the risk/benefit profile of these medications for the prevention of osteoporosis in those whose life expectancy can be measured in decades and whose immediate risk for fracture is not high.

Calcitonin

The hormone calcitonin is important for calcium regulation and bone metabolism. Salmon calcitonin has been shown to improve BMD at the spine and to inhibit bone turnover. The Prevent Recurrence of Osteoporotic Fractures study,[27] which demonstrated a significant reduction in the risk of new vertebral fracture in postmenopausal women with established osteoporosis, did not show an effect on nonvertebral fracture, had a dropout rate of 60%, and failed to demonstrate a dose-dependent effect on fracture rate, all of which limit confidence in study results.

Raloxifene

Raloxifene, a nonsteroidal benzothiophene, belongs to the class of medications known as selective estrogen receptor modulators. These compounds have estrogen-like effects on bone and lipids, but estrogen antagonist effects on the breast and uterus. In the Multiple Outcomes of Raloxifene Evaluation study, raloxifene was shown to prevent vertebral fractures but not nonvertebral fractures in postmenopausal women with osteoporosis. As with many of the treatments for osteoporosis, results were more impressive for women with previous fractures.[28] In a separate analysis, raloxifene was shown to reduce the incidence of breast cancer in postmenopausal women with osteoporosis.[29] Raloxifene does, however, significantly increase the risk of venous thromboembolism; therefore, raloxifene should be considered for women in whom combined effects of fracture reduction and breast cancer prevention outweigh the increased risk of venous thromboembolism.

Estrogen

Estrogen, either alone or combined with progesterone, has been shown to reduce bone loss and reduce the incidence of fractures of the hip and spine in postmenopausal women. The increased risk of adverse events, however, most notably stroke, but also (to varying degrees depending on nature of hormone therapy prescribed, age and menopausal status of the woman) uterine cancer, breast cancer, venous thromboembolism, coronary disease, cholecystitis, and dementia, suggest that for most women the risks of therapy outweigh the benefits.[30,31]

Parathyroid Hormone

Although (PTH) has been shown to increase lumbar spine bone mineral density and decrease the incidence of vertebral fractures, many questions remain about its optimal use.[32,33] PTH therapy is expensive and requires daily injections. There are also questions regarding its efficacy in patients previously treated with bisphosphonates (can it stimulate new bone formation in patients who have previously used bisphosphonates that are incorporated into bone) and regarding its timing and combination use with other agents. For instance, in postmenopausal women with osteoporosis, PTH plus alendronate was not better than monotherapy with either agent for increasing BMD at 12 months.[34] and in men with osteoporosis, PTH alone was more effective than PTH plus alendronate or alendronate alone for increasing BMD at the lumbar spine when alendronate was begun at baseline and PTH therapy was begun at the 6-month visit and continued for 30 months.[35]

Strontium Ranelate

Strontium ranelate, which decreases bone resorption and stimulates bone formation, has been shown to improve BMD and to reduce vertebral and nonvertebral fractures in postmenopausal women with osteoporosis.[36] Mild adverse events include diarrhea and headache. Strontium ranelate is considered an alternative first-line therapy for those in whom the bisphosphonates are contraindicated or poorly tolerated in Europe.[37] It has not yet been approved by the FDA for the treatment of osteoporosis. More experience with this new therapeutic agent will help to evaluate fully the benefit/

risk profile of strontium ranelate in the treatment of osteoporosis.

MONITORING OF TREATMENT

At present, there is no consensus as to whether and how the treatment of osteoporosis should be monitored. There is no evidence that repeated use of DXA testing or monitoring of serum biochemical markers has an impact on fracture risk for patients receiving treatment for osteoporosis. Compliance with prescribed medications, calcium, vitamin D, and exercise and attention to fall prevention should be emphasized by the care provider.

REFERENCES

1. Cummings SR, Melton LJ. Epidemiology and outcomes of osteoporotic fractures. *Lancet.* 2002;359:1761–1767.
2. Jagal S, Sherry P, Schatzker J. The impact and consequences of hip fracture in Ontario. *Can J Surg.* 1996;39:105–111.
3. Cauley JA, Thompson DE, Ensrud KC, Scott JC, Black D. Risk of mortality following clinical fractures. *Osteoporosis Int.* 2000;11:556–561.
4. Nelson HD, Helfand M, Woolf SH, Allan JD. Screening for postmenopausal osteoporosis: a review of the evidence for the U.S. Preventive Services Task Force. *Ann Intern Med.* 2002;137: 529–541.
5. Kern LM, Powe NR, Levine MA, et al. Association between screening for osteoporosis and the incidence of hip fracture. *Ann Intern Med.* 2005;142:173–181.
6. U.S. Preventive Services Task Force (USPSTF). Screening for Osteoporosis in Postmenopausal Women: Recommendations and Rationale. Agency for Healthcare Research and Quality, Rockville, MD; 2002. Available at: http://www.ahrq.gov/clinic/3rduspstf/osteoporosis/osteorr.htm. Accessed June 8, 2008.
7. National Osteoporosis Foundation. Physician's guide to prevention and treatment of osteoporosis. Washington, DC: National Osteoporosis Foundation; 1999. Available at: http://www.nof.org/physguide/diagnosis.htm. Accessed June 8, 2008.
8. Osteoporosis Prevention, Diagnosis and Therapy. NIH Consensus Statement Online 2000 March 27–29; 17(1): 1–36. Available at: http://consensus.nih.gov/2000/2000Osteoporosis111html.htm.
9. Cumming RG. Meta-analysis: bone mineral density measurement predicts risk for fractures in women. *ACP Journal Club.* 1996;125:48–49.
10. Marshall D, Johnell O, Wedel H. Meta-analysis of how well measures of bone mineral density predict occurrence of osteoporotic fractures. *BMJ.* 1996;312:1254–1259.
11. Siris ES, Miller PD, Barrett-Connor E, et al. Identification and fracture outcomes of undiagnosed low bone mineral density in postmenopausal women: results from the National Osteoporosis Risk Assessment. *JAMA.* 2001;286:2815–2822.
12. Cadarette SM, Jaglal SB, Kreiger N, et al. Development and validation of the Osteoporosis Risk Assessment Instrument to facilitate selection of women for bone densitometry. *Can Med Assoc J.* 2000;162:1289–1294.
13. Cadarette SM, Jaglal SB, Murray T, et al. Evaluation of decision rules for referring women for bone densitometry by dual-energy x-ray absorptiometry. *JAMA.* 2001;286: 57–63.
14. Lydick E, Cook K, Turpin J, et al. Development and validation of a simple questionnaire to facilitate identification of women likely to have low bone density. *Am J Manag Care.* 1998;4:37–48.
15. Siris ES, Chen YT, Abbott TA, et al. Bone mineral density thresholds for pharmacological intervention to prevent fractures. *Arch Intern Med.* 2004;164:1108–1112.
16. Silverman SL. Selecting patients for osteoporosis therapy. *Curr Osteoporosis Rep.* 2006;4:91–95.
17. Avenell A, Gillespie WJ, Gillespie LD, O'Connell DL. Vitamin D and vitamin D analogues for preventing fractures associated with involutional and post-menopausal osteoporosis. *Cochrane Database Syst Rev.* 2006;2:AN: 00075320-100000000-00018.
18. Whelan AM, Jurgens TM, Bowles SK. Natural health products in the prevention and treatment of osteoporosis: systematic review of randomized controlled trials. *Ann Pharmacother.* 2006;40: 836–849.
19. Cranney A, Welch V, Adachi JD, et al. Etidronate for treating and preventing postmenopausal osteoporosis. *Cochrane Database Syst Rev.* 2001;4: CD003376.
20. Liberman UA, Weiss SR, Broll J, et al. Effect of oral alendronate on bone mineral density and the incidence of fractures in postmenopausal osteoporosis. *NEJM.* 1995;333:1437–1443.
21. Harris ST, Watts NB, Genant HK, et al. For the Vertebral Efficacy with Risedronate Therapy (VERT) Study Group. Effects of risedronate treatment on vertebral and nonvertebral fractures in women with postmenopausal osteoporosis. A randomized controlled trial. *JAMA.* 1999;282:1344–1352.
22. Black DM, Cummings SR, Karpf DB, et al. Randomised trial of effect of alendronate on risk of fracture in women with existing vertebral fractures. Fracture Intervention Trial Research Group. *Lancet.* 1996;348:1535–1541.
23. Cranney A, Guyatt G, Griffith L, et al. Meta-analysis of therapies for postmenopausal osteoporosis. IX: Summary of meta-analyses of therapies for postmenopausal osteoporosis. *Endocr Rev.* 2002;23:570–578.
24. Rizzoli R. Long term outcomes of weekly biphosphonates. *Clin Orthop Rel Res.* 2006;443:61–65.
25. Cummings SR, Black DM, Nevitt MC, et al. Bone density at various sites for prediction of hip fractures. *Lancet.* 1993;341:72–75.
26. Bone HG, Hosking D, Devogelaer JP, et al. Ten years' experience with alendronate for osteoporosis in postmenopausal women. *NEJM.* 2004;350:1189–1199.
27. Chesnut CH, Silverman S, Andriano K, et al. A randomized trial of nasal spray salmon calcitonin in postmenopausal women with established osteoporosis: the prevent recurrence of osteoporotic fractures study. *Am J Med.* 2000;109:267–276.
28. Ettinger B, Black DM, Mitlak BH, et al. For the Multiple Outcomes of Raloxifene Evaluation (MORE) Investigators. Reduction of vertebral fracture risk in postmenopausal women with osteoporosis treated with raloxifene. Results from a 3-year randomized clinical trial. *JAMA.* 1999;282:637–645.
29. Cummings SR, Eckert S, Krueger KA, et al. The effect of raloxifene on risk of breast cancer in postmenopausal women. Results from the MORE randomized trial. *JAMA.* 1999;281:2189–2197.
30. Nelson HD, Humphrey LL, Nygren P, Teutsch SM, Allan JD. Postmenopausal hormone replacement therapy: scientific review. *JAMA.* 2002;228:872–881.
31. Farquhar CM, Marjoribanks J, Lethaby A, Lamberts Q, Suckling A. The Cochrane HT Study Group. Long term hormone therapy for perimenopausal and postmenopausal women. *Cochrane Database Syst Rev.* 2006;2: AN: 00075320-100000000-03165.
32. Crandall C. Parathyroid hormone for treatment of osteoporosis. *Arch Intern Med.* 2002;162:2297–2309.

33. Neer RM, Arnaud CD, Zanchetta JR, et al. Effect of parathyroid hormone on fractures and bone mineral density in postmenopausal women with osteoporosis. *NEJM.* 2001;344:1434–1441.

34. Black DM, Greenspan SL, Ensrud KE, et al. The effects of parathyroid hormone and alendronate alone or in combination in postmenopausal osteoporosis. *NEJM.* 2003;349:1207–1215.

35. Finkelstein JS, Hayes A, Hunzelman JL, et al. The effects of parathyroid hormone, alendronate, or both in men with osteoporosis. *NEJM.* 2003;349:1216–1226.

36. Meunier PJ, Roux C, Seeman E, et al. The effects of strontium ranelate on the risk of vertebral fracture in women with postmenopausal osteoporosis. *NEJM.* 2004;350:459–468.

37. Poole KE, Compston JE. Osteoporosis and its management. *BMJ.* 2006;333:1251–1256.

30

COMMON RHEUMATIC DISEASES IN THE ELDERLY

Beth L. Jonas, MD

Musculoskeletal pain in the elderly is frequently encountered in clinical practice. The list of conditions that cause pain is extensive and includes many self-limited conditions and those that are urgent and potentially disabling. A careful history-taking with attention to chronicity, preceding trauma, pattern of joint involvement, nature of the pain, factors that alleviate or exacerbate the pain, and any associated systemic symptoms can provide very useful diagnostic information. Joint pain may be from derangements in the joints themselves or in any of the supporting periarticular structures. In the elderly, these may coexist. Physical examination will allow further narrowing of the differential diagnosis. Attention should be paid to the presence of joint swelling and tenderness, bony deformities, joint range of motion (both passive and active), soft tissue tenderness, rashes, and subcutaneous nodules. The general medical examination is equally important to assess the presence of extraarticular disease in primary rheumatic conditions. In addition, numerous general medical problems may present with early musculoskeletal complaints, including thyroid disease, viral infections, and hematological malignancies. Laboratory studies and imaging studies can serve as an adjunct to the history and physical examination. Synovial fluid analysis, particularly in the case of a monoarthritis can be invaluable to rule out infection or confirm the diagnosis of a crystal-induced arthritis.

Evaluation and management of the elderly presents some unique challenges to the practitioner. Clinical presentation of disease may differ in older and younger adults and multiple comorbidities may make the workup challenging. Older adults may attribute symptoms to "getting old" and not seek medical attention until late in the course of the illness. Loss of functional status may lead to sleep disturbance, anxiety, and depression, further complicating the clinical presentation. In this chapter we will review the clinical presentation, diagnostic workup, and principles of management for the most common rheumatic conditions seen in the elderly.

OSTEOARTHRITIS

Introduction

Osteoarthritis (OA) is the most prevalent joint disorder in the United States and is the leading cause of disability. Advancing age is the strongest risk factor for the development of the disease. Data from the National Health Interview Survey estimates that 40% of men and 55% of women older than the age of 65 years have doctor-diagnosed arthritis with the majority of these cases from OA. Projected estimates for 2030, predict substantial increases in arthritis prevalence as well as arthritis-associated activity limitation. It is estimated that in 2030 there will be 67 million cases of arthritis, and more than half of these will be in the geriatric age group.[1] The aging population and the growing epidemic of obesity will contribute to the increasing burden of arthritis in our population.

OA was previously thought to be a consequence of normal aging; however, more recent evidence suggests that OA results from a complex interplay of numerous factors including genetic determinants, biochemical factors in the cartilage, mechanical forces, and local inflammation.[2] OA can be categorized as primary or secondary disease. Primary OA is an idiopathic disease that may be localized to a single joint area or have a more generalized presentation. The most common sites of involvement are the hands, knees, hips, feet, and spine. Less commonly involved joint groups are the shoulders, ankles, sacroiliac joints, and the wrists. Secondary OA may be a result of previous trauma, congenital diseases, calcium pyrophosphate deposition disease, primary inflammatory joint disorders (rheumatoid arthritis [RA], gout), osteonecrosis of the joints, or metabolic diseases (diabetes, thyroid disease, hemochromatosis, and acromegaly).

Clinical Presentation

The clinical presentation is one of joint pain that is localized and worse with activity. As the disease progresses, there is increasing pain, associated stiffness, and the development of rest pain or night pain. Night pain that occurs early in the course should raise the suspicion of a primarily inflammatory disease such as septic arthritis, RA, or a crystal-induced arthritis. A complete history-taking and physical examination is essential for the evaluation of any patient who presents with joint pain. Careful attention should be paid to rule out other causes of joint pain.

The physical examination reveals joint tenderness and crepitus from the irregular articulating surfaces. Bony enlargement may be appreciated due to osteophyte formation at the margins of the joint. Loss of the normal joint range of motion may be seen. Joint effusions may be present, but other signs of inflammation such as warmth and overlying erythema are usually absent. Synovial fluid analysis shows a non inflammatory joint fluid, with less that 2,000 cell/mm^3. The presence of crystals in the synovial fluid supports the diagnosis of gout or pseudogout. Other laboratory tests such as the WESR and C-reactive protein (CRP) are only indicated if there is a clinical suspicion for inflammatory arthritis. They are very sensitive tests that are frequently elevated in elderly patient with other comorbidities and are rarely helpful diagnostically.

Radiographs should be obtained and are helpful in establishing the diagnosis. In addition they are most important to rule out more serious causes of bony pain including fractures, infections, and tumors. Osteophyte formation and joint space narrowing are typical findings. Later in the course, joint space narrowing worsens and subchondral sclerosis and subchondral cyst formation may be seen. It should be noted that many elderly patients have radiographic evidence of OA, but may not be symptomatic. Because the currently available therapies are only effective in treating symptoms, these patients do not require any therapy.

Hands

OA of the hands is one of the most common presentations. Initially, pain predominates and the physical examination may be unremarkable. Over time, there is progressive bony enlargement of the joints, particularly the distal interphalangeal (Heberden nodes) and proximal interphalangeal ([PIP] Bouchard nodes) joints. The first carpometacarpal (CMC) joint is often involved and patients present with pain and swelling over that joint. This may lead to significant functional disability resulting from pain, weakness, and joint malalignment. Severe involvement of the first CMC joint may cause the characteristic squaring of that joint on physical examination. Inflammatory (or erosive) OA of the hands can occur and is characterized by severe pain, swelling, and progressive deformity of the hands. Because of the inflammatory nature of the presentation, it must be distinguished from psoriatic arthritis and RA.

Knees

OA of the knee presents with pain on weight-bearing, which is usually relieved with rest. Joint swelling may occur and if it is persistent or severe may lead to the formation of a Baker cyst. Most patients will have crepitus on examination and loss of range of motion occurs later in the course of the disease. Other causes of knee pain should be excluded including pes anserine bursitis, patellar malalignment, internal derangement of the knee, fracture of the bone, and referred pain from the femur, hip, or lumbar spine. Referred pain from the hip in the case of severe hip OA should be considered and careful hip examination may demonstrate groin pain or loss of hip range of motion.

Hips

OA of the hip typically presents with groin pain on ambulation. Pain that is located over the trochanteric bursa and is exacerbated by direct pressure is indicative of trochanteric bursitis and not hip OA. Pain in the posterior hip and/or buttock raises the concern for a lumbar radiculopathy. Progressive joint space loss and development of osteophytes leads to loss of range of motion of the hip. Progressive pain and functional limitations are seen late in the course.

Spine

Spinal involvement in OA is most common at the levels with the most spinal mobility. Osteophytes in the cervical spine may lead to pain and loss of cervical range of motion. Exuberant osteophytes may encroach on neural structures and lead to either spinal stenosis or narrowing of the neural foramina. Similarly, lumbar spondylosis may occur. Lumbar spinal stenosis may cause low back pain with radiation to the buttocks, which is worse on ambulation and relieved with rest.[3,4]

Therapeutic Approach

Nonpharmacological Management

The major goals of treating OA are to relieve pain and maintain functional status. Self-help classes have been advocated and are useful in educating patients about their disease and about exercise and other modalities that may relieve pain. Studies of these programs note only modest benefits.[3,4] Lifestyle modifications through exercise and weight control may provide some benefits to those patients who are able to comply with these therapies. In studies of older adults with knee OA, intensive weight loss has been associated with improvement in physical functioning, with the most improvement noted in those patients who lost the most weight.[5] An exercise program taking into account the burden of arthritis, current functional status, and other comorbidities can be invaluable for the elderly patient with OA. Consultation with physical and occupational therapists can aid in the development of an appropriate, structured, and individualized plan. Good supportive footwear is essential in the case of OA of the lower extremities and wedged insoles or custom fit orthotics can be very helpful.

Pharmacological Management

Currently, available therapies are aimed at controlling symptoms and do not alter the natural history of the disease. Acetaminophen in widely used for OA and has shown good efficacy. The recommended dose is 1,000 mg every 6 hours and is well tolerated in most people, although lower dosing (1,000 mg 3 times daily) may be advisable in the elderly. Hepatotoxicity can occur, but is usually seen only in patients with excessive alcohol consumption. Nonsteroidal antiinflammatory drugs (NSAIDs) have been shown to be more effective than acetaminophen for the treatment of OA,[6] but toxicity limits the use of NSAIDs in the elderly. Tramadol with or without acetaminophen relieves symptoms of OA, but the effects are modest.[7] Long-term treatment with opioid analgesics should be avoided if possible but may be necessary in some cases. Careful monitoring for side effects and drug interactions is important in the frail elderly.

Intraarticular steroids have been shown to be beneficial for OA of the knee[8] and the hip,[9] but the efficacy is usually short-lived and repeated injections are necessary. This approach can, however, be helpful for some patients with intermittent flare or those who are trying to put off joint replacement surgery as long as possible. Intraarticular hyaluronans are available and have shown benefit similar to intraarticular corticosteroids for knee OA.[10] Glucosamine sulfate is widely available over the counter and is used by many people with OA. Initial data on efficacy as a structure modifying drug was very promising,[11] but further studies have failed to show any significant benefits.[12]

Surgery

Arthroscopic debridement and joint lavage should be reserved for those patients with mechanical symptoms, shorter disease duration, and mild radiographic changes.[13,14] Ultimately, when conservative therapy fails, some patients with knee or hip OA may require joint replacement surgery. Total joint arthroplasty provides excellent pain relief and functional improvement in patients with advanced OA of the knee or hip. Careful medical workup should be performed in the elderly to assess perioperative risks, maximize medical status, and assist the orthopedic surgeons in evaluation and management of perioperative problems. Some patients with OA of the first CMC joint in whom conservative therapy has failed may be candidates for a suspension arthroplasty of the thumb.

RHEUMATOID ARTHRITIS

Introduction

RA is the most common inflammatory arthropathy in the general population with an overall prevalence of approximately 1%, and it has been estimated to be 2% in the population older than the age of 60 years.[15] The peak age of onset is in the 50s, and recent epidemiological studies have shown that the incidence and prevalence rate of RA increase to approximately the age of 85 years and then fall off.[16] Women are affected more frequently than men, although there has been a suggestion that there is a lower female predominance in elderly onset RA.[17] The etiology of RA is not completely understood but current thinking is that it is multifactorial with both genetic and environmental factors playing roles. There is a strong association with human leukocyte antigen class II alleles, particularly those containing the shared epitope, a conserved sequence that likely plays a role in antigen presentation. Among the geriatric population, clinicians are faced with caring for patients who have had lifelong RA that they take into their later years as well as elderly onset RA. Each of these patient populations presents unique challenges.

Clinical Presentation

RA is a chronic symmetrical polyarthritis with frequent systemic features. Early disease is characterized by morning stiffness, fatigue, and joint pain. As the disease progresses, synovitis is evident on physical examination. Frequently, the diagnosis is elusive in the early stages, so regular reevaluation is recommended. The joints of the hands (wrists, metacarpophalangeal, and PIP) and feet (metatarsophalangeal) are most commonly involved, but other patterns of joint involvement may occur. The majority of patients have an insidious onset over weeks to months but some patients may have an acute onset over days. Progressive involvement of other joints ensues in most patients and may include the cervical spine, shoulders, neck, elbows, knees, hips, and ankles. Extraarticular features may include Sjögren syndrome, episcleritis or scleritis, rheumatoid nodules, pleurisy, pulmonary fibrosis, and, in rare cases, rheumatoid vasculitis or Felty syndrome, which are associated with a poorer prognosis.

Laboratory evaluation may show a normochromic normocytic anemia, thrombocytosis, and elevation of the acute-phase reactants CRP and WESR. Monitoring the WESR or CRP in the elderly may be difficult, as numerous other factors may contribute to the elevation of the acute phase response. Anemia, infection, congestive heart failure, malignancy, and other systemic inflammatory conditions can interfere with interpretation of the results. The rheumatoid factor is a relatively insensitive marker in early disease as the prevalence of nonspecific autoantibodies increases with age. Therefore, the rheumatoid factor has a reduced diagnostic value in the elderly population. Antibodies directed against citrullinated peptides are more specific for RA,[18] and may be a more useful diagnostic tool in the elderly. Radiographic studies can be useful once the disease is established, but plain radiographs are frequently normal in early disease. Periarticular osteopenia and soft tissue swelling may indicate the presence of inflammatory joint disease, but they are relatively nonspecific signs for RA. The presence of marginal erosions is a specific marker and a poor prognostic sign. There is growing interest in the use of magnetic resonance imaging and ultrasound as diagnostic tools in RA because they may be more sensitive markers of joint damage before plain radiographic changes are seen.[19,20]

Established RA in the Elderly

Elderly patients with RA onset prior to the age of 65 years are likely to have had disease for some time. As a result, they have an advanced stage of the disease, having been affected for several decades. They are likely to have been exposed to numerous disease-modifying antirheumatic drugs (DMARDs) and may have undergone surgeries for medically resistant disease. The physical examination is characterized by varying degrees of disease activity with joint tenderness and swelling but evidence of joint damage is frequently evident. Ulnar deviation, flexion deformities of the elbows and knees, swan-neck, and boutonniere deformities may be seen. In general, patients with a longer disease duration have a higher burden of disease and greater functional limitations. Systemic manifestations associated with long-standing disease such as rheumatoid interstitial lung disease, peripheral neuropathy, vasculitis skin ulcers, and secondary amyloid can complicate the care of these patients. It is essential in the evaluation of these patients to determine the relative contribution of active disease and joint damage from previous disease activity as this will be the major factor in guiding the therapeutic approach.

Elderly Onset RA

Elderly onset RA is the development of RA in persons older than 65 years. The female predominance seen in younger onset RA may be less strong in EORA. Whether EORA is a distinct clinical entity from classic RA with a younger onset is not clear, but certain patterns of clinical manifestations have been described in this population. Severe morning stiffness and propensity for prominent involvement of the upper extremities has been described.[21] Marked synovitis of the shoulders, wrists, metacarpophalangeals, and PIPs with soft tissue swelling and loss of range of motion are seen. Typical deformities seen in long-standing RA are usually absent here. Patients with preexisting OA, particularly the inflammatory variant, can present a diagnostic challenge (Figure 30.1). It is increasingly common to see RA present in a patient with preexisting OA and the diagnosis may be delayed in that setting. Any change in the nature of the joint pain, pattern of joint involvement, emergence of new or more prolonged morning stiffness, or development of systemic features should warrant a careful investigation for EORA. An aggressive course may ensue in some patients and DMARD therapy is likely to improve the prognosis.

Therapy

The primary objectives of treatment are to control pain, maximize functional status, and prevent joint damage. Therapy of RA in the elderly is complicated because of comorbidities, changes in pharmacokinetics, drug interactions, and increased frequency of adverse drug reactions. In addition, although the prevalence of RA in the elderly population is increasing, the elderly are not well represented in controlled clinical trials.

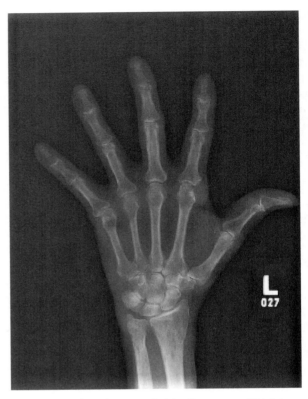

Figure 30.1. There is osteoarthritis of numerous IP joints as well as joint swelling and erosion of the 2nd MCP joint typical in appearance for rheumatoid arthritis.

Despite these factors, most elderly patients with RA can be treated safely and effectively with DMARDs (Table 30.1).

Therapies for RA can be divided into those that are symptom modifying and those that are disease modifying. NSAIDs and corticosteroids can be very helpful in alleviating the symptoms of RA but are not effective in slowing the progression of joint damage. The toxicity of NSAIDs usually limits their use in the elderly, so corticosteroids are often a better choice. Low-dose prednisone (7.5–10 mg daily) can be extremely beneficial and higher doses are not usually necessary. Care must be taken to minimize the dose of prednisone, and surveillance for common toxicities (osteoporosis, glucose intolerance, and cataracts) should be routinely performed. Local corticosteroid injections are effective in alleviating synovitis when only a few joints are active.

It is recommended that patients be started on DMARDs within 3 months of the onset of RA.[22] The earlier DMARDs are instituted, the better the chances are to limit damage from RA. The initial choice of a DMARD should be based on the severity of the inflammatory disease, the pace of the progression, and the presence or absence of erosive disease on radiographs. Other factors to consider in the elderly may include underlying renal or hepatic insufficiency, risk for infections, concomitant medication use, history of malignancy, and ability to understand and comply with the necessary monitoring. Age alone,

Table 30.1. Commonly Used Therapies for RA: Considerations in the Elderly

Drug	Dose	Precautions	Monitoring
NSAIDs		Hypertension GI ulceration/bleeding Fluid retention Contraindicated in renal impairment	Yearly CBC, LFTs, creatinine (more frequent in high risk patients)
Corticosteroids	Low dose <10mg/day	Glucose intolerance/diabetes Hypertension Weight gain Steroid induced osteoporosis Cataracts	BP, weight at each visit Yearly glucose Bone densitometry
Hydroxychloroquine	200–400 mg po QD	Nausea, epigastric pain Retinal toxicity (rare) Rash Myopathy (rare)	Annual dilated eye examination, visual field, and color vision monitoring
Sulfasalazine	1–3 g po QD in divided doses	Nausea, GI intolerance Hepatitis Myelosuppression (rare) Photosensitivity	CBC, urinalysis, chemistries at baseline. CBC every 2–4 weeks for the first 3 months, then Q 3 months thereafter
Methotrexate	15–25 mg po or SQ weekly	Myelosuppression Elevated LFTs Alopecia Pneumonitis (rare) Oral ulcers Immunosuppression Dose adjustment necessary for renal impairment	CBC, LFTs, creatinine at baseline and monthly for the first 6 months, then every 6–8 weeks thereafter. Baseline chest x-ray screen HCV Ab, HBsAg at baseline
Leflunomide	20 mg daily (10 mg/day if intolerant of 20 mg/day)	Elevated LFTs Diarrhea Alopecia Rash	Same monitoring as for methotrexate
Etanercept	50 mg SQ weekly	Injection site reactions(Etanercept and Adalimumab) Infusion Reactions (Infliximab) Risk for infections Reactivation of TB	PPD and chest x-ray before treatment Baseline CBC Screen for hepatitis B Update immunizations
Adalimumab	40 mg SQ Q week	Malignancy Demyelination (rare) Headache	
Infliximab	3 mg/kg at week 0, 2, and 6 then 3–10 mg/kg Q 4–8 weeks	Rashes Development of autoantibodies Use with caution in heart failure	
Abatacept	10 mg/kg Q month	Infusion reactions Risk for Infections Headaches Use with caution in COPD Malignancy	PPD and chest x-ray before treatment Update immunizations
Rituximab	1000 mg IV at day 1 and day 15	Infusion reactions Risk for Infections PML reported Abdominal pain/bowel obstruction Renal toxicity Use with caution in pulmonary or cardiac disease	Screen for hepatitis B and C Update immunizations

however, should not be a factor in proceeding with disease-modifying therapy.

Hydroxychloroquine (HCQ) and sulfasalazine (SSZ) are indicated for the treatment of early, mild, and nonerosive disease. Methotrexate (MTX) should also be considered in this setting when the pace of the disease is rapid or the patient has functional limitations. When erosive disease is documented at the outset, MTX should be instituted immediately unless there is a contraindication to therapy. Triple therapy with HCQ, SSZ, and MTX is used and, in general, combinations of therapy are more effective than monotherapy. Caution should be taken when instituting multiple new therapies and they should be sequentially added to assess for toxicity in the elderly. The starting dose of MTX should be 7.5 mg or 10 mg daily with lower doses used in patients with mild renal insufficiency. The dose should be escalated as tolerated up to 20–25 mg weekly. MTX should be avoided in patients with moderate or more severe renal disease (creatinine >2.0). If significant improvements are not seen, this is an indication to consider more intensive therapy. Leflunomide may be added to MTX, or in the absence of any appreciable response to the MTX, can be instituted as monotherapy or in combination with HCQ and/or SSZ. Frequent reassessment of the patient to ensure continued response to therapy as well as to monitor for drug toxicity is essential. Periodic radiographs are recommended to ensure that erosive disease has not progressed despite therapy. The goal of treatment is to maintain no evidence of disease because control of inflammation prevents radiographic and functional decline. When adequate control is not achieved with oral DMARDs, biological therapy should be instituted.

The initial biological therapy should be a tumor necrosis-α (TNFα) inhibitor. In general, this should be added to the baseline oral MTX therapy as the rate of radiographic progression has been shown to be improved when combination therapy is used. In patients intolerant of MTX, other oral DMARDS may be used in combination with a TNFα inhibitor or monotherapy may be prescribed. Numerous studies have shown TNFα inhibitors to be as effective in the elderly as they are in younger patients,[23–25] although one study showed no improvement in functional status despite improvement in disease activity scores.[25] The choice of a TNFα inhibitor is usually based on the patient's preferred route of administration and cost. The three currently available agents are equally efficacious. Although individual patients may respond better to one of the agents, there are currently no available methods of predicting likelihood of response to any given drug.

All patients should be screened for latent tuberculosis and therapy should be avoided in patients with a positive purified protein derivative of tuberculin test until treatment with isoniazid is instituted. Bacterial infections are a major concern in the elderly patient taking TNFα inhibitors, but at least one large study has shown no increased risk of infection in persons older than 65 years treated with TNFα inhibitors compared with MTX.[26] Immunizations should be reviewed and updated prior to institution of biological therapy and any patient who is immunosuppressed should not receive live vaccines. Routine immunization for influenza and pneumococcus is recommended. TNF inhibitors should be used with caution in patients with a history of malignancy, particularly leukemia and lymphoma.

If a patient does not respond to one TNFα inhibitor, it is reasonable to try another one because many patients will have a good response to the second agent. Inadequate response to TNFα inhibition can be treated with either abatacept or rituximab. As these are new agents, there are no data on the relative efficacy or safety of these agents in the elderly population, so caution is recommended. Combinations of biological therapy are not recommended because the efficacy is not enhanced and the toxicity resulting from infections is unacceptable.[27]

RA can be a very aggressive disease in the elderly. Early diagnosis and aggressive therapy tailored to the needs of the individual patient can significantly reduce disease activity and retard joint damage. Therapy of RA is a dynamic process and requires frequent reevaluation, monitoring, and medication adjustments.

POLYMYALGIA RHEUMATICA AND GIANT CELL ARTERITIS

Polymyalgia rheumatica (PMR) and giant cell arteritis (GCA) are common conditions that occur almost exclusively in persons older than age 50 years. They may be manifestations of the same disease process and they often coexist. They share common genetic markers and share a number of pathogenetic mechanisms including high levels of circulating interleukin-6; however, they usually have unique presentations.

POLYMYALGIA RHEUMATICA

Clinical Presentation

PMR is characterized by the gradual onset of symmetrical stiffness and pain in the shoulder and hip girdles. The pain is thought to be related to synovitis and/or bursitis of the large joints. The neck and torso may also be involved. Systemic complaints are very common and may include low-grade fevers, malaise and fatigue, anorexia, and weight loss. Peripheral joint involvement may occur with a propensity for the wrists but knee arthritis and generalized swelling of the hands and feet have also been described.[28] The physical examination is usually relatively unremarkable given the severity of the patients' complaints. There may be loss of active range of motion of the shoulders because of pain in the joint and proximal muscles, but passive range of motion and muscle strength is preserved.

There are no agreed on or validated criteria for the diagnosis of PMR. The diagnosis relies on the recognition of the clinical presentation of chronic stiffness and pain in the shoulder and pelvic girdle lasting at least 1 month with an elevated sedimentation rate of greater than 40 mm/h. The institution of prednisone at 15 mg/day is usually curative and the absence of a response should raise suspicion about the diagnosis. The diagnosis is frequently missed because of the nonspecific nature of the complaints, which are often ascribed to a known history of OA. In addition, a normal sedimentation rate has been described in up to 20% of patients with classic symptoms of PMR and appropriate response to low dose steroids.[29,30]

A wide variety of other diseases may mimic the clinical presentation, and the differential diagnosis of PMR is broad. PMR is often a diagnosis of exclusion. Patients with classic seropositive RA usually have a prominent symmetrical small joint synovitis that is only partially steroid responsive. There is considerable overlap with seronegative RA in the elderly population, which can have a benign course and be very sensitive to low-dose prednisone. Other diseases with a similar presentation may be hypothyroidism, bursitis/tendonitis, fibromyalgia, subacute bacterial endocarditis, and remitting seronegative symmetrical synovitis with pitting edema, polymyositis, and monoclonal gammopathies. Rarely, a paraneoplastic syndrome has been described but this responds to removal of the tumor.[31-33]

Therapy

Introduction of prednisone, 15 mg daily, is associated with rapid and often complete resolution of symptoms within a few days. When there is diagnostic uncertainty, a trial of steroids is often helpful in establishing the diagnosis. The diagnostic workup should continue in those patients who do not respond, with a particular focus on GCA and possible malignancy. Once symptoms are relieved, the patient should be maintained on the starting steroid dose for 4–6 weeks. After that, a long, slow steroid taper is recommended. Most patients require at least a year of steroid therapy. Rapid steroid tapering, as well as higher starting steroid dose, is associated with a higher rate of relapse.[34]

GIANT CELL ARTERITIS

GCA, also known as temporal arteritis, is a granulomatous vasculitis affecting large- and medium-sized arteries. The disease has a predilection to affect the extracranial branches of the carotid artery. It is the most common vasculitic syndrome in the elderly, with an incidence of 18.8 cases per 100,000 person-years in Olmstead County, Minnesota.[35] The incidence rate has been shown to be lower in the southern United States.[36]

Clinical Presentation

Patients with GCA typically present with headache, jaw claudication, scalp tenderness, and constitutional symptoms including fever. Occasionally a fever of unknown origin with failure to thrive and anemia without other more specific symptoms of GCA has been described.[37-39] Symptoms of PMR are present in approximately half of patients with GCA. The most worrisome complication of GCA is vision loss related to optic nerve ischemia from arteritis of the vessels of the ocular circulation.[40] The two symptoms most predictive of biopsy-proven GCA are jaw claudication and diplopia.[41] Limb claudication[42] and coronary ischemia[43,44] have been described because of involvement of the primary branches of the aorta. The physical examination is often normal but there may be nodularity, tenderness, or absent pulses in the temporal arteries. An elevated sedimentation rate is present in approximately 80% of patients. The elevated sedimentation rate with the compatible clinical features should suggest the diagnosis of GCA. Once the disease is considered, treatment with prednisone, 60 mg daily, should be rapidly instituted to prevent visual loss, and a temporal artery biopsy should be performed. Temporal artery biopsy is diagnostic in 50%–80% of cases. The larger the specimen, the better the yield, and it is recommended that the specimen be at least 3–5 cm in length and sampled at multiple levels. The sensitivity of the biopsy may decrease with steroid therapy and should be done as soon as possible after the start of corticosteroids.

Therapy

Corticosteroids are the mainstay of therapy in preventing visual complications and are associated with rapid improvement of other clinical symptoms including jaw claudication, PMR, and constitutional symptoms. There is some controversy regarding the optimal dose for GCA but most authors favor an initial dose of 60 mg/day. In patients who present with visual symptoms, some authors recommend pulse methylprednisolone at 1 g/day for 3 days, although there are no controlled studies. A clinical response is usually seen within the first few weeks and a slow steroid taper can usually begin after the first month of therapy. There is no standard prednisone tapering method and the rate of the taper should be driven by the patient's symptoms and the sedimentation rate if it was abnormal at the outset of the disease. The prednisone can usually be tapered down to 20 mg/day over the first 3 months, but after that, the taper should occur much more slowly. Many physicians will taper by 1 mg increments after a dose of 10 mg/day is reached. Relapses are common and may require an increase in steroid therapy. Most patients will require 2 years of corticosteroids and many patients will be able to discontinue therapy. There is currently no evidence that MTX or other immunomodulatory or cytotoxic therapies are as effective as steroid-sparing agents. Bisphosphonates should be used routinely in the elderly patient diagnosed with GCA to prevent steroid-induced osteoporosis.[45]

CRYSTAL-INDUCED ARTHRITIS

The two most common forms of crystal-induced arthritis are gout, caused by the deposition of monosodium urate, and pseudogout, caused by the deposition of calcium pyrophosphate dihydrate. The typical presentation is an acute self-limited episode of monoarthritis, but both diseases may cause polyarticular attacks, chronic arthritis, and destruction of cartilage and bone. Crystals are found in the synovium and synovial fluid during acute attacks and are associated with a brisk inflammatory response.

Table 30.2. Features of Gout in the Elderly

Associated with diuretic use

More frequent polyarticular onset

Involvement of the hand joints

Earlier development of tophi

Table 30.3. Clinical Features of Osteoarthritis

Age of Onset	>40
Joints involved (common)	1st CMC, DIPs, PIP, Knees, Hips, 1st MTP, cervical and lumbar spine
Symptoms	Joint pain, stiffness,
Physical exam	Tender, bony enlargement, loss of range of motion
Synovial fluid	Non-inflammatory, <2,000 cells, clear, normal viscosity
Radiographs	Joint space narrowing, subchondral sclerosis. osteophytes

GOUT

Gout is classically a disease of middle-aged men but there is an increasing incidence rate in men and women with advancing age. In one study, the highest gout prevalence (7.3%) was seen in men aged 75–84 years, and for the women, the prevalence continued to rise above the age of 85 years with a peak rate of 3%.[46] There is some evidence that the overall prevalence rate of gout in the elderly population is increasing over time.[47] Some factors that may contribute to that are increasing longevity, increased use of diuretics and low-dose aspirin, and comorbidities including hypertension, the metabolic syndrome, and cardiovascular disease.

There is a greater risk of gout in persons who consume more meat products and seafood; dairy products appear to be protective. These findings also correlate with increasing urate levels when the diet is high in meat or seafood or decreasing urate levels with increasing dairy product consumption.[48] Greater alcohol consumption, particularly beer, is also associated with an increased risk of incident gout.[49]

Hyperuricemia is associated with the onset of gout, although not all patients with hyperuricemia will develop joint inflammation. Hyperuricemia may result from decreased renal excretion or increased production of uric acid. In patients with primary gout, under excretion is seen in the majority (80%–90%) of cases. In elderly patients receiving diuretic therapy, hyperuricemia results from volume depletion with a decreased filtered load and enhanced tubular reabsorption of urate.[50]

Clinical Presentation

The initial attack is usually monoarticular and the lower extremity joints are most often affected. The monoarthritis is exquisitely painful and frequently is associated with inflammation of the surrounding skin, which is easily confused with a primary cellulitis. The classic presentation is involvement of the first metatarsophalangeal joint lasting from days to 2–3 weeks with a gradual resolution of inflammatory symptoms. Other frequently involved joints are the knee and ankle, although the first attack has been described in almost any joint. The initial attack is usually followed by an intercritical period that may last years. Most, but not all, patients will develop another attack. Over time, the attacks become more frequent, may become polyarticular, and are often associated with constitutional symptoms such as fever. Tophaceous deposits accumulate over the elbows, fingers, and other joint areas and a polyarticular

inflammatory arthritis may develop. This arthritis may be confused with RA, psoriatic arthritis, or inflammatory OA.

In the elderly, many patients present with a subacute or chronic polyarticular disease at the onset with fewer inflammatory signs and increased involvement of the hands (Table 30.3).[51] Older patients, particularly women on diuretic therapy, may be at risk for tophaceous disease without a preceding arthritis.[52] OA and gout often coexist and tophi may develop on Heberden or Bouchard nodes,[53] often leading to some diagnostic confusion. Tophi involving the finger pads, sometimes without arthritis,[54] has been described and has been associated with advanced age at onset, hyperuricemia, and impaired renal function.[55]

Diagnosis

The definitive diagnosis of gout requires demonstration of monosodium urate, strongly negatively birefringent crystals, in the synovial fluid by polarizing light microscopy. This is absolutely essential, particularly in the elderly, as gout can be easily confused with RA, OA, pseudogout, or a septic monoarthritis. Radiographic diagnosis of gout is difficult in the early stages of disease. Typical features of OA such as joint space narrowing, subchondral sclerosis, and osteophyte formation are common. In chronic gout, soft tissue tophi and central or periarticular erosions with sclerotic margins and overhanging edges may be seen.

Therapy

Treatment should be instituted as early as possible to achieve optimal results. The standard therapy for an acute attack of gout includes NSAIDs and colchicine, which are poorly tolerated in the elderly. Patients are at increased risk of adverse effects resulting from renal and hepatic impairment. The risk/benefit ratio should be carefully weighed and alternatives should be considered. NSAIDs should be avoided in patients with cardiac or renal failure, uncontrolled hypertension, and a history of peptic ulcer disease. When used, shorter-acting NSAIDs, such as ibuprofen, are preferred. Like NSAIDs, colchicine should not be used in the setting of renal or hepatic compromise. It has a very narrow therapeutic window with many patients developing toxicity before symptomatic benefit is achieved. Nausea, abdominal cramping, and diarrhea are very common and are dose limiting. In geriatric patients, corticosteroids are often the safest, most effective therapy for acute gout. They can be given by intraarticular route[56] in the case of a monoarthritis or systemically, either orally or intramuscularly, in the case of polyarticular disease.[57]

Once the acute attack is resolved, prophylactic therapy should be prescribed for patients who have had repeated acute attacks, have a polyarticular presentation, or who have tophaceous disease. Asymptomatic hyperuricemia is not an indication for treatment, and most authors agree that a single attack does not require long-term therapy. The goals of prophylactic therapy are to decrease the incidence and severity of acute attacks, decrease the bulk of tophi, and prevent future joint damage. The serum uric acid should be kept below 6 mg/dL. Low-dose colchicine (0.6 mg 1 or 2 times daily) may be effective in preventing acute attacks, but it does not lower serum urate. Allopurinol, a xanthine oxidase inhibitor, should be started in low dose (50–100 mg daily) and titrated up to reduce the serum concentration of uric acid to less than 6 mg/dL. Allopurinol dose should be adjusted based on the creatinine clearance. Allopurinol should not be started during an acute attack because it is likely to exacerbate the attack. Patients on chronic allopurinol therapy who develop an acute attack should be treated for acute gout and the allopurinol should be continued. Adverse reactions, most commonly rash, occur and may limit therapy. The allopurinol hypersensitivity syndrome is a rare, but potentially life-threatening complication of allopurinol therapy that has been described primarily in men with hypertension or renal insufficiency.[58] Uricosuric agents are generally poorly tolerated in the elderly and they have limited utility in the setting of renal impairment and use of low-dose aspirin. Newer agents, febuxostat and pegylated uricase, are currently under investigation and may be useful in patients who are intolerant to allopurinol.

In patients taking diuretics for control of hypertension, consideration should be given to discontinuing the diuretic in favor of another agent. Losartan and angiotensin–converting enzyme II inhibitor can help control the blood pressure and have been shown to have uricosuric properties.[59] Lifestyle modifications that have been shown to be beneficial include weight reduction, limiting alcohol consumption, limiting meat and seafood consumption, and increasing low-fat dairy consumption.

CALCIUM PYROPHOSPHATE DEPOSITION DISEASE

Clinical Presentation

Calcium pyrophosphate dehydrate deposition disease (CPPD) is a disease primarily of the elderly with an average age of onset of 70 years. CPPD crystal formation occurs in the articular and periarticular tissues and, unlike gout, does not usually form in the soft tissues. CPPD may have a number of unique clinical presentations and may mimic other rheumatic disease syn-

dromes. The term pseudogout refers to an acute arthropathy, which may be monoarticular or polyarticular and is most similar to gout. Chondrocalcinosis refers to calcium deposition in hyaline or fibrocartilage and is seen radiographically in many joints including the knee, hips, and hands. Chondrocalcinosis may be asymptomatic or associated with OA. A chronic polyarticular arthropathy has been described that looks most similar to RA. A systemic disease with fever, mental status changes, and leukocytosis has been described,[60] and should be considered in an elderly patient in whom infection has been ruled out. Rarely, involvement of the cervical spine with a cervical myelopathy has been reported, which may mimic RA.[61,62]

Diagnosis

The accurate diagnosis of CPPD remains a clinical challenge. Synovial fluid analysis should be performed. The fluid is usually inflammatory with cell counts of 10,000–20,000/μL. CPPD crystals are weakly positively birefringent crystals that can be seen under polarizing light but the sensitivity for the detection is very low in the typical clinical setting. The main differential diagnosis is with other crystal-induced arthropathies and infection. Radiographic studies often reveal chondrocalcinosis, but this is neither a sensitive nor specific marker for CPPD. Calcification of the menisci of the knees and of the triangular fibrocartilage at the wrist are the most common findings. Findings of OA frequently coexist with chondrocalcinosis. There are a number of metabolic disorders associated with CPPD including hemochromatosis, hypothyroidism, hyperparathyroidism, hypomagnesemia, hypophosphatasia, and familial hypocalciuric hypercalcemia. Studies to look for these disorders should be performed in patients diagnosed with pseudogout.

Therapy

Therapy of CPPD is usually unsatisfactory. In the case of an acute arthritis, the treatment is similar to gout. NSAIDs, colchicine, and corticosteroids may be used. Low-dose colchicine may play a role in prophylaxis of acute attacks but the evidence is limited.[63] There are currently no drugs available that alter the tissue levels of CPPD.

REFERENCES

1. Hootman JM, Helmick CG. Projections of US prevalence of arthritis and associated activity limitations. *Arthritis Rheum.* 2006;54:226–229.
2. Martel-Pelletier J, Lajeunesse D, Fahmi H, Tardif G, Pelletier JP. New thoughts on the pathophysiology of osteoarthritis: one more step toward new therapeutic targets. *Curr Rheumatol Rep.* 2006;8:30–36.
3. Warsi A, LaValley MP, Wang PS, Avorn J, Solomon DH. Arthritis self-management education programs: a meta-analysis of the effect on pain and disability. *Arthritis Rheum.* 2003;48:2207–2213.

4. vos-Comby L, Cronan T, Roesch SC. Do exercise and self-management interventions benefit patients with osteoarthritis of the knee? A metaanalytic review. *J Rheumatol.* 2006;33:744–756.

5. Miller GD, Nicklas BJ, Davis C, Loeser RF, Lenchik L, Messier SP. Intensive weight loss program improves physical function in older obese adults with knee osteoarthritis. *Obesity.* 2006;14:1219–1230.

6. Towheed TE, Maxwell L, Judd MG, Catton M, Hochberg MC, Wells G. Acetaminophen for osteoarthritis. *Cochrane Database Syst Rev.* 2006;1:CD004257.

7. Cepeda MS, Camargo F, Zea C, Valencia L. Tramadol for osteoarthritis: a systematic review and metaanalysis. *J Rheumatol.* 2007;34:543–555.

8. Arroll B, Goodyear-Smith F. Corticosteroid injections for osteoarthritis of the knee: meta-analysis. *BMJ.* 2004;328:869.

9. Lambert RG, Hutchings EJ, Grace MG, Jhangri GS, Conner-Spady B, Maksymowych WP. Steroid injection for osteoarthritis of the hip: a randomized, double-blind, placebo-controlled trial. *Arthritis Rheum.* 2007;56:2278–2287.

10. Leopold SS, Redd BB, Warme WJ, Wehrle PA, Pettis PD, Shott S. Corticosteroid compared with hyaluronic acid injections for the treatment of osteoarthritis of the knee. A prospective, randomized trial. *J Bone Joint Surg Am.* 2003;85:1197–1203.

11. Reginster JY, Deroisy R, Rovati LC, et al. Long-term effects of glucosamine sulphate on osteoarthritis progression: a randomised, placebo-controlled clinical trial. *Lancet.* 2001;357:251–256.

12. Towheed TE, Anastassiades T. Glucosamine therapy for osteoarthritis: an update. *J Rheumatol.* 2007;34:1787–1790.

13. Baumgaertner MR, Cannon WD Jr, Vittori JM, Schmidt ES, Maurer RC. Arthroscopic debridement of the arthritic knee. *Clin Orthop Rel Res.* 1990;253:197–202.

14. Novak PJ, Bach BR Jr. Selection criteria for knee arthroscopy in the osteoarthritic patient. *Orthop Rev* 1993;22(7):798–804.

15. Rasch EK, Hirsch R, Paulose-Ram R, Hochberg MC. Prevalence of rheumatoid arthritis in persons 60 years of age and older in the United States: effect of different methods of case classification. *Arthritis Rheum.* 2003;48:917–926.

16. Doran MF, Pond GR, Crowson CS, O'Fallon WM, Gabriel SE. Trends in incidence and mortality in rheumatoid arthritis in Rochester, Minnesota, over a forty-year period. *Arthritis Rheum.* 2002;46:625–631.

17. Kavanaugh AF. Rheumatoid arthritis in the elderly: is it a different disease? *Am J Med.* 1997;103(6A):40S–48S.

18. Avouac J, Gossec L, Dougados M. Diagnostic and predictive value of anti-cyclic citrullinated protein antibodies in rheumatoid arthritis: a systematic literature review. *Ann Rheum Dis.* 2006;65:845–851.

19. Hoving JL, Buchbinder R, Hall S, et al. A comparison of magnetic resonance imaging, sonography, and radiography of the hand in patients with early rheumatoid arthritis. *J Rheumatol.* 2004;31:663–675.

20. Szkudlarek M, Narvestad E, Klarlund M, Court-Payen, Thomsen HS, Ostergaard M. Ultrasonography of the metatarsophalangeal joints in rheumatoid arthritis: comparison with magnetic resonance imaging, conventional radiography, and clinical examination. *Arthritis Rheum.* 2004;50:2103–2112.

21. Glennas A, Kvien TK, Andrup O, Karstensen B, Munthe E. Recent onset arthritis in the elderly: a 5 year longitudinal observational study. *J Rheumatol.* 2000;27:101–108.

22. Guidelines for the management of rheumatoid arthritis: 2002 Update. *Arthritis Rheum.* 2002;46:328–346.

23. Fleischmann RM, Baumgartner SW, Tindall EA, et al. Response to etanercept (Enbrel) in elderly patients with rheumatoid arthritis: a retrospective analysis of clinical trial results. *J Rheumatol.* 2003;30:691–696.

24. Bathon JM, Fleischmann RM, Van der HD, et al. Safety and efficacy of etanercept treatment in elderly subjects with rheumatoid arthritis. *J Rheumatol.* 2006;33:234–243.

25. Genevay S, Finckh A, Ciurea A, Chamot AM, Kyburz D, Gabay C. Tolerance and effectiveness of anti-tumor necrosis factor alpha therapies in elderly patients with rheumatoid arthritis: a population-based cohort study. *Arthritis Rheum.* 2007;57:679–685.

26. Schneeweiss S, Setoguchi S, Weinblatt ME, et al. Anti-tumor necrosis factor alpha therapy and the risk of serious bacterial infections in elderly patients with rheumatoid arthritis. *Arthritis Rheum.* 2007;56:1754–1764.

27. Weinblatt M, Combe B, Covucci A, Aranda R, Becker JC, Keystone E. Safety of the selective costimulation modulator abatacept in rheumatoid arthritis patients receiving background biologic and nonbiologic disease-modifying antirheumatic drugs: a one-year randomized, placebo-controlled study. *Arthritis Rheum.* 2006;54:2807–2816.

28. Narvaez J, Nolla-Sole JM, Narvaez JA, Clavaguera MT, Valverde-Garcia J, Roig-Escofet D. Musculoskeletal manifestations in polymyalgia rheumatica and temporal arteritis. *Ann Rheum Dis.* 2001;60(11):1060–1063.

29. Helfgott SM, Kieval RI. Polymyalgia rheumatica in patients with a normal erythrocyte sedimentation rate. *Arthritis Rheum.* 1996;39:304–307.

30. Gonzalez-Gay MA, Rodriguez-Valverde V, Blanco R, et al. Polymyalgia rheumatica without significantly increased erythrocyte sedimentation rate. A more benign syndrome. *Arch Intern Med.* 1997;157:317–320.

31. Awadh B, Abdou NI. Rising erythrocyte sedimentation rate in a patient with treated polymyalgia rheumatica: colon cancer as an accidental association versus paraneoplastic syndrome. *J Clin Rheumatol.* 2006;12:102.

32. Tabata M, Kobayashi T. Polymyalgia rheumatica and thyroid papillary carcinoma. *Intern Med.* 1994;33:41–44.

33. Masin N, Buchard PA, Gerster JC. [Polymyalgia rheumatica and pulmonary cancer: paraneoplastic syndrome]. *Rev Rhum Mal Osteoartic.* 1992;59:153–154.

34. Kremers HM, Reinalda MS, Crowson CS, Zinsmeister AR, Hunder GG, Gabriel SE. Relapse in a population based cohort of patients with polymyalgia rheumatica. *J Rheumatol.* 2005;32:65–73.

35. Salvarani C, Crowson CS, O'Fallon WM, Hunder GG, Gabriel SE. Reappraisal of the epidemiology of giant cell arteritis in Olmsted County, Minnesota, over a fifty-year period. *Arthritis Rheum.* 2004;51:264–268.

36. Smith CA, Fidler WJ, Pinals RS. The epidemiology of giant cell arteritis. Report of a ten-year study in Shelby County, Tennessee. *Arthritis Rheum.* 1983;26:1214–1219.

37. Zenone T. Fever of unknown origin in adults: evaluation of 144 cases in a non-university hospital. *Scand J Infect Dis.* 2006;38:632–638.

38. Gonzalez-Gay MA, Garcia-Porrua C, mor-Dorado JC, Llorca J. Giant cell arteritis without clinically evident vascular involvement in a defined population. *Arthritis Rheum.* 2004;51:274–277.

39. Olopade CO, Sekosan M, Schraufnagel DE. Giant cell arteritis manifesting as chronic cough and fever of unknown origin. *Mayo Clin Proc.* 1997;72:1048–1050.

40. Hayreh SS, Podhajsky PA, Zimmerman B. Ocular manifestations of giant cell arteritis. *Am J Ophthalmol.* 1998;125:509–520.

41. Smetana GW, Shmerling RH. Does this patient have temporal arteritis? *JAMA.* 2002;287:92–101.

42. Brack A, Martinez-Taboada V, Stanson A, Goronzy JJ, Weyand CM. Disease pattern in cranial and large-vessel giant cell arteritis. *Arthritis Rheum.* 1999;42:311–317.

43. Lin LW, Wang SS, Shun CT. Myocardial infarction due to giant cell arteritis: a case report and literature review. *Kaohsiung J Med Sci.* 2007;23:195–198.

44. Eberhardt RT, Dhadly M. Giant cell arteritis: diagnosis, management, and cardiovascular implications. *Cardiol Rev.* 2007;15:55–61.

45. Saag KG, Emkey R, Schnitzer TJ, et al. Alendronate for the prevention and treatment of glucocorticoid-induced osteoporosis. Glucocorticoid-Induced Osteoporosis Intervention Study Group. *NEJM.* 1998;339:292–299.

46. Mikuls TR, Farrar JT, Bilker WB, Fernandes S, Schumacher HR Jr, Saag KG. Gout epidemiology: results from the UK General Practice Research Database, 1990–1999. *Ann Rheum Dis.* 2005;64:267–272.

47. Wallace KL, Riedel AA, Joseph-Ridge N, Wortmann R. Increasing prevalence of gout and hyperuricemia over 10 years among older adults in a managed care population. *J Rheumatol.* 2004;31:1582–1587.

48. Choi HK, Liu S, Curhan G. Intake of purine-rich foods, protein, and dairy products and relationship to serum levels of uric acid: the Third National Health and Nutrition Examination Survey. *Arthritis Rheum.* 2005;52:283–289.

49. Choi HK, Atkinson K, Karlson EW, Willett W, Curhan G. Alcohol intake and risk of incident gout in men: a prospective study. *Lancet.* 2004;363:1277–1281.

50. Scott JT, Higgens CS. Diuretic induced gout: a multifactorial condition. *Ann Rheum Dis.* 1992;51:259–261.

51. Ene-Stroescu D, Gorbien MJ. Gouty arthritis. A primer on late-onset gout. *Geriatrics.* 2005;60:24–31.

52. Macfarlane DG, Dieppe PA. Diuretic-induced gout in elderly women. *Br J Rheumatol.* 1985;24:155–157.

53. Foldes K, Petersilge CA, Weisman MH, Resnick D. Nodal osteoarthritis and gout: a report of four new cases. *Skeletal Radiol.* 1996;25:421–424.

54. Lopez Redondo MJ, Requena L, Macia M, Schoendorff C, Sanchez YE, Robledo A. Fingertip tophi without gouty arthritis. *Dermatology.* 1993;187:140–143.

55. Chopra KF, Schneiderman P, Grossman ME. Finger pad tophi. *Cutis.* 1999;64:233–236.

56. Fernandez C, Noguera R, Gonzalez JA, Pascual E. Treatment of acute attacks of gout with a small dose of intraarticular triamcinolone acetonide. *J Rheumatol.* 1999;26:2285–2286.

57. Groff GD, Franck WA, Raddatz DA. Systemic steroid therapy for acute gout: a clinical trial and review of the literature. *Semin Arthritis Rheum.* 1990;19:329–336.

58. Arellano F, Sacristan JA. Allopurinol hypersensitivity syndrome: a review. *Ann Pharmacother.* 1993;27:337–343.

59. Wurzner G, Gerster JC, Chiolero A, et al. Comparative effects of losartan and irbesartan on serum uric acid in hypertensive patients with hyperuricaemia and gout. *J Hypertens.* 2001;19:1855–1860.

60. Bong D, Bennett R. Pseudogout mimicking systemic disease. *JAMA.* 1981;246:1438–1440.

61. Finckh A, Van LD, Duvoisin B, Bovay P, Gerster JC. The cervical spine in calcium pyrophosphate dihydrate deposition disease. A prevalent case-control study. *J Rheumatol.* 2004;31:545–549.

62. Lin SH, Hsieh ET, Wu TY, Chang CW. Cervical myelopathy induced by pseudogout in ligamentum flavum and retro-odontoid mass: a case report. *Spinal Cord.* 2006;44:692–694.

63. Alvarellos A, Spilberg I. Colchicine prophylaxis in pseudogout. *J Rheumatol.* 1986;13:804–805.

31

Musculoskeletal Injuries in the Elderly

Joseph D. Zuckerman, MD, Aaron Schachter, MD

INTRODUCTION

Orthopedic trauma in the elderly patient presents both a medical and a surgical challenge. This growing population requires injury management tailored to specific patient needs. Injury treatment is based on patient factors, injury factors, and other special considerations to optimize outcome. The goal of injury treatment in the elderly patient is enabling return to preinjury functional status. This chapter will focus on the treatment of some of the more common injuries encountered in the elderly, including proximal humerus fractures, rotator cuff tears, wrist fractures, hip fractures, ankle fractures, and vertebral compression fractures.

PATIENT FACTORS

Preinjury Status

The goal of injury treatment in the elderly patient is a return to preinjury status. Therefore, a thorough history-taking that includes preinjury function is pivotal to guiding effective orthopedic care. The treatment goals of an independent community-dwelling ambulatory patient who sustains a hip fracture are different from those of an institutionalized nonambulatory patient. The former requires early operative intervention combined with aggressive postoperative rehabilitation, whereas the latter requires a less aggressive approach that provides for comfortable transfers and the ability to sit. Although the goal of each is to return to preinjury status, the approaches to each differ significantly.

Systemic Disease

Elderly patients often have preexisting medical comorbidities that influence musculoskeletal injury treatment. Cardiopulmonary disease is common in this population and affects the patient's ability to tolerate anesthetics, undergo surgery, and participate in a postoperative rehabilitation program. Cardiopulmonary disease is a major determinant of the American Society of Anesthesiologists preoperative risk assessment.[1]

The presence of neurological disorders such as Parkinson's disease, Alzheimer's disease, and previous cerebrovascular accident affect injury management. Profound Parkinson's disease associated with severe contractures and significant functional incapacity limits the treatment options for both fractures and soft tissue injuries.[2] Stroke patients are at an increased risk for fracture as a result of gait and balance problems, as well as osteopenia of the affected limbs. Fractures occurring in patients who have suffered a stroke usually occur on the affected side.[3,4]

Endocrinopathies, such as diabetes and thyroid disorders, are common in the elderly. Diabetic patients are considered immunocompromised and have microvascular disease that increases the risk of wound complications and infection following surgery.[5,6] Diabetics have greater risk of sustaining a fracture, longer time to fracture union, and poorer expected outcome of operative fracture fixation compared with age-matched nondiabetic patients.[5–8]

Bone Quality

Elderly patients frequently have osteopenic bone. Osteopenia is described as a decrease in bone mass caused by either osteoporosis (decreased bone density with normal mineralization) or osteomalacia (deceased mineralization with or without a change in density). Osteopenia is most commonly caused by senile osteoporosis, but also may be caused by other, treatable causes such as nutritional deficiencies, hyperparathyroidism, renal disease, tumors, and Cushing's disease.[9] A thorough medical evaluation should identify any of these treatable causes.

Osteopenia affects fracture management because osteopenic bone is at higher risk for delayed union and nonunion.

Additionally, osteopenic bone may affect the ability of the surgeon to achieve stable fixation during operative fracture fixation. Decreased pullout strength of traditional plate and screw constructs can lead to early failure of fixation. This problem is compounded by the osteopenia that develops during periods of immobilization. Several strategies can be used in an attempt to overcome this problem, namely bone graft, bone graft substitutes, methylmethacrylate cement, and new locked-plating systems.[10] Several preventive medical treatments for osteoporosis are currently available, such as bisphosphonate therapy and hormone replacement therapy.[11–15]

Osteomalacia in the elderly patient is often the result of nutritional deficiencies. This can be the result of malabsorption syndromes, aberrant metabolism of calcium, vitamin D, and phosphorus, or excessive use of phosphate-binding medications such as phenytoin or antacids. These conditions are generally treated medically by addressing the cause of the deficiency and providing increased dietary supplementation of the deficient metabolite.

Soft Tissue Quality

The most characteristic age-related change in skeletal muscle tissue is a loss of muscle mass secondary to a decrease in the size and/or number of muscle fibers.[16,17] Functional changes associated with aging are alterations in reaction time, strength, reflex time, coordination, speed, and endurance.[18,19]

As a result of aging, skin becomes more fragile and less tolerant of surgical intervention. These changes affect the treatment options considered. Age-related attritional changes can compromise soft tissue repair; aggressive surgical management requiring lengthy rehabilitation may not be warranted in patients with preexisting soft tissue compromise.

INJURY FACTORS

Polytrauma

Although patients older than age 65 years constitute a minority of the overall population, they also represent more than 28% of all fatal injuries in the United States.[20,21] For any operative injury, mortality and morbidity are greater in the geriatric patient. Traditional trauma rating systems used to triage patients and predict outcome are less reliable in the elderly.[22,23]

Recognition of skeletal injuries in the geriatric trauma patient requires vigilance. The presence of fractures should always be considered in high-energy trauma. Visceral injuries uncommonly occur without skeletal injury in the elderly trauma patient.[24] Long bone injuries should be immobilized to decrease hemorrhage and minimize the risk of fat embolization. The mortality rate of patients with acute and delayed complications of pelvic fractures (hemorrhage or sepsis) is 17% in cases of closed pelvic ring fractures and more than 80% in cases of open fractures.[21] Early stabilization of pelvic ring fractures and long bone fractures facilitates patient mobiliza-

tion, improves respiratory function, and, ultimately, results in improved outcomes.[25]

Open Fractures

Fractures in which the bone is exposed to the outside environment through a defect in the soft tissue cover are referred to as open fractures. Open fractures in the elderly, particularly those of the lower extremity, should be treated as limb-threatening injuries. Preexisting conditions such as vascular insufficiency, diabetes mellitus, atherosclerosis, osteopenia, and immunocompromise adversely affect the outcome of these injuries in the geriatric population. The basic tenets of open fracture management must be followed to optimize outcome in this population: timely and meticulous debridement of bone and soft tissue, fracture stabilization, bone grafting, and soft tissue coverage when necessary.[26,27]

Comminution

Low-energy fractures in the elderly patient often result in marked comminution, which is more commonly associated with high-energy trauma in the younger patient. This is often the result of relative weakness of osteopenic bone. Comminuted fractures in the geriatric population must be treated with special considerations in mind. The most important determinant of fracture stability is stable bony apposition at the fracture site. This may mean shortening of the bone to obtain a stable construct. Patients with evidence of osteoporosis should also be treated medically to improve bone stock and optimize chances of fracture healing.[28]

Intraarticular Fractures

Intraarticular fractures require a stable, anatomical reduction to prevent posttraumatic arthrosis and to allow for early range of motion. Early joint motion promotes articular cartilage healing.[29] Intraarticular fractures in an arthritic joint are generally unique to the elderly patient and may require primary prosthetic replacement. This is applicable in displaced intraarticular fractures of the hip and proximal humerus.

SPECIAL CONSIDERATIONS

Periprosthetic Fractures

The treatment of fractures about a total joint replacement is a challenging task. These fractures occur more frequently in women than men. Risk factors include osteopenia and previous revision surgery. Treatment of displaced periprosthetic fractures must be individualized.[30,31] The goals of treatment are early patient mobilization, preservation of limb alignment, and stability of the bone – implant interface. Nonsurgical management may result in limb malalignment and prolonged recumbency with associated pulmonary, genitourinary, and thromboembolic complications. Surgical management is

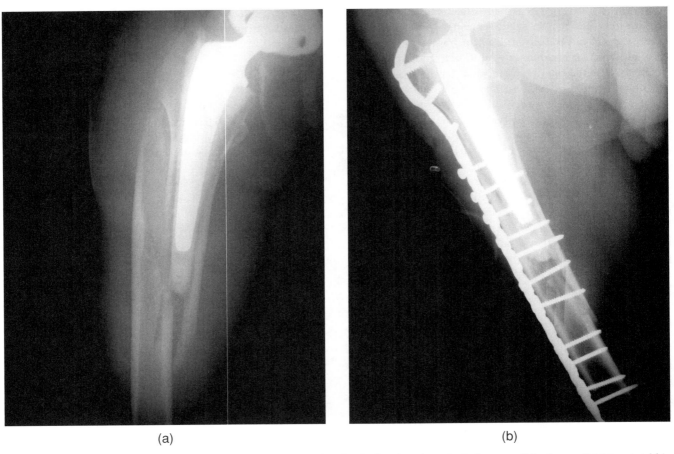

(a)   (b)

Figure 31.1. Preoperative (a) and postoperative (b) AP radiographs of a displaced periprosthetic fracture of the femur distal to a total hip replacement. The implant was stable in the femur and the decision was made to proceed with open reduction and internal fixation of the fracture while retaining the implant in the stable position. See color plates.

complicated by the presence of the implant, associated osteopenia, and implant instability. This often leads to difficult postoperative mobilization of the patient.

Periprosthetic fractures commonly occur at or near the end of an intramedullary portion of an implant (stem) and result in the loosening of the implant (Figure 31.1a,b). There is a high complication rate of treatment following periprosthetic fractures. Compared with fractures not near implants, there is a higher rate of nonunion, malunion, and infection. These rates are comparable to those of revision joint replacement.[32]

Pathological Fractures

The skeleton is the third most common site of metastatic disease. The incidence of bony involvement in patients with a known malignancy is reported to be between 12% and 70%.[33–35] Common primary malignancies that metastasize to the skeleton are lung, breast, renal, thyroid, and brain. Furthermore, primary malignancies and dyscrasias may involve the skeleton such as lymphoma, myeloma, and chondrosarcoma. The proximal femur is the most common location of pathological fracture and is involved in more than 50% of cases. This is

from the significant mechanical stresses that occur across the hip joint and proximal femur during ambulation.[36]

Treatments are, again, directed at early patient mobilization. Surgical treatment is the standard of care in neoplastic fractures, especially those of the femur.[37] The goals are to restore function, alleviate pain, facilitate nursing care, decrease hospital stays, and improve patient quality of life. Surgical contraindications are few but may include obtunded mental status, inability to tolerate the operative procedure, and life expectancy less than 1 or 2 months.

PREOPERATIVE CONSIDERATIONS

Absolute indications for operative fracture treatment are open fractures, compartment syndrome, and neurovascular compromise. Relative surgical indications include displaced intraarticular fractures in which acceptable reduction and alignment cannot be maintained and fractures that require stabilization to mobilize the patient out of bed. Fracture management in the elderly must take into consideration all of the injury factors, patient factors, and special considerations described previously.

All aspects must be considered to develop an individualized plan of care.

Timing of surgery in the elderly patient is controversial. Generally, surgery should be performed when all comorbid medical conditions are stabilized. Contradictory reports of timing and mortality have been reported in retrospective analyses.[38,39] A prospective study from our institution of 367 patients with hip fracture demonstrated that surgical delay of more than 2 days from hospital admission doubled the risk of patient death at 1 year when age, sex, and number of comorbidities were controlled.[40]

No significant difference has been demonstrated in survival rates in patients undergoing operative treatment of hip fractures with either regional or general anesthetics.[41,42] There has been demonstrated a reduced incidence of thromboembolic events (deep vein thrombosis, pulmonary embolus) after use of regional anesthetic.[43] Because pulmonary embolism is a significant cause of morbidity and mortality in the geriatric patient; regional anesthetic is generally preferred.

The goal of implant choice is to achieve a stable fracture construct with anatomical or near-anatomical alignment and/or reduction of articular surfaces to allow early mobilization and range of motion of the affected joint. Fracture impaction restores structural continuity, allows for force transmission across the fracture segment, and decreases the overall forces on the implant; all of which improve outcome and healing potential.

Intramedullary devices are the implant of choice for fractures in osteopenic bone when the location and fracture pattern are amenable. Intramedullary implants are closer to the mechanical axis of the bone and act as a load-sharing device, as opposed to load-bearing devices, such as plates.

HIP FRACTURES

Principles

Hip fractures in the elderly can be a life-threatening injury because of the impact on medical, functional, and psychological status of the patient. More than 250,000 hip fractures occur annually in the United States, which result in more than $9 billion in health care costs. Current age trends predict a doubling of the yearly incidence of hip fractures by the year 2050.[44–46]

The risk of a hip fracture increases with age, doubling every decade after the age of 50 years. Hip fractures occur most commonly in Caucasian women, followed by Caucasian men, and then African-American women and men. This may be from differences in bone density between these groups. Institutionalized patients are also at an increased risk for hip fracture, often with greater risk of mortality.[47–52]

Hip fractures usually occur from low-energy trauma. There are generally two types: intracapsular (femoral neck fractures) or extracapsular (intertrochanteric and subtrochanteric). Vascularity is compromised with intracapsular fractures. More than 90% of hip fractures in patients older than 65 years are femoral neck or intertrochanteric in origin, with a slight predominance for intertrochanteric fractures in very old patients.

Presentation and Management

Patients who have sustained a hip fracture present with the complaint of hip and groin pain with the inability to bear weight on the affected extremity after a fall. The affected extremity is usually positioned in external rotation and slight hip flexion. This position provides maximal capsular volume and the most comfort from the hematoma that develops in intracapsular fractures; in displaced extracapsular fractures, the displacement of the fracture results in a shortened and externally rotated position of the lower extremity. There will often be a noticeable leg length discrepancy. Evaluation should include a thorough neurovascular examination of the affected extremity as well as examination of all other extremities to exclude concomitant fracture. Neurological examination should include a determination of mental status and assess for a loss of consciousness associated with the fall. Medical consultation should be obtained at the time of presentation to optimize the patient medically for anticipated surgery. Injury radiographs, initial laboratory investigations, chest radiograph, and electrocardiogram should be performed. A baseline arterial blood gas level may be warranted because hip fractures carry a risk for thromboembolic phenomena. A Foley catheter should be placed to eliminate the need for positioning on a bedpan or use of a urinal to minimize patient discomfort. Orthogonal films should include a true anteroposterior (AP) and cross-table lateral (Figure 31.2a,b). Frog-leg laterals rotate through the fracture site, further displacing fracture fragments causing increased discomfort to the patient and the potential for further injury and should be avoided.

If a diagnosis of a hip fracture is suspected, but not confirmed by routine radiographs, further imaging studies are indicated. Traction-internal rotation AP views improve the visualization of the entire femoral head and neck. If further question remains, a technetium bone scan or magnetic resonance image should be obtained. A technetium bone scan requires 2–3 days after injury to minimize the risk of false-negative results, whereas a magnetic resonance image can be used to diagnose occult fracture accurately within 24 hours after injury.[53]

The preferred treatment of hip fractures is operative because it allows early mobilization, thereby decreasing the risk of cardiopulmonary events, urinary tract infections, decubitus ulcers, and the rate of mortality in the first year. It also minimizes the period of nonweightbearing, decreases the risk of nonunion/malunion, and increases the ease of transfer. Overall, operative management also decreases the cost of hip fractures when nonoperatively managed.[54]

The risk of thromboembolic complications (deep vein thrombosis or pulmonary embolism) is a concern and requires the use of preventive measures. Warfarin has historically been the gold standard for thromboprophylaxis. Currently, low-molecular-weight heparin has been used with good results and without the need for laboratory value monitoring.[55–57]

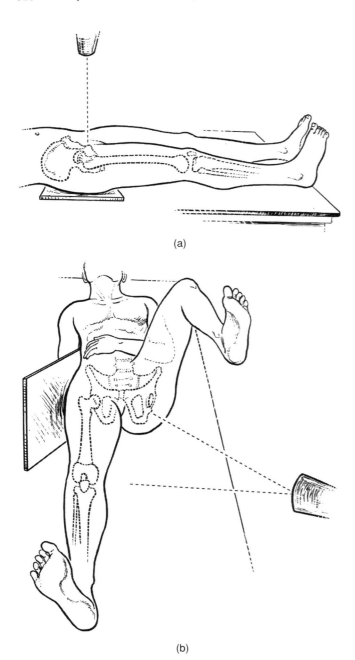

Figure 31.2. A sketch depicting the proper method of evaluating suspected hip fractures, demonstrating AP (a) and cross-table lateral (b) radiographs of a displaced fracture of the subcapital femoral neck in a patient with limited ambulatory capability. Fixation of these fractures is associated with a high incidence of avascular necrosis; therefore, this fracture was treated with hip hemiarthroplasty.

Low-molecular-weight heparin should be administered within 12 hours postoperatively. An inferior vena caval filter may be used when anticoagulation is contraindicated, or in patients at a high risk for recurrent thromboembolism.

Outcomes

The goal of surgical treatment of hip fractures is to restore the patient's functional status. At 1-year follow-up, 41% of patients will regain their preinjury ambulatory status, 40% will require increased assistance, and 8% will become nonambulatory.[58]

Mortality rates of patients with hip fractures are greater than age- and sex-matched controls.[38,59] The highest increase is seen in the first 6 months after injury and progressively decreases to that of age- and sex-matched controls at 1 year; however, 1-year mortality rates can be as high as 25%.[60]

Although the amount of time from injury to surgical treatment has been debated as a predictive factor, a prospective study from our institution, in which age, sex, and other comorbidities were controlled, demonstrated that a delay of surgical treatment for more than 2 days in patients who did not suffer from dementia and were ambulatory prior to injury doubled the 1-year mortality rate.[61]

Postoperative rehabilitation should use a weight bearing as tolerated program. Although some have recommended restricted weight bearing (or even nonweightbearing), in situations when fracture fixation is felt to be suboptimal, we believe that this has a very negative impact on the overall recovery and does not accomplish the intended goal of limiting forces across the hip (and therefore on the fracture fixation). Joint reaction forces across the hip are actually higher with nonweightbearing as opposed to toe-touch weight bearing.[62] When elderly patients are allowed immediate postoperative weight bearing as tolerated, they self-regulate the amount of weight on the injured extremity and will gradually increase the amount of weight bearing with time.[63,64] The approach encourages rather than limits their recovery of mobility and ambulation.

Femoral Neck Fractures

Fractures of the femoral neck are intracapsular, extraarticular fractures that occur between the femoral head and the intertrochanteric line. The location of these fractures has a significant impact on the primary blood supply to the femoral head. An extracapsular vascular ring at the base of the neck is formed by contributions from both the medial and lateral femoral circumflex arteries. This ring gives rise to a network of ascending vessels that terminate as bony perforatoring vessels in the femoral head (Figure 31.3a,b). These ascending vessels are at risk for injury from a neck fracture and are usually disrupted when the fracture is displaced (Figure 31.4a,b).

Although many classification systems have been developed to categorize fractures of the femoral neck, the most commonly used system is the Garden classification. Types I and II are nondisplaced fractures whereas types III and IV are displaced fractures (Figure 31.5).[65]

Osteonecrosis of the femoral head and nonunion following femoral neck increase in frequency as the degree of fracture displacement increases. Therefore, nondisplaced fractures (Garden types I and II) have rates of these complications between 5% and 10% whereas these rates are 20%–35% for displaced fractures (Garden types III and IV).[66–72] The presence of these complications is a common indication for revision surgery.

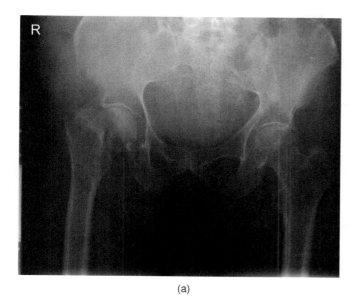

(a)

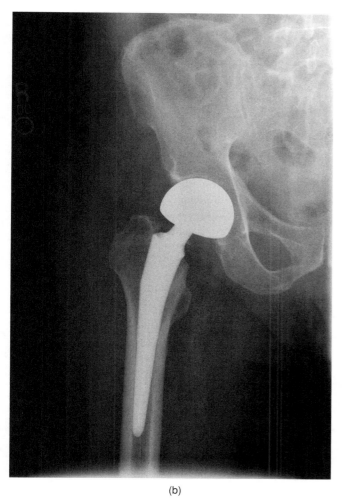

(b)

Figure 31.3. Preoperative (a) and postoperative (b) AP radiographs of a displaced fracture of the subcapital femoral neck in a patient with limited ambulatory capability. Fixation of these fractures is associated with a high incidence of avascular necrosis; therefore, this fracture was treated with hip hemiarthroplasty.

Intertrochanteric Hip Fractures

The intertrochanteric region is an extracapsular region of the hip lying between the greater and lesser trochanters. This is a region of metaphyseal bone that is rich in blood supply and a minimal risk of healing complications are associated with intracapsular fractures. The greater trochanter is a superolateral structure that serves as the insertion point for the hip abductors and short external rotators. The lesser trochanter is located distally at the posteromedial surface of the proximal femur and serves as the attachment site for the iliopsoas. The calcar femorale is a region of bone located along the posteromedial portion of the proximal femur and acts as a cortical strut to transmit the large forces across the intertrochanteric region.

Intertrochanteric hip fractures are classified as stable or unstable, based on whether the posteromedial buttress (calcar femorale) is intact or comminuted. This is determined on injury radiographs based on the position of the lesser trochanter. Stable fractures are characterized by an intact lesser trochanter on the distal fracture fragment, whereas unstable fractures demonstrate a displaced large lesser trochanteric fragment. A displaced large lesser trochanter is an indication of calcar comminution and an unstable fracture pattern.

Surgery is the treatment of choice for all intertrochanteric hip fractures. Although they have been most commonly treated with extramedullary devices, that is, a sliding hip screw, recently, an increasing number are being treated with cephalomedullary (intramedullary) devices (Figure 31.6a,b). Both methods are accepted forms of operative treatment and have demonstrated similar results and complications in recent prospective, randomized studies.[73–75] The indications and goals for nonoperative treatment are similar to those for femoral neck fractures.

ANKLE FRACTURES

The ankle joint is a modified hinge joint consisting of the lateral malleolus (distal fibula), the medial malleolus (distal tibia), the plafond (distal tibia), and the talus. Uniting these osseous structures are the lateral collateral ligaments, the deltoid ligaments, and the tibiofibular syndesmosis. The lateral collateral ligament is composed of three structures: the anterior talofibular ligament, the calcaneofibular ligament, and the posterior tibiofibular ligament. The deltoid ligament consists of an anterior, superficial portion that attaches to the navicular, sustentaculum tali, and the talus, whereas the stronger, deeper, posterior portion originates on the posterior colliculus of the medial malleolus, and inserts on the medial surface of the talus.

The clinical examination of a patient with a suspected ankle injury should include palpation of the aforementioned osseous and ligamentous structures. Swelling and ecchymoses should be noted. A neurovascular examination is mandatory, as is determining the ability to bear weight (patients are rarely able to bear weight on an unstable fracture).

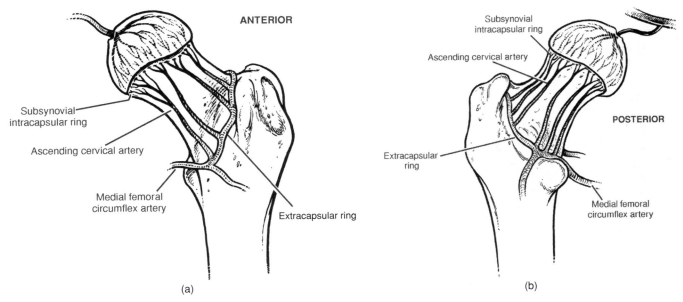

Figure 31.4. Vascular anatomy of the femoral neck.

Radiographic examination should include three views of the ankle: an AP view, a mortise view (20° internal rotation oblique), and a lateral view. Ankle fractures can include isolated lateral malleolus/distal fibula fractures, isolated medial malleolus fractures, fractures of both malleoli (bimalleolar), or both malleoli and the posterior portion of the tibial plafond (trimalleolar). Isolated fractures of the lateral malleolus should be evaluated with stress views to exclude the presence of a soft tissue injury that leads to ankle instability.[76]

The goal of treatment of ankle fractures in elderly patients is to restore the normal tibiotalar relationship while maintaining a congruous joint surface. Stable injuries, such as isolated lateral malleolus fractures, should be immobilized in the acute postinjury period with gradual return to weight bearing as tolerated with the use of a brace or fracture boot.

Bimalleolar injuries and fractures associated with talar displacement and joint incongruity are unstable and require operative fixation. Slight talar incongruity can lead to early posttraumatic arthritis.[77] The primary indication for operative treatment of an elderly patient with an ankle fracture is to obtain or maintain an anatomical relationship of the tibia, fibula, and talus, and thereby joint congruity.

The timing of operative treatment depends in large part on the condition of the soft tissue envelope. Ankle fractures and fracture-dislocations can be associated with significant swelling and the development of fracture blisters. When present, operative treatment should be avoided because of the risk of soft tissue sloughing following the surgical procedure. Surgery is best performed when swelling has subsided and skin wrinkles are present. At surgery, the skin should be handled atraumatically with little/no dissection of the subcutaneous tissues. This will minimize the risk of skin necrosis. Studies have demonstrated that in comparison to nonoperative treatment, operative management results in improved anatomical restoration, improved function, minimal pain, and restoration of stability.[78,79] There are, however, complications associated with operative treatment such as wound breakdown and loss of fixation that must be considered in operative planning.

PROXIMAL HUMERUS FRACTURES

Proximal humerus fractures are common in the elderly population. The proximal humerus is the third most common site of fracture and often occurs as a result of a low-energy mechanism, such as a fall from a standing position.

The current system used to classify fractures of the proximal humerus fractures was first described by Neer.[80,81] This classification divides the proximal humerus into four anatomical segments: the head, the shaft, the lesser tuberosity, and the greater tuberosity. A segment is considered displaced if it is displaced 1 cm or more, or angulated 45° or more from its anatomical position. Thus, these fractures are considered as one-part (minimally displaced), or as two-, three-, or four-part fractures. In addition, there are fracture-dislocations characterized by dislocation of the humeral head from the glenoid. The

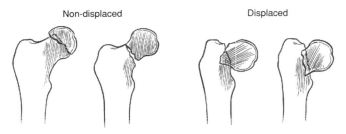

Figure 31.5. Garden classification of femoral neck fractures.

(a)

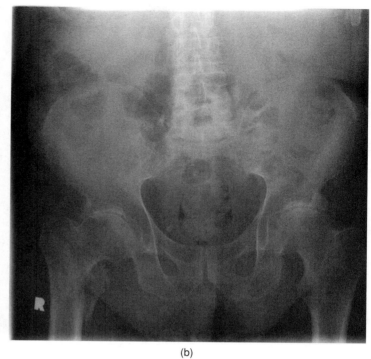
(b)

Figure 31.6. Preoperative (a) and postoperative (b) AP radiographs of an unstable intertrochanteric hip fracture. This fracture was fixed with a cephalomedullary device.

final group in this classification system is the articular surface or "head-splitting" fractures. This system is useful because it provides treatment and outcome guidelines based on fracture type.

Minimally displaced fractures account for approximately 80%–85% of all proximal humerus fractures. These fractures have an intact surrounding soft tissue envelope and can be expected to move as a single unit. These injuries are treated with an initial period of immobilization followed by early range of motion exercises.

There are different types of two-part fractures depending on the "part" involved. Surgical neck fractures can be impacted, angulated, separated, or comminuted. Closed reduction may be attempted but is generally not successful. The primary predictors of outcome in this patient group are age and initial displacement. Patients with three- and four-part fractures are at increased risk for osteonecrosis of the humeral head. Because of the potential disruption of the blood supply to the humeral head treatment options – internal fixation versus prosthetic replacement – are determined by patient factors (age and activity level) and fracture factors (bone quality, comminution, and presence of dislocation).

Prosthetic replacement is commonly performed for four-part fractures, fracture-dislocations, and head-splitting fractures (Figure 31.7a,b). The results of internal fixation in these fractures are generally poor because of a high incidence of osteonecrosis and posttraumatic arthrosis. Other indications for hemiarthroplasty include the late sequelae of these fractures

managed nonoperatively and include malunion, nonunion, and joint arthrosis.

Regardless of treatment approach, elderly patients with displaced proximal humerus fractures require a prolonged, supervised physiotherapy program to optimize functional outcomes. Minimally displaced one-part and adequately reduced two-part fractures can be expected to have good functional outcomes. Poor results may be related to compromise of the rotator cuff, malunion, nonunion, or osteonecrosis. Results of prosthetic replacement are predictable for pain relief, but is less consistent for functional recovery.

DISTAL RADIUS FRACTURES

Fractures of the distal radius represent the most common fracture that occurs in geriatric patients. The incidence of these injuries increases dramatically with age, particularly for women.[82] The age-related rate incidence parallels that seen for fractures of the proximal humerus and proximal femur and have been attributed to the presence of osteoporosis, as well as poor eyesight, impaired coordination, and decreased muscular strength.

Many classification systems have been developed to classify fractures of the distal radius. Most are based on fracture geometry, degrees of displacement and comminution, and concomitant injury to adjacent structures.[83] Unstable fractures are identified by marked comminution, greater than 1 cm of

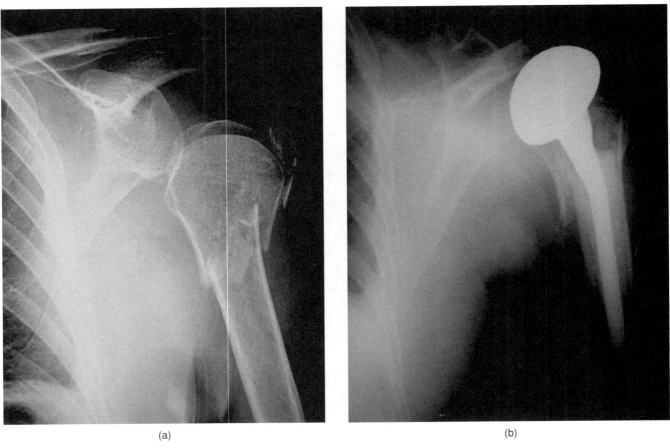

(a)   (b)

Figure 31.7. Preoperative (a) and postoperative (b) AP radiographs of a displaced 3-part fracture of the proximal humerus treated with prosthetic replacement. See color plates.

shortening, loss of palmar tilt, greater than 10° of dorsal tilt, and intraarticular displacement (Figure 31.8a,b). Unstable fractures account for 15%–25% of distal radius injuries in the geriatric population and are traditionally associated with poorer outcome.

Closed reduction and splint/cast application is the treatment of choice for most distal radius fractures in elderly patients. If closed reduction is successful, a cast should be applied for 6 weeks and radiographs should be performed weekly for 3–4 weeks to ensure that the reduction is maintained.

If closed reduction is not successful, operative intervention may be necessary, particularly when treating an active elderly patient with involvement of the dominant extremity. A large number of operative methods have been described, such as external fixation, percutaneous pin fixation, and internal

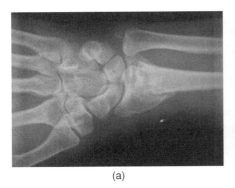
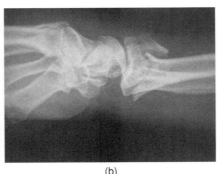
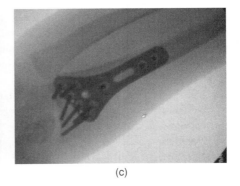

(a)   (b)   (c)

Figure 31.8. AP (a) and lateral (b) radiographs of an unstable distal radius fracture demonstrating significant shortening and comminution as well as loss of radial inclination and palmar tilt. This fracture underwent operative fixation and was repaired using open reduction and internal fixation with an anterior plate (c).

plate fixation. The choice is often surgeon dependent, and each option has its own specific risk/benefit profile.

The results of the treatment of distal radius fractures can be quite dependent on patient factors, treatment method, and quality of reduction. Minimally displaced fractures treated in cast immobilization generally do well with minimal loss of preinjury function. Surgical fixation of displaced fractures demonstrates good to excellent results in 70%–90% of patients with comminuted, unstable fractures.[84] In low-demand elderly patients, however, closed treatment of displaced fractures may yield acceptable functional results despite a cosmetic deformity.[85] Ultimately, the treatment of each patient should be individualized and should be based on not only fracture type but also presence of comorbidities, preinjury functional status, and hand dominance.

VERTEBRAL COMPRESSION FRACTURES

Vertebral compression fractures often result from a low-energy trauma (i.e., a simple fall or even just sitting down in an awkward or forceful manner) in the setting of osteoporotic bone and have become almost synonymous with osteoporosis. Jensen et al.[86] have estimated that 44% of women aged 70 years or older have vertebral compression fractures. Older patients with vertebral compression fractures are at an increased risk for developing other osteoporotic fractures, such as those of the distal radius, proximal femur, and proximal humerus.

Vertebral compression fractures often occur in the midthoracic spine. When vertebral collapse occurs over several adjacent segment, kyphosis (humpback deformity) or scoliosis (lateral compression deformity) may develop.

Vertebral compression fractures may present as an incidental finding; however, most are associated with the acute onset of pain. The location of the pain is typically midline in the thoracolumbar spine but may be referred to the lumbosacral area. If a neurological deficit is present, metastatic disease, infection, and Paget's disease must be included in the differential diagnoses.

Physical examination demonstrates decreased spinal range of motion, kyphotic deformity, and midline spinal tenderness to palpation. Radiographic evaluation should include standing AP and lateral radiographs. If the patient is too uncomfortable to stand, then supine radiographs may be obtained. A bone scan can be helpful in differentiating old fractures from acute ones. A computed tomography scan can be helpful for evaluating the integrity of the posterior elements and to identify more severe injuries, such as burst fractures, that can compromise the spinal canal and cause compression of the neural elements.

Historically, a nonoperative approach has been the mainstay for the treatment of vertebral compression fractures. The protocol should involve a short period of rest combined with appropriate analgesia followed by mobilization. Casts and orthoses may be used for comfort, although they may be poorly tolerated.

Recent advances in the use of vertebroplasty have changed the management of compression fractures. Vertebroplasty con-sists of the percutaneous insertion of a large gauge cannula into the vertebral body. Liquid bone cement is then injected into the vertebra. The cement gradually hardens and serves to stabilize the fracture and prevent further collapse. Concerns about potential extravasation of cement into surrounding structures was one of the reasons for the development of vertebral kyphoplasty. This procedure is performed by percutaneous insertion of a balloon tamp to create a cavity within the vertebral body followed by the injection of cement to maintain vertebral height. Recent studies have demonstrated that compared with traditional nonoperative treatment of vertebral compression fractures, kyphoplasty provides improved pain relief, restoration of vertebral height, less disability, shorter duration of hospital stay, and improved return to function.[87]

CONCLUSION

Orthopedic injuries are responsible for significant morbidity and mortality in the geriatric population. As life expectancy continues to increase, the prevalence of these problems will most also likely increase. The ideal treatment should focus on prevention of predisposing risk factors to these injuries, such as osteoporosis and falls. The primary goals of treatment are to provide analgesia, allow as close to immediate patient mobilization as possible, and return the patient to his/her preinjury level of function. Treatment should include patient education and rehabilitation to optimize outcome. Each treatment plan should be individualized based on patient factors, injury factors, and the other mitigating variables presented previously that are unique to each patient, situation, and injury.

REFERENCES

1. Owens WD, Felts JA, Spitznagel EL Jr. ASA physical status classifications: a study of consistency of ratings. *Anesthesiology.* 1978;49:239–243.
2. Bloem BR, Grimbergen YA, Cramer M, Willemsen M, Zwinderman A. Prospective assessment of falls in Parkinson's disease. *J Neurol.* 2001;248:950–958.
3. McClure J, Goldsborough S. Fractured neck of femur and contralateral intracerebral lesions. *J Clin Pathol.* 1986;39:920–922.
4. Soto-Hall R. Treatment of transcervical fractures complicated by certain common neurological conditions. In: Reynolds FC, ed. *Instructional Course Lectures XVII.* Vol 17. St Louis: CV Mosby; 1960:117–120.
5. Loder RT. The influence of diabetes mellitus on the healing of closed fractures. *Clin Orthop.* 1988;232:210–216.
6. Ganesh SP, Pietrobon R, Cecilio WA, Pan D, Lightdale N, Nunley JA. The impact of diabetes on patient outcomes after ankle fracture. *J Bone Joint Surg Am.* 2005;87:1712–1718.
7. Ahmed LA, Joakimsen RM, Berntsen GK, Fonnebo V, Schirmer H. Diabetes mellitus and the risk of non-vertebral fractures: the Tromso study. *Osteoporos Int.* 2006;17:495–500.
8. Egol KA, Tejwani NC, Walsh MG, Capla EL, Koval KJ. Predictors of short-term functional outcome following ankle fracture surgery. *J Bone Joint Surg Am.* 2006;88:974–979.

9. Lane JM, Vigorita VJ. Osteoporosis. *J Bone Joint Surg Am.* 1983;65:274–278.

10. Fulkerson E, Egol KA, Kubiak EN, Liporace F, Kummer FJ, Koval KJ. Fixation of diaphyseal fractures with a segmental defect: a biomechanical comparison of locked and conventional plating techniques. *J Trauma.* 2006;60:830–835.

11. Bonnick SL, Shulman L. Monitoring osteoporosis therapy: bone mineral density, bone turnover markers, or both? *Am J Med.* 2006;119(4 Suppl 1):S25–S31.

12. Emkey RD, Ettinger M. Improving compliance and persistence with bisphosphonate therapy for osteoporosis. *Am J Med.* 2006;119(4 Suppl 1):S18–S24.

13. Cramer JA, Silverman S. Persistence with bisphosphonate treatment for osteoporosis: finding the root of the problem. *Am J Med.* 2006;119(4 Suppl 1):S12–S17.

14. Sammartino A, Cirillo D, Mandato VD, Di Carlo C, Nappi C. Osteoporosis and cardiovascular disease: benefit-risk of hormone replacement therapy. *J Endocrinol Invest.* 2005; 28(10 Suppl):80–84.

15. Gass M, Dawson-Hughes B. Preventing osteoporosis-related fractures: an overview. *Am J Med.* 2006;119(4 Suppl 1):S3–S11.

16. Kalu DN, Masoro EJ. The biology of aging, with particular reference to the musculoskeletal system. *Clin Geriatr Med.* 1988;4:257–267.

17. Tomonaga M. Histochemical and ultrastructural changes in senile human skeletal muscle. *J Am Geriatr Soc.* 1977;25:125–131.

18. McCarter R. Effects of age on contraction of mammalian skeletal muscle. *Aging.* 1978;6:1–21.

19. Murray MP, Duthie EH Jr, Gambert SR, et al. Age-related differences in knee muscle strength in normal women. *J Gerontol.* 1985;40:275–280.

20. Broos PL, Stappaerts KH, Rommens PM, et al. Polytrauma in patients of 65 and older: injury patterns and outcomes. *Int Surg.* 1988;73:119–122.

21. Martin RE, Teberian G. Multiple trauma and the elderly patient. *Emerg Med Clin North Am.* 1990;8:411–420.

22. DeMaria EJ, Kenney PR, Merriam MA, et al. Survival after trauma in geriatric patients. *Ann Surg.* 1987;206:738–743.

23. Horst HM, Obeid FN, Sorensen VJ, et al. Factors influencing survival of elderly trauma patients. *Crit Care Med.* 1986;4:681–684.

24. Oreskovich MR, Howard JD, Copass MK, et al. Geriatric trauma: Injury patterns and outcome. *J Trauma.* 1984;4:565–572.

25. Bone L, Bucholz R. The management of fractures in the patient with multiple trauma. *J Bone Joint Surg Am.* 1986;68:945–949.

26. Gustilo RB, Simpson L, Nixon R, et al. Analysis of 511 open fractures. *Clin Orthop* 1969;66:148–154.

27. Gustilo RB, Anderson JT. Prevention of infection in the treatment of one thousand and twenty-five open fractures of long bones: Retrospective and prospective analyses. *J Bone Joint Surg Am.* 1976;58:453–458.

28. Cornell CN, Lane JM, Poynton AR. Orthopedic management of vertebral and long bone fractures in patients with osteoporosis. *Clin Geriatr Med.* 2003;19:433–455.

29. Salter RB, Dimonds DF, Malcolm BW, et al. The biological effect of continuous passive motion on the healing of full-thickness defects of articular cartilage. An experimental investigation in the rabbit. *J Bone Joint Surg Am.* 1980;62:1232–1251.

30. Scott RD, Turner RH, Leitzes SM, et al. Femoral fractures in conjunction with total hip replacement. *J Bone Joint Surg Am.*1975;57:494–501.

31. Zickel RE, Fietti VG Jr, Lawsing JF, et al. A new intramedullary fixation device for the distal third of the femur. *Clin Orthop* 1977;125:185–191.

32. Johansson JE, McBroom R, Barrington TW, et al. Fracture of the ipsilateral femur in patients with total hip replacement. *J Bone Joint Surg Am.* 1981;63:1435–1442.

33. Clain A. Secondary malignant disease of bone. *Br J Cancer* 1965;19:15–29.

34. Jaffe HL. *Tumors and Tumorous Conditions of Bones and Joint.* Philadelphia: Lea & Febiger; 1958.

35. Parrish FF, Murray JA. Surgical treatment for secondary neoplastic fractures: A retrospective study of ninety-six patients. *J Bone Joint Surg Am.* 1970;52:665–686.

36. Harrington KD. Impending pathologic fractures from metastatic malignancy: Evaluation and management. In: Anderson LD, ed. American Academy of Orthopaedic Surgeons *Instructional Course Lectures XXXV.* St Louis: CV Mosby; 1986:357–381.

37. Harrington KD, Sim FH, Enis JE, et al. Methylmethacrylate as an adjunct in internal fixation of pathologic fractures: experience with three hundred and seventy-five cases. *J Bone Joint Surg Am.* 1976;58:1046–1055.

38. Sexson SB, Lehner JT. Factors affecting hip fracture mortality. *J Orthop Trauma.* 1987;1:298–305.

39. Kenzora JE, McCarthy RE, Lowell JD, et al. Hip fracture mortality: Relation to age, treatment, preoperative illness, time of surgery, and complications. *Clin Orthop.* 1984;186:45–56.

40. Zuckerman JD, Skovron ML, Koval KJ, et al. Postoperative complications and mortality associated with operative delay in older patients who have a fracture of the hip. *J Bone Joint Surg Am.* 1995;77:1551–1556.

41. Davis FM, Woolner DF, Frampton C, et al. Prospective, multicentre trial of mortality following general or spinal anaesthesia for hip fracture surgery in the elderly. *Br J Anaesth.* 1987;59:1080–1088.

42. Valentin N, Lomholt B, Jensen JS, et al. Spinal or general anaesthesia for surgery of the fractured hip? A prospective study of mortality of 578 patients. *Br J Anaesth.* 1986;58:284–291.

43. Modig J, Borg T, Karlstrom G, et al. Thromboembolism after total hip replacement: role of epidural and general anesthesia. *Anesth Analg.* 1983;62:174–180.

44. Brody JA. Commentary: prospects for an ageing population. *Nature.* 1985;315:463–466.

45. Frandsen PA, Kruse T. Hip fractures in the county of Funen, Denmark. Implications of demographic aging and changes in incidence rates. *Acta Orthop Scand.* 1983;54:681–686.

46. Praemer A, Furner S, Rice DP, eds. *Musculoskeletal Conditions in the United States 1992.* Park Ridge, IL: The American Association of Orthopaedic Surgeons; 1992.

47. Greenspan SL, Myers ER, Kiel DP, et al. Fall severity and bone mineral density as risk factors for hip fractures in ambulatory elderly. *JAMA.* 1994;271:128–133.

48. Hinton RY, Lennox DW, Ebert FR, et al. Relative rates of fracture of the hip in the United States: geographic, sex, and age variations. *J Bone Joint Surg Am.* 1995;77:695–702.

49. Hinton RY, Smith GS. The association of age, race, and sex with the location of proximal femoral fractures in the elderly. *J Bone Joint Surg Am.* 1993;75:752–759.

50. Garraway WM, Stauffer RN, Kurland LT, O'Falba WM. Limb fractures in a defined population. I: frequency and distribution. *Mayo Clin Proc.* 1979;54:701–707.

51. Johnell O, Sernbo I. Health and social status in patients with hip fractures and controls. *Age Ageing.* 1986;15:285–291.

52. Uden G, Nilsson B. Hip fracture frequent in hospital. *Acta Orthop Scand*, 1986;57:428–430.

53. Rizzo PF, Gould ES, Lyden JP, Asnis SE. Diagnosis of occult fractures about the hip. Magnetic resonance imaging compared with bone-scanning. *J Bone Joint Surg Am*. 1993;75:395–401.

54. Parker MJ, Myles JW, Anand JK, et al. Cost-benefit analysis of hip fracture treatment. *J Bone Joint Surg Br*. 1992;74:261–264.

55. Colwell CW, Spiro TE, Trowbridge AA, et al. Use of enoxaparin, a low-molecular weight heparin, for the prevention of deep venous thrombosis after elective hip replacement. A clinical trial comparing efficacy and safety. Enoxaparin Clinical Trial Group. *J Bone Joint Surg Am*. 1994;76:3–14.

56. Geerts WH, Jay RM, Code KI, et al. A comparison of low-dose heparin with low-molecular weight heparin as prophylaxis against venous thromboembolism after major trauma. *NEJM*. 1996;335:701–707.

57. Merli GJ. Update deep venous thrombosis and pulmonary embolism prophylaxis in orthopaedic surgery. *Med Clin North Am*. 1993;77:397–412.

58. Koval KJ, Skovron ML, Aharonoff GB, et al. Ambulatory ability after hip fracture: a prospective study in geriatric patients. *Clin Orthop*. 1995;310:150–159.

59. White BL, Fischer WD, Lauren C. Rates of mortality for elderly patients after fracture of the hip in the 1980s. *J Bone Joint Surg Am*. 1987;69:1335–1340.

60. Aharonoff GB, Koval KJ, Skovron ML, Zuckerman JD. Hip fractures in the elderly: predictors of one-year mortality. *J Orthop Trauma*. 1997;11:162–165.

61. Zuckerman JD, Skovron ML, Koval KJ, et al. Postoperative complications and mortality associated with operative delay in older patients who have a fracture of the hip. *J Bone Joint Surg Am*. 1995;77: 1551–1556.

62. Frankle VH, Burstein AH, Lygre L, Brown RH. The telltale nail. *J Bone Joint Surg Am*. 1971;53:1232.

63. Koval K, Friend KD, Aharonoff GB, Zuckerman JD. Weightbearing after hip fracture: a prospective series of 596 geriatric hip fracture patients. *J Orthop Trauma*. 1996;10:526–530.

64. Koval K, Sala DA, Kummer FJ, Zuckerman JD. Postoperative weightbearing after a fracture of the femoral neck or an intertrochanteric fracture. *J Bone Joint Surg Am*. 1988;80:352–356.

65. Barnes R, Brown JT, Garden RS, Nicoll EA. Subcapital fractures of the femur. A prospective review *J Bone Joint Surg Br*. 1976;58:2–24.

66. Schmidt AH, Swiontkowski Mf. Femoral neck fractures. *Orthop Clin North Am*. 2002;33:97–111.

67. Cobb AG, Gibson PH. Screw fixation of subcapital fractures of the femur: a better method of treatment. *Injury*. 1986;17:259–264.

68. Garden RS. Malreduction and avascular necrosis in subcapital fractures of the femur. *J Bone Joint Surg Br*. 1971;53:183–197.

69. Stromqvist B, Hansson LI, Nilsson LT, et al. Hook-pin fixation in femoral neck fractures: a two-year follow-up study of 300 cases. *Clin Orthop*. 1987;218:58–62.

70. Bently G. Treatment of non-displaced fractures of the femoral neck. *Clin Orthop*. 1980;152:91–101.

71. Calder SJ, Anderson GH, Jagger C, et al. Unipolar or bipolar prosthesis for displaced intracapsular hip fractures in octogenarians. *J Bone Joint Surg Br*. 1996;78: 391–394.

72. Keating JF, Grant A, Masson M, et al. Randomized comparison of reduction and fixation, bipolar hemiarthroplasty, and total hip arthroplasty. Treatment of displaced intracapsular hip fractures in healthy older patients. *J Bone Joint Surg Am*. 2006;88:249–260.

73. Hardy DC, Descamps PY, Krallis P, et al. Use of an intramedullary hip-screw compared with a compression hip-screw with a plate for intertrochanteric femoral fractures. A prospective, randomized study of one hundred patients. *J Bone Joint Surg Am*. 1998;80:618–630.

74. Adams CI, Robinson CM, Court-Brown CM, McQueen MM. Prospective randomized controlled trial of an intramedullary nail versus dynamic screw and plate for intertrochanteric fractures of the femur. *J Orthop Trauma*. 2001;15:394–400.

75. Crawford CH, Malkani AL, Cordray S, Roberts CS, Sligar W. The trochanteric nail versus the sliding hip screw for intertrochanteric hip fractures: a review of 93 cases. *J Trauma*. 2006;60:325–328; discussion 328–329.

76. McConnell T, Creevy W, Tornetta P 3rd. Stress examination of supination external rotation-type fibular fractures. *J Bone Joint Surg Am*. 2004;86:2171–2178.

77. Ramsey PL, Hamilton W. Changes in tibiotalar area of contact caused by lateral talar shift. *J Bone Joint Surg Am*. 1976;58:356–357.

78. Beauchamp CG, Clay NR, Thexton PW. Displaced ankle fractures in patients over 50 years of age. *J Bone Joint Surg Br*. 1983;65:329–332.

79. Ali MS, McLaren AN, Routholamin E, O'Connor BT. Ankle fractures in the elderly: nonoperative or operative treatment. *J Orthop Trauma*. 1987;1:275–280.

80. Neer CS II. Displaced proximal humeral fractures: Part I. Classification and evaluation. *J Bone Joint Surg Am*. 1970;52:1077–1089.

81. Neer CS II. Displaced proximal humeral fractures. Part II. Treatment of three-part and four-part displacement. *J Bone Joint Surg Am*. 1970;52:1090–1103.

82. Alfram P, Bauer G. Epidemiology of fractures of the forearm. *J Bone Joint Surg Am*. 1970;52:1090–1103.

83. Fryckman G. Fractures of the distal radius including sequelae. *Acta Orthop Scand Suppl*. 1967;180:1–153.

84. Rozental TD, Blazar PE. Functional outcome and complications after volar plating for dorsally displaced, unstable fractures of the distal radius. *J Hand Surg Am*. 2006;31:359–365.

85. Young BT, Rayan GM. Outcome following nonoperative treatment of displaced distal radius fractures in low-demand patients older than 60 years. *J Hand Surg Am*. 2000;25:19–28.

86. Majd ME, Farley S, Holt RT. Preliminary outcomes and efficacy of the first 360 consecutive kyphoplasties for the treatment of painful osteoporotic vertebral compression fractures. *Spine J*. 2005;5:244–255.

87. Prather H, Van Dillen L, Metzler JP, et al. Prospective measurement of function and pain in patients with non-neoplastic compression fractures treated with vertebroplasty. *J Bone Joint Surg Am*. 2006;88:334–341.

32

FOOT HEALTH FOR THE ELDERLY: PODOGERIATRIC OVERVIEW

Arthur E. Helfand, DPM

INTRODUCTION

Foot problems in the older patient are prevalent and are major factors in podalgia, limitation of mobility, developmental functional disability, impairment, ambulatory dysfunction, gait imbalance, as a causative factor in falls, and increased pain and discomfort. Foot disorders in the older patient are related to the aging process, systemic diseases and/or disorders, focal changes in the foot, and/or complications associated with other medical problems, especially those associated with degenerative joint change and deformity, neurosensory, peripheral arterial, and sensory deficits. Chronic foot conditions limit independence and the quality of life and increase the potential for marked limitation of activity, a fall, hospitalization, and limb loss. The goals of a geriatric foot health program include prevention, detection, assessment, treatment, and management.

ASSESSING AND IDENTIFYING FOOT AND RELATED DISORDERS IN THE OLDER PATIENT

In many instances, because foot, ankle, and related problems are the primary complaint, the patient may seek foot care initially. Preventing complications is essential and a comprehensive approach includes assessment, assessment protocols, risk stratification, practitioner education, patient education, lifelong surveillance, appropriate footwear and orthotics as indicated, medical and surgical management of foot conditions, as well as continuing medical and podiatric management.

Comprehensive podogeriatric assessment and risk factor stratification includes identifying those individuals who are most at-risk, and developing proper prevention and management strategies. A comprehensive assessment and risk stratification process was developed for The Pennsylvania Department of Health under contract with the Temple University, School of Podiatric Medicine. A copy of the Protocol (Helfand

Index) is attached as Appendix A. The validated protocol permits practitioners to complete a diagnostic assessment and risk stratification procedure that includes primary clinical elements. The protocol also includes risk stratification procedures for peripheral arterial disease, neurological deficits, sensory deficits, Medicare's class findings, onychia dystrophies, onychomycosis, mechanical and pressure keratosis, and ulceration.

Medicare excludes certain foot care services that are defined as the treatment of flat foot conditions and the prescription of supportive devices: the treatment of subluxations of the foot, and routine foot care (including the cutting or removal of corns, calluses, the trimming of nails), and other routine hygienic care.

The exemption for "routine foot care," permits coverage for patients with peripheral vascular and neurosensory deficits and includes the following systemic diseases and disorders, as examples:

Peripheral vascular conditions and diabetes
Diabetes mellitus*
Arteriosclerosis obliterans
Buerger disease
Chronic thrombophlebitis*
Peripheral neuropathies involving the feet
Associated with malnutrition and vitamin deficiency*
    Malnutrition
    Alcoholism
    Malabsorption
    Pernicious anemia
Associated with carcinoma*
Associated with diabetes mellitus*
Associated with drugs or toxins*
Associated with multiple sclerosis*
Associated with uremia (chronic renal disease)*
Associated with traumatic injury

Associated with leprosy and neurosyphilis
Associated with hereditary disorders
    Hereditary sensory radicular neuropathy
    Angiokeratoma corporis diffusum (Fabry)
    Amyloid neuropathy

When the patient's condition is one of those designated by an asterisk, routine care is covered only if the patient is under the active care of a doctor of medicine or osteopathy for a documented risk disease. Other significant systemic risk criteria include coagulopathies and immunodeficiencies associated with chemotherapy, human immunodeficiency syndrome, and acquired immunodeficiency syndrome.

The severity of one of these systemic diagnoses that would lead to a consideration of Medicare coverage involves documentation of clear evidence of significant circulatory changes defined as Class Findings. The patient must present with one class A finding; two class B findings; or one class B and two class C findings.

Class A Finding:
    Nontraumatic amputation of foot or integral skeletal portion there
Class B Findings:
    Absent posterior tibial pulse
    Absent dorsalis pedis pulse
    Advanced trophic changes (at least three of the following):
        Decrease or absence of hair growth
        Nail thickening
        Skin discoloration
        Thin and shiny skin texture
        Rubor or redness of skin
Class C Findings:
    Claudication
    Temperature changes (cold feet)
    Edema
    Paresthesia (abnormal spontaneous sensations in feet)
    Burning

The classification for onychomycosis also includes documentation of mycosis and/or dystrophy causing secondary infection and/or pain that results or would result in marked limitation of ambulation, which includes, but is not limited to discoloration, hypertrophy, subungual debris, onycholysis, secondary infection, and limitation of ambulation and pain.

Coverage was also extended for the evaluation and management of at-risk diabetic patients with sensory neuropathy, resulting in a loss of protective sensation that includes the following:

Diagnosis of loss of protective sensation
Patient history
Physical examination consisting of findings regarding at least the following elements:
    Visual inspection of the forefoot, hindfoot, and web spaces

Evaluation of protective sensation
Foot structure and biomechanics
Vascular status
Skin integrity
Recommendations for footwear
Patient education

Medicare's Durable Medical Equipment program also provides coverage for "therapeutic shoes" with custom and/or customized multidensity insoles for the at-risk diabetic patient. The coverage criteria include one or more of the following:

A history of partial or complete amputation of the foot
History of previous foot ulceration
History of preulcerative callus
Peripheral neuropathy with evidence of callus formation
Foot deformity
Poor circulation

The assessment should include the treatment or management plan, podiatric referral, patient education, medical referral, vascular studies, clinical laboratory studies, special footwear needs, imaging, (plain radiography [weight and nonweight bearing studies], computed tomography [CT], bone scan, magnetic resonance [MR] imaging, bone density), and other prescriptions and/or referrals.

The examination may also indicate the need for expanded vascular, dermatological, neurological, and biomechanical evaluation that includes foot type, angulations, muscle power, contractions, and other deformities that affect both weight bearing and nonweight bearingability (e.g., hip contraction increases pressure on ipsilateral heel).

Other studies that may be indicated to assess clinically and stratify risk include the use of Doppler evaluation; pulse volume recording; ankle-brachial index; oscillometer; laser radiometer; skin surface thermometer and scanner; Duplex ultrasound with color flow imaging; digital subtraction angiography, MR angiography; C-128 tuning fork; biothesiometer; vibration threshold meter; percussion hammer; neurological hammer; Babinski hammer; monofilament sensory testing such as Semmes-Weinstein, Norton, or West; Tip Therm, two-point discriminator; goniometer (foot and ankle and digital); and ultraviolet light (Wood light).

PSYCHOSOCIAL CONSIDERATIONS

With the projected increase in the number of older persons, the changes in living arrangements including more than 55 residential communities, continuing care retirement communities, long-term care facilities and other forms of living arrangements, mental status change, cognitive issues, and depression become important considerations. The foot is more than a single purpose locomotor accessory. From a psychosocial sense, the foot is utilized to demonstrate hostility, such as kicking an individual or object. The foot may also be the site of unconsciously chosen expressions of deeper emotional feelings and inadequacies. In addition, the foot and primarily the musculoskeletal structures are often a focus for psychosomatic problems associated with depression, loneliness, and isolation. For example, suggesting to older patients that considering the condition of their feet, one cannot understand how they can walk, may be all that is needed to significantly limit ambulation, develop a social dependence, and increase the cost of care.

The prevalent physical manifestations in the foot associated with mental health disorders in older patients include hysterical paralysis, psychogenic tremors, localized neurodermatitis, pruritus, and hyperhidrosis. Covariant conditions that are affected by emotional disorders result in exacerbation of the disease or disorders such as gout, diabetes mellitus, obesity, vascular insufficiency, psoriasis, urticaria, and atopic dermatitis.

When an older patient presents with inappropriate clinical complaints and symptoms that are not demonstrable as an actual foot disorder, neglect, or as a manifestation of organic pathology, the potential for emotional transfer should be considered. The foot may provide more than a primary focus for an emotional or psychiatric disorder, it may prove to be exclusive. The older patient may be using his or her foot complaint as a cry for "help" and as a means to seek attention, expecting relief through some form of physical treatment. When such treatment fails to bring relief, the patient usually reacts emotionally by blaming the doctor or other professional staff, feeling hopeless, dejected, and may even project hostility. The patient may also react somatically, by increasing symptoms and complaints. Foot problems with psychogenic components usually represent some form of anxiety neurosis. They can also manifest as neurotic or psychotic depression, schizophrenia, involutional psychosis, or as a manifestation of organic brain syndrome. Patients with dementia or Alzheimer's disease may present with serious changes as a result of neglect and the inability to recognize that a problem even exists. With added obesity, the patient may not even be able to see his or her feet. With our changing society and longevity, the potential to manage foot problems associated with challenged mental impairments, drug, and alcohol abuse, must now be considered in planning for foot care for the elderly in mental health programs.

PRIMARY FOOT PROBLEMS AND THEIR MANAGEMENT

The management of foot problems in older patients has as its primary goals the reduction of pain, improvement of the functional capacity of the patient, and maintaining that restored function to provide comfort for the patient to live life to the end.

Disorder of the Toenails

The onychial changes that occur are the result of a new disease, the residuals of long-term disease, injury, and/or functional modification. Onychial degeneration, hypertrophy, deformity, trophic changes, and keratin dysplasia are more prevalent in the older patient.

Onychia, an inflammation of the posterior nail wall and/or nail bed, is usually precipitated by local trauma or pressure, and/or as a complication of systemic diseases, such as diabetes mellitus. It is an early indicator of infection. Mild erythema, swelling, and pain are the most prevalent findings. Treatment should be directed to removing all pressure from the area and the use of tepid saline compresses. With systemic complications, antibiotics as well as imaging may be indicated to detect bone change. Lambs wool, tube foam, or shoe modifications should be considered to reduce pressure to the toe and nail. If not managed early, paronychia may develop including abscess and infection of the posterior nail wall. The infection progresses proximally with deeper structure involvement. The potential for osteomyelitis is greater in the presence of diabetes mellitus and peripheral arterial disease, with an increased risk of necrosis, gangrene, and the potential for amputation. Management includes drainage, culture and sensitivity, radiographs and scans as appropriate, saline compresses, and appropriate systemic antibiotics.

Deformities of the toenails result from repetitive microtrauma, degenerative changes, or disease. For example, the continued friction of the toe nails over the years, against the interior toe box of the shoe is sufficient trauma to produce onychauxis (thickening). Onychorrhexis, an accentuation of normal ridging, trophic changes, and longitudinal striations, is present when related to disease and/or nutritional etiology. When debridement is not completed on a periodic basis, the nail structure hypertrophies and continues to thicken and becomes markedly deformed (onychogryphosis). Onychogryphosis or 'Rams Horn Nail' may be complicated by fungal infection. The resultant disability can limit mobility and place the patient at risk of falling. Pain is usually associated with pressure and the deformity. In addition, traumatic avulsion of the toenail becomes more prevalent. The exaggerated curvature (onychodysplasia) may penetrate the skin, with resultant infection and ulceration. Management should be directed toward periodic debridement, including dermabrasion. The degree of onycholysis (freeing of the nail from the anterior edge) and onychoschizia (splitting), help determine the level of debridement. With excess pressure and deformity, the nail grooves may become keratotic. Debridement and the use of mild keratolytics and emollients provide home care strategies. When onycholysis, subungual debris, and keratosis develop, discomfort and pain increase. With sensory impairment, assessment and management may be deferred until complications are present.

The elderly diabetic usually exhibits some form of onychopathy or nail changes such as onychorrhexis, onychophosis, deformity, hypertrophy, onychodysplasia (incurvation or involution), subungual hemorrhage (nontraumatic) onycholysis (freeing from the distal segment), onychomadesis (freeing from the proximal segment), autoavulsion, and onychomycosis. Similar clinical findings are present in patients with vascular insufficiency, coagulopathies, cardiac disease, chronic renal failure, chronic obstructive pulmonary disease, and immuno-suppression that increase the risk of infection, necrosis, gangrene, and potential amputation.

The most prevalent nonbacterial infection of the toenails is onychomycosis. By definition onychomycosis is a chronic and communicable infectious disease and clinically it may appear as distal subungual, white superficial, proximal subungual, total dystrophic, or as candida onychomycosis. In the white superficial form, changes appear on the superior surface of the toenail and generally do not invade the deeper structures, unless left untreated. In the distal, proximal, and total dystrophic manifestations, the nail bed, as well as the nail plate are involved. There is usually some degree of onycholysis (freeing of the nail from the distal edge) and subungual keratosis. Because of the chronic nature of this condition, the posterior nail wall, eponychium, and nail plate demonstrate xerotic, keratotic, and hypertrophic changes. Candida is prevalent in patients with chronic mucocutaneous manifestation.

The patient usually presents with a chronic infection involving one or more of the nail plates. The entire thickness of the nail plates are usually involved with resultant hypertrophy and deformity. Pain is related to pressure and/or secondary bacterial infection. Mycotic onychia, autoavulsion, subungual hemorrhage, a foul, musty odor, and degeneration of the nail plate are shared findings. Management includes systemic and topical antifungals, keratolytic agents, debridement, and surgical removal. Because of chronicity, matrix involvement, hypertrophy, deformity, the residuals are usually not reversed in the older patient. In addition, multiple drug use for disease and vascular impairment may impair or contraindicate systemic management. Periodic debridement along with, the application 20%–50% urea to aid in debridement, systemic terbinafine hydrochloride or itraconazole, and topical fungicides such as ciclopirox provide the best approach to management.

Ingrown toenails (onychocryptosis) are usually the end result of deformity and related to improper prior care. When the nail penetrates the skin, an abscess, and infection result. If not managed early, ulcerative periungual granulation tissue may form, which complicates treatment. Deformity and involution (onychodysplasia) also provide a complicating factor. In the early stages, a wedge-shaped segment of nail can be removed, drainage established, with follow-up saline compresses and antibiotics used as indicated. Preventive measures should be used to prevent reoccurrence. When granulation tissue is present, excision, fulguration, desiccation, or the use of caustics, such as silver nitrate (75%) and astringents are used to reduce the granulation tissue. In all cases, removal of the penetrating nail is primary. Partial excision of the nail plate and matrix can be completed utilizing regional anesthetic followed by excision and chemical cautery of the matrix area with CP phenol. Postoperative management includes appropriate dressings and preparations to manage the chemical cauterization.

The excessive medial–lateral curvature of the nail plate because of onychodysplasia results in incurvation, involution, or pincer deformity that appears "C" shaped distally. The pressure of the nail plate on the nail bed and folds produces ony-chophosis (hyperkeratosis in the nail folds) and discomfort, with complaints similar to an ingrown toenail. The condition may precipitate pressure ulcerations and infection. When this condition is severe, partial or total excision of the nail plate and matrix should be considered to avoid future complications.

Subungual heloma, when present, is usually associated with a subungual exostosis, spur, or hypertrophy of the tufted end of the distal phalanx. Initial treatment consists of debridement of the hyperkeratosis, protection of the toe involved, and the use of a shoe with a high toe box. Excision of the osseous deformity may be required if the condition cannot be managed in a conservative manner. With suspected bone pathology, radiographs properly positioned to isolate the area of pathological entity will provide an appropriate diagnostic approach. Subungual ulceration and melanoma are two important diagnostic differentials.

There are also other onychopathies that are associated with cutaneous and systemic diseases that also should be considered in older persons. The most prevalent include onychatrophia (atrophy), onychia sicca (dryness), onychexallis (degeneration), diabetic onychopathy, subungual abscess, periungual verruca, onychophyma (painful degeneration with hypertrophy), onychophyma (hemorrhagic), onychoclasis (cracking), onychomalacia (softening), onychoptosis (shedding), subungual spur, hemorrhage, Beau lines (transverse growth cessation), pterygium (hypertrophy of eponychium), and diabetic hypertrophic onychodystrophy.

PRIMARY DERMATOLOGICAL DISORDERS

The skin as an organ system may fail and respond slowly toward improvement. Changes include hair loss, atrophy of soft tissue, dryness, pigmentation, hemosiderin deposition and stasis, hyperkeratosis (hypertrophy and hyperplasia), keratin dysfunction, arterial insufficiency, and ulceration.

Xerosis and excessively dry skin are associated with older patients. A lack of hydration, lubrication, and degenerative processes are contributing factors. Keratin dysfunction is associated with xerosis. Fissures develop as a result of dryness and stress. When present on the heel, a potential hazard exists for the development of ulceration. Initial management includes the use of an emollient following hydration and a mild keratolytic. A plastic or soft heel cup can assist in minimizing trauma and reduce the potential for complications.

Pruritus is usually more severe in the colder weather. It is related to dryness, scaliness, decreased skin secretions, keratin dysfunction, environmental changes, and defatting of the skin that is usually aggravated by the use of warm foot soaks. Scratching and excoriations are also clinical findings. Chronic tinea, allergic, neurogenic, and/or emotional dermatoses should be considered as part of the differential diagnosis. Management includes hydration, lubrication, protection, topical steroids if indicated, and judicious use of antihistamines. If excoriations are infected, antibiotics should be utilized early on as indicated.

For hyperhidrosis and bromidrosis if local in etiology, topical hydrogen peroxide, isopropyl alcohol, and astringents may be utilized to control excessive perspiration and odor. Neomycin powder will help control the odor by reducing the bacterial decomposition of perspiration. Recommendations on footwear and stocking modifications should be considered. Shoe component contact dermatitis may also be a factor. In winter and colder climates, dampness can predispose the patient to the vasospastic complications.

Contact dermatitis is associated with reactions to chemicals used in shoe construction, such as nickel, footwear fabrics, and/or stockings. Skin lesions and clinical findings are limited and usually bilateral in distribution. Skin testing can identify the primary irritant. Management includes removing the primary irritant, mild wet dressings, and the use of topical steroids.

Stasis dermatitis is associated with venous insufficiency and chronic ulceration with dependent edema. Management includes elevation, mild wet dressings, topical steroids, antibiotics as indicated, and supportive measures needed to manage the venous disease. With pyoderma and superficial bacterial infections antibiotics should be considered as indicated. Tinea if present requires antifungal therapy.

Tinea pedis is many times an extension of onychomycosis, which serves as a focus of infection. It is more common in warmer climates with the chronic keratotic type more prevalent. Poor foot hygiene and the inability to view one's feet may motivate the patient to seek care only when the condition becomes clinically significant. The wide variety of topical medications available can usually control this condition. Antifungal solutions and/or creams (water washable or miscible) are usually easier for the patient to remove. Foot hygiene is an essential preventive strategy.

Solitary and/or hemorrhagic bullae are related to shoe trauma and friction or related to systemic diseases such as diabetes mellitus. Management is directed toward eliminating pressure, protection, and drainage when appropriate. Supportive dressings and shoe modifications should be used as appropriate. Gait changes in older individuals magnify many of the foot to shoe incompatibilities that can result in local foot lesions. Hemorrhagic and bullae related to diabetes mellitus are early ulcerative indicators.

Other common dermatological manifestations include those associated with atopic dermatitis; nummular eczema; neurodermatitis; psoriasis; painful or painless wounds; slow or nonhealing wounds; trophic, diabetic, or peripheral vascular ulceration; necrosis; skin color changes, such as cyanosis or rubor; excessive pigmentation and discoloration; verruca; maceration; hematoma; preulcerative changes; and ulceration noting perfusion, extent, depth, infection, and sensation, which are managed based on their etiology, symptoms, and clinical signs.

ULCERATIONS

The mechanical factors that are risk factors for ulceration include: body mass, tissue trauma, weight diffusion, weight dispersion, pathomechanics, biomechanics, and imbalance. In addition, force, compression stress, tensile stress, shearing stress, friction, elasticity, fluid pressure, ambulatory speed, and the weight of the individual are all important considerations.

The management of ulcerations in the older patient depends on the etiology and usually occurs as a complication associated with diabetes mellitus, peripheral arterial disease, infection, and trauma or a combination of multiple etiologies, including foot deformities. For the patient with diabetes mellitus, neuropathy, and/or peripheral arterial disease, early management can prevent limb loss. General principles include supportive measures to reduce trauma and pressure to the ulcerated area, such as dressings, wound care, orthoses, shoe modifications, and special shoes and braces, such as surgical shoes, healing or wound care sandals, flap closure shoes, extra depth shoes, rocker soles, half-soles, wedge shoes, night splints, foot and heel suspension devices, ankle foot orthosis, foot drop braces, CAM walkers®, cast walkers with removable insole segments, Charcot-resistant orthopedic walker, multidensity total contact insoles and/or orthoses, total contact casts, cast walkers, and custom molded shoes. Patient awareness, temperature monitoring, and ambulatory aids, such as canes, crutches, walkers, wheelchairs, also assist in pressure reduction. Other methods include the use of orthoses and/or shoe last changes and/or the use of pads, bars, wedges, and other modifications. Increasing the sole thickness and using shock-absorbing material, such as a Vibram or ripple sole can be of assistance.

The prevention and control of infection and maintaining a clean, healthy base to permit healing are essential. Cultures, biopsy, ulcer measurement, and imaging (x-ray, MR images, CT scans) initially to establish a baseline and rule out bone change are important issues. Granulation tissue, the color and consistency of drainage, sinus formation, fluctuation, and edema are important clinical indicators. The early evaluation of diabetics for neuropathic osteoarthropathy (Charcot) is essential. Topical debriding agents can be used and should be monitored. The debridement of keratosis when indicated is essential to prevent roofing of the ulcer. With infection, considering early hospital admission for patients in metabolic disarray, those who are febrile, and those who have questionable compliance is important. Targeted antibiotics should be utilized as indicated. The use of physical modalities and measures such as low-voltage therapy (contractile currents) and exercises can assist in improving the local vascular supply to the ulcer and in helping to establish a clean base. Pressure ulcers of local origin are usually associated with a bony prominence, biomechanical abnormality, external trauma, or are the result of stress associated with gait change. Atrophy of soft tissue and the residuals of arthritis provide a focus for the development of ulcerations. Those associated with systemic disease are usually related to neuropathic change and vascular insufficiency, as with diabetes mellitus. Management focuses on identifying the underlying diagnosis, local supportive measures, adequate treatment of the related systemic diseases and efforts to minimize the potential for osteomyelitis, and maintaining the ambulatory status of the patient for as long as possible. Older patients who avoid the use of foot wear at home, because of their inability to bend, expose themselves to the potential of foreign bodies and foot injury. For example, animal hairs will appear as keratotic plugs and require debridement and/or excision to relieve pain. Left untreated, these lesions ulcerate.

With peripheral vascular diseases, such as venous diseases and peripheral arterial diseases, vascular consultation and studies such as ultrasound, CT angiography, and MR angiography should be considered as indicated. The relationship to diabetes mellitus and cardiovascular disease is also important. Other special studies to also be considered include duplex ultrasound with color flow imaging, Doppler studies, ankle brachial index, and distal subtraction angiography. Additional considerations include percutaneous transluminal angioplasty, stent implantation, cryoplasty, peripheral cutting balloon, and laser-assisted angioplasty.

HYPERKERATOSIS

The many forms of hyperkeratotic lesions, such as tyloma (callous) and heloma (corn) and their varieties, such as hard, soft, vascular, neurofibrous, seed, and subungual are prevalent. Intractable keratoma, eccrine poroma, porokeratosis, and verruca must be differentiated from these keratotic lesions, although each may present initially as a hyperkeratotic area. The biomechanical and pathomechanical factors that create these problems are those associated with stress, that is, compressive, tensile, and/or shearing. Soft tissue atrophy and plantar fat pad displacement and atrophy increase pain and limit ambulation. Contractures, gait changes, deformities (hammertoes, hallux valgus, and metatarsal prolapse), and the residuals of arthritis are all additional factors that need to be considered in management. The incompatibility of the foot type (inflare, straight, or outflare) to the shoe last is another factor to be considered. It is important to recognize that there is usually not one factor but a multiplicity of conditions including skin tone, elasticity, and keratin dysfunction that result in the development of keratotic lesions in the elderly. Their management is not routine and the term management signifies a period of continuing care, similar to other chronic conditions. The prevalent sites for the development of hyperkeratotic lesions include digital areas, plantar metatarsal heads, marginal calcaneal, and with deformities such as hammertoes, digital rotations, contractures, hallux valgus, bunion, tailor's bunion, and those that form as space replacement.

Foot deformities, soft tissue atrophy, biomechanical, and pathomechanical deformities are precipitating factors to foot to shoe last incompatibilities that produce excessive pressure on segments of the foot. Management and treatment of hyperkeratotic lesions should be directed toward the functional needs of the patients and on their activity needs for daily living. Considerations include debridement, padding, emollients, shoe modifications, as well as shoe last changes, orthoses, and surgical revision as indicated. Materials to provide soft tissue replacement, weight dispersion, and weight diffusion are also

indicated. Long-standing keratotic lesions represent a hyperplastic and hypertrophic pathological entities that may persist even when weight bearing is removed. Hyperkeratotic lesions are a form of body protection to pressure and are symptoms of an abnormal state. If permitted to persist, enlarge, and condense, they become primary irritants. With pressure such as weight bearing and ambulation, and local avascularity, ulceration can be resultant sequelae. Pressure ulcers in the foot usually begin with subkeratotic hemorrhage. Once debrided and managed properly, they usually heal but may be repetitive, unless adequate measures are instituted to reduce the pressure to the localized areas of ulceration. Even with all measures, the problem may persist due to residual deformity and systemic diseases that may require surgical intervention.

FOOT DEFORMITIES

Feet are fairly rigid structures both static and dynamic. The foot itself is in the shape of a modified rectangle and bears weight in a triangular pattern. The transmission of weight starts at heel strike, proceeds anteriorly along the lateral segment of the foot, medially across the metatarsal heads, to the first metatarsal segment of the foot for the push off phase of the gait cycle. Life's activities, the aging process, occupation, and the social needs of society produce many morphological variations in both the structure and function of the feet and related structures, in keeping with Wolff's and Davis' Laws as the body adapts to the stress placed on it. To a great degree, the inability to adapt to stress is a precipitating factor in the development of inflammation and pain. The environment, flat hard surfaces, shock absorption, repetitive microtrauma, obesity, as well as aging, magnify discomfort and pain. It is these mechanical and systemic stressors that have their greatest change in older patients, who cannot adapt to the residuals of deformity and aging itself.

There are a variety of residual foot deformities that can be present in multiple combinations in the elderly. These include hallux valgus, hallux varus, splay foot, hallux flexus, digiti flexus (hammertoe), digiti quinti varus, overlapping toes, underriding toes, prolapsed metatarsal heads, pes cavus, pes planus, pronation, hallux limitus, hallux rigidus, and biomechanical and pathomechanical abnormalities. Foot deformities create functional impairment relating to gait and footwear selection.

Treatment consists of both nonsurgical and surgical considerations. Bilateral weight and nonweightbearing radiographic studies are indicated when management is considered from both a static and dynamic phase. Age itself should not be the final determining factor in considering surgery. Consideration must also be given to the patient's ability to adapt to change in relation to ambulation, for to have an anatomically corrected joint and a patient who cannot ambulate without pain defeats the treatment needs of the elderly. Conservative modalities include shoe last changes, shoe modifications, orthoses, digital braces, physical modalities, exercises, and mild analgesics for pain. Residual deformities with stress precipitate inflammatory changes such as periarthritis, bursitis, myositis, synovitis, neuritis, tendonitis, sesamoiditis, and plantar myofascitis, for example, which need to be managed medically, physically, and mechanically to keep the patient ambulatory and pain free.

Fractures of the foot and toes may be the result of direct trauma and/or stress related to bone loss (osteopenia and osteoporosis). The progressive loss of muscle mass and atrophy of soft tissue, decreased function, and inactivity predisposes the older patient to the potential of a fracture. Most uncomplicated and closed fractures that are in good position can be managed with the use of a surgical shoe and supportive dressings, as long as the joints distally and proximally are immobilized. Silicone molds can be utilized for digital fractures and their use maintains position through healing, permitting the patient to maintain proper hygiene.

Shoe modifications that can be considered for the elderly include mild calcaneal wedges to limit motion and alter gait; metatarsal bars to transfer weight; Thomas heels to increase calcaneal support; long shoe counters to increase midfoot support and control foot direction; heel flares to add stability; shank fillers or wedges to produce a total weight bearing surface; steel plates to restrict motion; and rocker bars to prevent flexion and extension. Additional internal modifications include longitudinal arch pads, wedges, bars, lifts, and tongue or bite pads. The available orthoses include the rigid, semirigid and flexible varieties; using materials such as plastic, leather, laminates, polyurethane, sponge, or foam rubber; and Korex, felt, latex, wood flour, Plastazote, Aliplast, and silicone to provide support, reduce pressure, and provide for weight diffusion and weight dispersion.

LONG-TERM CARE GUIDELINES

Foot care and/or podiatric services should be organized and staffed in a manner designed to meet the foot health needs of patient/residents. A consulting podiatrist should provide the foot health service that includes consultation, assessment, management, surveillance, and education, as a member of the staff. The foot health program should be an integral part of the facility's total health care program and written policies and procedures should be developed to serve as a guide for foot care. The quality and appropriateness of podiatric services should be included in the overall quality assurance program, consistent with other practitioner/professional services.

A program of professional, in-service, and patient education should form a part of a total geriatric program for long-term care. This same program can be utilized for ambulatory care, home care, hospice, and other related programs. An example of the content includes the following:

A. The relationship of foot problems to the total older patient includes: needs; ambulation and independence; risk diseases; factors that modify foot care in society and health care; Medicare and Medicaid; mental health considerations; long-term care; and rehabilitation.
B. Primary foot care includes assessment and examination; toenail diseases and disorder; skin diseases and disorders; hyperkeratotic disorders; foot orthopedic, biomechanical, and pathomechanical changes; foot deformities associated with aging; risk diseases, such as diabetes mellitus, degenerative and rheumatoid arthritis, gout, peripheral arterial and vascular diseases, and other related conditions; management; footwear and related considerations; care delivery; and interdisciplinary coordinated care.
C. Foot Health Education

CONCLUDING REMARKS

Foot pain in the older patient reduces the physical and mental aspects of the quality of life as well as mobility, and limits independent living. Patient education, assessment, risk stratification, continuing surveillance, and management are critical factors for patient care. Foot impairment, including diseases and disorders of the foot, are prevalent in the older individual and impact general health. The early recognition of change, management, and referral as indicated significantly improves the quality of life, ensures dignity, and helps maintain self-esteem for older citizens.

APPENDIX A

TEMPLE UNIVERSITY SCHOOL OF PODIATRIC MEDICINE
Podogeriatric Assessment and Chronic Disease Protocol

THE FOO
& ANKLE
INSTITUT

Date of Service _____   MR # _____

Patient Name _____   Date of Birth _____   Social Security # _____

Address _____   City _____   State _____   Zip Code _____

Sex M   F   Race B W A L N/A   Weight _____ lbs   Height _____ in   Marital Status M S W D Sep

Name of Primary Physician/Health Care Facility _____   Date of Last Visit _____

HISTORY OF PRESENT ILLNESS

___Swelling of Feet ___Infections ___Duration
___Painful Feet ___Cold Feet ___Context
___Hyperkeratosis ___Other ___Modifying Factors
___Onychial Changes ___Location ___Associated Signs & Symptoms
___Bunions ___Quality
___Painful Toe Nails ___Severity

PAST HISTORY

___Heart Disease ___Thyroid ___Hypercholesterol
___High Blood Pressure ___Allergy ___Gout
___Arthritis ___Diabetes Mellitis* ___History: Smoking: OH
___* Circulatory Disease ___IDDM ___NIDDM ___Family - Social

SYSTEM REVIEW

___Constitutional ___Hematologic ___Neurologic
___ENT ___Card / Vasc ___Endocrine
___Eyes ___Musculo-Skeletal ___GI
___Skin / Hair ___GYN ___Immunlogic
___Respiratory ___Lymphatic
___Psychiatric ___GU

MEDICATIONS

DERMATOLOGIC

___* Hyperkeratosis ___Onychodystrophy ___Hematoma
___Onychauxis B-2-b ___* Cyanosis ___Rubor
___Infection ___Xerosis ___* Preulcerative
___* Ulceration ___Tinea Pedis ___Discolored
___Onychomycosis ___Verruca

FOOT ORTHOPEDIC

___* Hallux Valgus ___* Pes Valgoplanus ___* Prominent Met Head
___* Anterior Imbalance ___* Pes Cavus ___* Charcot Joints
___* Digiti Flexus ___* Hallux Rigidus Limitus
___* Pes Planus ___* Morton's Syndrome Bursitis ___Other

VASCULAR EVALUATION

___* Coldness C-2 ___* Night Cramps ___* Amputation
___* Trophic Changes B-2-a ___* Edema C-3 ___* AKA BKA FF T A-1
___* DP Absent B-3 ___* Claudication C-1 ___Atrophy B-2-d
___* PT Absent B-1 ___Varicosities

NEUROLOGIC EVALUATION

___* Achilles ___* Paresthesia C-4 ___* Burning C-5
___* Vibratory ___Superficial Plantar ___Other
___* Sharp / Dull ___* Joint Position

RISK CATEGORY - NEUROLOGIC

___- 0 = No Sensory Loss ___* 2 = Sensory Loss & Foot Deformity
___* I = Sensory Loss ___* 3 = Sensory Loss, Hx Ulceration & Deformity

RISK CATEGORY - VASCULAR

___ 0 - 0 No Change ___* I - 4 Ischemic Rest Pain
___* I - 1 Mild Claudication ___* II - 5 Minor Tissue Loss
___* I - 2 Moderate Claudication ___* III - 6 MajorTissue Loss
___* I - 3 Severe Claudication

CLASS FINDINGS

___A1 Nontraumatic Amputation ___B2e Skin Color (rubor or redness)
___B1 Absent Posterior Tibial ___B3 Absent Dorsalis Pedis
___B2 Advanced Trophic Changes ___C1 Claudication
___B2a Hair Growth (decrease or absent) ___C2 Temperature Changes (cold)
___B2b Nail Changes (thickening) ___C3 Edema
___B2c Pigmentary Changes (discoloration) ___C4 Paresthesia
___B2d Skin Texture (thin, shiny) ___C5 Burning

Onychomycosis: Documentation of mycosis/dystrophy causing secondary infection and/or pain which result or would result in marked limitation of ambulation.

Discoloration   Onycholysis
Hypertrophy   Secondary Infection
Subungual Debris Limitation of Ambulation and Pain

CLASSIFICATION OF MECHANICAL OR PRESSURE HYPERKERATOSIS

Grade	Description
0	No Lesion
1	No specific Tyloma Plaque, but diffuse or pinch Hyperkeratotic tissue present or in narrow bands.
2	Circumscribed, Punctate oval, or circular, well defined thickening of Kertinized Tissue
3	Heloma Milliare or Heloma Durum with no associated Tyloma
4	Well defined Tyloma Plaque with a definite Heloma within the Lesion
5	Extravasation, Maceration and early breakdown of structures under the Tyloma or Callus Layer
6	Complete breakdown of structure of Hyperkeratotic Tissue, Epidermis, extending to superficial Dermal involvement

PLANTAR KERATOMATA PATTERN

LT 1 2 3 4 5   RT 1 2 3 4 5

ULCER CLASSIFICATION

Grade - 0 - Absent Skin Lesions
Grade - 1 - Dense Callus but not Pre-Ulcer or Ulcer
Grade - 2 - Preulcerative Changes
Grade - 3 - Partial Thickness (Superficial Ulcer)
Grade - 4 - Full Thickness (deep) Ulcer but no involvement of Tendon, Bone, Ligament or Joi
Grade - 5 - Full Thickness (deep) Ulcer with involvement of Tendon, Bone, Ligament or Joint
Grade - 6 - Localized Infection (Abscess or Osteomyelitis)
Grade - 7 - Proximal spread of Infection (Ascending Cellulitis or Lymphadenopathy)
Grade - 8 - Gangrene of Forefoot only
Grade - 9 - Gangrene of Majority of Foot

ONYCHIAL GRADES AT RISK

Grade I Normal   Grade IV Hypertrophic
Grade II Mild Hypertrophy   Deformed
Grade III Hypertrophic   Onychogryphosis
         Dystrophic   Dystrophic
         Onychauxis   Mycotic
         Mycotic   Infected
         Infected
         Onychodysplasia

FOOTWEAR SATISFACTORY   **HYGIENE SATISFACTORY**
   Yes   No   Yes   No

STOCKINGS: Nylon   Cotton   Wool   Other   None

ASSESSMENT

PLAN

___Podiatric Referral ___Medical Referral ___Vascular Studies ___Imaging
___Patient Education ___Special Footwear ___Clinical Lab ___Rx

BIBLIOGRAPHY

1. *Diabetic Foot Disorders – A Clinical Practice Guideline.* Park Ridge, IL: American College of Foot and Ankle Surgeons; 2000.
2. American Diabetes Association. Preventive foot care in people with dabetes. *Diabetes Care.* 2003;26(Suppl):S78–S79.
3. Armstrong DG, Lavery LA. *Clinical Care of the Diabetic Foot.* Alexandria, VA: American Diabetes Association; 2005.
4. Birrer RB, Dellacorte MP, Grisafi PJ. *Common Foot Problems in Primary Care.* 2nd ed. Philadelphia: Henley & Belfus; 1998.
5. Bolton AJM, Connor H, Cavanagh, PR. *The Foot in Diabetes.* 3rd ed. Chichester: John Wiley & Sons Ltd; 2000.
6. Bowker JH, Pfeifer MA. *Levin and O'Neal's The Diabetic Foot.* 6th ed. St. Louis: Mosby; 2001.
7. Collet BS. Foot problems. *The Merck Manual of Geriatrics.* 3rd ed. Chapter 56. Whitehouse Station, NJ: Merck Research Laboratories; 2000:544–557.
8. Dauber R, Bristow I, Turner W. *Text Atlas of Podiatric Dermatology.* London: Martin Dunitz; 2001.
9. Edmonds ME, Foster AVM, Sanders LJ. *A Practical Manual of Diabetic Footcare.* Malden, MA: Blackwell Publishing; 2004.
10. Evans JG, Williams FT, Beattie BL, Michel JP, Wilcock GK. *Oxford Textbook of Geriatric Medicine.* 2nd ed. Oxford: Oxford University Press; 2000.
11. Gabel LL, Haines DJ, Papp KK. *The Aging Foot: An Interdisciplinary Perspective.* Columbus, OH: The Ohio State University, College of Medicine and Public Health, Department of Family Medicine; 2004.
12. Gallo JJ, Busby-Whitehead J, Rabins PV, Silliman, RA, Murphy JB. *Reichel's Care of the Elderly, Clinical Aspects of Aging.* 5th ed., Philadelphia: Lippincott Williams & Wilkins; 1999.
13. Helfand AE, Jessett DF. Foot problems. In: Pathy MSJ, Sinclair AJ, and Morley JR, eds. *Principles and Practice of Geriatric Medicine.* 4th ed. Chichester: John Wiley & Sons; 2006.
14. Helfand AE. Geriatric footwear. *Podiatr Manage.* 2000;20:103–108.
15. Helfand AE. Assessing the Older Diabetic Patient. Compact Disc. Pennsylvania Diabetes Academy, Pennsylvania Department of Health, Temple University, School of Medicine, Office for Continuing Medical Education, Temple University, School of Podiatric Medicine, Harrisburg PA, December, 2001.
16. Helfand AE. Foot problems. In: Mezzy MD, ed. *The Encyclopedia of Elder Care* New York: Springer; 2001:267–272.
17. Helfand AE. Podiatric medicine. In: Mezey MD, ed. *The Encyclopedia of Elder Care* New York: Springer; 2001:412–414.
18. Helfand AE. Disorders and diseases of the foot. In: Cobbs EL, Duthie ED, Murphy JB, eds. *Geriatric Review Syllabus, A Core Curriculum in Geriatric Medicine.* 6th ed. Malden MA: Blackwell Publishing; 2006.
19. Helfand AE. Clinical podogeriatrics: assessment, education, and prevention. *Clin Podiatr Med Surg.* 2003:20(3):540–541.
20. Helfand AE. Clinical assessment of podogeriatric patients. *Podiatr Manage.* 2004;23:145–152.
21. Helfand AE. Foot problems in older patients: a focused podogeriatric assessment study in ambulatory care. *J Am Podiatr Med Assoc.* 2004;94:293–304.
22. Helfand AE. *Public Health and Podiatric Medicine – Principles and Practice.* 2nd ed. Washington, DC: American Public Health Association; 2006.
23. Helfand AE. *Foot Health Training Guide for Long-Term Care Personnel.* Baltimore: Health Professions Press; 2007.
24. Levy LA, Hetherington VJ. *Principles and Practice of Geriatric Medicine.* 2nd ed. Brooklandville, MD: Data Trace Publishing Co; 2006.
25. Lorimer D, French G, O'Donnell M, Burrow JG. *Neale's Disorders of the Foot, Diagnosis and Management.* 6th ed. New York: Churchill Livingstone; 2002.
26. Merriman LM, Turner W. *Assessment of the Lower Limb.* 2nd ed. New York: Churchill Livingstone; 2002.
27. Robbins JM. *Primary Podiatric Medicine.* Philadelphia: W. B. Saunders; 1994.
28. Turner WA, Merriman LM. *Clinical Skills in Treating the Foot.* 2nd ed. Edinburgh: Churchill Livingstone; 2005.

33

GERIATRIC DERMATOLOGY

James Studdiford, MD, Brooke E. Salzman, MD, Amber Tully, MD

INTRODUCTION

Dermatological conditions are common among the elderly as the occurrence of many skin diseases increases with aging and cumulative environmental exposures, most notably, ultraviolet radiation (UVR). The prevalence of skin diseases rises steadily throughout life.[1] Various biological and physiological changes in the skin of older people account for an increased susceptibility to disease. In addition, many skin conditions observed more commonly in the elderly are the result of a higher prevalence of systemic diseases that affect skin such as diabetes, vascular insufficiency, and various neurological conditions. Furthermore, the increased incidence of some skin disorders in the elderly may be a consequence of reduced local skin care because of decreased mobility or functional impairment.[2]

Caring for skin conditions in the elderly requires an awareness of cutaneous changes associated with aging and chronic UVR exposure, as well as knowledge of common tumors, inflammatory diseases, and infections seen in older persons. As elderly persons represent the fastest growing segment of the population, providers will encounter dermatological conditions associated with aging more and more frequently. Because geriatric patients are living longer today than in the past, the likelihood of their developing skin conditions is substantial.[3] Moreover, the current cohort of aging individuals, namely the "baby boomers" are anticipated to present with increasing rates of many skin conditions including skin cancer, as they are believed to have had greater UVR exposure compared with prior generations without the early benefit of currently available sunscreens.[4]

This chapter first reviews the clinical and histological skin changes associated with aging, distinguishing between intrinsic aging and photoaging, and then discusses skin conditions and tumors that are commonly encountered by practitioners in primary care.

Aging Skin

Aging is a complex, multifactorial process, resulting in many changes in the skin that affect its function as well as appearance. Skin aging is generally broken down into two components, intrinsic aging and photoaging. Intrinsic aging refers to changes in skin over time alone, whereas photoaging describes skin changes attributable to chronic exposure to UVR. Distinguishing the two processes permits analysis of their relative contributions to the appearance of aged skin as well as the occurrence of dermatological disease; however, aged skin is the result of both processes superimposed on one another.

Intrinsic aging of skin is characterized by dryness, roughness, laxity, fine wrinkling, and skin atrophy.[5,6] There is also an increased incidence of neoplasms, both benign and malignant.[5,6] Age-related structural skin changes affect various components of skin and are summarized in Table 33.1. Losses in skin functions associated with such changes are listed in Table 33.2 and Table 33.3.

Epidermis

Age-related structural skin changes involve various components of skin including the epidermis, dermis, and subcutaneous tissue. Histologically, there is uniform flattening of the dermal–epidermal junction, with a reduced number of interdigitations, or rete ridges, between the dermis and epidermis. As a result, there is diminished contact between the two layers causing them to separate more easily, as manifested by the tendency of elderly skin to tear and the higher occurrence of blistering in older adults.[2,6]

The outer layer of the epidermis is the stratum corneum that helps provide a barrier between the internal and external world. With aging, the stratum corneum becomes more susceptible to damage and is slower to recover from such damage. Age-associated reductions in stratum corneum lipid

Table 33.1. Histological Features of Aging Skin

Epidermis	Dermis	Subcutaneous Tissue	Appendages
Flattened dermal–epidermal junction	Atrophy	Overall decrease	Decreased number of hair follicles
Fewer melanocytes	Fewer fibroblasts	Change in distribution	Loss of hair bulb melanocytes
Fewer Langerhans cells	Fewer and fragmented elastic fibers		Decreased number of sweat glands
Decreased keratinocyte proliferation	Fewer blood vessels		Abnormal nail plates
Reduced lipids	Less collagen		
Less filaggrin	Fewer mast cells		

Information from references,[6,7] and [14].

levels contribute to this increased susceptibility. Slower recovery from damage with aging is a consequence of decreased proliferation of epidermal cells, or keratinocytes. The epidermal turnover rate declines approximately 30%–50% between the third and eighth decades.[2,6] Clinically, this results in slower wound healing rates in aged skin. In addition, slower epidermal turnover rates can delay the clearance of substances that contact the epidermis.[7]

In aging skin, various cellular components of the epidermis decline, affecting skin appearance and function. For instance, there is a prominent decrease in the epidermal protein, filaggrin, which can cause elderly skin to appear dry and flaky, especially over the lower extremities.[2,6] Filaggrin is required for binding of keratin filaments into macrofibrils. Its relative deficiency in aged skin not only causes increased scaliness but may also affect the barrier function of skin.[2,6]

In addition, the number of active melanocytes per unit surface area of skin decreases by approximately 10%–20% per decade, reducing the body's protective barrier against UVR.[2,6,8] The number of melanocytic nevi also decreases progressively with age and are rarely observed in persons older than age 80 years.[8]

Furthermore, with aging, there is a 20%–50% reduction in the number of epidermal Langerhans cells, the immune cells responsible for antigen presentation.[2,6,9] This decrease in Langerhans cells contributes to the observed age-associated decline in cutaneous immune responsiveness. Variations in the production of interleukins and cytokines with aging also contribute the skin's declining immunological function.[9] The decreased immune responsiveness with aging results in an increased susceptibility to infections and an increased incidence of neoplasms.[9]

Additionally, vitamin D production is limited in the elderly, as the level of epidermal 7-dehydrocholesterol (the immediate biosynthetic precursor to vitamin D) per unit of skin surface area appears to decrease approximately 75% with aging.[6] This contributes to vitamin D deficiency in older adults along with other factors including insufficient dietary intake of vitamin D, insufficient sun exposure, and use of sunscreens.

Dermis

The dermis of aging skin decreases in thickness by approximately 20%, which is usually more pronounced in photodamaged skin.[6] In the dermis of elderly skin, there is a significant reduction in dermal vascularity and cellularity. The regression of vascular beds in aged skin is particularly noteworthy and is thought to underlie many of the physiological alterations in older skin, including decreases in temperature, thermoregulation, inflammatory response, absorption, wound healing, sweat response, and a subdued clinical presentation of many cutaneous diseases.[7] Basal and peak cutaneous blood flow is reduced by approximately 60%, which can be observed in the pallor of aged skin.[2,6]

The number of cells in the dermis including fibroblasts, macrophages, and mast cells decreases with aging. Reductions in mast cells with aging by approximately 50% account for the decreased incidence of urticaria in older adults.[6]

In the dermis of elderly skin, there are significant changes in the connective tissue stroma. The amount of dermal collagen and elastic fibers declines. Fibers also become fragmented, disorganized, and calcified. Such changes contribute to the laxity, loss of resilience, and finely wrinkled appearance of aged skin.[7]

Subcutaneous Fat

With aging, there are changes in the amount and distribution of subcutaneous fat. Subcutaneous fat protects the body from trauma and it plays a role in thermoregulation by limiting conductive heat loss. With aging, there is a relative decrease in subcutaneous fat on the face and hands, but a relative increase on the thighs and abdomen.[6] The overall volume of subcutaneous fat declines with age. The loss of this protective padding

Table 33.2. Functions of Skin that Decline with Age

Barrier function	Cell replacement
Wound healing	DNA repair
Elasticity	Vitamin D production
Inflammatory responsiveness	Thermoregulation
Immunological responsiveness	Sensory perception
Protection from UV light	Absorption
Chemical clearance	Mechanical protection
Sweat production	Sebum production

Information from references,[6,7] and [14].

results in increased susceptibility of pressure-prone surfaces as well as an increased risk of hypothermia.[7]

Appendages: Glands, Hair, and Nails

There is a reduction in the overall number of eccrine sweat glands in aged skin together with a decline in the functional capacity of the remaining glands.[6] Impairment of evaporative heat loss because of decreased sweating and attenuated dermal vasculature leads to an increased risk of heat stroke during hot weather. There is also a decline in apocrine gland size and function with age that is a consequence of the age-associated decrease in hormone levels.[6] This results in a decrease in body odor and, therefore, the need for antiperspirants and deodorants. Although sebaceous glands increase in size with aging, there is a decrease in sebum production, which may contribute to dry skin in older adults.

The rate of hair growth on the scalp declines with aging along with the diameter of individual terminal hairs. A greater percentage of hairs are in the telogen or resting stage. Graying of hairs occurs because of the progressive loss of functional melanocytes from the hair follicle bulb.[8] Hair substantially grays in approximately 50% of persons by age 50 years.[6,7] Not all hair shows a decrease of growth with aging. In older women, there is an increase in hair on the lip and chin. Older men may lose scalp and beard hair, but have an increased growth of hair over their ears, eyebrows, and nostrils.

The rate of nail growth declines by an average of 35% between the ages of 20 and 80 years.[7] Nails can become grossly thickened and distorted, which may indicate a fungal infection (onychomycosis). Because of the decrease in nail growth rates in the elderly, treatments for fungal diseases in the nail need to be longer. Nails in older individuals become more dry, brittle, and dull appearing. They also appear more flat or concave instead of convex. Longitudinal striations with ridging and beading often form on the nail plate.[6]

Photoaging

Photoaging, or dermatoheliosis, accounts for an overwhelming proportion of clinical changes in skin and remains the culprit for more than 90% of skin changes that people associate with "old" appearing skin as well as most skin cancers. Photoaging is the consequence of chronic exposure to UVR and therefore affects the sun-exposed areas of skin. The UV spectrums responsible for photodamage are UVA (320–400 nm) and UVB (290–320 nm) irradiation, as UVC (200–290 nm) radiation is generally blocked by the ozone layer.[10] Although UVB radiation primarily causes sunburn, suntanning, and photocarcinogenesis, UVA radiation also plays a large role in skin damage and photoaging.[2] UVA radiation is also responsible for most drug photosensitivity reactions, such as those observed in patients taking thiazide diuretics, tricyclic antidepressants, certain hypoglycemic agents, and antibiotics.[10]

Photoaged skin is characterized by fine and coarse wrinkling, roughness, dryness, laxity, dyspigmentation (mottled hyperpigmentation and brown macules), and telangiectases.[4,8] Photoaged skin loses its normal sheen and progressively develops a sallow, yellow hue. There is also an increased development of benign and malignant neoplasms on photoaged skin. Photoaged skin may be hypertrophic or atrophic, depending on the patient's complexion and the severity of sun damage. Cigarette smoking significantly exacerbates photoaging, and in particular, the severity of wrinkling.

Histologically, changes associated with photoaged skin include epidermal cell dysplasia and atypia, decreased number of Langerhans cells, irregular distribution of melanocytes, accumulation of abnormal elastic fibers, dilated and tortuous blood vessels, and a low-grade inflammatory dermal infiltrate.[2,4,6] Loss of immunological and inflammatory responsiveness is greater than that caused by intrinsic aging alone.

Strategies to prevent photodamage include sun avoidance, sun-protective clothing, and sunscreens. Because damage from photoaging is cumulative, preventive measures are of greatest benefit if started during childhood. Furthermore, there are indications that sun exposure during childhood may be particularly significant in the development of skin cancer in later life. Still, preventive measures can achieve substantial clinical improvement in older patients with already damaged skin. For instance, regular sunscreen use in older patients with photodamaged skin has been shown to decrease the frequency of new actinic keratoses, a common premalignancy of the skin, allow regression of established lesions, and reduce risk of developing squamous skin cancer.[10–13] There is, as yet, no convincing evidence that sunscreen use reduces the risk of basal cell skin cancer or melanoma.[13]

Sunscreens with a sun protection factor of greater than or equal to 15 should be applied on sun-exposed areas (Grade B);[13] however, use of high sun protection factor sunscreens should not lead individuals to extend the duration of sun exposure as skin damage can occur long before sunburn appears.[13] Patients should avoid sun exposure when UVR is strongest, which is around midday. Because sunscreens can also block UV-induced vitamin D formation in the skin, elderly patients should be advised to consume vitamin D–fortified products or supplements (Grade B).[2,6]

Table 33.3. Histological and Biological Features of Aging Skin with their Affect on Skin Function or Appearance

Histological or Biological Feature	Affect on Skin Function or Appearance
Flattened dermal–epidermal junction	Less contact between layers
	Skin tears more easily
	Greater tendency to blister
Reduced lipid levels in stratum corneum	Decline in barrier function of epidermis
Reduced keratinocyte proliferation/reduced cell turnover	Slower wound healing
	Decreased clearance of substances in contact with epidermis
Decreased filaggrin	Increased scaliness
	Decline in barrier function of epidermis
Reduced melanocytes	Reduced protection from UVR
Reduced Langerhans cells	Decreased immune responsiveness
	Increased susceptibility to infections and incidence of neoplasms
Reduced epidermal 7-dehydrocholesterol	Reduced vitamin D production
Reduced dermal vascularity	Decreases in temperature, thermoregulation, inflammatory response, absorption, wound healing, and sweat response
	Muted clinical presentation of disease
	Skin pallor
Reduced dermal fibroblasts	Reduced synthesis of extracellular matrix
Reduced mast cells	Decreased urticaria
Reduced dermal collagen	Skin laxity, loss of resilience, and wrinkles
Reduced elastin/disorganized elastin	Skin laxity, loss of resilience, and wrinkles
Reduced subcutaneous fat	Decrease in thermoregulation
	Increased risk of pressure sores

Information from references,[6,7] and [14].

Other agents have been found to benefit photoaged skin. Topical retinoid acid, also termed tretinoin, has been the most studied and commonly used. Topical retinoids have been shown both clinically and histologically to improve skin changes associated with photodamage (Grade A).[12,14] Clinical benefits include modest improvements in overall skin appearance, skin dyspigmentation, wrinkling, and roughness.[15–17] Several weeks of treatment are required before clinical improvement is appreciated. Patients should be warned that topical retinoids often cause a mild dermatitis associated with erythema, peeling, and stinging. Such irritation declines with continued use. Retinoid preparations can be applied less frequently (i.e., every other day or every few days) until tolerance improves.

Alpha-hydroxy acids (AHAs) have also been shown to benefit modestly photoaged skin. AHAs are compounds derived from dairy products (lactic acid), fruit (malic acid, citric acid), or sugar cane (glycolic acid). Topical treatment of photodamaged skin with AHAs has been reported to result in subtle clinical improvements in wrinkling, roughness, and hyperpigmentation (Grade B).[2,14,18]

Additionally, numerous oral and topically applied antioxidants have been investigated for their ability to prevent or reverse clinical signs associated with photoaging by modifying oxidative stress and free radical production (Grade C).[2] Examples of antioxidants include, but are not limited, to vitamin C (ascorbic acid), vitamin E (tocopherols), β-carotene, coenzyme Q_{10}, and α-lipoic acid.[14] More clinical trials are needed to substantiate their benefit. Other therapies for photoaged skin include various chemical peels, oral and topical hormonal therapy, topical application of growth factors and cytokines, collagen injections, injections with botulinum toxins, resurfacing techniques such as microdermabrasion and microablation, rhytidectomy (face-lift), and various forms of laser surgery.[4] Patients should be advised that the healing time for many skin procedures tends to be longer than that for younger adults.

BENIGN SKIN LESIONS

Benign proliferative skin lesions are very common among the elderly. These lesions form as early as the third decade of life and increase in number with age. Although most of these benign conditions do not require treatment, it is important for primary care physicians to be able to recognize these lesions and distinguish them from potentially malignant tumors.

Acrochordons

Acrochordons, commonly called skin tags, are flesh-colored or hyperpigmented 1–5 mm papules (Figure 33.1). These lesions are often pedunculated and occur most commonly in skin folds or areas subject to frequent friction, such as the neck, groin, axilla, or around the eyes.[19] Twenty-five percent of adults have at least one acrochordon, with the lesions occurring more commonly in the elderly, women, the obese, and persons with acromegaly.[20]

A skin biopsy of these lesions would reveal thinned epidermis and fibrous stroma with capillaries.[20] Skin tags tend to be asymptomatic but may become painful if torn, thrombosed, or irritated. They do not require removal unless they are painful or for cosmetic reasons.

Office removal is a simple procedure. If pedunculated, the lesion can be excised with minimal pain using sharp scissors and no anesthesia. Larger lesions can be removed in a similar fashion, after application of a local anesthetic, by electrocautery or cryosurgery. Histological confirmation is generally not

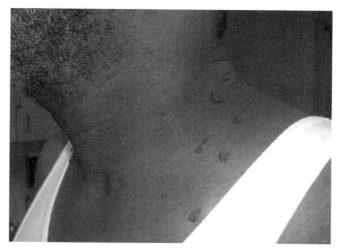

Figure 33.1. Acrochordons. Pedunculated, fleshy, benign, papules on the neck of this patient

necessary; however, in cases in which lesions around the eyelids resemble skin tumors such as seborrheic keratosis, melanocytic nevi, neurofibromas, or molluscum contagiosum, tissue confirmation should be obtained.[20]

Cherry Angiomas

Cherry angiomas, or hemangiomas, are smooth red to violaceous vascular papules ranging in size from 0.5 to –5.0 mm (Figure 33.2).[20] The lesions are primarily found on the trunk.

Figure 33.2. Cherry angioma. Symetrical erythematous benign vascular lesion found on this patient's trunk. See color plates.

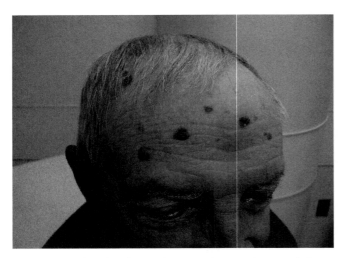

Figure 33.3. Seborrheic keratosis. Hyperpigmented, cratered plaque with a classic "stuck on" appearance on this patient's forehead. See color plates.

Cherry angiomas may begin to appear at age 30 years and increase in number with age. Differential diagnosis includes angiokeratoma, pyogenic granuloma, telangiectasias, nodular melanoma, and metastatic carcinoma.

Diagnosis is clinical and skin biopsy is seldom required. Histological examination will show dilated capillaries lined by flattened endothelial cells with edematous stroma. Reassurance remains the mainstay of treatment. If patients request removal for cosmetic reasons, cherry angiomas can be ablated using laser surgery, electrocautery, or simple excision. Lesions may be related to hormone production.[20] If rapid appearance of numerous lesions occurs, investigation for possible occult malignancy (particularly cancers such as pancreatic, gastric, or pulmonary) may be warranted.[20]

Keratoacanthomas

Keratoacanthomas (KAs) are rapidly growing, dome-shaped, red papules with central keratin-filled craters. They occur most commonly in Caucasian persons aged 50–70 years. These lesions appear on the face, neck, dorsal hands, and sun-damaged extremities. KAs develop quickly over 2–4 weeks and may be tender during their proliferative phase.

It can be difficult clinically to distinguish KAs from invasive squamous cell carcinoma. KAs are much faster growing than squamous cell carcinomas and will regress slowly over 6–12 months, if left untreated. Still, all lesions should be removed via excisional biopsy or shave biopsy and presumed cancerous until pathological composition is confirmed. Recurrent lesions proved benign may be treated with 5-flourouracil used topically or injected intralesionally.[21] Lesions usually resolve in approximately 6 weeks.

Human papilloma virus (HPV) has been identified as a possible cause of keratoacanthomas, but the etiology is still unknown. UVR and chemical exposures have also been implicated as possible risk factors for KA development.

Seborrheic keratoses

Seborrheic keratoses (SKs) are the most common benign epithelial tumors seen in the elderly population (Figure 33.3). The hyperpigmented, verrucous lesions have a characteristic "stuck-on" appearance. They begin as small brown macules, progress to a 1–3-mm papules or plaques, then to the larger 1–6-cm lesions. SKs can frequently occur as multiple lesions, are often hereditary, and usually spare the lips, palms, and soles. Lesions can be pink, white, brown, or black in color. The color may even vary within a single lesion, which may make them suspicious for melanoma.

SKs occurring in areas of friction may become inflamed and irritated. Lesions can be removed for cosmetic purposes or if symptomatic by curettage, cautery, or liquid nitrogen. Rarely, biopsy is indicated to rule out melanoma.

Solar Lentigines

Solar lentigines are well-circumscribed 1–3-cm brown macules that occur as a result of localized proliferation of melanocytes caused by chronic sun exposure (Figure 33.4).[21] These benign lesions are common in Caucasian persons older than 40 years and are seen on the forehead, cheeks, nose, dorsa of the hands, forearms, upper back, chest, and shins.

Differential diagnosis includes café-au-lait macule, early seborrheic keratosis, solar-pigmented actinic keratosis, and lentigo maligna. Skin biopsy reveals irregular elongation of the rete ridges, basal layer keratinocyte hyperpigmentation, and a large number of junctional melanocytes.[20] Clinical appearance and history of chronic sun exposure make the diagnosis. Lentigines with discrete areas of hyperpigmentation, hypopigmentation, thickening, or with irregular borders should undergo biopsy. Avoidance of sun or the use of sunscreens best prevents these lesions. No treatment is indicated, but patients with multiple solar lentigines should have close surveillance for skin cancer. If patients desire removal for cosmetic reasons, azelaic acid, glycolic peels, or hydroquinone solutions may be applied topically for several weeks to reduce hyperpigmentation.[20]

INFLAMMATORY SKIN CONDITIONS

Pruritus and Xerosis

Pruritus and xerosis are the two most common skin complaints among the elderly.[22] Both of these conditions occur in 50%–75% of people older than age of 65 years and are the cause of multiple physician visits each year.[22] Pruritus may be caused by xerosis, inflammatory skin conditions, or medication side effects. Occasionally, pruritus may occur in the absence of skin findings. Psychological stressors, anxiety, and depression may also be associated with pruritus. Patients should be asked about environmental exposures and situational stressors that may trigger itching. Certain systemic diseases such as renal impairment, liver disease, anemia, thyroid

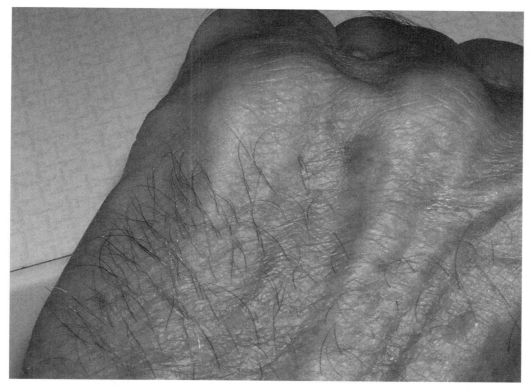

Figure 33.4. Solar lentigo. Localized proliferation of melanocytes caused by chronic sun exposure, expressed as a circumscribed brown macule on the dorsal surface of the hand. See color plates.

disease, and lymphoma may cause itching and should be considered.[19]

The scratch–itch cycle can lead to excoriations, infection, trauma, and lichenification of the skin. Underlying skin disease and/or infection should be identified before symptomatic treatment for pruritus is initiated. Emollients, calamine lotion, oatmeal baths, milk baths, and chamomile preparations have all been reported to give relief in various types of pruritus.[22]

Xerosis is a common skin finding in the aging population. The stratum corneum has increased transepidermal water loss as the skin ages, leading to decreased moisture and lipid biosynthesis.[22] Excessive bathing, the use of strong detergents or soaps, alcohol-based bathing products, and 3-hydroxy-3-methyl-glutaryl-Coenzyme A reductase inhibitors may exacerbate dry skin.[6] Dry skin may become easily irritated and pruritic, leading to inflammatory skin conditions. Xerosis is treated by hydrating skin with moisturizers and avoiding environmental insult.

Asteatotic Eczema

Asteatotic eczema (or dermatitis) is a common superficial inflammatory disease of the skin. Although most atopic skin diseases begin during childhood, eczema can occur in older patients with no history of skin disease.[23] Atrophy of sebaceous glands with decreased sebaceous production, decreased free fatty acids in the stratum corneum, and decreased water storage in the skin predisposes the elderly skin to drying and thinning.

Affected skin areas are dry, pruritic, and erythematous with overlying excoriation, crusting, scaling, and lichenification. Legs, arms, and hands are most frequently affected. Flares tend to be worse during winter months when elderly individuals spend lots of time in low-humidity heated homes. The disease may also be exacerbated by use of diuretics and antiandrogen medications.

Aging of the skin may lead to more widespread eruption of eczematous lesions. Eczema is a disease characterized by flares and remissions. As such, the therapeutic approach must be tailored to the state of disease (Table 33.4).[24] The first step is to identify and eliminate offending agents, such as dry air, strong soaps, mechanical abrasions, irritants, and chemicals. Over-the-counter petrolatum-based emollients or prescription strength lactic acid are recommended to help hydrate the skin and remove scales. These must be applied frequently and liberally. Topical steroids should be used with caution, given the elderly are predisposed to fragile skin and easy bruising. Oral steroids and antihistamines are reserved for severe cases because of their side-effect profile and potential interaction with many medications. Other therapies include UV light therapy, azathioprine, cyclosporine, tacrolimus, and low-dose methotrexate (Grade B).[23]

Table 33.4. Treatment Options for Asteatotic Eczema[16]

Treatment	Use	Benefit	Potential Side Effects*
Emollients: Eucerin Cream Aveeno Lotion	First-line use for mild eczema and adjunctive therapy with other treatment	Decreased dryness and itching, reducing penetration of skin by irritants	Mild burning with application, residue on skin
Topical Steroids See Table 33.5	First-line for moderate-to-severe eczema; use only low-potency steroid on the face, neck, and intertriginous areas; use steroids only in bursts of 1 or 2 wks	Reduced itching, inflammation, and length of outbreak	Local effects: irreversible skin thinning, striae, telangiectasias Systemic effects: Cushing's syndrome, suppression of hypothalamic-pituitary-adrenal axis
Oral Steroids	Reserved for severe flares	Decreased itching, erythema, and infiltration	Increased appetite, psychosis, dyspepsia, hypertension, osteoporosis, adrenal suppression, Cushing's syndrome
Antihistamines	Adjunctive therapy for symptom relief	Improvements in itching and sleep	Drowsiness, anticholinergic toxicity, photosensitivity, tinnitus
Tacrolimus	Moderate-to-severe eczema unresponsive to topical steroids	Reduced itching, inflammation, and improved skin appearance	Skin burning with application, may cause photosensitivity, long-term safety unknown

* Most common side effects listed.

Bullous Pemphigoid

The loss of dermal–epidermal adhesion in the elderly predisposes them to blistering disorders. Bullous pemphigoid is an autoimmune blistering disease primarily occurring in patients older than 60 years. Autoantibody interaction with bullous pemphigoid antigen at the basal surface of keratinocytes causes blisters to form.[6] Prodromal symptoms of pruritus accompanied by urticarial lesions, erythema, and small plaques may precede the bullae by several weeks. Plaques turn red and bullae appear on their surface. The large tense blisters contain clear or hemorrhagic exudates. The bullae are firm and have a negative Nikolsky sign (they do not extend into normal skin with firm pressure), which distinguishes bullous pemphigoid from the rare pemphigus vulgaris. Lesions commonly occur on the abdomen, groin, and flexor surfaces and rarely involve the mucous membranes. The bullae are often clustered but may present in different stages.[25] The lesions may remain intact for a week before rupturing. Healed lesions often result in hyperpigmented postinflammatory skin changes.

Diagnosis is made based on clinical presentation, but confirmatory skin biopsy is recommended. Biopsy will reveal subepidermal bulla with eosinophilic infiltrates within the dermis. Immunofluorescence demonstrates immunoglobulin G and compliment C3 deposition within the basement membrane.[20]

Untreated bullous lesions may regress spontaneously or rapidly spread. Bullous pemphigoid is a chronic disease characterized by exacerbations and remissions. Pruritus associated with the blisters can be treated with nonsedating antihistamines. Localized disease may be treated with topical class I steroids twice daily until 2 weeks after lesions have healed. Systemic prednisone, 40–60 mg/day, may be needed in addition to topical therapy in more severe cases (Grade B).[26] Oral steroids should be slowly tapered after all lesions have cleared. Steroids should always be used with caution in the elderly because these patients are at high risk of corticosteroid-associated complications including diabetes, gastrointestinal bleeding, hypertension, osteoporosis, immunosuppression, and psychosis.

Recently, the use of dapsone, alone or as adjuvant therapy with antiinflammatory agents has been reported to be effective in producing remission in a dose ranging between 100 and 200 mg daily (Grade C).[26] Other agents with antiinflammatory properties that have been used are minocycline or tetracycline with nicotinamide. If dapsone and prednisone fail, immunosuppressive agents such as azathioprine, methotrexate, chlorambucil, cyclosporine, cyclophosphamide, and mycophenolate mofetil may be necessary. Methotrexate at a dose of 5–10 mg/wk has been used as an efficacious steroid-sparing agent in the elderly population with bullous pemphigoid (Grade C).[27] It has been reported that intravenous immunoglobulin therapy induced a long-term clinical remission in patients who had refractory bullous pemphigoid (Grade C).[26] The clinical course of bullous pemphigoid varies dramatically. The 1-year mortality rate of 19% is primarily because of treatment complications such as prolonged immunosuppression associated with steroid treatment or secondary systemic infection.[20] It is important to institute timely diagnosis and treatment of this disorder to improve the patient's chance for remission. Treatment side effects must also be closely monitored.

Lichen Simplex Chronicus

Lichen simplex chronicus is localized plaque formation secondary to repeated scratching or rubbing of the skin (Figure 33.5). The lesions tend to be violaceous to erythematous and scaly with prominent skin lines. The lower legs,

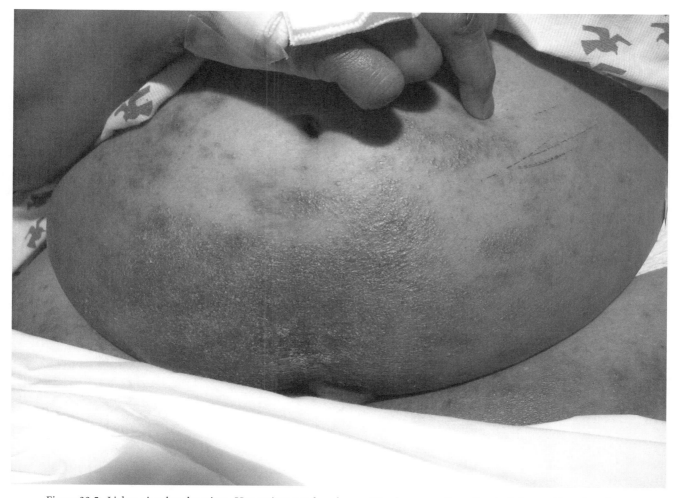

Figure 33.5. Lichen simplex chronicus. Hyperpigmented, scaly, pruritic plaques on the patient's abdomen. See color plates.

wrists, ankles, posterior scalp, and folds behind the ears are most commonly affected. The plaques tend to stabilize over time with little change in color or size.

Tinea infections may resemble lichen simplex chronicus and potassium hydroxide scraping should be done to rule out infection if there is strong clinical suspicion. Treatment first begins with helping the patient to stop scratching or rubbing the affected area. Topical or intralesional steroids can be used in addition to antihistamines to control the symptoms. Tar preparations and phototherapy have been used if other treatment options fail. Anxiety and stress play a large role in aggravating this condition. Reducing stressors or precipitating factors can ameliorate this condition.

Psoriasis

Psoriasis is a chronic papulosquamous disease resulting in sharply demarcated erythematous plaques covered by an adherent silvery scale (Figure 33.6). If the scale is removed, punctate bleeding points are revealed, known as Auspitz sign. Fewer than 3% of persons with psoriasis develop the disease after the age of 60, and many patients with the disease have improvement of

symptoms as they age because of the decreased mitotic potential of the skin cells.[6] The cause of this disorder is not well understood, but abnormal T-lymphocyte function has been implicated.

Plaque psoriasis is the most common type and is characterized by patches on the scalp, trunk, and limbs and may be worse in areas of physical trauma (Köbner phenomenon), such as the belt line. Guttate psoriasis is characterized by small red dots on the trunk that frequently appear after an upper respiratory infection, particularly streptococcal pharyngitis. These lesions tend to resolve with antistreptococcal antibiotic therapy. Nail psoriasis may cause pits in the nails, which may become yellow and thickened, eventually leading to onycholysis.

Psoriatic arthritis affects approximately 5% of those with skin symptoms.[20] It is a monoarticular seronegative arthritis most commonly affecting the distal interphalangeal, knee, and foot joints. Treatment of the skin condition often results in improvement of the arthritis.

The diagnosis of psoriasis is usually clinical but punch biopsy may be performed to confirm diagnosis. Tests for rheumatoid factor and erythrocyte sedimentation rate are usually normal. Uric acid levels may be elevated in psoriasis,

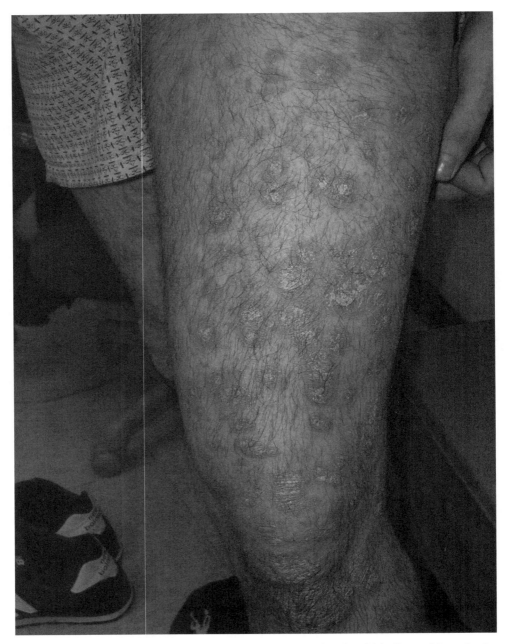

Figure 33.6. Psoriasis. Inflamed, edematous skin lesions covered with a thick silvery white scale. See color plates.

causing confusion with gout. Treatment includes topical tar preparations, topical corticosteroids, and topical retinoids. For recalcitrant cases and cases involving more than 20% of body surface, phototherapy with UVB or photochemotherapy UVA, and cytotoxic agents such as methotrexate and cyclosporine may be used (Grade C).[28]

Rosacea

Rosacea is a chronic inflammatory disorder characterized by erythema, telangiectasias, papules, and pustules erupting on the cheeks, forehead, and nose. This disorder usually presents between the fourth and sixth decade of life and is more common in women. Rosacea can be exacerbated by stress, hormonal fluctuations, spicy foods, alcohol, and sunlight.

There are four subtypes of rosacea, which help guide treatment options. Subtype one is characterized by mild facial erythema. These patients may respond to topical metronidazole or azelaic acid.[29] Breneman et al[30] compared the efficacy of once-daily use of metronidazole 1% cream with placebo and demonstrated significant reductions in inflammatory lesions at 4 weeks in the group using metronidazole (Grade B). In patients who do not respond to metronidazole, vascular laser or intense pulse light can be used. In subtype two, patients have

Table 33.5. Topical Steroid Preparations

Potency	Steroid Preparation	Strength
Very high	Clobetasol propionate	Cream or ointment 0.05%
	Halobetasol propionate	Cream or ointment 0.05%
High	Betamethasone dipropionate	Cream or ointment 0.05%
	Betamethasone valerate	Ointment 0.1%
	Fluocinolone acetonide	Cream 0.2%
	Halcinonide	Cream or ointment 0.1%
Medium	Betamethasone valerate	Cream 0.1%
	Fluocinolone acetonide	Cream or ointment 0.025%
	Hydrocortisone valerate	Cream or ointment 0.2%
	Triamcinolone acetonide	Cream, ointment, or lotion 0.1% or 0.025%
Low	Hydrocortisone	Cream, ointment, lotion 1%–2.5%

papules and pustules in addition to erythema. Treatment with a combination of topical and systemic antibiotics is indicated.[31] In subtype three severe irreversible thickening of the skin and nose (rhinophyma) occurs. This is more common in men. Treatment is with systemic antibiotics combined with ablative lasers. Patients with subtype four have ocular symptoms of conjunctivitis, eye pain, blepharitis and/or increased lacrimation. These patients should be treated with systemic antibiotics and artificial tears, and they should be referred to an ophthalmologist.

Seborrheic Dermatitis

Seborrheic dermatitis is a common chronic dermatosis characterized by erythema and scaling of the scalp, central face, and/or anterior chest. Lesions are yellow and greasy, forming coalescing patches or plaques. They tend to flare in areas where the sebaceous glands are most active.

The exact etiology of seborrheic dermatitis is unknown, but the yeast species, *Malassezia*, has been correlated with outbreaks of lesions.[32] The elderly tend to have flares of disease related to stress, sleep deprivation, fatigue, and climate changes. Diagnosis can be made based on clinical appearance. Differential diagnosis includes psoriasis, rosacea, tinea infection, atopic dermatitis, and candidiasis.[32]

Seborrheic dermatitis of the scalp can be treated with topical steroids (Grade C).[32] Antidandruff shampoos containing ketoconazole, ciclopirox, selenium sulfide, salicylic acid, coal tar, or zinc pyrithione used daily and left on for several minutes improve success of treatment and decrease recurrence (Grade B).[31] Facial breakouts can be treated with topical calcineurin inhibitors, tacrolimus ointment, or pimecrolimus cream (Grade B).[32] Recalcitrant facial breakouts can be treated with once-daily ketoconazole in addition to once-daily desonide,

for a 2-week period (Grade B).[32] Oral antifungal medications are rarely indicated.

Stasis Dermatitis

Stasis dermatitis is an inflammatory condition that occurs secondary to venous stasis from vascular insufficiency (Figure 33.7). Fifteen to 20 million people older than the age of 50 years are thought to be affected by stasis dermatitis.[33] As blood vessels age there is decreased competence of valves resulting in pooling of the blood in the lower extremities leading to edema, varicose veins, and hyperpigmentation.

Stasis dermatitis is an eczematous dermatitis commonly affecting the lower legs and ankles. The skin appears erythematous, hyperpigmented, scaly, and fissured. Pruritus and itching can lead to excoriated skin that is prone to infection and ulcer formation. Severe exudative inflammation should be treated with a wet dressing applied for 10–20 minutes twice daily.[20] Topical antibiotic ointment can be used to treat superficial open lesions, and oral antibiotics are reserved for more severe infections. Short term use of topical corticosteroids will help relieve pruritus. Alleviation of dryness is critical in maintaining skin integrity, which can be achieved by using petrolatum-based emollients applied twice daily. After an acute flare is treated, frequent elevation of the legs and use of compression stockings are the mainstays of therapy.

INFECTIOUS SKIN CONDITIONS

Cellulitis

Cellulitis is an acute, expanding, suppurative skin infection that involves the dermis and subcutaneous tissue (Figure 33.8). The most common causative agents are group A *Streptococcus* and *Staphylococcus aureus* (*S. aureus*). Erysipelas, on the other hand, is a more superficial form of cellulitis, with prominent raised borders and a distinct lymphatic involvement, which is often referred to as "peau d'orange." The etiology is almost always group A *Streptococcus*.

The timely diagnosis of cellulitis is based on the recognition of the distinctive clinical pattern, which is described as spreading, hot, red and painful. The location is often in proximity to an ulcer, eczematoid dermatitis or an interdigital erosion secondary to tinea pedis.[34] Cellulitis also commonly involves an edematous limb, secondary to compromise of either the lymphatic or venous circulation. The postmastectomy patient who has lymphedema secondary to axillary node dissection and radiation is at greater risk of ipsilateral upper extremity cellulitis (Grade B).[35] Likewise, coronary artery grafting procedures requiring saphenous venectomy put the cardiac patient at significant risk for recurrent leg cellulitis (Grade B).[36]

More direct precipitants of cellulitis include animal or human bites, intravenous catheters, intravenous drug abuse, and exposure to freshwater (*Aeromonas hydrophila*) seawater (*Vibrio vulnificus*) pathogens. Older individuals with cirrhosis are especially prone to the latter organism.[37] Certain patients

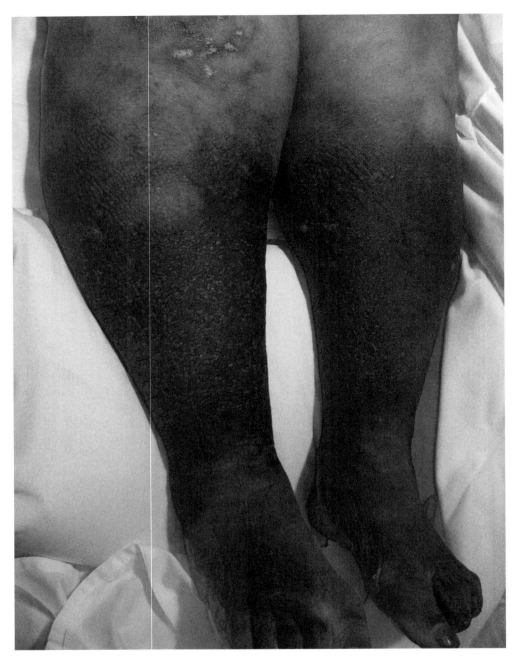

Figure 33.7. Stasis dermatitis. Hyperpigmented, thickened, edematous skin and subcutaneous tissue bilaterally on this patient's lower extremities. See color plates.

are especially prone to cellulitis secondary to pneumococ-cal bacteremia including immunocompromised patients with diabetes mellitus, alcoholism, systemic lupus erythematosus, nephrotic syndrome, or dermatological cancers as well as those who have undergone splenectomy. Thus blood cultures should be promptly drawn in such patients if cellulitis develops.[38] At the time of initial examination, the clinician should exam-ine for crepitant cellulitis, indicating a gas-forming organism (clostridia, bacteroides, or peptostreptococci) as well as exten-sive necrosis associated with gangrenous cellulitis (possibly

indicating mucormycosis in immunocompromised patients). These last two conditions should prompt early radiological examination and surgical consultation.

The history provided by the geriatric patient with cel-lulitis generally includes a prodrome of malaise, fever, and chills followed by the development of a red, hot, edematous, poorly demarcated area, most commonly located on the lower extremity. The clinician should be aware of atypical presenta-tions in the elderly including delirium, anorexia, or lethargy. Additional inquiry should focus on prior episodes of cellulitis

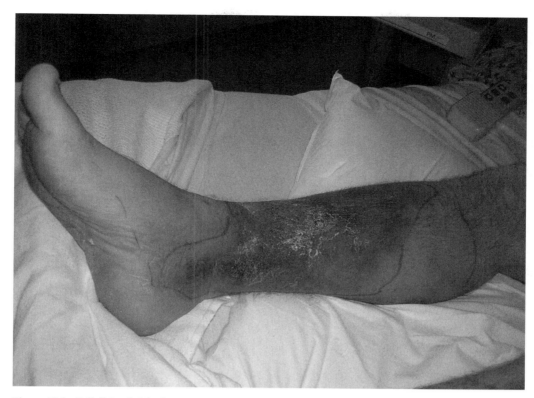

Figure 33.8. Cellulitis of right lower extremity. Erythematous, hyperpigmented, edematous, tender, warm pretibial skin in a patient with venous insufficiency. Pen lines indicate original and current border of infection. See color plates.

with progressive venous insufficiency and lymphedema exacerbated by dependency, paraplegia, or congestive heart failure. A concerning history of pain out of proportion to the extent of the cellulitis in a toxic patient should sound the alarm for possible necrotizing fasciitis.[39] This clinical presentation requires prompt surgical consultation for emergency fasciotomy.[40]

The physical examination should focus on stability of the vital signs and establishment of the perimeter of the cellulitis by tracing it with a magic marker (Figure 33.8). A portal of entry should be sought by inspecting for a "weeping" dermatitis, an abrasion, an ulcer, or interdigital tinea pedis. The clinician should also examine for associated conditions such as deep vein thrombosis and local abscesses. Culture of the latter is especially important to establish the presence of a specific bacterial etiology such as methicillin-resistant *S. aureus* (MRSA), which may require additional antibiotic treatment. It is also important in the elderly patient to expand the differential diagnosis to include gout, fixed drug eruption, giant urticaria, erythema nodosum, and erythema migrans (Lyme borreliosis).[41]

The treatment of cellulitis is often empiric because of the difficulty in establishing the microbiological etiology (see Table 33.6). Attempts at culturing infected skin with needle aspirations or punch biopsies of the advancing border of cellulitis have not proven helpful for determining the etiology. For instance, the former technique yields a likely pathogen in only 29% of cases, whereas the latter is positive in approximately 33% of the cases (Grade D).[42,43]

Bacteremia occurs infrequently in patients with cellulitis. In a study involving 272 patients, blood cultures were positive in only 4%.[44] Of the positive isolates, group A *Streptococcus* and *S. aureus* together comprised 66%.

In addition to microbiological studies for cellulitis, the following radiological investigations may be indicated: plain x-rays (rule out gas formation or foreign bodies), ultrasound (to demonstrate local collections of drainable pus), Doppler studies (to rule out deep vein thrombosis), and magnetic resonance imaging (to establish the diagnosis of necrotizing fasciitis or osteomyelitis).

The majority of older patients with community-acquired cellulitis are treated with empiric antibiotic therapy to provide coverage against *Streptococcus* and *S. aureus*. Outpatient therapy is generally sufficient for mild, uncomplicated cases. Hospitalization for intravenous antibiotics is recommended for patients with severe cellulitis as manifested by fever, rapidly spreading lesions, and significant comorbidities such as major organ failure, immunocompromise, or asplenia. Antibiotic treatments are summarized in Table 33.4.[45,46]

The outpatient treatment of MRSA skin infection is generally surgical with incision and drainage of the associated furuncle or abscess whenever possible. For lesions less than 5 cm in size this is usually all that is necessary; however, larger lesions with associated cellulitis often require hospitalization for more extensive surgical drainage and intravenous antibiotic therapy. Table 33.4 lists inpatient and outpatient antibiotic therapies

Table 33.6. Antibiotic Treatments for Cellulitis

Cellulitus	Location and Type of Treatment	Antibiotic	Dose	Duration of Treatment	Strength of Recommendation
Uncomplicated	Outpatient, oral	Cephalexin	500 mg q 6 h	5–10 day	Grade B[45]
		Dicloxacillin	500 mg q 6 h		
		Augmentin	500/125 mg tid		
		Azithromycin	500 mg initial dose, then 250 mg q day		
	Inpatient, IV	Penicillin G	1–2 million unit q 6 h	With clinical improvement, can switch to oral	Grade B[45]
		Cephazolin	1.0 g q 8 h		Grade B[46,47]
		Nafcillin	2.0 g q 4 h		
		PCN allergic			
		Vancomycin	1.0 g q 12 h		
		Linezolid	600 mg q12 h		
MRSA	Outpatient	Clindamycin	300 mg q 6 h	5–10 day	Grade B[45]
		Bactrim	2 DS tabs bid		
		Doxycycline	100 mg bid		
		Linezolid	600 mg bid		
	Inpatient	Vancomycin	1.0 g q 12 h	With clinical improvement, can switch to oral	Grade B[46,47]
		Linezolid	600 mg q 12 h		
Prophylaxis for recurrent cellulitis	Outpatient	Penicillin G	250 mg bid	Several months	Grade C[49]
		Erythromycin	250 mg bid		

for MRSA.[45,46] Regarding linezolid, it is important to note that its use is limited because of expense and hematological toxicities.[47]

The diabetic patient with cellulitis complicated by foot ulcer deserves special attention. This entity is generally associated with long-standing sensory neuropathy followed by excessive, unappreciated trauma. It is often complicated by peripheral arterial insufficiency. Additional assessment of deep ulcers for associated osteomyelitis or abscess should be considered. Multiple pathogens, including MRSA, aerobic Gram-negative bacilli and anaerobes necessitate broad spectrum antibiotic coverage (ampicillin/sulbactam, imipenem-cilastatin, or meropenem).[48] Adjunctive treatment considerations should include debridement of the ulcer, relief of pressure-related trauma, and peripheral vascular evaluation.

In addition to antibiotics, the comprehensive care of the geriatric patient with cellulitis includes cool saline compresses, elevation of the affected limb, and immobilization. It is also standard care to document regression of the perimeter of the cellulitis, resolution of the fever, and the presence or absence of any local collection of pus. Any dermal port of entry should be identified and treated accordingly. This would include the use of antifungals for interdigital tinea pedis, topical steroids for the patient with eczema, and compression stockings or Unna boots for patients with venous insufficiency. Long-term prophylactic antibiotic treatment for recurrent episodes of cellulitis in the

same anatomical location has been successful in some cases (Table 33.4).[49]

In summary, cellulitis in the geriatric population requires prompt evaluation and detailed decision making. Grampositive organisms, *S. aureus,* and *Streptococcus* spp. are the most common offenders. Antibiotic therapy is most often selected on an empiric basis. The diabetic patient with a foot ulcer mandates special attention to establish a microbiological diagnosis and rule out osteomyelitis. The warning signs for gas gangrene and necrotizing fasciitis should be sought in severely ill patients. Portals of entry should be routinely identified and treated. Chronic venous insufficiency and lymphedema of an extremity can be mechanically reduced using elevation, support stockings, and compression sleeves. Long-term antibiotic therapy is a consideration for recurrent bouts of cellulitis.

Herpes Zoster

Herpes zoster, or shingles, is a reactivation of the varicella zoster virus (VZV) and is characterized by an acute vesicular eruption occurring in a dermatomal distribution (Figure 33.9). It most commonly resides in the sensory dorsal root ganglion following the primary VZV infection, chickenpox. Zoster is most often an illness of older adults, and is associated with a waning of cell-mediated immunity.[50] The latter parallels the aging process and becomes progressively diminished in adults older than

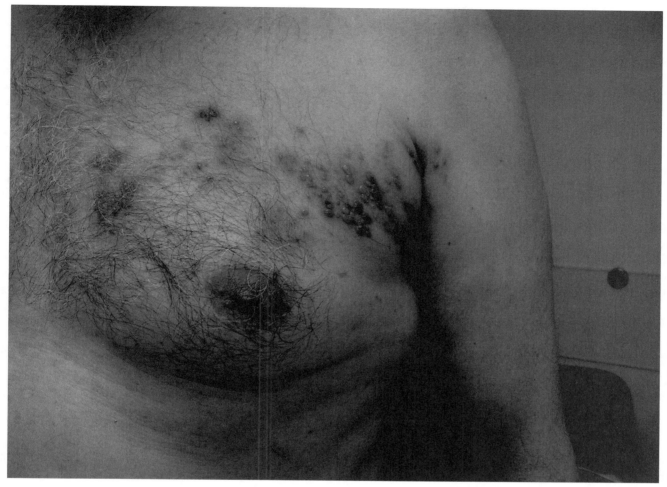

Figure 33.9. Herpes zoster of the left T2 and T3 dermatomes. Groups and clusters of vesicles on an erythematous, edematous base. See color plates.

60 years. In predisposed persons zoster may be triggered by electrocautery, trauma, corticosteroids, local irradiation, and surgery (especially neurosurgery).[51,52]

The cumulative lifetime incidence of herpes zoster in the United States is 10%–20% of the population; the highest incidence is found in the elderly group.[50,53] A second episode will be experienced by 4% of the population.[54] In the course of 1 year, a family physician will diagnose four cases of herpes zoster, and over a 3-year span will see at least one case of postherpetic neuralgia (PHN).[55]

The natural history of herpes zoster includes a prodrome, an acute phase, and occasionally a chronic pain syndrome (PHN). The prodrome is heralded by several days of malaise, fever, and stabbing pain in the dermatomal distribution. The thoracic and lumbar areas are most commonly involved. During the acute phase, grouped vesicles or bullae appear in a dermatomal pattern, which may become hemorrhagic or pustular over the next 3–5 days. The lesions gradually crust over by 7–10 days as infectiousness diminishes. In most cases complete resolution takes place over 3–4 weeks. If the acute episode does not resolve then PHN develops, which is a burning, neuropathic pain or

allodynia (dysesthesia after light touch over the affected dermatome). Most experts temporally define PHN as pain that persists for longer than 1 month after the resolution of the rash. This may occur in 10%–15% of patients. Those older than age 60 years comprise 50% of patients with PHN.[56,57]

Extracutaneous complications of zoster include PHN (7.9%), bacterial superinfection (2.3%), ocular complications (1.6%), motor neuropathy (0.9%), meningitis (0.5%), and herpes oticus (0.2%).[58] The ominous occurrence of herpes zoster ophthalmicus stems from reactivation of latent virus in the trigeminal ganglion involving the V1 dermatome. Involvement of the frontal branch can result in ocular complications (corneal ulcers, keratitis, scleritis, uveitis, neuritis, and glaucoma) in 50%–72% of patients.[59] The clinician should look for Hutchinson sign, papules, or vesicles on the tip and side of the nose, which involves the dermatome supplied by the nasociliary branch of the ophthalmic nerve and portends corneal involvement in 75% of cases.[60] Early initiation of antiviral therapy can be sight saving.[61] Another ominous cranial neuropathy that can result in deafness, the Ramsay–Hunt syndrome (Herpes Zoster Oticus), is marked by the triad of ear pain, ipsilateral facial paralysis, and vesicles in the area of the auditory meatus.[62]

The differential diagnosis of herpes zoster in the prodromal phase, which is characterized by severe pain without rash, can be confusing. Depending on the dermatome, possibilities include acute entities in diverse organ systems such as cardiac, central nervous system, or pleural disease. The multiple etiologies of an acute abdomen must also be considered. The eruption of zoster itself must be distinguished from other herpetic infections, allergic contact dermatitis, insect bites, burns, and other skin infections.

The diagnosis of zoster in the older patient is generally based on the characteristic appearance of the vesicular lesion in a dermatomal distribution in the setting of antecedent prodromal pain. In questionable cases, a Tzanck smear utilizing Wright stain looking for multinucleated giant cells is often useful. A viral culture to distinguish VZV from herpes simplex can be performed but these are costly and technically difficult. A more sensitive test is the direct immunofluorescence assay that distinguishes VZV from herpes simplex (Grade B).[63]

Prompt antiviral treatment of herpes zoster in the elderly patient promotes rapid healing of lesions, diminishes severity and extent of acute pain, and lessens complications, especially PHN. Treatment should be initiated within 72 hours of the onset of the vesicular dermatomal eruption. Late exceptions to this timeframe can be made for those at increased risk of PHN who still show signs of ongoing vesicle formation even after 72 hours.

Acyclovir (ACV) has been shown to be effective in randomized controlled trials (RCTs) in a dosage of 800 mg five times daily.[64] In patients older than 50 years, ACV proved more effective than placebo both in terms of reducing the acute pain and diminishing PHN by 46% after 6 months (Grade A).[65,66]

Valacyclovir (which is converted in vivo to ACV) has three to five times the bioavailability of ACV. The simpler dosing schedule (1 g three times daily) allows for improved compliance. In a clinical trial involving patients older than 50 years of age with acute herpes zoster, valacyclovir was superior to ACV in terms of resolution of the acute pain (38 days vs. 51 days for the ACV group) and reduction of the duration of PHN at 6 months (19% vs. 26% for the ACV group) (Grade A).[67]

Famciclovir (500 mg three times daily) has proved superiority over placebo in an RCT of patients who were age 50 years or older. The rate of healing of acute lesions was accelerated and the duration of PHN (63 vs. 163 days on placebo) was reduced in the famciclovir recipients (Grade A).[68]

All three antiviral agents are beneficial in the outpatient treatment of herpes zoster in the older population. Ease of administration and improved pharmacokinetics favor valacyclovir and famciclovir over ACV. There are indications for intravenous administration of ACV (10 mg/kg, three times daily for 7 days) for critically ill patients with ophthalmic zoster, disseminated zoster, transplant recipients, and patients with advanced acquired immunodeficiency syndrome. Although these drugs are safe and well tolerated, dose adjustments must be made if the creatinine clearance falls below 60 mL/min, which often occurs in the elderly patient.[69]

Corticosteroid therapy, combined with ACV, has been studied in two RCTs for the treatment of acute zoster.[70,71] Statistically significant benefit was demonstrated in the reduction of acute pain and the rate of healing of acute lesions in the group receiving the combination therapy;[71] however, there was no difference in PHN at 6 months. The authors noted that corticosteroid therapy is contraindicated in patients at risk for steroid toxicity (diabetes mellitus, glaucoma, hypertension, and gastritis). Therefore, consideration for corticosteroids in combination with antiviral therapy should be reserved for the reduction of the intensity and duration of pain in the acute phase only (Grade C).[71]

PHN is especially problematic for the elderly patient with a reported incidence as high as 43% in some populations older than 50 years.[72] It is known that the timely administration of antivirals during the acute phase of herpes zoster does reduce the duration of PHN. Other therapeutic approaches including antivirals combined with tricyclics or anticonvulsants administered early in the acute phase have been unsuccessful and are not recommended (Grade D).[73,74] Evidence-based treatment is lacking for PHN of less than 6 months duration, which in most cases resolves spontaneously.[75] For PHN extending beyond this 6-month timeframe a practice parameter, written by the American Academy of Neurology, endorses tricyclic antidepressants, gabapentin, pregabalin, opioids, and lidocaine patches, as treatments that are more effective than placebo (Grade B).[76] A second earlier systematic review made similar recommendations and also included intrathecal steroid therapy as a consideration for severe refractory cases (Grade B).[77]

The most optimistic development in the last few years has been the pioneering and testing of a zoster vaccine (Oka/Merck VZV vaccine), which has been shown to reduce both the incidence of acute zoster and postherpetic complications in the elderly population.[75] This vaccine is designed to boost the cell-mediated immunity for VZV in the seropositive elderly patient population. The Shingles Prevention Study Group, as reported by Oxman and colleagues, conducted a nationwide 3-year RCT to study the effectiveness of the vaccine among 38,000 men and women who were 60 years of age or older. After a 3-year follow-up the incidence of herpes zoster and PHN was reduced in the vaccinated group by 50% and 67%, respectively (Grade A).[75] The Food and Drug Administration recently approved the vaccine, Zostavax (Merck), which is intended for use in immunocompetent patients older than 60 years to reduce the incidence of herpes zoster and its complications.

In summary, primary care providers should be able to make a confident clinical diagnosis and render timely antiviral therapy for uncomplicated herpes zoster infections. The addition of corticosteroids to the antiviral regimen may be useful during the acute phase of the zoster outbreak. In the elderly patient the clinician should be especially alert for ocular complications, widely disseminated disease, and secondary bacterial infections. The recently approved zoster vaccine is safe and effective, and should provide protection for patients older than age 60.

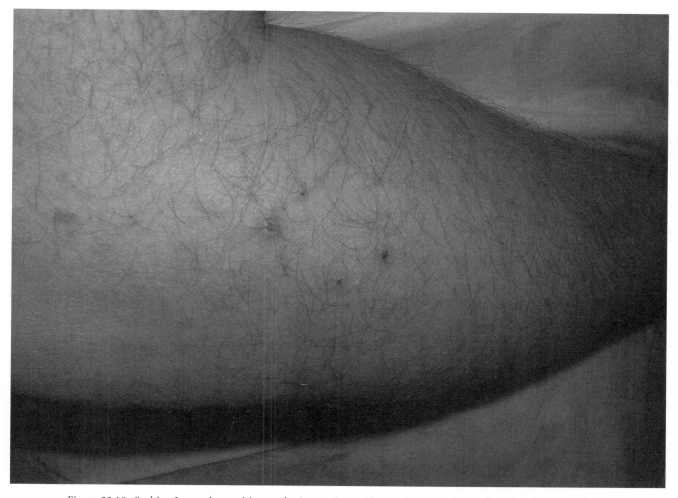

Figure 33.10. Scabies. Intensely pruritic papules in a patient with a prolonged scabies infestation. See color plates.

Scabies

Scabies is a commonly encountered infestation in the geriatric population. It is highly contagious and characterized by intensely pruritic, serpiginous burrows, and papules typically located in the finger webs, wrists, axillae, external genitalia, nipples, and buttocks (Figure 33.10). The incidence is notably rising in the institutionalized, debilitated, vulnerable nursing home patient.[78] The prevalence is in excess of 300 million cases annually. The definitive pathogenesis is a type IV hypersensitivity reaction to the mites, *Sarcoptes scabiei*, their eggs, saliva, or scybala (feces). Classic scabies involves the invasion of 10–15 adult mites on a host, whereas the highly contagious form, known as "crusted or keratotic" or "Norwegian scabies," can represent an infestation with literally thousands to millions of mites. The latter cases are generally found in mental institutions, homeless shelters, and understaffed nursing homes.[79] Often such patients can serve as the index patient for scabies epidemics.[80]

The differential diagnosis of scabies is extensive. It is important to consider other dermatological conditions such as atopic dermatitis, pruritus secondary to metabolic disease, impetigo, delusional parasitosis, prurigo nodularis, vasculitis, papular urticaria, and secondary syphilis. Definitive diagnosis rests in identifying the mite or its scybala on microscopic examination. Skin scrapings are obtained by scraping the lateral edge of a suspicious burrow or papule. The skin sample is then covered with mineral oil and examined under the low power of a light microscope. A clinical diagnosis can be made based on the classic history of intense pruritus, especially at night, and typical skin findings in the setting of crowded living conditions or sexual exposure.

Treatment should be prescribed for infected individuals and their close physical and sexual contacts after the mite, its eggs, or excreta have been identified, or a clinical diagnosis has been established. Of the available topical treatments in the United States, 5% permethrin cream (Elimite or Acticin) is the first-line therapy that has the endorsement of the Centers for Disease Control and Prevention (CDC) (Grade A).[81] Application at bedtime should scrupulously cover head-to-toe, including scalp, hands, groin, and under nails and should be left on for 8–12 hours. A repeated treatment is recommended

1 week later. Lindane 1% cream is considered a second- or third-line alternative;[80] however, it is associated with neurotoxic side effects (seizures, vertigo, and irritability) that has limited its use. The CDC recommends crotamiton 10% cream as a second-line topical agent or, in some circumstances, oral therapy with ivermectin (200 μg/kg).[81] Because topical treatments are inconvenient and poorly tolerated by some elderly patients, oral ivermectin is an acceptable alternative. The findings of one randomized trial comparing ivermectin with 5% permethrin demonstrated that a single dose of ivermectin resulted in a cure rate of 70% compared with one application of permethrin, which had a 98% cure rate. A second dose of ivermectin, however, given 2 weeks later, boosted the cure rate to 95% (Grade A).[82] Thus, the success rates of the two treatments are similar with the ease of administration favoring oral ivermectin. This may be especially useful for some elderly patients for whom the inconvenience and cost of topical applications of permethrin may represent a barrier to treatment. Another possible indication for ivermectin is in the immunocompromised patient with "crusted" or "Norwegian scabies." In addition to keratolytics and antimite agents such as permethrin, ivermectin in repeated dosages can be useful.[83] Because it is a potential neurotoxin, ivermectin should not be administered to adults who may not have an intact blood–brain barrier. Ivermectin does not yet have FDA approval for treatment of scabies.[83]

An assessment of response to therapy for scabies should routinely be made at 14 and 28 days. If continued pruritus remains a problem, then an alternative diagnosis, such as irritative dermatitis, should be sought or a relapse of scabies should be considered and treated accordingly.

In summary, scabies is a common problem in the elderly. In addition to the index patient, household members and sexual contacts should be treated even if they are asymptomatic. The CDC has approved permethrin cream as first-hand therapy with crotamiton cream, or oral ivermectin, as suitable alternatives.

Onychomycosis

Onychomycosis is an inclusive term describing fungal infections of the nail caused by dermatophytes (tinea unguium) in the majority of cases, but other fungi including nondermatophyte molds and *Candida* may be implicated. The majority of cases are caused by the dermatophyte species, *Trichophyton rubrum*. The geriatric population is especially vulnerable to these infections because of decreased epidermal regeneration and a diminished rate of nail growth.[84] A Canadian study, focusing on patients presenting for care in the offices of one family doctor and three dermatologists, found the prevalence of onychomycosis to be 8%.[85]

The classic physical finding is a brownish-yellow or whitish discoloration caused by the deposition of keratinaceous debris at the distal or lateral edge of the nail (Figure 33.11). This typical presentation of tinea unguium is termed distal and lateral

subungual onychomycosis. In a retrospective Italian study of 4,046 cases of nail fungus, 98% were distal.[86] With the accumulation of extensive subungual keratotic material, the distal nail plate separates from the bed, predisposing to secondary bacterial invasion. This is especially pernicious for elderly diabetic or immunocompromised patients who are subject to recurrent cellulitis with the threat of osteomyelitis and limb loss.

The positive documentation of fungi is necessary prior to the initiation of expensive, long-term antifungal therapy. This is important because other etiologies of nail dystrophy can mimic onychomycosis in 50% of cases.[85] The differential diagnosis should include psoriasis, irritant dermatitis, trauma, senile ischemia or onychogryphosis, lichen planus, and Reiter syndrome. Mycological confirmation should be sought for definitive diagnosis by using one or several of the following: potassium hydroxide examination, culture (on Sabouraud medium), or nail plate biopsy with period acid–Schiff stain.[87] The latter is the most reliable technique.

In addition to debridement of dystrophic nails, costly and lengthy courses of oral antifungal medications are available. These should be reserved for patients with complications of tinea unguium including recurrent cellulitis, paronychia, pain from pressure on the nail bed, and disfiguring physical appearance.

Successful therapy for tinea unguium almost always requires an oral antifungal agent (see Table 33.7). The older drug, griseofulvin, was associated with a disappointing cure rate of 25% after 1 year of therapy, and now has limited use.[88] It has been replaced by newer therapies including itraconazole and terbinafine. Itraconazole, a fungistatic azole, can be administered in a fixed dosage or by pulse dosing. Terbinafine is administered in a dosage of 250 mg/day for 2–3 months depending on the site of infection. Dosing schedules for both drugs are listed in Table 33.7. Long-term mycological cure rates were superior with terbinafine compared with itraconazole according to one review study (Grade B).[89]

In addition to indications for prescribing antifungal agents, the clinician should be aware of drug interactions and laboratory monitory. Itraconazole is a potent inhibitor of CYP3A4 and can be associated with a number of serious drug–drug interactions. On the other hand, terbinafine is linked to a few minor interactions and there are no drugs that are contraindicated for concomitant use. Liver function tests should be performed at baseline and again at 4 and 8 weeks when prescribing a course of itraconazole. These tests should be monitored only once at 6 weeks when ordering a 3-month course of terbinafine.

In summary, tinea unguium occurs more frequently in older individuals who are at greater risk for significant complications, including cellulitis, osteomyelitis, and loss of limb. Laboratory confirmation of fungal infection is required prior to authorization of extended antifungal therapy by most U.S. insurance companies. According to most head-to-head studies, terbinafine appears superior to itraconazole in terms of long-term clinical outcomes.[90] Terbinafine also has a better safety profile with fewer serious drug interactions.

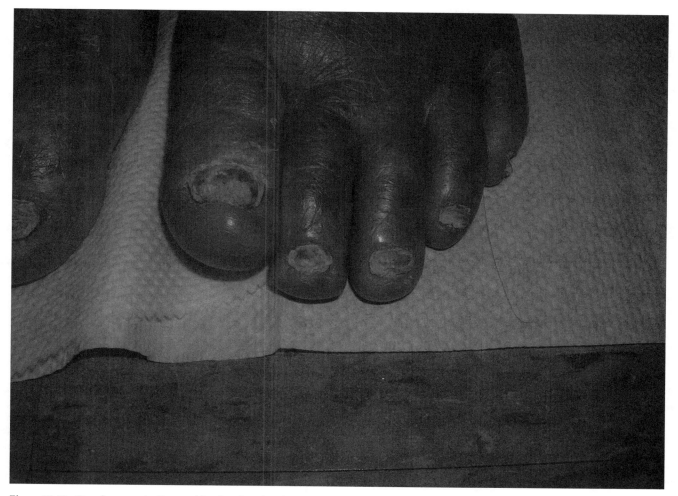

Figure 33.11. Onychomycosis. Dystrophic, discolored nails with an accumulation of white keratinaceous debris under the distal and lateral nail plate. See color plates.

SKIN CANCERS

Cancer of the skin (including melanoma and nonmelanoma skin cancer) is the most common of all cancers, probably accounting for more than 50% of all cancers.[91] The number of premalignant and malignant skin cancer cases has increased dramatically in the last two decades secondary to increased UVR exposure, an aging population, and increased detection.[92] It is estimated that there will be more than 1 million cases of nonmelanoma cancers diagnosed in the year 2006.[91] Most of these cancers, approximately 800,000–900,000 are basal cell cancers. Squamous cell cancers account for approximately 200,000–300,000 cancers. Melanoma accounts for approximately 4% of skin cancer cases, but causes a large majority of skin cancer deaths. Death from nonmelanoma skin cancers is uncommon, causing approximately 1,000–2,000 deaths per year.[91] Early recognition of premalignant and malignant skin lesions can prevent significant morbidity and mortality.

Although a total-body skin examination by a clinician is the most commonly advocated screening test for skin can-

cer, there are no randomized trials or case-control studies that have shown that screening is associated with improved clinical outcomes such as reduced morbidity and mortality from skin cancer, even in high-risk patients (Grade I).[93] The American Cancer Society recommends skin examination as part of a cancer-related checkup every 3 years for people between 20 and 40 years, and on a yearly basis for anyone older than 40 years.

Although benefits from screening are unproved, clinicians should be aware that fair-skinned men and women older than 65 years, patients with atypical moles, patients with more than 50 moles, and patients with a family history of melanoma represent groups that are at substantially increased risk for melanoma. Clinicians should remain alert for skin lesions with malignant features noted in the context of physical examinations performed for other purposes. Asymmetry, border irregularity, color variability, diameter greater than 6 mm (A, B, C, and D), or rapidly changing lesions are features associated with an increased risk of malignancy. Suspicious lesions should undergo biopsy (Grade A).

Table 33.7. Oral Antifungal Agents for Tinea Unguium

Itraconazole

Fixed dosing

Fingernail: 200 mg/day for 6 wk

Toenail: 200 mg/day for 12 wk

Pulsed dosing

Fingernail: 200 mg bid for 1 wkmo for 2 mo

Toenail: 200 mg bid for 1 wkmo for 3 mo

Terbinafine

Fingernail: 250 mg/day for 2 mo

Toenail: 250 mg/day for 3 mo

Premalignant Lesions

Actinic keratoses, also known as solar keratoses, affect 60% of light-skinned individuals older than 40 years of age.[92] They are regarded as precursors to squamous cell cancers, and as such, are the most common premalignant skin lesions; however, a growing body of evidence suggests that actinic keratoses may actually represent early squamous cell carcinomas. The development of actinic keratoses is related to chronic UVR exposure and associated with an increased risk for basal cell carcinoma and malignant melanoma. Although actinic keratoses are considered premalignant lesions, the majority resolve without treatment; however, approximately 60% of squamous cell carcinomas develop from actinic keratoses.[92]

Actinic keratoses appear as poorly circumscribed, sometimes scaly, erythematous papules or plaques on sun-exposed areas such as the face, ears, and dorsum of the hands and arms. They usually feel rough and are more often easily palpated than seen. Some may have an overlying thick, hard growth known as a cutaneous horn. Lesions on the lips are called actinic cheilitis.

Actinic keratoses are usually treated to prevent progression to squamous cell carcinoma and to decrease discomfort. They respond to a variety of locally destructive treatments including cryotherapy with liquid nitrogen, topical acids, topical 5-fluorouracil, or excision. When there is diffuse disease, topical 5-fluorouracil can be effective. Creams or solutions of 5-fluorouracil can be applied once or twice a day over the entire sun-damaged area for approximately 2 weeks until the onset of tender, red, and ulcerated skin. Treatment is then discontinued, and healing occurs over another few weeks. Other therapies include peels, laser resurfacing, curettage, and photodynamic treatments.

Bowen's disease is a form of squamous cell carcinoma. It is a localized squamous cell carcinoma in situ. Sun exposure usually underlies the development of Bowen's disease; however, other etiologies include arsenic exposure and HPV. Lesions consist of persistent, erythematous, scaly plaques with well-defined margins. Treatments are similar to those for AKs.

Lentigo maligna, or Hutchinson freckle, are premalignant lesions that may give rise to lentigo maligna melanoma. Lentigo maligna consist of pigmented macules, usually greater than 1 cm in diameter with irregular borders on sun-exposed skin. Lesions gradually expand in a superficial growth phase. Nodule development indicates conversion to malignant melanoma. The risk of conversion to melanoma by age 75 is approximately 1%–2%.[6] Treatment options include cryotherapy or laser therapy; however, both procedures have high recurrence rates.

Malignant Lesions

Basal Cell Cancer

Basal cell carcinoma is the most common skin cancer and is responsible for approximately 75% of skin cancers diagnosed each year.[91] Its incidence is increasing worldwide by up to 10% a year.[94] White individuals in North America have a lifetime risk of approximately 30% of developing a basal cell carcinoma.[94] Although mortality from basal cell carcinomas is low, this malignancy causes considerable morbidity and burden on health care services.[95] Risk factors for basal cell carcinoma include fair complexion, light hair and eye color, freckling or sunburn in childhood, family history of skin cancer, immunosuppression, exposure to radiation, and ingestion of arsenic.[94]

Basal cell carcinomas are derived from the basal layer of keratinocytes, which is the deepest cell layer of the epidermis. They usually develop in sun-exposed areas, with 80%–85% on the head and neck.[94] Basal cell carcinoma is slow growing. It is highly unusual for a basal cell cancer to spread to lymph nodes or to distant parts of the body. If a basal cell cancer is left untreated, however, it can invade underlying tissues and destroy bone or cartilage, especially around the eyes, nose, and ears.[96] Patients with a history of basal cell cancer are at increased risk for subsequent skin cancers.[94]

The hallmark of basal cell carcinoma is a waxy, translucent, or pearly appearing papule (Figure 33.12).[96] These lesions typically have rolled edges and telangiectasias on the surface. As they enlarge, they can develop an ulcerated center called a rodent ulcer. The clinical subtypes are described as nodular or cystic, pigmented, sclerosing or morpheic, or superficial, each having slightly different characteristics. Pigmented basal cell carcinomas can easily be confused with melanoma. Sclerosing or morpheic basal cell carcinomas can appear as flat, atrophic lesions with indistinct borders. They are often the most aggressive subtype.[94]

Enlarging or symptomatic lesions that are not clearly benign should be excised or undergo biopsy to determine appropriate treatment (Grade A). Raised lesions can be sampled easily with a simple superficial shave biopsy. Small lesions may be entirely excised with a punch biopsy. An elliptic excision may be selected in areas in which tissue loss and cosmesis with a linear scar is acceptable. Large lesions or flat lesions can be sampled with a punch biopsy. Pigmented or lesions suspicious for melanoma should be completely excised (Grade A).[96]

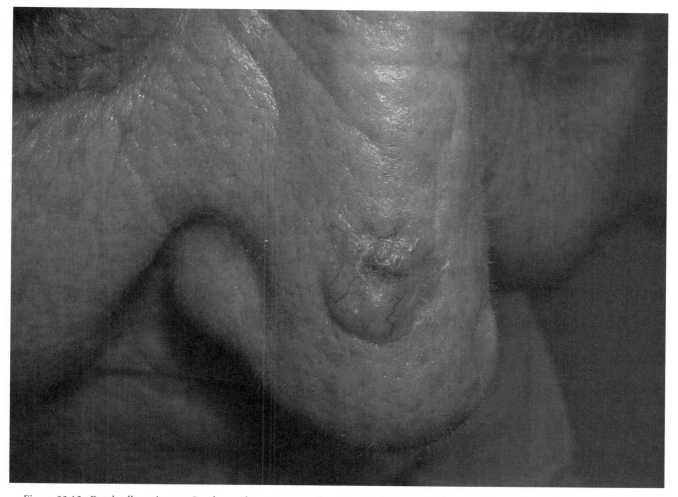

Figure 33.12. Basal cell carcinoma. Pearly, erythematous papule with raised edges and telangectasias on the surface. See color plates.

Basal cell cancers are usually treated with simple excision or electrodesiccation and curettage (Grade A). Other treatments include cryotherapy, photodynamic therapy, radiotherapy, and topical use of 5-fluorouracil or imiquimod (Aldara). Evidence-based guidelines have not been developed because of difficulty comparing outcomes data when results are not reported uniformly.[97] The choice of treatment options is based on multiple variables, such as patient factors (age, sex, and general health), tumor characteristics (size, location, and histological subtype), as well as the treating physician's preference and available resources.[98]

High-risk basal cell carcinomas are best treated with Mohs micrographic surgery to eradicate the tumor, prevent recurrence, and spare tissue (Grade A). Mohs micrographic surgery is a specialized technique utilizing serial sections for histological analysis until all margins are clear. Indications for Mohs micrographic surgery include high-risk anatomical location (eyelids, nose, ears, lips, genitalia, and fingers), large tumors (≥20 mm in diameter), recurrent tumors after previous excision or destruction, tumors occurring in sites of previous radiation therapy, tumors with aggressive histological patterns, tumors in immunosuppressed patients, and tumors with clinically indistinct margins or with positive margins after resection.[98,99]

Squamous Cell Cancer

Squamous cell cancer is the second most common skin cancer and accounts for approximately 10%–30% of all skin cancers.[91] They commonly appear on sun-exposed areas of the body such as the face, ear, neck, lip, and dorsum of the hands. Squamous cell cancers arise from more superficial layers of keratinocytes in the epidermis. Keratinocyte damage leading to squamous cell cancer results from repeated exposure to UVR, especially in susceptible persons. Sixty percent of squamous cell carcinoma lesions arise from existing actinic keratoses.[92] Squamous cell carcinoma can also develop in scars or skin ulcers. Common risk factors for the development of squamous cell cancer include advanced age, light complexion, and chronic sun exposure. Other risk factors include immunosuppression, environmental exposures to arsenic, thermal burns, radiation treatment or x-rays, and chronic infection with oncogenic HPV subtypes.

Squamous cell carcinoma lesions typically grow slowly and superficially; however, they tend to be more aggressive than basal cell cancers. Squamous cell carcinoma lesions are more likely to invade local tissues beneath the skin. Although uncommon, squamous cell carcinomas are slightly more likely to spread to lymph nodes or distant parts of the body. They may metastasize approximately 2%–5% of the time.[6]

Squamous cell carcinomas may have a variety of appearances, and any nonhealing nodule or plaque should arouse suspicion. Squamous cell cancers can be scaly like actinic keratoses, but they tend to be thicker, larger, and more erythematous. Lesions may be described as a patch, plaque, or nodule. Their surface may be keratotic, ulcerated, or crusted. The borders often are irregular and bleed easily.[96]

Squamous cell carcinomas usually are treated with the same modalities as basal cell cancers; however, studies examining various treatments for squamous cell carcinomas are lacking.

Melanoma

Although melanoma accounts for only 4% of all skin cancers, it is responsible for 80% of deaths from skin cancer.[100] Furthermore, only 14% of patients with metastatic melanoma survive for 5 years.[100] Melanoma is the sixth leading cause of cancer death in the United States. The incidence of melanoma increases by 4.1% per year, faster than any other malignancy.[101]

Melanoma is much more common in Caucasians than in nonCaucasians. The most significant risk factors for melanoma are a family history of melanoma, multiple benign or atypical nevi, and a previous melanoma.[100] Other risk factors for the development of melanoma have been identified, including exposure to UVR (especially during childhood), sun sensitivity, white skin, fair complexion, light eyes, tendency to freckle, large congenital nevi, and immunosuppression.[101] Although sun exposure is a risk factor for melanoma, cutaneous melanomas can arise in areas of the body not exposed to the sun.

There are four types of melanoma, the incidence of all of which increase with age. The four types include superficial spreading, nodular, lentigo maligna, and acral-lentiginous. Superficial spreading melanoma accounts for approximately 60%–70% of all melanomas and is the most common form in the elderly.[6]

Suspicious lesions should undergo biopsy, optimally with an excisional biopsy with 1–2-mm borders (Grade A). Shave biopsies should not be used if melanoma is suspected because prognosis is related to tumor thickness at the time of excision rather than to histological type (Grade D). An incisional or punch biopsy is appropriate when the suspicion for melanoma is low, when the lesion is large, or when it is impractical to perform an excision (Grade B).[102]

The Breslow thickness of a tumor is measured from the top of the viable epidermis to the point of deepest invasion. Depth of less than 0.76 mm is associated with a 96% 5-year survival rate, whereas tumor depth of more than 4 mm is associated with 47% 5-year survival rate.[92] Other factors associated with poor prognosis include advanced age, anatomical site, male sex, and ulceration.[92] In the elderly, melanoma tends to be diagnosed at a later stage and is more likely to be lethal than it is in the general population.[93] As metastatic melanoma is usually fatal,

cure depends on early diagnosis and excision while the tumor has not deeply invaded the dermis.

After melanoma is confirmed, patients must undergo complete excision of the tumor or tumor site (Grade A). Resection is curative for local disease. After wide excision, treatment depends on staging. Staging systems grade the local lesion, nodes, and metastases to determine the treatment approach. Long-term prognosis and recurrence rates correlate closely with thickness of local tumor at time of diagnosis. Patients who are diagnosed with nonulcerated melanoma less than 1 mm deep are unlikely to have nodal metastasis. Thicker melanomas, at least 1 mm deep, are suspect for possible lymph node metastases. Any palpable local lymph node gives cause for regional lymph node dissection. If no nodes are palpable, the benefit of sentinel, elective, or complete lymph node dissection approaches have not been proved, and are considered experimental.[92] Sentinel lymph node biopsy has, however, become the standard of care for nodal staging in patients with intermediate thickness melanoma (1–4 mm) and clinically negative nodes. Patients with metastatic tumor in the sentinel lymph node and those who have clinically evident nodal metastasis often undergo therapeutic lymph node dissection of the entire draining nodal basin. When there are metastases, the prognosis is poor, and the treatment options do not typically afford a great deal of extension of life. Therapies include chemotherapy, immunotherapy with vaccines and immune system stimulators, and radiation for local palliation.[92]

REFERENCES

1. Kligman AM, Koblenzer C. Demographics and Psychological Implications for the Aging Population, *Dermatol Clin.* 1997;15:549–553.
2. Yaar M, Gilchrest BA. Aging of skin, In: Freedberg IM, Eisen AZ, Wolff K, Austen KF, Goldsmith LA, Katz SI, eds. *Fitzpatrick's Dermatology in General Medicine.* 6th ed. New York: McGraw-Hill;2003:1386–1398.
3. Dewberry C, Norman RA. Skin cancer in elderly patients. *Dermatol Clin.* 2004;22 (1): 93–96.
4. Glogau RG. Physiologic and Structural Changes Associated with Aging Skin, *Dermatol Clin.* Vol. 15, No.4, Oct 1997, pp 555–559.
5. Chung JH, Hanft VN, Hang S. Aging and photoaging, *J Am Acad Dermatol.* 2003;49:690–697.
6. Gilchrest BA, Chiu N. Aging and the Skin. Chapter 122 In: Beers MH, Berkow R, eds. *The Merck Manual of Geriatrics.* 3rd ed. Whitehouse Station, NJ, Merck and Co, Inc, 2000.
7. Balin AK. Skin disease. In: Evans JG, Williams TF, Beattie BL, Michel J-P, Wilcock GK, eds. *Oxford Textbook of Geriatric Medicine.* 2nd ed. Oxford: Oxford University Press; 2000:721–738.
8. Castanet J, Ortonne J-P. Pigmentary changes in aged and photoaged skin. *Arch Dermatol.* 1997;133:1296–1299.
9. Sunderkotter C, Kalden H, Luger TA. Aging and the skin immune system. *Arch Dermatol.* 1997;133:1256–1262.
10. Danahy JF, Gilchrest BA. Geriatric dermatology. In: Gallo JJ, Busby-Whitehead J, Rabins PV, Silliman RA, Murphy JB, eds. *Reichel's Care of the Elderly, Clinical Aspects of Aging.* 5th ed. Philadelphia: Lippincott Williams & Wilkins; 1999:513–524.
11. Thompson SC, Jolley D, Marks R. Reduction of solar keratoses by regular sunscreen use. *NEJM.* 1993;329 (16):1147–1151.

12. Gendler EC. Topical Treatment of the aging face, *Dermatol Clin.* 1997;15:561–567.

13. Gallagher RP. Sunscreen protection: sunscreens in melanoma and skin cancer prevention. *Can Med Assoc J.* 2005;173(3):244–245.

14. Rabe JH, Mamelak AJ, McElgunn PJ, Morison WL, Sauder SN. Photoaging: mechanisms and repair. *J Am Acad Dermatol.* 2006;55 (1): 1–19.

15. Olsen EA, Katz HI, Levine N, Nigra TP, Pochi PE, Savin RC, et al. Tretinoin emollient cream for photodamaged skin: results of 48-week, multicenter, double-blind studies. *J Am Acad Dermatol.* 1997;37: 217–26.

16. Gilchrest BA. A review of skin ageing and its medical therapy. *Br J Dermatol.* 1996;135:867.

17. Kang S, Fisher GJ, Voorhees JJ. Photoaging and topical tretinoin. *Arch Dermatol.* 1997;133:1280–1284.

18. Stiller MJ, Bartolone J, Stern R, Smith S, Kollias N, Gillies R, Drake LA. Topical 8% glycolic acid and 8% lactic acid creams for the treatment of photodamaged skin: a double-blind vehicle-controlled clinical trial. *Arch Dermatol.* 1996;132 (6): 631–636.

19. Gay C, Thiese M, Garner E. Geriatric dermatology. *Clin Fam Pract.* 2003; 5 (3):771–789.

20. Habif T. *Skin Disease.* 2nd ed. Philadelphia: Elsevier; 2005.

21. Fitzpatrick T. *Color Atlas and Synopsis of Clinical Dermatology.* 4th ed. New York: McGraw-Hill; 2001.

22. Roberts W. Dermatologic problems of older women. *Dermatol Clin.* 2006;24:271–280.

23. Schaffrali F. Experience with low-dose methotrexate for the treatment of eczema in the elderly. *J Am Acad Dermatol.* 2003;48:417–419.

24. Williams H. Atopic dermatitis. *NEJM.* 2005;352:2314–2324.

25. Kazandjian D, Okulicz J. Skin tears? *Am J Med.* 2006;119:657–659.

26. Sami N. Blistering diseases in the elderly: diagnosis and treatment. *Dermatol Clin.* 2004;22:73–86.

27. Paul MA, Jorizzo JL, Fleischer AJ, White WL. Low-dose methotrexate treatment in elderly patients with bullous pemphigoid. *J Am Acad Dermatol.* 1994;31:620–625.

28. Shupack J, Abel E, Bauer E. Cyclosporine as maintenance therapy in patients with severe psoriasis. *J Am Acad Dermatol.* 1997;36:423–432.

29. Pelle MT. Rosacea: II. Therapy. *J Am Acad Dermatol.* 2004;51:499–512.

30. Breneman DL, Stewart D, Hevia O, Hino PD, Drake LA. A double-blind, multicenter clinical trial comparing efficacy of once-daily metronidazole 1 percent cream to vehicle in patients with rosacea. *Cutis.* 1998;61:44–47.

31. Gupta AK. Seborrheic Dermatitis. *Dermatol Clin.* 2003;21:401–412.

32. Schwartz R, Janusz C, Janniger C. Seborrheic dermatitis: an overview. *Am Fam Physician.* 2006;74:125–130

33. Theodosat A. Skin diseases of the lower extremities in the elderly. *Dermatol Clin.* 2004;22:13–21.

34. Swartz MN. Clinical practice. Cellulitis. *New Engl J Med.* 2004;350:905.

35. Simon MS, Cody RL. Cellulitis after axillary lymph node dissection for carcinoma of the breast. *Am J Med.* 1992;93:543–548.

36. Baddour LM, Bisno AL. Non-group A beta-hemolytic streptococcal cellulitis: association with venous and lymphatic compromise. *Am J Med.* 1985;79:155–159.

37. Fernandez JM, Serrano M, De Arriba JJ, Sanchez MV, Escribano E, Ferraras P. Bacteremic cellulitis caused by non-01, non-0139 *Vibrio cholerae*: report of a case in a patient with hemochromatosis. *Diagn Microbiol Infect Dis.* 2000;37:77–80.

38. Parada JP, Maslow JN. Clinical syndromes associated with adult pneumococcal cellulitis. *Scand J Infect Dis.* 2000;32:133–136.

39. Bisno AL, Cockerill FR III, Bermudez CT. The initial outpatient-physician encounter in group A streptococcal necrotizing fasciitis. *Clin Infect Dis.* 2000;31:607–608.

40. Wall DB, Klein SR, Black S, de Virgilio C. A simple model to help distinguish necrotizing fasciitis from nonnecrotizing soft tissue infection. *J Am Coll Surg.* 2000;191:227–231.

41. Swartz MN. Cellulitis and subcutaneous tissue infections: In: Mandell GL, Bennett JF, Dolin R, eds. *Principles and Practice of Infectious Diseases.* 5th ed. Philadelphia: Churchill Livingstone; 2005:1172–1194.

42. Kielhofner MA, Brown B, Dall L. Influence of underlying disease process on the utility of cellulitis needle aspirates. *Arch Intern Med.* 1988;148:2451–2452.

43 Hook EW III, Hooton TM, Horton CA, Coyle MB, Ramsey PG, Turck M. Microbiologic evaluation of Cutaneous cellulitis in adults. *Arch Intern Med.* 1986;146:295–297.

44. Sigurdsson AF, Gudmundsson S. The etiology of bacterial cellulitis as determined by fine-needle aspiration. *Scand J Infect Dis.* 1989;21:537–542.

45. Gilbert DN, Moellering RC, Eliopoulos, GM, Sande MA. The Sanford guide to antimicrobial therapy 2006. *Antimicrob Ther.* 2006;(36):38–41.

46. Swartz MN. Clinical practice. Cellulitis. *New Engl J Med.* 2004;350:909.

47. Stevens DL, Herr D, Lamperis H, Hunt JL, Batts DH, Hafkin B. Linezolid versus vancomycin for the treatment of methicillin-resistant *Staphylococcus aureus* infections. *Clin Infect Dis.* 2002;34:1481–1490.

48. Lipsky BA. Evidence-based antibiotic therapy of diabetic foot infections. *FEMA Immunol Med Microbiol.* 1999;26:267–276.

49. Kremer M, Zuckerman R, Avraham Z, Raz R. Long-term antimicrobial therapy in the prevention of recurrent soft-tissue infections. *J Infect.* 1991;22:37–40.

50. Schmader K. Herpes zoster in older adults. *Clin Infect Dis.* 2001;32:1.

51. Burke VL, Steele RW, Beard OW, et al. Immune responses to varicella-zoster in the aged. *Arch Intern Med.* 1982;142:291.

52. Arvin AM, Pollard RB, Rasmussen LE, Merigan TC. Cellular and humoral immunity in the pathogenesis of recurrent herpes viral infections in patients with lymphoma. *J Clin Invest.* 1980;65: 869.

53. Straus SE, Ostrove JM, Inchauspe G, et al. NIH conference. Varicella-zoster virus infections. Biology, natural history, treatment, and prevention. *Ann Intern Med.* 1988;108:221.

54. Donahue JG, Choo RW, Manson JE, Platt R. The incidence of herpes zoster. *Arch Intern Med.* 1995;155:1605.

55. Helgason S, Sigurdsson JA, Gudmundsson S. The clinical course of herpes zoster: a prospective study in primary care. *Eur J Gen Pract.* 1996;2:12–16.

56. Rowbotham M, Harden N, Stacey B, et al. Gabapentin for the treatment of postherpetic neuralgia. *Arch Intern Med.* 1997;157:1217.

57. Choo PW, Galil K, Donahue JG, et al. Risk factors for postherpetic neuralgia. *Arch Intern Med.* 1997;157:1217.

58. Galil K, Choo PW, Donahue JG, Platt R. The sequelae of herpes zoster. *Arch Intern Med.* 1997;157:1209.

59. Pavan-Livingston D. Herpes zoster ophthalmicus. *Neurology.* 1995;45:S50.

60. Liesegang TJ. Diagnosis and therapy of herpes zoster ophthalmicus. *Ophthalmology.* 1991;98:1216.

61. Severson EA, Baratz KH, Hodge DO, Burke JP. Herpes zoster ophthalmicus is Olmsted county, Minnesota: have systemic

antivirals made a difference? *Arch Ophthalmol.* 2003;121: 386.

62. Robillard RB, Hilsinger RL, Adour KK. Ramsey Hunt facial paralysis: clinical analyses of 185 patients. *Otolaryngol Head Neck Surg.* 1986;95:292.

63. Dahl H, Marcoccia J, Linde A. Antigen detection: the method of choice in comparison with virus isolation and serology for laboratory diagnosis of herpes zoster in human immunodeficiency virus-infected patient. *J Clin Microbiol.* 1997;35:345–349.

64. Huff JC, Bean B, Balfour HH, et al. Therapy of herpes zoster with oral acyclovir. *Am J Med.* 1988;85(Suppl 2A):84–88.

65. Wood MJ, Kay R, Dworkin RH, et al. Oral acyclovir therapy accelerates pain resolution in patients with herpes zoster: meta-analysis of placebo controlled trials. *Clin Infect Dis.* 1996;22:341.

66. Jackson JL, Gibbons R, Meyer G, Inouye L. The effect of treating herpes zoster with oral acyclovir in preventing postherpetic neuralgia. *Arch Intern Med.* 1997;157:909.

67. Beutner KR, Friedman DJ, Forszpaniak C, Andersen PL, Wood MJ. Valaciclovir compared with acyclovir for improved therapy for herpes zoster in immunocompetent adults. *Antimicrob Agents Chemother.* 1995;39:1546–1553.

68. Tyring S, Barbarash RA, Nahlik JE, et al. Famciclovir for the treatment of acute herpes zoster: effects on acute disease and postherpetic neuralgia a randomized, double-blind, placebo-controlled trial. *Ann Intern Med.* 1995;123:89–96.

69. Beutner KR. Clinical management of herpes zoster in the elderly patient. *Compr Ther.* 1996;22:183–186.

70. Wood MJ, Johnson RW, McKendrick MW, Taylor J, Mandal BK, Crooks J. A randomized trial of acyclovir for 7 days and 21 days with and without prednisone for treatment of acute herpes zoster. *NEJM.* 1994;330:896–900.

71 Whitley RJ, Weiss H, Gnann JW, et al. Acyclovir with and without prednisone for the treatment of herpes zoster: a randomized, placebo-controlled trial. *Ann Intern Med.* 1996;125;376–383.

72. Brown GR. Herpes zoster: correlation of age, sex, distribution, neuralgia, and associated disorders. *South Med J.* 1976; 69: 576–578.

73. Dworkin RH, Perkins FM, Nagasako EM. Prospects for the prevention of postherpetic neuralgia in herpes zoster patients. *Clin J Pain.* 2000; 16(Suppl 2):S90–S100.

74. Bowsher D. The effects of pre-emptive treatment of postherpetic neuralgia with amitriptyline: a randomized, double-blind, placebo-controlled trial. *J Pain Symptom Manage.* 1997;13:327–331.

75. Oxman MN, Levin MJ, Johnson GR, Schmader KE, Straus SE, Gelb LD, et al, with the Shingles Prevention Study Group, A vaccine to prevent herpes zoster and postherpetic neuralgia in older adults. *NEJM.* 2005;352 (22):2271–2284.

76. Dubinsky RM, Kabbani H, El-Chami Z, et al. Practice parameter: treatment of postherpetic neuralgia: an evidence-based report of the Quality Standards Subcommittee of the American Academy of Neurology. *Neurology.* 2004;63:959.

77. Alper BS, Lewis PR. Treatment of postherpetic neuralgia: a systematic review of the literature. *J Fam Pract.* 2002;51:121.

78. Gimenez Garcia R, de la Lama Lopez-Areal J, Avellaneda Martinez C. Scabies in the elderly. *J Eur Acad Dermatol Venereol.* 2004;18:105–107.

79. Fitzpatrick TB, Johnson RA, Wolff K. *Color Atlas and Synopsis of Clinical Dermatology, Common and Serious Disease.* 4th ed. New York: McGraw Hill; 2001.

80. Chosidow O. Clinical Practices: Scabies. *NEJM.* 2006; 354 (16): 1718–1727.

81. Scabies fact sheet. Atlanta: Centers for Disease Control and Prevention, 2005. Available at: http://www.cdc.gov/ncidod/dpd/parasites/scabies/factsht_scabies.htm. Accessed June 10, 2008.

82. Usha V, Gopalakrishnan-Nair TV. A comparative study of oral ivermectin and topical permethrin cream in the treatment of scabies. *J Am Acad Dermato.l* 2000;42:236–240.

83. MeinKing TL, Taplin D, Jermida JL, Pardo R, Kerdel FA. The treatment of scabies with ivermectin. *NEJM.* 1995;333:26–30.

84. Weinberg JM. Fungal diseases of the skin. In: Demiss DJ, ed. *Conn's Current Therapy 2002.* 54th ed. Philadelphia: WB Saunders; 2002:827–829.

85. Gupta AK, Jain HC, Lynde CW, et al. Prevalence and epidemiology of onychomycosis in patients visiting physicians' offices: a multicenter canadian survey of 15,000 patients. *J Am Acad Dermatol.* 2000;43:244.

86. Romano C, Gianni C, Difonzo EM. Retrospective study of onychomycosis in Italy: 1985–2000. *Mycoses.* 2005;48:260.

87. Gupta AN. Onychomycosis in the elderly. *Drugs Aging.* 2000;16:397–407.

88. Scher RK. Onychomycosis: therapeutic update. *J Am Acad Dermatol.* 1999;40:S21.

89. Crawford F, Young P, Godfrey C. et al. Oral treatments for toenail onychomycosis: a systematic review. *Arch Dermatol.* 2002;138:811.

90. Sigurgeirsson B, Olafsson JH, Steinsson JB, et al. Long-term effectiveness of treatment with terbinafine vs. itraconazole in onychomycosis: a 5-year blinded prospective follow-up study. *Arch Dermatol.* 2002;138:353.

91. American Cancer Society. Cancer Reference Information. Available at: http://www.cancer.org/docroot/CRI/CRI_2x.asp?sitearea = &dtz39. Accessed June 10, 2008.

92. Gay C, Thiese MS, Stulberg DL. Malignant tumors of the skin in the maturing adult, *Clin Fam Pract.* 2003;5(3):757–770.

93. Berg AO. Screening for Skin Cancer: Recommendations and Rationale, U.S. Preventive Services Task Force, Guidelines from Guide to Clinical Preventive Services. 3rd ed. (2000–2003), April 1, 2001.

94. Wong CSM, Strange RC, Lear JT. Basal cell carcinoma. *BMJ.* 2003;327:795–798.

95. Housman TS. Skin cancer is among the most costly of all cancers to treat for the Medicare population. *J Am Acad Dermatol.* 2003;48:425–429.

96. Stulberg DL, Crandell B, Fawcett RS. Diagnosis and treatment of basal cell and squamous cell carcinomas. *Am Fam Physician.* 2004;70:1481–1488.

97. Thissen M, Neumann M, Schouten LJ. A systematic review of treatment modalities for primary basal cell carcinomas. *Arch Dermatol.* 1999;135:1177–1183.

98. Leibovitch I, Huilgol SC, Selva D, Richards S, Paver R. Basal cell carcinoma treated with Mohs surgery in Australia III: outcome at 5-year follow-up, *J Am Acad Dermatol.* 2005;53:(3):452–457.

99. Bowen GM, White GL, Gerwels JW. Mohs micrographic surgery. *Am Fam Physician.* 2005;72:845–848.

100. Miller AJ, Mihm MC. Mechanisms of disease: melanoma *NEJM.* 2006;355:51–65.

101. Rager EL, Bridgeford EP, Ollila DW. Cutaneous melanoma: update on prevention, screening, diagnosis, and treatment. *Am Fam Physician.* 2005;72:269–276.

102. Sober AJ, Chuang TY, Duvic M, et al. Guidelines of care for primary cutaneous melanoma. *J Am Acad Dermatol.* 2001;45:579–586.

34

Pressure Ulcers: Practical Considerations in Prevention and Treatment

Mary H. Palmer, PhD, RN-C, FAAN, Jan Busby-Whitehead, MD

INTRODUCTION

The 2004 death of actor/director, Christopher Reeve, at the age of 52 years from heart failure secondary to an infected pressure ulcer underscores the importance of effective pressure ulcer prevention, treatment, and management strategies.[1] Septic infections are associated with pressure ulcers and age-adjusted mortality rate calculations are 3.79 per 100,000 population (95% confidence interval [CI] 3.77–3.81).[2] The incidence of pressure ulcers vary greatly. In the acute care setting, incidence ranges from 0.4%–38% and in nursing homes prevalence rates range from 2%–23.9%.[3]

Pressure ulcers add significantly to health care costs and patient suffering. Beckrich and Aronovitch[4] estimated that pressure ulcers cost the U.S. health care system $5–$8 billion (1999 dollars). Patients describe, "endless pain," isolating themselves from others, and fear of odors emanating from pressure ulcers.[5]

More than 95% of pressure ulcers develop on the lower half of the body with the greatest number in the heaviest part, the pelvic girdle.[6] Approximately one quarter of adult Americans have a pressure ulcer at the time of their death.[7] Because of the high prevalence and incidence of pressure ulcers and their complications, costs to the health care system, pain and suffering for affected adults, and caregiver burden, efforts are being made to reduce pressure ulcer rates. One of the goals of Healthy People 2010 is to "reduce the proportion of nursing home residents with current diagnosis of pressure ulcers."[8]

The purpose of this chapter is to discuss evidence-based literature regarding the prevention and treatment of pressure ulcers in older adults and the need for an interdisciplinary team approach in pressure ulcer care.

BACKGROUND

Skin, the body's largest organ, comprises 10%–15% of body weight and serves to maintain thermoregulation, prevent infection and water loss, and act as a protective covering to underlying tissues and structures of the human body.[9] The skin also mirrors the health of the human organism, and the concept of skin failure has been proposed.[9] In this chapter, acute skin failure was defined as an event that occurs during a critical illness in which skin and underlying tissue die.[9] For example, a person not considered at risk for pressure ulcer formation could experience an event such as sepsis, trauma, or myocardial infarction whereby volume depletion results in low blood pressure, which would affect blood flow to the skin. In such events, body parts may be subjected to prolonged pressure that occludes blood flow to tissue; localized ischemia can occur and overt changes to the skin can result.[10] In addition, development of pressure ulcers is related to immobility and malnutrition.[9]

In addition to changes in a person's medical condition, other factors play a role in pressure ulcer development. In a study with nursing home residents admitted without a pressure ulcer but with a Braden scale score of less than or equal to 17 (indicating risk of developing a pressure ulcer), the amount of direct care time by registered nurses was associated with fewer pressure ulcers.[11] Therefore, factors beyond characteristics of the person can influence the development of pressure ulcers.

Pressure ulcers are considered a quality indicator of nursing care in the acute-care setting.[12] In addition, long-term care facilities must ensure that "a resident who enters the facility without pressure sores does not develop pressure sores unless the individual's clinical condition demonstrates that they were unavoidable."[13]

Table 34.1. Pressure Ulcer Stages

Stage I	Intact skin with nonblanchable redness of a localized area usually over a bony prominence. Darkly pigmented skin may not have visible blanching; its color may differ from the surrounding area.
Stage II	Partial-thickness loss of dermis presenting as a shallow open ulcer with a red pink wound bed, without slough. May also present as an intact or open/ruptured serum-filled blister.
Stage III	Full-thickness tissue loss. Subcutaneous fat may be visible but bone, tendon, or muscle are not exposed. Slough may be present but does not obscure the depth of tissue loss. May include undermining and tunneling.
Stage IV	Full-thickness tissue loss with exposed bone, tendon, or muscle. Slough or eschar may be present on some parts of the wound bed. Often include undermining and tunneling.
Unstageable	Full-thickness loss in which the base of the ulcer is covered by slough (yellow, tan, gray, green, or brown) and/or eschar (tan, brown, or black) in the wound bed.

Definitions and Stages

Pressure ulcers have been called pressure sores, bedsores, and decubitus ulcers and have been described in the medical literature for more than three centuries. A sixteenth century surgeon, Ambrose Paré, proposed that removing the cause, relieving the pain, and providing nutrition and rest were the first steps in healing.[4,15] Pressure ulcers are defined as, "localized injury to the skin and/or underlying tissue usually over a bony prominence, as a result of pressure, or pressure in combination with shear and/or friction. A number of contributing or confounding factors are also associated with pressure ulcers; the significance of these factors is yet to be elucidated."[16]

Pressure ulcers are classified by stage. The most commonly used staging system, the National Pressure Ulcer Advisory Panel (NPUAP) classification system, uses four stages that are based on depth and color of the lesion.[6] Pigment variation in the population, however, requires color definitions for darkly pigmented skin, especially for stage I pressure ulcers.[6] In addition to the four stages, the NPUAP provides a definition for an unstageable pressure ulcer, "full thickness loss in which the base of the ulcer is covered by slough (yellow, tan, gray, green, or brown) and/or eschar (tan, brown or black) in the wound bed Table 34.1.[16]

Nonblanchable redness with intact skin is classified as a stage I pressure ulcer. Assessment of nonblanchable redness is difficult in dark pigmented skin and interrater reliability is often questioned. Two methods can be used to assess nonblanchable redness. One method involves using a finger to press the skin and, if it does not blanch when the pressure is removed,

it is considered nonblanchable redness. The second method involves the use of a transparent disk that is pressed over the area and nonblanchable redness is considered present if the skin, viewed through the disk after pressure is released, does not blanch. Research indicates that the use of the transparent disk is the preferred method.[17] Darkly pigmented skin may not visibly blanch but will show variation in pigmentation from surrounding tissue.[16] Nonblanching redness has been found to be associated with the development of stage II or higher pressure ulcers in surgical patients.[18]

Recent research has demonstrated that some pressure ulcer development involves injury to deep tissues while the skin remains intact.[19] The NPUAP, however, provided a definition for suspected deep tissue injury: "purple or maroon localized area of discolored intact skins or blood-filled blister due to damage of underlying soft tissue from pressure and/or shear. The area may be preceded by tissue that is painful, firm, mushy, boggy, warmer or cooler as compared to adjacent tissue."[16] This type of injury can occur after prolonged immobilization and evolve into a stage IV pressure ulcer (Figure 34.1).[9]

Epidemiology of Pressure Ulcers

Although pressure ulcers are considered to be a significant clinical problem, their prevalence and incidence are not precisely known because different methodologies and definitions have been used across studies. This variability makes comparisons among studies difficult. Nonresponse bias, which occurs when patients may be unable or unwilling to join a study, can influence reported prevalence rates. By calculating nonresponse bias in prevalence studies, it is possible to obtain comparable data. Achieving high response rates is the ideal as the range of possible prevalence rates will be smaller with high response rates.[20]

In the United States, the prevalence and incidence of pressure ulcers has been estimated in different care settings. The range of incidence was 0.4%–38% in general acute care; 2.2%–23.9% in nursing homes, and 0%–17% in home care.[21] An overall estimate of pressure ulcer incidence in nursing home residents is 11%.[23] Whittington and Briones estimated that 2.5 million pressure ulcers are treated in U.S. hospitals annually.[23] The cumulative incidence of pressure ulcers in hip fracture patients at the third day of hospitalization was 6.2% (95% CI 5.4%–7.1%). The majority of pressure ulcers were classified as stage II and located in the sacral area or heel.[24] Racial differences in pressure ulcer incidence have been reported. The incidence of stage II, III, and IV pressure ulcers in black nursing home residents was 0.56 per person-year with compared with 0.35 per person-year for whites.[25] Black nursing home residents have fewer stage I pressure ulcers identified than white nursing home residents, perhaps because of the difficulty in detecting nonblanchable erythema in dark pigmented skin.[26]

The European Pressure Ulcer Advisory panel established a standardized methodology to determine prevalence rates among hospitalized patients. Findings indicated that

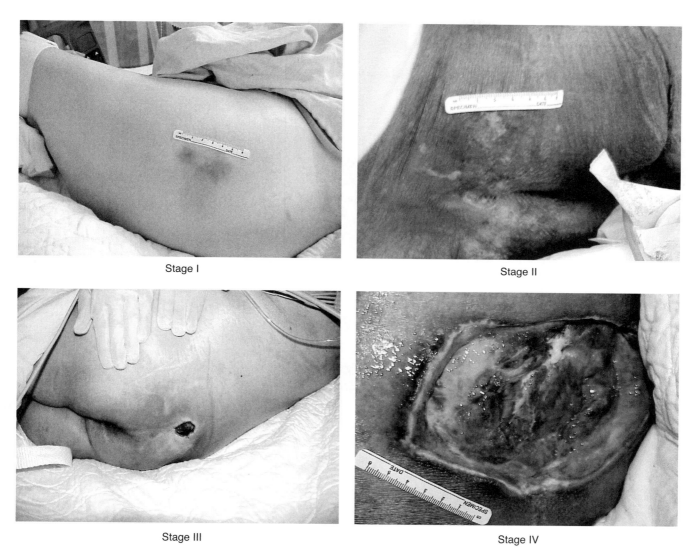

Stage I

Stage II

Stage III

Stage IV

Figure 34.1. Photos of stages I to IV. See color plates.

prevalence rates varied within German hospitals by type of service: surgical/orthopedic, medical, or geriatric (2004 prevalence: 28.2%, 17.3%, and 59.3% respectively).[27] In nursing home residents with a Braden score of less than or equal to 17, which was the cutoff score used to identify residents at risk of developing a pressure ulcer, 29% developed a new pressure ulcer during a 12-week period.[28] In a German study, 53% of hip fracture patients had a stage I or II pressure ulcer at the time of hospital discharge.[29]

Few current data are available regarding the remission or cure rates of pressure ulcers. An instrument to measure pressure ulcer healing for stage II to IV pressure ulcers, the Pressure Ulcer Scale for Healing, has been developed.[30] This instrument (can be accessed at www.npuap.org/push3-0.htm) helps to quantify several parameters: surface area as measured by length multiplied by width of the pressure ulcer, exudate amount, and tissue type. This instrument offers an alternative to a practice known

as reverse staging. The current position by the NPUAP is that a healed stage IV ulcer should be classified as a healed stage IV pressure ulcer rather than using a reverse staging technique such as classifying it as a stage 0.[31] Despite such recommendations, some clinicians continue to use reverse staging to indicate healing has occurred.

Costs of Pressure Ulcers

Few current data are available on the cost effectiveness of primary prevention interventions for pressure ulcers. Once a pressure ulcer exists, however, treatment and care are costly. The presence of a stage II pressure ulcer has been associated with increased hospital costs and duration of stay.[32] Hospitals incur costs of approximately $125–$200 for each stage I and stage II pressure ulcer and $14,000–$23,000 (1999 dollars) for each stage III and stage IV pressure ulcer.[4] In addition to direct financial costs in caring for pressure ulcers other complications, such as nosocomial infections and sepsis, related to pressure ulcers increase health care costs.[4,32]

Quality of Life

Few data are available about the effect of pressure ulcers on the quality of life of the affected adult. Pressure ulcer pain has been documented in the literature as both acute and chronic. Because pressure ulcers themselves can cause pain, as can pressure ulcer treatment, use of a visual analog scale to document pain should be incorporated into care. Administration of oral or local analgesics may be necessary prior to pressure ulcer treatments.[33,34] It is not inconceivable that the unsightly nature of the pressure ulcer and the associated odors that may emanate from them would cause psychological distress. Depending on the location of the pressure ulcer, comfortable body positioning and mobility may be impeded. More research about the effects of pressure ulcers on quality of life from the patient, family member, and formal caregiver perspective is needed.

Pathophysiology of Pressure Ulcers

Tissue injury can be superficial, deep, or a combination of both. Injury to the skin and deep tissue can occur within 2 hours,[7] and clinically detectable pressure ulcers can develop within 2–6 hours.[35] Emerging evidence indicates that deep tissue injury may occur under intact skin but the current staging systems do not sufficiently encompass these types of lesions.[19] Pressure to skin over bony prominences, such as the sacrum, heels, trochanters, femoral condyles, malleoli, or ischial tuberosities, may occlude capillary blood flow and lead to tissue death.[35] Shearing forces and friction also traumatize open skin, cause ischemia, and lead to tissue damage.[36] This can occur when a supine person is raised to a greater than 30° angle or when a patient is pulled up in bed without the use of a pull sheet.

A mechanism of ischemia/reperfusion injury has been proposed. Return of perfusion to ischemic tissue helps the return of function but it also elicits an acute inflammatory response as evidenced by the activation of neutrophils, which in turn releases reactive oxygen species. The reactive oxygen species affects cellular function as well as cytotoxic proteins.[37]

Bacterial colonization can occur as early as 48 hours in an open wound.[38] Anaerobic bacteria also colonize these wounds. Enzymes released by bacteria break down protein that could otherwise aid wound healing.[36] Fluids from chronic wounds exhibit increased protease levels and proinflammatory cytokine levels as well as decreased levels of growth factors.[38] An impaired healing response in older adults with pressure ulcers may be a result of the interplay among several intrinsic and extrinsic factors including ischemic and oxidant stress, metabolic disruptions, prolonged application of uneven pressure to tissue, and exposure to shearing forces and friction.[38,39]

Table 34.2. Pressure Ulcer Risk Factors and Correlates

Intrinsic Risk Factors and Correlates

    Immobility or reduced mobility[42,82]

    Sensory impairment[42,82]

    Acute illness[82]

    Level of consciousness[82]

    Vascular disease[82]

    Severe or chronic illness or terminal illness[82]

    History of pressure ulcers[82]

    Malnutrition and dehydration[42,82]

    Moisture/Incontinence[42,83]

    Race[25]

    Dry skin[54]

Extrinsic Risk Factors and Correlates

    Shearing forces[42]

    RN staffing levels[11]

    Intraoperative factors – hypothermia, support surface[39]

The intraoperative phase has been investigated as a time of potential tissue damage. Several factors may place tissue at risk. These include 1) hypothermia, which may lead to hypoxia and reduced oxygen skin tension; 2) decreases in blood pressure, and thus blood flow to tissue under pressure during anesthesia; 3) surgical trauma; and 4) surgical positioning that prolongs uneven pressure on body parts.[39]

Risk Factors and Correlates

Many risk factors for the development of pressure ulcers have been identified. These include immobility or reduced mobility, sensory impairment, acute illness or trauma, alteration in level of consciousness, vascular disease, history of pressure ulcers, malnutrition, dehydration, and excessive moisture on the skin such as incontinence. See Table 34.2 for a list of risk factors and correlates. In neurologically impaired patients, increased sacral temperature has also been identified as a predictor of pressure ulcers in the sacral area with the sacral temperature increasing by 1.2°C in the 24–96 hours before the pressure ulcer develops.[40] Researchers conducting this study also noted that measurement of sacral temperature could help clinicians detect tissue damage in darkly pigmented skin.

Factors related to pressure ulcer prevalence extrinsic to the human organism include nursing staff levels and staff skill mix.[41] The exact mechanism of the effect of skills mix on patient outcomes and quality of care is not completely understood but registered nurse supervision is assumed to improve implementation of prevention interventions. In another study, increased time spent by registered nurses in direct care in nursing homes also led to decreased pressure ulcer development.[11]

BRADEN SCALE FOR PREDICTING PRESSURE SORE RISK

Patient's Name _____ Evaluator's Name _____ Date of Assessment

SENSORY PERCEPTION ability to respond meaningfully to pressure-related discomfort	**1. Completely Limited** Unresponsive (does not moan, flinch, or grasp) to painful stimuli, due to diminished level of con-sciousness or sedation. OR limited ability to feel pain over most of body	**2. Very Limited** Responds only to painful stimuli. Cannot communicate discomfort except by moaning or restlessness OR has a sensory impairment which limits the ability to feel pain or discomfort over 1/2 of body.	**3. Slightly Limited** Responds to verbal commands, but cannot always communicate discomfort or the need to be turned. OR has some sensory impairment which limits ability to feel pain or discomfort in 1 or 2 extremities.	**4. No Impairment** Responds to verbal commands. Has no sensory deficit which would limit ability to feel or voice pain or discomfort.
MOISTURE degree to which skin is exposed to moisture	**1. Constantly Moist** Skin is kept moist almost constantly by perspiration, urine, etc. Dampness is detected every time patient is moved or turned.	**2. Very Moist** Skin is often, but not always moist. Linen must be changed at least once a shift.	**3. Occasionally Moist:** Skin is occasionally moist, requiring an extra linen change approximately once a day.	**4. Rarely Moist** Skin is usually dry, linen only requires changing at routine intervals.
ACTIVITY degree of physical activity	**1. Bedfast** Confined to bed.	**2. Chairfast** Ability to walk severely limited or non-existent. Cannot bear own weight and/or must be assisted into chair or wheelchair.	**3. Walks Occasionally** Walks occasionally during day, but for very short distances, with or without assistance. Spends majority of each shift in bed or chair	**4. Walks Frequently** Walks outside room at least twice a day and inside room at least once every two hours during waking hours
MOBILITY ability to change and control body position	**1. Completely Immobile** Does not make even slight changes in body or extremity position without assistance	**2. Very Limited** Makes occasional slight changes in body or extremity position but unable to make frequent or significant changes independently.	**3. Slightly Limited** Makes frequent though slight changes in body or extremity position independently.	**4. No Limitation** Makes major and frequent changes in position without assistance.
NUTRITION <u>usual</u> food intake pattern	**1. Very Poor** Never eats a complete meal. Rarely eats more than 1/3 of any food offered. Eats 2 servings or less of protein (meat or dairy products) per day. Takes fluids poorly. Does not take a liquid dietary supplement OR is NPO and/or maintained on clear liquids or IV's for more than 5 days.	**2. Probably Inadequate** Rarely eats a complete meal and generally eats only about 1/2 of any food offered. Protein intake includes only 3 servings of meat or dairy products per day. Occasionally will take a dietary supplement. OR receives less than optimum amount of liquid diet or tube feeding	**3. Adequate** Eats over half of most meals. Eats a total of 4 servings of protein (meat, dairy products per day. Occasionally will refuse a meal, but will usually take a supplement when offered OR is on a tube feeding or TPN regimen which probably meets most of nutritional needs	**4. Excellent** Eats most of every meal. Never refuses a meal. Usually eats a total of 4 or more servings of meat and dairy products. Occasionally eats between meals. Does not require supplementation.
FRICTION & SHEAR	**1. Problem** Requires moderate to maximum assistance in moving. Complete lifting without sliding against sheets is impossible. Frequently slides down in bed or chair, requiring frequent repositioning with maximum assistance. Spasticity, contractures or agitation leads to almost constant friction	**2. Potential Problem** Moves feebly or requires minimum assistance. During a move skin probably slides to some extent against sheets, chair, restraints or other devices. Maintains relatively good position in chair or bed most of the time but occasionally slides down.	**3. No Apparent Problem** Moves in bed and in chair independently and has sufficient muscle strength to lift up completely during move. Maintains good position in bed or chair.	

Total Score

Figure 34.2. Braden scale.

Prevention of Pressure Ulcers

Screening patients at risk for the development of pressure ulcers is central to patient care. A widely used screening tool, the Braden scale, has six subscales that measure sensory perception level, skin moisture, level of physical activity, mobility, nutrition, friction, and shear.[42] This scale was not designed to be used perioperatively or as a method to evaluate pressure ulcer healing.[43] The sensitivity and specificity of this scale are 57.1% and 67.5%, respectively.[44] Scores on the Braden scale range from 6 to 23 and the lower the score the higher the risk of pressure ulcer development.[42] This tool has high interrater reliability for registered nurses (Pearson r = 0.99, agreement 88%).[42] Although the tool tends to overpredict pressure ulcer risk,[45] the assignment of risks is as follows: 19–23 not at risk, 15–18 mild risk, 13–14 moderate risk, 10–12 high risk, and a score of 9 or lower indicates very high risk.[42] In people of color, a score of 18 or below on the Braden scale was accu-

rate in predicting pressure ulcers.[46] See Figure 34.2 for the Braden scale. A systematic literature review concluded that the Braden scale offers the best balance between sensitivity and specificity. The Braden scale and the Norton scale (a scale that measures five domains: physical condition, mental condition, activity, mobility, and incontinence) are highly correlated, 0.73 using the kappa statistic,[47] and are more accurate than clinical judgment alone in predicting pressure ulcer development.[44] In home health agencies, clinical judgment was the most commonly used method to assess pressure ulcer risk; only 21% of home health agencies used a validated assessment tool, thus at risk patients may have been missed by agencies that rely on clinical judgment.[48]

Because identification of at risk individuals is the first step in the prevention, use of an evidence-based, systematic approach to patients is essential. Adherence to published pressure ulcer guidelines has been lacking in nursing homes. The highest implementation rate for a guideline element was 61%

performance of a standardized risk assessment for pressure ulcers.[49] In the past, few nursing homes have used validated assessment tools.[50] The Resident Assessment Protocol, however, identifies intrinsic risk factors, information about skin condition, and other factors that can increase the risk of developing a pressure ulcer.[51] In addition risk factors that may be modifiable or removable should be identified using this instrument.

People who sit for long periods of time may not be able to shift their position and an increased risk of pressure ulcer development exists for this population.[52] A validated tool, the Wheelchair Seating Discomfort Assessment tool, consists of 31 items, is self-administered, and takes approximately 5 minutes to complete. This tool helps to assess discomfort from seating and the location and intensity of the discomfort in individuals with sensation who sit for 8 hours or more.[53] Thus, it may be useful in helping to identify individuals experiencing discomfort and providing them assistance to alleviate that discomfort.

A systematic review of literature on prevention of pressure ulcers found that repositioning the individual, use of supportive surfaces, optimizing nutritional status, and moisturizing the sacral area are promising prevention interventions.[54]

Repositioning is considered the cornerstone of pressure ulcer prevention because repositioning relieves or eliminates interface pressure for the maintenance of microcirculation. A turning schedule of every 2 hours is recommended.[54] Support surfaces, such as mattresses, pads and cushions, relieve pressure exerted on subcutaneous tissues by body weight when the body part presses against a chair or bed's surface. These support surfaces may be static (like a mattress) or dynamic (whereby pressure under the body is varied mechanically). The use of doughnut cushions for sitting patients is not recommended.[55]

Although evidence is limited, impaired nutritional status should be improved through nutritional supplements to help prevent the development of pressure ulcers. Sacral dryness is a risk factor for pressure ulcer development and moisturizers are a relatively inexpensive, therefore application of moisturizers to the sacral area is recommended.[54]

Treatment of Pressure Ulcers

Many clinical guidelines are available for the prevention and treatment of pressure ulcers. The National Guideline Clearinghouse provides a comprehensive listing at its website: www.guideline.gov. The American Medical Directors Association (AMDA website: www.amda.com) guidelines on pressure ulcers include the following recommendations. 1) *Recognition* of pressure ulcers by determining the history of pressure ulcers, identifying pressure ulcers through a skin inspection, documenting presence of a pressure ulcer, and administering a risk assessment tool such as the Braden scale. Consideration of risk factors and comorbidities that may contribute to the risk of pressure ulcer development should occur as well. 2) *Diagnosis* of a pressure ulcer by using a classification system with weekly reassessments. 3) *Treatment* involving a multidisciplinary team

and including the prevention of further pressure ulcer development and specific interventions for stage II–stage IV pressure ulcers.[56]

As with prevention of pressure ulcers, repositioning to relieve pressure over bony prominences is a cornerstone of pressure ulcer treatment. Protection from pressure by keeping the head of the bed at lowest degree of elevation to avoid shearing and friction may prevent further pressure ulcer development.

The maintenance of a clean wound base is important for healing. The goal is to create an environment for healing to occur. Nonirritating, neutral cleansers with minimal trauma via mechanical or chemical means should be used.[55] Initially debridement may include removal of necrotic material via mechanical, enzymatic, or surgical means. Mechanical removal occurs through wet-to-dry dressings, wound irrigation, or whirlpool.[55] Enzymatic debridement involves the application of a dressing that allows exogenous enzymes to remove necrotic material.[55] Because dry skin can increase the risk of pressure ulcer development, application of moisture to maintain moisture balance is considered important.[55] Surgical debridement is indicated for timely removal of necrotic tissue.[57]

In one study, the application of a body wash and skin protectant was found to significantly reduce the incidence of stage I and stage II pressure ulcers when these products were incorporated into skin care protocols.[58] The use of moist dressings to remove slough and nutritional supplementation that ensures 30 kcal/kg of body weight in long-term care has been found to be effective in promoting wound healing for stage II, stage III, and stage IV pressure ulcers.[43] A systematic review was conducted to investigate the comparative efficacy of various pressure ulcer wound cleaning solutions but no evidence to support a specific wound cleansing solution or technique was found.[59]

For stage II–stage IV pressure ulcers, provision of a moist dressing promotes the division and migration of dermal and epidermal cells across the wound surface, thus enhancing healing.[60] Many types of dressings are used for this function including those that are films, foams, hydrogels, and collagen dressings. Dressings are classified into two broad categories. A wound contact dressing is placed into the wound and the wound's depth, presence of undermined areas, and volume of exudate are considered in the dressing selection. The other category is cover dressings. These dressings are flat and are placed over the wound.[61] See Table 34.3 for discussion of dressing types. The important principle for dressings is the maintenance of a protected moist environment in the wound.[55] A guideline for pressure ulcer treatment recommends dressings that minimize additional pressure, shear, friction, and skin irritation.[55]

Infection is a frequent complication for pressure ulcers and will undermine healing. Debridement remains an important goal to remove necrotic and bacteria-laden tissue to create a wound base for healing. Evidence exists that systemic antibiotics do not decrease wound bacterial levels.[55] Antibiotic administration should rely on wound culture determination. In

Table 34.3. Options for Pressure Ulcer Dressings

Pressure Ulcer Type*	Description	Objective	Options
Shallow (stage II)	Dry with no to minimal exudate	Create or retain moisture; protect from infection	Cover with transparent film, thin hydrocolloid, or thin polyurethane foam
			Wrap with nonadherent gauze dressing
	Wet with moderate to large exudate	Absorb exudates, facilitate autolysis, maintain moisture, protect from infection	Cover with alginates, hydrocolloid with or without paste or powder, or polyurethane form
			Wrap with gauze dressing or absorptive contact layer
Deep (stages III and IV)	Dry, with no to minimal exudate	Fill cavities, create or maintain moisture, protect from infection	Fill with hydrocolloid hydrogel or damp gauze
			Cover with transparent thin film, polyurethane foam, or gauze pad
	Wet, with moderate to large exudate	Fill cavities, absorb exudates, maintain moisture, protect from infection	Fill with hydrocolloid paste, calcium alginates, hydrofibers, or foam
			Cover with transparent thin film, polyurethane foam

* Dressings are not usually needed for stage I pressure ulcers.

cases of suspected osteomyelitis, magnetic resonance imaging should be performed. In a recent meta-analysis, magnetic resonance imaging was found superior to white blood cell counts, plain radiography, and Technetium-99m bone scanning.[62]

For nonhealing pressure ulcers at stage II, stage III, and stage IV, topical negative pressure techniques have been used. Negative pressure has also been called subatmospheric pressure, vacuum-assisted wound closing, vacuum pack, and sealed-surface wound suction.[60] With topical negative pressure dressings suction is created to draw off fluids from the wound surface. The goal of this technique is to provide protection against contamination and a physiological milieu that promotes healing.[63] A systematic research review found weak evidence for topical negative pressure as opposed to saline dressings in healing wounds.[60]

Surgical treatment is the final treatment of choice for a nonhealing wound. The goals of the surgical procedure include healing of the wound or definitive closure of the wound.[55] The principle underlying surgical procedures that lead to wound healing by exploring, unroofing, and treating sinuses or cavities is that tissue not exposed to treatment agents cannot respond to these therapeutic agents.[55] The principle for surgical procedures to provide wound closure is pressure reduction. Bony prominences and fibrotic bursa cavities are removed so soft tissue compression is eliminated.[55]

Pressure Redistribution Interventions

Relieving and redistributing pressure is the cornerstone to any pressure ulcer prevention and management program. One goal in pressure ulcer prevention includes reducing the magnitude and duration of pressure between the person and the body-supporting surface. The NPUAP defined a support surface as,

"a specialized device for pressure redistribution designed for the management of tissue loads, microclimate, and/or other therapeutic functions (i.e., any mattresses, integrated bed systems, mattress replacements, overlays, or seat cushions or seat cushion overlays)."[64] Two pressure redistribution mechanisms are used to relieve pressure. One involves devices designed to distribute pressure over a large area. These include mattresses, cushions, and specialized beds. Another mechanism involves devices that apply alternating pressure. See Table 34.4 for features of support surfaces. Devices that alternate pressure include mattresses and overlays. Evidence from a meta-analysis indicates that patients lying on ordinary foam mattresses were more likely to develop pressure ulcers than those lying on a higher specification mattress.[21] The range of costs for these products varies considerably.

Nutritional Intervention

Little systematic evidence exists on the effectiveness of enteral and parenteral nutrition on the prevention of pressure ulcers.[65] Several nutritional guidelines are available and they generally include recommendations for conducting a nutritional assessment, which includes weighing the patient, reviewing food and fluid intake, and investigating unexplained weight loss. Other recommendations include recognizing the effects of malnutrition, correcting an underfed status by designing a diet based on 35 kcal/kg, 1.0–1.5 g/kg of protein and 1 mL/kcal of fluids, and evaluating the effects of a nutritional intervention.[66] High-protein oral nutritional supplements were found effective in reducing the risk of pressure ulcer development[67] and in pressure ulcer healing.[68] Little high-quality research is available to guide clinical practice including providing vitamin C supplementation to promote wound healing.[69] No evidence from

Table 34.4. Features of Support Surfaces

Support Surfaces	Definitions
Air fluidized	A feature of a support surface that provides pressure redistribution via a fluidlike medium created by forcing air through beads as characterized by immersion and envelopment.
Alternating pressure	A feature of a support surface that provides pressure redistribution via cyclic changes in loading *and unloading* as characterized by frequency, duration, amplitude, and rate of change parameters.
Lateral rotation	A feature of a support surface that provides rotation about a longitudinal axis as characterized by degree of patient turn, duration, and frequency.
Low air loss	A feature of a support surface that provides a flow of air to assist in managing the heat and humidity (microclimate) of the skin.
Zone	A segment with a single pressure redistribution capability.
Multizoned surface	A surface on which different segments can have different pressure redistribution capabilities.

randomized clinical trials exists that dietary zinc supplementation is effective in promoting wound healing.[70] Limited evidence exists that for some people nutritional support via tube feeding achieves positive nitrogen balance may be indicated.[55]

Other Therapies

Electromagnetic therapy for pressure ulcer treatment has been studied, although a systematic review concluded that at present no evidence exists supporting the benefit of this therapy.[71] The use of therapeutic ultrasound for pressure ulcer healing has also been investigated and no systematic evidence exists regarding the benefits of this treatment. The authors of both systematic reviews noted that further research is needed.[72]

Results of a meta-analysis on the use of electrical stimulation on chronic wound healing indicated that increased wound healing occurred. The proposed mechanism of electrical stimulation on healing is that it restarts or accelerates wound healing by stimulating fibroblasts and increasing the migration of neutrophils and macrophages.[73]

Surgical closure of pressure ulcers is indicated when bacterial colonization is less than 10^5 colonies, albumin level of greater than 3.5 g/mL, and risk of recurrence is minimal.[74] Flap reconstruction is performed for stage III and IV pressure ulcers. Few data are available to evaluate the long-term patient outcomes of this intervention.

Pain Management

People with pressure ulcers experience acute and chronic pain from these wounds. Words patients use to describe pain from

a pressure ulcer include: burning, shooting, sharp, aching, cutting, and hot.[75] Pain is caused by irritation of nerve endings in and around the pressure ulcer.[34] Pain is also caused by pressure ulcer treatment such as debridement or pressure applied to the wound from dressings.[34] Many times pain is not addressed as a part of wound care in hospitalized patients, and differences in pain levels are observed in racial groups with nonwhites reporting more pain.[76] Thus, pain should be assessed using a validated tool such as the McGill Pain Scale and treated prior to dressing changes or other treatment interventions including repositioning and pressure relief.

Pain is a recurrent theme in the lives of many people with pressure ulcers.[5] Pain may be from the wound itself, but also from dressing changes and the technique of the caregiver doing the dressing change.[77] To relieve pain, the affected person may reduce movement and mobility,[5] thus compounding the risks of immobility to skin and other tissues. Because pressure ulcer pain may not respond well to oral analgesia, topical treatment has been tested.[34] In a small pilot study with hospice patients, diamorphine gel was applied to the pressure ulcer daily and when compared with a placebo gel, it provided statistically significant pain relief in 1–2 hours after its application.[78] Dutch researchers found strong evidence for the effectiveness of diamorphine gel, benzydamine gel, and eutectic mixture of local anaesthetic-cream for pressure ulcer pain relief.[34]

End-of-Life Interventions

At the time of their death, 24% of Americans have a stage II or higher pressure ulcer.[7] Despite best care practices, intractable pressure ulcers may occur and are considered part of the dying process.[7] A pear-shaped pressure ulcer with irregular borders may appear on the sacrum in the late stages of the dying process.[79] Because wound healing is not the goal and it is not feasible for a person close to death, dressings that alleviate pain and cause little discomfort should be used to cover the wound. The goals of palliative wound care are symptom management and improvement of the quality of life.[79] Support of family caregivers is especially important as they may believe that pressure ulcers are a sign of neglect. Family members may need assistance to understand the stages of the dying process and accept that care activities change according to the stages. When death is imminent, repositioning to prevent pressure ulcers and food and oral fluids to sustain life may be discontinued. Measures to maximize dignity and comfort should continue until death occurs.

Interdisciplinary Team Approach

The prevention and the treatment of pressure ulcers are complex interventions requiring the expertise of multiple disciplines. Some health care organizations have adopted the six sigma approach.[77] This approach, originally developed by Motorola, aims to improve productivity, profitability, and quality. The six sigma process includes five phases: defining the problem, measuring performance, analyzing the problem to uncover root causes, improving the situation, and providing for sustainability of improvements in operations.[80] Thus, the inclusion of several disciplines is necessary.[57] Quality improvement initiatives in nursing homes have demonstrated that the incidence of stage III and stage IV pressure ulcers can be reduced.[81]

Primary or consultative medical management by physicians, nurse practitioners, or physician assistants of comorbid conditions such as diabetes mellitus and circulatory diseases to achieve maximal disease and symptom control is needed. Nutritionists, nurses, and rehabilitation specialists provide key expertise to create a comprehensive care plan. In addition, surgeons may be needed to perform debridement, and infectious disease specialists may be needed to provide aggressive treatment of deep infections.[57]

Communication among clinicians, other health care professionals, and family caregivers about the goal and expected outcomes of treatment interventions is essential in the implementation and evaluation of successful interdisciplinary care.

Summary and Conclusions

The complex interactions between intrinsic and extrinsic factors that lead to pressure ulcer development are becoming better understood. Promotion of good skin health and prevention of pressure ulcers remain essential to reducing the impact of pressure ulcers on the health and well-being of older adults. Education of health care providers, patients, and family members is necessary to change and maintain practice standards that optimize patient outcomes. Research that includes standardized definitions, rigorous methods, and adequate sample sizes is needed to expand the existing foundation of knowledge regarding pressure ulcer prevention, treatment, and management in all health care settings.

REFERENCES

1. Harris S. Reeve's Death Highlights Dangers of Bedsores. The Hilltop Online. Available at: http://media.www.thehilltoponline.com/media/storage/paper590/news/2004/10/29/LifeStyle/Reeves.Death.Highlights.Dangers.Of.Bedsores-786421.shtml. Accessed June 13, 2008.
2. Redelings MD, Lee NE, Sorvillo F. Pressure ulcers: more lethal than we thought? *Adv Skin Wound Care.* 2005;18:367–372.
3. National Pressure Ulcer Advisory Panel, National Pressure Ulcer Advisory Board. Pressure ulcers in America: prevalence, incidence, and implications for the future. An executive summary of the National Pressure Ulcer Advisory Panel monograph. *Adv Skin Wound Care.* 2001;14:208–215.
4. Beckrich K, Aronovitch SA. Hospital-acquired pressure ulcers: a comparison of costs in medical vs. surgical patients. *Nurs Econ.* 1999;17:263–271.
5. Hopkins A, Dealey C, Bale S, Defloor T, Worboys F. Patient stories of living with a pressure ulcer. *J Adv Nurs.* 2006;56:345–353.
6. Maklebust J. Pressure ulcers: the great insult. *Nurs Clin North Am.* 2005;40:365–389.
7. MacLean D. Preventing & managing pressure sores. Caring for the ages volume. *Caring for the Ages,* 2003;4(3):34–37.
8. Office of Disease Prevention and Health Promotion. Healthy People 2010 Available at: http://www.healthypeople.gov. Accessed June 13, 2008.
9. Langemo DK, Brown G. Skin fails too: acute, chronic, and end-stage skin failure. *Adv Skin Wound Care.* 2006;19:206–211.
10. Bansal C, Scott R, Stewart D, Cockerell CJ. Decubitus ulcers: a review of the literature. *Int J Dermatol.* 2005;44:805–810.
11. Horn SD, Buerhaus P, Bergstrom N, Smout RJ. RN staffing time and outcomes of long-stay nursing home residents: pressure ulcers and other adverse outcomes are less likely as RNs spend more time on direct patient care. *Am J Nurs.* 2005;105:58–70; quiz 71.
12. Hart S, Bergquist S, Gajewski B, Dunton N. Reliability testing of the National Database of Nursing Quality Indicators pressure ulcer indicator. *J Nurs Care Qual.* 2006;21:256–265.
13. CMS Manual System: Publication 100–07 State Operations Provider Certification, D.o.H.H. Services, Editor. 2004:Nov.12., Centers for Medicare & Medicaid Services. Available at: www.cms.hhs.gov/SurveyCertificationGenInfo/downloads/SCLetter05-17.pdf.
14. Levine JM. Historical notes on pressure ulcers: the cure of Ambrose Pare. *Decubitus.* 1992;5:23–24, 26.
15. Levine JM. Historical perspective on pressure ulcers: the decubitus ominosus of Jean-Martin Charcot. *J Am Geriatr Soc.* 2005;53:1248–1251.
16. National Pressure Ulcers Advisory Panel. Pressure Ulcer Stages, 2007. Available at: http://www.npuap.org. Accessed June 13, 2008.
17. Vanderwee K, Grypdonck MH, De Bacquer D, Defloor T. The reliability of two observation methods of nonblanchable erythema, Grade 1 pressure ulcer. *Appl Nurs Res.* 2006;19:156–162.
18. Nixon J, Cranny G, Bond S. Skin alterations of intact skin and risk factors associated with pressure ulcer development in surgical patients: a cohort study. *Int J Nurs Stud.* 2007;44(5):655–663. Epub 2006 Apr 24.
19. Ankrom MA, Bennett RG, Sprigle S, et al. Pressure-related deep tissue injury under intact skin and the current pressure ulcer staging systems. *Adv Skin Wound Care.* 2005;18:35–42.
20. Lahmann N, Halfens RJ, Dassen T. Effect of non-response bias in pressure ulcer prevalence studies. *J Adv Nurs.* 2006;55:230–236.
21. National Pressure Ulcer Advisory Panel. Pressure ulcers in America: prevalence, incidence, and implications for the future. An executive summary of the National Pressure Ulcer Advisory Panel monograph. *Adv Skin Wound Care.* 2001;14:208–215.
22. Bergstrom N. The Braden scale for predicting pressure sore risk: reflections on the perioperative period. *J Wound Ostomy Continence Nurs.* 2005;32:79–80.
23. Whittington KT, Briones R. National Prevalence and Incidence Study: 6-year sequential acute care data. *Adv Skin Wound Care.* 2004;17:490–494.
24. Baumgarten M, Margolis DJ, Localio AR, et al. Pressure ulcers among elderly patients early in the hospital stay. *J Gerontol A Biol Sci Med Sci.* 2006;61:749–754.
25. Baumgarten M, Margolis D, van Doorn C, et al. Black/White differences in pressure ulcer incidence in nursing home residents. *J Am Geriatr Soc.* 2004;52:1293–1298.
26. Rosen J, Mittal V, Degenholtz H, et al. Pressure ulcer prevention in black and white nursing home residents: a QI initiative of enhanced ability, incentives, and management feedback. *Adv Skin Wound Care.* 2006;19:262–268.

27. Gunningberg L. EPUAP Pressure Ulcer Prevalence Survey in Sweden: a two-year follow-up of quality indicators. *J Wound Ostomy Continence Nurs.* 2006;33:258–266.

28. Horn SD, Bender SA, Ferguson ML, et al. The National Pressure Ulcer Long-Term Care Study: pressure ulcer development in long-term care residents. *J Am Geriatr Soc.* 2004;52:359–367.

29. Houwing R, Rozendaal M, Wouters-Wesseling W, et al. Pressure ulcer risk in hip fracture patients. *Acta Orthop Scand.* 2004; 75:390–393.

30. Stotts NA, Rodeheaver GT, Thomas DR, et al. An instrument to measure healing in pressure ulcers: development and validation of the pressure ulcer scale for healing (PUSH). *J Gerontol A Biol Sci Med Sci.* 2001;56:M795–M799.

31. NPUAP, NPAB. The Facts about Reverse Staging in 2000. 2000.cited 2006 December 21]; Available from: www.woundsupport.com/docs/HTML/education/documents/Facts_about_Reverse_Staging_in_2000.pdf.

32. Allman RM, Goode PS, Burst N, Bartolucci AA, Thomas DR. Pressure ulcers, hospital complications, and disease severity: impact on hospital costs and length of stay. *Adv Wound Care.* 1999;12:22–30.

33. Freeman K, Smyth C, Dallam L, Jackson B. Pain measurement scales: a comparison of the visual analogue and faces rating scales in measuring pressure ulcer pain. *J Wound Ostomy Continence Nurs.* 2001;28:290–296.

34. de Laat EH, Scholte op Reimer WJ, van Achterberg T. Pressure ulcers: diagnostics and interventions aimed at wound-related complaints: a review of the literature. *J Clin Nurs.* 2005;14:464–472.

35. Lyder CH. Pressure ulcer prevention and management. *JAMA.* 2003;289:223–226.

36. Gupta S, Baharestani M, Baranoski S, et al. Guidelines for managing pressure ulcers with negative pressure wound therapy. *Adv Skin Wound Care.* 2004;17(Suppl 2):1–16.

37. Sener G, Sert G, Ozer Sehirli A, et al. Melatonin protects against pressure ulcer-induced oxidative injury of the skin and remote organs in rats. *J Pineal Res.* 2006;40:280–287.

38. Mustoe TA, O'Shaughnessy K, Kloeters, O. Chronic wound pathogenesis and current treatment strategies: a unifying hypothesis. *Plast Reconstr Surg.* 2006;117(7 Suppl):35S–41S.

39. Scott EM, Buckland R. Pressure ulcer risk in the peri-operative environment. *Nurs Stand.* 2005;20:74, 76, 78 passim.

40. Sae-Sia W, Wipke-Tevis DD, Williams DA. Elevated sacral skin temperature (T(s)): a risk factor for pressure ulcer development in hospitalized neurologically impaired Thai patients. *Appl Nurs Res.* 2005;18:29–35.

41. Dellefield ME. Organizational correlates of the risk-adjusted pressure ulcer prevalence and subsequent survey deficiency citation in California nursing homes. *Res Nurs Health.* 2006;29:345–358.

42. Braden BJ, Maklebust J. Preventing pressure ulcers with the Braden scale: an update on this easy-to-use tool that assesses a patient's risk. *Am J Nurs.* 2005;105:70–72.

43. Bergstrom N, Horn SD, Smout RJ, et al. The National Pressure Ulcer Long-Term Care Study: outcomes of pressure ulcer treatments in long-term care. *J Am Geriatr Soc.* 2005;53:1721–1729.

44. Pancorbo-Hidalgo PL, Garcia-Fernandez FP, Lopez-Medina IM, Alvarez-Nieto C. Risk assessment scales for pressure ulcer prevention: a systematic review. *J Adv Nurs.* 2006;54:94–110.

45. Brown SJ, The Braden Scale. A review of the research evidence. *Orthop Nurs.* 2004;23:30–38.

46. Maklebust J, Sieggreen MY, Sidor D, et al. Computer-based testing of the Braden Scale for Predicting Pressure Sore Risk. *Ostomy Wound Manage.* 2005;51:40–42, 44, 46 passim.

47. Agostini JV, Baker DI, Bogardus ST. *Prevention of Pressure Ulcers in Older Patients, in Making Health Care Safer: A Critical Analysis of Patient Safety Practices.* Shojania KG, Duncan BW, McDonald KM, Wachter RM, eds. Evidence Report/ Technology Assessment No. 43, AHRQ Publication No. 01-E058, July 2001:301–306.

48. Bergquist S. The quality of pressure ulcer prediction and prevention in home health care. *Appl Nurs Res.* 2005;18:148–154.

49. Saliba D, Rubenstein LV, Simon B, et al. Adherence to pressure ulcer prevention guidelines: implications for nursing home quality. *J Am Geriatr Soc.* 2003;51:56–62.

50. Wipke-Tevis DD, Williams DA, Rantz MJ, et al. Nursing home quality and pressure ulcer prevention and management practices. *J Am Geriatr Soc.* 2004;52:583–588.

51. Mor V. A comprehensive clinical assessment tool to inform policy and practice. Applications of the minimum data set. *Med Care.* 2004;42(4 Suppl):III50–III59.

52. Anton L. Pressure ulcer prevention in older people who sit for long periods. *Nurs Older People.* 2006;18(4):29–35.

53. Crane BA, Holm MB, Hobson D, et al. Test-retest reliability, internal item consistency, and concurrent validity of the wheelchair seating discomfort assessment tool. *Assist Technol.* 2005;17:98–107.

54. Reddy M, Gill SS, Rochon PA. Preventing pressure ulcers: a systematic review. *JAMA.* 2006;296:974–984.

55. Whitney J, Phillips L, Aslam R, et al. Guidelines for the treatment of pressure ulcers. *Wound Repair Regen.* 2006;14:663–679.

56. American Medical Directors Association (AMDA) Clinical Practice Guidelines. Pressure Ulcers. Columbia, MD: American Medical Directors Association; 1996:16.

57. Niezgoda JA, Mendez-Eastman S. The effective management of pressure ulcers. *Adv Skin Wound Care.* 2006;19(Suppl 1):3–15.

58. Thompson P, Langemo D, Anderson J, Hanson D, Hunter S. Skin care protocols for pressure ulcers and incontinence in long-term care: a quasi-experimental study. *Adv Skin Wound Care.* 2005;18:422–429.

59. Moore ZE, Cowman S. Wound cleansing for pressure ulcers. *Cochrane Database Syst Rev.* 2005;4:CD004983.

60. Evans D, Land L. Topical negative pressure for treating chronic wounds. *Cochrane Database Syst Rev.* 2001;1:CD001898, DOI: 10.1002/14651858.CD001898.

61. Doughty D. Dressings and more: guidelines for topical wound management. *Nurs Clin North Am.* 2005;40:217–231.

62. Kapoor A, Page S, Lavalley M, Gale DR, Felson DT. Magnetic resonance imaging for diagnosing foot osteomyelitis: a meta-analysis. *Arch Intern Med.* 2007;167:125–132.

63. Fette A. Treatment of pressure ulcers with topical negative pressure versus traditional wound management methods: a research sampler. *Plast Surg Nurs.* 2005;25:176–180.

64. NPUAP, N P A B (2006) Support Surface Standards Initiative: Terms and Definitions. Available at www.npuap.org/PDF/NPUAP%20S3I%20Terms%20and%20Definitions%5B1%5D.pdf

65. Langer G, Knerr A, Kuss O, Behrens, J, and Schlomer GJ. Nutritional interventions for preventing and treating pressure ulcers. *Cochrane Database Syst Rev.* 2003;4:CD001735. DOI: 10.1002/14651858.CD001735.pub2.

66. Schols JM, de Jager-v d Ende MA. Nutritional intervention in pressure ulcer guidelines: an inventory. *Nutrition.* 2004;20:548–553.

67. Stratton RJ, Ek AC, Engfer M, et al. Enteral nutritional support in prevention and treatment of pressure ulcers: a systematic review and meta-analysis. *Ageing Res Rev.* 2005;4:422–450.

68. Lee SK, Posthauer ME, Dorner B, Redovian V, Maloney MJ. Pressure ulcer healing with a concentrated, fortified, collagen protein hydrolysate supplement: a randomized controlled trial. *Adv Skin Wound Care*. 2006;19:92–96.

69. Gray M, Whitney JD. Does vitamin C supplementation promote pressure ulcer healing? J Wound Ostomy Continence Nurs. 2003;30:245–249.

70. NPUAP, N P A B. Nutritional Support for Patients. Question # 501 What is the role of nutritional support for patients in the preventions and treatment of pressure ulcers? Frequently Asked Questions.cited 2006 December 21]; Available from: www.ame-medical.com/faq_pressure_ulcers.pdf

71. Olyaee Manesh A, Fleming K, Cullum NA, and Ravaghi H. Electromagnetic therapy for treating pressure ulcers. *Cochrane Database Syst Rev*. 2006;(2):CD002930. DOI: 10.1002/14651858.CD002930.pub3.

72. Baba-Akbari Sari A, Flemming K, Cullum NA, Wollina U. Therapeutic ultrasound for pressure ulcers. *Cochrane Database Syst Rev*. 2006:CD001275. DOI: 10.1002/14651858.CD001275.pub2.

73. Gardner SE, Frantz RA, Schmidt FL. Effect of electrical stimulation on chronic wound healing: a meta-analysis. *Wound Repair Regen*. 1999;7:495–503.

74. Wilhelmi B, Neumeister M. Pressure Ulcers, Surgical Treatment and Principles. eMedicine from WebMD: http://www.emedicine.com/plastic/topic462.htm

75. Rastinehad, D. Pressure ulcer pain. *J Wound Ostomy Continence Nurs.*2006. 33(3):252–257.

76. Stotts NA, Puntillo K, Bonham Morris A et al. Wound care pain in hospitalized adult patients. *Heart Lung*. 2004;33:321–332.

77. Spilsbury K, Nelson A, Cullum N, et al. Pressure ulcers and their treatment and effects on quality of life: hospital inpatient perspectives. *J Adv Nurs*. 2007;57:494–504.

78. Flock P. Pilot study to determine the effectiveness of diamorphine gel to control pressure ulcer pain. *J Pain Symptom Manage*. 2003;25:547–554.

79. Schim SM, Cullen B. Wound care at end of life. *Nurs Clin North Am*. 2005;40:281–294.

80. Courtney BA, Ruppman JB, Cooper HM. Save our skin: initiative cuts pressure ulcer incidence in half. *Nurs Manage*. 2006;37:36, 38, 40 passim.

81. Lynn J, West J, Hausmann S, et al. Collaborative clinical quality improvement for pressure ulcers in nursing homes. *J Am Geriatr Soc*. 2007; 55(10):1663–1669.

82. NICE, N C C f N a S C, Clinical Guideline 7: Pressure ulcer prevention: pressure ulcer risk assessment and prevention, including the use of pressure-relieving devices (beds, mattresses and overlays) for the prevention of pressure ulcers in primary and secondary care. 2003: October, National Institute for Clinical Excellence. Available at www.nice.org.uk/nicemedia/pdf/CG7_PRD_algorithm.pdf

83. Bergquist S. Subscales, subscores, or summative score: evaluating the contribution of Braden Scale items for predicting pressure ulcer risk in older adults receiving home health care. J Wound Ostomy Continence Nurs. 2001;28:279–289.

35

Anemia and Other Hematological Problems of the Elderly

Inna Sheyner, MD, Karen Travis Stover, MPH, MSN, ARNP, CS

GENERAL OVERVIEW OF ANEMIA IN THE ELDERLY

Definition of Anemia

The word anemia is derived from the Greek language and means "bloodlessness" (an = not; haimia = blood). In 1968, the World Health Organization defined anemia as hemoglobin of less than 13 g/dL in males and hemoglobin less than 12 g/dL in females.[1] Those values are widely used for epidemiological studies. These thresholds may not reliably delineate high and low risks of adverse outcomes in elderly patients. In fact, improved overall health measures generally appear to correlate with higher hemoglobin levels, up to the level of approximately 14 g/dL.[2] Increased risk of mortality and functional impairment in women 65 and older was associated with hemoglobin levels of 13.5 g/dL and lower.[3]

Epidemiology of Anemia in Aging Population

The prevalence of anemia in community-dwelling persons increases with age. In persons between 61 and 75 years of age, the prevalence of anemia is between 8% and 15%. Beyond age 75, the prevalence varies from 16% to 26%.[4] In a group of nearly 4,000 adults older than the age of 70 years, anemia was present in 9% of those aged 71–74 years and in 41% of men and 21% of women older than the age of 90.[5] The prevalence of anemia is even higher in residents in long-term care, affecting 31.4%–49% of nursing home residents.[6]

Aging of the Population

Population aging, the process by which older individuals become a proportionally larger share of the total population, was one of the most distinctive demographic events of the twentieth century. It will remain important throughout the twenty-first century. In the United States individuals aged 65 years and older represents 12% of the population, this proportion is projected to increase to 20% by 2030.[7] Because the prevalence of anemia increases with age,[2] this substantial expansion of the oldest segment of our population has profound implications for public health and preventive and clinical medicine.

Consequences of Anemia in the Elderly

Especially in the elderly, anemia is frequently thought of as a marker for disease rather than a clinical problem in its own right. Recent data, however, indicate that anemia is an independent risk factor for disease-related morbidity, mortality, functional impairment (basic and instrumental activities of daily living), falls, and deterioration in quality of life.[2,8–12] Hypoxia of the brain because of anemia can increase risk of delirium from medications in older individuals with anemia.[13] Risk of dementia has been demonstrated to be higher among patients with anemia, and anemic individuals with normal mental status were more likely than nonanemic patients of the same age to develop dementia over 5 years.[14]

Production of Red Blood Cells

Production of the red blood cells ([RBCs] erythropoiesis) is an orderly process that leads to the production of mature erythrocytes.[15] Trough proliferation and differentiation of stem cells in the bone marrow are driven by a variety of factors (stimulatory and inhibitory) and reticulocytes are released into the circulation. Within 1 day, reticulocytes transition into mature RBCs that circulate for 100–120 days, at which time they are removed from circulation by macrophages in the spleen and other reticuloendothelial tissues.[16] The major positive stimulatory factor is erythropoietin. It is

Table 35.1. Most Common Causes of Anemia in Elder Community Dwellers

1. IDA: 20%
2. ACD: 20%
3. Megaloblastic anemia: 14%
4. Anemia of CKD: 8%
5. Unexplained anemia: 38%

Table 35.2. Most Common Causes of Anemia in Residents of Long-Term Care Institutions

1. IDA: 23%
2. ACD: 18%
3. Anemia of CKD: 6%
4. Myelodysplasia: 5%
5. Unexplained anemia: 45%

produced by the kidney and circulates to the bone marrow where it stimulates erythrocytosis.[17] Several cytokines, such as tumor necrosis factor-α (TNF-α), interferon-γ, and interleukin-6 may induce bone marrow suppression of erythropoiesis and erythropoietin secretion; they also may disrupt iron metabolism.[18,19]

CLASSIFICATIONS OF ANEMIA

Two general approaches can be used to identify the cause of anemia: A kinetic approach based on the direct mechanism responsible for the reduction in hemoglobin level or a morphological approach based on RBC size and reticulocyte response to the reduced hemoglobin level.

1. Kinetic approach
   a. Decreased RBC production (hypoproliferative anemia) because of: absence of nutrients (iron, B12, folate) because of inadequate dietary intake, malabsorption (pernicious anemia, sprue), or iron loss (bleeding), bone marrow disorders (aplastic anemia, pure RBC aplasia, myelodysplasia, tumor infiltration), bone marrow suppression (chemotherapeutic agents and other drugs, irradiation). Reduced level of trophic hormones (erythropoietin in chronic kidney disease (CKD), thyroid hormone in hypothyroidism, and androgens in hypogonadism) AACD (now more commonly referred to as anemia of chronic inflammation)
   b. Increased RBC destruction hemolytic anemia (congenital or acquired)
   c. Blood loss (obvious or occult)
2. Morphological approach
   a. Microcytic anemia (mean corpuscular count [MCV] <80 fL). Three most common causes of microcytosis in clinical practice are iron deficiency, α or β thalassemia minor, and anemia of chronic inflammation
   b. Normocytic anemia (MCV between 80 and 100 fL) can be present in systemic disorders and in anemia of chronic renal disease
   c. Macrocytic anemia (MCV >100 fL) can be present in any condition causing marked reticulocytosis, such as folate or cobalamin deficiency, medications, alcohol

abuse, liver disease, hypothyroidism, myelodysplastic syndrome, and acute leukemia)

Most Common Causes of Anemia in the Elderly

Data from the Third National Health and Nutrition Examination Survey (NHANES III; 1988 to 1994)[4] found that in older community dwellers in the United States, the most common types of anemia were iron deficiency anemia (IDA) and anemia of chronic disease (ACD), with each present in approximately 20% of the population. Other anemias were less prevalent: megaloblastic anemia (14%), chronic kidney disease (8%), and mixed anemia of chronic kidney disease (CKD) and anemia of chronic disease. The prevalence of unexplained anemia was 34% (See Table 35.1.). Other terms used are unspecified anemia or idiopathic anemia. Interest in the causes of unexplained anemia remains high. Most likely numerous factors are involved, including failure of precursor cells coupled with decline in stimulatory factors such as erythropoietin and testosterone in addition to decline in renal functions and low levels of inflammation.

In residents of long-term care institutions, the most common forms of anemia are iron deficiency anemia (23%), anemia of chronic disease (13%), anemia of kidney disease (6%), and myelodysplasia (5%). The cause of anemia was unexplained in 45% of persons (See Table 35.2.).

EVALUATION OF THE ELDERLY PATIENT WITH ANEMIA

Anemia is never normal and every patient with anemia should be evaluated. Different methods and algorithms are available for assessment of anemia in the elderly and the specificity of those methods continues to be debated. In general, the assessment method should be informative, simple, and minimally invasive. The workup should be directed toward answering the following important questions.

- Has there been blood loss (recent or remote)?
- Is there evidence for increased RBC destruction (hemolysis)?
- Is the bone marrow suppressed?
- Is the patient iron deficient? If so, why?

- Is the patient deficient in folic acid or vitamin B-12? If so, why?[20]

The workup should start with a detailed history-taking that should cover several important components.

- History of anemia (recent anemia is almost always an acquired disorder, lifelong anemia is more likely to be a congenital disorder)
- Evidence of bleeding (tarry stools, blood in the urine, vomiting blood, coughing blood)
- Evidence of decreased oxygen delivery, such as dyspnea, decreased functional performance, worsening of congestive heart failure and angina symptoms
- Preexisting medical conditions, which can cause or contribute to anemia
- Complete list of medications including herbal preparations
- Assessment of nutritional status
- History of colonoscopy

The physical examination should be directed toward the severity of the patient's condition and signs of organ or multisystem involvement. Several assessment components (such as heart rate and postural hypotension) can be interpreted incorrectly in the elderly patient due to preexisting orthostatic hypotension and treatment with β blockers.

Although evaluation for pallor and jaundice is a standard part of the physical examination, it may not be very accurate. The sensitivity and specificity for pallor in the palms, nail beds, face, or conjunctivae as predictors for anemia varies from 19% to 70% and from 70% to 100%, respectively.[21,22]

Jaundice may be difficult to detect under artificial (nonfluorescent) lighting conditions and even under optimal conditions it can be missed in as many as 42% of the patients with a total serum bilirubin concentration of 2.5 mg/dL. Lymphadenopathy and splenomegaly could point toward a hematological malignancy. Despite its limitations, the role of the physical examination cannot be underestimated in the evaluation of anemic patients.[23]

Initial Laboratory Evaluation

Initial testing of the anemic patient should start with a complete blood count (CBC). In some medical centers white blood cell (WBC) differential, platelet count, and reticulocyte count are not part of the routine CBC; these may have to be ordered separately.

WBC count and differential can offer clues to the specific abnormality.

- Increased absolute neutrophil count can be present in infection.
- Increased absolute monocyte count can be present in myelodysplasia.
- Increased absolute eosinophil count can be present in certain types of parasitic infections and allergic states.

- Decreased absolute neutrophil count can follow chemotherapy.
- Decreased absolute lymphocyte count can be present in human immunodeficiency virus (HIV) infection or following treatment with corticosteroids.

Neutrophil hypersegmentation (presence of more than 5% of neutrophils with five or more lobes or presence of one or more neutrophils with six or more lobes) is classically associated with impaired DNA synthesis, as seen in disorders of vitamin B12 and folic acid deficiency.

Platelet count can also provide important information. Thrombocytopenia occurs in the variety of disorders associated with anemia, including hypersplenism, marrow involvement with malignancy, autoimmune platelet destruction, sepsis, and folate or vitamin B12 deficiency. High platelet counts may reflect myeloproliferative disease, chronic iron deficiency, inflammatory, infectious, or neoplastic disorders.

Pancytopenia is a combination of anemia, thrombocytopenia, and leukopenia. Presence of pancytopenia narrows the differential diagnosis to disorders such as aplastic anemia, folate or vitamin B12 deficiency or hematological malignancy.

Iron deficiency evaluation is indicated when the history (hematochezia or tarry stools, hematuria, hemoptysis) or preliminary laboratory data (low MCV, low mean corpuscular hemoglobin, high RBC distribution width) support this diagnosis. Determination of serum ferritin is the best screening test for iron deficiency, even though the level can be spuriously elevated by the coexistence of inflammation. Calculation of transferrin saturation was the time honored method to differentiate between iron deficiency and chronic inflammation, but its value is diminished by the multiple other factors that may influence both iron and transferrin level.[19] More recently, the determination of the soluble transferrin receptor has been introduced to assist in the interpretation of ferritin levels of 200 ng/mL or lower. Elevated levels of soluble transferrin receptor are characteristic of iron deficiency anemia (IDA).[24] This test, however, is not yet widely available. Also characteristic of iron deficiency are hypochromic reticulocytes and low reticulocyte hemoglobin.

Hemolysis evaluation should be considered in the patient with a rapid fall in hemoglobin concentration, reticulocytosis, and/or abnormally shaped RBC (spherocytes or fragmented RBCs) on the peripheral smear. Assessment of lactate dehydrogenase (LDH) and haptoglobin levels can assist in the diagnosis. The combination of an increase in LDH and a reduction of haptoglobin is 90% specific for diagnosing hemolysis, whereas the combination of a normal LDH and serum haptoglobin greater than 25 mg/dL is 92% sensitive for ruling out hemolysis.[25]

Bone marrow examination generally offers little additional diagnostic information in the more common forms of anemia. It is an invasive procedure with possible complications such as excessive bleeding, infection, pain, and adverse reaction to the use of intravenous sedation. This procedure should be reserved for patients with an uncertain diagnosis and suspected aplastic anemia, myelodysplasia, bone marrow replacement with malignancy, or myeloproliferative disorder. Another consideration is that in elderly patients, the procedure may be further complicated by comorbid conditions that preclude optimal positioning during the examination.

MOST COMMON FORMS OF ANEMIA IN THE ELDERLY

Iron Deficiency Anemia

One of the most common causes of anemia in the elderly is IDA.[26]

The gold standard for this diagnosis is the presence of decreased iron stores in the bone marrow aspirate.[27]

In iron deficiency, there is a decrease in the amount of iron available for metabolic process. The manifestation of iron deficiency can occur in several stages. First there is depletion of iron stores; therefore, less iron is available for hemoglobin synthesis. Eventually, the iron and hemoglobin deficiencies are so severe that iron-deficient red cell production occurs. Most of the body's iron is stored in the hemoglobin. Approximately 30% of iron is also stored as ferritin and hemosiderin in the bone marrow, spleen, and liver.[28] The main cause of IDA is chronic bleeding from cancer, diverticuli, or angiodysplasia. Gastrointestinal tract abnormality can be identified in more than half of elderly patients with IDA.[29]

In old age iron deficiency may have other causes, including decreased absorption of iron because of achlorhydria,[30] or increased circulating concentration of hepcidin. Hepcidin, a protein synthesized in the liver, whose production is stimulated by interleukin-6, prevents the absorption of iron from the duodenum.[31]

Iron malabsorbtion can also be present in patients with celiac disease and approximately 70% of those with autoimmune atrophic gastritis or *Helicobacter pylori* infection.[32]

The diagnosis of IDA in the elderly is often difficult due to presence of multiple abnormalities.[33] Serum ferritin level is considered the best single test for the diagnosis of iron deficiency because its concentration is proportional to the total body iron stores;[34] however, in the elderly, serum ferritin level is not a reliable test because level increases with age,[35] as well as chronic disorders and malignancy, which are common in the elderly.[36]

Treatment should be directed toward the correction of the cause (bleeding, treatment of the celiac disease or *H. pylori* infection) and/or iron supplementation. If oral absorption is complicated for a variety of reasons, parenteral supplementation should be considered.

Anemia of Chronic Disease

Anemia of chronic disease is the second most prevalent anemia after IDA and occurs in patient with acute or chronic inflammation.[37] The condition has thus been termed "anemia of inflammation."

The hallmark of ACD is the development of disturbance of iron homeostasis, with increased uptake and retention of iron within cells of the reticuloendothelial system and low serum iron levels. This leads to subsequent limitation of iron for adequate erythropoiesis despite normal total body iron.[38]

Inflammatory cytokines (such as interleukin-1, interleukin-6, and TNF-α) can contribute to abnormal iron homeostasis and development of anemia in several ways: by suppression of RBC precursor development,[39] by suppression of the erythropoietin production,[40] and by inhibition of recycling of iron due to production of hepcidin.[41,42]

ACD is a normochromic, normocytic anemia with mild-to-moderate decline in serum hemoglobin. Reticulocyte count is low to normal, indicating underproduction of RBCs. Serum iron level is low with normal-to-elevated whole-body iron. Transferrin levels remain normal or only slightly decreased. The soluble transferrin receptor is a truncated fragment of the membrane receptor that is increased in IDA, when the availability of iron for erythropoiesis is low.[24] In contrast, levels of soluble transferrin receptors in ACD are not significantly different from normal because transferrin receptor expression is negatively affected by inflammatory cytokines.[43] Compared with patients who have ACD alone, patients with ACD and concomitant IDA more frequently have microcytes, and their anemia tends to be more severe. The ratio of the concentration of soluble transferrin receptors to the log of the ferritin level may also be helpful.[44] A ratio of less than 1 suggests ACD, whereas a ratio of more than 2 suggests absolute iron deficiency coexisting with ACD. Measurement of erythropoietin levels is useful only in anemic patients with hemoglobin levels of less than 10 g/dL because erythropoietin levels at higher hemoglobin concentrations remains well within the normal range.[45]

The therapeutic approach in ACD is treatment of the underlying disease. In cases in which this is not possible, alternative strategies are necessary.[46] Treatment options include transfusions, iron therapy, and erythropoietic agents.

Blood transfusions are widely used as a rapid and effective therapeutic intervention. Transfusions are especially helpful in the context of severe anemia (hemoglobin <8.0 g/dL) and concomitant conditions such as coronary artery disease with angina or pulmonary disease with worsening dyspnea. Blood transfusion therapy has been associated with increased survival rates in anemic patients with myocardial infarction.[47] It is important to understand that existing guidelines for the management of ACD in patients with cancer or CKD do not recommend long-term blood transfusion therapy in their management algorithms because of the risks associated with long-term transfusions, such as iron overload and sensitization to human leukocyte antigens that may occur in patients before renal transplantation.[48]

Iron therapy is also challenging in patients with ACD. Oral iron is poorly absorbed because of the downregulation of absorption in the duodenum.[49] Only a fraction of the absorbed iron will reach the sites of erythropoiesis because of the diversion of iron into the reticuloendothelial system mediated by cytokines. Current data indicate that patients with ACD and absolute iron deficiency should receive supplemental iron therapy.[50–52] Iron therapy should also be considered for patients who are unresponsive to therapy with erythropoietic agents because of functional iron deficiency that develops under conditions of intense erythropoiesis.[53] Iron therapy is currently not recommended for patients with ACD who have a high or normal ferritin level, owing to possible adverse outcomes in this setting.[43]

Erythropoietic agents for patients with ACD are currently approved for use in patients with cancer who are undergoing chemotherapy, patients with CKD, and patients with HIV infection who are undergoing myelosuppressive therapy.[54] Twenty-five percent of patients with myelodysplastic syndrome will respond to therapy with erythropoietic agents,[52] 80% of patients with multiple myeloma,[53] and up to 95% of patient with rheumatoid arthritis and CKD.[50] Erythropoietic agents work by counteracting the antiproliferative effects of cytokines,[54] along with the stimulation of iron uptake and heme biosynthesis in erythroid progenitor cells.[37] Accordingly, poor response to treatment is associated with increased level of cytokines and poor iron availability.[55]

Anemia of Kidney Disease

Anemia is usually observed when the glomerular filtration rate (GFR) falls below 60 mL/min/1.73 m^2 and worsens as both renal function and erythropoietin production decline. In a multicenter study in Canada, the prevalence of anemia was found to be approximately 25% in patients with creatinine clearance greater than 50 mL/min.[56] By the time a patient reaches a GFR of 15–29 mL/min/1.73 m^2, approximately 44% of patients are anemic (anemia defined as a hemoglobin of $\leq$12 g/dL in men and $\leq$11 g/dL in women), and by stage 5 CKD approximately 90% of patients are anemic. In older persons, the serum creatinine often fails to represent the true status of kidney function. This is called "masked renal disease" and occurs because older persons have often lost lean tissue mass and therefore have a lower production of creatinine than younger persons. GFR can be calculated by using either the Cockcroft–Gault or the modification of diet in renal disease (MDRD) formulas.

Cockcroft–Gault formula: creatinine clearance = 140-age (years) $\times$ weight (kg)/serum creatinine (mg/dL) $\times$ 72. For females, multiply results by 0.85.[57] MDRD GFR calculator can be found online at: www.nkdep.nih.gov/professionals/gfr_calculators/index.htm.[58]

The treatment of anemia in patients with kidney disease was transformed by the cloning of erythropoietin in 1983 by Lin and colleagues and its commercial availability in 1989. Before this, anemia was either untreated or various maneuvers, such as repeated blood transfusions or the use of anabolic steroids, were the mainstay, especially among dialysis patients. Presently, treatment for anemia in both pre–end-stage renal disease and

end-stage renal disease patients is strongly recommended. Erythropoietin is a 30,400-D glycoprotein, rich in sialic acid, whose production is regulated by reduced oxygenation of the kidney. It has minimal side effects including occasionally high blood pressure or seizures. Antibodies can result in pure RBC dysplasia. Erythropoietin-like agents have been shown to increase hemoglobin not only in patients with CKD, but also in ACD and in very high doses in patients with myelodysplasia. The 2006 revised Kidney Disease Quality Outcomes Initiative guidelines recommend that hemoglobin levels be maintained at or above 11 g/dL in all patients with CKD and that hemoglobin levels not be routinely maintained above 13 g/dL.[59] The U.S. Food and Drug Administration has stated that physicians should adjust the dose of erythropoiesis-stimulating agents (ESAs) to maintain the lowest hemoglobin level necessary to avoid the need for transfusions and monitor patients' hemoglobin levels to ensure they do not exceed 12 g/dL. In March 2007, a new black box warning was issued, describing this recommendation based on results of new studies in patients with CKD as well as patients with cancer and those undergoing orthopedic surgery.[60] Based on this new labeling change and warning, it is likely that lower hemoglobin levels may be recommended and that physicians will be reluctant to maintain hemoglobin levels in the 11.0–12.0 g/dL range that has been generally accepted for many patients with CKD, although the implications of this announcement remain unclear.

The availability of iron can limit the hemoglobin response following treatment with erythropoietin in patients with cancer-related anemia as well as those with renal failure. Iron deficiency frequently develops quickly in treated patients who have borderline iron levels at the onset of therapy. Even patients with adequate iron stores may have difficulty adequately mobilizing iron to respond to erythropoietin therapy due to cytokine-mediated inhibition of the transfer of iron from macrophages to the developing erythrocytes. Iron should be given during ESA therapy to maintain a transferrin saturation of $\geq$20% and a serum ferritin level of $\geq$100 ng/mL. Parenteral iron given concomitantly with an ESA may augment erythropoiesis by providing iron in an easily bioavailable form.[48] The observed increase in erythropoiesis seen when using ESAs in combination with parenteral iron needs to be balanced against the potential risk of aggravating total body iron overload.

Macrocytic Anemia

On a blood smear, macrocytic anemias are characterized by large RBCs withan MCV above 100 fL. Conditions causing the production of macrocytic RBCs are broadly grouped into those associated with megaloblastic (folate or cobalamin deficiency) or normoblastic (alcoholism, liver disease, hypothyroidism, and certain medications) RBC precursors.

The incidence and prevalence of vitamin B12 deficiency increases with age. The most common cause of B12 deficiency is the inability to digest B12 in food due to decreased gastric secretion of hydrochloric acid and pepsin. Vitamin B12 deficiency is treated by vitamin B12 supplementation, parentally or orally. An intramuscular dosage of 1,000 µg daily for 7 days, then 1,000 µg weekly for 4 weeks, followed by 1,000 µg monthly is the most commonly used regimen. Treatment with 1,000–2,000 µg of oral crystalline B12 can be as successful as intramuscular injections.[61] A response to therapy characterized by an increase in reticulocytosis often occurs within a week of the initiation of therapy.

Excessive alcohol consumption is a common cause of macrocytosis. Even before anemia appears, 90% of alcoholics have macrocytosis (MCV between 100 and 110 fL).[62] This abnormality can be induced by regular ingestion of 80 g of alcohol each day (one bottle of wine). Alcohol-induced macrocytosis occurs even though patients are folate and cobalamin replete and do not have liver disease. Abstinence from alcohol results in resolution of the macrocytosis within 2–4 months, thus confirming the diagnosis.[63]

Liver disease, particularly if caused by alcohol, is another common cause of macrocytosis and is frequently accompanied by target cell formation. The mechanism is not known but increased lipid deposition on RBC membranes, similar to that seen in hyperlipidemia, may be involved.

Virtually all patients with the myelodysplastic syndrome will have macrocytic anemia at presentation. In the early stages, myelodysplastic syndrome may be the cause of an apparently idiopathic macrocytic anemia, especially in elderly patients.[64]

Evaluation should be initiated in patients with an MCV above 100 fL. It should begin with a focused history-taking including the extent of alcohol use, exposure to antimetabolites and other medications, nutritional status, and the possible presence of liver disease. Unless the history clearly points to the diagnosis, routine laboratory testing consists of examination of the blood smear, reticulocyte count, and analysis of serum for cobalamin, folate, thyroid-stimulating hormone, liver function, and protein electrophoresis for the rare case of multiple myeloma.

Hemolytic Anemias

Hemolysis is the destruction or removal of RBCs from the circulation before their normal life span of 120 days. Although hemolysis may be a lifelong asymptomatic condition, it presents as anemia when production of the RBCs cannot match the pace of RBCs destruction. Hemolysis can manifested as jaundice, cholelithiasis, or isolated reticulocytosis.

There are two mechanisms of hemolysis. *Intravascular hemolysis* is the destruction of RBCs in the circulation with the release of cell contents into the plasma; it can be caused by mechanical trauma from a damaged endothelium, complement fixation, or infectious agents that may cause direct membrane degradation and cell destruction. *Extravascular hemolysis* is the removal and destruction of RBCs with membrane alteration by the macrophages of the spleen and liver.

Hemolytic anemias can also be divided into hereditary or acquired. Newly diagnosed hemolytic anemia in the elderly most likely will be acquired. Among acquired anemias, the most common are immune mediated and microangiopathic (due to mechanical disruption of RBCs in circulation). Immune hemolytic anemia is mediated by antibodies directed against antigens on the RBC surface. Microspherocytes on a peripheral smear and a positive direct antiglobulin test are the characteristic findings. Immune hemolytic anemia is classified as autoimmune, alloimmune, or drug induced, based on the antigen that stimulates antibody- or complement-mediated destruction of RBCs. Autoimmune hemolytic anemia is mediated by autoantibodies and further subdivided according to their maximal binding temperature. Warm hemolysis refers to immunoglobulin (Ig)G autoantibodies, which maximally bind RBCs at a body temperature of 37°C (98.6°F). In cold hemolysis, IgM autoantibodies (cold agglutinins) bind RBCs at lower temperatures (0–4°C/32–39.2°F). When warm antibodies attach to RBCs surface antigens, the IgG-coated RBCs are partially ingested by macrophages of the spleen, leaving microspherocytes, the characteristic cells of autoimmune hemolytic anemia. These spherocytes are trapped in the splenic sinusoids and then removed from circulation.[65] Cold autoantibodies (IgM) temporarily bind to the RBC membrane, activate complement, and deposit complement factor C3 on the cell surface. These C3-coated RBCs are cleared slowly by the macrophages of the liver (extravascular hemolysis).[66] The direct antiglobulin test, also known as the direct Coombs test, demonstrates the presence of antibodies or complement on the surface of RBCs and is the hallmark of autoimmune hemolysis.[67] A number of commonly prescribed medications (penicillin, ampicillin, rifampin, isoniozid, insulin, and ibuprofen) can induce production of both types of antibodies.[68] Certain infections (infectious mononucleosis, mycoplasma pneumonia, and HIV) can induce both warm and cold autoimmune anemia.[69]

The anemia of hemolysis is usually normocytic, although a reticulocytosis can cause elevated measurements of MCV because of the large size of the reticulocyte (average 150 fL).[70] Review of the peripheral blood smear is an important step in the evaluation of anemias, including hemolytic anemia. A characteristic laboratory feature of hemolysis along with anemia is reticulocytosis, which is a normal response of the bone marrow to the loss of RBCs. In healthy bone marrow reticulocytosis should be evident within 3–5 days after a decline in hemoglobin.

The destruction of the RBCs leads to a release of hemoglobin and LDH into the circulation. Hemoglobin is converted into unconjugated bilirubin in the spleen or may be bound in the plasma by haptoglobin. The haptoglobin–hemoglobin complex is rapidly cleared by the liver. The aforementioned events will result in elevated LDH, elevated unconjugated bilirubin, and low haptoglobin levels.[25] In cases of severe intravascular hemolysis, the binding capacity of haptoglobin is exceeded rapidly and free hemoglobin is filtered by the glomeruli, causing red brown urine with urine dipstick positive for blood without RBCs.

Conclusion

Anemia is very common in older patients and is associated with decreased survival, functional dependence, and several geriatric syndromes including dementia, delirium, depression, and falls. In approximately 33% of cases, the cause of anemia is not obvious and may be the result of several contributing factors.

Evaluation of anemia should be initiated for hemoglobin levels of 13 g/dL for men and 12 g/dL for women. Further studies are necessary to clarify the afoementioned parameters.

The management of anemia consists of eliminating the causes and replenishing the missing factors. What remains to be determined is whether pharmacological correction of anemia in the elderly with recombinant erythropoietin can slow disease progression, reduce morbidity, improve quality of life, and prolong survival. This question should be answered in randomized controlled trials in the future.

CHRONIC MYELOPROLIFERATIVE DISEASES

Classic myeloproliferative diseases include polycythemia vera (PV), essential thrombocythemia (ET), myelofibrosis, and chronic myeloid leukemia (CML). This group of diseases shares several distinct features. They are clonal disorders of hematopoiesis that arise in a hematopoietic stem cell or early progenitor cell. They are characterized by the dysregulated production of a particular lineage of mature myeloid cells with fairly normal differentiation. They exhibit a variable tendency to progress to acute leukemia, usually of the myeloid variety. The individual myeloproliferative disorders are characterized clinically by the proliferation of a single predominant myeloid cell type, resulting in an excess of erythrocytes in PV, excess platelets in ET, and an excess number of neutrophils in CML.

Polycythemia Vera

PV is a chronic myeloproliferative disorder characterized by an increased RBC mass, which leads to hyperviscosity and increased risk of thrombosis. The median age of patients diagnosed with PV is 60 years; approximately 7% of patients are diagnosed before age 40 years. Median survival in untreated patients is 6–18 months; with treatment, median survival is more than 10 years.[71] Patients may present with complaints of pruritus after bathing, burning pain in the distal extremities (erythromelalgia), gastrointestinal disturbances, or nonspecific complaints such as weakness, headaches, or dizziness. Other patients are asymptomatic and are diagnosed after an incidental finding of an elevated hemoglobin and/or hematocrit level on a routine blood count. In making the diagnosis of PV, the physician must first exclude a secondary erythrocytosis.[72] Once a secondary cause is ruled out, the diagnosis of PV is determined using a combination of major and minor criteria defined by the Polycythemia Vera Study Group. Although new diagnostic modalities have been developed, these criteria remain the standard method of diagnosis. Major diagnostic criteria include increased RBC mass, normal oxygen saturation, and the presence of splenomegaly.[73] There is no single treatment for PV. Thrombosis is the major cause of morbidity and mortality; therefore, treatment is aimed at the prevention of thrombotic events. Examples of thrombotic events include arterial and venous thrombosis, cerebrovascular accident, deep venous thrombosis, myocardial infarction, peripheral arterial occlusion, and pulmonary infarction. Phlebotomy is the mainstay of treatment, the goal of which is to reduce hyperviscosity by decreasing the hematocrit level to less than 45% in white men and 42% in African-Americans and women.[71] Several myelosuppressive agents have been used for treatment of PV including hydroxyurea, recombinant interferon-α2b, radioactive phosphorus, and busulfan. The preferred agent is hydroxyurea, which is less leukemogenic and is an effective bone marrow suppressant.[74] Because the of incidence of leukemia associated with treatment with radioactive phosphorus peaks after 7 years of treatment, it is reasonable to recommend the use of radioactive phosphorus in elderly patients, especially if life expectancy is less than 10 years.[71] The current lack of evidence correlating thrombocytosis with thrombosis in PV does not support the potential therapeutic value of the use of anagrelide, an area that needs additional evaluation.[71] Inhibiting platelet function with aspirin remains another possibility for treatment and has been tested in several studies. High-dose aspirin in PV has been discouraged because of the previously demonstrated association with an increased incidence of gastrointestinal hemorrhage.[75] The effectiveness of low-dose aspirin in reducing the incidence of thrombosis in PV was planned to be tested in approximately 1,800 patients over a 5-year follow-up period in a multicenter double-blind randomized European trial.[76] Because of poor enrollment, accrual to the study was stopped early and follow-up was confined to a period of 12 months. Results obtained in 518 evaluable patients showed aspirin significantly lowered the combined risk of cardiovascular death, nonfatal myocardial infarction, nonfatal stroke, pulmonary embolism, or major venous thrombosis, and aspirin significantly reduced the combined rate of major or minor thrombosis. The study was insufficiently powered to detect significant differences between aspirin and placebo in the rates of any bleeding, major bleeding, or minor bleeding.[77]

Chronic Myeloid Leukemia

CML is a rare disease worldwide. It represents 14% of all leukemia and 20% of adult leukemia. The annual incidence is 1.6 cases per 100,000 adults with a slight male preponderance. The median age at diagnosis is 65 years.[78] CML was the first malignancy determined to be caused by a chromosomal abnormality after the discovery of a minute chromosome (now known as the Philadelphia chromosome,) which was found to result from at (9;22) reciprocal chromosomal translocation.[79] The clinical hallmark of CML is the uncontrolled production of maturing granulocytes, predominantly neutrophils but also eosinophils and basophils. The disease has a triphasic clinical course: a chronic phase, which is present at the time of diagnosis in approximately 85% of patients; an accelerated phase, in which neutrophil differentiation becomes progressively impaired and leukocyte counts are more difficult to control with myelosuppressive medications; and blast crisis, a condition resembling acute leukemia in which myeloid or lymphoid blasts fail to differentiate.[79] The clinical findings at diagnosis of CML vary among reported series. Up to 50% of patients are asymptomatic, with the disease initially suspected from review of routine blood tests.[79,80] Among symptomatic patients, systemic symptoms such as fatigue, malaise, weight loss, excessive sweating, abdominal fullness, and bleeding episodes due to platelet dysfunction are common. Acute gouty arthritis may also present at this time due to overproduction of uric acid.[80] Treatment of CML has changed dramatically over the recent years because of development of tyrosine kinase inhibitors. Until recently, interferon-α and stem cell transplantation were the only therapeutic options for patients with CML. Treatment decisions remain complex and require involvement of an experienced oncologist. Available treatment options include:

- Administration of first and second generation oral tyrosine kinase inhibitors (e.g., imatinib, dasatinib, and nilotinib), which have become the initial treatment of choice
- Stem cell transplantation, which is of high importance in younger patients
- Other agents (e.g., hydroxyurea, interferon-α with or without cytarabine, busulfan, and homoharringtonine[81]

Acute Myeloid Leukemia

Acute myeloid leukemia (AML) or acute nonlymphocytic leukemia refers to a hematopoietic neoplasm involving cells of the myeloid line. AML is characterized by a clonal proliferation of myeloid precursors with reduced capacity to differentiate into more mature cellular elements. As a result, there is an accumulation of leukemic forms in the bone marrow, peripheral blood, and other tissues, with a marked reduction in RBCs, platelets, and neutrophils. The increased production of malignant cells, along with reduction in these mature elements, results in a variety of systemic symptoms, anemia, bleeding, and an increased risk of infection.

Approximately 11,000 individuals are diagnosed with AML annually in the United States. The median age at presentation is 65 years.[82] The incidence of AML increases with age and is almost 10 times greater among persons older than 65 years of age. If left untreated, AML usually results in death within a few months of diagnosis.[83]

Presenting symptoms are usually related to pancytopenia (anemia, neutropenia, and thrombocytopenia) and include easy fatigue, cognitive impairment, infections, bleeding (gingival bleeding, ecchymosis, and epistaxis). Combination of these symptoms is common.[84]

Treatment of AML may differ among younger and older adults. Although there is no clearly accepted definition of younger compared with older adults when dealing with AML, in most studies, "older adult" has been variously defined as older than 55, 60, or 65 years. Increasing age and comorbid conditions are poor prognostic factors in patients with AML. Many of these patients are unable to tolerate intensive chemotherapy and its complications.[85] In addition patients with comorbid conditions such as cardiac, pulmonary, hepatic, or renal disorders suffer greater acute toxicity from chemotherapy. At present, a reasonable standard regimen for many older patients is 7 days of continuous infusion with cytarabine plus 3 days of daunorubicin.[86]

Chronic Lymphocytic Leukemia

Chronic lymphocytic leukemia (CLL) is the most common form of leukemia in adults in the western world, representing almost 25% of all leukemia. The median age at diagnosis is 70 years, with 81% of patients being diagnosed at age 60 years or older.[87] The cause of CLL is unknown. It is the only leukemia not associated with previous exposure to ionizing radiation, drugs, or chemicals. Epidemiological studies have shown that the risk of CLL is increased in relatives of patients with CLL.[88]

Approximately 50% of patients with CLL are asymptomatic at the time of presentation and are found to have an isolated peripheral lymphocytosis on laboratory work obtained for unrelated reasons.[89] Constitutional symptoms are present in approximately 15% of patients at diagnosis with night sweats, weight loss, and fatigue being the most frequently reported complaints.[90]

The most common finding on physical examination is lymphadenopathy, present in 50%–90% of patients. Lymph node enlargement may be generalized or localized; the size of enlarged nodes may be as small as a few millimeters in diameter or as large as orange. The most commonly affected sites are cervical, supraclavicular, and axillary. The spleen is the second most frequently enlarged organ. It is usually painless and nontender on palpation with a smooth firm surface.[90] Enlargement of the liver can be present in 15%–25% of the cases. It is nontender on palpation with a firm smooth surface. Infiltration with B-CLL cells may occur in any organ but the skin is the most commonly involved nonlymphoid organ and this is present in less than 5% of the cases.[91] The indications for initiation of therapy for CLL are those recommended by the National Cancer Institute–sponsored Working Group.[92] Criteria for therapy include B symptoms (fevers, night sweats, or weight loss), progressive enlargement of lymph nodes, hepatosplenomegaly, obstructive adenopathy, development of or worsening thrombocytopenia and anemia, immune hemolysis or thrombocytopenia not responsive to corticosteroids, and rapid lymphocyte doubling time. If treatment is indicated, the traditional approach is to administer chlorambucil plus corticosteroids. Treatment with the purine analog fludarabine, alone, or in combination with other agents (e.g., chlorambucil, cyclophosphamide, rituximab), produces a higher response rate than alkylating agent regimens or combination regimens, although such treatment has not yet been shown to prolong overall survival and are associated with greater toxicity.[93]

Thrombocytopenia

The normal platelet count in adults ranges from 150,000–450,000/μL, with mean values of 237,000 and 266,000/μL in males and females, respectively.[94] Thrombocytopenia is defined as a platelet count less than 150,000/μL (150×10^9/L), although 2.5% of the population will have a platelet count lower than this. Thrombocytopenia is not usually detected clinically (see later) until the platelet count has fallen to levels significantly below 100,000/μL. The major mechanisms for a reduced platelet count are decreased production and increased destruction. Two additional mechanisms include dilutional or distributional thrombocytopenia. Platelet production by bone marrow can be impaired when the bone marrow is suppressed or damaged. In the case of bone marrow suppression there will be evidence of decreased production of RBCs and WBCs (pancytopenia). Causes of bone marrow suppression include viral infections (rubella, mumps, varicella, parvovirus, hepatitis C, Epstein–Barr virus), chemotherapy or radiation therapy to the sites of platelet production (as in total nodal irradiation), direct alcohol toxicity, and vitamin B12 and folate deficiencies.

Increased platelet destruction is seen in number of conditions, including idiopathic thrombocytopenic purpura and systemic lupus erythematosis. The mechanism is presumed to be due to the presence of autoimmune antiplatelet antibodies. In posttransfusion or posttransplantation thrombocytopenia, there is alloimmune destruction. Increased platelet destruction occurs in disseminated intravascular coagulation, thrombotic thrombocytopenic purpura (TTP), and antiphospholipid syndrome after administration of certain medications (heparin, quinine, quinidine, and valproic acid). Physical destruction of platelets can occur during cardiopulmonary bypass and in large aortic aneurysms.[95] Distributional thrombocytopenia can be caused by splenomegaly. In healthy adults, approximately one third of circulating platelets are sequestered in the spleen. In patients with splenomegaly, up to 90% of platelets can be sequestered in the spleen, although total platelet mass and overall platelet survival remain relatively normal. Patients with cirrhosis, portal hypertension, and splenomegaly may have a significant degree of thrombocytopenia but rarely have clinical bleeding because their total platelet mass is usually normal.[96] Dilutional thrombocytopenia can occur in patients with massive blood loss and transfusion of 20 units or more of packed RBC in a 24-hour period because of absence of viable platelets in packed RBC products.[97] Patients with thrombocytopenia may be asymptomatic and thrombocytopenia may initially be detected on a routine CBC. The most common clinical presentation of thrombocytopenia is mucosal or cutaneous bleeding. Mucosal bleeding may be manifested as epistaxis and gingival bleeding. Bleeding into the skin is manifested as petechiae or superficial ecchymosis.

Immune Thrombocytopenic Purpura

Immune thrombocytopenic purpura (ITP) is an immune disorder characterized by a low platelet count and mucocutaneous bleeding. It can be primary (idiopathic thrombocytopenic purpura) or secondary due to an underlying disorder such as systemic lupus erythematosis, the antiphospholipid syndrome, CLL, lymphoma, infection with HIV and hepatitis C, and therapy with curtain drugs. ITP can be acute or chronic.

A presumptive diagnosis of ITP is made when the history, physical examination, CBC and examination of a blood smear do not suggest other etiologies for the isolated thrombocytopenia. In older patients (>60 years of age), bone marrow aspiration can be recommended to rule out myelodysplastic syndrome.[98] For patients with presumed ITP, severe thrombocytopenia, and/or clinical bleeding, urgent hematological consultation is a priority. For asymptomatic patients with modest degrees of thrombocytopenia, consultation is less urgent but should be pursued should treatment be required in the future. Treatment decisions are complex and should be shared between the clinician and the patient. Factors that should be taken into account include presence or absence of severe bleeding, risk for trauma given the patient's age, occupation, and lifestyle, and comorbid medical conditions that can increase risk of bleeding. Standard practice is to initiate treatment with prednisone, 1 mg/kg orally given as a single daily dose. The duration of initial prednisone treatment is determined by the platelet count response. If the platelet count recovers promptly to normal, the prednisone dose is tapered and discontinued; there is no standard regimen for tapering the prednisone dose.[98]

Thrombotic Thrombocytopenic Purpura

TTP is an acute syndrome with abnormalities in multiple organ systems. It occurs primarily in adults with the annual incidence in the United States estimated at 4–11 cases per million people.[99] Prompt recognition of TTP is important because the disease responds well to plasma exchange treatment but is associated with a high mortality rate when untreated.[100] Patients are diagnosed primarily by the presence of thrombocytopenia and microangiopathic hemolytic anemia without another clinically apparent cause, and most have some neurological and renal abnormalities.

Plasma exchange is the only treatment of TTP for which there are firm data on effectiveness.[100] The American Association of Blood Banks, the American Society for Apheresis, and the British Committee for Standards in Haematology recommend daily plasma exchange with replacement of 1.0–1.5 times the predicted plasma volume of the patient as standard therapy for TTP.[101,102] The British guidelines recommend that plasma exchange therapy be continued for a minimum of 2 days after the platelet count returns to normal ($>150,000/cm^3$), and they also recommend the use of glucocorticoids for all patients with TTP.

REFERENCES

1. WHO Technical Report Series. *Nutritional anemias.* 1968;405:5–37.
2. Penninx BW, Pahor M, Cesari M, Corsi AM, Woodman RC, Bandinelli S. Anemia is associated with disability and decreased physical performance and muscle strength in the elderly. *J Am Geriatr Soc.* 2004: 52 (5):719–724.
3. Chaves PH, Ashar B, Guralnik J, Fried LP. Looking at the relationship between hemoglobin concentration and prevalent mobility difficulty in older women. Should the criteria currently used to define anemia in older people should be reevaluated? *J Am Geriatr Soc.* 2002 Jul: 50(7):1257–1264.
4. Guralnik JM, Eisenstaedt RS, Ferrucci L, Klein HG, Woodman RC. Prevalence of anemia in persons 65 years and older in the United States: evidence for a high rate of unexplained anemia. *Blood* 2004;104:2263–2268.
5. Salive ME, Cornoni-Huntley J, Guralnik JM. Anemia and hemoglobin levels. *Principles of Geriatric Medicine. Am Geriatr Soc.* 1992;40:489–496.
6. Artz AS, Fergusson D, Drinka PJ, et al. Mechanisms of Unexplained Anemia in the Nursing Home. *J Am Geriatr Soc.* Mar 2004;52(3):423–427.
7. US Census Bureau, 2004, "US Interim Projections by Age, Sex, Race and Hispanic Origin" www.census.gov/ipc/www/usinterimproj. Internet release date March 18, 2004.
8. Nissenson AR, Goodnough LT, Dubois RW. Anemia: not just an innocent bystander? *Arch Intern Med.* 2003;163:1400–1404.
9. Kikuchi M, Inagaki T, Shinagawa N. Five-year survival of older people with anemia: variation with hemoglobin concentration. *J Am Geriatr Soc.* 2001;49:1226–1229.
10. Zakai NS, Katz R, Hirsch C, et al. A prospective study of anemia status, hemoglobin concentration, and mortality in an elderly cohort: The Cardiovascular Health Study. *Arch Intern Med.* 2005; 165:2214–2220.
11. Dharmarajan TS, Norkus EP. Mild anemia and the risk of falls in older adults from nursing home and the community. *J Am Med Dir Assoc.* 2004;5:395–400.
12. Ershler WB. Association of anemia with health-related quality of life and functional status in an ambulatory, geriatric population. Annual Scientific Meeting of the Gerontological Society of America, Washington, DC. 2004.
13. Balducci L. Epidemiology of anemia in the elderly: Information on diagnostic evaluation. *J Am Geriatr Soc.* 2003;51(Suppl): S2–S9.
14. Pandav RS, Chandra V, Dodge Hiroko H, DeKosky S, Ganguli M. Hemoglobin levels and alzheimer disease: an epidemiologic study in India. *American Journal of Geriatric Psychiatry.* 12(5):523–526, September/October 2004.
15. Perry C, Soreq H. Transcriptional regulation of erythropoiesis: fine tuning of multi-domain elements. *Eur J Biochem.* 2002; 269:3607–3618.
16. Rosse W. The spleen as a filter. *N Engl J Med.* 1987; 317:704–706.
17. Ebert BL, Bunn HF. Regulation of the erythropoietin gene. *Blood* 1999; 94:1864–1877.
18. Krafte-Jacobs B, Levetown ML, Bray GL, Ruttimann UE, Pollack MM. Erythropoietin response to critical illness. *Crit Care Med.* 1994;22:821–826.
19. Rogiers, P, Zhang, H, Leeman, M, et al. Erythropoietin response is blunted in critically ill patients. *Inten Care Med.* 1997; 23:159–162.
20. Schrier, SL. Approach to the adult patient with anemia. January 2008. Up-to-Date Online Version 16.1.
21. Nardone DA, Roth KM, Mazur DJ, et al. Usefulness of physical examination in detecting the presence or absence of anemia. *Arch Intern Med.* 1990;150.
22. Hung OL, Kwon NS, Cole AE, et al. Evaluation of the physician's ability to recognize the presence or absence of anemia, fever, and jaundice. *Acad Emerg Med.* 2000;7.
23. Ruiz MA, Saab S, Rickman LS. The clinical detection of scleral icterus: observations of multiple examiners. *Mil Med.* 1997;162.
24. Punnonen K, Irjala K, Rajamaki A. Serum transferring receptor and its ratio to serum ferritin in the diagnosis of iron deficiency. *Blood* 1997;89:1052–1057.
25. Marchand A, Galen RS, Van Lente F. The predictive value of serum haptoglobin in hemolytic disease. *JAMA* 1980; 243:1909–1911.
26. Ania BJ, Suman VJ, Fairbanks VF, Rademacher DM, Melton LJ III. Incidence of anemia in older people: an epidemiologic study in a well defined population. *J Am Geriatr Soc.* 1997;45:825–831.
27. Fairbanks VF, Beutler E. Iron deficiency. In *Williams Hematology*, 6th Edition. Edited by: Beutler E, Lichtman MA, Coller BS, Kipps, TJ, Seligsohn, V. New York: McGraw-Hill Medical Publishing Division; 2001:447–470.
28. Bridges KR, Seligman PA. Disorders of iron metabolism. In: Blood: Practice and Principles of Hematology. Handin, RI, Lux, SE, Stossel, TP, Eds. Part 7: Red Blood Cells, Chapter 49, p 1433–1472. JB Lippincott Co. Phil, PA, 1995.
29. Joosten E, Ghesquiere B, Linthoudt H, et al. Upper and lower gastrointestinal evaluation of elderly inpatients who are iron deficient. *Am J Med.* 1999;107:24–29.
30. Annibale B, Capurso G, Chistolini A, D'Ambra G. Gastrointestinal causes of refractory iron deficiency anemia in patients without gastrointestinal symptoms. *Am J Med.* 2001;111.
31. Nemeth E, Tuttle MS, Powelson J, et al. Hepcidin regulates iron efflux by binding to ferroportin and inducing its internalization. Science, Dec 17 2004; 306(5704): 2051–2053.
32. Hershko C, Hoffbrand AV, Keret D. et al. Role of autoimmune gastritis, Helicobacter pylori and celiac disease in refractory or unexplained iron deficiency anemia. *Haematologica* 2005; 90.
33. Guyatt GH, Patterson C, Ali M, Singer, J, Levine, M, Turpie, I, Meyer, R. Diagnosis of iron-deficiency anemia in the elderly. *Am J Med.* 1990;88(3):205–209.
34. Krause JR, Stolc V. Serum ferritin and bone marrow biopsy iron stores, II: correlation with low serum iron and Fe/TIBC ratio less than 15%. *Am J Clin Pathol.* 1980;74:461–464.
35. Casale G, Bonora C, Migliavacca A, Zurita IE, de Nicola P. Serum ferritin and aging. *Age Ageing.* 1981;10:119–122.
36. Witte DL. Can serum ferritin be effectively interpreted in the presence of the acute-phase response? *Clin Chem.* 1991;37:484–485.
37. Weiss G. Pathogenesis and treatment of anaemia of chronic disease. *Blood Rev.* 2002;16:87–96.
38. Alvarez-Hernandez X, Liceaga J, McKay IC, Brock JH. Induction of hypoferremia and modulation of macrophage iron metabolism by tumor necrosis factor. *Lab Invest.* 1989;61:319–322.
39. Means RT Jr. Recent developments in the anemia of chronic disease. *Curr Hematol Rep.* 2003;2:116–121.
40. Jelkmann W. Proinflammatory cytokines lowering erythropoietin production. *J Interferon Cytokine Res.* 1998;18:555–559.

41. Nemeth E, Rivera S, Gabayan V, et al. IL-6 mediates hypoferremia of inflammation by inducing the synthesis of the iron regulatory hormone hepcidin. *J Clin Invest.* 2004;113(9):1271–1276.

42. Laftah AH, Ramesh B, Simpson RJ, et al. Effect of hepcidin on intestinal iron absorption in mice. *Blood* 15 May 2004;103(10):3940–3944.

43. Weiss G. Iron and immunity: a double-edged sword. *Eur J Clin Invest.* 2002;32(Suppl 1):70–78.

44. Miller CB, Jones RJ, Piantadosi S, Abeloff MD, Spivak JL. Decreased erythropoietin response in patients with the anemia of cancer. *NEJM.* 1990;322:1689–1692.

45. Goodnough LT, Bach RG. Anemia, transfusion, and mortality. *NEJM.* 2001;345:1272–1274.

46. Brugnara C. Iron deficiency and erythropoiesis: new diagnostic approaches. *Clin Chem.* 2003;49:1573–1578.

47. Andrews NC. Anemia of inflammation: the cytokine-hepcidin link. *J Clin Invest.* 2004;113:1251–1253.

48. Auerbach M, Ballard H, Trout JR, et al. Intravenous iron optimizes the response to recombinant human erythropoietin in cancer patients with chemotherapy-related anemia: a multicenter, open-label, randomized trial. *J Clin Oncol.* 2004;22:1301–1307.

49. Rizzo JD, Lichtin AE, Woolf SH, et al. Use of epoetin in patients with cancer: evidence-based clinical practice guidelines of the American Society of Clinical Oncology and the American Society of Hematology. *J Clin Oncol.* Oct 1 2002; 20(19):4083–4107.

50. NKF-K/DOQI. Clinical practice guidelines for anemia of chronic kidney disease: update 2000. *Am J Kidney Dis.* 2001;37(Suppl 1):S182–S238. [Erratum. *Am J Kidney Dis.* 2001;38:442.]

51. Kletzmayr J, Sunder-Plassmann G, Horl WH. High dose intravenous iron: a note of caution. *Nephrol Dial Transplant.* 2002;17:962–965.

52. Thompson JA, Gilliland DG, Prchal JT, et al. Effect of recombinant human erythropoietin combined with granulocyte/macrophage colony-stimulating factor in the treatment of patients with myelodysplastic syndrome. *Blood* 2000;95:1175–1179.

53. Ludwig H, Fritz E, Kotzmann H, Hocker P, Gisslinger H, Barnas U. Erythropoietin treatment of anemia associated with multiple myeloma. *NEJM.* 1990;322:1693–1699.

54. Means RT Jr, Krantz SB. Inhibition of human erythroid colony-forming units by gamma interferon can be corrected by recombinant human erythropoietin. *Blood* 1991;78:2564–2567.

55. Goodnough LT, Skikne B, Brugnara C. Erythropoietin, iron, and erythropoiesis. *Blood* 2000;96:823–833.

56. Gomez JM, Carrera F. What should the optimal target hemoglobin be? *Kidney Int.* 2002; 80(Suppl):39–43.

57. Cockcroft DW, Gault MH. Prediction of creatinine clearance from serum creatinine. *Nephron.* 1976; 16(1):31–41.

58. Levey AS, Greene T, Kusek JW, Beck GL. MDRD Study Group. A simplified equation to predict glomerular filtration rate from serum creatinine (abstract) *J Am Soc Nephrol* 2000 Sep; 11.

59. NKF-K/DOQI. Clinical practice guidelines for anemia of chronic kidney disease. *Am J Kidney Dis.* 2006;47(Suppl 4).

60. Warnings: Increased Mortality, Serious Cardiovascular and Thromboembolic Events and Tumor progression. Procrit (Epoetin alfa) www.fda.gov/cder/foi/label/2007/103234s5158lbl.pdf. 1–8–07.

61. Jacques PF, Rosenberg IH, Rogers G, et al. Serum total homocysteine concentrations in the third National Health and Nutrition Examination Survey (1991–1994): population references ranges and contribution of vitamin status to high serum concentrations. *Ann Intern Med,* 1999, 131, 331–339.

62. Seppä K, Sillanaukee P, Saarni M. Blood count and hematologic morphology in nonanemic macrocytosis: Differences between alcohol abuse and pernicious anemia. *Alcohol* 1993;10.

63. Hoffbrand V, Provan D. ABC of clinical haematology. Macrocytic anaemias. *BMJ.* 1997;314.

64. Anttila P, Ihalainen J, Salo A, Heiskanen M, Juvonen E, Palotie A. Idiopathic macrocytic anaemia in the aged: Molecular and cytogenetic findings. *Br J Haematol.* 1995; 90:797–803.

65. Maedel L, Sommer S. *Morphologic Changes in Erythrocytes.* Vol. 4. Chicago: American Society for Clinical Pathology Press; 1993: slides 50, 52, 66.

66. Engelfriet CP, Overbeeke MA, von dem Borne AE. Autoimmune hemolytic anemia. *Semin Hematol.* 1992;29:3–12.

67. Jefferies LC. Transfusion therapy in autoimmune hemolytic anemia. *Hematol Oncol Clin North Am.* 1994;8:1087–1104.

68. Schwartz RS, Berkman EM, Silberstein LE. Autoimmune hemolytic anemias. In: Hoffman R, Benz EJ Jr, Shattil SJ, et al., eds. *Hematology: Basic Principles and Practice.* 3rd ed. Philadelphia: Churchill Livingstone; 2000.

69. Gehrs BC, Friedberg RC. Autoimmune hemolytic anemia. *Am J Hematol.* 2002;69:258–271.

70. Walters MC, Abelson HT. Interpretation of the complete blood count. *Pediatr Clin North Am.* 1996;43:599–622.

71. Tefferi A. Polycythemia vera: a comprehensive review and clinical recommendations. *Mayo Clin Proc.* 2003;78:174–194.

72. Tefferi A. Diagnosing polycythemia vera: a paradigm shift. *Mayo Clin Proc.* 1999;74:159–162.

73. Berlin NI. Polycythemia vera: diagnosis and treatment 2002. *Expert Rev Anticancer Ther.* 2002;2:330–336.

74. Michiels JJ, Barbui T, Finazzi G, Fuchtman SM, Kutti J, Rain JD. Diagnosis and treatment of polycythemia vera and possible future study designs of the PVSG. *Leuk Lymphoma* 2000;36:239–253.

75. Tartaglia AP, Goldberg JD, Berk PD, Wasserman LR. Adverse effects of antiaggregating platelet therapy in the treatment of polycythemia vera. *Semin Hematol.* 1986; 23:172–176.

76. Landolfi R, Marchioli R. European collaboration on low-dose aspirin in polycythemia vera (ECLAP): a randomized trial. *Semin Thromb Hemost.* 1997;23.

77. Landolfi R, Marchioli R, Kutti J, et al. Efficacy and safety of low-dose aspirin in polycythemia vera. *N Engl J Med.* 2004; 350:114–124.

78. Jemal A, Tiwari RC, Murray T, et al. *Cancer statistics, 2004. CA Cancer J Clin.* 2004;54:8–29.

79. Faderl S, Talpaz M, Estrov Z, et al. The biology of chronic myeloid leukemia. *N Engl J Med.* 1999; 341:164–172.

80. Savage DG, Szydlo RM, Goldman JM. Clinical features at diagnosis in 430 patients with chronic myeloid leukaemia seen at a referral centre over a 16-year period. *Br J Haematol.* 1997; 96.

81. Kantarjian HM, Cortes J, Guilhot F, et al. Diagnosis and management of chronic myeloid leukemia: a survey of American and European practice patterns. *Cancer* 2007; 109:1365–75.

82. O'Donnel MR. Acute leukemia. In: Pazdur R, Coia LR, Hoskins WJ, Wagman LD, eds. *Cancer Management: A multidisciplinary Approach.* 8th ed. Manhasset, NY: CMP Healthcare Media, Oncology Publishing Group; 2004:747–772.

83. Lang K, Earle CC, Foster T, Dixon D, Van Gool R, Menzin J. Trends in the treatment of acute myeloid leukaemia in the elderly. *Drugs Aging.* 2005;22(11):943–955.

84. Meyers CA, Albitar M, Estey E. Cognitive impairment, fatigue, and cytokine levels in patients with acute myelogenous leukemia or myelodysplastic syndrome. *Cancer* 2005;104.

85. Wahlin A, Markevarn B, Golovleva I, Nilsson M. Prognostic significance of risk group stratification in elderly patients with acute myeloid leukaemia. *Br J Haematol.* 2001; 115.

86. Mayer RJ, Davis RB, Schiffer CA, et al. Intensive postremission chemotherapy in adults with acute myeloid leukemia. *Cancer and Leukemia Group B. N Engl J Med.* 1994; 331:896–903.

87. Diehl LF, Karnell LH, Menck HR. The American College of Surgeons Commission on Cancer and the American Cancer Society. The National Cancer Data Base report on age, gender, treatment, and outcomes of patients with chronic lymphocytic leukemia. *Cancer* 1000;86:2684–2692.

88. Faguet GB. Chronic lymphocytic leukemia: an updated review. *J Clin Oncol.* 1994;12:1974–1990.

89. Molica S, Levato D. What is changing in the natural history of chronic lymphocytic leukemia? *Haematologica.* 2001;86:8–12.

90. Pangalis GA, Vassilakopoulos TP, Dimopoulou MN, et al. B-chronic lymphocytic leukemia: practical aspects. *Hematol Oncol.* 2002;20:103–146.

91. Robak E, Robak T. Skin lesions in chronic lymphocytic leukemia. *Leuk Lymphoma.* 2007;48.

92. Cheson BD, Bennett JM, Grever M, et al. National Cancer Institute-sponsored Working Group guidelines for chronic lymphocytic leukemia: revised guidelines for diagnosis and treatment. *Blood* 1996; 87(12):4990–4997.

93. Shanafelt TD, Byrd JC, Call TG, Zent CS, Kay NE. Narrative review: initial management of newly diagnosed, early-stage chronic lymphocytic leukemia. *Ann Intern Med.* 2006;145:435–447.

94. Buckley MF, James JW, Brown DE, et al. A novel approach to the assessment of variations in the human platelet count. *Thromb Haemost.* 2000;83:480–484.

95. Malouf MA, Milliken S, Glanville AR. Successful management of profound thrombocytopenia after lung and heart–lung transplantation. *J Heart Lung Transplant.* 2000;19.

96. Aster RH. Pooling of platelets in the spleen: role in the pathogenesis of "hypersplenic" thrombocytopenia. *J Clin Invest.* 1966;45.

97. Leslie SD, Toy PTCY. Laboratory hemostatic abnormalities in massively transfused patients given red blood cells and crystalloid. *Am J Clin Pathol.* 1991;96.

98. George JN, Woolf SH, Raskob GE, et al. Idiopathic thrombocytopenic purpura: a practice guideline developed by explicit methods for the American Society of Hematology. *Blood* 1996; 88(3)1–2.

99. Terrell DR, Williams LA, Vesely SK, et al. The incidence of thrombotic thrombocytopenic purpura-hemolytic uremic syndrome: all patients, idiopathic patients, and patients with severe ADAMTS-13 deficiency. *J Thromb Haemost.* 2005;3:1432–1436.

100. Rock GA, Shumak KH, Buskard NA, et al. Comparison of plasma exchange with plasma infusion in the treatment of thrombotic thrombocytopenic purpura. *NEJM.* 1991;325:393–397.

101. Allford SL, Hunt BJ, Rose P, Machin S. Guidelines on the diagnosis and management of the thrombotic microangiopathic haemolytic anaemias. *Br J Haematol.* 2003;120:556–573.

102. Smith JW, Weinstein R. Therapeutic apheresis: a summary of current indication categories endorsed by the AABB and American Society for Apheresis. *Transfusion* 2003;43:820–822.

36

Cancer in the Elderly

Danielle Snyderman, MD, Christopher Haines, MD, Richard Wender, MD

INTRODUCTION

Cancer is a major public health problem with a disproportionate impact on older adults. The lifetime risk of developing cancer is 1 in 2 for men and 1 in 3 for women.[1] Seventy-six percent of all cancers occur in patients older than the age of 55. From 2000 to 2003 the median age of cancer at time of diagnosis was 67 years. During this time, the median age at death was 73 years old.[2] There are epidemiological differences based on ethnicity, with African-Americans having both the highest cancer incidence and mortality. Factors accounting for differences are multifactorial and a topic of ongoing research.[3] The overall health care costs associated with cancer were estimated to have been $219.2 billion in 2007.[1] As the size of the elderly population continues to increase, all health care professionals can expect to care for a steadily increasing number of older patients with cancer.

Cancer and Aging

Although principally a geriatric disease, under no circumstances should cancer be considered a normal consequence of aging. The relationship between cancer biology and the biology of aging is multidimensional and has yet to be fully understood. The incidence of some cancers such as breast, prostate, and colon increases with advancing age, whereas others such as cervical cancer are less frequent. The increasing prevalence of cancer with advancing age is thought to result from the accumulation of damaging genetic events and mutations that occur over time, the decline of DNA repair mechanisms over time, and the decline in cellular immunity.[4,5] Additionally, the aggressiveness of cancer with advancing age can vary. Malignancies such as acute myelogenous leukemia, and lymphomas tend to be more aggressive with advancing age, most likely secondary to particular histological subtypes of the disease that appear to be age dependent. Breast cancer may have an indolent course in the elderly, an example of age-associated decline in tumor aggressiveness that may be due to impaired tumor angiogenesis in older patients, although older adults still die of this disease. Various aging processes can affect cancer presentation and management including decreased homeostatic reserve, altered pharmacodynamics and pharmacokinetics, and declining adaptability.[6]

Principles of Cancer Screening

Screening recommendations in older adults are still subject to controversy and therefore a consensus has not been reached. Walter and Covinsky provided a framework for evaluating screening in the elderly population that includes consideration of life expectancy, benefit of screening, potential harms of screening, and values and preferences of each patient.[7] These items should be considered in the context of the overall purpose of screening tests, which is to reduce morbidity and mortality. Even when large randomized studies have found screening tests to be efficacious, they have systematically excluded older patients, making it difficult to extrapolate benefit seen in younger adults to geriatric patients. Given this limitation, an additional consideration for screening in the elderly is to improve function and quality of life.[8] Screening is subject to bias with lead-time bias and length-time bias each having significance in older adults. Lead bias occurs when the underlying disease cannot be altered by treatment. In the unscreened population, the diagnosis is not made until clinical symptoms are present. The screened population is given a diagnosis in the asymptomatic period. Screening does not alter time of death. It only allows patients to know about their disease earlier. Because of length-time bias, screening is more likely to detect slower-growing tumors and less likely to detect faster-growing tumors, thus producing the impression that individuals found with screening do better than those who are found through symptoms. This has relevance in the geriatric population who may have several comorbidities that may compete with the cancer diagnosis. Prostate cancer and breast cancer in older adults are examples of diseases that may be affected by length-time bias.[9] Lead-time and length-time biases are potential sources of harm when screening the elderly for cancer. In general, it can be concluded that a patient with a life expectancy of less than 5 years is unlikely to benefit from cancer screening.[7]

Comprehensive Geriatric Assessment and Geriatric Oncology

Epidemiological studies have shown that the geriatric population has been undertreated with regard to all oncological care compared with those younger than 65 years. Historically, patients were determined to be "elderly" when they reached the age of 65 years (retirement age, Medicare eligible). Yet the elderly are not adequately defined solely by chronological age. Rather, ongoing emphasis has been placed on physiological age as a determinant of how elderly patients are defined. As aging is multifaceted and highly individual, a standardized approach to evaluate each patient has been increasingly recognized and encouraged by geriatricians and oncologists over the past decade. Comprehensive geriatric assessment (CGA) is a multidisciplinary-based tool to address this need and has been utilized when estimating life expectancy and candidacy for treatment in older patients with a cancer diagnosis.[10] The International Society of Geriatric Oncology recommends the use of CGA in the evaluation of older patients with cancer to detect unaddressed problems and improve functional status and, possibly, survival.[11] Until recently, the use of the CGA in older patients was recommended based on the expectation that it would eventually be shown to improve outcomes. There is now increasing data showing the ability of the CGA intervention in reducing morbidity and mortality.[12] This evidence has prompted further research in the development of a comprehensive evaluative tool that can guide interventions improving quality cancer care in older adults. Elements of a CGA are detailed in Chapter 2, "Assessment of the Older Patient."

Principles of Management

Advanced age is not in itself a contraindication to cancer therapy. Making evidence-based decisions in elderly patients may be difficult due to their limited inclusion in randomized trials. When guiding a patient through treatment decisions, it is important to consider whether the patient is able to tolerate life-prolonging treatment and whether treatment will improve symptoms and quality of life. Elective surgery does not appear to be associated with a higher mortality rate, although postsurgical complications and duration of hospital stay can increase with age. Radiation therapy is generally well tolerated by older patients and new methods of delivery, such as hyperfractionated radiation therapy are also showing promise in this age group. Chemotherapy should be considered in patients for whom cure,

survival, or palliation may be achieved; however, it should be noted that age associated pharmacological changes may alter tolerance of chemotherapeutics. Older patients are at increased risk for myelosuppression, mucositis, anemia-related fatigue, cardiomyopathy, and neuropathy.

Prevention

Even though age, one of the major risk factors for development of cancer, is not modifiable, cancer is a potentially preventable disease. Screening, as discussed above, remains controversial as a form of secondary prevention in the elderly. Much emphasis has been placed on primary prevention and its potential benefits for older adults. It has been estimated that two thirds of cancer deaths in the United States can be linked to smoking, lack of exercise, and obesity.[13] Nine modifiable risk factors are responsible for one third of cancers worldwide. After smoking and alcohol, overweight/obesity is the third most common cause of cancer-related death in developed countries.[14] Smoking cessation is the single most important preventable public health measure in decreasing the incidence of lung and other cancers in the elderly. Overall health benefit of smoking cessation even in the oldest old has been established.[15] Chemoprevention is an example of primary prevention that targets neoplastic transformation at its earliest form. Classes of chemopreventive agents such as selective estrogen receptor modulators (SERMs) may play a therapeutic role for selected elderly patients in prevention of breast cancer. Ongoing studies continue to determine their role in cancer prevention.

LUNG CANCER

Epidemiology

Lung cancer remains the leading cause of cancer death in the United States. The American Cancer Society estimates 215,020 cases of lung cancer will be diagnosed in 2008.[1] At the time of diagnosis, most patients older than 65 years are found to have stage III or IV disease and a median survival of 9–10 months. More than 80% of lung cancer diagnoses are non-small cell lung cancer (NSCLC), with the median age of diagnosis being 68 years. The remainder of lung cancers is composed of the small cell type, which occurs almost exclusively in smokers.[16] The overall 10-year survival rate is 7% and survival rate decreases with advancing age (5-year survival rate for patients <50 is 10% compared with 5% in patients >70).[17] Small cell lung cancer (SCLC) is characterized by rapid doubling time, high growth fraction, and early development of metastases.[18] Although most solid tumors utilize a tumor node metastasis (TNM) staging system because of its yield of prognostic information, it has not been useful in aiding in prognosis and management of SCLC. Therefore, a two-stage system categorizes SCLC into limited disease (tumor confined to one hemithorax and ipsilateral nodes) and extensive disease (tumor not confined to one hemithorax and/or presence of malignant effusions). Most long-term survivors are derived from the limited-disease group.

Table 36.1. Professional Organizations' Recommendations for Lung Cancer Screening

American Academy of Family Physicians[19]	■ **Recommends against** the use of chest x-ray and/or sputum cytology in asymptomatic persons for lung cancer screening
American Cancer Society[20]	■ **Does not recommend** lung cancer screening for asymptomatic individuals at risk for lung cancer
	■ However, high-risk patients and their physicians may decide evidence is sufficient to warrant screening with spiral CT on an individual basis
USPSTF[21]	■ Fair evidence that LDCT, chest x-ray, sputum cytology, or a combination of these tests can detect lung cancer earlier than in an unscreened population, *but*
	■ Poor evidence that any screening modality decreases mortality and screening poses significant risk of harm to patients
	■ **Insufficient evidence to recommend for or against** screening in asymptomatic patients
	■ Level I recommendation

In general, SCLC is a highly aggressive malignancy. Without treatment, median time of survival is 2–4 months.

Screening and Prevention

No major professional associations recommend screening for lung cancer because the benefit has not been established in any group including high-risk older smokers (Table 36.1).

The development of the low-dose helical computed tomography (LDCT) scanning to detect nodules as small as a few millimeters has sparked new interest in lung cancer screening. The sensitivity of LDCT for detection of lung cancer is four times that of chest x-ray and is six times more likely to detect stage I (potentially curable cancers).[22] The potential drawbacks of LDCT as a method of lung cancer screening include more false positives, greater radiation exposure, and increased costs ($200–$300). An important concern about screening for lung cancer is the risk of overdiagnosis and subsequent overtreatment without detection of advanced tumors or a change in the mortality rate, suggesting increased diagnoses of indolent tumors.

There is fair evidence that screening with LDCT detects lung cancer at an earlier stage but a decrease in mortality has not yet been demonstrated in randomized trials. In a recent study of annual screening in high-risk patients, most cancers detected were early stage, many of which were curable with surgery, suggesting promise for this method of screening asymptomatic patients.[23] Survival times for the group of individuals detected through the LDCT screens far exceed historical rates, although the study was not a randomized trial, and it lacked a specific control group. In fact, an analysis of several screening trials confirmed that more small cancers are found through screening but argued that the mortality rates in these series matched the

rates expected in the absence of screening.[24] Several ongoing trials are aimed at helping to elucidate the impact of lung cancer screening on mortality. Currently three randomized clinical trials are underway including the National Lung Screening Trial which randomly assigned patients between the ages of 55 and 74 years old to either lung cancer screening with CT or with chest radiographs and is powered to detect a 20% reduction in lung cancer mortality resulting from differences in methods of screening. The final analysis is expected to be released in 2012 after 8 years of data collection.[25]

Because of poor yield of secondary prevention for lung cancer, the value of primary prevention, mainly smoking cessation, should be emphasized. Cancer risk is dependent on quantity and duration of tobacco use. It has been demonstrated that quitting at any age decreases risk of developing lung cancer.[26] This confirms that the risk of developing lung cancer is a greater function of tobacco exposure than of increasing age. Although lung cancer screening holds potential promise, smoking prevention and cessation programs will continue to have by far the largest impact. The interventions that contribute to tobacco use prevention are known. Increasing the cost of tobacco products, enforcing clean indoor air laws and policies, limiting access to tobacco, particularly for young people, decreasing tobacco advertising, and increasing aggressive counter advertising are proven methods to reduce tobacco utilization.

Paraneoplastic Syndromes

SCLC is most commonly associated with endocrinological and neurological paraneoplastic syndromes. They are defined as nonmetastatic systemic effects that accompany malignant disease. The exact mechanism by which they occur is not understood. At times the symptoms of the paraneoplastic syndrome may precede the diagnosis of the malignancy, occur late in disease, or be a sign of disease recurrence. The most prevalent syndrome is the syndrome of inappropriate antidiuretic hormone secretion, affecting 40%–70% of patients with SCLC. The syndrome usually resolves within 3 weeks of completion of combination chemotherapy, but it has a tendency to recur. Increased serum and tissue levels of adrenocorticotropic hormone can cause Cushing's syndrome, uncommon in lung cancer, but characterized by weakness, hyperglycemia, edema, confusion, and hypokalemic alkalosis. Neurological paraneoplastic syndromes include Lambert–Eaton syndrome, a rare disorder of the neuromuscular junction that resembles myasthenia gravis. Hypercalcemia is more common in NSCLC.[27]

Management

Surgery

Surgery is generally the treatment of choice in early (stages I–III) NSCLC. Cure is unlikely in patients with NSCLC who do not undergo surgery. Although older patients are less likely to be treated with surgery, advanced age (>75 years) is not correlated with short-term or long-term postoperative results in lung cancer patients who are in good clinical condition prior to surgery.[28] Older patients are more likely to have medical problems that may preclude surgery but age alone should not determine their candidacy. Choice of surgery method is also important in minimizing risk. Lobectomy or wedge resection is preferred over pneumonectomy. Patients older than 70 years have been noted to have more complications following pneumonectomy with a three times increased risk of death compared with younger patients with comparable disease and risk. Respiratory function is the most accurate predictor of mortality in older patients.[29]

Radiation Therapy

Radiation therapy is the most commonly offered treatment to elderly patients with early stage lung cancer. Radiation therapy, given with curative intent, is often given to patients who are not candidates for or choose not to undergo surgery. Survival rates are inferior to those who have surgery. Thoracic radiation is equally tolerated in older and younger populations with age having no effect on symptoms such as nausea, vomiting, dyspnea, weakness, or esophagitis.[30] Older patients have been shown to be more likely to experience weight loss. Thus, nutritional status should be assessed in patients who are being considered for radiation therapy as it has been shown that weight loss is an independent predictor of mortality in community-dwelling older adults.[31] In locally advanced lung cancer, the survival benefit of concurrent chemotherapy and radiation therapy over sequential therapy in the population at large has been demonstrated but is associated with increased risk of short-term toxicity in the older lung cancer patient.[32] If it is thought that toxicities outweigh the benefit of concurrent chemotherapy and radiation, older patients ineligible for surgery may derive the most benefit from radiation alone. For patients with incurable disease, radiation has proved to

be useful in palliation of symptoms including hemoptysis and thoracic pain.[33]

Thoracic radiation therapy has been shown to improve survival moderately for SCLC patients with limited disease but the benefit has not been proven in patients older than age 70 years. Additionally, there is a potential for toxicity; however, the added potential of increased survival may justify this more aggressive treatment approach in patients with good performance status. The timing of the delivery of radiation therapy is controversial. Concurrent (given at the same time) or alternating (given on days chemotherapy is not) therapies are appealing because these treatment schedules have been hypothesized to improve survival outcomes but the data are not consistent. If radiation is chosen in an elderly patient, it should not be given concurrently (but rather, sequentially) with chemotherapy because the risk of esophageal and bone marrow toxicity is accentuated in the elderly.[18] Radiation in the setting of extensive disease only plays a palliative role.

Prophylactic Cranial Irradiation

Central nervous system (CNS) metastases in SCLC are common. In patients who achieve a complete remission after therapy, nearly 50% still progress to develop brain metastases in the next 2 years. When brain metastases are present, they are rarely curable by chemotherapy or radiation. This is the framework for the rationale that moderate doses of radiation to the brain in patients without CNS involvement may prevent future overt metastatic disease. Prophylactic cranial irradiation (PCI) has been shown to decrease metastases as well as have a modest improvement in 3-year survival rates (5%).[34] There has been concern about neurotoxicity, memory deficits, and quality of life in patients receiving PCI. Although the evidence is not conclusive, administering chemotherapy after completion of the radiation course decreases the risk of neurocognitive impairment. On the basis of outcome data, PCI is recommended for patients with limited-stage disease in whom a complete response is achieved after chemotherapy (Level of recommendation: A). Patients with extensive disease in whom a complete response is achieved after treatment may also be offered PCI after full discussion of risks and benefits. (Level of recommendation: C: fair evidence, small benefit).[35] PCI is not recommended in patients with multiple comorbidities, a poor performance status, or impaired baseline cognitive function.

Chemotherapy

Randomized studies show that fit older patients with advanced NSCLC benefit from chemotherapy. The Elderly Lung Cancer Vinorelbine Italian Study Group compared single-agent vinorelbine with best supportive care in patients older than the age of 70 years. Vinorelbine provided both a survival advantage and a symptomatic advantage over best supportive care. Adverse effects included constipation, neuropathy and fatigue.[36] An assessment of quality of life during this study also showed an advantage in the chemotherapy treated group. The Multicenter Italian Lung Cancer in the Elderly Study trial was the largest study conducted in elderly patients with NSCLC.

Patients older than 70 years were randomized to receive single-agent vinorelbine, single-agent gemcitabine, or the combination of the two agents. The results did not show a significant advantage for the nonplatinum-based doublet over the single agent but did demonstrate increased toxicities with the agents combined.[37] From this study and the Elderly Lung Cancer Vinorelbine Italian Study Group study, it was concluded that single-agent therapy should be the standard therapy in elderly patients with advanced NSCLC. Functional status and a patient's comorbid status prior to lung cancer diagnosis aid in treatment decisions. Although not proven by randomized trials, patients with a poor functional status because of comorbidities may be good candidates for single-agent therapy. On the other hand, patients with no prior major comorbidities may benefit from more aggressive chemotherapy with platinum-based combination therapy. Additionally, chemotherapy has offered a survival advantage when administered to elderly patients who have undergone resection.[38]

With surgery being a very rare option in SCLC, combination chemotherapy remains the cornerstone of management of SCLC with a response rate of 70%–80% in limited disease (compared with 60%–70% in extensive disease). Despite its responsiveness to chemotherapy, SCLC is characterized by a high recurrence rate within 2 years of treatment and poor overall survival. In limited-disease SCLC, the median survival is 12–16 months with up to 5% being considered cured. In extensive-disease SCLC, the median survival is 9–11 months with virtually no survivors after 5 years.[39] For patients with limited-stage disease, standard chemotherapy consists of four–six cycles of etoposide and cisplatin with or without thoracic irradiation. Patients in whom complete remission is achieved may be offered prophylactic brain irradiation.

For patients with extensive-stage disease, a combination platinum-based chemotherapy regimen is recommended. Several retrospective studies evaluated multiple prognostic factors including age in elderly patients treated with standard combination chemotherapy regimens. There was no statistical difference in survival based on age and only a marginal difference based on performance status.[40] No studies resulted in inferior response rates for overall survival for older patients (>70 years). These treatments generally lead to greater toxicity in older adults compared with younger adults. Single-agent chemotherapy is not an adequate substitution for combination therapy in older patients with SCLC because of findings in randomized studies showing inferior survival with single-agent chemotherapy.[41,42]

Supportive Care

Given the aggressiveness of lung cancer, providers, patients, and caregivers place greater emphasis on quality-of-life considerations. This is particularly important in patients for whom the disease is incurable. Besides proper analgesia and oxygen therapy, supportive care may include palliative radiotherapy, which is effective in short-term control of thoracic and bone pain as well as in decreasing CNS metastases. A focus on the emotional care of the patient and caregivers should be emphasized as well. Depression in the setting of lung cancer can be missed, as symptoms may be mistaken for those secondary to the cancer itself.

COLON CANCER

Epidemiology

Colorectal cancer is the third most common malignancy in the United States with approximately 148,610 new cases of large bowel cancers being diagnosed each year. Of these cases, greater than 70% are localized in the colon with the remainder being in the rectum.[43] In 2008, it is estimated that 49,960 Americans will die of colorectal cancer, accounting for approximately 9% of all cancer deaths. Colon cancer ranks second to lung cancer as a cause of cancer death.[1]

Age is a major risk factor for the development of colorectal cancer, with 90% of cases occurring after the age of 50 years. The median age of diagnosis of colorectal cancer is 71.1 years of age.[2] The lifetime risk of developing colorectal cancer is 1 in 18, a risk that increases with age regardless of race or sex. The increased risk of colorectal cancer with aging may be linked to the observation that more than 80% of colorectal cancers arise from adenomatous polyps. Ten percent of polyps larger than 1 cm become malignant after 10 years and nearly 25% after 20 years.[44] The prevalence of polyps increases with age; 50% of patients older than 75 have polyps.[45]

Risk Factors

Risk factors also include a personal or family history of sporadic cancers or adenomatous polyps, inflammatory bowel disease, diabetes mellitus, and cigarette smoking. Individuals with ulcerative colitis are at particularly high risk for colon cancer, even if the disease is clinically quiescent and must undergo screening far more frequently, beginning 8 years after developing this disease in conjunction with pancolitis or 12–15 years after the onset of left-sided disease.[1] Prophylactic colectomy is a reasonable step in appropriate candidates. Several rare familial syndromes, such as familial adenomatous polyposis and hereditary nonpolyposis colon cancer also confer very high risk and require early and intensive screening or prophylactic colectomy depending on results of genetic testing. In family members testing positive for the gene causing familial adenomatous polyposis, screening should be performed regularly, and colectomy should be considered when polyps are found. Patients with hereditary nonpolyposis colon cancer should undergo colonoscopy every 1–2 years beginning at age 20–25 years, or 10 years earlier than the youngest age of colon cancer diagnosis in the family; whichever comes first.[46] The role of diet and additional environmental factors has not been fully determined.[47] Two large prospective studies have shown an association of obesity with higher risk of colon cancer, a relationship that is probably, although not definitively, causal.[48,49] Although a family history of colorectal cancer is a known risk factor for developing colorectal cancer, a prospective study examining the strength of this association concluded that the risk is significant in younger people but does not predict cancer risk in patients older than 65 years.[50]

Screening

The U.S. Preventive Services Task Force (USPSTF) strongly recommends that clinicians screen average-risk men and women 50 years of age or older for colorectal cancer (A recommendation).[51] What remains uncertain is the optimal means by which to screen and the age at which to stop screening.

The major screening tests currently recommended by the American Cancer Society to detect polyps or colorectal cancer are yearly fecal occult blood test (FOBT) utilizing either guaiac-based or immunochemical testing methodology, sigmoidoscopy every 5 years, the combination of FOBT and sigmoidoscopy, double-contrast barium enema every 5 years, and colonoscopy every 10 years. Medicare covers these methods of screening in patients older than age 50 years. The current evidence does not support choosing one test over another. Evidence demonstrates that all tests are effective but differ in sensitivity, specificity, cost, and safety. Cost-effectiveness models have been calculated for yearly FOBT, sigmoidoscopy every 5 years, and colonoscopy every 10 years, each of which falls within usual cost-effectiveness thresholds.

Fecal Occult Blood Testing with Immunochemical Technology, or Guaiac-Based Technology

The only randomized prospective trials of colon cancer screening utilized FOBT. The Minnesota trial demonstrated that colon cancer mortality is reduced by 33% with annual testing and 16% with biannual testing.[52] All individuals who test positive for blood in the stool must have a colonoscopy to gain the protective benefit. Advantages of this method of screening include low cost, high safety, easy availability, and support through high-quality evidence. The actual sensitivity and specificity of these stool-based testing strategies vary depending on the type of test used. Tests that have at least a 50% sensitivity for cancer are available and should be used. This strategy may be particularly important in older individuals with comorbidities for whom colonoscopy carries a higher risk.

Sigmoidoscopy

A 60-cm sigmoidoscopy can only reach to the splenic flexure. A cross-sectional analysis of colonoscopy screening found one half of all advanced adenomas and cancers in the proximal region would be missed on sigmoidoscopy examination.[53] One recent colonoscopy series estimates that a strategy of sigmoidoscopy screening followed by colonoscopy for individuals in whom a polyp is found would detect approximately 75% of advanced polyps.[54] As individuals age, a higher percentage of polyps and colon cancer are found on the right side of the colon, a clinical observation that argues against the use of sigmoidoscopy alone.

Colonoscopy

A benefit of colonoscopy as a screening method is its long-lasting protective effects if negative. A case-control study, in which almost half of the patients were older than 70 years, demonstrated that patients who died of colon cancer were less likely to have had a colonoscopy in the prior 10 years.[55] Screening colonoscopy in patients older than age 80 has been shown to have only 15% of the expected gain in life expectancy in younger patients.[56] Although colonoscopy is the most sensitive and specific (>90% for both) of colorectal screening tests, it has remained uncertain whether these attributes translate into reduced colorectal cancer mortality. Complications from colonoscopy include perforation (1/1,000), serious bleeding (3/1,000), and cardiorespiratory events from intravenous anesthetics (5/1,000).[57] There is an increased risk of perforation with increasing age and presence of two or more comorbidities.[58] The procedure itself can be more difficult in older adults due to changes in bowel elasticity and increased presence of diverticulosis.[59] Challenges related to the bowel preparation are especially salient in older patients including volume depletion and electrolyte abnormalities, as well as an increased risk of falls when patients try to get to the bathroom quickly.

In summary, the choice of screening method remains individualized depending on patient preference, functional status, and comorbidities. The proved mortality benefit in FOBT results in part from the sequence of a positive FOBT leading to colonoscopy for visualization of the entire colon. Sigmoidoscopy is generally less valuable in the older population due to the increasing incidence of right-sided neoplasms with advancing age. In patients who can tolerate the procedure, colonoscopy may be most appropriate because of its long-lasting protective effect. Every patient should be offered an evidence-based screening option and systems to help schedule and implement performance are critically important.

When to Stop Screening

Although there is good evidence supporting screening patients older than age 50 years for colorectal cancer, there are no data to guide the decision to stop screening. Even though the yield of screening would be higher with advancing age because of a higher incidence of colon cancer, it is difficult to extrapolate the proved benefit in younger patients because older patients may receive less benefit and face greater risk. Advancing age, inflammatory bowel disease, and a history of multiple or large colorectal adenomas all increase the risk of developing and dying from colon cancer, which increases the chance to benefit from screening. The benefits, however, may be limited as a result of competing causes of death. Although the three trials evaluating FOBT included a small number of individuals up to 80 years old and had a proved benefit in decreasing colorectal cancer mortality, there was no subgroup analysis for older patients.[60] Evidence suggests it takes at least 5 years to see a mortality benefit from screening, so it is reasonable to conclude that there is little value in screening if the life expectancy of the patient is estimated to be less than this.

Clinical Presentation and Diagnosis

Colon cancer is asymptomatic in early stages. As the disease progresses, symptoms vary depending on the location of the tumor. Older patients are more likely to present with right-sided lesions that are large, fungating, bleeding masses that cause iron deficiency anemia, weakness, and fatigue.[61] Right-sided masses do not usually cause obstruction but can grow large enough to allow palpation on examination. Left-sided masses are usually "napkin-ring" obstructive lesions causing obstruction, rectal bleeding, and altered bowel habits. When an elderly patient reports rectal bleeding or has occult blood in the stool, complete evaluation of the colon and rectum is indicated. Colonoscopy has become the diagnostic gold standard because it allows visualization of the entire colon and biopsy areas of concern.

Staging and Survival Rates

The TNM staging system is now the most commonly used staging system in colon cancer and serves to predict likelihood of 5-year survival.[1,62]

Table 36.1. TMN Staging System

Stage	TNM Classification	5-y Survival Rate
I	T1, N0, M0	
	T2, N0, M0	93%
IIA	T3, N0, M0	85%
IIB	T4, N0, M0	72%
IIIA	T1, N1, M0	
	T2, N1, M0	83%
IIIB	T3, N1, M0	
	T4, N1, M0	64%
IIIC	Any T, N2, M0	44%
IV	Any T, any N, M1	8%

Treatment

Surgery

Older patients with colon cancer are more likely to have comorbid conditions, present with advanced stage disease, undergo emergency surgery, and less likely to receive curative surgery than their younger counterparts.[63] Outcomes following colorectal cancer surgery can be favorable even in the oldest old group. Selected elderly patients benefit from surgery because a large proportion survives for 2 or more years, independent of age. Given that colon cancer survival following emergency surgery is associated with worse outcomes in older patients because of advanced tumor stage and poor physical health at time of presentation, careful assessment of the older patient for elective surgery should be considered and candidacy should not be determined based on age alone.[64]

Adjuvant Therapy

Although adjuvant chemotherapy is standard for colon cancer patients following surgery, this treatment modality has been controversial in patients older than 70 years because of concerns regarding toxicities and uncertain efficacy. It has been observed that older patients with stage II or III colon cancer are offered adjuvant therapy less often than younger patients.[65] In a pooled analysis of seven randomized studies including more than 3,000 patients with stage II–III disease undergoing 5-fluorouracil (5 FU)-based adjuvant chemotherapy showed a positive effect on both survival time and time to recurrence. No significant relationship was established between age and efficacy of treatment. Elderly patients did not experience increased toxicity compared with younger patients except for an increase in leukopenia in one study.[66]

Chemotherapy for Recurrent or Advanced Disease

Fluorinated pyrimidines (5-FU) represent the backbone of colon cancer therapy. 5-FU is given as an infusion usually in combination with leucovorin. For patients with advanced colorectal cancer this treatment combination reduces the size of the tumor by 50% or more in approximately 20% of patients and prolongs the median survival rate from 6 months (for those untreated) to 11 months.[67]

BREAST CANCER

Breast cancer is a common diagnosis in older women. In 2008, an estimated 182,460 breast cancer cases in women will be diagnosed in the United States.[1] The incidence of breast cancer increases with age; nearly half the cases arise in women 65 years and older. Most patients spanning all age groups present with stage I or II breast cancer, whereas the oldest old (>85 years) are more likely to present with metastases.[68] As many as half of the patients older than 65 years, who present with breast cancer die from the disease, accounting for a significant cause of morbidity and mortality in the geriatric population. A multidisciplinary approach to breast cancer in older patients includes understanding of the distinctive characteristics of breast cancer, detection of early disease, and management options specific to this patient population.

Characteristics of Breast Cancer in Older Women

Although infiltrating ductal carcinoma remains the most common subtype of breast cancer in both younger and older women, breast cancer in the elderly population has distinctive biological and clinical characteristics. Older women are more likely to have less aggressive tumors and a more favorable

Table 36.2. Professional Organizations Recommendations for Stopping Breast Cancer Screening

Organization	Recommendation	Comments
American Cancer Society[77]	**No upper age limit**; instead cessation is function of comorbidity	Recommends annual mammogram, CBE, and monthly SBE
American Geriatric Society[78]	**Offer up until the age of 85 years in women with life expectancy of greater than 4 y** who would pursue treatment	Screening mammography every 1–2 y until age 75 then every 3 years.
USPSTF[79]	**Uncertain precise age at which to stop screening** Class C recommendation	Lack of clinical evidence to recommend for or against screening in women older than 70 years
American College of Physicians[79]	**Upper age limit of 75 years**	Based on data that 80% of mortality benefit is reached by this age

biological tumor profile. It has been shown that for tumors of similar size, the prevalence of axillary lymph node involvement decreased with the age of the patient after age 55 years.[69] Additionally, older breast cancer patients have been noted to have a longer detectable preclinical period, a higher percentage of estrogen receptor positive (ER+) cells, and are more likely to harbor moderately well differentiate tumors, characteristics that may improve survival.[70] The proportion of ER+ tumors continues to increase even within the older-than-65 cohort, with 87% of patients aged 65–74 years having ER+ tumors, compared with 91% of patients aged 85 years and older.[71]

Detection and Screening

The presentation of breast cancer does not differ significantly in the older population. The most common symptom of breast cancer remains a painless mass. Pain, thickening, nipple discharge, and swelling are all symptoms that should be actively pursued in older women. The breasts become less dense as women age, making the clinical examination easier. Additionally, an abnormal mammogram has greater sensitivity and specificity with increasing age.[72] A diagnosis is ultimately made using tissue sampling by either core or excisional biopsy.

Given the distinctive characteristics of breast cancer in the elderly, screening older women for early breast cancer could potentially improve survival. Yet evidence for a mortality benefit from screening beyond age 70 years has not been proved by randomized controlled trials. Early diagnosis of breast cancer in the elderly may not decrease mortality due to competing causes of death. Patients with three or more comorbidities are 20 times more likely to die of a cause other than breast cancer within 3 years.[73] The number of patients one needs to screen with mammography to prevent one breast cancer–related death is estimated at 242 for the average 70-year-old woman and 533 for the average 80-year old.[71] A study on cost effectiveness concluded that if all women received idealized treatment, the benefits of mammography beyond age 79 years would be too low relative to cost to justify continued screening.[74] Although

the increased sensitivity and specificity of mammograms in older patients would purport a theoretical benefit to screening, a potential increased rate of detection of ductal carcinoma in situ (DCIS) may lead to overtreatment due to its uncertain malignant potential and management controversy.[75]

Because of a lack of evidence for utility of screening for breast cancer in older women, no consensus on screening has been reached. (See summary of professional organization recommendations in Table 36.2.) Although no data show efficacy for the clinical breast examination, the American Geriatrics Society (AGS) recommends annual clinical breast examination. The examination is covered by Medicare and takes little physician time. It may be of added value in older women with arthritis and/or neuropathies who may not be able to participate in breast self-examination or do not wish to undergo mammography. Breast self-examination, although neither endorsed nor discourage by AGS because of its marginal benefit, increases women's awareness of their breast health.[76]

Primary and Secondary Prevention

Primary prevention of breast cancer involves modification of known risk factors for disease. The strongest risk factor for breast cancer is age. Historical risk factors for breast cancer also include family history, early menarache, late age at birth of first child, late age of menopause, and a personal history of benign breast disease. These risk factors cannot be modified in elderly patients. Because it is an estrogen dependent disease, breast cancer is an ideal candidate for chemoprevention. Tamoxifen, a SERM, is the only medication approved by the FDA as chemoprevention in high-risk patients. The use of tamoxifen, however, has been associated with increased risk of thromboembolic events after 5 years of use. Additionally, an increased risk of endometrial cancer, hot flushes, cerebrovascular accidents, and vaginal bleeding has been noted with use of tamoxifen. The development of endometrial cancer in large clinical trials has been reported to occur at a rate that is two–seven times greater than that observed in untreated women.[80–83] Because of the side-effect profile of tamoxifen, the USPSTF recommends against routine use of SERMs for the primary prevention of breast cancer in women at low or average risk for breast cancer (recommendation D). Discussion of chemoprevention in patients who are at high risk for the development of breast cancer and low risk for adverse effects of chemoprevention is recommended by the USPSTF (recommendation B).

Despite tamoxifen's proven effectiveness, its side-effect profile has prompted further investigation into other SERMs and their potential use in chemoprevention. The Study of Tamoxifen and Raloxifene trial was the first head-to-head randomized trial comparing the efficacy and safety of both drugs in reducing breast cancer risk in postmenopausal patients. The study involved nearly 20,000 women (41% of women in the study were >60 years) at increased risk of developing breast cancer (without a personal history of breast cancer) and randomly assigned them to either receive raloxifene or tamoxifen over a 5-year period. Both drugs were shown to reduce risk of developing invasive breast cancer by 50% but raloxifene was not as effective in reducing risk of developing noninvasive breast cancer. The raloxifene group was found to have a more favorable side-effect profile with 36% fewer uterine cancers and 29% fewer deep vein thromboses.[84]

Management of the Older Patient with Breast Cancer

Ductal Carcinoma In Situ

DCIS is a precancerous condition, which is characterized by abnormal cells that have not invaded the surrounding breast tissue. Although DCIS can present as a palpable mass, it is usually asymptomatic and presents as calcifications on a screening mammogram. With the increasing rates of mammography use, incidence of carcinoma in situ (most common of which is DCIS) has also increased, accounting for approximately 20% of breast cancers. There are several different histological subtypes; the comedo subtype poses the greatest risk of aggressiveness and recurrence after treatment.[85] The goals of treatment of DCIS include controlling local disease and preventing progression to invasive cancer. In the past, the mainstay of therapy for women with DCIS was mastectomy; however, studies suggest that breast conservation is appropriate for many women with DCIS. A large randomized trial demonstrated that radiotherapy along with lumpectomy, compared with lumpectomy alone, decreases the likelihood of recurrence.[86] Prospective trials have also looked at the role of hormonal therapy in addition to lumpectomy and radiation therapy. In one randomized study, tamoxifen was shown to decrease risk of recurrence but this reduction was not replicated in another randomized trial. Neither trial proved a survival benefit with use of tamoxifen.[87,88] Both studies demonstrated tamoxifen-related toxicities and emphasized the importance of using a patient's comorbidities and a comprehensive discussion of risk–benefit ratio of hormonal therapy.

What makes the management of DCIS difficult is that some patients go on to develop malignancy whereas others do not, and currently, there is no prognostic capability to determine the

risk of each individual patient. In a study of breast-conserving surgery with and without radiation, only 1.6% of deaths were attributable to breast cancer in more than 800 women after a mean follow-up of 8 years.[89] This is particularly salient in the older population who often do present with comorbidities that carry a greater mortality risk than the DCIS.

Management of Early Stage Breast Cancer

Surgery in Primary Management (Stage I and IIA, IIB Disease)

Surgery is the mainstay of curative therapy for breast cancer. Many retrospective studies have demonstrated significant undertreatment by disease stage of breast cancer patients older than the age of 65 years. Options for surgical management of the primary tumor include breast-conserving surgery plus radiation therapy, mastectomy plus reconstruction, and mastectomy alone. Breast-conserving therapy (lumpectomy, axillary dissection, and breast irradiation) has been shown to be equal in efficacy to more extensive surgical options without significant differences in overall 20-year survival.[90,91] The literature suggests that surgery in older women is safe and is without increased risk compared with younger cohorts.[92] The main factor influencing morbidity is not age but the presence of comorbidity. Mortality rates after breast cancer surgery in octogenarians and nonagenarians have been shown to be 0.5%.[93] Despite evidence of efficacy and safety of surgery in this age group, older patients are being offered less aggressive treatment than their younger counterparts. Even when older women are undergoing breast-conserving therapy, they are less likely to have axillary dissection, postoperative radiation, and chemotherapy.[94]

Nodal status is one of the most important indicators of prognosis in early stage breast cancer. Although often omitted in the assessment of older women, axillary surgery plays a role in either determining nodal disease control or in accurately staging the tumor, which aid in determination of adjuvant therapy. Addressing the latter, women with node positive ER+ breast cancer may be candidates for chemotherapy in addition to hormone therapy. Also, in postmenopausal women, those with four or more positive lymph nodes may be offered postmastectomy radiation therapy. Despite its surmised usefulness in determining therapy options, axillary node dissection remains a controversial topic in breast cancer management in the elderly because full axillary clearance increases morbidity whereas the omission of axillary surgery puts the patient at increased risk of nodal disease.[95] Meanwhile, whether omission of axillary surgery adversely affects survival is a matter of intense debate.

The sentinel lymph node technique (SLNT), an axillary node sampling technique using injection of a tracer material into the skin and breast mass and subsequent monitoring of uptake in a small number of axillary nodes, has recently been developed as an alternative to axillary node dissection. SLNT is associated with a lower rate of arm morbidity, such as lymphedema, that can have a negative impact on functional status and quality of life. The SLNT biopsy's impact on survival in comparison to full axillary dissection has yet to be proved.[96]

Although research into the debate surrounding axillary lymph node assessment continues, it is reasonable to recommend axillary lymph node dissection in all patients with clinically positive nodes. Axillary lymph node assessment via SLNT could be considered in patients who have a clinically negative axilla, ER-tumor, and whose health status would make them eligible for chemotherapy. Axillary assessment can be omitted in women with a small (≤2 cm) tumor and clinically node-negative breast cancer who will be treated with adjuvant hormonal therapy. Additionally, axillary assessment should be considered in women with large ER+ tumors who are not eligible for breast-conserving therapy.

Role of Tamoxifen in Primary Management

Enthusiasm surrounded the introduction of tamoxifen in the 1980s as a sole treatment effective in the geriatric population. A recent Cochrane review analyzing surgery compared with primary endocrine therapy in operable primary breast cancer in women older than 70 concluded that primary endocrine therapy is inferior to surgery (with or without endocrine therapy) for the local control of breast cancer in medically fit older women. Surgery was not shown to improve overall survival significantly, although patients treated with tamoxifen alone had more local progression than those treated surgically.[97] This study supported previous data demonstrating 81% of elderly women treated with primary tamoxifen appear to develop progressive disease after 12 years of follow-up compared with 38% with mastectomy alone.[98] Given significant local relapse rates, sole tamoxifen therapy should be reserved for patients with highly selective ER+ breast cancer who are not deemed surgical candidates or for those patients who choose not to pursue surgery.

Adjuvant Radiotherapy

Radiotherapy following breast conservative therapy is considered a standard component of treatment. Radiation therapy delivered over 4–6 weeks in this setting has been found to decrease recurrence rates, permit preservation of cosmetically satisfactory breast, and have a small increase in survival compared with lumpectomy alone.[99] Radiation therapy is generally well tolerated and provides good cosmetic results even in older women. Observational studies have shown that for older women with early breast cancer radiotherapy has been associated with decreased risk of a second ipsilateral breast cancer.[100] The value of postoperative radiotherapy has been questioned as the risk of local recurrence is lower in older women and the benefit of radiotherapy declines with advancing age. A randomized study of women older than age 70 years who received tamoxifen and radiotherapy compared with tamoxifen alone following lumpectomy demonstrated no significant differences in mastectomy for local recurrence, risk for distant metastases, or overall survival.[101] Additionally, the demand of daily transportation for older patients to receive radiotherapy may preclude this as a viable option in this patient population. As a

potential alternative to daily radiotherapy, weekly hypofractionated radiotherapy has been studied in retrospective series and can be considered particularly in women with ER- tumors who would not benefit from adjuvant hormone therapy.[102] Partial breast irradiation (limiting the radiation to the tumor bed rather than the entire breast) and more rapid fractionation schedules are also being explored as possible alternatives to radiotherapy.

Adjuvant Hormonal Therapy

A large meta-analysis of The Early Breast Cancer Trial Collaborative Group provided 15-year follow-up data on recurrence and survival of 145,000 women with early breast cancers who participated in 194 randomized clinical trials of adjuvant systemic therapies. A meta-analysis demonstrated that 5 years of adjuvant tamoxifen therapy in known ER+ women results in a 50% proportional reduction in recurrence risk and a decrease of mortality by 33%. The 15-year cumulative reduction in mortality is more than twice as great as at 5 years after diagnosis. The study also proved an increased benefit of a 5-year course of tamoxifen compared with a two-year treatment regimen.[103] The data have not supported use of tamoxifen for longer than 5 years. The benefits of tamoxifen have been proven regardless of age and nodal status. Women with ER- tumor status do not benefit from tamoxifen. Based on clear benefits, every woman with ER+ early breast cancer larger than 1 cm should be offered hormone therapy.

The potential toxic profile of tamoxifen contributed to the studies looking at aromatase inhibitors as adjuvant hormonal agents. Newer data have supported that aromatase inhibitors are as effective or more effective in decreasing risk of disease relapse and death in breast cancer patients and a 42% decreased risk of developing breast cancer in the contralateral breast.[104] Although long-term benefit has not yet been shown with aromatase inhibitors, as it has with tamoxifen, a more favorable side-effect profile has led to increased use. Preliminary reports do show long-term use with this class of hormonal therapy is associated with increased likelihood of development of osteoporosis. Thus, for women with a history of osteoporosis and/or fracture the prevalence of which is significant in older women who are deemed candidates for adjuvant hormone therapy, tamoxifen is currently preferred over the aromatase inhibitors.

Chemotherapy

Compared with the widespread acceptance of adjuvant chemotherapy in premenopausal breast cancer patients, this line of treatment is more controversial in the older patient population for several reasons. The risk of chemotherapy increases with increasing age due to an increased number of comorbidities and a decline in organ function. Another factor complicating treatment decisions is that the relative efficacy of chemotherapy is reduced with age. In the Early Breast Cancer Trial Collaborative Group trials there was a statistically significant reduction in recurrence and breast cancer–specific mortality in the adjuvant chemotherapy group across all ages, but the absolute magnitude of benefit was three times greater in younger women. In addition, the data in the group of women age 70 years and older were limited as this group only comprised 4% of the population in the meta-analysis, therefore leading to insufficient data showing the benefit of chemotherapy in this age group.[103] ER status also contributes to older women receiving adjuvant chemotherapy less frequently than their younger counterparts because the benefit of chemotherapy is less pronounced in ER+ patients than ER- patients. Chemotherapy has been associated with a reduction in mortality in older patients with ER-, lymph node–positive breast cancers.[105]

In general, the International Consensus Group for the Primary Treatment of Breast Cancer recommends offering chemotherapy to patients with tumors larger than 1 cm in size that are hormone nonresponsive. For ER+ tumors that have unfavorable histopathological features, are larger than 2 cm and/or involve three or more lymph nodes, and/or overexpress HER2/neu (confers high risk), chemotherapy can be recommended. The consensus group no longer gives the age limit of 70 years in their recommendations.[106] The decision to use chemotherapy in older patients is complex and in addition to considering the tumor's hormone responsiveness and nodal status, providers should consider the patient's life expectancy, comorbidities, and functional status. An internet-based tool (Adjuvantonline.com) serves to assist in estimating prognosis in the setting of chemotherapy. It calculates risk of relapse and/or death in women with early stage breast cancer based on age and comorbidities and can be used to provide the foundation on which risks, benefits, and patient preferences for chemotherapy can be discussed.

Management of Locally Advanced Breast Cancer (Stage III)

Elderly patients with cancers larger than 5 cm or with multiple clinically positive nodes may be candidates for preoperative treatment with hormonal therapy if the tumor is shown to be ER+ or with chemotherapy if it is ER-. This provides the theoretical advantage of shrinking the tumor such that the patient now becomes a candidate for breast-conserving therapy. Studies that have shown successful downstaging of tumors have focused on a younger patient population.[107] Even so, no studies have been able to show that preoperative systemic therapy improves survival over surgery followed by systemic therapy. For elderly patients with large initial lesions who wish to pursue breast-conserving surgery, the decision to proceed with neoadjuvant therapy remains an individualized decision neither supported nor refuted by randomized clinical studies.

Management of Metastatic Disease (Stage IV)

All treatment of metastatic breast cancer is palliative. The 5-year survival rate across all age groups in women diagnosed with metastatic disease is approximately 20%. Even though the overall survival of patients with metastatic disease is usually 2–3 years, approximately 10% of patients experience breast

cancer as a chronic disease and may live 10 years or more. Quality of life and palliation of symptoms remain the cornerstone of management that serve to guide health care providers' care to these patients. In the absence of rapidly progressive or immediate life-threatening disease, hormonal therapy (in patients who are antiestrogen naïve) using tamoxifen or aromatase inhibitors should be considered in patients with hormone receptor–positive tumors. In patients whose disease progresses while receiving antiestrogen therapy, alternative hormonal therapies may be considered in patients who are hormone receptor positive, whereas chemotherapy may be considered for patients whose tumors are hormone receptor negative. Bisphosphonates are recommended for all patients with lytic bone disease. Treatment of women with metastatic disease must be decided after performing individualized assessment of risks and benefits, quality-of-life issues, and comorbidities. The clinician and other members of the health care team play an instrumental role in facilitating end-of-life preferences with the patient and her family.

Care of Breast Cancer Survivors

Because of the combined effect of life expectancy continuing to increase in the general population and the relative success of breast cancer treatment, more and more elderly patients are breast cancer survivors. Recommendations for follow-up care will aid providers in treating such patients. Risk of recurrence after primary treatment of breast cancer continues for at least 15 years. Appropriate breast cancer follow-up care in the adjuvant setting includes regular history-taking, physical examination, and mammography. History-taking and physical examinations should be performed every 3–6 months for the first 3 years, every 6–12 months for years 4 and 5, and annually thereafter. For those who have undergone breast-conserving surgery, a posttreatment mammogram should be obtained 1 year after the initial mammogram and at least 6 months after completion of radiation therapy. Following this, unless otherwise indicated, an annual mammogram should be obtained.[108,109] Often follow-up care is delivered by both the oncologist and primary care provider and rates of mammography are higher in patients who benefit from this care than those who only saw one of the physicians (not both).[110] It is important for providers to recognize the potential for adverse effects following breast cancer treatment including lymphedema following axillary node dissection, symptoms of heart failure following specific chemotherapeutic agents, and side effects of estrogen deprivation secondary to tamoxifen use. Of equal importance is a continued emphasis on the cancer survivor's emotional care and other medical problems. A recent study showed that elderly cancer patients had more functional limitations than women who had never been diagnosed with cancer; data that suggests the diagnosis of cancer impacts women long after successful treatment.[111] Comprehensive follow-up care of a breast cancer survivor also includes addressing issues of quality of life, emotional health, adherence to oral therapies, and spiritual well-being.

Table 36.3. Screening Recommendation from Professional Organizations

Organization	General Recommendation	Comment
USPSTF[117]	Insufficient evidence to recommend for or against screening	Unlikely to benefit: age older than 70–75 and/or life expectancy less than 10 y
American Urological Association[119]	Annual screening in average-risk* men starting at age 50 in patients with life expectancy of 10 y	Unlikely to benefit: age older than 70–75 and/or life expectancy less than 10 y
American Cancer Society[120]	Annual screening should be offered to average-risk* men starting at age 50 in patients with life expectancy of 10 years	Unlikely to benefit: age older than 70–75 and/or life expectancy less than 10 y

* High-risk men (those of African American heritage or with a first-degree family relative with prostate cancer) can be offered screening at age 40.

PROSTATE CANCER

Epidemiology

Prostate cancer is the most common malignancy and the second most common cause of cancer death in men. The American Cancer Society estimated that 186,320 men will be diagnosed with and 28,600 men will die of prostate cancer in 2008.[1] The incidence of prostate cancer increases with age with 80% of all prostate cancer occurring in men older than the age of 65. Autopsy studies reveal that prior to age 40 approximately 29% of men show microscopic evidence of disease and this increases to as many as 65% of men by age 70.[112] The lifetime risk of developing the disease is approximately 16%, whereas the risk of dying from prostate cancer is 3%, supporting the notion that most men with prostate cancer die with the disease rather than of it.[113]

In addition to advancing age, African-American race is a risk factor for prostate cancer. Among African-American men, prostate cancer occurs at an earlier age, is more advanced at time of diagnosis, and is associated with higher mortality rates. Men with a family history of prostate cancer in a first-degree relative have more than a twofold risk of developing the disease and this risk increases with each relative affected. Theorized increased risk associated with vasectomy has not been proved.

Screening Controversy

Prostate cancer can be characterized as a disease marked by high prevalence and relatively low mortality. Although there has been a decline in prostate cancer mortality since the advent of prostate-specific antigen (PSA) screening, screening programs remain controversial because to date, no randomized, controlled trial has provided evidence that screening for prostate cancer at any age (directly) decreases disease-specific mortality. Nevertheless, a preponderance of data from epidemiological trends strongly indicates that screening with PSA has led to a dramatic decline in prostate cancer mortality rates for those populations who are offered screening around the world.

Age-adjusted prostate cancer mortality rates in the United States have now dropped to levels last seen in the 1940s and for Caucasian men are at the lowest rate recorded since data tracking began. A similar dramatic reduction in prostate cancer mortality has been observed in the Austrian state of Tyrol where an organized screening program was offered to all eligible men with no offer of screening in all other Austrian states. Investigators observed a threefold adjusted decrease in prostate cancer mortality rates in Tyrol compared with in the rest of Austria.[114]

One of the important challenges confronting clinical decision making is identifying those men who are at significant risk of dying of their prostate cancer and aggressively treating that group of men and withholding aggressive therapy from those men who are unlikely to die of their prostate cancer. Regardless of the biological characteristics of the cancer, an important predictor of cancer mortality, those men who are very old and those men with serious comorbidities are less likely to die of their prostate cancer. Evidence has shown that the median time taken from diagnosis to death from prostate cancer for men with nonpalpable disease approximates 17 years, although disease aggressiveness and natural history are variable.[115] The current recommendations reflect the controversy and uncertainty regarding prostate cancer screening. (Refer to Table 36.3. for summary of recommendations.) All organizations recommend that physicians discuss with their patients the uncertain benefits and possible harms of screening and individual preferences should be taken into account.

Perhaps even more salient in the geriatric population is when to stop screening. It will be particularly difficult to prove a mortality benefit because of the exclusion of patients older than the age of 75 years from randomized clinical trials.[116] Major guidelines agree that men who have less than a 10-year life expectancy or who are older than age 70–75 years are unlikely to benefit from screening.[117] The average life expectancy for a 75-year-old man is 10.3 years. Despite these recommendations, in the Veterans Affairs medical system, 56% of men older than 70 years had a PSA performed in 2003. Screening rates not only remain high despite advancing age, they also are offered to older men in poor health at rates similar to those in good health. In the Veterans Affairs study, in men older than 85, 34% of men in good health and 36% in poor health were screened with a PSA.[118]

Another disadvantage of screening is the screening tools themselves.[121] The postulated benefit of screening is the high sensitivity of the PSA allowing detection of malignancy at an early stage, therefore enhancing the likelihood of curative therapy for disease confined to the prostate. An elevated PSA alone does not translate directly into a diagnosis of prostate cancer. Approximately 25% of biopsies reveal prostate cancer, a similar rate of positive biopsy as seen in women with abnormal mammograms.[122] The PSA can be elevated in cancer as well as in benign prostatic hypertrophy, prostatitis, recent ejaculation, and minor trauma. False positives may lead to heightened patient anxiety, unnecessary biopsies, and increased costs. Routine annual digital rectal examination (DRE) screening alone has not been shown to reduce mortality from prostate cancer.[123] DRE of the prostate gland allows palpation of the posterior surfaces of the lateral lobes, the site in which cancer commonly begins; however, there are areas of the prostate that cannot be reached, and subsequently, DRE alone can miss up to 40% of cancer diagnoses.[117]

It is reasonable to conclude that those older than 80 years and men older than 70 with serious comorbidities are least likely to benefit from screening. This is because even if screening is ultimately proven to reduce prostate cancer mortality, lead-time estimates and studies of untreated localized prostate cancer suggest that only men who are likely to live 10–20 years could expect to receive such a survival benefit. Conversely, because of the increasing life expectancy of men in the United States, select older patients with few comorbidities may benefit from early detection and treatment of prostate cancer, and thus PSA screening should be extended to such men.

Symptoms

Prior to the advent of the PSA, most prostate cancers presented with an abnormal DRE of a hard, irregular, and nodular gland and/or urinary symptoms. Now the diagnosis of prostate cancer is often made when the patient is asymptomatic and is found to have an elevated PSA prompting further workup. When a patient does present with symptoms, they may include nocturia, urinary frequency, dribbling, and hesitancy; although these symptoms represent an overlap that is seen with benign prostate hypertrophy. Less frequently patients present with symptoms of metastatic disease such as bone pain, pathological fractures, and rarely spinal cord compression.[124,125]

Diagnostic Tests

A prostate biopsy is considered to be the gold standard for diagnosis of prostate cancer. What remains uncertain is how to interpret screening test results to determine candidacy for biopsy.

Prostate biopsy is recommended for all patients with a PSA greater than 10 ng/mL because chance of malignancy in this situation is greater than 50%. In these patients, the likelihood of the malignancy extending beyond the prostate is increased 24–50 fold.[126]

There is a high rate of false positives in patients who have a PSA between 4–10 ng/mL, evidenced by only one in five biopsies revealing cancer. These data support continued research regarding PSA testing, including age-specific PSA and PSA velocity, to help interpret intermediate ranges of PSA. The optimal management of patients with PSA less than 4 ng/mL is less clear because most would have negative biopsies. There have been data suggesting a substantial number of men with prostate cancer do have PSA of 4 ng/mL or less at time of diagnosis.[127] Perhaps the most important finding has been the emergence of PSA velocity, defined as the rate of rise of PSA in a defined period, as a more powerful predictor of the presence of cancer than the absolute value of the test. Using a PSA velocity of 0 75 ng/mL rise per year to determine the need for biopsy would improve detection accuracy even in men with total PSAs as low as 2.5 ng/mL. Percentage of free PSA and complexed PSA are also emerging as tests that can enhance PSA accuracy.[128]

A recent multidisciplinary consensus panel put forth guidelines and recommendations targeted toward patients older than the age of 75 years. Their recommendations include not only considering the serum PSA but they also recommend using tools to evaluate the patient's comorbidities and functional status prior to pursuing further evaluation. Eastern Cooperative Oncology Group performance status (0–2 recommended), Karnofsky Performance Scale score ($\geq$70 recommended) and activities of daily living or instrumental activities of daily living scales are recommended tools for functional assessment. A deficit in either an activities of daily living or instrumental activities of daily living score should prompt further evaluation, as it can be suggestive of a comorbidity that could impact treatment decisions.[129]

Staging, Prognosis, and Principles of Treatment

Based on biopsy results, stage and grade of the prostate cancer can be determined and are essential in determining prognosis and management of each patient.

Grade refers to the histological appearance of prostate cancer and represents the cancer's aggressiveness. The Gleason system is generally used with a score of 2–4 representing well differentiated, 5–7 being moderately differentiated, and 8–10 being poorly differentiated. A higher Gleason score (>7) represents a higher-grade cancer and therefore a worse prognosis.

Stage refers to the extent of the spread of the disease (confined to gland, locally invasive, or metastatic) based on PSA, DRE, and biopsy results. Two staging classification systems are used: TNM and Jewett–Whitmore (stages A, B, C, and D). Previously, radionuclide bone scans and CT scans were routinely used to evaluate the extent of prostate cancer. Not all men, however, need to undergo additional imaging because spread to other organs can be estimated based on PSA and grade. In an asymptomatic patient with a PSA of 10 ng/mL or less and Gleason score of less than 6, a bone scan can be omitted because risk of skeletal metastases is rare.[130] Staging CT scans of the abdomen and pelvis can be useful in patients who are being considered for external beam radiation therapy (EBRT) to determine portals of treatment and for patients with PSA greater than 10 ng/mL and Gleason score greater than 6 who have a higher likelihood of lymph node metastases.[131]

Disease that has spread beyond the seminal vesicles and lymph nodes is not appropriate for radiation or radical prostatectomy (RP). Meanwhile, there has been much discussion surrounding the method of treatment for early low-grade prostate cancer. Patients with moderately-to-well differentiated tumors that are small in volume (≤0.5 mL) are not likely to die of their disease. The 5-year survival rate for patients with prostate cancer at all stages is 98%, a statistic that is representative of the slow-growing nature of the malignancy and the shift toward earlier diagnosis over the past 15 years. Compared with the 34% survival rate for patients with undifferentiated tumors, the 10-year disease-free survival for patients with minimal disease is 87%, which closely mirrors the natural life expectancy for elderly men. Age is considered a key prognostic factor in determining treatment. Current guidelines recommend potentially curable treatment for patients with an estimated life expectancy of greater than 10 years.[132,133] This rule of thumb of 10 years is based on the rationale that men with a life expectancy of less than 10 years are more likely to die of unrelated causes whereas men with a life expectancy of greater than 10 years are more likely to die of the prostate cancer.

Management of Localized Prostate Cancer

An ongoing debate surrounds the optimal treatment for men with locally confined prostate cancer at any age. The controversy is intensified in older patients. In general, older patients and patients with a life expectancy of less than 10 years with moderately differentiated cancer will most likely not benefit from aggressive management of their disease. One population-based cohort study showed that although aggressive treatment of prostate cancer in men older than 75 years was associated with a slight increase in disease-specific survival rates, it was also more likely to have a negative impact on quality of life including symptoms of urinary leakage, bowel function, and patient concern regarding sexual function.[134] New findings from an observational cohort study of nearly 45,000 men aged 65–80 years suggest elderly men who received treatment with either radiation therapy or RP for localized prostate cancer (well or moderately differentiated tumors) survived significantly longer than men who received conservative management after 12 years of follow-up.[135] Although these results are encouraging when considering the spectrum of treatment options in older men with prostate cancer, the results are based on observational data that are subject to concerns about selection bias and confounders. These results need to be validated by randomized trials to inform better treatment decisions.

Additionally, management of prostate cancer is based on risk stratification to predict likelihood of disease recurrence and disease-specific survival. Patient preference can be used in addition to risk stratification tools to help guide treatment decisions.[136] By understanding the nuances of treatment options, the primary care provider can be instrumental in facilitating discussions among the patient, family, urologist, and radiotherapist. The three standard treatment options for men with organ-confined prostate cancer are conservative management, RP, and radiation therapy.

Conservative Management

Conservative management, also known as active surveillance, with or without androgen ablation for symptomatic disease is a common option for elderly patients. The advantage of conservative management is the avoidance of overtreatment of indolent cancer and the potential side effects from treatment. The limitation of conservative management is that treatment is deferred until the cancer progresses, which will occur in a percentage of patients who pursue this treatment option. Once cancer progression does occur, only palliative therapies can be initiated. Patients may develop symptoms from the prostate cancer and die of the disease. Patients who choose conservative management should be followed up every 6 months with a DRE and PSA level.

A meta-analysis of men aged 55–75 years treated conservatively showed that patients with a Gleason score between 2 and 4 and 5 and 6 had a relatively small risk of dying of prostate cancer whereas those with a Gleason scores of 7 and 8–10 were more likely to have died of prostate cancer at 15-year follow-up than of other causes.[137,138] An update of the data after 20 years showed that few men with low-grade tumors developed progression leading to death. Additionally, most men with high-grade tumors died of prostate cancer regardless of their age at time of diagnosis.[139]

The ideal candidates for conservative management are men older than the age of 70 who have medical comorbidities that reduce life expectancy to less than 10 years, and those who present with organ-confined, low-grade cancer.

Radical Prostatectomy

RP involves surgical removal of the entire prostate gland and seminal vesicles. Generally, RP should be considered for patients with moderately and poorly differentiated localized prostate cancer (strength of recommendation B, AFP, SORT).[140] A trial of men with clinically localized prostate cancer (median age 65 +/− 5 years) randomized patients to either RP or conservative management with a median follow-up of 6.2 years. The study showed RP reduced disease-specific mortality, but there was not a significant difference between surgery and conservative management with regard to overall survival.[141] More recently, survival results from the study at 8.2 years concluded RP is associated with statistically significant reductions in disease-specific mortality, overall mortality, and distant metastases compared with conservative management. The reduction in disease-specific mortality in the RP group had the greatest benefit in patients younger than 65 years.[142,143] The Veterans Affairs Prostate Cancer Intervention vs. Observation trial comparing RP with conservative management in more than 700 men is currently underway but is not expected to be completed until 2009.[142,144]

The most common adverse events associated with RP include erectile dysfunction and urinary symptoms. Erectile dysfunction occurs in more than 50% (ranging to 90%) of patients after RP. Patients are also at risk for stress incontinence with estimated rates ranging from 15% to 65%. Obstructive urinary symptoms and retention can occur because of bladder neck contractures. The risk of developing these symptoms increases with comorbidities and advanced age.[145,146] The risk of outlet obstruction, however, is higher in the untreated group.

Lack of consensus from randomized studies in juxtaposition with the individuality of each case illustrates the complexity of treatment decisions, the importance of discussing alternative therapy, and individual patient preferences. Generally, RP is an option presented to patents younger than 70 years, although it can be said that the best candidates for RP are those with a 10-year life expectancy and few comorbidities.

Radiotherapy

External and interstitial radiation are both options for the treatment of localized prostate cancer. EBRT involves daily radiation treatments for 5–8 weeks. The cure rate following EBRT is comparable to RP at least for the first 5–8 years.[147] Some argue that after 10 years the outcome with EBRT is not as favorable as RP, because of incomplete tumor destruction, albeit recurrences are thought to occur infrequently. Whether long-term results are inferior after radiotherapy compared with RP remains unresolved because of the lack of randomized controlled direct comparison trials.

Complications following EBRT include urinary dysfunction (pain, burning, and urgency) in 5%–30% of men and impotence in up to 40% of men.[148] Impotence rates are similar to those following RP but can be delayed in EBRT. The risk of long-term bowel symptoms including tenesmus and fecal soiling is highest following EBRT compared with the risk following other methods of treatment.[149]

Interstitial brachytherapy is another alternative for organ-confined diseased. This procedure involves ultrasound-guided placement of permanent radioactive seeds (iodine-125 or palladium-103) into the prostate gland. The advantage of brachytherapy over EBRT is the convenience, requiring a one-time insertion in an outpatient setting, usually performed under light general anesthetic. Permanent brachytherapy used as monotherapy is indicated in patients with low-risk cancers.[128] Urinary symptoms may be more frequent and men with preexisting urinary discomfort should be cautioned. Brachytherapy may not be appropriate in patients with a large prostate (>50–60 g) and significant preexisting urinary symptoms. Impotence is also a risk with brachytherapy but may be slightly lower than that in RP or EBRT.

Locally Advanced Disease and Metastatic Disease

Manifestations of metastatic and advanced prostate cancer may include anemia, bone marrow suppression, weight loss, pathological fractures, spinal cord compression, pain, hematuria, ureteral and/or bladder outlet obstruction, urinary retention, chronic renal failure, urinary incontinence, and symptoms relating to bone or soft tissue metastases. The goal of treatment for management of locally advanced prostate cancer is to reduce the risk of metastatic spread and prolong survival. For locally advanced disease, the treatment of choice has been EBRT. Studies have suggested the improvement in progression-free survival with the addition of androgen deprivation therapy (ADT) for these patients. ADT, aimed to eliminate cancer growth stimulation, has been considered the primary approach to treating the patient with metastatic prostate cancer. It is effective in reducing bone pain and, although it is not curative, it can modestly prolong survival.[150] Orchiectomy and luteinizing hormone–releasing hormone agonists are equally effective in reducing androgens to castration levels. Chemotherapy for the treatment of hormone-refractory prostate cancer has been reserved for the treatment of severe bone pain. Although recently, docetaxel-based therapy has demonstrated an extension in survival for men who have hormone-refractory metastatic prostate cancer.[151]

Palliative Care of the Patient with Prostate Cancer

Even though many men with prostate cancer may ultimately die of a coexisting comorbidity, symptoms from prostate cancer are a major source of morbidity in elderly men. The most common site of prostate metastases is bone, occurring in 80% of men with advanced prostate cancer.[152] Bone metastasis is an important clinical problem given its propensity to cause the patient significant pain and have a negative impact on quality of life. The goal of management of pain from bony metastatic disease is palliation and prevention of complications such as spinal cord compression and fractures.

Use of Bisphosphonates

As hormone therapy has become a mainstay of treatment for advanced prostate cancer, it has been discovered that a drawback of ADT is a loss in bone mass over time and an increased risk of osteoporotic fracture.[153] There are four theoretical benefits for the use of bisphosphonates in men with advanced prostate cancer: delaying skeletal progression, protecting the bone from loss in density that can accompany treatment with ADT, direct antitumor effects, and palliation of bone pain. The use of zoledronic acid is recommended in men with hormone-refractory prostate cancer and bone metastases to decrease the frequency of skeletal events, although evidence of its benefit is limited and expert consensus has not been reached. The only bisphosphonate currently approved by the FDA is zoledronic acid. A recent Cochrane review evaluated the role of bisphosphonates in palliation of symptoms related to advanced prostate cancer. There was no statistically significant difference between the bisphosphonate group and the control group in terms of prostate cancer death, disease progression, radiological response, and PSA response.[154] Yet, there remains promise of potential benefit of palliation and the review highlights a need for ongoing research in this area.

PRINCIPLES OF SYMPTOM MANAGEMENT AND PALLIATIVE CARE IN CANCER PATIENTS

Whether or not patients decide to undergo cancer-specific treatment, it is particularly important to address and offer symptom-specific care from the time of cancer diagnosis until death. (Further details on palliative care are discussed in chapter 44). Fatigue can be a common symptom in elderly cancer patients and may be addressed with treatment modalities including education, exercise when tolerated, treatment of possible underlying anemia, and screening and treatment of depression. Pain affects approximately 80% of cancer patients prior to death.[155] The American Geriatrics Society developed guidelines for the management of chronic, persistent pain in elderly patients and these can be applied to cancer patients.[156] Pain management can be approached by using the World Health Organization ladder, although it is accepted that opioids are the first-line choice for moderate-to-severe cancer-related pain.[157] It is important to screen for depression in elderly cancer patients. This poses a diagnostic difficulty for health care providers because at times it can be difficult to discern between symptoms of depression and symptoms of the cancer itself. There is also an association between depression and comorbidity as well as a relationship between depression and pain. Use of the Geriatric Depression Scale can be helpful in screening elderly cancer patients. Psychosocial support for patients and their caregivers is critical and can aid in communication that is essential for palliation. End-of-life care including discussion and information about advanced directives and goals of care should begin early in the setting of the cancer diagnosis.

REFERENCES

1. American Cancer Society. Cancer Facts and Figures 2008. Available at: http://www.cancer.org/docroot/stt/stt_0.asp. Accessed June 19, 2008.
2. Ries LAG, Harkins D, Krapcho M, et al. eds. *SEER Cancer Statistics Review, 1975–2003.* Available at: http://seer.cancer.gov/csr/1975_2003/. Accessed June 19, 2008.
3. National Institute on Aging. Ongoing Initiative: Cancer, Aging, Race and Ethnicity. Available at: http://www.nia.nih.gov/AboutNIA/StrategicPlan/ResearchGoalsHD.htm. Accessed June 19, 2008.
4. Ershler, W. Cancer: disease of the elderly. *J Support Oncol.* 2003;1(Suppl 2):5–10.
5. Pompei P, Murphy JB, eds. *Geriatrics Review Syllabus: A Core Curriculum in Geriatric Medicine.* 6th ed. New York: American Geriatrics Society; 2006:479–488.
6. White HK, Cohen HJ. The older cancer patient. *Med Clin North Am.* 2006;90:967–982.
7. Walter LC, Covinsky KE. Cancer screening in elderly patients. A framework for individualized decision making. *JAMA.* 2001;285:2750–2756.
8. Parks SM, Hsieh C. Preventive health care for older patients. *Prim Care Clin Office Pract.* 2002;29:599–614.
9. Gates T. Screening for cancer: evaluating the evidence. *Am Fam Physician.* 2001;63:513–522.
10. Monfardini S, Ferrucci L, Fratino L, et al. Validation of a multidimensional evaluation scale for use in elderly cancer patients. *Cancer.* 1996;77:395–401.
11. Extermann M, Aapro M, Bernabei R, et al. Use of comprehensive geriatric assessment in older cancer patients: recommendations from the task force on CGA of the International Society of Geriatric Oncology. *Crit Rev Oncol Hematol.* 2005;55:241–252.
12. Extermann M, Hurria A. Comprehensive geriatric care for older patients with cancer. *J Clin Oncol.* 2007;25:1824–1831.
13. Costanza ME, Li FP, Finn LM, et al. Cancer prevention: strategies for practice. In: Lenhard RE Jr, Osteen RT, Gansler T, eds. *Clinical Oncology.* Atlanta: American Cancer Society; 2001:55–74.
14. Goodarz D, Vander Hoorn S, Lopez AD, et al. Causes of cancer in the world: comparative risk assessment of nine behavioural and environmental risk factors. *Lancet.* 2005; 366:1784–1793.
15. Burns DM. Cigarette smoking among the elderly: disease consequences and benefits of cessation. *Am J Health Promot.* 2000;14:357–361.
16. Hurria A, Kris M. Management of lung cancer in older adults. *CA Cancer J Clin.* 2003;53:325–341.
17. Fry WA, Phillips JL, Menck HR. Ten-year survey of lung cancer treatment and survival in hospitals in the United States: a national cancer data base report. *Cancer.* 1999;86:1867–1876.
18. Rossi A, Maione P, Colantuoni G, et al. Treatment of small cell lung cancer in the elderly. *Oncologist.* 2005;10:399–411.
19. Collins L, Haines C, Perkel R. Enck R. Lung cancer: diagnosis and management. *Am Fam Physician.* 2007;75:52–64.
20. Smith RA, Cokkinides V, Eyre HJ. American Cancer Society guidelines for the early detection of cancer, 2006. *CA Cancer J Clin.* 2006;56:11–25.
21. U.S. Preventive Services Task Force. *Lung Cancer Screening: Recommendation Statement.* May 2004. Agency for Healthcare Research and Quality, Rockville, MD. Available at: http://www.ahrq.gov/clinic/3rduspstf/lungcancer/lungcanrs.htm. Accessed June 19, 2008.
22. Henschke CI, McCauley DI, Yankelevitz DF, et al. Early lung cancer action project: overall design and findings from baseline screening. *Lancet.* 1999;354:99–105.
23. Henschke CI, Yankelevitz DF, Libby DM, Pasmantier MW, Smith JP, Miettinen OS. Survival of patients with stage I lung cancer detected on CT screening. *NEJM.* 2006;355:1763–1771.
24. Bach PB, Jett JR, Pastorino U, Tockman MS, Swensen SJ, Begg CB. Computed tomography screening and lung cancer outcomes. *JAMA.* 2007;297:953–961.
25. National Lung Screening Trial. National Cancer Institute. Available at: http://www.cancer.gov/nlst/what-is-nlst. Accessed June 19, 2008.
26. Bach PB, Kattan MW, Thornquist MD, et al. Variations in lung cancer risk among smokers. *J Natl Cancer Inst.* 2003;95:470–478.
27. Beckles M, Spiro S, Colice G, et al. Initial evaluation of the patient with lung cancer: symptoms, signs, laboratory tests, and paraneoplastic syndromes. *Chest.* 2003;123:97S–104S.
28. Sawada S, Komori E, Nogami N, et al. Advanced age is not correlated with either short-term or long-term postoperative

results in lung cancer patients in good clinical condition. *Chest.* 2005;128:1557–1563.

29. Leo F, Scanagatta P, Baglio P, et al. The risk of pneumonectomy over the age of 70. A case-control study. *Eur J Cardio-Thorac Surg.* 2007;31:779–782.

30. Pignon T, Gregor A, Schaake Koning C, et al. Age has no impact on acute and late toxicity of curative thoracic radiotherapy. *Radiother Oncol.* 1998;46:239–248.

31. Newman AB, Yanez D, Harris T, et al. Weight change in old age and its association with mortality. *J Am Geriatr Soc.* 2001;49:1309–1318.

32. Langer CJ, Hsu C, Curran W, et al. Do elderly patients (pts) with locally advanced non-small cell lung cancer (NSCLC) benefit from combined modality therapy? A secondary analysis of RTOG 94–10. I. *J Radiat Oncol Biol Phys.* 2002; 51(Suppl 1):20–21.

33. Numico G, Russi E, Merlano M. Best supportive care in non-small cell lung cancer: is there a role for radiotherapy and chemotherapy? *Lung Cancer.* 2001;32:213–226.

34. PCIOC, G Cranial irradiation for preventing brain metastases of small cell lung cancer in complete remission. *Cochrane Database Syst Rev.* 2000;4,CD002805.

35. Simon GR, Turrisi A, American College of Chest Physicians. Management of small cell lung cancer: ACCP evidence-based clinical practice guidelines (2nd edition). *Chest.* 2007;132(3 Suppl):324S–39S.

36. The Elderly Lung Cancer Vinorelbine Italian Study Group. Effects of vinorelbine on quality of life and survival of elderly patients with advanced non-small-cell lung cancer. *J Natl Cancer Inst.* 1999;91:66–72.

37. Gridelli C, Perrone F, Gallo C, et al. Chemotherapy for elderly patients with advanced non-small-cell lung cancer: the Multi-center Italian Lung Cancer in the Elderly Study (MILES) phase III randomized trial. *J Natl Cancer Inst.* 2003;95:362–372.

38. Pepe C, Hasan B, Winton T. Adjuvant chemotherapy in elderly patients: an analysis of National Cancer Institute of Canada Clinical Trials Group and Intergroup BR.10. *J Clin Oncol.* 2006;24(Suppl):7009.

39. Ihde DC. Chemotherapy of lung cancer. *NEJM.* 1992;327:1434–1441.

40. Shepherd FA, Amdemichael E, Evans WK, et al. Treatment of small cell lung cancer in the elderly. *J Am Geriatr Soc.* 1994;42:64–70.

41. Girling, DJ. Comparison of oral etoposide and standard intravenous multidrug chemotherapy for small cell lung cancer: a stopped multicentre randomized trial. Medical Research Council Lung Cancer Working Party. *Lancet.* 1996;348:563–566.

42. Souhami RL, Spiro SG, Rudd RM, et al. Five day oral etoposide treatment for advanced small cell lung cancer; randomized comparison with intravenous chemotherapy. *J Natl Cancer Inst.* 1997;89:577–580.

43. Jermal A, Siegel R, Ward E, et al. Cancer Statistics, 2006. *CA Cancer J Clin.* 2006;56:106.

44. Stryker SJ, Wolff BG, Culp CE, Libbe SD, Ilstrup DM, MacCarty RL. Natural history of untreated colonic polyps. *Gastroenterology.* 1987;93:1009–1013.

45. Winawer SJ, Shike M. Prevention and control of colorectal cancer. In: Grewenwald P, Kramer BS, Weed DL, eds. *Prevention and Control.* New York: Marcel-Dekker; 1995:537–560.

46. Winawer S, Fletcher R, Rex D, et al, and for the U.S. Multisociety Task Force on Colorectal Cancer Colorectal cancer screening and surveillance: Clinical guidelines and rationale – Update based on new evidence. *Gastroenterology.* 2003;124:544–560.

47. Willett WC. Diet and cancer: an evolving picture. *JAMA.* 2005;293:233–234.

48. Martinez ME, Giovannucci E, Spiegelman D, Hunter DJ, Willett WC, Colditz GA. Leisure-time physical activity, body size, and colon cancer in women. Nurses' Health Study Research Group. *J Natl Cancer Inst.* 1997;89:948–955.

49. Giovannucci E, Ascherio A, Rimm EB, Colditz GA, Stampfer MJ, Willett WC. Physical activity, obesity, and risk for colon cancer and adenoma in men. *Ann Intern Med.* 1995;122:327–334.

50. Fuchs CS, Giovannucci EL, Colditz GA, et al. A prospective study of family history and the risk of colorectal cancer. *NEJM.* 1994;331:1669–1674.

51. U.S. Preventive Services Task Force. Screening for Colorectal Cancer: Recommendations and Rationale. July 2002. Agency for Healthcare Research and Quality, Rockville, MD. Available at: http://www.ahrq.gov/clinic/3rduspstf/colorectal/colorr.htm. Accessed June 19, 2008.

52. Mandel JS, Bond JH, Church TR, et al. Reducing mortality from colorectal cancer by screening for fecal occult blood: Minnesota Colon Cancer Control Study. *NEJM.* 1993;328:1365–1371.

53. Imperiale TF, Wagner DR, Lin CY, Larkin GN, Rogge JD, Ransohoff DF. Risk of advanced proximal neoplasms in asymptomatic adults according to the distal colorectal findings *NEJM.* 2000;343:169–174.

54. Lieberman DA, Weiss DG, Bond JH, Ahnen DJ, Garewal H, Chejfec G. Use of colonoscopy to screen asymptomatic adults for colorectal cancer: Veterans Affairs Cooperative Study 380. *NEJM.* 2000;343:162–168.

55. Muller AD, Sonnenberg A. Protection by endoscopy against death from colorectal cancer a case-control study among veterans, *Arch Intern Med.* 1995;155:1741–1748.

56. Lin O, Kozarek R, Schembre D, et al. Screening colonoscopy in very elderly patients: prevalence of neoplasia and estimated impact on life expectancy *JAMA.* 2006;295:2357–2365.

57. Winawer SJ, Fletcher RH, Miller L, et al. Colorectal cancer screening. *Gastroenterology.* 1997;112:594–642.

58. Gatto NM, Frucht H, Sundararajan V, et al. Risk of perforation after colonoscopy and sigmoidoscopy: a population-based study. *J Natl Cancer Inst.* 2003;95:230–236.

59. Waye JD. Completing colonoscopy. *NEJM.* 2000;95:2681–2682.

60. Walter, LC, Lewis CL, Barton MB. Screening for colorectal, breast and cervical cancer in the elderly: a review of the evidence. *Am J Med.* 2005;118:1078.

61. Yamaji Y, Mitsushima T, Ikuma H, et al. Right-side shift of colorectal adenomas with aging. *Gastrointest Endoscop.* 2006;63:453–458.

62. Greene FL, Balch CM, Flemming JD, et al. *AJCC Cancer Staging Handbook.* 6th ed. New York: Springer; 2002.

63. Simmonds PD, Best L, George S, et al. Colorectal Cancer Collaborative Group. Surgery for colorectal patients in elderly patients: a systematic review, *Lancet.* 2000;356:968–974.

64. Runkel NS, Schlag P, Schwarz V, Herfarth C. Outcome after emergency surgery for cancer of the large intestine. *Br J Surg.* 1991;78:183–188.

65. Mahoney T, Kuo YH, Topilow A, Davis JM. Stage III colon cancers: why adjuvant chemotherapy is not offered to elderly patients. *Arch Surg.* 2000;185:182–185.

66. Sargent J, Goldberg RM, Jacobson SD, et al. A pooled analysis of adjuvant chemotherapy for resected colon cancer in elderly patients, *NEJM.* 2001;345:1091–1097.

67. Meyherhardt J, Mayer R. Systemic therapy for colon cancer. *NEJM.* 2005;352:476–487.

68. Yancik R, Wesley MN, Ries LA, et al. Effect of age and comorbidity in postmenopausal breast cancer patients aged 55 years and older. *JAMA.* 2001;285:885–892.

69. Holmberg L, Lindgren A, Norden T, et al. Age as a determinant of axillary node involvement in invasive breast cancer. *Acta Oncol.* 1992;31:533–538.

70. McCarty KS Jr, Silva JS, Cox EB, et al. Relationship of age and menopausal status to estrogen receptor content in primary carcinoma of the breast. *Ann Surg.* 1983;197:123–127.

71. Holmes C, Muss H. Diagnosis and treatment of breast cancer in the elderly. *CA Cancer J Clin.* 2003; 53:227–244.

72. Carney PA, Miglioretti DL, Yankaskas BC, et al. Individual and combined effects of age, breast density, and hormone replacement therapy use on the accuracy of screening mammography. *Ann Intern Med.* 2003;138:168–175.

73. Satariano WA, Ragland DR. The effect of comorbidity on 3 year survival of women with primary breast cancer. *Ann Intern Med.* 1994;120:104–110.

74. Mandelblatt JS, Schechter CB, Yabroff KR, et al. Toward optimal screening strategies for older women. Costs, benefits, and harms of breast cancer screening by age, biology, and health status. *J Gen Intern Med.* 2005;20:487–496.

75. Fonseca R, Hartmann LC, Peterson LA, et al. Ductal carcinoma in situ of the breast. *Ann Intern Med.* 1997;127:1013–1022.

76. O'Malley MS, Fletcher SW. USPSTF. Screening for breast cancer with self breast examination: a critical review. *JAMA.* 1987;257:2196–2203.

77. Smith RA, Saslow D, Sawyer KA, et al. American Cancer Society guidelines for breast cancer screening: update 2003. *CA Cancer J Clin.* 2003;53:141–169.

78. American Geriatrics Society (AGS) Position Statement Breast Cancer Screening In Older Women AGS Clinical Practice Committee. 1999. Available at: http://www.americangeriatrics.org/products/positionpapers/brstcncr.shtml. Accessed June 19, 2008.

79. Humphrey LL, Helfand M, Chan BKS. Breast cancer screening: a summary of the evidence for the U.S. Preventive Services Task Force. *Ann Intern Med.* 2002;137:347–360.

80. Fornander T, Rutqvist LE, Cedermark B, et al. Adjuvant tamoxifen in early breast cancer: occurrence of new primary cancers. *Lancet.* 1989;1(8630):117–120.

81. Magriples U, Naftolin F, Schwartz PE, et al. High-grade endometrial carcinoma in tamoxifen-treated breast cancer patients. *J Clin Oncol.* 1993;11:485–490.

82. Fisher B, Costantino JP, Redmond CK, et al.: Endometrial cancer in tamoxifen-treated breast cancer patients: findings from the National Surgical Adjuvant Breast and Bowel Project (NSABP) B-14. *J Natl Cancer Inst.* 1994;86:527–537.

83. Van Leeuwen FE, Benraadt J, Coebergh JW, et al. Risk of endometrial cancer after tamoxifen treatment of breast cancer. *Lancet.* 1994;343:448–452.

84. Wickerham DL, Costantino JP, Vogel V, et al. The study of tamoxifen and raloxifene (STAR): initial findings from the NSABP P-2 breast cancer prevention study. *J Clin Oncol.* 2006;24(Suppl):3708–3709.

85. Frykberg ER, Bland KI. Overview of the biology and management of ductal carcinoma in situ cancer of the breast. *Cancer.* 1994;74:350–361.

86. Early Breast Cancer Trialists' Collaborative Group: Favourable and unfavourable effects on long-term survival of radiotherapy for early breast cancer: an overview of the randomised trials. *Lancet.* 2000;355:1757–1770.

87. Fisher B, Dignam J, Wolmark N, et al. Tamoxifen in treatment of intraductal breast cancer: National Surgical Adjuvant Breast and Bowel Project B-24 randomized controlled trial. *Lancet.* 1999;353:1993–2000.

88. Houghton J, George WD, Cuzick J, Duggan C, Fentiman IS, Spittle M. Radiotherapy and tamoxifen in women with completely excised ductal carcinoma in situ of the breast in the UK, Australia, and New Zealand: randomized controlled trial. *Lancet.* 2003;362:95–102.

89. Fisher B, Dignam J, Wolmark N, et al. Lumpectomy and radiation therapy for the treatment of intraductal breast cancer: findings from National Surgical Adjuvant Breast and Bowel Project B-17. *J Clin Oncol.* 1998;16:441–452.

90. Early Breast Cancer Trialists' Collaborative Group. Effects of radiotherapy and surgery in early breast cancer: an overview of the randomized trials. *NEJM.* 1995;333:1444–1455.

91. Fisher B, Anderson S, Bryant J, et al. Twenty-year follow-up of a randomized trial comparing total mastectomy, lumpectomy, and lumpectomy plus irradiation for the treatment of invasive breast cancer. *NEJM.* 2002;347:1233–1241.

92. Kemeny MM, Busch-Devereaux E, Merriam LT, et al. Cancer surgery in the elderly. *Hematol Oncol Clin North Am.* 2000;14:169–192.

93. Damhuis R, Meurs C, Meijer W. Postoperative mortality after cancer surgery in octogenarians and nonagenarians: results from a series of 5,390 patients. *World J Surg Oncol.* 2005;3:71.

94. Gajdos C, Tartter PL, Bleiweiss IJ, Lopchinsky RA, Bernstein JL: The consequences of under-treating breast cancer in the elderly. *J Am Coll Surg.* 2001;192:698–707.

95. Martelli G, Miceli R, De Palo G, et al. Is axillary lymph node dissection necessary in elderly patients with breast carcinoma who have a clinically uninvolved axilla. *Cancer.* 2003;97:1156–1163.

96. Lyman GH, Giuliano AE, Somerfield MR, et al. American Society of Clinical Oncology guideline recommendations for sentinel lymph node biopsy in early-stage breast cancer. *J Clin Oncol.* 2005;23:7703–7720.

97. Hind D, Wyld L, Beverley CB, Reed MW. Surgery versus primary endocrine therapy for operable primary breast cancer in elderly women (70 years plus). *Cochrane Database Syst Rev.* 2006;CD004272.

98. Kenny FS, Robertson JFR, Ellis IO, Elston CW, Blamey RW. Long-term follow-up of elderly patients randomised to primary tamoxifen or wedge mastectomy as initial therapy for operable breast cancer. *Breast.* 1998;7:335–339.

99. Vinh-Hung V, Verschraegen C. Breast-conserving surgery with or without radiotherapy: pooled analysis for risks of ipsilateral breast tumor recurrence and mortality. *J Natl Cancer Inst.* 2004;96:115.

100. Smith BD, Gross CP, Smith GL, Galusha DH, Bekelman JE, Haffty BG. Effectiveness of radiation therapy for older women with early breast cancer. *J Natl Cancer Inst.* 2006;98:681–690.

101. Hughes KS, Schnaper LA, Berry D, et al. Lumpectomy plus tamoxifen with or without irradiation in women 70 years of age or older with early breast cancer. *NEJM.* 2004;351:971–977.

102. Ortholan, C, Hannoun-Levi, JM, Ferrero JM, et al. Long-term results of adjuvant hypofractionated radiotherapy in breast cancer in elderly patients. *Int J Radiat Oncol Biol Phys.* 2005;61;154.

103. Early Breast Cancer Trialists' Collaborative Group (EBCTCG). Effects of chemotherapy and hormonal therapy for early breast cancer on recurrence and 15 year survival: an overview of the randomized trials. *Lancet.* 2005;365:1687–1717.

104. Howell A, Cuzick J, Baum M, et al. Results of the ATAC (Arimidex, Tamoxifen, Alone or in Combination) trial after completion of 5 years' adjuvant treatment for breast cancer. *Lancet.* 2005;365:60–62.

105. Giordano SH, Duan Z, Kuo Y-F, Hortobagyi GN, Goodwin JS. Use and outcomes of adjuvant chemotherapy in older women with breast cancer. *J Clin Oncol.* 2006;24:2750–2756.

106. Goldhirsch A, Glick JH, Gelber RD, et al. Meeting highlights: International expert consensus on the primary therapy of early breast cancer 2005. *Ann Oncol.* 2005; 16: 1569.

107. Fisher B, Brown A, Mamounas E, et al. Effect of preoperative chemotherapy on local-regional disease in women with operable breast cancer: Findings from National Surgical Adjuvant Breast and Bowel Project B-18. *J Clin Oncol.* 1997;15:2483–2493.

108. Khatcheressian J, Wolff A, Smith TJ, et al. American Society of Clinical Oncology 2006 Update of the Breast Cancer Follow-Up and Management Guidelines in the Adjuvant Setting. *J Clin Oncol.* 2006;24: 5091–5097.

109. Lash TL, Fox MP, Buist DSM, et al. Mammography Surveillance and Mortality in Older Breast Cancer Survivors. *J Clin Oncol.* 2007;25:3001–3006.

110. Etim A, Schellhase K, Sparapani R, et al. Effect of model of care delivery on mammography use among elderly breast cancer survivors. *Breast Cancer Res Treat.* 2006;96:293–299.

111. Sweeney C, Schmitz KH, Lazovich D, Virnig BA, Wallace RB, Folsom AR. Functional limitations in elderly female cancer survivors. *J Natl Cancer Inst.* 2006;98:521–529.

      Smith RA, Cokkinides V, Eyre HJ. American Cancer Society guidelines for the early detection of cancer 2005. *CA Cancer J Clin.* 2005;55: 31–44.

112. Wilson SS, Crawford ED. Screening for prostate cancer: current recommendations. *Urol Clin N Am.* 2004;31:219–226.

113. Crawford ED. Epidemiology of prostate cancer. *Urology.* 2003;62:3–12.

114. Bartsch G, Horninger W, Klocker H, et al. Decrease in prostate cancer mortality following introduction of prostate specific antigen (PSA) screening in the Federal State of Tyrol, Austria, 1993–1999. *Eur J Cancer.* 2001;37(Suppl 6):S364.

115. Horan AH, McGehee M. Mean time to cancer-specific death of apparently clinically localized prostate cancer: policy implications for threshold ages in prostate-specific antigen screening and ablative therapy. *BJU Int.* 2000;85:1063–1066.

116. Hoffman RM. Viewpoint: limiting prostate cancer screening. *Ann Intern Med.* 2006;144:438–440.

117. U.S. Preventive Services Task Force. Screening for prostate cancer: recommendations and rationale. *Ann Intern Med.* 2002;137:915–916.

118. Walter LC, Bertenthal D, Lindquist K, Konety BR. PSA screening among elderly men with limited life expectancies *JAMA.* 2006;296:2336–2342.

119. Prostate specific antigen (PSA) best practice policy. American Urological Association. *Oncology* 2002;14:267–272.

120. American Cancer Society. ACS cancer detection guidelines: prostate cancer. Available at: http://www.cancer.org/docroot/PED/content/PED_2_3X_ACS_Cancer_Detection_Guidelines.

121. Gates T, Beelan M, Hershey C. Cancer screening in men. *Prim Care Clin Office Pract.* 2006;33:115–138.

122. Thompson IM, Ankerst DP, Chi C, et al. Assessing prostate cancer risk: results from the Prostate Cancer Prevention Trial. *J Natl Cancer Inst.* 2006;98:529–534.

123. Schroder FH, van der Maas P, Beemsterboer P, et al. Evaluation of the digital rectal examination as a screening test for prostate cancer. Rotterdam section of the European Randomized Study of Screening for Prostate Cancer. *J Natl Cancer Inst.* 1998;90:1817–1823.

124. Penson DF, Litwin MS. The physical burden of prostate cancer. *Urol Clin North Am.* 2003;30:305–313.

125. Pompei P, Murphy JB, eds. *Geriatric Review Syllabus. A Core Curriculum in Geriatric Medicine.* 6th ed. New York: American Geriatrics Society; 2006:423–429.

126. Catalona WJ, Smith DS, Ratliff TL, et al. Measurement of prostate-specific antigen in serum as screening test for prostate cancer. *NEJM.* 1991;324;1156.

127. Thompson IM, Goodman PJ, Tangen CM, et al. The influence of finasteride on the development of prostate cancer. *NEJM.* 2003;349:215.

128. National Comprehensive Cancer Network (NCCN) guidelines. Available at: http://www.nccn.org/professionals/physician_gls/default.asp. Accessed June 19, 2008.

129. Konety BR, Sharp VJ, Raut H, Williams RD. Screening and management of prostate cancer in elderly men: the Iowa prostate cancer consensus. *Urology.* 2008;71(3):511–514.

130. Abuzallouf S, Dayes I, Lukka H. Baseline staging of newly diagnosed prostate cancer: a summary of the literature. *J Urol.* 2004;171:2122.

131. Partin AW, Kattan MW, Subong EN, et al. Combination of prostate specific antigen, clinical stage, and Gleason score to predict pathologic stage of localized prostate cancer: a multi-institutional update. *JAMA.* 1997;277:1445.

132. Aus G, Abbou CC, Pacik D, et al. EAU guidelines on prostate cancer. *Eur Urol.* 2001;40:97–101.

133. Scherr D, Swindle PW, Scardino PT. National Comprehensive Cancer Network guidelines for the management of prostate cancer. *Urology.* 2003;61(2 Suppl 1):14–24.

134. Hoffman R, Barry M, Stanford, J, et al. Health outcomes in older men with localized prostate cancer: results from the Prostate Cancer Outcomes Study. *Am J Med.* 2006;119:418–425.

135. Wong YN, Mitra N, Hudes G, et al. Survival associated with treatment vs observation of localized prostate cancer in elderly men. *JAMA.* 2006; 296:2683–2693.

136. D'Amico AV, Whittington R, Malkowicz SB, et al. Biochemical outcome after radical prostatectomy, external beam radiation therapy, or interstitial radiation therapy for clinically localized prostate cancer. *JAMA.* 1998;280:969–974.

137. Albertson PC, Hanley JA, Gleason DF, Barry MJ. Competing risk analysis of men aged 55–74 years at diagnosis managed conservatively for clinically localized prostate cancer. *JAMA.* 1998;280:975–980.

138. Albertson, PC, Fryback DG, Storer BE, Kolon TF, Fine J. Long term survival among men with conservatively treated localized prostate cancer. *JAMA.* 1995;274:626–631.

139. Albertson PC, Hanley JA, Fine J. 20 year outcomes following conservative management of clinically localized prostate cancer. *JAMA.* 2005;293:2095–2101.

140. Bhatnager K. Treatment options for prostate cancer: evaluating the evidence. *Am Fam Physician.* 2005;71:1915–1922.

141. Holmberg L, Bill-Axelson A, Helgesen F, et al. A randomized trial comparing radical prostatectomy with watchful waiting in early prostate cancer. *NEJM.* 2002;347:781–789.

142. Chodak GW, Warren KS. Watchful waiting for prostate cancer: a review article. *Prostage Cancer Prostat Dis.* 2006;9:25–29.

143. Axelson B, Holmberg L, Ruutu M. Radical prostatectomy versus watchful waiting in early prostate cancer. *NEJM.* 2005;352:1977–1984.

144. Wilt TJ, Brwaer MK. The Prostate Cancer Intervention versus Observation trial (PIVOT) *Oncology.* 1997;11:1133–1139.

145. Althof SE. Quality of life and erectile dysfunction. *Urology.* 2002;59:803–810.

146. Krane RJ. Urinary incontinence after treatment for localized prostate cancer. *Mol Urol.* 2002;4:279–286.

147. Kanamaru H, Arai Y, Moroi S, et al. Long-term results of definitive treatment in elderly patients with localized prostate cancer. *Int J Urol.* 1998;5:546.

148. Hamilton AS, Stanford JL, Gilliland FD, et al. Health outcomes after external-beam radiation therapy for clinically localized prostate cancer: results from the prostate cancer outcomes study. *J Clin Oncol.* 2001;19:2517.

149. Potosky AL, Legler J, Albertsen PC, et al. Health outcomes after prostatectomy or radiotherapy for prostate cancer: results from the Prostate Cancer Outcomes Study. *J Natl Cancer Inst.* 2000;92:1582–1592.

150. Robson M, Dawson N. How is androgen-dependent metastatic prostate cancer best treated? *Hematol Oncol Clin North Am.* 1996;10:727.

151. Petrylak DP.: Chemotherapy for androgen-independent prostate cancer. *World J Urol.* 2005;23:10–13.

152. Carlin BI, Andriole GL. The natural history, skeletal complications, and management of bone metastases in patients with prostate carcinoma. *Cancer.* 2000;88:2989–2994.

153. Smith MR. Diagnosis and management of treatment related osteoporosis in men with prostate carcinoma. *Cancer.* 2003;97(Suppl 3):789–795.

154. Yuen KK, Shelley M, Sze WM, Wilt T, Mason MD. Bisphosphonates for advanced prostate cancer. *Cochrane Database Syst Rev* 2006 Issue 4 CD006250.

155. Levy MH. Pharmacologic treatment of cancer pain. *NEJM.* 1996;335:1125.

156. American Geriatrics Society Panel on Persistent Pain in Older Persons. Management of persistent pain in older persons. *J Am Geriatr Soc.* 2002;50:S205–S224.

157. Grond S, Zech D, Schug SA, et al. Validation of World Health Organization Guidelines for cancer pain relief during the last days and hours of life. *J Pain Sympt Manage.* 1991;6:411–422.

37

EYE PROBLEMS OF THE AGED

Omesh P. Gupta, MD, MBA, William Tasman, MD

OCULAR DISORDERS OF AGING

Approximately 80 million Americans experience visual impairment and more than 3 million Americans 40 years and older are legally blind.[1] The rate of visual impairment and blindness is highest in the geriatric population. In a population-based study, the rate of visual impairment in individuals 80 years and older was 15–30 times greater than individuals 40–50 years old.[2] In addition, because many are unaware of their eye disease, otherwise healthy patients 65 years and older should have a comprehensive eye examination every 1–2 years.[3]

Ophthalmologists are in the unique position of being able to provide not only primary eye care, but also comprehensive medical and surgical eye care for the elderly. Preventing blindness is an important factor in assisting an elderly person to function autonomously and to lead a productive life. Blinding disorders can cause significant personal, familial, and societal burdens. A thorough ophthalmological evaluation allows for diagnosis and potential treatment of common and uncommon eye diseases.

EYELIDS AND LACRIMAL SYSTEM

The function of the eyelids is to protect the surface of the globe. The eyelids are composed of an anterior lamella consisting of the cilia, dermis, orbicularis oculi muscle, and lid retractors (Figure 37.1A). The tarsal plate, which is composed of dense connective tissue, and the palpebral conjunctiva constitute the posterior lamella (Figure 37.1B).

The function of tear film is to provide the cornea with 1) lubrication and protection; 2) a smooth optical surface; 3) antimicrobial properties; and 4) necessary nutrients. The tear film is composed of three layers: lipid, aqueous, and mucinous layers. The meibomian glands, sebaceous glands, and apocrine glands produce the lipid layer of the tear film. The aqueous portion is produced by the lacrimal and accessory lacrimal glands. Conjunctival goblet cells produce the mucinous layer of the tear film, which adheres to the superficial conjunctival and corneal surfaces. The tears first drain into the upper and lower lid puncta through the canaliculi and nasolacrimal sac and into the nose.

Eyelid Structural Changes Associated with Aging

Dermatochalasis is the most common eyelid change observed in the elderly. It is characterized by a progressive laxity of the delicate eyelid skin and can cause visual impairment by obstructing the superior visual field. Dermatochalasis may be associated with blepharoptosis, or drooping of the upper lid due to levator aponeurotic dehiscence or disinsertion. Myogenic disorders, such as myasthenia gravis, are less commonly associated with ptosis but these disorders are characterized by asymmetrical, variable ptosis.

A variety of conditions can develop from horizontal lid laxity. Lagophthalmos, or inability to close the lids completely, can produce chronic ocular irritation and dry eye symptoms. Entropion, the inward rotation of the eyelid margins, may result from involutional changes or cicatrizing processes of the conjunctiva, such as Stevens–Johnson syndrome or ocular cicatricial pemphigoid. This may be accompanied by trichiasis, or malpositioned eyelashes. Ectropion, the outward rotation of the lid margin, may be a consequence of involutional, cicatricial, paralytic, or inflammatory processes of the skin, orbicularis oculi muscle, or lid retractors. These eyelid malpositions may produce tearing and ocular discomfort secondary to mechanical irritation or exposure keratopathy. The treatment of these structural changes is generally surgical.

Structural changes can also be a common cause of chronic tearing. It can be caused by obstruction of any portion of the lacrimal tract. Stenotic puncta or lacrimal sac obstruction can often be observed with inspection and palpation. Involutional

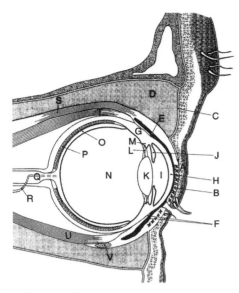

Figure 37.1. Cross-section anatomy of the eye, orbit, and eyelids. A, B, posterior lamellae of eyelid; C, orbital septum; D, orbital fat; E, superior fornix and conjunctiva; F, inferior fornix and conjunctiva; G, sclera; H, cornea, I, anterior chamber; J, iris; K, lens; L, zonular fibers; M, ciliary body and muscle; N, vitreous body; O, retina; P, choroid; Q, optic nerve; R, central retinal artery; S, levator muscle; T, superior rectus muscle; U, inferior rectus; and V, inferior oblique muscle. (from *Reichel's Care of the Elderly*, 5th ed. Used by permission.)

stenosis of the nasolacrimal duct is the most common type of nasolacrimal duct obstruction in elderly persons.[4] The treatment for lacrimal tract obstruction depends on its anatomical location. Stenotic puncta may be enlarged with a simple snip procedure, whereas lacrimal sac and nasolacrimal duct obstructions usually require silicone intubation and dacryocystorhinostomy. This procedure requires creating a bony ostium between the sac and the nasal cavity. The most common reason for tearing is aqueous hyposecretion or tear film abnormalities. The proper workup for tearing should include examination of the lids and tear film for dry eyes, blepharitis, trichiasis, and lid malpositions.

Eyelid Neoplasms

Basal cell carcinoma (BCC) is the most common malignancy of eyelid skin, accounting for more than 90% of eyelid tumors. Risk factors include fair skin and ultraviolet exposure, especially in southern climates. The upper lids are the most frequent location and medial canthal involvement has the worst prognosis. Typically, the lesion is painless and slow growing. The color of BCC ranges from light to dark brown and has the appearance of a nodular ulcer with raised rolled borders (rodent ulcer). It may also appear as a diffuse indurated tan plaquelike lesion (morpheaform) with ulcerated areas or nodules interspersed throughout the lesion. Its can be associated with ectropion, entropion, dimpling of skin, or loss of eyelashes. Metastasis is rare. The diagnosis is made with an excisional biopsy.

The treatment of BCC is generally surgical. The technique of Mohs' micrographic surgery, the careful stepwise excision

and microscopic monitoring of the surgical margins, produces a lower recurrence rate than other methods.[5] Chemotherapy is an alternative treatment for unresectable tumors.

Squamous cell carcinoma (SCC) of the eyelid accounts for fewer than 5% of malignant eyelid tumors. Contrary to BCC, SCC most commonly occurs in the lower lid and can grow fairly rapidly with extension into surrounding structures. It may arise in areas of actinic keratosis and may resemble other benign lid lesions or BCCs. Metastasis occurs in only 0.5% of SCCs that arise from sun-damaged skin, although metastasis may be more common in tumors that arise from chronically inflamed areas.[6] Lesions appear flat with mild erythema and overlying telangiectasias, and scaling is often present. As the tumor grows, it often forms an ulcer with surrounding induration and loss of eyelashes can occur. Excision with frozen section examination of the margins is the treatment of choice.

Sebaceous cell carcinoma, like the superficial variant of BCC, is thought to be multicentric in origin and exhibits pagetoid or horizontal spread. It is often found in the elderly, but can have a variable clinical presentation. Chronic, unilateral blepharitis is a highly suspicious sign of this disorder. The tumor arises from the meibomian glands, glands of Zeis, and sebaceous glands and is best diagnosed by examining a full-thickness lid biopsy. The prognosis of sebaceous cell carcinoma is worse than that of BCC or SCC, with a mortality rate of 20% or more secondary to metastasis.[7] The treatment includes excision, including possible orbital exenteration and radiation therapy.

Common nonmalignant tumors of the eyelids include seborrheic keratosis, actinic keratosis, and keratoacanthoma. Seborrheic keratosis appears as an elevated, light brown, greasy plaque on the skin. These lesions can be inherited in an autosomal dominant fashion. Actinic keratosis is associated with surrounding inflammatory changes in the skin and is considered a premalignant lesion that may progress to SCC.[8] Excessive sun exposure is a risk factor. Keratoacanthoma is a large, round, elevated lesion with a central depressed core of keratin. It can develop rapidly over several weeks and be mistaken for SCC. Consequently, these lesions are treated with simple excision and should always be examined histopathologically.

Blepharitis

Blepharitis is an extremely common condition characterized by inflammation of the anterior eyelid margin or by meibomian gland dysfunction of the posterior lids. It is frequently associated with dry eye syndrome, a dysfunction in aqueous secretion and/or tear film that leads to ocular surface irritation. Both entities occur most commonly in elderly patients, and dry eye syndrome is more common in women than in men. Patients with blepharitis and dry eyes complain of burning, foreign body sensation, redness, mild itching, and tearing. These symptoms worsen in the evening and are exacerbated by prolonged reading or wind exposure. Patients with keratoconjunctivitis sicca associated with autoimmune processes, such as Sjögren syndrome, may have severe pain, photophobia, and blurry vision.

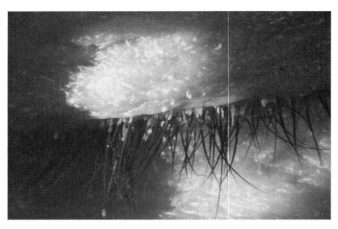

Figure 37.2. Anterior blepharitis. Clinical external photograph demonstrating crusting on eyelids and collarettes on eyelashes. See color plates.

Blepharitis may be secondary to infectious or noninfectious causes. Organisms that inhabit the eyelids can also produce inflammation of the lids and cornea. It is important to recognize and treat blepharitis because it is a common cause of ocular complaints and can lead to endophthalmitis following intraocular surgery.

The most common infectious cause of blepharitis is *Staphylococcus*. Signs of anterior staphylococcal blepharitis include collarettes, or material deposited at the base of the eyelashes, as well as broken or absent cilia (madarosis) (Figure 37.2). Mucopurulent discharge, hordeolum, chronic conjunctivitis, and corneal changes are often noted. The treatment for staphylococcal blepharitis includes lid hygiene and topical antibiotics. Lid hygiene consists of scrubbing the eyelid margins with dilute baby shampoo or a commercial preparation. A washcloth followed by a thorough rinsing with warm water can loosen eyelash crust. Warm compresses may be applied to the lids with a clean washcloth. Lid hygiene should be performed each morning as part of the patient's daily routine. An antibiotic ointment, such as erythromycin or bacitracin, should be applied to the lids before bedtime for at least 6 weeks. Eyelid cultures are usually unnecessary, but should be performed when the condition is severe.

Noninfectious types of blepharitis include seborrheic blepharitis and meibomitis. Patients with seborrheic blepharitis may exhibit oily lid margins, crusting of the lashes, conjunctivitis, and seborrheic dermatitis. Meibomitis is characterized by thickened irregular lid margins with inflammation around the orifices of the glands on the posterior eyelid surface. When expressed, the material within the glands may have a thick consistency. Meibomitis is associated with chalazia and acne rosacea. The treatment for noninfectious blepharitis includes lid hygiene, warm compresses, and systemic doxycycline for 6–8 weeks, or longer if necessary.

Patients with dry eye syndrome present with mild conjunctival injection, a low tear meniscus, and an abnormal tear breakup time, or a shortened interval between the blink and the separation of the tear film. The rose bengal stain and Schirmer test are sometimes used to evaluate patients with keratoconjunctivitis sicca. Treatment includes artificial tear preparations, lubricating ointment at bedtime, and punctal occlusion. Humidifiers and side shields on glasses can be useful. A tarsorrhaphy can minimize exposure in patients with severe disease.

CONJUNCTIVA

Conjunctivitis is a common condition in all age groups; it may be classified as acute or chronic and infectious or noninfectious. It generally does not cause structural damage to the eye, but certain organisms, such as *Neisseria gonorrhoeae*, if untreated may invade the cornea and cause blindness. The symptoms are nonspecific and include irritation, discharge, photophobia, and itching. The conjunctiva is typically diffusely erythematous, and a follicular or papillary response may be discernible in the palpebral conjunctiva by slit-lamp examination.

Patients with bacterial conjunctivitis have copious mucopurulent discharge. Although the disease is generally self-limited, cultures should be obtained. Treatment includes a topical broad-spectrum antibiotic agent, such as erythromycin or bacitracin ointment, for 5–7 days. The antibiotic regimen may be modified according to results from culture and sensitivity testing. Any patient with gonococcal or meningococcal infection should be followed daily and treated systemically with intravenous antibiotic therapy because of the rapid and destructive clinical course of these infections.

Patients with adenoviral conjunctivitis, the most common viral infection, may have associated upper respiratory tract flulike symptoms. The discharge is more watery than that associated with bacterial infections, but can have extreme crusting of lashes in the morning. The disease is self-limited, typically lasting up to 10 days. Preauricular lymphadenopathy and rapid progression with bilateral spread are characteristic of epidemic keratoconjunctivitis. This condition affects the corneal epithelium resulting in photophobia and blurry vision. It is highly contagious and may be contracted in health care environments. Viral conjunctivitis does not require therapy except lubricants and symptomatic relief with cool compresses. Severe cases may require topical steroids under the care of an ophthalmologist because these agents can cause cataracts and glaucoma.

Allergic conjunctivitis is characterized by itching and a stringy white mucous discharge. These patients commonly have concurrent seasonal allergic symptoms. Cold compresses and topical nonsteroidal agents or antihistamine preparations help to relieve itching. Environmental control of the offending allergen and systemic antihistamines are the most effective therapies. In severe cases, topical steroids can also be used under the care of an ophthalmologist.

In addition to conditions previously discussed, the differential diagnosis of chronic conjunctivitis includes systemic diseases such as Stevens–Johnson syndrome or ocular cicatricial pemphigoid. Other causes are occult neoplasm (SCC or sebaceous cell carcinoma), molluscum contagiosum, retained foreign body, eyelid abnormalities, chronic dacryocystitis, topical medications such as glaucoma medications, or orbital processes such as arteriovenous shunt or thyroid disease. Conjunctival lymphoma can masquerade as chronic conjunctivitis, but patients often present with chronic redness and rarely discomfort. Because it classically appears as a "salmon-patch," thorough examination of the conjunctiva, especially superior and inferior fornices, should be performed. If a neoplastic or cicatricial systemic process is suspected, a conjunctival biopsy should be performed.

CORNEA

The cornea (Figure 37.1H) is the major refracting surface of the eye. Its transparency allows transmission of light to the retina, and it provides structural integrity to the globe. The cornea consists of five layers: epithelium, Bowman membrane, stroma, Descemet membrane, and endothelium. The endothelium functions as a metabolic pump by transporting fluid across its surface and keeping the cornea dehydrated and clear. The number of endothelial cells and the pumping ability of the endothelium decrease with age. Corneal edema may result from the loss of endothelial cells. The normal decrease in endothelial cells due to aging is usually insufficient to cause corneal edema unless there is underlying dystrophy or trauma secondary to intraocular surgery.

Fuchs dystrophy, first described in 1910, is characterized by corneal epithelial and stromal edema associated with endothelial changes called guttata, which are warty excrescences on Descemet membrane. The endothelial cells overlying the guttata are abnormal or absent, producing a thickened basement membrane. It is more common in women than in men and is bilateral but may be asymmetrical. Patients are initially asymptomatic. Symptoms of early stromal edema include blurry vision in the morning that clears throughout the day as the evaporation from the ocular surface leads to stromal dehydration. As the endothelial function decreases over time, the visual acuity decreases and epithelial edema or bullae may occur, causing pain and tearing. The treatment of Fuchs endothelial dystrophy begins with topical hyperosmotic agents for morning stromal edema and may progress to therapeutic contact lens discomfort caused by corneal epithelial edema and ruptured bullae. If further corneal decompensation occurs and visual rehabilitation is required, corneal transplantation can be a very successful therapeutic option.

Persons who have had cataract extraction with intraocular lens implantation may develop progressive corneal stromal edema with epithelial swelling similar to the changes seen in Fuchs dystrophy. This condition, known as pseudophakic bullous keratopathy, requires a corneal transplantation for improvement of vision. The development of improved cataract surgical techniques and intraocular lens implants has dramatically decreased the incidence of pseudophakic bullous keratopathy.

Infectious diseases of the cornea are another cause of decreased vision and pain and should always be suspected in persons who complain of a sudden onset of red eye, photophobia, and tearing. Contact lens wearers are susceptible to microbial keratitis, specifically *Pseudomonas* and *Acanthamoeba* infections. Staphylococcal infections are associated with blepharitis and may lead to peripheral corneal infiltrates that progress slowly, while Gram-negative bacterial infections progress rapidly and may lead to corneal perforation. *Acanthamoeba* is a ubiquitous protozoan organism found in soil, swimming pools, hot tubs, and lake water. Fungal keratitis is most common in southern climates and immunocompromised persons. Herpes simplex and varicella zoster infections may cause corneal anesthesia and scarring. Varicella zoster infections also produce pain and vesicular skin lesions in a dermatomal distribution and may involve all the structures of the eye and surrounding orbit.

The management of most corneal infections includes Gram and Giemsa staining of material obtained by scraping the bed of the ulcer as well as culture and sensitivity testing. Fortified broad-spectrum antibiotics prepared from intravenous medications and/or topical fluoroquinolones may be applied topically up to every 15 minutes initially. Modification of the treatment regimen is based on culture results and clinical response. Corneal biopsy may be necessary to diagnose fungal or *Acanthamoeba* infections. Prolonged topical therapy is usually successful, but surgical treatment may be necessary in severe cases. Herpes simplex keratitis is treated with topical antiviral agents. Oral acyclovir may be helpful in treating and preventing recurrent keratitis. Acute varicella zoster infections are treated for 7–10 days with oral medications: acyclovir 800 mg five times daily, famciclovir 500 mg three times daily, or valacyclovir 1 g three times daily to minimize ocular complications.[9] Steroids can exacerbate herpetic infections because of their immunosuppressive effect. Consequently, topical steroids should only be administered under the care of an ophthalmologist for any patient presenting with a red eye.

Indications for corneal transplantation include corneal scarring from trauma or herpetic infections, severe keratoconus, and corneal dystrophies involving the deeper layers of the stroma. Corneal grafts have a success rate approaching 90%; however, the success rate decreases if the underlying pathology includes inflammatory or infectious diseases. These conditions, such as herpes simplex keratitis, may induce corneal neovascularization and increase the rate of graft rejection.[10] Superficial corneal scarring or anterior basement membrane corneal dystrophies may be an indication for phototherapeutic or superficial keratectomy. Partial-thickness lamellar corneal transplantation can be used for conditions that only involve either the anterior or posterior corneal surface.

PRESBYOPIA AND CATARACTS

Presbyopia is the most common ocular condition affecting the aging population. Presbyopia develops in the aging eye when accommodation for near focusing becomes weakened. This usually begins in the mid-40s and progresses with age. Accommodation of the normal eye is produced by the ciliary muscle, which contracts and causes a change in the shape and, therefore, the power of the crystalline lens (Figure 37.1M). The lens also becomes more rigid with aging and may play a part in the decreased ability to accommodate. Subsequently, patients need visual aids, usually reading glasses or bifocals. Because traditional intraocular lens implants are also rigid, patients require reading glasses following cataract surgery. Recently intraocular lens implants have been designed with some ability to accommodate. Selected patients now have the potential to see clearly at distance as well as at near without glasses following cataract surgery.

The lens is behind the iris and supported by zonular fibers that arise from the internal layers of the eye (Figure 37.1K and L). The lens consists of several layers and becomes thicker with age. Cataract is defined as an opacity in the lens that develops with aging. At present there is no medical therapy to prevent the formation or progression of cataract in an otherwise healthy eye. The development of cataracts is a multi-faceted progressive process that is not well understood. Two fundamental processes seem to occur in the lens to produce cataract. The lens cortex may become overhydrated leading to aggregation of lens proteins. The resulting changes cause deterioration to the highly organized structure of the lens. Oxidative damage and photo oxidation over decades of chronic exposure may contribute to the development of a cataract.[11] There is no concrete evidence in humans that supplemental antioxidants will slow the progression of cataract formation. Poor nutrition producing deficiencies of trace minerals and certain vitamins has also been found to cause experimental cataract in animals, but the role in human cataractogenesis is uncertain.

Other than aging, some specific entities may cause cataracts in the older patient. In particular, diabetes mellitus is associated with early onset and a higher incidence of cataracts. Large osmotic shifts in a patient's fluid balance, commonly noted during hyperglycemic episodes, have been reported to produce reversible or irreversible cataracts because of swelling of the lens fibers. Blunt trauma, electrical shock, or ionizing radiation can also cause cataracts. Last, many drugs have been linked to cataract progression. Long-term topical or systemic corticosteroid use often leads to posterior subcapsular cataract changes. Chlorpromazine, amiodarone, phenothiazides, and others have been implicated in cataract formation.

Most patients with cataractous changes have a combination of opacities in the nuclear and cortical layers. Nuclear sclerosis occurs as the number and density of lens fibers increases and produces a gradual decline in visual acuity. Initially the change may manifest as a myopic shift, in which patients can read without glasses again and a change in eyeglass prescription is necessary. The progressive yellowing of the lens causes poor hue discrimination. Cortical cataract changes often appear as spoke-shaped opacities; they impair vision to varying degrees. Posterior subcapsular cataract tends to be more prevalent in a somewhat younger population and patients chronically taking corticosteroids. Visual difficulty and glare symptoms are found in bright light with both cortical and posterior subcapsular changes.

Cataract Surgery

The prevalence of cataracts in Americans between the ages of 65 and 74 years is approximately 50%.[11,12] The prevalence increases to 70% in Americans older than age 75 years. In 2001, approximately 1.6 million cataract extractions were performed on Medicare recipients.[13] This procedure was the fourth largest allowed charge by Medicare and comprised nearly 27% of all allowed charges by ophthalmologists. Nonsurgical management of cataract entails accurate refraction and eyeglass correction. Eventually the vision does not improve significantly with a change in lens prescription. Once optical modalities no longer meet the patient's needs, the patient may be offered cataract surgery based on an ophthalmologist's evaluation and the patient's need and motivation.

The technological advances in cataract surgery over the past two decades have been enormous. Extracapsular cataract extraction and phacoemulsification are microsurgical techniques that remove the cataract and leave the posterior lens capsule intact so that an intraocular lens may be implanted in the native lens capsule. Intraocular lens implants are small disc-shaped pieces of polymethylmethacrylate, acrylic, silicone, or hydrogel that are manufactured with differing powers. The power of the implant is determined by the optical properties of each patient's eye, which is measured with sophisticated instruments. Almost all cataract surgery is done on an outpatient basis with local anesthetic and mild intravenous sedation. Adequate wound healing and stabilization occur by 4–8 weeks. Ideally following cataract surgery, distance glasses are not required because refractive error is taken into account with intraocular lens power selection.

Visual acuity after cataract surgery is 20/40 or better in 97% of patients without coexisting ocular pathology. Patients have significant improvement in their quality of life and overall visual function, such as nighttime and daytime driving, community and home activities, mental health, and life satisfaction.[14] In addition, patients who undergo necessary cataract surgery in both eyes report greater subjective improvement than patients who undergo surgery in one eye alone.[15,16]

Complications that follow cataract surgery have been well described. The most common complication is opacification of the posterior lens capsule in approximately 20%–30% of patients. This can be cleared with a laser procedure even months to years later. Retinal detachment is one of the more serious sequelae following cataract surgery with a lifetime incidence as high as 0.7%. Cystoid macular edema following cataract surgery may cause temporary and sometimes permanent visual impairment but is less common with modern techniques. Secondary glaucoma, hyphema, intraocular lens dislocation, endophthalmitis, and expulsive choroidal hemorrhage are all rare complications, but can be sight threatening when they occur.

Vitreoretinal Complications of Cataract Surgery

Bacterial Endophthalmitis

Bacterial endophthalmitis is a true emergency and one of the most feared complications of intraocular surgery. This most commonly occurs after cataract surgery and, in particular, within 2 weeks of the surgery date. Less than 1 in 1,000 surgeries are complicated by acute bacterial endophthalmitis.[17] The most common causative organism is the colonizer of skin and conjunctiva, *Staphylococcus epidermidis*. Less commonly, *Staphylococcus aureus*, streptococcal species, and Gram-negative bacteria are identified.

Patients typically present with acute eye pain and loss of vision. Anterior chamber inflammation may be associated with a hypopyon (layered leukocytes). Immediate referral to an ophthalmologist is necessary if this condition is suspected. Surgical removal of the vitreous body with instillation of intravitreal antibiotics and steroids has been successful in treating this condition.

Cystoid Macular Edema

Cystoid macular edema is characterized by intraretinal edema. Patients present with a gradual loss in central vision. It most commonly occurs after cataract surgery, typically 6–10 weeks postoperatively. Approximately, 75% cases of cystoid macular edema improve spontaneously. Steroid drops, nonsteroidal antiinflammatory drops, and periocular steroids may be useful in cases that do not spontaneously improve.

GLAUCOMA

Glaucoma is the second most common cause of blindness in the United States. Among African Americans it is the leading cause of blindness. In the United States, 1 in 10 elderly African Americans and 1 in 50 elderly Caucasians have glaucoma. Of the 2.2 million people who develop glaucoma, approximately half are unaware of their disease.[18] The known risk factors include high intraocular pressure; Native American, African or Hispanic descent; age; diabetes; hypertension; vascular disease; and family history. Glaucoma is not a single disease but rather a group of diseases with common findings. Glaucoma is intraocular pressure that is too high for the health of the optic nerve, which leads to characteristic optic atrophy and visual field loss. Once the damage occurs, it is irreversible. Consequently, early detection and treatment are essential to prevent loss of visual function.

Intraocular pressure is the function of three features of the eye: the rate of aqueous fluid production by the ciliary body (Figure 37.1M), the resistance to aqueous outflow through the trabecular meshwork in the anterior chamber angle (Figure 37.1I), and the venous pressure of the episcleral veins. Current glaucoma therapy targets one or more of these pathophysiological mechanisms. In most eyes, elevated intraocular pressure is caused by an increased resistance to outflow through the trabecular meshwork; however, an elevated intraocular

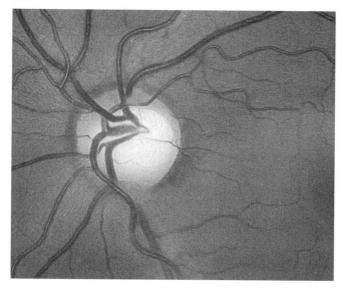

Figure 37.3. Glaucomatous cupping of the optic nerve. A thin rim is noted along the inferior portion of the optic nerve. An associated nerve fiber layer defect also is present. See color plates.

pressure does not cause glaucoma, rather a multifactorial genetic tendency contributes to the development of glaucoma.

Routine direct ophthalmoscopy of the optic disc in all adult patients by the primary care physician can help identify suspected glaucoma. Although the ratio of cup/disc varies, usually a ratio of 0.3 in Caucasians and 0.5 in African Americans is considered normal. The optic discs should be symmetrical. Larger cups should raise the suspicion of glaucoma, especially vertically oval cups that have a cup/disc ratio greater than 0.6 (Figure 37.3). The disc rim should have uniform thickness throughout its temporal portion, without notches, localized atrophy, or splinterlike hemorrhages. Intraocular pressure measurements should be a part of the routine physical examination of adults older than 40 years. Intraocular pressure of 21 mm Hg or less is considered to be "normal;" however, glaucoma may develop with levels of intraocular pressure in the "normal" range, so called low-tension glaucoma. Primary care physicians should become comfortable in the use of a tonometer for routine examinations as well as for ophthalmic emergencies. Handheld devices are user-friendly, but costly. Patients should be referred to an ophthalmologist for routine ophthalmic care including intraocular pressure measurement and evaluation of the optic disc cup.

During routine comprehensive examinations, the ophthalmologist takes a medical and family history and performs an examination that includes several tests to screen for glaucoma. This includes Goldmann applanation tonometry, gonioscopy (a mirrored lens examination of the anterior chamber angle), and dilated fundus examination with detailed evaluation of the optic disc and nerve fiber layer. Patients who have risk factors for glaucoma may undergo visual field testing by automated or manual methods.

Open-angle glaucoma has no obvious macroscopic mechanical restriction to outflow, whereas angle-closure glaucoma has an impediment to outflow because of mechanical blockage by the peripheral iris (Figure 37.1J). Open-angle glaucoma is the most common form of glaucoma in the United States and primary open-angle glaucoma (POAG) constitutes 70% of glaucoma in adults.

POAG is asymptomatic until late in the course of the disease when near-total loss of the visual field becomes obvious to the patient. Elevated intraocular pressure is a chronic condition and often does not produce any sensation of pain or discomfort. Known as the thief of sight, glaucomatous field loss develops slowly and initially affects the peripheral and paracentral fields without affecting the central visual acuity. Patients may not detect any visual change until the disease is far advanced. The diagnosis of POAG is made by finding characteristic optic cupping and typical visual field changes in the presence of an open, normal-appearing angle.

Pigmentary glaucoma, pseudoexfoliation glaucoma, and steroid-induced glaucoma are other types of open-angle glaucoma. Patients who are taking systemic or topical steroids for any condition may develop high intraocular pressure and glaucoma. Even skin creams containing steroids that are used near the eye may cause steroid-induced glaucoma, if used on a continuing basis. The steroids modify the intracellular structure of the trabecular meshwork cells and increase the resistance outflow. This effect may or may not be reversible.

Although acute angle-closure glaucoma occurs in only 0.1% of people older than age 40 years in the United States, it is a true emergency. Anatomically narrowed anterior chamber angle depth predisposes a patient to acute angle-closure glaucoma. Moderate-to high-hyperopia, Asian decent, and female sex are all known risk factors. The peak prevalence is between 55 and 70 years of age.[19]

The anterior chamber depth decreases normally with age because of the growth of the lens. In patients who already have a narrow chamber angle, the iris becomes apposed to the anterior surface of the lens. This impedes the normal flow of aqueous fluid from its production site behind the iris to the drainage site in the trabecular meshwork. The pressure builds up behind the iris, causing the peripheral iris to bow forward and further obstruct aqueous outflow. Aqueous fluid production continues and the rapid rise in pressure causes severe pain.

The unilateral presentation of pain and redness is sudden in onset, can be excruciating, and may be attributed to sinus pain or headache. Other symptoms include blurred vision especially when dark, haloes around lights, and nausea and vomiting. Fewer than 5% of patients have bilateral attacks, although narrow angles are a bilateral condition. On examination, the anterior chamber may appear shallow and the pupil is moderately dilated and nonreactive.

The attack often occurs in the evening during periods of dim illumination when the pupil becomes moderately dilated and has the greatest surface contact with the anterior lens. Rarely, a dense, swollen neglected cataract precipitates angle-closure glaucoma. Patients who have narrow angles and have undergone pharmacological dilation may develop angle-closure glaucoma as the dilation slowly wanes and the iris becomes arrested in mid-dilation. Certain common medications predispose patients with narrow angles to angle closure, including medications with anticholinergic side effects, such as decongestants, tricyclic antidepressants, and antispasmodics.

Patients with a suspicious clinical appearance and elevated intraocular pressure should be referred to an ophthalmologist immediately. Gonioscopy can confirm a closed angle in the involved eye and a narrow angle in the other eye. The goals of treatment are first to lower the intraocular pressure as rapidly as possible with medical treatment and then relieve the angle obstruction definitively with a laser iridectomy. The hole in the iris provides an alternative channel for aqueous flow into the anterior chamber. The iris settles back and relieves the outflow obstruction. It protects against further attacks of angle-closure glaucoma and should be performed in both eyes.

Chronic angle-closure glaucoma may develop in patients who have chronic apposition of the iris against the trabecular meshwork or are chronically treated with predisposing medications. Laser iridectomies may relieve the iris apposition, but damage that occurred during the glaucomatous attack may result in a mixed open and closed angle form of glaucoma.

The goal of glaucoma treatment is to lower intraocular pressure to a safe level and prevent further damage to the optic nerve and visual field. Medical therapy is usually the initial treatment in the United States. Topical glaucoma medications all have the potential for systemic side effects because they are drained through the nasolacrimal duct system and absorbed by the nasal mucosa. Nevertheless, patients often do not attribute systemic symptoms to their eye drops. Primary care physicians should question their patients about ophthalmic medications (Table 37.1).

Beta-blockers have been the first-line of therapy since their introduction in 1978. They lower intraocular pressure by reducing aqueous fluid production and are administered once or twice a day. Beta-blockers are well tolerated but contraindicated in patients with congestive heart failure, bradycardia, or pulmonary disease. Newer medications have a lower potential for systemic side effects.

Adrenergic α_2-agonists are approved for long-term use and perioperatively for laser surgery. Apraclonidine and brimonidine have minimal systemic side effects and are potent inhibitors of aqueous fluid production. They have made ophthalmic laser procedures safer by reducing the risk of postoperative pressure elevations. They are not contraindicated in patients with cardiovascular or pulmonary disease and may be safer than β-blockers in the geriatric population.

Prostaglandin analogs lower intraocular pressure by increasing uveoscleral outflow and have minimal systemic side effects. This once-a-day drop is becoming a common fistline therapy for glaucoma patients of any age. Topical carbonic anhydrase inhibitors have fewer systemic side effects than the oral medications but are less potent. The oral carbonic anhydrase inhibitors acetazolamide (Diamox) and methazolamide (Neptazane) lower intraocular pressure by reducing aqueous fluid production up to 50%. The systemic side effects of the oral drugs often limit their use, especially in older patients. For

Table 37.1. Systemic Side Effects of Glaucoma Medications

Drugs	Side Effects
Topical β-Blockers	
Nonselective: Timolol (Timoptic, Betimol), Levobunolol (Betagan), Metipranolol (OptiPranolol), Carteolol (Ocupress)	Bradycardia, heart block, bronchospasm, impotence, lethargy, central nervous system disturbance, exacerbates myasthenia gravis, and masks hypoglycemia
Cardioselective: Betaxolol (Betoptic)	Same side effects, but less bronchospasm
Adrenergic α₂-agonists	
Brimonidine (Alphagan), Apraclonidine (Iopidine)	Allergy, dry mouth, lethargy, headache, miosis
Cholinergic agents	
Anticholinesterases: Echothiophate (Phospholine Iodide)	Cataracts, can cause acute poisoning by overdose: sweating, gastrointestinal disturbances, bradycardia, respiratory paralysis
Direct Acting: Pilocarpine (Salagen), Carbachol (Isopto Carbachol)	Headache, accommodative spasm, miosis, can cause acute poisoning by overdose: sweating, salivation, nausea, tremor, hypotension
Carbonic Anhydrase Inhibitors	
Topical: Dorzolamide (Trusopt), brinzolamide (Azopt)	Metallic taste, paresthesias, malaise, weight loss
Oral, IV: Acetazolamide (Diamox), Methazolamide (Neptazane)	Side effects of topical medications in addition to metabolic acidosis, renal lithiasis, hypokalemia, diarrhea, agranulocytosis, aplastic anemia, thrombocytopenia
Prostaglandin Analogs	
Latanoprost (Xalatan), Bimatoprost (Lumigan), Travoprost (Travatan), Unoprostone (Rescula)	Hyperemia, eyelash growth, iris pigmentation, cystoid macular edema

decades cholinergic agents have been used to treat glaucoma by increasing the outflow of aqueous fluid, but because of their ocular side effects, these drugs are rarely used today.

Laser trabeculoplasty is applied by directing a small, focused argon or diode laser at the trabecular meshwork. The desired result is an improvement in outflow facility and reduction in intraocular pressure. Studies in patients with POAG have shown laser trabeculoplasty to be safe and effective, although there is a decline in success rate from year 1 (60%) to year 4 (44%).[20] Current practice in the United States is to offer laser trabeculoplasty prior to glaucoma filtration surgery.

Glaucoma filtration surgery is usually offered after medical and laser therapies fail to provide adequate control of the glaucoma. The most common surgery for POAG entails the creation of a fistula from the anterior chamber of the eye to the subconjunctival space. Finally, eyes in which multiple surgeries have failed may undergo implantation of an artificial aqueous drainage device or a cyclodestructive procedure.

VITREOUS AND RETINA

The neurosensory retina is composed of nine layers with millions of photoreceptors to capture light rays and convert them into electrical impulses (Figure 37.1O). As the eye ages, a host of conditions can affect the vitreoretinal interface, the retinal circulation, the retinal pigment epithelial choroidal complex, and the optic nerve. Most of these conditions may result in moderate-to-severe visual loss.

Posterior Vitreous Detachment

Posterior vitreous detachment (PVD) is a very common condition that occurs in approximately 75% of patients older than 65 years of age. The vitreous, a jellylike substance, occupies 80% of the volume of the eye (Figure 37.1N). PVD occurs when liquefaction of the vitreous body occurs to the point that it separates from the retina. This process may be subclinical for many years but may begin to develop symptoms as the vitreous continues to liquefy.

Patients often present with symptoms of flashes and floaters. Photopsias, or flashes of light, are often described as arc-shaped, "lightning bolts" in the peripheral field. These flashes can be subtle and only noticed when in a dim or dark environment. Flashes are caused by traction of the vitreous on the retina, which creates an electrical stimulus. Floaters are also common and are caused by opacities in the vitreous body. It may represent aggregation of the vitreous gel, blood, or pigment from the retina. The most obvious floater is the separation of the vitreous from the optic nerve. Known as a Weiss ring, it may appear to the patient to be an insect or cobweb.

Approximately 10% of patients with acute PVD symptoms have a retinal tear. Vitreous hemorrhage may also occur in patients undergoing vitreous liquefaction and may be present without a tear in 5% of PVDs. If a blood vessel is torn during vitreous separation, the vitreous cavity can fill with blood and result in a dramatic decrease in vision. The risk of retinal tear is approximately 65% in these cases.

Rhegmatogenous Retinal Detachment

Retinal detachment secondary to a tear or hole (rhegma) in the retina is typically seen in persons older than 50 years. The incidence of occurrence is highest in patients who have had cataract extraction or who have myopia. The mechanism of hole or tear formation is detachment of the posterior vitreous from the surface of the retina.

Symptoms of retinal detachment include a decline in central vision if the macula is involved. More commonly, a peripheral visual field defect is detected by the patient as a curtain or shade over part of the visual field. Examination of the retina by binocular indirect ophthalmoscopy is the most important way to identify retinal tears and detachment. Techniques for repair of retinal detachments include photocoagulation, pneumatic retinopexy, scleral buckling, and pars plana vitrectomy (removal of the vitreous gel) with intraoperative laser of the retinal tear(s). Rapid referral to an ophthalmologist is indicated if a retinal detachment is suspected, so that immediate intervention may improve the chances of saving central and peripheral vision.

Macular Hole

Idiopathic macular hole is a partial or complete hole in the neurosensory retina located in the fovea and results in loss of central vision to the 20/60–20/400 range. Average age of onset is 67 years of age and the prevalence is 1 in 3,000. Formation of macular holes may result from vitreoretinal traction caused by the separation of the posterior vitreous. The chance of a bilateral condition is 5% if the vitreous is already separated in the fellow eye. Vitrectomy surgery may improve central visual acuity in patients affected with this disorder.[21]

Idiopathic Epiretinal Membrane

Epiretinal membrane (cellophane maculopathy) is typically seen in patients older than age 50 years and occurs in both eyes in 20% of cases. It is thought to be secondary to a posterior vitreous detachment. After the vitreous detaches, small dehiscences in the internal limiting membrane of the retina cause glial cells to proliferate on the surface of the retina. Retinal distortion may result from contraction of the epiretinal membrane. Epiretinal membranes may also result in loss of normal retinal capillary integrity that may lead to cystoid macular edema. In general when visual acuity drops to 20/100 or worse, surgical removal of the epiretinal membrane can be performed by pars plana vitrectomy in an attempt to improve vision.[21]

RETINAL VASCULAR DISORDERS

Diabetic Retinopathy

After 15 years of type II diabetes mellitus, patients have a significant risk of diabetic retinopathy or maculopathy. Consequently, retinopathy commonly develops in type II diabetics older than

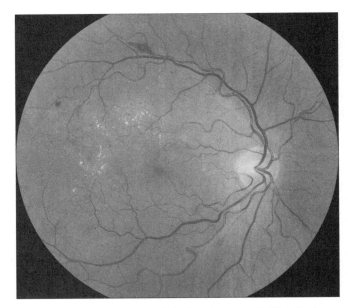

Figure 37.4. Nonproliferative diabetic retinopathy. Diffuse dot hemorrhages, microaneurysms, and hard exudate are noted throughout the fundus. See color plates.

age 50. Type II diabetics should be examined yearly by an ophthalmologist for evidence of retinopathy starting at the time of diagnosis. The earliest signs of diabetic retinopathy include microaneurysms, dot and blot hemorrhages, cotton wool spots (retinal nerve fiber layer infarcts), and venous beading (Figure 37.4). Proliferative diabetic retinopathy is evidenced by the formation of new retinal blood vessels on the surface of the retina and in the vitreous cavity. These fragile abnormal blood vessels cause vitreous hemorrhages and exert traction on the retina causing retinal detachments.

Diabetes can affect central visual acuity as well. Abnormal retinal capillaries can form microaneurysms that can leak serous or lipid exudate and result in macular edema. Macular edema is the most common cause of loss of vision in type II diabetics. Laser photocoagulation has proved beneficial for the treatment of proliferative diabetic retinopathy and maculopathy.[22,23] The goal of laser photocoagulation in proliferative diabetic retinopathy is to halt the progression of new blood vessels. Pars plana vitrectomy is an important technique for clearing the vitreous cavity of blood and removing the fibrovascular scaffold that results in retinal detachment by traction.[24]

Retinal Vein Occlusion

Retinal vein occlusion can either affect the central retinal vein or a distal branch. Symptoms include loss of central vision and visual field defects. Associated systemic conditions include hypertension, diabetes, cardiovascular disease, and arteriosclerosis. Blood dyscrasias, dysproteinemias, and vasculitides all may result in central retinal vein occlusion (CRVO). Acute changes on fundus examination show tortuous veins, superficial hemorrhages, retinal edema, and cotton wool spots. In

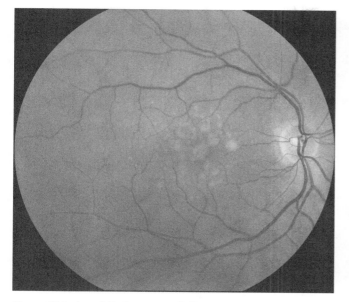 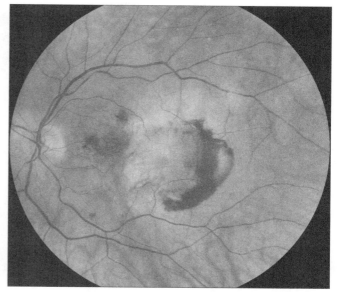

Figure 37.5. A and B. Dry AMD (left).: Hard and soft drusen are noted in the center of the macula. Exudative AMD (right): Subretinal hemorrhage and exudate denote a choroidal neovascularization. See color plates.

CRVO, these changes are observed throughout the fundus, but only a sector of the retina is involved in cases of branch retinal vein occlusions. Invariably the site of occlusion is at an arteriovenous crossing site. The prognosis for vision is poor in patients with CRVO. Only 10% of eyes with ischemia have a visual acuity better than 20/400. Laser photocoagulation offers proven benefit for the two major complications, macular edema and retinal neovascularization.[25,26] Loss of vision is typically due to macular edema. Retinal neovascularization can result in vitreous hemorrhage and glaucoma.

Retinal Artery Occlusion

Acute retinal artery occlusion results in infarction of the inner retina secondary to an embolus or an intraluminal thrombus. Patients typically present with sudden, painless loss of vision and have visual field defects. The retina becomes white, edematous, and a cherry red spot may be present in cases of central retinal artery occlusion. Cholesterol emboli arise from the carotid arteries, platelet-fibrin emboli from large vessel arteriosclerosis, and calcific emboli from cardiac valves. Evaluation and management of patients is focused on the embolic workup. Carotid noninvasive testing and cardiac echography are important tests in this evaluation.

Giant cell arteritis (GCA) is a rare cause of retinal artery occlusion but should always be considered in patients in their seventies or older, since it can be bilateral. An erythrocyte sedimentation rate (ESR) should be obtained in patients. Signs of embolic disease affecting other organ systems (e.g., stroke) should be sought if retinal emboli are suspected as the etiology of the retinal infarct. Carotid noninvasive studies and color Doppler imaging are also useful in assessing flow through the carotid, ophthalmic, and retinal circulations.

CHOROIDAL DISORDERS

Age-Related Macular Degeneration

Age-related macular degeneration (AMD) is the leading cause of legal blindness in the United States. Approximately 6.3 million people are projected to develop AMD in 2030 compared with 1.7 million in 1995. Persons older than 60 years of age are at greatest risk and the prevalence of this disorder increases with age. Approximately 2% of patients older than 65 years have severe unilateral loss of vision (worse than 20/200) because of this disorder. Its hallmark is the loss of central vision with deterioration of the macula, the highly sensitive portion of the retina responsible for central vision.

Two forms of AMD occur, the dry type in 85% of eyes and the wet type in 15%. Sudden visual loss can occur when the dry form of AMD converts to the wet, or exudative, form. Some dry forms may be characterized by drusen deposits under the retina (Figure 37.5A). The majority of patients with dry AMD have mild visual impairment. Choroidal neovascularization, or abnormal vessel growth under the retina, is the characteristic finding in wet AMD (Figure 37.1P and 37.5B). These complexes result in hemorrhage, lipid exudates, or serous exudate in the macula.

For many years, laser photocoagulation was the only treatment with proved benefit for the choroidal neovascular sequelae of this disorder.[27] Recently, antivascular endothelial growth factor treatments have been shown to be beneficial in the treatment of choroidal neovascularization.[28–30] This revolution in treatment has dramatically changed the visual prognosis of patients with AMD. In some patients, laser photocoagulation slows the progression of visual loss. Some of the newer antivascular endothelial growth factor treatments have demonstrated stabilization or even improvement in visual acuity.

Low-vision aids, particularly magnifiers, telescopes, and computers, can always be helpful for persons with loss of central vision.

OPTIC NERVE DISORDERS

Giant Cell Arteritis/Arteritic Ischemic Optic Neuropathy

GCA is a systemic disease that most commonly presents with weight loss but also can present with headache, scalp tenderness, jaw claudication, malaise, and proximal muscle weakness. GCA is a primary vision-threatening disorder that affects the optic nerve and causes an anterior (arteritic) optic neuropathy. Preauricular tenderness or an enlarged temporal artery may be signs of temporal arteritis. An elevated ESR and C-reactive protein as well as a low platelet count can support the suspicion of GCA, but the diagnosis is made based on history and clinical examination. Biopsy should also be performed if the diagnosis of GCA is entertained as nearly 10% of patients with this condition have a normal ESR.

If the diagnosis is suspected, high-dose intravenous steroids should be administered immediately. The role of steroids is to protect against the sequelae of other organ disease, including visual loss in the unaffected eye. Temporal artery biopsy should be performed within 2 weeks of initiating steroid therapy because pathological features can change with duration of treatment.

Nonarteritic Ischemic Optic Neuropathy

Nonarteritic ischemic optic neuropathy is an infarction of the optic nerve that occurs in patients older than 50 years of age. It is associated with hypertension and diabetes mellitus, but collagen vascular disorders can also cause nonarteritic ischemic optic neuropathy. There is an acute loss of vision that is not associated with pain. Vision may vary from normal to no light perception. Patients may present with partial edema of the optic nerve head and hemorrhages within the nerve fiber layer. Vision is rarely fully recovered. There is no proved treatment for this condition.

REFERENCES

1. *Vision Problems in the U.S.: Prevalence of Adult Vision Impairment and Age-Related Eye Disease in America.* Bethesda: National Eye Institute, 2002.
2. Tielsch JM, Sommer A, Witt K, et al. Blindness and visual impairment in an American urban population. The Baltimore Eye Survey. Arch Ophthalmol. 1990;108:286–290.
3. Comprehensive Adult Eye Examination. In: *American Academy of Ophthalmology.* San Francisco: American Academy of Ophthalmology; 1996.
4. Tantenbaum MMC. Lacrimal drainage system. In: Tasman W JE, ed. *Duane's Clinical Ophthalmology.* Philadelphia: Lippincott; 2006:Vol 4, Chapter 13.
5. Rubin AI, Chen EH, Ratner D. Basal-cell carcinoma. *NEJM.* 2005;353:2262–2269.
6. Vaughn GJ DR, Gayre GS. Eyelid malignancies. In: Yanoff M DJ, Augsburger JJ, eds. *Ophthalmology.* Philadelphia: Mosby; 2004:Chapter 93.
7. Jacobiec FA. Sebaceous tumors of the ocular adnexa. In: Albert DA, Jacobiec FA, eds. *Principles and Practice of Ophthalmology.* Philadelphia: Saunders; 1994.
8. Marks R. Who benefits from calling a solar keratosis a squamous cell carcinoma? *Br J Dermatol.* 2006;155:23–26.
9. Pepose JS. The potential impact of the varicella vaccine and new antivirals on ocular disease related to varicella-zoster virus. *Am J Ophthalmol.* 1997;123:243–251.
10. Vail A, Gore SM, Bradley BA, et al. Clinical and surgical factors influencing corneal graft survival, visual acuity, and astigmatism. Corneal Transplant Follow-up Study Collaborators. *Ophthalmology.* 1996;103:41–49.
11. Kuszak JR A-GK, Costello MJ. Pathology of Age-Related Human Cataracts. In: Tasman W, Jaeger, ed. *Duane's Clinical Ophthalmology.* Philadelphia: Lippincott, 2006.
12. Klein BE, Klein R, Lee KE. Incidence of age-related cataract: the Beaver Dam Eye Study. *Arch Ophthalmol.* 1998;116(2):219–225.
13. Gillis K. Physician Marketplace Report: *Medicare Physician Payment Schedule Services for 2001 – A Summary of Claims Data.* Center for Health Policy Research: American Medical Association; 2003.
14. Brenner MH, Curbow B, Javitt JC, et al. Vision change and quality of life in the elderly. Response to cataract surgery and treatment of other chronic ocular conditions. *Arch Ophthalmol.* 1993;111:680–685.
15. Busbee BG, Brown MM, Brown GC, Sharma S. Cost-utility analysis of cataract surgery in the second eye. *Ophthalmology.* 2003;110:2310–2317.
16. Javitt JC, Brenner MH, Curbow B, et al. Outcomes of cataract surgery. Improvement in visual acuity and subjective visual function after surgery in the first, second, and both eyes. *Arch Ophthalmol.* 1993;111:686–691.
17. Javitt JC, Vitale S, Canner JK, et al. National outcomes of cataract extraction. Endophthalmitis following inpatient surgery. *Arch Ophthalmol.* 1991;109:1085–1089.
18. American Academy of Ophthalmology Preferred Practice Committee. *Primary Open Angle Glaucoma.* San Francisco: American Academy of Ophthalmology; 2005.
19. Coleman AL, Brigatti L. The glaucomas. *Minerva Med.* 2001;92:365–379.
20. Weinand FS, Althen F. Long-term clinical results of selective laser trabeculoplasty in the treatment of primary open angle glaucoma. *Eur J Ophthalmol.* 2006;16:100–104.
21. Tranos PG, Ghazi-Nouri SM, Rubin GS, et al. Visual function and subjective perception of visual ability after macular hole surgery. *Am J Ophthalmol.* 2004;138:995–1002.
22. Anonymous. Photocoagulation treatment of proliferative diabetic retinopathy: the second report of diabetic retinopathy study findings. *Ophthalmology.* 1978;85:82–106.
23. Early Treatment Diabetic Retinopathy Study Research Group. Photocoagulation for diabetic macular edema. Early Treatment Diabetic Retinopathy Study report number 1. *Arch Ophthalmol.* 1985;103:1796–1806.
24. The Diabetic Retinopathy Vitrectomy Study Research Group. Early vitrectomy for severe vitreous hemorrhage in diabetic retinopathy. Two-year results of a randomized trial. Diabetic Retinopathy Vitrectomy Study report 2. *Arch Ophthalmol.* 1985;103:1644–1652.

25. Branch Vein Occlusion Study Group. Argon laser photocoagulation for macular edema in branch vein occlusion. *Am J Ophthalmol.* 1984;98:271–282.

26. Branch Vein Occlusion Study Group. Argon laser scatter photocoagulation for prevention of neovascularization and vitreous hemorrhage in branch vein occlusion. A randomized clinical trial. *Arch Ophthalmol.* 1986;104:34–41.

27. Macular Photocoagulation Study Group. Argon laser photocoagulation for neovascular maculopathy. Five-year results from randomized clinical trials. *Arch Ophthalmol.* 1991;109:1109–1114.

28. D'Amico DJ, Patel M, Adamis AP, et al. Pegaptanib sodium for neovascular age-related macular degeneration: two-year safety results of the two prospective, multicenter, controlled clinical trials. *Ophthalmology.* 2006;113:1001 e1–6.

29. Michels S, Rosenfeld PJ, Puliafito CA, et al. Systemic bevacizumab (Avastin) therapy for neovascular age-related macular degeneration twelve-week results of an uncontrolled open-label clinical study. *Ophthalmology.* 2005;112:1035–1047.

30. Rosenfeld PJ, Schwartz SD, Blumenkranz MS, et al. Maximum tolerated dose of a humanized anti-vascular endothelial growth factor antibody fragment for treating neovascular age-related macular degeneration. *Ophthalmology.* 2005;112:1048–1053.

38

Geriatric Ear, Nose, and Throat Problems

Clarence (Fred) Gehris, MD, Leonard Proctor, MD, Lauren G. Collins, MD

It is important to check carefully for a number of problems among elderly patients, who may be unaware of the insidious development of hearing loss, balance deficits, or intraoral or pharyngeal cancers. Unsuspected balance deficiencies may be putting the patient at risk for falls. Nasal obstruction may be dismissed by the patient; however, inspection may reveal easily treatable problems such as benign polyps or life-threatening disease such as a neoplasm.

OUTER EAR

The anterior and posterior surfaces of the pinna are common sites for actinic keratoses and skin cancers.[1] The eardrum, especially the pars flaccida, is a common location for an occult cholesteatoma (see later). If cerumen obstructs the examiner's view it can be removed by direct manipulation or by irrigation with clean[2] water at body temperature, provided there is no eardrum perforation. Alternatively, instilling mineral oil will soften and lubricate the impaction, making removal easier and more comfortable. Cerumen impaction can usually be avoided by keeping the ear oily (by adding a couple of drops of mineral oil weekly) and keeping soapy water away from the ear canal.

Swelling of the external auditory canal associated with purulent secretions indicates an external otitis. External otitis should be treated[3,4] by applying eardrops containing an antibiotic (typically polymyxin and neomycin combined with hydrocortisone) in an acidic solution. Cortisporin, Coly-mycin or VoSoL are commonly used preparations. Drops should be applied three times daily. It is important that a) the canal orifice should be cleared of secretions and debris before the application and b) the patient's head must be adjusted so that the ear canal is tilted upward. When the canal is significantly swollen, a methylcellulose or cotton wick should be inserted into the canal to reduce swelling and help conduct the medication into the canal. Aluminum subacetate solution is especially helpful in such cases because it is astringent as well as antibacterial. Domeboro Otic is a convenient commercial preparation. Systemic antibiotics should usually be avoided in the management of external otitis.

A rare but important disorder of the outer ear is herpes zoster oticus, which may produce a localized rash that is often limited to the ear canal.[4] The vestibular nerve may be severely affected by concomitant inflammation, producing a picture of acute vestibular neuronitis (see later). There may also be hearing loss and facial weakness (Ramsay Hunt syndrome).[5,6] Early administration of antiviral medication, such as valacyclovir 1,000 mg three times daily is indicated and prednisone (1 mg/kg/day) should be added if facial paralysis or hearing loss occur.[4]

Malignant external otitis is a rare but aggressive and potentially fatal infection of tissues surrounding the external auditory canal most commonly caused by *Pseudomonas aeruginosa*. The usual victims are elderly patients with diabetes and immunocompromised patients.[4,6] The hallmark finding is granulation tissue in the floor of the ear canal at the bony–cartilaginous junction.

MIDDLE EAR

Problems within the middle ear are reflected in the appearance of the eardrum. A bulging reddened or yellowish drum accompanied by pain suggests a purulent otitis media. Systemic antibiotics are indicated; in some cases, myringotomy may be required to relieve pain and avoid permanent damage to the eardrum. A history of earache followed by purulent discharge and subsidence of pain associated with absence of tenderness when the pinna is pulled strongly suggests spontaneous rupture of the eardrum. Similar symptoms associated with a serous discharge may be spontaneous drainage from bullous myringitis.[4] Chronic purulent discharge is a sign of chronic otitis media, which may lead to serious complications.[7,8] When a drum perforation is present, treatment can follow the protocol for external otitis, except that it is best to avoid the use of ototoxic antibiotic drops.[9] Instead, use Cipro HC or Floxin.

A dull appearance of the drum, especially coupled with a chalky white appearance of the malleus handle indicates middle ear fluid. Dark stripes on the drum indicate fluid with air bubbles, signifying partial or intermittent function of the eustachian tube. Eustachian tubal blockage will usually resolve spontaneously, although application of nasal decongestants may sometimes be required. Persistent blockage should prompt a careful examination of the nasopharynx with an endoscope to check for a possible neoplasm or other lesion in this area. Sometimes the eustachian tube is patulous,[10] in which case symptoms can be confusing. The patient may report a very annoying feeling of pressure and autophony (hearing his or her own voice louder than usual).

When examining the eardrum, it is important to check the upper part of the drum, the pars flaccida, for the presence of a cholesteatoma.[11] A cholesteatoma is a skin-lined pouch that may present as white debris associated with the orifice of a small hole or depression. This is a benign but progressively expansive lesion that should be treated early by surgery.[11] Untreated, serious complications can occur, including fistulization of the labyrinth, meningitis, or damage to the ossicles or facial nerve.[12,13]

AUDITORY DISORDERS

Hearing loss is common in the geriatric population and may have a significant impact on the quality of life of older patients. Hearing loss in a cognitively impaired or depressed patient is often unrecognized and may be an important factor in reduced functionality.[14] Individuals with significant hearing loss have difficulty ignoring competing speech, and conversation becomes progressively more frustrating when several people are talking concurrently. Inappropriate conversational responses may lead to embarrassment or a perceived rejection by peers or family and a withdrawal from social interactions. This in turn can reduce mental and physical activity and lead to loneliness or depression. Fortunately, the adverse psychological and practical effects of hearing loss can be largely reversed through auditory rehabilitation, which may include education, hearing aids, assistive listening devices, or cochlear implants.[15,16]

Presbycusis

Hearing loss that has no disease-specific diagnosis and is simply associated with aging ("presbycusis") is thought to result primarily from degenerative changes in the inner ear.[16] These changes result in a degradation and slowing of the auditory signal. Some degenerative organic changes also occur in the central projections of the auditory system and are largely secondary to the losses within the cochlea.[17] The diminution in microcirculation to the cochlea that accompanies aging contributes to these degenerative changes.[18]

Sudden Sensorineural Hearing Loss

Sudden sensorineural hearing loss in most cases is idiopathic. The incidence is estimated at 5–20 per 100,000 per year, with a peak in the sixth decade.[19] Patients typically present with unilateral hearing loss that develops in less than 12 hours; patients may report an associated fullness or tinnitus, and vertigo can be expected in approximately 40% of cases.[19] Sudden sensorineural hearing loss is an emergency and should be evaluated by an otolaryngologist on an urgent basis. Administration of prednisone or valacyclovir may be indicated.

Specific Disorders Causing Hearing Loss

There are a number of specific conditions associated with hearing loss that should be considered, such as impacted cerumen, otitis media, and labyrinthitis.[6] Otosclerosis, a benign disease of the bone surrounding the inner ear, may cause conductive hearing loss.[20] A number of systemic diseases, including hypertension, impaired glucose metabolism, kidney disorders that alter fluid and electrolyte metabolism, hyperlipoproteinemia, and thyroid disorders, also have potential deleterious effects on hearing.[15,21] Infectious causes of hearing loss include measles, mumps, Rocky Mountain Spotted Fever, syphilis, and Lyme disease.[19]

Autoimmune inner ear disease may produce a rapidly progressive sensorineural hearing loss (SNHL) with a course usually extending over a period of weeks or months.[22] Both ears are affected but hearing loss may initially be unilateral for months. Autoimmune factors may be detected in the blood, but diagnosis of autoimmune inner ear disease is based on clinical evaluation, audiometric demonstration of progressive SNHL, and a positive response to corticosteroids.[22] Disorders which may produce a similar progressive SNHL include Cogan's syndrome, Vogt-Koyanagi-Harada disease, Wegener' granulomatosis, syphilis, and systemic vasculitides such as polyarteritis nodosa.

Ototoxicity from various antibiotics and other drugs[9,19,23–25] is insidious and can produce a profound deafness. Potentially ototoxic drugs include streptomycin, neomycin, kanamycin, gentamicin, tobramycin, amikacin, netilmicin, sisomicin, cisplatin, carboplatin, furosemide, bumetanide, salicylates, quinine, erythromycin, azithromycin, and vancomycin. Risk factors for ototoxicity include the combined administration of more than one potentially ototoxic drug, bacteremia, fever, diminished renal or hepatic function, and the presence of an inherited mitochondrial mutation.[25]

Of note, hearing loss may progress (or even begin) after drug treatment has been discontinued[25] and careful attention should be paid to administration of ototoxic medications. Several medications given along with potentially ototoxic drugs may have a protective effect.[23,26] For example, aspirin can significantly attenuate the risk of gentamicin-induced hearing loss.[26]

Central Auditory Disorders

The most pervasive auditory problem among the elderly is diminishing ability to understand speech, especially in the presence of noise. Although this results primarily from changes in the cochlea (reduced sensitivity to higher frequencies), changes in the central nervous system may also contribute. In some cases, individuals have a much poorer ability to understand speech than their threshold audiogram would predict.[27] This condition has been referred to as "central auditory processing disorder" (CAPD).[21,27] Humes[28] found that the prevalence of CAPD is probably less than 10% of patients suffering from presbycusis. Seventy to 90% of presbycusis results from peripheral hearing loss, with cognitive factors accounting for the rest.[28] This is important information for patients, because it is presumably less discouraging to learn that one's ear is malfunctioning than to learn that one's brain is doing so. Other aging changes will adversely affect the ability to understand speech. For example, Bellis and Wilber[29] has pointed out the implications of age-related atrophy in certain regions of the corpus callosum, which is important in gauging communicative intent, speech perception in noise, sustained attention, auditory verbal learning and memory, and other functions associated with speech processing.

The concept of CAPD can also lead to some confusion when dealing with patients who have various cognitive impairments such as Alzheimer's disease or dementia. In such cases specialized auditory testing (see later) can be helpful in establishing the site of auditory impairment.

Tinnitus

Tinnitus is a common problem in older patients. Tinnitus is an expected accompaniment of hearing loss from acoustic trauma, aging, or ototoxic drugs, but it is also associated with Ménière's disease, acoustic neuroma, and other auditory disorders. Tinnitus is more common among patients suffering from anxiety and depression and may be a side effect of a wide variety of drugs.[30] Tinnitus that is pulsatile should be investigated carefully because it may indicate the presence of a vascular lesion.[31] Fitting the patient with a hearing aid usually has an immediate beneficial effect on tinnitus.[32] Patients will benefit greatly by understanding that tinnitus is a benign condition caused by disharmonious nervous activity and by the suggestion that the condition will probably become less intense and less frequently noticeable as time goes by. More active intervention through counseling, medication, or other methods may be indicated in some cases.[33]

EVALUATION AND MANAGEMENT OF HEARING LOSS

An initial estimate of hearing acuity can be achieved by asking the patient to close his eyes and indicate when he hears a tuning fork, rubbed fingers, or spoken voice as they are brought closer to his ear. When hearing impairment is suspected, diagnostic audiological tests[15] should be administered. Such tests provide objective quantifiable information that is important for two reasons: 1) a site-of-lesion diagnosis must be established to search rationally for treatable diseases such as acoustic neuroma or conductive hearing loss from stapedial fixation, and 2) they are needed to evaluate the patient's rehabilitative potential.

An important test for elderly persons is the speech discrimination score, which is the percentage of phonetically balanced words that are correctly identified when they are presented at a loudness that is well above threshold. Another key test is the determination of the patient's threshold for hearing tones at various frequencies. Tones are presented through earphones (air conduction threshold) or by a vibrator applied to the mastoid process (bone conduction threshold). Results are plotted on a chart (audiogram) where the loudness in decibels required for detection of tones at 500, 1,000, 2,000, 4,000, and 8,000 cycles/sec are shown. Each ear is tested separately. Specific patterns are suggestive of specific diagnoses. A more pronounced loss at lower frequencies is consistent with Ménière's disease. A loss in the higher frequencies is typical in an elderly population and results in difficulty hearing higher frequency speech cues such as "s" and "t," which in turn leads to degradation in understanding speech. The more sophisticated hearing aids can differentially amplify specified frequencies and have proven very helpful in such cases. The use of bilateral hearing aids helps sort out and reject competing speech and other irrelevant sounds through sound localization.[15]

In some cases there is an abnormal sensitivity to increments of loudness, a condition termed "recruitment." This phenomenon is common in Ménière's disease but is also seen in many patients with presbycusis. Recruitment can be demonstrated by the Short Increment Sensitivity Index test or by the loudness balance test (perceived loudness of a tone is compared between the affected ear and the unaffected ear). Patients with a narrow range of comfortable loudness are helped by using hearing aids that dampen excessively loud sounds.

The reflex contraction of the stapedius muscle to loud tones presented in the same or opposite ear can be evaluated by monitoring the acoustical impedance of the middle ear. This test provides helpful information about the physical condition of the middle ear compartment, drum and ossicles and also indicates the status of the stapedius reflex arc (auditory nerve, brainstem interneurons, and facial nerve).

Auditory system responses to acoustical clicks can be detected by computerized signal averaging from electrodes placed in the outer ear canal[15] and can be useful in evaluating patients suspected of suffering from Ménière's disease, acoustic neuromas, and demyelinating disorders. Electrocochleography is an analysis of the signals during the first 10 ms, representing neural activity within the cochlea and auditory nerve. The auditory brainstem response includes signals from the brainstem as well as the signals previously noted.

DISORDERS OF BALANCE

A gradual deterioration of many of the structures in the peripheral and central vestibular system occurs with aging.[34–42] Concomitant reductions in vision, proprioception, muscle strength, and joint mobility may produce a cumulative negative impact on older patients' sense of equilibrium and stability, increasing their risk of falls.[43,44] With aging, there is a diminution in the vascular supply to the labyrinth[18] and concomitant degenerative changes in the otoconia, vestibular neuroepithelium, vestibular nerve, and central vestibular projections. There is also a decrease in the number and structural integrity of the otoconia.[38] Fragmented otoconial debris can become displaced into the semicircular canals, causing positional balance disturbances.[34,42,45] Histological studies have demonstrated a gradual decline in the number of neurons in the vestibular nerve and neuronal loss in the descending, medial, and lateral vestibular nuclei.[46] Cell loss in the cerebellar vermis[39] indicates that some of the central connections of vestibular projections within the cerebellum are also affected by aging.

Benign Positional Vertigo

Benign positional vertigo (BPV) is the most common cause of acute vertigo. It is caused by displaced otoconia within one or more of the semicircular canals.[34,38,42,47,48] Patients report recurrent brief episodes of vertigo that appear with changes in head position relative to gravity, such as looking up, lying down, or rolling over in bed.

Vestibular Neuronitis

Vestibular neuronitis usually produces a single episode of severe vertigo that gradually subsides over a period of 3–5 days.[49] Patients typically report awakening with severe vertigo associated with nausea, vomiting, and difficulty walking. The causative lesion, a presumed viral inflammation of the vestibular nerve, is usually unilateral, with strong "paralytic" nystagmus beating away from the involved ear during the first day and a tendency to fall or veer toward the affected side.[50] Vertigo, nystagmus, and dysequilibrium often subside promptly because of central nervous system compensation. Caloric responses are severely depressed or absent on the affected side[50] but they will often recover with time. Recurrent attacks are rare.[51]

Ménière's Disease

Ménière's disease is associated with vertigo that lasts 2–12 hours, but episodes are recurrent, accompanied by tinnitus, aural fullness, and fluctuating hearing loss. Rarely, drop attacks can occur and can mimic stroke.[52] Etiology has not been established. Serial audiometric assessments are of key importance in establishing the diagnosis.

Migrainous Vertigo

Migrainous vertigo is another common cause of vertigo and should be suspected even when positional vertigo or intermittent auditory symptoms are present.[53–58] A temporal pattern and duration of vertigo episodes that is not typical of known inner ear or vestibular nerve syndromes should raise suspicion. Headache and visual symptoms may be unassociated with vertiginous attacks.[53–55] When migrainous vertigo is positional, it can be distinguished from BPV by the short duration of attack episodes, frequent recurrences, manifestation early in life, migrainous symptoms during episodes with positional vertigo, and atypical positional nystagmus.[56,58]

Acoustic Tumor

Acoustic tumors may present as unilateral sensorineural hearing loss. As the tumor enlarges, patients may report vertigo, headache, facial numbness, pain, ataxia, and other neurological symptoms. A suspicion of acoustic tumor should be high when unilateral sensorineural hearing loss is associated with evidence of vestibular weakness or paralysis by caloric testing. Diagnosis is established through computed tomography or enhanced magnetic resonance imaging. Early diagnosis of acoustic nerve tumors is important because of the comparatively low morbidity and mortality of surgical removal if the tumor is small.

Labyrinthitis

Serous labyrinthitis may be associated with otitis media,[6] labyrinthine fistula,[59] autoimmune disorder,[22] or infectious disease.[24] Purulent labyrinthitis is rare. When bacteria invade the inner ear, the result is typically a rapid and profound deafness associated with absent responses to vestibular stimulation in the involved ear.[19]

Labyrinthine Fistula

Patients reporting vertigo in response to loud sound (Tullio phenomenon[60]) or caused by coughing, straining, or touching their ear may be suffering from labyrinthine fistula. Erosion of a semicircular canal may occur spontaneously (superior canal dehiscence syndrome[59]) or secondary to trauma, an expanding cholesteatoma, or from syphilitic involvement of the temporal bone.

Drug Toxicity

Drug toxicity may also cause paresis or paralysis of the vestibular reflexes.[61] The damage is usually bilateral and irreversible. Patients with bilateral vestibular paralysis may report that the world appears to bob or shift when they move their head quickly (oscillopsia). Tobramycin, gentamicin, streptomycin, kanamycin, and cisplatinum are the most common potentially vestibulotoxic drugs.[25] A subset of patients with a certain mito-chondrial mutation[25] are at particularly high risk for drug toxicity.

Central Disorders

A number of central disorders may damage the vestibular system as well. These include neoplastic or demyelinating disease,[53,57,58] cerebellar degeneration, Arnold–Chiari malformation, and cerebrovascular disease that affects the brainstem or cerebellum.[53,57]

CLINICAL EVALUATION OF BALANCE DISORDERS

When evaluating any patient with vertigo the first step should be to establish the anatomical site of the disturbance. Acute vertigo can be caused by life-threatening events such as hemorrhage or infarction within the posterior cranial fossa[53,57,58,62] as well as lesions affecting the inner ear or vestibular nerve. The presence of neurological signs or headache should prompt examination with magnetic resonance imaging. When disorders of the inner ear or vestibular nerve are the source of acute or chronic imbalance or vertigo, the pattern and character of symptoms alone may be enough to establish a diagnosis. For example, recurrent episodes of clear vertigo (an illusion of movement of self or environment) that only appear with changes in head position relative to gravity (looking up, lying down, or rolling over in bed) and last only for 5 to 30 seconds are almost conclusively diagnostic of benign positional vertigo. A brief physical examination[63] is usually sufficient to determine the site of the lesion. It should be noted that absence of vertigo does not rule out involvement of the peripheral vestibular system.

Spontaneous or gaze-evoked nystagmus can be very helpful in establishing a diagnosis. Patients with recurrent symptoms should ask someone to look at their eyes during an attack to see if nystagmus is present. Nystagmus is almost always "paralytic" (beating away from the involved ear) during or immediately after the onset of unilateral disease affecting the inner ear or vestibular nerve.[51,52,63] Nystagmus is rarely "irritative" (beating toward the involved ear) during the acute phase of a lesion but may be seen very briefly at the very outset of a Ménière attack or for a couple of hours during the initial stages of infectious labyrinthitis. Because of compensatory central nervous system mechanisms, spontaneous nystagmus rapidly declines after an acute lesion. For example, on the first day of an acute vestibular paresis or paralysis from vestibular neuronitis there is usually an obvious nystagmus that beats away from the involved ear in all directions of gaze. Later, the nystagmus is only seen on lateral gaze away from the involved ear. Thereafter, it is necessary to take away the patient's opportunity for visual fixation to detect the nystagmus. This is done by using +20 diopter lenses (Frenzel goggles) or by electronystagmography with eyes closed or video-oculography (see later). Several weeks or months after an acute severe lesion there may

occur a moderate "recovery nystagmus" beating toward the affected ear. This is seldom detectable without removal of the opportunity for visual fixation. To test for labyrinthine fistula, loud sound or alternating positive and negative pressure applied to the outer ear canal may induce vertigo and possibly nystagmus.

Weakness of the vestibuloocular reflex (which stabilizes the eyes during head movement) can be detected by tests that are analogous to the knee jerk test (instead of stretch receptors stimulated by elongation of a tendon, hair cells are stimulated by displacement of fluid in a semicircular canal). In the head-thrust test,[49,62,63] the patient's eyes are observed while the examiner rapidly rotates the patient's head in a single horizontal thrust. The patient focuses on the examiner's nose while the examiner rotates his head from a rightward- or leftward-displaced position to a center position, with a very abrupt stop. If there is a weakness, there will be a "catch-up" saccade (a quick return of the eyes from a position off-target).

Another method for detecting a weakened vestibuloocular reflex is to compare the patient's visual acuity on a standard eye chart with and without head shaking. Ask the patient to read down the chart as far as possible and note which line is still clear to him. Next, ask him again to read down the chart while you rotate his head back and forth rapidly in a horizontal plane. With a normal vestibuloocular reflex there should be a difference of only one or two lines in the patient's performance under the two conditions. When weakness of the vestibuloocular reflex is suspected, the caloric test is a useful measure to confirm and quantify this finding (see later).

To test for the presence of BPV the patient is brought quickly from an upright sitting position with his head rotated 45° to either the right or left to a recumbent position.[36,47,49,64–66] This test effectively rotates the head in the plane of a pair of vertical canals; for example, with the head turned to the left the left posterior and right anterior canals are stimulated. The maneuver is more reliable when the patient's head is hyperextended but care must be exercised in patients with problems that limit neck movement; fortunately, the test is still effective when hyperextension is not accomplished.[34] If there are free-floating otoconia within the semicircular canal ("canal lithiasis') or adherent to the cupola ("cupola lithiasis') their gravity-driven movement will cause movement of the endolymph–cupola system. Because this movement is the specific mechanism that excites the vestibuloocular reflex, a nystagmus appropriate to the canal involved will be induced (rotatory/up-beating toward the brow in the case of the posterior canal). The posterior canal is most commonly involved, but different patterns of nystagmus should alert the examiner to involvement of other canals.[34,37] Also, it must be kept in mind that positional vertigo and nystagmus can be a sign of central nervous system disease.[57,61] Suspicion should be aroused of a central lesion if positional nystagmus is purely vertical, sustained, not accompanied by vertigo, or does not subside with repeated testing or therapeutic maneuvers.

To assess inner ear balance, it is also useful to perform the tandem Romberg test. For this maneuver, the patient stands in a corner, facing outward (in this way he will be supported should he fall backward) with arms folded and eyes closed for 60 sec. If this is accomplished, he is then asked to narrow his base of support by moving one foot slightly forward or even standing heel-to-toe. Normal individuals exhibit a progressively reduced competence on this test over time.[67] Finally, gait, touch, position sense, rapid alternating movements, and strength should be evaluated along with a general neurological assessment.[44,58,62]

LABORATORY TESTING OF BALANCE REFLEXES

One of the most valuable features of laboratory testing is the ability to remove the patient's opportunity for visual fixation, thereby revealing or enhancing a latent or weak spontaneous nystagmus. This is done by observing and recording eye movements with infrared video recordings behind blackout goggles, or behind closed lids, using electronystagmography with electrodes placed near the eyes. A printed record of eye movements is provided for detailed analysis, along with scores that indicate the intensity of any nystagmus that is detected. Demonstrating the presence and direction of positional nystagmus is another useful feature of this technique.

Responses to caloric stimulation of the lateral semicircular canals provide a means for detecting weakness of this vestibular receptor. The caloric test is of key importance because it provides a means for evaluating each ear independently. In this test, convection displacement of endolymph within the canal is induced by establishing a temperature gradient across the canal. The fluid displacement simulates the inertial displacement caused by rotatory head movement and induces a nystagmus whose intensity reflects the sensitivity of the vestibuloocular reflex. Interpretation of the caloric test is based primarily on a comparison of responses from the two sides (there should be less than a 20% difference in nystagmus intensity). Absolute values of nystagmus velocity below about 6°/sec indicate a weakened response and increases or diminution in responses over time above 40°/sec are pathologically significant.[68] Quantitative information can be elucidated about the patient's ability to maintain upright posture by using dynamic posturography.[45,67] In this test, the patient stands on a movable platform within a movable visual surround. Test conditions are manipulated to challenge the patient's ability to respond to unstable conditions or perturbations in his support base or in the visual panorama. The test evaluates both motor control and sensory organization. Posturography is not only useful for diagnosis; it is very helpful in evaluating and following patients during vestibular rehabilitation.

TREATMENT OF BALANCE DISORDERS

For some disorders, treatment can be offered that is aimed directly at eliminating or controlling the underlying disorder, such as surgical removal of an acoustic neuroma, repair of a labyrinthine fistula, or treatment of labyrinthitis, autoimmune disease, or migraine. Fortunately, when weakening or loss of vestibular function is stable, symptoms usually subside spontaneously. For example, in vestibular neuronitis, compensatory changes within the central vestibular reflex system normally allow full function to be established within a few weeks. Meanwhile, symptomatic treatment of vertigo and nausea with sedatives, antiemetics, and antivertiginous drugs may be helpful during an acute attack.[49] Vestibular exercises designed to improve ocular stability and balance[69,70] and psychological support[71] can accelerate recovery after a peripheral vestibular lesion and should be started as early as possible. Although steroid treatment of vestibular neuronitis has generally not been recommended, recent studies[72] have indicated that methylprednisolone may provide improved recovery. Vestibular rehabilitation is useful when symptoms are persistent or when recovery of performance is incomplete.[69,70] Maintenance of good balance is important in all older adults through physical activity and programs such as Tai Chi, dancing, and participation in active sports.[72]

Benign Positional Vertigo

BPV usually resolves spontaneously.[70] If it does not, simple maneuvers can be applied to move the offending otoconia out of the semicircular canals.[34,45,47,64–66] When torsional, geotropic nystagmus suggests involvement of the posterior canal, the Epley,[34,45,65] Semont,[65] or Gans[64] maneuvers can be performed. During these maneuvers, the patient's head is first rotated in the plane of the affected canal, allowing the vertigo and nystagmus to appear and subside. Then the patient's head is rotated in a plane that is orthogonal to the first rotational plane to move the otoconia out of the affected canal back into the vestibule of the labyrinth. Care must be exercised to avoid potentially harmful neck extension.[64] When horizontally directed nystagmus is observed (implying involvement of the lateral semicircular canal), the patient is rotated 360° around his vertical axis (termed the barbecue rotation).[65]

Ménière's Disease

Definitive treatment for Ménière's disease has not been established.[73,74] In most cases, the initial management of Ménière's disease should be expectant with inclusion of sedatives, antiemetics, and antivertiginous drugs to control symptoms during an attack. It is important to provide patient education and counseling.[50] If symptoms do not improve spontaneously, a low-salt diet and possibly use of diuretics may be helpful.[75] When attacks of vertigo and associated symptoms are severe and persistent, surgical intervention[73] aimed at weakening or eliminating the vestibular reflex on the affected side can be considered.[9,76] It is very important for patients to understand the pathophysiology behind their symptoms, especially those with a chronic recurrent inner ear balance disorder such as Ménière's disease.[70] An interactive discussion, spread over several visits is usually required.

Vestibular Ototoxicity

Vestibular ototoxicity can be avoided by a) judicious selection and use of potentially toxic drugs, b) screening for susceptibility[38] through careful evaluation of family history, and c) monitoring vestibular and auditory function during administration. It also may be possible to coadminister agents that will serve a protective function. At present there is experimental evidence favoring a wide spectrum of such agents.[36]

NASAL AND SINUS CONDITIONS

Changes in the structure and physiology of the nose, septum, turbinates, and sinuses contribute to a number of nasal and sinus conditions found in the elderly. Drooping of the nasal tip accompanied by recession of periodontal tissues alters the external nasal valve and leads to disturbance of nasal airflow. Diminished secretion and thickening of nasal mucus, in combination with the desiccating effect of many medications, creates the sensation of postnasal drainage. Viscous and ropey, but clear drainage material may be seen draped from the uvula to the edge of the soft palate. Desiccation of nasal membranes may also lead to complaints of nasal stuffiness or blockage. Excessive desiccation also contributes to epistaxis. Most nosebleeds occur in Little's area, generally visible on the septum just inside the nasal vestibule, where crusting, clotting, and erythema are usually visualized. Because many elderly patients are receiving chronic aspirin therapy or antithrombotics, epistaxis can be severe. Treatment may require cauterization or packing with gauze or synthetic sponges. All of the conditions related to dryness respond favorably to moisturization with saline spray. Saline gels are also available and have a longer period of effectiveness. Application of petroleum jelly or antibiotic ointment is controversial, as conjectured aspiration and subsequent chemical pneumonitis is a concern.

Rhinitis

Rhinitis is a common condition in the elderly. Common causes include viral illness, allergy, and vasomotor (nonallergic) rhinitis. Perennial nonallergic rhinitis describes a condition that is sometimes confused with allergic rhinitis. The condition is distinguished from allergic rhinitis in that it represents a response to irritating substances or conditions including changes in temperature, humidity, barometric pressure, or substances that may create direct irritation of the trigeminal nerve endings in the nasal passages. Treatment, however, is similar to that of allergic rhinitis with intranasal steroid sprays being the gold standard.

Sinusitis

Acute sinusitis is characterized by persistent upper respiratory infection (>7–10 days), congestion, mucopurulent drainage, cough, and sometimes fever, headache, and facial pain. On the other hand, chronic sinusitis (symptoms lasting ≥8–12 weeks) is denoted by persistent nasal obstruction, purulent nasal and posterior pharyngeal discharge, postnasal drip and cough, as well as facial fullness or headache, fatigue, hyposmia, and fetor oris. Location of head or face pain may indicate which sinuses are involved. The frontal sinuses produce pain above the eyes. The ethmoid sinuses may cause pain between or behind the eyes. Maxillary sinusitis is associated with pain in the face and teeth, whereas the sphenoid sinuses cause pain at the top, back, or sides of the head. *Streptococcus pneumonia*, *Haemophilus influenza*, and *Moraxella catarrhalis* are the most common pathogens. Treatment of the various sinusitis entities beings with assessing the patient's environment, reducing exposure to allergens and environmental irritants; and antibiotic treatment of infections. For more complicated cases, surgery is directed at opening crucial areas for drainage, particularly the ostiomeatal drainage tracts. The surgery is facilitated by the use of shavers, image-guided navigation, and balloon sinuplasty.[77]

Gustatory Rhinorrhea

One problem that is most often seen in the elderly is called gustatory rhinorrhea. Patients with this condition report copious clear rhinorrhea coming from the anterior nasal passage when they sit down to eat. The pathophysiological mechanism for this is not completely understood; however, symptoms may respond to ipratropium bromide nasal spray. Occasionally, Robinul (glycopyrrolate) in saline may be used to pretreat the patient 30–60 minutes before sitting down to a meal.

Nasal Polyps

Nasal polyps are pale, grapelike growths usually attached to the middle meatus. When enlarged, they may protrude out the nostril or below the edge of the soft palate orally. They are often found in association with tinnitus or atopic conditions and often interfere with olfaction. Unless dramatic blockage is evident, treatment may be initiated with nasal steroid spray. Any unusual appearance to a nasal polyp should raise suspicion of a neoplasm and surgical removal may be necessary. Epistaxis in association with a visualized mass should also prompt removal.

DISORDERS OF SMELL AND TASTE

Healthy elderly persons have a diminished capacity to identify, discriminate, and remember odors. Disorders of smell and taste, and difficulty with identifying various odors may create a potentially dangerous situation if patients are unable to smell gas leaks, smoke, or other alarming odors in a timely manner. The majority of disorders of smell are secondary to rhinitis, polyps, or sinusitis. Alzheimer's disease, Parkinson's disease, and multiple sclerosis are also associated with smell and taste disorders. Hypothyroidism, vitamin deficiency, trauma, and tumors of the sinonasal cavities may also affect the ability to smell. Smoking also diminishes the acuteness of olfaction. Several medications may interfere with the ability to smell including lipid-lowering agents, calcium channel blockers, antidepressants, and opiates. Treatment of anosmia or microsomia is directed at the underlying cause. Alarms are now available that can notify a patient of gas leak and, of course, smoke alarms and carbon monoxide detectors are also recommended.

Salt, sweet, sour, and bitter are the only true taste senses and depend on taste receptors primarily in the tongue but also in the palate and pharynx. These receptors may be diminished through a variety of disorders including autoimmune disease and infection as well as various medications.

ORAL CAVITY

A careful examination of the oral cavity in older patients is important. Various pigmentary changes may be noted including: amalgam tattoo, which is dental amalgam material under a healed mucosal laceration; melanosis (physiological pigmentation, often seen as dark patches of the oral mucosa): brownish pigmentation with Addison's disease; bronze pigmentation with hemochromatosis; yellow/gray pigmentation with xanthomatosis disease; black pigmentation with bismuth; and, violaceous macules with Kaposi sarcoid. Oral candidiasis is a relatively common condition seen in older patients, particularly those who are taking inhaled steroids or antibiotic therapy, and for those with a history of radiation therapy.[78] Treatment is with topical or systemic antifungals. Leukoplakia may be found on a careful oral examination; it is a whitish hyperkeratotic lesion that may or may not be associated with dysplastic changes. Lichen planus may present as a reticular branching pattern of leukoplakia usually on the buccal mucosa. Erosive lichen planus has a 10%–15% chance of developing into squamous carcinoma and should be treated with topical steroids. Hairy tongue results from hyperplasia of the fungiform papillae of the tongue; it may be black, blue, brown, or white, depending on microflora and nicotine staining, and is often associated with candidal overgrowth. Fordyce granules are benign, painless, pinpoint yellow nodules occurring bilaterally in the posterior buccal mucosa.[78] Macroglossia should raise suspicion of amyloidosis or myeloproliferative disease. Pernicious anemia, iron-deficiency anemia, folic acid deficiency, diabetic neuropathy, or malignant disease may cause a burning tongue.

SWALLOWING DISORDERS

Swallowing disorders disproportionately affect elderly patients. The most common cause of swallowing disorders is laryngopharyngeal reflux or gastroesophageal reflux disease, sometimes with stricture, and cerebrovascular accidents. Left-sided cerebrovascular accidents often lead to difficulties during the oral phase of swallowing including problems in initiating the swallow and delay of propulsion of bolus through the oral cavity. In contrast, patients with right-sided cortical strokes tend to have problems with the pharyngeal phase of swallowing resulting in pharyngeal residue and aspiration tendency.

Other neurological conditions should also be considered in patients with swallowing dysfunction, particularly if there is an accompanying voice abnormality. Motor neuron disease can present with swallowing difficulty as an initial symptom with reduced lingual control and reduced labial palatal movements. Parkinson's disease has a typical pattern of swallowing problems including repetitive tongue pumping to initiate the oral stage of swallowing, delayed pharyngeal swallow, and pharyngeal residue. In addition, a number of general medical conditions including rheumatoid arthritis, diabetic neuropathy, and polymyositis can lead to swallowing difficulties as a consequence of their disease process.

Cancers of the head and neck comprise approximately 5% of all cancers and are a relatively common cause of swallowing dysfunction in the elderly. The majority of these cancers are squamous cell carcinomas; risk factors include smoking, alcohol, and poor oral hygiene. Clinicians must carefully evaluate neck masses, hoarseness, dysphagia, otalgia (ear pain), and unexplained weight loss. In the past, early (T-1) lesions of the larynx have been treated primarily with radiation therapy whereas more extensive lesions have been treated by partial or total laryngectomy with neck dissection. Since the early 1990s, evidence supports concurrent chemoradiation. Positron emission tomography scanning is now used to follow cancer patients and to detect metastases or reoccurrences earlier.[79] Placement of percutaneous endoscopic gastrostomy may significantly improve a patient's nutritional status during treatment of head and neck cancer and enable patients to have a better quality of life during and after treatment. Nonetheless, head and neck cancers remain potentially disfiguring, life altering or fatal, with a significant impact on quality of life. Prevention in the form of smoking cessation, moderation of alcohol intake, and attention to oral hygiene should be encouraged.

Evaluation

The traditional means of evaluating dysphagia, namely the barium swallow has been largely supplanted by the modified barium swallow, which provides a wider range of data for evaluation and may be used to initiate therapy at the same time. Functional endoscopic evaluation of swallowing, functional endoscopic evaluation of sensory competence, and transnasal esophagoscopy are all available for direct examination and evaluation of the swallowing mechanism in real time with video documentation. Unsedated transnasal esophagoscopy allows video-documented examination and biopsy of the esophagus, nasal passages, nasopharynx, oropharynx, hypopharynx, and larynx. Application of CO_2 laser by flexible fiberoptic cable and pulsed dye laser allows treatment of many lesions, including carcinomas, polyps, granulomas, webs, strictures, and Reinke edema.

VOICE DISORDERS

Some characteristics of the aging voice include altered pitch, roughness, breathiness, weakness, and tremulousness. As many as 10%–15% of elderly individuals have vocal dysfunction. Dysfunctions may be classified into those that are part of the aging process and those associated with other pathological entities.

A number of structural changes to the vocal folds may contribute to the changes in voice in older men and women. Decreased amounts of collagen fibers and decreased density of these fibers and fibrosis of the vocal ligaments result in thinner vocal cords that vibrate more rapidly, contributing to the vocal fold atrophy, glottal gap, and higher fundamental frequency commonly observed in aged men. In contrast, vocal fold edema noted in older women adds mass to the vocal folds and may decrease the fundamental frequency of older women's voices. Surface irregularities can also prevent complete approximation of the cords and result in breathiness and reduced vocal intensity. Aging laryngeal muscles also undergo some degree of atrophy. Increased amounts of connective tissue and fatty infiltration are found interspersed among the degenerating fibers. Reduction in vocal fold moisture may contribute to a slowing of the mucosal wave and vocal difficulties. Medications are common offenders of mucosal drying including diuretics, steroid inhalers, sedatives, and antidepressants with anticholinergic side effects. Improved function can be readily achieved by careful withdrawal and/or substitution of drugs and the use of mucolytics.

Some of the perceived acoustic characteristics of geriatric voice such as tremulousness, weakness, and pitch variability are suggestive of neuromuscular impairment of laryngeal control. Dysphonia may be the presenting symptom of some neurological disorders such as essential tremor and Parkinson's disease. In Parkinson's disease, the voice is low in volume, breathy, and monotonic and the ability to read rapidly is reduced. Postoperative recurrent laryngeal nerve dysfunction after anterior cervical fusion or thyroidectomy is also well known. The treatment normally involves intensive treatment for reflux as well as possible laryngoplasty, either through injection of filler substance in the vocal cord or by actual surgical repositioning of portions of the laryngeal framework.

Videostroboscopy is an essential prerequisite examination to these procedures; it can identify lesions not seen on mirror examination, as well as subtle neurological signs not visible on mirror or fiberoptic examination. Voice therapy can be initiated at the first videostroboscopic examination, during which time recommendations for further treatment are developed.

REFERENCES

1. Quaedvlieg PJ, Tirsi E, Thissen MR, Krekels GA. Actinic keratosis: how to differentiate the good from the bad ones? *Eur J Dermatol.* 2006;16:335–339.
2. Grandis JR, Hirsch BE, Yu VL. Simultaneous presentation of malignant external otitis and temporal bone cancer. *Arch Otolaryngol. Arch Otolaryngol. Head Neck Surg.* 1993;119:687–689.
3. Osguthorpe JD, Nielsen DR. Otitis externa: Review and clinical update. *Am Fam Physician.* 2006;74:1510–1516.
4. Ruckenstein MJ. Infections of the external ear. In: Cummings CW, Flint PW, Harker LA, et al, eds. *Otolaryngology Head & Neck Surgery.* 4th ed. Philadelphia: Elsevier/Mosby; 2005:2929–2987.
5. Kuhweide R, Van de Steene V, Vlaminck S, Casselman JW. Ramsay Hunt syndrome: pathophysiology of cochleovestibular symptoms. *J Laryngol Otol.* 2002;116:844–848.
6. Hyden D, Akerlind B, Peebo M. Inner ear and facial nerve complications of acute otitis media with focus on bacteriology and virology. *Acta Otolaryngol.* 2006;126:460–466.
7. Dubey SP, Larawin V. Complications of chronic suppurative otitis media and their management. *Laryngoscope.* 2007;117:264–267.
8. Hafidh MA, Keogh I, Walsh RM, Walsh M, Rawluk D. Otogenic intracranial complications. A 7-year retrospective review. *Am J Otolaryngol.* 2006;27:390–395.
9. Kaplan DM, Hehar SS, Bance ML, Rutka JA. Intentional ablation of vestibular function using commercially available topical gentamicin-betamethasone eardrops in patients with Meniere's disease: further evidence for topical eardrop ototoxicity. *Laryngoscope.* 2002;112:689–695.
10. Grimmer JF, Poe DS. Update on eustachian tube dysfunction and the patulous eustachian tube. *Curr Opin Otolaryngol Head Neck Surg.* 2005;13:277–282.
11. Chole RA, Sudhoff HH. Chronic otitis media, mastoiditis and petrositis. In: Cummings CW, Flint PW, Harker LA, et al, eds. *Otolaryngology Head & Neck Surgery.* 4th ed. Philadelphia: Elsevier/Mosby; 2005:2988–3012.
12. Quaranta N, Cassano M, Quaranta A. Facial paralysis associated with cholesteatoma: a review of 13 cases. *Otol Neurotol.* 2007;28:405–407.
13. Smith JA, Danner CJ. Complications of chronic otitis media and cholesteatoma. *Otolaryngol Clin North Am.* 2006;39:1237–1255.
14. Allen HN, Burns A, Newton V, et al. The effects of improving hearing in dementia. *Age Aging.* 2003;32:189–193.
15. Weinstein BE. *Geriatric Audiology.* New York: Thieme, 2000.
16. Gates GA, Mills JH. Presbycusis. *Lancet.* 2005;366:1111–1120.
17. Frisina RD, Walton JP. Age-related structural and functional changes in the cochlear nucleus. *Hear Res.* 2006;216–217:216–223.
18. Seidman MD, Quirk WS, Shirwany NA. Mechanisms of alterations in the microcirculation of the cochlea. *Ann NY Acad Sci.* 1999;884:226–232.
19. Arts HA. Sensorineural hearing loss: evaluation and management in adults. In: Cummings CW, Flint PW, Harker LA, et al, eds. *Otolaryngology Head & Neck Surgery.* 4th ed. Philadelphia: Elsevier/Mosby; 2005:3535–3561.
20. Derks W, De Groot JA, Raymakers JA, Veldman JE. Fluoride therapy for cochlear otosclerosis? an audiometric and computerized tomography evaluation. *Acta Otolaryngol.* 2001;121:174–177.
21. Jerger J, Mahurin R, Pirozzolo F. The separability of central auditory and cognitive deficits: Implications for the elderly. *J Am Acad Audio.* 1990;1:116–119.
22. Rauch SD, Ruckenstein MJ. Autoimmune inner ear disease. In: Cummings CW, Flint PW, Harker LA, et al, eds. *Otolaryngology Head & Neck Surgery.* 4th ed. Philadelphia: Elsevier/Mosby; 2005:2933–2943.
23. Selimoglu E. Aminoglycoside-induced ototoxicity. *Curr Pharm Des.* 2007;13:119–126.

24. Schacht J, Hawkins JE. Sketches of otohistory. Part 11: Ototoxicity: drug-induced hearing loss. *Audiol Neurootol.* 2006;11:1–6.

25. Rybak LP. Vestibular and auditory toxicity. In: Cummings CW, Flint PW, Harker LA, et al, eds. *Otolaryngology Head & Neck Surgery.* 4th ed. Philadelphia: Elsevier/Mosby; 2005:2933–2943.

26. Chen Y, Huang WG, Zha DJ, et al.Aspirin attenuates gentamicin ototoxicity: from the laboratory to the clinic. *Hear Res.* 2007;226:178–182.

27. Stach BA, Spretnjak ML, Jerger J. The prevalence of central presbyacusis in a clinical population. *J Am Acad Audiol.* 1990;1:109–115.

28. Humes L, Christopherson L, Cokely, C. *Central Auditory Processing Disorders in the Elderly: Fact or Fiction?* St. Louis: Mosby Year Book; 1992:Chapter 11.

29. Bellis TJ, Wilber LA: Effects of aging and gender on interhemispheric function. *J Speech Lang Hear Res.* 2001;44:246–263.

30. Robinson SK, Viirre ES, Stein MB. Antidepressant therapy in tinnitus. *Hear Res.* 2007;226:221–231.

31. Sonmez G, Basekim CC, Ozturk E, Gungor A, Kizilkaya E. Imaging of pulsatile tinnitus: a review of 74 patients. *Clin Imaging.* 2007;31:102–108.

32. Zagolski O: Management of tinnitus in patients with presbycusis. *Int Tinnitus J.* 2006;12: 175–178.

33. Caffier PP, Haupt H, Scherer H, Mazurek B. Outcomes of long-term outpatient tinnitus-coping therapy: psychometric changes and value of tinnitus-control instruments. *Ear Hear.* 2006;27:619–627.

34. Jackson LE, Morgan B, Fletcher JC Jr, Krueger WW. Anterior canal benign paroxysmal positional vertigo: an underappreciated entity. *Otol Neurotol.* 2007;28:218–222.

35. Lopez L, Honrubia V, Baloh RW. Aging and the human vestibular nucleus. *J Vestib Res.* 1997;7:77–85.

36. Rogers J, Zornetzer SF, Blooom FE: Senescent pathology of the cerebellum: Purkinje neurons and their parallel fiber afferents. *Neurobiol Aging.* 1981;2:15–25.

37. Glick R, Bondareff W. Loss of synapses in the cerebellar cortex of the senescent rat. *J Gerontol.* 1979;34:818–822.

38. Ross MD, Johnsson LG, Peacor D, Allard LF. Observations on normal and degenerating human otoconia. *Ann Otol Rhinol Laryngol.* 1976;85:310–326.

39. Hall TC, Miller AKH, Corsellis JAN: Variations in the human Purkinje cell population according to age and sex. *Neuropathol Appl Neurobiol.* 1975;1:267–292.

40. Engstrom H, Bergstrom B, Rosenhall U. Vestibular sensory epithelia. *Arch Otolaryngol.*1974;100:411–418.

41. Rosenhall U. Degenerative changes in the aging human vestibular geriatric neuroepithelia. *Acta Otolaryngol.*1973;76:208–220.

42. Schuknecht HF: Cupulolithiasis. *Arch Otolaryngol.* 1969;90:765–778.

43. Buatois S, Gueguen R, Gauchard GC, Benetos A, Perrin PP. Posturography and risk of recurrent falls in healthy non-institutionalized persons aged over 65. *Gerontology.* 2006; 52:345–352.

44. Rubino FA. Gait disorders. *Neurologist.* 2002;8:254–262.

45. Epley JM. Human experience with canalith repositioning maneuvers. *Ann NY Acad Sci.* 2001;942:179–191.

46. Alvarez JC, Diaz C, Suarez C, et al.Aging and the human vestibular nuclei: morphometric analysis. *Mech Aging Dev.* 2000;114:149–172.

47. Aw ST, Todd MJ, Aw GE, McGarvie LA, Halmagyi GM. Benign positional nystagmus. A study of its three-dimensional spatio-temporal characteristics. *Neurology.* 2005;65:1897–1905.

48. Parnes LS, McClure JA. Free-floating endolymph particles: a new operative finding during posterior semicircular canal occlusion. *Laryngoscope.* 1992;102:988–992.

49. Baloh RW. Vestibular neuritis. *NEJM.* 2003;328:1027–1032.

50. Proctor LR, Perlman H, Lindsay J, Matz G. Acute vestibular paralysis in herpes zoster oticus. *Ann Otol Rhinol Laryngol.* 1979;88:303–310.

51. Huppert D, Strupp M, Theil D, Glaser M, Brandt T: Low recurrence rate of vestibular neuritis: a long-term follow-up. *Neurology.* 2006;67:1870–1871.

52. Ballester M, Liard P, Vibert D, Hausler R. Meniere's disease in the elderly. *Otol Neurotol.* 2002;23:73–78.

53. Seemungal BM. Neuro-otological emergencies. *Curr Opin Neurol.* 2007;20:32–39.

54. Brantberg K, Trees N, Baloh RW. Migraine-associated vertigo. *Acta Otolaryngol.* 2005;125:276–279.

55. Lempert T, Neuhauser H. Migrainous vertigo. *Neurol Clin.* 2005;23:715–730.

56. von Brevern M, Radtke A, Clarke AH, Lempert T. Migrainous vertigo presenting as episodic positional vertigo. *Neurology.* 2004;62:469–472.

57. Baloh RW. Episodic vertigo: central nervous system causes. *Curr Opin Neurol.* 2002;15:17–21.

58. Solomon D. Distinguishing and treating causes of central vertigo. *Otolaryngol Clin North Am.* 2000;33:579–601.

59. Minor LB. Labyrinthine fistulae: pathobiology and management. *Curr Opin Otolaryngol Head Neck Surg.* 2003;11:340–346.

60. Backous DD, Minor LB, Aboujaoude ES, Nager GT. Relationship of the utriculus and sacculus to the stapes footplate: anatomic implications for sound-and/or pressure-induced otolith activation. *Ann Otol Rhinol Laryngol.* 1999;108:548–553.

61. Proctor LR. Vestibular disability from aminoglycoside induced vestibular paralysis. *Johns Hopkins Med J.* 1982;151:162–163.

62. Delaney KA. Bedside diagnosis of vertigo: value of the history and neurological examination. *Acad Emerg Med.* 2003;10:1388–1395.

63. Goebel JA. The ten-minute examination of the dizzy patient. *Semin Neurol.* 2001;21:391–398.

64. Roberts RA, Gans RE, Montaudo RL. Efficacy of a new treatment maneuver for posterior canal benign paroxysmal positional vertigo. *J Am Acad Audiol.* 2006;17:598–604.

65. Sekine K, Imai T, Sato G, Ito M, Takeda N. Natural history of benign paroxysmal positional vertigo and efficacy of Epley and Lempert maneuvers. *Otolaryngol Head Neck Surg.* 2006;135:529–533.

66. Salvinelli F, Trivelli M, Casale M, et al.Treatment of benign positional vertigo in the elderly: a randomized trial. *Laryngoscope.* 2004;114:827–831.

67. Peterka RJ, Black FO. Age-related changes in human posture control: sensory organization tests. *J Vestib Res.* 1990;73–85.

68. Proctor L, Glackin R, Shimizu H, Smith C, Lietman P. Reference values for serial vestibular testing. *Ann Otol Rhinol Laryngol.*1986;95:83–90.

69. Macias JD, Massingale S, Gerkin RD. Efficacy of vestibular rehabilitation therapy in reducing falls. *Otolaryngol Head Neck Surg.* 2005;133:323–325.

70. Wrisley DM, Pavlou M. Physical therapy for balance disorders. *Neurol Clin.* 2005;23:855–874.

71. Andersson G, Asmundson GJ, Denev J, Nilsson J, Larsen HC. A controlled trial of cognitive-behavior therapy combined with

vestibular rehabilitation in the treatment of dizziness. *Behav Res Ther.* 2006;44:1265–1273.

72. Strupp M, Zingler VC, Arbusow V, et al.Methylprednisolone, valacyclovir, or the combination for vestibular neuritis. *NEJM.* 2004;351:354–361.

73. Goycoolea MV, ed. Surgical treatment of incapacitating peripheral vertigo. *Otolaryngol Clin North Am.* 1994;27(2).

74. Brinson GM, Chen DA, Arriaga MA. Endolymphatic mastoid shunt versus endolymphatic sac decompression for Meniere's disease. *Otolaryngol Head Neck Surg.* 2007;136:415–421.

75. Thirlwall AS, Kundu S. Diuretics for Meniere's disease or syndrome. *Cochrane Database Syst Rev.* 2006;3:CD003599.

76. Cohen-Kerem R, Kisilevsky V, Einarson TR, Kozer E, Koren G, Rutka JA. Intratympanic gentamicin for Meniere's disease: a meta-analysis. *Laryngoscope.* 2004;114:2085–2091.

77. Bolger WE, Brown CL, Church CA, et al. Safety and outcomes of balloon catheter sinusotomy: a multicenter 24-week analysis in 115 patients. *Otolaryngol Head Neck Surg.* 2007;157: 10–20.

78. Lee KJ, ed. *Essential Otolaryngology.* 8th ed. 2003:448–450. McGraw Hill, New York, NY.

79. Gordin A, et al.The role of FDG-PET/CT imaging in head and neck malignant conditions: impact on diagnostic accuracy and patient care. *Otolaryngol Head Neck Surg.* 2007;137:130–137.

39

Geriatric Dentistry

Allen D. Samuelson, DDS

Recent research has forged a link between oral health and systemic health such that the relationship can no longer be ignored. Periodontitis and the attendant inflammatory response and byproducts have been linked to cardiovascular disease, preterm low-birth-weight infants, and have relationships to diabetic control and severity.[1-6] It is incumbent on the practicing physician to have a basic knowledge of the oral and maxillofacial region as well as the pathological changes likely to occur. Oral disease such as periodontitis and dental caries, specifically root surface caries, is particularly prevalent in the elderly population. The baby boomer generation will present challenges to the medical health care system and to those delivering dental care. The rate of edentulism for those older than age 65 years has dropped from 40% in the 1980s to approximately 20% in the beginning of the twenty-first century. This number is expected to decrease further in the coming years.[7-11] There will be a large increase in retained teeth over the next few decades. Dental caries and periodontitis therefore will be present in many of these patients due to the presence of teeth.[7-11]

INTRODUCTION

As the initial portion of the aero-digestive tract, the maxillofacial structures form an important, interrelated complex of skin, mucosa, joints, bones, glandular tissues, vessels, ligaments, tendons, nerves, and teeth. These structures work together to allow an individual to speak, masticate, provide for facial expression, swallow, breathe, and allow for immunological and physical protection. Importantly, these structures also provide facial support and esthetics that are critical to self-esteem. Richly innervated and vascular, the oral cavity serves as a front line of defense in the protection of the individual as well as serving as the means for nutritional intake so the body can properly repair itself. There are a multitude of diseases that can affect one or more of these structures and therefore effect change or

loss of function resulting in loss or diminished happiness in the individual. Discomfort, dysfunction, or malformations in this region can severely affect an individual's ability to thrive.

A variety of prosthetic devices can also be present in the mouth such as fixed or removable prostheses, implants, jaw positioning and protective devices, orthodontic hardware, and obturators for developmental, functional, esthetic, traumatic, or pathological deformations. The elderly patient more than likely will have one or more of these devices in their mouth. These devices may fit and function very well or very poorly. They can also fatigue and need repair or replacement.

The general or geriatric physician is in a good position to screen for these problems by including a brief history and oral and maxillofacial examination within the framework of their routine general physical examination. The time-honored history and techniques of inspection, palpation, percussion, and auscultation are certainly valid when examining the maxillofacial structures and oral cavity. This chapter serves as an introduction to the general characteristics, basic anatomy, and age-related changes that can be expected in the oral cavity and maxillofacial region.[12-20]

ORAL MUCOSA

General Characteristics and Anatomy

Mucosa is the lining epithelium and connective tissue of the oral cavity and has similar functions to that of the skin in that it serves as a barrier for protection of underlying structures. There are differing levels of mucosal thickness and keratinization depending on location. There are three distinct types of mucosa present in the oral cavity: masticatory, lining, and specialized. The gingiva and hard palate are lined with masticatory mucosa that is well keratinized. The gingival and other periodontal tissues will be discussed later in the chapter. Masticatory mucosa does not stretch and serves to bear the forces and

435

friction of mastication. The soft palate, ventral tongue, floor of mouth, and the alveolar and buccal mucosa are all nonkeratinized and designed to stretch and allow for movement of the underlying muscular and bony tissues. The mucosa on the dorsum of the tongue and vermillion border of the lips is known as specialized mucosa. The tongue is coated with taste buds and papillae of various types (foliate, fungiform, filiform, circumvallate) and the vermillion border, only present in humans, serves as a transitional zone between skin and mucosa on the lips. All mucosal tissues should be moist, pink or red in color, without ulcerations, masses, inflammation, clefting, or defect. Depending on the skin tones of the individual, racial pigmentation may be present in various areas of the mucosal surfaces, including the tongue. The tongue should be clean and pink without staining or overly hyperplastic papillae. The mucosal tissues present over residual ridges, where teeth were once present and lost to disease or trauma, should be smooth, pink, firm, and without ulcerations.

Age-Related Changes

Although there are conflicting data as to exactly how aging affects the oral mucosa it is generally agreed that change does occur. The lining mucosal tissues in older adults are thinner, smoother, and dryer than younger cohorts. There are studies that indicate nutritional factors such as iron or B-vitamin deficiencies and not age per se may be the cause of the abovementioned changes. The floor of the mouth and ventral tongue can exhibit varicosities. The tongue mucosa may likewise become thinner with loss of filiform papillae. Sun exposure can cause changes in the vermillion border, specifically a loss of distinct delineation. Burning mouth syndrome is manifested by painful mucosa with no apparent etiology. The most worrisome mucosal lesion is that of oral cancer. There are many types of cancerous lesions that may occur in the oral cavity including melanoma, squamous cell carcinoma, and various sarcomas: the most common being squamous cell carcinoma. Squamous cell carcinoma can appear as a white, red, or mixed lesion, generally firm and painless. Common regions of occurrence are the floor of the mouth, ventral tongue, and palatal tissues. Mucosal changes of note with certain medications include xerostomia, lichenoid (resembling lichen planus), direct mucosal injury as with antineoplastic medications and radiation, gingival hyperplasia, and allergy. Xerostomia is particularly worrisome as it causes oral discomfort and, with the lack of the buffering capacity and lubrication of saliva, places the teeth at risk for dental caries that will be discussed later. Multiple systemic diseases may manifest in the oral structures including diabetes mellitus, Crohn's disease, leukemia, and lymphoma.

Examination Techniques

The oral mucosa should be inspected with good lighting. Make certain that all prosthetic devices have been removed from the mouth prior to the examination. The lips and buccal and labial mucosa should be inspected for macules, papules, ulcerations, or other abnormalities. The hard and soft palate can likewise be inspected. These structures can also be palpated using the bimanual technique or with a single digit to detect intramucosal masses or tenderness over any region. Residual ridges bearing a prosthetic device such as a denture should be inspected and palpated for irritation, reactive lesions, or other pathological entity. In patients who abuse tobacco and alcohol, please note that the risk for oral cancerous lesions are elevated.

JOINTS AND OSTEOLOGY

General Characteristics and Anatomy

The maxilla and mandible articulate via the temporomandibular joint (TMJ). This bilateral, complex structure defined as a ginglymoid diarthrodial joint allows for many of the functions listed in the introductory paragraph. This joint is unique in that it allows for translation and rotation in two axes. A fibrocartilaginous disc is interposed between the condylar head of the mandible and the fossa in the skull base. The TMJ should display a good range of motion laterally and in protrusion without limitations, deviations, pain, dysfunction, or noise. The average maximum voluntary opening for the human mouth is approximately 50–55 mm and for lateral movements approximately 10–11 mm. The teeth, known as gomphoses or immobile joints, will be discussed later in the chapter.

The maxillofacial osteology is complex. There are a multitude of bones working in concert for the survival, protection, and function of the individual. There are several foramina where nerves, blood vessels, and lymphatics exit. The mandible and maxilla are the primary bony structures of concern in this chapter. The mandible and maxilla are intramembranous bones in that they are formed by ossification of the mesenchymal tissues in the developing fetus and newborn. There should be facial symmetry and these bones, along with others, should provide for good support of the facial soft tissues. Several muscles of mastication have their origin and insertion on the maxilla and mandible to allow for the motor functions listed in the introductory paragraph. Located within several bones of the maxillofacial region are sinus cavities of various sizes. The maxillary sinus is located within the maxillary bones and should be healthy and pain free. Intraorally, all bony tissue should be covered with nonulcerated lining or masticatory mucosa unless a recent dental extraction has occurred. There may be protuberances of bone on the buccal or lingual of the alveolus. These rock-hard, immobile structures are generally normal and are termed exostoses or tori.

Age-Related Changes

The TMJ may develop pain related to arthritis or other functional disturbances. Arthritic changes can cause pain, deviations, and limitations of motion. Noises, such as clicking, popping, or crepitations within the joint can signal displacement or distortion of the articular disc mentioned previously.

Many of the changes that occur in the peripheral skeleton and joints occur in the maxillofacial region. Periosteal expansion, thinning of cortical bone, and gradual loss of trabecular bone can cause fragility and loss of support for the dental structures. If teeth are lost then there is loss of alveolar bone. This loss continues throughout life and can become severe and make prosthetic reconstruction difficult. Osteoporosis can be a risk factor for the development of periodontal disease.

Examination Techniques

The bones of the maxillofacial region should be inspected for symmetry and masses. They can be palpated to note masses, tenderness, or fracture. The sinus cavities, particularly the maxillary sinus, can be percussed to evaluate pain and transilluminated to evaluate for mucosal changes indicative of sinusitis. The TMJ can be inspected for range of motion, deviations, or other dysfunction. The TMJ can also be palpated for tenderness, and clicks, pops, or crepitations. The TMJ can be auscultated directly anterior to the tragus of the ear to evaluate for joint sounds. Intraorally, the bony structures of the maxilla and mandible can be inspected and palpated to note any pathological entities.

MUSCLES OF MASTICATION AND FACIAL EXPRESSION

General Characteristics and Anatomy

There are two major muscle groups in the maxillofacial region: the muscles of facial expression innervated by cranial nerve VII (facial nerve with five branches) and the muscles of mastication innervated by cranial nerve V (trigeminal nerve with three main divisions and several branches). These structures work together to accomplish the functions listed in introductory paragraph. There are numerous muscles of facial expression that should work symmetrically to provide for facial animation. The muscles of mastication act to depress, elevate, rotate, and translate the mandible to allow for a full range of mobility free of limitations, deviations, or pain. The major depressors of the mandible are the lateral (external) pterygoid, digastrics, and the temporalis muscles. The major elevators of the mandible are the medial (internal) pterygoid, masseter, and temporalis.

Age-Related Changes

Certainly, generalized weakness may occur as a patient ages. Myofacial pain is manifested as muscle pain in the maxillofacial region. Generally the patient states that the "side of their face is sore or tender" and does not necessarily point directly to the joint itself. Bell palsy affects the muscles of facial expression and will manifest as palsy or as an asymmetrical disfigurement.

Examination Techniques

The muscles of facial expression can be inspected for symmetry during facial animation or in a static pose. One peculiarity of note is that occulomotor nerve (III) opens the eye and the facial nerve (VII) closes the eyelid. The muscles of mastication can be inspected for symmetry and palpated for masses or to examine for tenderness. The muscles of mastication can be palpated extraorally and intraorally and strength can be tested by having the individual biting a tongue depressor. Range of motion can be evaluated as well.

NERVES

General Characteristics and Anatomy

The maxillofacial complex is richly innervated via the 12 pairs of cranial nerves as well as the cervical nerves. These nerves should provide for motor, sensory, proprioceptive, and autonomic functions without pain, dysesthesia, paresthesia, or dysfunction. The major nerve providing sensory and motor input in the maxillofacial region is the trigeminal. The trigeminal is divided into three divisions: ophthalmic, maxillary, and mandibular. As previously discussed, the facial nerve provides for facial expression and contributes to the taste response. The facial nerve also supplies secretory fibers to both the submandibular and sublingual salivary glands. Taste response is completed by contributions from the vagus and glossopharyngeal nerves. Branches of the glossopharyngeal nerve also supply the secretory fibers to the parotid gland.

Age-Related Changes

Trigeminal neuralgia (TN) is a relatively common cause of facial pain in the elderly. The pain is characterized by a trigger point, generally intraorally, with subsequent severe, lancinating pain of a few seconds to minutes duration. TN may be an early sign of multiple sclerosis in some patients. Postherpetic neuralgia due to previous infection with the herpes zoster virus is a severely debilitating illness and is difficult to treat.

Examination Techniques

The neurological examination portion of the dental physical examination includes the 12 pairs of cranial nerves. Motor, sensory, and autonomic function can be examined with relative ease. The muscles of facial expression can be examined by inspecting the face for symmetry during facial animation and in static pose. The muscles of mastication can be tested by having the patient bite on a tongue depressor and the physician attempts to remove it from the mouth. Sensation can be assessed by swiping a wisp of cotton in the region of each division of the trigeminal nerve. Autonomic function can be assessed subjectively by a query about mouth dryness and objectively by examining the mouth directly.

GLANDULAR TISSUE

The primary glandular tissues of note are the major and minor salivary glands and lymphatic tissues. The salivary glands serve to produce sufficient amounts of saliva for food bolus preparation, assist in taste, provide initial enzymatic breakdown of food, provide immunological protection against microorganisms, and lubricate the oral mucosa. Salivary glands contain mucous cells, serous cells, or a combination. Serous cells produce watery saliva and mucous cells produce saliva thicker in quality. Major salivary glands include the parotid, submandibular, and sublingual. There are also many minor or accessory salivary glands. The parotid glands are located laterally in the face near the anterior aspect of the tragus and below the lobe of the ear. The submandibular and sublingual gland is located in the floor of the mouth. The minor salivary glands are located in the labial mucosa and palate. Lymphatic tissues such as the tonsils, adenoids, and accessory tissues are present in the mouth. There are also lymphoid tissues present within the salivary glands as well.

Age-Related Changes

Age-related changes include xerostomia from a variety of causes including medications, Sjögren syndrome, and radiation to the head and neck. There are typically more ductal cells in the older adult rather than acinar cells and therefore possibly less salivary production. Calcifications within the gland called sialoliths can block salivary flow leading to swelling, pain, stasis, and infection. Xerostomia can lead to difficulty with eating, speaking, and prosthetic retention. Lacking the buffering capacity of saliva when xerostomic, the teeth are at high risk for caries. Lymphoma may manifest as a palatal swelling or other swelling about the head and neck.

Examination Techniques

Salivary glands can be inspected for symmetry and swelling by examining the face from the anterior. The tissues in the mouth can be inspected for swellings and asymmetry. The glands can be palpated extraorally for masses or tenderness. Intraorally, if the mirror or tongue depressor being used sticks to the mucosa, this may indicate dryness or xerostomia. Also, if you suspect xerostomia, you can administer the cracker test. Obtain a saltine cracker to investigate whether the patient can adequately chew and swallow it. If not, xerostomia may be a problem. One may also attempt to "milk" the glands to assess patency and flow from the parotid duct located in the buccal mucosa bilaterally opposite the upper molar teeth or the submandibular duct, located in the anterior floor of the mouth. Likewise the anterior lip can be everted, dried with a 2 × 2 gauze, and inspected for flow from the minor salivary glands evident as discreet beads of saliva. Bimanual palpation of the floor of the mouth can be performed to assess symmetry and locate masses or tenderness.

VESSELS

The oral and maxillofacial region is rich in blood supply provided mainly from branches of the external carotid and basilar arteries. The arteries of the head and neck should display a normal pulse without bruits.

Age-Related Changes

Changes that occur in the vascular system include skin, mucosal, and rarely intraosseous. Telangiectasia and angiomas may occur on the skin of the face and neck. Intraorally, the most frequent finding is caviar tongue or lingual varicosities. Intraosseous lesions such as arteriovenous malformation can be present. Although rare, tooth removal in the area of an arteriovenous malformation may cause life-threatening blood loss. Temporal arteritis and headaches of various causes are relatively common.

Examination Techniques

Inspection extraorally, intraorally, radiographically may reveal lesions indicative of vascular pathology. Palpation may reveal mucosal lesions involving the vascular system.

PERIODONTIUM

Three important structures comprise the periodontium: alveolar bone, periodontal ligament, and gingival tissues. Alveolar bone is present in both the mandible and maxilla, and forms the housing for the teeth. Alveolar bone contains both cortical and cancellous bone. Alveolar bone provides firm support for the teeth, the interface being designated a gomphosis or immobile joint. Surrounding each tooth at the root area is the periodontal ligament, which provides a cushioning effect for the teeth upon occlusion. The ligament runs in several different orientations counterbalancing vertical and lateral forces placed on the teeth. The gingiva surrounding the teeth is composed of masticatory and lining mucosa and serves to protect the underlying bony and dental structures. The tissues immediately adjacent to the teeth are masticatory and keratinized and the gingiva below this tissue is lining mucosa and nonkeratinized.

Age-Related Changes

Gingivitis and periodontitis are the two most prominent diseases of the periodontium. These are inflammatory in nature and the extreme result is tooth looseness or loss. Gingivitis manifests the cardinal signs of inflammation in the gingiva. Periodontitis is an inflammatory-mediated destruction of the periodontium and manifests as bone loss, loose teeth, and generally inflamed gingival tissues. Other presentations of gingival or periodontal disease may occur such as acute necrotizing ulcerative gingivitis, aggressive periodontitis, and periodontal abscess. There may indeed be substantial bone loss in the apparent absence of local factors (plaque, calculus). Poor control of diabetes and immune deficits also can be contributing factors to the exacerbation of periodontal disease. Systemic illnesses such as leukemia can affect the appearance of the gingival tissues generally manifesting as hyperplasia, friability, and hemorrhage.

Examination Techniques

The periodontium can be inspected for loss, abscesses, purulence, bleeding, and general inflammation. The periodontium can be palpated as well for masses or tenderness. Oral cancerous lesions can also occur on the gingival tissues.

TEETH

There are 20 primary or milk teeth and 32 adult or permanent teeth. There can be additional teeth known as supernumerary. One or more primary teeth can occasionally be retained into adulthood, especially if there is no permanent successor. Teeth are designated as central incisors, lateral incisors, cuspids (canines), 1st and 2nd bicuspids (premolars), and 1st, 2nd, and 3rd molars. There are several methods for numbering teeth with the military designation being the most common in the United States. The teeth are numbered 1–32 beginning in the upper right, proceeding to the upper left, continuing in the lower posterior left, and proceeding to the lower posterior right. Anterior and posterior are general positional designations for teeth such as the 1st molar, which is the most posterior tooth present. Positional designations for individual teeth are mesial, distal, lingual (toward the tongue), and facial (toward the cheek) or buccal such as the cavity is located on the mesial of the central incisor mesial being that surface toward the center of the mouth. There are four separate layers of various mineral compositions in dental structure: enamel (90% mineral and the hardest substance in the human body), dentin (70% mineral), cementum (50% mineral), and pulpal tissue (0% mineral composed of nerves, blood vessels, and lymphatics). Teeth generally exhibit a white, yellow, or light gray hue of varying chromas. Teeth may also take on the color of the restorative material used to repair lost tooth structure. The teeth should all be present and occlude or fit together smoothly on closing with no interferences. The upper teeth are generally slightly facial to the lower teeth. Teeth should be clean with minimal plaque, tarter (calculus), or food debris.

Age-Related Changes

Although poor oral hygiene may be present at any age, an elderly individual may be more prone to this because of loss of manual dexterity, visual deficit, or cognitive decline. Teeth may be lost due to caries, periodontitis, or fracture. As a result of loss of teeth a poor occlusal or interdigitating relationship may occur, leading to tipped, rotated, or increased spacing between teeth.

Beside dental caries and periodontal disease, a variety of factors can lead to tooth structure loss including: attrition, abrasion, erosion, and abfraction. Attrition is loss of tooth structure due to tooth-to-tooth contact. Abrasion is loss if tooth structure due to dietary or environmental materials, for example, sand, course dietary components, tobacco, and so forth.

Examination Techniques

The teeth should be inspected for the presence of calculus, plaque, and food debris. Plaque only requires approximately 24 hours to form and tarter (calculus) can form in as few as 3 days. The teeth can indeed be inspected for caries, wear, and fractured cusps or other tooth components. The teeth can be palpated for tenderness or looseness. A tongue blade may be used to push on the teeth from several directions for this assessment. The teeth can be percussed to assess for tenderness as well. To assess for tooth fracture, a tongue blade may be applied over the tooth in question and a bite force can be applied to elicit any tenderness. The general occlusion of the teeth can be assessed by having the patient bite the teeth together. Normally there is an overjet and overbite and the teeth fit together evenly and symmetrically.

PROSTHETICS

A variety of prosthetic devices may be present in the mouth. These devices may be permanently affixed to the mouth or removable. Appliances may be worn to aid in mastication and for esthetics. These appliances should be well adapted and not painful. Appliances may be worn to aid in protecting the dentition due to grinding or bruxism, position the jaw in a certain way, or to straighten the teeth. Implants affixed to the jaw should be immobile and function well . Any prosthetic devices should allow for smooth, symmetrical, and pain-free closure and functioning. All prosthetic devices used for whatever purpose should be clean and free of plaque, calculus, or food debris.

Age-Related Changes

There are myriad prosthetic devices that may be present in the mouth for a variety of reasons. It is critical for the patient to be followed closely by their dental professional if they wear a prosthetic device. Often times, however, there is minimal follow-up and the device may become ill fitting because of changes and loss of oral structures. Fixed prosthetics, if preventive measures are not in place, can gather plaque, calculus, and suffer from recurrent or new caries around the device at the margins between the prosthesis and the natural tooth. Abutment teeth for bridges can become loose for a variety of reasons. The fit and function of removable devices can change because of a loss of alveolar bone, which occurs throughout life once teeth have been extracted. The prosthesis, being acrylic or metal, will not adapt to these changes and can become ill fitting with time. Nutritional deficiencies can affect the tissues' response to trauma from prosthetic devices. Poor oral and prosthesis hygiene may be present. Prosthetic devices can gather plaque, calculus, and infectious organisms (fungus as well). Oral mucosal lesions can be associated with removable prosthetic devices: epulis and papillary hyperplasia. Generally, both the prosthesis and the attendant tissue must be treated for full resolution.

Examination Techniques

Removable prosthetic devices should be removed on examination of the mouth. They should be inspected for cleanliness and integrity. Once placed in the mouth, they should be inspected for proper general fit and function. Of course a subjective history from the patient may also alert the practitioner to potential problems with the prosthesis. Fixed devices (crowns, bridges, implants, etc.) should be inspected for cleanliness and the condition of the periodontium surrounding them.

CASE STUDIES

The following brief cases demonstrate important circumstances or findings where a referral to a general dentist is warranted or serious consequences may follow.

Case 1: Approach to the Patient with a Maxillofacial Swelling

A 75-year-old white man presents to your office on referral from the Assistant Director of Nursing at a local nursing home. The patient has a 101°F temperature and is tachycardic. He has refused food and drink for approximately 1.5 days. He has a history of dementia but has become somewhat combative with acute mental status changes in the past day. He has a large swelling in the right facial region and on intraoral examination, has trismus and multiple grossly carious teeth.

Swellings in the maxillofacial region can be due to a number of conditions: tumors, salivary gland infection, and infection due to dental or periodontal disease. A good rule of thumb is that a swelling in the maxillofacial region is odontogenic in origin until proven otherwise. Maxillofacial infections can be extremely dangerous and can result in death. Trismus and airway compromise can complicate therapy as well. Pain alone may not be indicative of frank infection. Pain along with swelling, drainage, and perhaps constitutional symptoms indicate serious infection. Referral to a general dentist, oral and maxillofacial surgeon, or depending on patient symptoms, the emergency department is mandatory. If signs of infection are obvious, such as submandibular or cervical adenitis, fever, swelling, pain, purulence, or laboratory studies are consistent with a bacterial infection, an empiric decision by the physician to place the patient immediately on an antibiotic regimen, most typically penicillin in the nonallergic patient, would be prudent along with an appropriate narcotic or nonnarcotic analgesic. Too often, dental consultation is not readily available in the nursing home setting and or even in the hospital emergency room.

Case 2: Approach to the Patient with Osteoporosis

A 62-year-old white woman presents to your office on self-referral for a complete physical examination. After a complete examination and a bone scan you find that she suffers from osteoporosis. You note, upon brief oral examination, that there is poor oral hygiene, dental caries, and gingival appearance, which is indicative of periodontal disease. A bisphosphonate medication will be prescribed for her to prevent sequelae of this disease. A referral to a general dentist is appropriate to control and remove sources of infection or potential infection.

Bisphosphonate-associated osteonecrosis of the jaws (BONJ) is associated with the use of both oral and intravenous bisphosphonate-medications and is a relatively recently identified phenomenon. Because of the metabolic actions of bisphosphonate medications, spontaneous or trauma-induced osteonecrosis may occur. Oral bisphosphonates present the lowest risk for developing BONJ, especially those patients who have take the medication for less than 3 years. Because of the severe, debilitating nature of BONJ, it is mandatory that the patient receive a dental screening so that a preventive regimen can be instituted along with the removal of potential sources of infection.[11]

Case 3: Approach to the Patient with Intraoral Bleeding

An 85-year-old black woman with a history of dementia is examined by you in the nursing home and found to have a mouth full of bright red blood. The nurse relates that the patient was seen by a local dentist several hours ago. Multiple dental extractions were performed with the insertion of dentures.

Realizing that a drop of blood in saliva can tinge the whole mouth red, you are nonetheless impressed with the rapidity with which the mouth seems to be filling with blood from what appears to be an indeterminable site. Identification of the source of bleeding must be determined to avoid disastrous consequences. Good lighting and suction are essential. Dentures should be removed and moist 4 × 4 gauzes sponges can be placed either by manual pressure or by the patient biting on the gauze. After several minutes the gauze can be removed and the area of bleeding can be identified if it has not already been controlled by direct pressure. If it appears that a single extraction site is responsible for the hemorrhage, further pressure with gauze pads or even iodoform gauze pushed into the extraction site can usually arrest even the most stubborn bleeding. If many sites are bleeding you might want to consider an altered coagulation state due to anticoagulation medication or a coagulopathy. The treating dentist should be consulted and your timely intervention might prove to be definitive.

SUMMARY AND RECOMMENDATIONS

Oral health is intimately related to systemic health and directly related to quality of life. Frail, homebound, and institutionalized older adults are particularly susceptible to oral health problems and should be screened carefully at the initial medical visit. Nursing homes are required by law to have a contract with a dentist or assist in locating a dentist for their clients.[21] All adults should be reminded that proper nutrition, oral hygiene, and habit cessation, especially tobacco products, are critical to maintaining good oral health. As in all medical specialties, prevention and patient education are paramount. All adult patients should, therefore, be screened or evaluated by an oral health professional so that optimal health can be achieved and maintained.

REFERENCES

1. Glick, M, ed.. The oral-systemic disease connection: an update for the practicing dentist. *JADA*. 2006;137 (Suppl):1S–40S.
2. Paquette DW, Nichols T, Williams RC. Oral inflammation, CVD, and systemic disease. *Connections: Oral Syst Health Rev.* 2005;1(1).
3. Paquette DW. Periodontal disease and the risk for adverse pregnancy outcomes. *Grand Rounds Oral Syst Med. Grand Rounds Oral Syst Med.* 2006;1:14–24.
4. Moritz AJ, Mealey, BL. Periodontal disease, insulin resistance, and diabetes mellitus: a review and clinical implications. *Grand Rounds Oral Syst Dis.* 2006;1:13–20.
5. DePaola DP, (guest ed.). Proceedings and Consensus Opinion form the Global Oral and Systemic Health Summit. *Grand Rounds Suppl.* 2007;1–20.
6. Beck JD, Slade G, Offenbacher S. Oral disease, cardiovascular disease and systemic inflammation. *Periodontology.* 2000;23:110–120.
7. Satcher D (Surgeon General United States of America). Oral Health in America: A Report of the Surgeon General. May, 2000.
8. Beltrán-Aguilar ED, Barker LK, Canto MT, et al. Surveillance for dental caries, dental sealants, tooth retention, edentulism, and enamel fluorosis – United States, 1988–1994 and 1999–2002. *MMWR* 2005;54:1–44.
9. Vargas CM, Kramaraow E, Yellowitz J. Oral health of older americans. Centers for Disease Control and Prevention Aging Trends No. 3, March, 2001.
10. Holm-Pederson P, and Löe H, eds. *Textbook of Geriatric Dentistry.* 4th ed. New York: McGraw Hill; 1999.
11. Hazzard WR, Blass JP. *Principles of Geriatric Medicine and Gerontology.* New York: McGraw-Hill Professional; 2003.
12. Wade, ML, Suzuki, JB. Issues related to diagnosis and treatment of bisphosphonate-induced osteonecrosis of the jaws. *Grand Rounds Oral Syst Dis.* 2007;2:46–53.
13. Bhaskar SN. *Orban's Oral Histology and Embryology.* 10th ed. Philadelphia: C.V. Mosby; 1986.
14. Ten Cate AR. *Oral Histology Development, Structure, and Function.* 2nd ed. Philadelphia: C.V. Mosby; 1985.
15. Regezi JA, Sciubba JJ. *Oral Pathology Clinical-Pathologic Correlations.* Philadelphia: W.B. Saunders; 1989.
16. Montgomery RL. *Head and Neck Anatomy with Clinical Correlations.* New York: McGraw-Hill; 1981.
17. Hollinshead HW. *Anatomy for Surgeons: The Head and Neck.* Baltimore: Williams & Wilkins; 1982.
18. Okeson JP. *Management of Temporomandibular Disorders and Occlusion.* 4th ed. Philadelphia: Mosby; 1998:234–309.
19. Sheiham A. Oral health, general health, and quality of life. *Bull World Health Organ.* 2005;83(9). [Editorial]
20. Matear DW. Demonstrating the need for oral health education in geriatric institutions. *Probe.* 1999;33:66–71.
21. Federal Nursing Home Reform Act from the Omnibus Budget Reconciliation Act of 1987 (OBRA 1987).

40

Surgical Principles in the Aged

Susan Galandiuk, MD, FACS, Hiram C. Polk, Jr., MD, FACS

The massive increase in the geriatric population has been more than paralleled by a vast increase in the number of patients older than the age of 65 years, or indeed, over any such benchmark, who now seek both elective and emergency surgical care. We discuss the topic of *emergency* surgery separately near the end of this chapter, because this is such a complex issue that involves by definition issues of life or death, especially in those without treatment. In the United States, 85,000 patients seek *elective* surgery every working day. A high proportion of these (approximately 50%) are Medicare beneficiaries, that is, older than the age of 65 years. Therefore, the practice of all surgical specialties in most countries is becoming, in fact, more and more a practice of geriatric surgery.

SURGEON–PATIENT COMMUNICATION ISSUES

Profoundly important ethical issues are involved, especially for the elderly who may be impaired and/or with an issue regarding informed consent. One of the most important principles is that the surgeon and the patient have a serious discussion and reach a real agreement about the goals of care. The surgeon should always inquire as to the presence of an advance directive from all older patients, which provides an important entry for discussion in a variety of areas.

This discussion really gets cast into bold relief when the presence of a living will and variably interpreted do not resuscitate orders exist. Under these circumstances, it is essential that the patient and a (preferably the) responsible family member, if at all possible, and the surgeon seriously discuss the patient's interpretation of the living will and the do not resuscitate standard. Be certain that the patient and the family understand that the performance of an elective operation may countermand the presence of the do not resuscitate orders in some circumstances.

This situation can be so complicated that the presence of a staff person from the surgeon's office or from the hospital during this discussion is frequently advised. On many occasions, the patient's personal physician or geriatrician, as well as a medical social worker, may well want to participate in this conversation and all reach a concurrence as to the patient's preferences and newly understood goals of treatment. It is never pleasant, but, in some cases, increasingly important to talk about unlikely events: death or serious complications after elective operations. For example, in a recent study sponsored by the Center for Medicare and Medicaid Services in the United States, we examined the care of 5,285 patients undergoing elective operations in Kentucky in 2004.[1] Although death was uncommon (n = 32), readmission was more common and reoperation was also common. A little more than half these patients were Medicare or Medicaid beneficiaries. So, these likely or unlikely events must be put into clear-cut perception for the patient and family.

Another issue of common misunderstanding is the likelihood of temporary nursing home or rehabilitative facility care. A large number of patients and their families in the United States have come to the conclusion that this is not a desired end-of-life circumstance, and they have difficulty accepting a similar kind of facility as a useful transition back toward preoperative status. The availability of occupational therapy and physical therapy in a familiar setting, euphemistically called home health care, has its own advantages and disadvantages. These *need* to be discussed up front, depending on the procedure and the patient,

Issues related to vision and hearing impairment in older patients are a critical part of care, but these are an especially important part of assessment and understanding of their preoperative status as well. Throughout a patient's care, whether in the hospital or not, prevention of falls and other untoward

Table 40.1. Life Expectancy Tables (U.S.)

Life Expectancy

Age (yrs)	2002	2004
65	16	19
75	10	12
85	5	–
90	4	–

Table basis: both sexes U.S. population.

events is absolutely crucial as are measures to clarify time of day or night and the day and date.

OPERATIVE RISK ASSESSMENT

This teamwork scenario, however, focuses back on the surgeon and anesthesiologist when one begins to consider, develop, and make more objective the assessment of operative risk for a given patient.[2] Huge advances have been made in this field during the last decade, particularly through the Veterans Affairs Medical Centers in the United States, where a program called the National Surgical Quality Improvement Project has been implemented and associated with improved results, correlating closely with improved operative risk assessment.[3] This can be enhanced by the additional use of the Charlson–Kilmore morbidity index which, although developed for other purposes, has very real meaning and value in this setting. Operative risk assessment is a complicated process, one that requires careful extrapolation of life expectancies (Table 40.1) in the absence of coexisting diseases purely based on the patient's age.[5] We choose to reemphasize the enormous value of good communication between the surgeon and the anesthesiologist. One simple issue is the presence of severe degenerative arthritis of the cervical spine, and the problem it creates with elective peroral endotracheal intubation. There can be many other issues. It is critical that the surgeon and anesthesiologist have a detailed review of and understanding about the goals of therapy, including the complexity of preoperative assessment. We have had an uncommonly good experience with one surgical specialty and anesthesiology in one of our participating hospitals. This formal cooperation contributed to our quality improvement effort, and there are few situations that can create a better environment than such ideal communication and agreement on goals of therapy between the anesthesiologist and the surgeon and, most especially, involving the patient as well.[6] If a medical specialty consultation, such as endoscopy or pulmonary medicine, is needed, it is much more valuable if this is provided by a physician who already knows the patient.

ACCURATE MEDICATIONS AND PERIOPERATIVE CARE

We have already mentioned the importance of fall prevention and the recognition of cervical spine arthritis in patients who may choose to undergo elective operations. One of the most memorable events of the senior author's long career in surgery was a session only 2 years ago, in which a number of the busiest surgical specialists from multiple specialties in our region of the United States discussed, in a no-holds-barred fashion, the most pressing issues in real-world surgical practice. Interestingly enough, these were not issues related to reimbursement for care or professional liability insurance, but rather focused on the importance of and difficulty in obtaining an accurate list of medications prescribed for and taken by their elderly patients.[7] The massive professional effort, called medication reconciliation in the United States, is a case in point. This, however, will take years to come to pass. Meanwhile, any surgeon undertaking an elective operation will be haunted by problems concerning what the patient understands as medication and what is not medication. For example, low-dose aspirin and a whole variety of herbs and other health supplements are not considered medications by patients and are frequently not conveyed to surgeons. The propensity for operating on an elderly patient with medication-induced hypocoagulability is a real danger.

The need to acquire a careful and complete history is essential, both on the part of the patient and from the closest caregiver and/or relative. This is all the more important because of the need to withdraw medications that may alter blood coagulation well in advance of an elective procedure and because of the need for surgeons and the entire perioperative team to understand the potential for patients' withdrawal syndromes. Although such data have been widely publicized, we found that in 2004 as many as 30% of patients who were already receiving β-blockers for hypertension or other cardiac indications and were undergoing elective operations did not have their medications continued![8] In this very same study, we found that patients who did not have their β-blockers continued were twice as likely to develop a myocardial infarct and, if they had one, were three times as likely to die of it. Although understanding and perception of issues such as β-blockade continuation can never be complete, it has been well publicized as a dramatic finding of our clinical study of elective surgery in 2004.[9] Furthermore, the withdrawal syndromes associated with other medications' termination can be profound, such as with some anxiolytic drugs (Table 40.2).

Finally, there is major difficulty with a diminished therapeutic range for most drugs, which, in some part, may be due to the diminished lean muscle mass in many elderly patients. This is a constant concern for both the anesthesiologist and surgeon.

In the discussion of operative risk, one of the most complex issues is assessment of coexisting illness, its degree of medical compensation, and its impact on the patient's personal life expectancy.[10] Perhaps the most dramatic example of an

Table 40.2. Drugs Frequently Causing Confusion

Morphine sulfate

- Dilaudid
- Meperidine
- Oxycodone
- Hydrocodone

Drugs associated with withdrawal symptoms

- Alprazolam
- Diazepam
- Alcohol

Table 40.3. Unsuspected Adverse Surgical Risk Factors[1,3,9]

Serum albumin count	<2 mg/dL
White blood cell count	>11,000/dL
Impaired functional status	Wheelchair, any cause
Unknown or unrecalled medications that interfere with coagulation	

age-associated condition would be the rather linear impairment of renal function and what it might mean under conditions of hypovolemia, shock, oliguria, and/or transfusion, which may lead to hemoglobin deposition in the distal renal tubules. The other side of that coin, that is, renal tubular lavage by the administration of substantial volumes of so-called balanced salt solution, is the ease with which elderly patients can be pushed into congestive failure by what are standard intravenous fluid loads in many anesthesiology and surgery units around the world. To avoid tremendous danger, one must be sure to ascertain that the fluid infusion rate stays proportionate to urine output, and the drugs are constantly reassessed according to the patient's weight, age, and status of recovery. Nevertheless, the chemically diuresed hypertensive patient is a dramatic case in point in the dangerous use of urine output as a sign of sufficient resuscitation. Remember the frail elderly patient may not have enough body mass to generate 30 mL of urine per hour postoperatively.

A less dramatic but more common error in estimation of operative risk attends the diagnosis of remote, recurrent, or persistent cancer. For example only, assume gangrenous cholecystitis in an 80-year-old woman with an associated history of one of the following:

a) colon cancer treated 4 years ago but now associated with bilobar hepatic metastases and impaired liver function, or
b) a hormonally responsive breast cancer with bone metastases now in remission a year after treatment with a tamoxifen-like drug, or
c) a squamous cancer of the tonsil treated by irradiation 4 years ago, but with large bilateral metastases to cervical lymph nodes but no systemic metastases.

The first patient has a life expectancy of 100 days; gangrenous cholecystitis deserves surgical treatment; chronic biliary colic probably does not. The second patient may live for several years and could even respond again to newer therapies; she should undergo operation. The third patient may live a year, but with severe pain and difficulty in swallowing, creating

a much less clear choice than for the other two scenarios, even given the usual futility of bilateral neck dissections in terms of disease care.

OTHER FACTORS

We have found the addition of epidural and/or regional anesthetic extremely valuable in elderly patients, particularly because such may allow the surgical team to avoid and/or minimize the use of opioids, which are so associated with confusion and diminution of respiratory drive. In the same vein, the frequently used mechanical bowel preparation in many forms of intestinal surgery is especially dangerous to a patient who has often been on diuretics and may be marginally hypokalemic before operation. The phosphosoda preparations are especially dangerous. Because urinary output is often a critical measure of resuscitation early in a patient's recovery, indwelling catheters are often the norm. One constantly needs to be aware that the elderly patient, especially if male, is more likely to need this catheter for a longer period of time before he begins to void normally, because of temporary prostatic hypertrophy. Similarly, when inserting these catheters for this reason, a Coudé tip catheter may be necessary. Postoperative medications such as Hytrin® or Flomax® may be required.

A critical keystone of elective surgical management in elderly patients is the early mobilization of the patient and a constant awareness of fall prevention. Further points of importance are the observations covered in Table 40.3 that reflect not yet widely recognized enhanced operative risks.

A recent in-depth review of these matters once again emphasizes the unalterable impact of age on major surgical complications and deaths.[11] The time between when the patient is seen in the surgeon's office and an elective procedure is scheduled is often several weeks in duration. This frequently allows low-grade purely intercurrent infections to develop. We have found that preoperative nursing assessment frequently ascertains the suspicion of such an infection that has been missed by the surgeon 1 or 2 weeks before.[3] To the same end, we have found that one of the most deadly observations in routine laboratory testing is a white blood cell count of 11,000 or greater. We think these points are especially dangerous to older patients, who are more prone to infections. These patients, then, come to an elective operation with an intervening event of some mild infectious nature, which is thrown into bold relief by the elevated white count and the nurse's recognition that an infection has intervened. This should be a red flag for all concerned and all such elective operations should be delayed.

We hold that venous thromboembolic events are much less common than presently suggested; we found 15 pulmonary emboli in 5,285 prospectively studied selective operations in 2004, all nonfatal. Accordingly, we tend to use elastic stockings, mechanical devices, and little else, although we are in a minority among surgeons.

This is much like the dramatic increase in operative risk for individuals who have low albumin. It has become legendary in American medicine that our principal federal government program does not routinely reimburse for testing for albumin as part of preoperative assessment, but it is one of the most dramatic predictors of the likelihood of postoperative death studied, primarily in a different government-funded ordered system.[1] The significance of a low albumin may represent anything from significant hepatic parenchymal disease to simple poor nutrition. Regardless, it has a dramatic effect on surgical outcome and should usually be ordered.

Another issue seen in the aging patient is the presence of mechanical devices, which have often prolonged life significantly. Whether one is talking about improving the quality of life, such as occurs with total hip and knee replacement, or actually prolonging life with pacemakers and cardiac valve replacement; all these mechanical devices are extraordinarily prone to colonization following bacteremia, even the relatively mild bacteremia that may follow an elective operation. Special attention to the timing and dose of antibiotic prophylaxis around all such procedures in patients with such indwelling foreign bodies is essential. The dose and timing are critical but prophylactic antibiotic duration beyond 48 hours is, on balance, harmful.

Trauma in the elderly has an entirely different face than the closed femur fracture typically seen in an infirm older woman with a litany of comorbidities. First is the frequency with which trauma intensive care unit beds are filled with older patients: It is no longer the purview of the young, largely male nighttighter. The populational increase in older patients is paralleled by increases in morbidity and reduced awareness due to cervical osteoarthritis and limited fields of peripheral vision. Full-speed automobile impacts are often the norm. This chapter is an emphasis on priorities, and trauma now needs the skills of an on-the-scene geriatrician. The physiological resiliency of youth no longer facilitates resuscitation. Pump failure regularly compounds hypovolemia, and urinary output is no longer an acceptable index of adequate replenishment of blood loss. Diagnoses must be much more precise, and errors of recognition are no better tolerated than delays in appreciation of complications. The desire to avoid unnecessary treatment morbidity in an imaging-dependent medical system does not mandate uniform conservatism; an experienced laparoscopist can help, but a negative laparotomy is much better tolerated than an unrecognized slow, but ongoing, intraabdominal bleeding. The issues of living wills, preexisting physical, mental, and emotional health, and medication reconciliation must be done in minutes, but

is often complicated by late-to-arrive or geographically remote next-of-kin and interfamily discord over a mixture of medical and nonmedical issues.

If there is one lesson that dominates after a lifetime of care for trauma victims, it is that the active senior citizen with an array of injuries can frequently return to a very good quality of life provided that definitive care is cogently planned and technically well conducted. Amidst generalizations, it is vital that the patient be informed of the health status of a spouse who may well have been in the same accident. A more modern version is that the secret of caring for the patient is to care about the patient, be it multisystem trauma or a chronic illness.

Finally, the patient who comes in an impaired functional status: The use of a wheelchair, even for partial assistance, is another critical marker of substantially increased operative risk that needs to be included in all aspects of a patient's evaluation. Paraplegia as an indicator for wheelchair use is especially ominous.

A decubitus ulcer is a disaster in any patient, especially an older one. Protection begins in the operating theater with special attention to thin skin and all pressure points, notably the heels. Special postoperative mattresses are helpful, but the surgeon and patient's physician can set a good standard by turning the patient every day to look for early signs of pressure injury to the skin.

SUMMARY

The care of the elderly about to undergo a major surgical procedure is nothing more than a textbook recital of all the problems that exist in overall surgical practice. This group of patients, however, often has impaired physiological reserves, multiple associated illnesses, and, in many cases, a wide array of both indicated and unindicated medications. It represents the best interest of the patient, the immediate family, and the surgeon or anesthesiologist, as well as the geriatrician, that these issues all be assessed carefully, repeatedly, and exactly.

REFERENCES

1. Polk HC Jr. Surgical quality and safety: the patient comes first. *Am Surg.* 2007;73:538–542.
2. Polk HC. The mathematics of clinical judgment: including an evaluation of operative risk. In: Polk HC, Gardner B, Stone HH, eds. *Basic Surgery.* 5th ed. St. Louis: Quality Surgical Publishing; 1995:10–26.
3. Khuri SF, Daley J, Henderson W, et al. The Department of Veterans Affairs' NSQIP: the first national, validated, outcome-based, risk-adjusted, and peer-controlled program for the measurement and enhancement of the quality of surgical care. *Ann Surg.* 1998;228:491–507.
4. Charlson ME, Pompei P, Ales KL, et al. A new method of classifying prognostic comorbidity in longitudinal studies: development and validation. *J Chronic Dis.* 1987;40:373–383.
5. Linn BS, Linn MW, Gurel L. Physical resistance and longevity. *Gerontol Clin.* 1969; 11:362.

6. Galandiuk S, Rao MK, Heine MF, Scherm MH, Polk HC Jr. Mutual reporting of process and outcomes enhances quality outcomes for colon and rectal resections. *Surgery.* 2004;136:833–841.

7. Shively EH, Heine MJ, Schell RH, et al.Practicing surgeons lead in quality care, safety, and cost control. *Ann Surg.* 2004;239:752–760.

8. Galandiuk S, Mahid SS, Polk HC Jr, Turina M, Rao M, Lewis JN. Differences and similarities between rural and urban operations. *Surgery.* 2006; 140:589–596.

9. Richardson JD, Cocanour CS, Kern JA, et al. Perioperative risk assessment in elderly and high-risk patients. *J Am Coll Surg.* 1994;199:133–146.

10. Polk HC Jr, Cheadle WG, Franklin GA. Principles of preoperative preparation. In: Townsend CM, Evers GM, eds. *Sabiston's Textbook of Surgery: The Biological Basis of Modern Surgical Practice.* 16th ed. Philadelphia: WB Saunders; 2001:163–170.

11. Turrentine FE, Wang H, Simpson VB, Jones RS. Surgical risk factors, morbidity, and mortality in elderly patients. *Am Coll Surg.* 2006;203:865–877.

41

REHABILITATION IN OLDER ADULTS

Kenneth Brummel-Smith, MD

INTRODUCTION

One of the distinguishing aspects of geriatrics is attention to the person's functional abilities. Rehabilitation is the process by which patients who have lost function can recover them, or adapt to the loss function to be more independent. Because independence is held in such high value by older people, rehabilitation should be seen as the foundation of good geriatric care. From a physician's perspective, rehabilitation is sometimes seen as the province of the discipline of physical medicine and rehabilitation (PM&R). However, there are many circumstances when rehabilitation interventions are provided to older people without the involvement of a PM&R specialist, and the primary care physician, geriatrician, nurse practitioner or physician assistant may be working closely with other rehabilitation team members. Hence, all providers who care for older people should have a working knowledge of rehabilitation.[1]

Rehabilitation of older adults is increasingly applied to two populations: those who acquire a disability late in life, and more recently, those who have lived with a disability much of their lives and are now aging. The latter group includes those with spinal cord injuries, traumatic brain injury, and a variety of birth injuries and genetic causes of disability. If the trend towards lessening of disability in the older population continues, it would be expected that the group who are aging with a disability will expand.

FUNCTION AND DISABILITY

The World Health Organizations framework for health and disability is the International Classification of Functioning, Disability and Health (ICF).[2] The ICF stresses health and functioning, rather than disability. This is an important concept in geriatrics. Having a disability does not mean that one is unhealthy or sick. It is clear that a diagnosis alone does not predict service needs, length of hospitalization, level or site of care, or, importantly, functional outcomes. One person with a stroke may be totally dependent, whereas another can resume normal daily activities. Under the ICF model, functioning and health can be viewed from an individual, an institutional, and the societal levels. In this way, it can be determined how health conditions (diagnoses or injuries) interact with what external conditions (the personal environment or the available resources), and what needs to be done to optimize the individual's function.

In ICF, disability and functioning are viewed as outcomes of interactions between *health conditions* (diseases, disorders and injuries) and *contextual factors*. Among contextual factors are external *environmental factors* (for example, social attitudes, architectural characteristics, legal and social structures, as well as climate, terrain and so forth); and internal *personal factors*, which include sex, age, coping styles, social background, education, profession, past and current experience, overall behavior pattern, character and other factors that influence how disability is experienced by the individual. The ICF model is biopsychosocial and holistic, and includes a number of components which must be attended to in rehabilitation (Table 41.1).

IMPACT OF COMORBID CONDITIONS

The presence of comorbid conditions can greatly affect the rehabilitation process in an older person. Multiple chronic illnesses are common in the older adult. Over 500,000 persons in the United States have more than one chronic illness. Twenty percent of the older population has more than[4] chronic conditions.[3] Comorbid conditions can affect access to rehabilitation services, the course of treatment, or increase the risk of interventions. Multiple comorbid conditions predict both the overall functional change in rehabilitation and the rate at

Table 41.1. WHO Interventional Classification of Functioning, Disability, and Health (ICF) Components

- **Body Functions** are physiological functions of body systems (including psychological functions).
- **Body Structures** are anatomical parts of the body such as organs, limbs and their components.
- **Impairments** are problems in body function or structure such as a significant deviation or loss.
- **Activity** is the execution of a task or action by an individual.
- **Participation** is involvement in a life situation.
- **Activity Limitations** are difficulties an individual may have in executing activities.
- **Participation Restrictions** are problems an individual may experience in involvement in life situations.
- **Environmental Factors** make up the physical, social and attitudinal environment in which people live and conduct their lives.

which those gains are reached.[4] It is crucial that all older persons receiving rehabilitation receive a comprehensive assessment (see Chapter 2) at the onset of rehabilitation in order to identify all conditions affecting the patient. Furthermore, physicians should ensure that all comorbid medical conditions are appropriately treated during rehabilitation. Uncontrolled blood pressure or diabetes, cardiac arrhythmias, intercurrent infections, and other medical problems can delay participation in the rehabilitation program or retard progress towards the patient's goals.

Cognitive ability is important in rehabilitation. Rehabilitation is essentially a learning process. The exact degree of cognitive impairment which limits a person's capacity to participate is not clear. Clearly, delirium should be recognized and resolved before rehabilitation begins. Mild levels of dementia do not appear to significantly interfere with rehabilitation, as long as the patient can remember the training from one day to the next.[5] The ability to follow two-stepped commands is often seen as important. A screening test, such as the Mini-Mental State exam is usually used, though more extensive neuropsychological testing may be needed.[6] The person must also have the ability to recognize his or her deficits. Hence, those with severe neglect, or lack of awareness of their deficits, may have difficulty benefiting from rehabilitation. Those with mild levels of cognitive impairment may be provided rehabilitation in skilled nursing facilities where the pace may be less rapid.

Pre-existing cardiac or pulmonary conditions can affect exercise capacity and influence the rehabilitation course. Many conditions which lead to disability, such as stroke or hip fracture, significantly stress the cardiopulmonary systems during walking training. The energy cost of walking with a hemiplegic gait may be 35% above normal, while walking with a below-the-knee prosthesis is 10% to 40% above normal.[1] These concerns must be balanced against the risk of immobility. For that reason, close medical attention and physiologic monitoring is preferable over avoiding rehabilitation for fear of an adverse event.

Depression is common in persons who have acquired a new disability and is especially common after a stroke. Its negative effect on rehabilitation outcome is well documented.[7] All patients being considered for rehabilitation should screened using standardized instruments such as the Geriatric Depression Scale. In complex cases consultation by a psychologist or psychiatrist may be necessary. Treatment of depression has been shown to improve rehabilitation outcomes.[8]

Other comorbid conditions which are important to be aware of during rehabilitation include osteoarthritis, peripheral vascular disease, diabetes, and COPD. In addition, polypharmacy is a difficult problem when dealing with the patient with multiple comorbid conditions. One the one hand, adequate attention to multiple medical conditions may optimize the chances of rehabilitation being successful. On the other hand, the risk of adverse drug events increases with the number of medications. A general rule would be to stop or replace any medication thought to be directly interfering with the rehabilitation. Commonly psychotropic drugs are in this category. Similarly, any medication which is being used for a condition that is no longer active can be stopped temporarily. Finally, because pain is a significant hindrance to exercise, adequate pain control is essential.

Secondary complications are common in rehabilitation and often are related to lack of mobility. Close monitoring by all team members is needed. Pressure sores are frequently seen in immobilized patients, and depending on bodily placement, can interfere or even halt the rehabilitation program. Likewise, pneumonia is a risk with bed rest and certain disabling conditions, such as stroke. Incontinence may be a premorbid condition or may begin after a disabling condition occurs. Constipation and fecal impaction also are common and may be missed if attention to a bowel program is not paid. These problems are addressed in other chapters but the main concern is to try to prevent them from occurring and to treat them quickly if they do occur in spite of preventive efforts.

REIMBURSEMENT FOR REHABILITATION

Medicare covers a variety of methods for providing rehabilitation. Coverage for services in a Medicare-certified inpatient rehabilitation hospital or unit is provided if the patient can participate in 3 hours of more of therapy per day (sometime called the "3-hour rule"). Medicare coverage may not extend to every condition which causes disability so in-patient units typically screen patients for admission very carefully. There must be daily physician coverage, 24-hour nursing care, and an interdisciplinary team of nurses and therapists. Coverage is paid on a prospective basis, but rather than being based on diagnoses it is based on functional levels using the Functional Independence Measure (FIM).[9]

Many older patients, especially those with multiple comorbid conditions can not participate in 3 hours of therapy per day. A Medicare-certified skilled nursing facility with a dedicated rehabilitation staff can provide effective rehabilitation. Physicians do not have to see the patient daily but must be available for emergency care, as well as supervise the rehabilitation interventions. Reimbursement is also prospective based upon the Resource Utilization Groups (RUG III).

Other settings for rehabilitation include outpatient facilities. Some cities have Certified Outpatient Rehabilitation Facilities (CORF). Medicare also pays for home-health based rehabilitation to "homebound" patients. Services must be prescribed and recertified every 60 days. Home health is also under prospective payment, using the Outcome and Assessment Information Set (OASIS).

Medicare Health Maintenance Organizations (HMO) are required to provide at least the same options for rehabilitation as standard Medicare. However, there is evidence that some HMO shift resource use to lower levels of care, with poorer outcomes.[10]

TEAM WORK

Rehabilitation is provided by a number of different disciplines working together as a team (See Table 41.2). In inpatient settings, there is often an interdisciplinary team, where team members meet regularly to discuss the cases and plan the care of the patient. In most other settings, the members of the multidisciplinary team work with the patient individually and communicate with one another through the medical record or by electronic means. There is little empirical evidence of the value of one type of team over the other.

Primary care providers often have interactions with rehabilitation providers. A physician's approval is usually required for approval of rehabilitation services. Team members need to practice good communication to deliver the best outcomes for their patients. It is important that each show respect for the expertise provided by the other. Interdisciplinary team care depends on asking questions, challenging each other's assumptions and having a professional interchange.

Medical rehabilitation equipment prescriptions require physician certification for reimbursement. Certain items, such as orthoses, wheel chairs, and prostheses usually require the evaluation by a rehabilitation therapist, orthotist (when applicable) and a physiatrist to ensure proper utilization and fit of the device. The most important member of the team – the patient – must agree to the use and value of the device.

The team should work to create a rehabilitation plan which includes measurable goals. The patient and the family must be involved in the setting of these goals. Regular updates should be provided, with note of progress towards those goals. The physician should carefully evaluate the initial goals to ensure they have a reasonable chance of being achieved. In general, the newer and less severe the disability, the greater the likelihood

Table 41.2. Members of the Rehabilitation Team

Primary Physician	*Social Worker*
Rehabilitation nurse	Rehabilitation counselor/ psychologist
Occupational therapist	Psychiatrist
Physical therapist	Pharmacist
Speech and language pathologist	Orthotist
Nutritionist	Recreation therapist
Physiatrist (specialist in Physical Medicine and Rehabilitation)	

of a goal being achieved. Long standing functional deficits are unlikely to be improved significantly in rehabilitation.

If the patient stops progressing, it is important to discuss why that might be. Beware of a too sudden acceptance of a statement that the patient has "plateaued." Failure to progress could result from untreated medical conditions, poorly managed pain, unrecognized depression, or drug side effects. The physician, nurse practitioner or physician assistant should carefully conduct a new assessment of the patient before determining rehabilitation interventions should cease.

ASSISTIVE DEVICES

Mobility

Devices to promote safer or more independent mobility are the most common form of assistive device. All devices must be seen as acceptable to the patient or the device will not be used. A properly fitted walker is not useful if the patient keeps it in the closet. Canes, walkers, crutches and wheelchairs come in a myriad of types and many have very specialized uses. In general, an evaluation of the patient by a physical therapist should be considered before prescribing any of these. All devices must be properly sized to fit each patient. The handles of canes, walkers and crutches should be set at the height of the patient's greater trochanter. Generally this is measured from the floor to the bend of the wrist, with the patient's arms hanging loosely at the side, or with the arm bent at 20 to 30 degrees when holding the cane at the side (Figure 41.1).

Canes are useful when minimal additional support is needed. Single point canes are inherently unstable and no more than 15%–20% of body weight should be applied to them. The cane should be used on the side opposite to the problem. For example, a person with arthritis of the right hip would hold the cane in the left hand. The cane is advanced when the opposite foot swings forward. Canes are especially helpful for persons with neuropathy because the cane provides additional proprioceptive input through the upper extremities, which are generally less affected in neuropathy, and by creating a 3-point base of support. Three- or four prong canes are often preferred by patients because they stand up when not being used and more

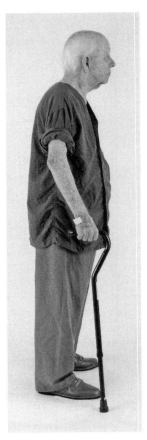

Figure 41.1. Proper fitting of a cane. The cane should just reach the greater trochanter. A measurement can be made from the floor to the bend of the patient's wrist.

weight can be applied to them. However, the multiple prongs can lead to instability in uneven surfaces, such as outdoors. (Figure 41.2).

Crutches are not often used in geriatric rehabilitation. They may be difficult to control for a frail older person, brachial plexus injuries can occur from improper fitting or use, and wrist or hand arthritis may interfere with their use. Forearm support attachments can be added when hand arthritis prevents use of the standard handles.

There are numerous types of walkers, each of which have specific uses. They are often prescribed for those with poor balance and coordination, weakness, and weight-bearing restrictions. All walkers provide a very wide base of support. Pickup walkers (no wheels) are used primarily after major lower extremity surgeries. They promote an abnormal and inefficient gait. Front-wheeled walkers are helpful with weakness and poor balance. A somewhat more normal gait occurs, but turning and maneuvering is often compromised. They provide dual protection for patients with Parkinson's disease – the absence of rear wheels lessens the risk of festination while the forward body position prevents backward instability. Three- or four-wheeled walkers ("rollators") promote a much more efficient gait and

are often seen as more desirable by the patient. They are, however, less stable than front-wheeled walkers and cannot accept significant body weight being applied. They usually have brakes which can be set and a seat for rest periods. Baskets are often added to allow carrying objects. Patients must have good hand function to actuate the brakes and good sensory and cognitive function to use the walker safely. The three-wheeled walker is useful when the patient must frequently move it in and out of a car (Figures 41.3 & 41.4).

Wheelchairs can be used just for transporting patients or for self-transportation. The standard hospital transport wheelchair should not be used by patients for self-transportation. The proper wheelchair includes customization of height and width, presence of foot rests, back height and style, seating surface, and wheel type. Armrests must be removable if the patient needs to make transfers from the bed to the wheelchair using a sliding board. Brake handle extensions are sometimes required

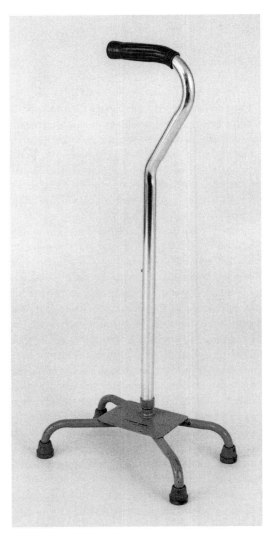

Figure 41.2. Four-prong cane. This device is used when the patient must place additional weight on the cane.

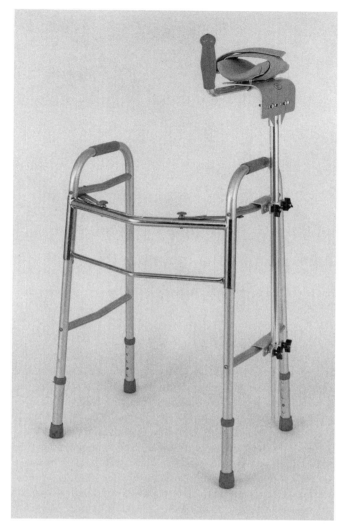

Figure 41.3. Pick-up walker with forearm rest attachment. The arm rest attachment is used when patients have arthritis or weakness in the wrist.

if the patient has arthritis or weakness. Because of all these considerations, a physical therapist evaluation to evaluate the patient's needs and prescribe the correct combination of features is required (Figure 41.5).

Many older patients ask their physicians for power-operated wheelchairs and scooters. In addition, direct-to-consumer advertising may influence patients to ask for them. A difficult balance of benefits and risks must be addressed. Unnecessary use of a powered vehicle may lead to worsening strength, endurance and balance. On the other side, the use of such a device may lead to greater social involvement and improved quality of life. Ideally, unless the patient is truly unable to manage mobility with standard devices, they should be used only for negotiating longer distances and the patient should use other devices for household mobility. In addition, sensory and cognitive problems may lead to unsafe usage. If a powered-wheelchair or scooter is to be prescribed the patient should receive training

in its use, and the equivalent of a "behind-the-wheel" drivers test.

Self-Care Devices

There are a large number of devices which can be used to assist in activities of daily living. It is not acceptable to simply provide the patient with one or more of these tools. The patient should receive instruction in their proper use. Usually it is the occupational therapist who provides this training.

Tools which can be used to dress more independently include dressing hooks, sock donners, long-handled shoe horns, "reachers" (a mechanical extension used to pick up objects on the floor or in high cabinets), and clothes hooks (Figures 41.6, 41.7 & 41.8). Bathing devices include long-handled brushes, mirrors that are tilted towards the floor for people who do personal grooming in a wheelchair, shower hose extensions, and either tub seats (for those persons with adequate balance and stability) or tub benches (for patients who need an extra measure of safety). Toilet adaptations include a raised toilet seat for persons with weak hip extensors, or arm attachments to the toilet ("Versaframe") (Figure 41.9). There are a number of devices useful in the kitchen, such as levers to assist

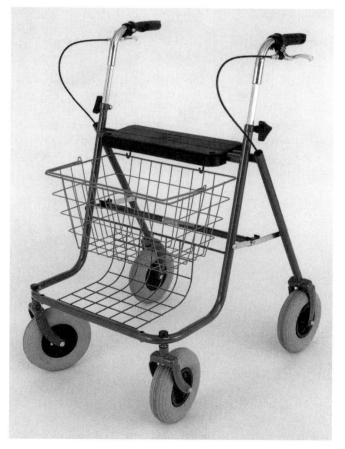

Figure 41.4. Four-wheeled rolling walker (Rollator). This walker provides for the most normal gait.

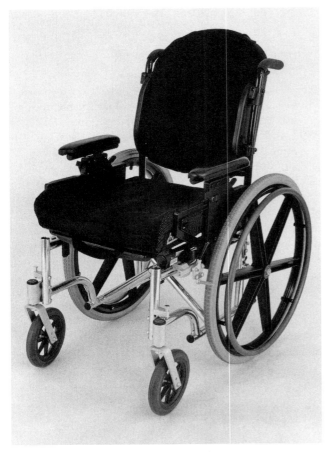

Figure 41.5. Special fitted wheelchair. A seat and back designed to prevent pressure sores and promote proper positioning.

with opening jars, a variety of adapted eating utensils (rocker knives, swivel spoons, utensils with built-up handles), and special plates and plate guards (Figures 41.10, 41.11 & 41.12). Medicare generally covers personal adaptive equipment.

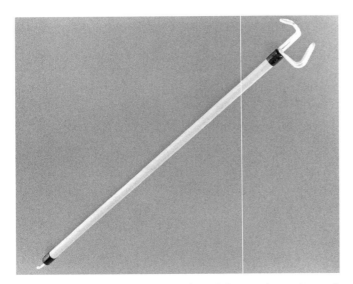

Figure 41.6. Dressing hook. A simple tool that can be used to pull off socks or help in putting on shirts.

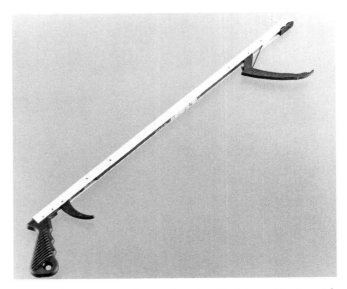

Figure 41.7. Reacher used to reach up to objects in a cabinet or pick things up from the floor.

Housing modifications are also important in rehabilitation. Doors must be wide enough to accommodate walkers and wheelchairs. Ideally the home should be on a single floor. If a ramp is needed to enter the house, the length of the ramp is generally 12 inches of run for every one inch of rise. Hence, a set of stairs 4 feet high would require a ramp 48 feet long. Bathrooms often need to be modified to allow independent use of the tub or access to the sink, particularly if the patient uses a wheelchair for mobility. Similarly, the kitchen may need modifications. For patients with limited endurance, a high stool to sit on while preparing food or cleaning dishes is helpful. Medicare generally does not cover housing modifications and many older people with disabilities may need to seek alternative accessible housing.

REHABILITATION OF COMMON GERIATRIC PROBLEMS

Stroke

Stroke is the most common condition for which older people receive medical rehabilitation services. Over 700,000 Americans have a stroke each year.[11] Early interventions (such as thrombolytic therapy) to limit the acute stroke may be beneficial, but may not be appropriate in very old patients. In addition, many older patients present too late (>3 hours after onset) to benefit from such interventions. Forty percent of stroke patients are left with moderate functional impairment and 15% to 30% with severe disability.[12] Hence, rehabilitation is the most important intervention.

A number of studies have shown that stroke rehabilitation units provide better outcomes than routine medical care. In general, the more intensive the rehabilitation program, the better the outcome.[13,14,15] Some studies have shown improved

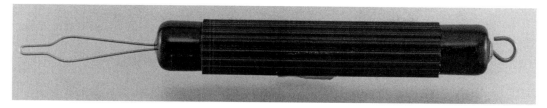

Figure 41.8. Button hook. The loop is passed through the button hole, then hooked over the button and pulled through.

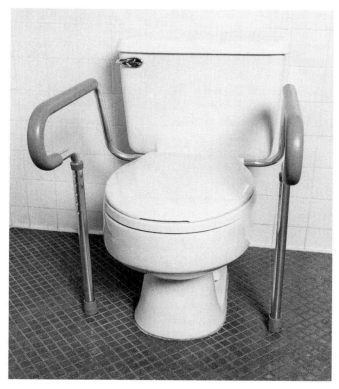

Figure 41.9. Arm attachments for the toilet. Allows those with weak hip extensors to push up with the arms to rise from the toilet.

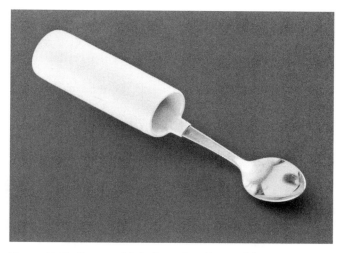

Figure 41.11. Spoon with built-up handle. Used by persons with weak hand strength.

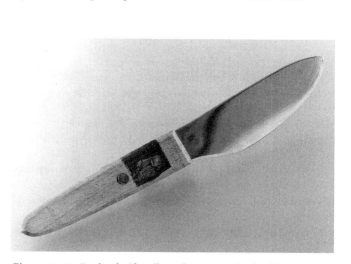

Figure 41.10. Rocker knife. Allows for cutting food with one hand.

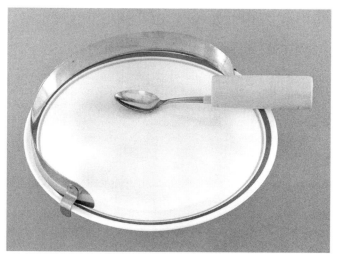

Figure 41.12. Plate guard. Assists with scooping food onto the spoon or fork.

Table 41.3. Predictors of Positive Rehabilitation Outcomes in Stroke

Less severe paralysis

Little neglect

Able to follow more than a single step command

Less receptive aphasia

Good cognition

Less sensory deficits

outcomes in skilled nursing facilities that are rehabilitation oriented.[16] These improved outcomes are reductions in mortality, and ADL dependency. The positive effects appear to extend to those over age 75, and are more likely seen when the rehabilitation services are targeted to those with intermediate severity of deficits. Long term costs savings and lessening burden on the family have also been demonstrated in studies.[17]

Often it is difficult to predict shortly after the stroke whether the patient will benefit from rehabilitation. Those likely to improve and be more independent are shown in Table 41.3. Neglect is the absence of awareness, usually from a right parietal lobe stroke. It is not a lack of sensation. It can be detected by using the technique of "double simultaneous stimulation." In this test, the examiner independently assess light touch sensation on each side of the patient's body, then, without warning the patient, simultaneously stimulates both sides of the patient's body at the same time and asks which side is felt. The patient with intact sensation, but neglect will report he (or she) feels it only on the side without neglect. Patients in rehabilitation need to be able to follow directions to participate in exercises and learn new methods for doing activities. A person with a productive aphasia (motor or Broca's aphasia) may have difficulty speaking but usually can understand instructions. With receptive aphasia (sensory or Wernicke's aphasia), the person often cannot understand instructions, making rehabilitation training difficult. Cognition is very important, but the question is what is "good enough" to participate? There are no agreed upon standards but the usual geriatric assessment of cognition using the Mini-Mental State Exam will suffice. Patients with mild levels of dementia have been shown to make gains in rehabilitation.[18] While patients often focus on motor function recovery (e.g., walking) as a sign of improvement, sensory function probably plays a bigger role in achieving independent activities.

Recovery of lost function in stroke is a combination of natural recovery processes, improvements produced by the rehabilitation process, and adaptations made by the patient to be more independent using newly learned techniques and equipment. There are generally three time periods that signal the course of improvements. By one week after the stroke most people who recover already show some significant improvement. If there has been no motor or sensory improvement by 1 week, the prognosis is more guarded. By one month 70%–80% of native

neurologic recovery is complete. Of course, the patient still may make many gains in independence through the training process. After six months virtually all motor recovery is complete. Swallowing dysfunction, speech capabilities, and sensory function may gradually improve over a considerably longer time.

Many team members are involved in a stroke rehabilitation program. The nurse is perhaps the most important member of the team. In addition to providing primary nursing services, he or she ensures secondary complications don't develop (e.g., preventing pressure sores by frequent turning and skin care), ensures techniques learned in therapy are practiced, providing range of motion (ROM) exercises, training family members care-giving skills, and patient education. Nursing staff are also involved in preventing and treating common bowel and bladder problems, such as incontinence or urinary retention. Foley catheters should be removed as soon as possible to facilitate mobility and practice at ADL. Full discussion of incontinence and bowel problems is found in chapters 25 and 26. The physical therapist works with the patient to improve sitting and standing balance, strengthening and conditioning, testing and extending ROM, mobility training, and fitting and teaching the patient use of orthoses.

ADL training, teaching the patient the use of assistive devices, and cognitive training are the purview of the occupational therapist. A speech and language pathologist is often involved to conduct a swallowing assessment, dysphagia rehabilitation, and provide language and communication training. Because of the high incidence of post-stroke depression, the services of a rehabilitation counselor or psychologist are invaluable. They assist the patient with adjustment to disability, depression management, and cognitive assessment. The social worker may provide counseling, assessment of social support needs, referral to community resources, and discharge planning. Finally, the physician must closely manage the patient's medical conditions and pay particular attention to reducing the chance of further strokes by risk reduction interventions, such as controlling blood pressure or hyperglycemia, evaluating the need for lipid lowering agents, and making decisions about anticoagulation.

The stroke patient is at great risk for the development of secondary complications and all members of the team must be vigilant to prevent them from occurring. Pressure sores start within two hours when the person is completely immobilized. Frequent turning, avoiding elevating the head of the bed and pulling the patient across bed sheets, and close, regular observation of the skin is needed. Contractures are a fixed shortening of the muscles and tendons, due to lack of movement. They begin early in the course and must be prevented by doing passive range of motion exercises. Once the person has been trained, he or she can self-administer these exercises. Deep venous thrombosis is a concern as long as the person is not walking. Probably the majority of stroke survivors have some DVT. Subcutaneous low-dose unfractionated, or low-molecular weight heparin, are probably the most effective treatments but have a risk of causing bleeding. Aspirin may be used when anticoagulation risk is too high. Intermittent compression is also useful but interferes with mobility. Deconditioning sets in whenever someone is not regularly exercising. A gradually rising morning heart rate may be an early indication. Exercise is the treatment. Subluxation of the shoulder may occur naturally after a stroke, but is promoted when the hemiparetic arm is pulled on or left to lie under the person's body. Regular range of motion keeps the shoulder limber and subluxation will usually remit if the person regains muscle tone in the shoulder. Depression occurs in up to 70% of dominant hemisphere strokes. Assessment is more difficult in the presence of aphasia and sometimes patients, family and providers believe that depression is a normal consequence of going through such a major loss in life. However, depression adversely affects outcomes, and treatment has been shown to improve outcomes.[19] The evidence for the prevention and management of stroke complications is discussed in the VA/DOD Stroke Rehabilitation Guidelines.[20]

Specific rehabilitation interventions for stroke have been the subject of two major evidence-based reviews. The most recent, developed by the Department of Veterans Affairs and the Department of Defense, reviews initial assessment and rehabilitation treatment in both inpatient and outpatient settings.[20] Recommendations with Level I evidence include the delivery of post-stroke care in a multidisciplinary rehabilitation setting or stroke unit, early patient assessment via the NIH Stroke Scale,[21] early initiation of rehabilitation therapies, swallow screening testing for dysphagia, an active secondary stroke prevention program, and proactive prevention of venous thrombi. Standardized assessment tools should be used to develop a comprehensive treatment plan appropriate to each patient's deficits and needs. Medical therapy for depression or emotional lability is strongly recommended. A speech and language pathologist should evaluate communication and related cognitive disorders and provide treatment when indicated. The patient, caregiver, and family are essential members of the rehabilitation team and should be involved in all phases of the rehabilitation process. These recommendations build upon the earlier stroke rehabilitation guidelines published by the Agency for Health Care Policy and Research in 1995.[17]

Traditionally, rehabilitation for stroke was seen as primarily oriented to prevention of secondary disabilities while natural recovery occurred, and in teaching the patient new methods for conducting ADL and IADL with the residual disability. However, there is some evidence that aggressive therapeutic interventions may facilitate recovery of neurologic function. The Bobath approach is based on the theory of proprioceptive neuromuscular facilitation which is used to restore motor control.[22] One of the newest techniques is constraint-induced therapy, whereby the patient's functional extremity is prevented from being used in order to force use of the affected extremity. In animal models, this type of intervention has produced biologic evidence of neural regeneration. A randomized trial is underway to investigate its utility in humans.[23] Another new technique being tested is using suspended body weight support to provide gait training on a treadmill. The patient does not have to fear falling. A recent Cochrane review found no

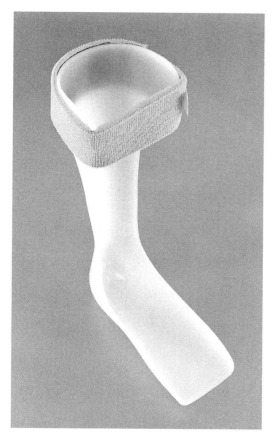

Figure 41.13. Polyethylene ankle-foot orthosis (AFO). Useful for persons with foot drop or weakness after a stroke.

statistically significant effect of treadmill training but individual randomized trials have shown benefits.[24] Finally, electrical stimulation is being studied to determine whether motor recovery can be facilitated. In summary, it is clear that physical therapy interventions are beneficial in stroke recovery, there is insufficient evidence to say that any one approach is preferable over others.[25]

Orthotics, sometime called braces, are often needed by stroke patients. An orthotic is named according to the joints it crosses. The most common type of brace used after stroke is an ankle-foot-orthosis (AFO). There are two major types of AFO – a polyethylene, molded plastic brace and a metal AFO (Figures 41.13 & 41.14). They help to stabilize the ankle joint, including ankle plantar flexion and dorsiflexion, and mediolateral stability at the ankle. In addition, AFOs provide exert an influence on the knee during ambulation because of their effect on the ankle. Extension of the knee is facilitated by plantar flexion of the ankle and dorsiflexion of the ankle leads to flexion of the knee. During gait and weight bearing, AFOs exert effects on the knee, foot, and ankle, and have been shown to decrease the incidence of ankle contracture in patients with hemiparesis.[26]

The molded AFOs are often preferred by patients because they are easier to don and do not "look medical." A metal

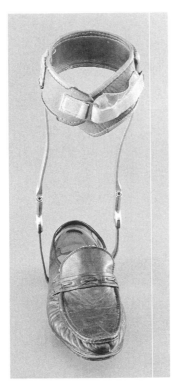

Figure 41.14. Metal ankle-foot orthosis (AFO). Used for persons needing support for ankle instability.

AFO may be prescribed if there is neuropathy because there are fewer points on skin contact or spasticity. However, the choice of which type would be guided by the patient's physical disabilities and a physical therapist, orthotist, and often a specialist in physical medicine and rehabilitation is usually need to choose the correct device. Some older patients are reluctant to switch from one type to the other if they are used to using it, in spite of the medical indications.

Upper extremity splints are sometimes used to control position in a paralyzed extremity. Unlike orthoses, they don't directly enhance function. However, in order to prevent flexion contractures of the fingers or wrist, a volar splint may be prescribed for use during sleep. The occupational therapist usually makes this recommendation.

Spasticity is a common complication of stroke and can significantly impede functional ability. Fortunately, many patients progress out of a spastic phase. It is sometimes alleviated by simple repositioning. Lower extremity spasticity may actually facilitate walking. Still, a significant number of stroke survivors will have spasticity of the affected muscle groups. Stretching and range of motion exercises are often very helpful. Traditionally, this complication was treated with centrally acting medications such as benzodiazepines or baclofen. But these often cause sedation or confusion in older patients, and were not very effective in spasticity due to stroke. More recently, botulinum toxin injections, performed by a physiatrist, are sometimes useful.

Dysphagia

Swallowing problems are common sequelae of a stroke. The patient usually exhibits a "wet hoarseness" whereby a gurgling sound may be heard while talking. The patient often complains of coughing while eating, and especially when drinking liquids. The evaluation begins with a bedside evaluation by the speech and language pathologist by observing the patient attempt to swallow small amounts of liquids. If the patient can swallow, they should be encouraged to have a normal diet. Routine use of supplements has not been supported by randomized trials and may actually increase the risk of death.[27]

If there is concern, an endoscopic or radiographic evaluation of swallowing function will be obtained. If there are problems swallowing the major concerns are obtaining adequate nutrition and hydration, prevention of aspiration, and medication administration.

One of the difficult questions in dysphagia is the use of artificial nutrition and hydration through a feeding tube. Feeding tubes do not prevent aspiration but they do facilitate delivery of nutrients. The critical decision is what is the goal of care? Often, the decision about a feeding tube must be made relatively early in the post-stroke course. The amount of functional recovery that will occur is uncertain in the early stages, but malnutrition and dehydration reduce the chance of successful rehabilitation outcomes. On the other hand, it is not clear that feeding tubes significantly improve outcomes in stroke.[28] Most patients are willing to accept a feeding tube if the duration of use is expected to be short and the goal is improvement in functional abilities. Later, if swallowing function does not return, a decision can be made whether to maintain the tube based upon the patient's goals of care.

HIP FRACTURE

Hip fractures are the most common traumatic cause leading to rehabilitation interventions. The incidence of hip fractures is 1289 per 100,000 by age 80 years.[29] Two main types of fractures occur: 1) intracapsular, which include fractures of the femoral neck in the subcapital or transcervical areas, and 2) extracapsular, which include intertrochanteric and subtrochanteric fractures. Early repair is associated with reduced mortality and complications, but only if the patient is medical stable when undergoing surgery. Hence, patients should be quickly stabilized medically before proceeding to the surgery suite.[30] Antibiotic prophylaxis should be provided to all patients.

Type of surgery is determined by type of fracture, though post-surgical exercise recommendations by orthopedists often vary widely. Recent evidence that early ambulation also leads to better outcomes, even with "pins." Patients who have compression screws or implanted hip arthroses can usually be allowed to weight bear fully by the second post-operative day. In general, older patients should be told to weight bear to their tolerance for pain.[31] Very few older people can "toe-touch" weight bear. The only time weight bearing should be restricted is when the repair is unstable. These patients have a high risk of never walking again.[32] Physical therapy has been shown to affect outcomes and should start early, even before full ambulation is allowed. Long-term outpatient therapy can improve physical function and reduce disability.[33]

From the geriatric care provider's perspective, the postoperative rehabilitation period is the most important. The patient must be carefully monitored for delirium, which occurs in up to 65% of patients. It is often difficult to recognize when the patient is presenting with a withdrawn and apathetic appearance, and the patient may be mistaken for having low motivation to participate in rehabilitation. Adequate control of pain will both lessen the risk of delirium and improve the patient's ability to participate in exercise.[34] Patients who have had a hip replacement must be taught to make safe transfers and bed positions, as hip flexion greater than 90 degrees and significant adduction of the hip can lead to dislocations. In spite of the fact that most hip fractures in older patients are related to osteoporosis a surprising number of patients are not treated for this condition.[35] No patient with a hip fracture should leave the hospital without an assessment for the presence of osteoporosis and a decision about whether treatment should be offered.

AMPUTATION

Amputations are common complications of diabetes, peripheral vascular disease and neuropathy in older persons. The incidence is 50–100/100,000 hospital admissions. From a functional standpoint a below-the-knee (BK) amputation is preferable over an above-the-knee (AK) amputation. The energy cost of walking with a BK prosthesis is 35% increased over normal walking. While significant, most elderly patients can tolerate this increase in energy costs. Hence, the vast majority of older patients with unilateral BK amputation regain independent ambulation with a prosthesis. On the other hand walking with an AK amputation requires 80–100% increased energy cost. Few elderly patients with an AK amputation regain independent ambulation even with a prosthesis.

If the amputation is elective, pre-operative education and training is important. The patient can learn range of motion and quadriceps strengthening exercises. This is very important to prevent the development of flexion contractures of the knee, which may interfere with later use of a lower extremity prosthesis. Upper body strengthening can also start before the operation. It's helpful to start bicycle training or upper extremity ergometer training to improve cardiovascular status. If patients can tolerate it, having them lie on their stomach will help extend the hips and knees and prevent flexion contractures.

A temporary prosthesis is often fitted very soon after surgery to promote ambulation and prevent deconditioning. The patient must receive training in stump care, wrapping, and transfers. After six or more weeks, once the stump has healed, the older patient is often provided a permanent prosthesis. Almost all older patients will also need training in the use

of a wheelchair for traveling longer distances. Stump care is part of patient education and chronic disease self-management training. Successful adaptation to use of the prosthesis is associated with careful attention to stump care.

There are some relative contraindications to the provision of a prosthesis. Persons with such poor cognition that they can not learn how to safely manage their stump and don their prosthesis should probably not be provided one. Those with severe deficits in sensation, or those with severe arthritis or peripheral vascular disease in the contralateral leg may develop serious complications when using a prosthesis. Flexion contractures of the hip or knee will also prevent use of a prosthesis. It is very important to check for its development using direct observation and measurement of extension with a goniometer. When lying in bed, it's very easy to think the knee is fully extended when it is not.

PARKINSON'S

The evidence that physical therapy interventions are useful in the routine care of patients with Parkinson's disease is slim.[36] However, PT evaluation can be helpful in determining equipment needs and training the patient in proper use of a walker and a home exercise program.[37] Training may also help with movement initiation and counter acting the flexed posture.[38,39] It is important to choose assistive devices carefully. For instance, one probably would like to avoid the use of canes, non-wheeled pick-up walkers, and perhaps even four-wheeled walkers. Because of the flexed and internally rotated posture of the upper extremities, canes can cause tripping. Pick up walkers may promote retropulsion, while 4-wheeled walkers may allow the patient to walk too fast if there is festination. A front-wheeled walkers is probably the best mobility device as it forces the patient to keep the center of gravity forward (thereby preventing backwards falls) but also provides enough drag to prevent festination. Recently, evidence has shown that regular exercise may prevent decline so all patients should be encouraged to exercise regularly.[40] A recumbent stationary bicycle is a useful device as it is safe, provides good cardiac stimulation and the circular movements are conducive to balance.

Other rehabilitation therapists may have a role in helping people with Parkinson's disease stay independent. An occupational therapy home consultation may be helpful for home modifications. Whether speech therapy is helpful in Parkinson's disease is controversial.

SUMMARY

Rehabilitation is the process for helping older persons with disability regain lost function or enhance declining abilities. It should be considered in any situation where the older person has experienced a change in functional abilities. It usually requires two or more multidisciplinary team members. Medicare reimbursement is available for rehabilitation interventions as long as the patient can demonstrate improvements in function as a result of the treatment.

REFERENCES

1. Hoenig H, Nusbaum N, Brummel-Smith K. Geriatric rehabilitation: State of the art. *J Am Geriatr Soc*, 1997;45:1371–1381.
2. http://www.who.int/classifications/icf/en. Accessed November 13, 2008.
3. Bodenheimer T, Wagner EH, Grumbach K. Improving primary care for patients with chronic illness. *JAMA* 2002;288:1775–1779.
4. Patrick L, Knoefel F, Gaskowski P, Rexroth D. Medical comorbidity and rehabilitation efficiency in geriatric inpatients. *J Am Geriatr Soc* 2001;49:1471–1477.
5. Huusko TM, Karppi P, Avikainen V, et al. Randomised, clinically controlled trial of intensive geriatric rehabilitation in patients with hip fracture: Subgroup analysis of patients with dementia. *BMJ* 2000;321:1107–1111.
6. Cristian A. The assessment of the older adult with a physical disability: a guide for clinicians. *Clin Geriatr Med* 2006;22:221–238.
7. Patrick L, Knoefel F, Gaskowski P, Rexroth D. Medical comorbidity and rehabilitation efficiency in geriatric inpatients. *J Am Geriatr Soc* 2001;49:1471–1477.
8. Cole MG, Elie LM, McCusker J, Bellavance F, Mansour A. Feasibility and effectiveness of treatments for post-stroke depression in elderly inpatients: systematic review. *J Geriatr Psychiatry Neurol*. 2001;14:37–41.
9. Brummel-Smith K. Assessment in Rehabilitation, in Comprehensive Geriatric Assessment, Beck J, Osterweil D, Brummel-Smith K, Beck J, (eds), McGraw-Hill, Philadelphia, 2000, pp. 155–158.
10. Kramer AM, Kowalsky JC, Lin M, et al. Outcome and utilization differences for older persons with stroke in HMO and fee-for-service systems. *J Am Geriatr Soc.* 2000;48:726–734.
11. American Heart Association Heart and Stroke Statistics Update 2007, www.americanheart.org, accessed 2/15/07.
12. Bates B, Choi JY, Duncan PW, et al. Veterans Affairs/Department of Defense clinical practice guideline for the management of adult stroke rehabilitation care. *Stroke* 2005;36:2049–2056.
13. Cifu DX, Stewart DG. Factors affecting functional outcome after stroke: a critical review of rehabilitation interventions. *Arch Phys Med Rehabil.* 1999;80(5 suppl 1):S35–S39.
14. Stroke Unit Trialists' Collaboration. Organised inpatient (stroke unit) care for stroke. Cochrane Database Syst Rev. 2002(1):CD000197.
15. Evans RL, Connis RT, Hendricks RD, Haselkorn JK. Multidisciplinary rehabilitation versus medical care: a meta-analysis. *Soc Sci Med.* 1995;40:1699–1706.
16. Murray PK, Singer M, Dawson NV, Thomas CL, Cebul RD. Outcomes of rehabilitation services in nursing home residents. *Arch Phys Med Rehabil* 2003;84:1129–1136.
17. Gresham GE, Duncan PW, Staşon WB, et al. Post Stroke Rehabilitation. Clinical Practice Guideline No. 16. Rockville, MD: U.S. Department of Health and Human Services. Public Health Service, Agency for Health Care Policy and Research. AHCPR Publication No. 1995:95-0662.
18. Ruchinskas RA, Singer HK, Repetz NK. Cognitive status and ambulation in geriatric rehabilitation: Walking without thinking? *Arch Phys Med Rehabil* 2000;81:1224–1228.
19. Teasell RW, Mersky H, Deshpande S. Antidepressants in rehabilitation. *Phys Med Rehabil Clin North Am* 1999;10:237–253.
20. www.oqp.med.va.gov/cpg/STR/STR_base.htm, accessed 2/13/07.
21. www.strokecenter.org/trials/scales/nihss.html, accessed 2/13/07.
22. Paci M. Physiotherapy based on the Bobath concept for adults with post-stroke hemiplegia: a review of effectiveness studies. *J Rehabil Med.* 2003;35:2–7.
23. Wittenberg GF, Chen R, Ishii K, et al. Constraint-induced therapy in stroke: magnetic-stimulation motor maps and cerebral activation. *Neurorehabil & Neural Repair.* 2003;17:48–57.
24. Moseley AM, Stark A, Cameron ID, Pollock A. Treadmill training and body weight support for walking after a stroke. Cochrane Database of Systematic Reviews. 4, 2006, Art. No.: CD002840. DOI: 10.1002/14651858.CD002840.pub2.
25. Pollock A, Baer G, Pomeroy V, Langhorne P. Physiotherapy treatment approaches for the recovery of postural control and lower limb function following stroke. Cochrane Database of Systematic Reviews. 4. 2006.
26. Shah MV. Rehabilitation of the older adult with stroke. *Clin Geriatr Med* 2006;22:469–489.
27. Dennis MS, Lewis SC, Warlow C. FOOD Trial Collaboration. Routine oral nutritional supplementation for stroke patients in hospital (FOOD): a multicentre randomized controlled trial. *Lancet* 2005;365:755–763.
28. Dennis MS, Lewis SC, Warlow C. FOOD Trial Collaboration. Effect of timing and method of enteral tube feeding for dysphagic stroke patients: a muticentre randomized controlled trial. *Lancet* 2005;365:764–772.
29. Gullberg B, Johnell O, Kanis JA. World-wide projections for hip fracture. *Osteoporosis Int* 1997;7:407–413.
30. Beaupre LA, Jones CA, Saunders LD, et al. Best practices for elderly hip fracture patients. A systematic overview of the evidence. *J Gen Intern Med* 2005;20:1019–1025.
31. Koval KJ, Friend KD, Aharonoff GB, et al. Weight bearing after hip fracture: a prospective series of 596 geriatric hip fracture patients. *J Orthop Trauma* 1996;10:526.
32. Burns RB, Moskowitz MA, Ash A, et al. Do hip replacements improve outcomes for hip fracture patients? *Med Care* 1999;37:285–294.
33. Binder EF, Brown M, Sinacore DR, et al. Effects of extended outpatient rehabilitation after hip fracture. A randomized controlled trial. *JAMA* 2004;292:837–846.
34. Morrison RS, Magaziner J, McLaughlin MA, et al. The impact of post-operative pain on outcomes following hip fracture. *Pain* 2003;103:303–311.
35. Bellantonio S, Fortinsky R, Prestwood K. How well are community-living women treated for osteoporosis after hip fracture? *J Am Geriatr Soc* 2001;49:1197–1204.
36. Deane KHO, Jones D, Playford ED, et al. Physiotherapy versus placebo or no intervention in Parkinson's disease. Cochrane Database of Systematic Reviews. 2001, Issue 3. Art. No.: CD002817. DOI: 10.1002/14651858.CD002817.
37. Hirsch MA, Toole T, Maitland CG, Rider RA. The effects of balance training and high-intensity resistance training on persons with idiopathic Parkinson's disease. *Arch Phys Med Rehabil* 2003;84:1109–1117.
38. Bergen JL, Toole T, Elliott RG, et al. Aerobic exercise intervention improves aerobic capacity and movement initiation in Parkinson's disease patients. *Neurorehabilitation* 2002;17:161–168.
39. Villianl T, Pasquetti P, Magnolfi S, et al. Effects of physical training on straightening-up processes in patients with Parkinson's disease. *Disability & Rehabil* 1999;21:68–73.
40. Chen H, Zhang SM, Schwarzschild MA, et al. Physical activity and the risk of Parkinson's disease. *Neurology* 2005;64:664–669.

42

COMMUNITY-BASED LONG-TERM CARE

Nasiya N. Ahmed, MD, Randal W. Scott, MSW, MBA, Mindy J. Fain, MD

Community-based long-term care encompasses a wide array of medical and nonmedical diagnostic, preventive, therapeutic, rehabilitative, personal, social, supportive, and palliative services in a variety of settings for individuals who have lost some capacity for self-care because of a chronic illness or physical, cognitive, or emotional impairment.[1] Some of the support services allow the patient to remain at home (including adult daycare, home health services, home medical care, and telemedicine), whereas other services require a change of residence (such as assisted living, adult care homes, and continuing-care retirement communities). The goal of care is to build on interprofessional expertise and teamwork to promote the optimally independent level of physical, social, and psychological functioning in the least restrictive environment.

In 2003, approximately 7 million older adults (aged 65 years or older) needed some form of long-term care. During the past several years, there has been a trend toward community-based services, moving away from institutional care such as nursing homes. Most patients with chronic health problems prefer to remain at home or in a homelike setting, and only approximately 20% of older adults who require long-term care reside in nursing homes. This shift was formalized by the Olmstead Decision (July 1999) in which the U.S. Supreme Court upheld the right of individuals to receive care in the community instead of in an institution whenever possible.[2]

Community-based long-term care services involve attending to the patient's medical and psychosocial needs, bringing together those services necessary to maintain or improve the patient's clinical status, preventing acute exacerbations of chronic illness, and avoiding unnecessary and costly emergency room visits and acute hospitalizations. The services include assistance with activities of daily living (ADLs) and instrumental activities of daily living (IADLs). In addition, the care seeks to maintain the patient's safety and provide comfort and assurance. It may entail hands-on or supervisory human assistance, assistive devices, and technology such as computerized medication reminders and emergency alert systems.

Case/care managers are often the point of entry to in-home and community-based services and are responsible for the determination of the patient's needs. Case manager services may be provided by the physician, nurse, social worker, private consultant, or the patient. A key component of such management involves a review of an individual's socioeconomic, environmental, psychological, and physical health challenges, and the development of a care plan for services or treatment. Comprehensive geriatric assessment, a multidimensional and multidisciplinary process, embodies a formal approach to optimize matching the patient's needs with available resources and to provide effective and quality care. The areas to identify, in determining level of care or resources needed, are outlined in Table 42.1.

The role of the physician in long-term care is vital because these patients are among those with the greatest need for quality medical services. Whether or not the physician assumes the formal role of the case manager, he or she will most likely be responsible for authorizing and supervising complex medically necessary plans of care, advocating for the patient, and promoting a collaborative interdisciplinary team effort. Physicians play an essential role in certifying patient eligibility for Medicare-funded home health care (HHC), including nursing care, rehabilitative therapies, and hospice care. Medicare has assigned billing codes specifically for physicians who coordinate long-term care services under Medicare. Physicians also provide a critical consultative function for community-based services funded by other sources.

Formal community-based long-term care may be more cost-effective than institutional care, although this has not been proven.[3] Community-based care enables elderly persons with disabilities to live more independently and may reduce the probability of institutionalization; however, the downside

Table 42.1. Useful Assessments to Determine the Level of Care or Resources

Domain	Areas to Be Evaluated
Function	ADLs
	IADLs
	Medication use and adherence
Cognition	Mental status
	Decision-making capacity
	Health literacy
Psychosocial	Mood
	Culture, beliefs, and preferences
Nutritional	Access to food, assistance with preparation
Caregiver	Availability and willingness to perform tasks
	Types of tasks required
	Physical health and emotional capability
Environment	Safety for patient care, including electricity and fire safety
	Comfort and functionality, including needed adaptations
Community	Access to emergency services
	Availability of supportive resources
Financial	Available funding (private or public)
	Impact on family

Adapted with permission from Medical Management of the Home Care Patient: Guidelines for Physicians. (1998). American Medical Association. Chicago, IL.

is that some communities only offer an incomplete continuum of care, potentially leaving the patient isolated and vulnerable.

HOME CARE

Home care is defined by the American Medical Association as "the provision of equipment and services to the patient in the home for the purpose of restoring and maintaining his or her maximal level of comfort, function and health . . . and is a collaborative effort of the patient, family, and professionals."[4] Home care includes a wide array of services: HHC, home medical care, telemedicine monitoring, technologically intensive services, hospice care, and long-term supportive care, such as home-delivered meals.[5] Between 5% and 10% of all patients in a typical medical practice receive home care services.

HHC is among the fastest growing service industries in the United States. Medicare skilled HHC was initially designed to provide acute and postacute care following hospitalization, but the industry exploded through the 1990s because of liberalization of the benefit, a rapidly aging population, and pressures on hospitals to discharge patients early under prospective

payment. The 1997 Balanced Budget Act limited Medicare spending by refocusing goals of care and services; as a result, reimbursement to home health agencies was dramatically reduced.

HHC includes skilled nursing care, health monitoring, dispensing of medications, physical and other rehabilitative therapies, personal care, homemaker services, and instructing patients and family members about correct patient care. With recent technological advances, HHC diagnostic and therapeutic procedures may include intravenous antibiotics, transfusions, chemotherapy, dialysis, enteral and parenteral nutrition, and mechanical ventilation. The use of telemonitoring systems offers the options of telehome care and "electronic house calls" that may assist with specialized chronic disease management programs. HHC may be provided by one of the 6,900 Medicare-certified home health agencies (in 2003) or other agencies.

The older patient in need of HHC often has complex medical problems and functional impairments. The indications for a patient referral include advanced age, frailty, multiple comorbidities, frequent emergency room visits or hospitalizations, functional disability, or impaired psychosocial functioning. A series of assessments is required to determine medical necessity, including the acuity of the problem, underlying comorbidities, the severity of the patient's functional disability and homebound status, and potential interventions. This process includes a determination of the appropriate level of care and services, and the patient and/or caregiver's ability to implement the plan of care.

HHC reimbursement options include Medicare, Medicaid, private insurance, managed care, the Older Americans Act, and self-paid. Medicare-covered services are part-time, intermittent, skilled services that are limited to homebound patients. This care must be ordered by a physician, provided by a nurse, physical therapist, or speech therapist, and must be appropriate to the patient's illness and/or injury. Other services, such as those provided by a social worker or home health aide, may be reimbursed but only when the patient is receiving care from one of the three core skilled services. Reimbursement models other than Medicare may include considerations of cost-effectiveness, patient prognosis, and the opportunity to achieve certain outcomes of care. This may include care for patients who are not homebound, but who require services such as infusion therapy.

Most primary care physicians will be involved in the certification and oversight of complex home care plans for their homebound patients. Medicare policy requires that the skilled HHC service must be determined to constitute "reasonable and necessary care," and the goals of care must be defined. The physician is required to determine the frequency and duration of skilled services. The ability of the patient and caregiver to learn and carry out certain tasks is critical, and the physician should include the expertise of the HHC nurse and other interdisciplinary team members in the determination of the plan of care.

The efficacy of HHC in specific prevention and assessment programs is well known, including optimizing home safety, enhancing education, and in the identification of common geriatric issues that would otherwise go unrecognized.[6] Additionally, a wide range of home-based interdisciplinary programs has been developed to optimize the management of patients with advancing chronic illness, and there is evidence that specifically targeted programs can improve outcomes for high-risk conditions such as congestive heart failure.[7] A recent study examined the long-term beneficial effects of team home-based intervention for a heterogeneous group of chronically ill patients, demonstrating fewer hospital admissions and reduced health care costs.[8] Although evidence concerning the effectiveness of HHC is accumulating, further investigation is needed.

Home medical care refers to the provision of medical care by a physician or other primary care provider, such as a physician's assistant or nurse practitioner, in the home as part of an ongoing office-based practice, a hospital-based program, or a free-standing practice. The categories of intervention include preventive, diagnostic, therapeutic, rehabilitative, and long-term maintenance. Indications for a home medical visit include advanced age, multiple comorbidities, homebound status with impaired functioning, frequent emergency department visits or recurrent acute hospitalizations, and determination of patient values and goals of care.

The number of homebound elders with difficulty accessing primary medical care continues to rise, and their care is disproportionately managed in the emergency room or the acute care setting. These vulnerable, elderly, homebound patients may receive care at home through home visits or "house calls." Although house calls are now more financially feasible for clinicians, few physicians provide home care because of perceived poor reimbursement, time-inefficiencies, and concerns about safety, liability and legal issues, and lack of equipment.

There are a few examples of successful home-based primary care programs embedded in academic medical centers, including the Mt. Sinai Visiting Doctors Program established in 1995, which is recognized for its leadership in teaching, research, and clinical care.[9] Other models of home-based primary care programs, including affiliations with community health systems and visiting nurse associations, have demonstrated improvements in medication and health management, improved patient and caregiver education, decreased hospitalization and emergency room utilization, and increased satisfaction.[10]

The cost-effectiveness of medical home care remains controversial. The VA Home-based Primary Care Program is a national model of interdisciplinary care for homebound veterans with multiple medical, functional, and psychosocial problems and is part of the continuum of Veterans Administration programs providing comprehensive and coordinated care. The effectiveness of this program of team-managed primary care was examined in a multisite, randomized controlled trial. It demonstrated improved caregiver quality-of-life measures, satisfaction with care, and a 22% reduction in hospital readmissions at 6 months. It did not, however, substitute for other forms of care, and resulted in 6% higher costs at 6 months, and 12% higher costs at 12 months.[11] Further studies will assist in determining the replicability of the model as well as its application to other populations.

The recent development by the Home-based Primary Care Quality Initiative of a comprehensive set of evidence-based process quality indicators for homebound seniors provides a quality framework to evaluate home-based primary medical care.[12] Despite a burgeoning homebound elderly population, home-based primary care practices have been slow to develop and have gained little institutional support outside of the Veterans Administration system or as part of the Program of All-Inclusive Care for the Elderly (PACE).

Hospital-at-home provides treatment of an acute medical problem in the home by health care professionals. This alternative was prompted by both the need to cut medical care costs and the high rate of functional decline, iatrogenic illness, and other adverse events that elders experienced during acute hospitalization. There are several definitions of hospital-at-home, including blends of skilled nursing and medical services, as well as avoidance of, or only short-term, hospitalization.

This heterogeneity precludes a clear evaluation of the effects of hospital-at-home as compared with inpatient care. A Cochrane Systematic Review assessed the effects of hospital-at-home compared with inpatient hospital care, and included 22 trials representing various models of care.[13] The review noted that although clinical outcomes appeared to be the same, and patient satisfaction at home may be higher, there was little evidence of economic benefit, and the burden on caregivers at home can be high.

A recent study evaluated a hospital-at-home model that replaced acute hospital care for certain older adults with selected acute medical problems: community-acquired pneumonia, exacerbations of heart failure and/or chronic obstructive pulmonary disease, or cellulitis.[14] The model included daily physician visits at home, one-on-one home nursing care for an extended period, and 24-hour physician coverage for urgent clinical conditions. This study suggested that hospital-at-home can be both feasible and efficacious for older patients with common medical conditions, resulting in lower costs, fewer clinical complications such as incident delirium, as well as higher patient and family satisfaction.

HOSPICE CARE

Hospice is a palliative and supportive care program for terminally ill patients and their families, with the goal of providing a comfortable and dignified death at home. The hospice movement, which began in the United States with the first inpatient hospice opening in 1975, was a reaction to the belief that burgeoning technology and pursuit of a cure were interfering with the humanitarian care of the dying patient. In 1983, the Medicare Hospice Benefit (MHB) was established.

The MHB was funded as a capitated system with rules for eligibility and covered services; it serves as a guideline for hospice services provided by other payers. The key elements of the MHB are outlined in Table 42.2. All inpatient hospices that

Table 42.2. Hospice Care Benefit Eligibility and Services

Requirements for Elected Hospice Care Benefit	Hospice Services Provided for the Terminal Illness and Related Conditions
Patient is eligible for Medicare Part A	Physician care
Patient is certified by 2 physicians as having a terminal disease with a prognosis of 6 months or less, if the illness runs its normal course	Nursing care
	Volunteers
Patient agrees to palliative care for terminal diagnosis	Medical equipment and supplies
	Medications
Patient receives care from a Medicare-approved hospice program	Home health aid and homemaker services
	Physical, occupational, speech pathology
Patient elects the hospice benefit and waives all rights to Medicare Payments for services for the terminal illness and related conditions	Social worker services
	Dietary counseling
	Spiritual counseling and grief/loss counseling
	Short-term hospital or respite care
	Other reasonable services identified by team

Adapted with permission from, Hospice Payment System Fact Sheet. (2006). Medicare Learning Network, Centers for Medicare and Medicaid Services, Nov, ICN: 006817.

accept Medicare payments are required to have a comprehensive outpatient hospice service.

Today approximately 90% of patients in hospice receive their care at home by an interdisciplinary team with expertise in the physical, psychological, social, and spiritual needs of the dying patient and family. Routine hospice home care is also an option for patients residing in other places such as assisted living facilities (ALFs), adult care homes, and nursing homes. Although hospice care does not require a primary caregiver in the home, additional support is often needed as death nears. Inpatient respite hospice care is available, as well as continuous home care for brief periods in a crisis that would otherwise lead to an inpatient hospice admission.

On admission to the hospice program, the patient, doctor, and interdisciplinary team develop a plan of care that identifies the patient's goals of care and services. Importantly, no Medicare regulation specifies which interventions are "palliative," and each hospice has its own guidelines, a decision determined by both philosophical and financial considerations. Some controversial potentially palliative treatments include parenteral fluids, enteral feeding, radiation therapy, blood cell transfusions, chemotherapy, and antibiotics.

The MHB requires that the patient have an anticipated survival of less than 6 months. Cancer is the most common referring diagnosis, and patients with dementia are markedly underrepresented in hospice care. For patients with advanced chronic disease, difficulties with prognostication often result in late referrals by the physician. The National Hospice Organization has developed general criteria for referral for hospice, and guidelines for prognosis in chronic disease such as heart, pulmonary, stroke, dementia, renal disease, and liver disease.

Although very few studies have been done, research shows that home hospice does improve quality of life. Symptoms are more adequately controlled and patients are able to maintain a higher level of function. They have lower scores for pain, nausea, shortness of breath, and restlessness, and also have a higher level of functioning and interaction with family members.[15] Furthermore, studies show that when physical symptoms are controlled, patients are able to concentrate on their emotional and spiritual needs at the end of life.

As our population continues to age, hospice care, especially at home, will increase in demand as an essential part of the continuum of care. There are no federal guidelines outlining quality-of-care measurements or requirements. The creation of national standards, increased education regarding hospice care, and the development of a subspecialty in palliative medicine will improve hospice services and fully integrate it into the health care system in this country.

ADULT DAYCARE PROGRAMS

Adult daycare programs serve a wide variety of frail and disabled persons who need assistance or supervision during the day. The program offers relief to family members or caregivers, and allows them the freedom to go to work and handle personal business, or provides respite from the strain of caregiving. More than 3,500 adult day centers are operating in the United States. Half of participants have some cognitive impairment and 59% require assistance with two or more ADLs.[16] There are three types of daycare models: a social model, a medical model, and a special purpose model that serves the need of a particular comorbid illness (for example, dementia). Medical models focus on skilled health care and rehabilitative services; some have workshops for memory improvement and incontinence.

These centers generally provide supervision, a meal and snacks, recreation, and health care/monitoring to adults with physical, mental, or social impairments. Participants do not require 24-hour institutional care, yet are not capable of full-time, independent living. Notably, most daycare services do not offer transportation, although special needs municipal transportation may be available.

Funding for adult daycare is fragmented and changing. The sources of funding vary from fee-for-service, Medicaid, Older Americans Act, and various state sources. Adult daycares cannot receive funding from Medicare or Medicaid unless medical services are provided. Because of the poor funding, adult daycare services can be costly to the patient. Daily fees vary, but are almost always less than the cost of a home health visit.

Although families and patients report positive experiences with adult daycare, few studies have been done showing its benefits. A Cochrane review showed that daycare appeared to be more effective than no treatment when comparing morbidity, mortality, and dependency; however, daycare services were not more beneficial when compared with other comprehensive home elderly services.[17] In stroke patients, studies have shown that daycare hastened functional recovery and reduced outpatient visits without increasing costs; studies also have shown a reduction in hospitalizations and institutionalizations.[18]

There are no national quality measures available to benchmark standards for adult day services, but studies are underway to build a baseline of quality indicators to encourage national comparison. Guidelines for adult daycare are available at www.aspe.hhs.gov/daltcp/reports/adultday.htm.

Residential Care Facilities

Residential care facilities (RCFs) include facilities variously known as adult care, personal care, adult board and care homes, or domiciliary care homes; adult congregate living facilities, or assisted-living facilities (ALFs). RCFs were designed as less expensive, and often more appropriate, alternatives to nursing home placement for older persons with chronic care needs. Although both nursing homes and RCFs provide housing and care to elders with disabilities, a number of important characteristics differentiate them, such as 1) their philosophical orientations, 2) the knowledge and skills of workers, 3) limitations on the types of services provided, 4) limitations on the needs of the residents, and 5) the degree of regulation by federal and state governments.

The numbers of RCFs and RCF residents are growing rapidly. There are an estimated 45,000 RCFs serving nearly a million people, a substantial gain from earlier estimates.[19] Whereas RCFs were originally designed to serve elders with uncomplicated needs and few medical problems, the increased

acuity level of residents in nursing homes is having a "downstream" impact. RCFs now commonly provide services to elders with complicated and unstable mental and physical problems, and many cater specifically to individuals with dementia.

Just as RCFs were designed to be different from nursing homes, their regulation was also designed differently. Unlike nursing homes, where the U.S. Centers for Medicare and Medicaid Services sets the standards that qualify a facility for federal Medicare/Medicaid funding, states are the primary regulators of RCFs. Across states, there are no generally agreed upon standards for care and no consensus about which RCFs should be licensed. States establish their own requirements and may provide little oversight or protection for residents. Overall, changes in the long-term care system have resulted in large numbers of physically and mentally disabled elders receiving care in what is a largely unregulated industry.

ALFs and adult board and care homes are two examples in the continuum of Residential Care Facilities.

ALFs originally were designed to serve those who needed care intermediate between independent living and skilled nursing facilities (SNFs.) The National Center for Assisted Living estimates that there are approximately 33,000 assisted-living residences housing approximately 800,000 people. ALFs may offer individual houses, town houses, condominiums, or apartments that often incorporate disability features and assistive technology. They can be located in freestanding facilities or on a campus with other facilities.

Assisted living traditionally has provided meals and special diets, housekeeping, recreational, social, and educational activities, transportation, emergency help, and only limited assistance with ADLs and personal care. More and more ALFs are offering many levels of care, including more ADL and IADL assistance, as well as nursing care. The services offered vary from institution to institution, but laws in most states require ALFs to provide 24-hour staff, help with ADLs and IADLs, some health-related services, social services, recreational services, meals, housekeeping/laundry, and transportation. Consequently, ALFs are beginning to blur the line between community and institutionally based long-term care. Generally, there is no medical director or physician employed by the ALF.

Seniors living in ALFs usually are fairly independent, but there are no definite guidelines. The average age of residents in an ALF is 75 years but more than 50% of residents are older than 85 years. Comorbidities and dependencies vary among residents, but 25% have moderate-to-severe dementia, 33% have urinary incontinence, 51% needed assistance with bathing, 77% received assistance with medications, 93% need help with IADLs, and 81% need help with at least one of their ADLs. Although these percentages seem high, they are similar to those for patients living at home and being cared for by family members and home services, although not as severe as nursing home patients.[20]

Traditionally, assisted-living costs are not covered by Medicare, Medicaid, or private insurance; however, resources vary from state to state. Fairly recently, the Deficit Reduction Act temporarily allowed minimal Medicaid funding for nonnursing home care including ALFs. Residency in ALFs can be costly, ranging from $1500–$6000/month depending on the quality and services provided.

Regulation of ALFs is relatively limited, primarily because the facilities usually are not recipients of federal or state funding. Those regulations that exist, such as staffing, are enacted by the states. No specific standardized measures of quality of care are in effect yet. One study adapted the observable indicators of Nursing Home Care Quality Instrument to fit residential care facilities; this showed some promise as a potential set of guidelines on which to base quality care measurements.[21] ALFs can choose to be accredited by the Joint Commission on the Accreditation of Healthcare Organizations but few pursue this. In 2001, the U.S. Senate Special Committee on Aging commissioned a comprehensive national report that called for widespread quality improvements in assisted living and provided guidelines for both federal and state policy and state regulations.

Adult board and care homes are designed to serve older adults who require supervision and some personal care, but few onsite medical services. They are privately operated and are often converted single-family homes. State law and local zoning regulations determine the exact number of residents allowed (approximately 2–20).

Board and care homes typically provide a basic room (may be shared), meals, some assistance with daily activities, custodial help (including reminders to take medications, laundry, housekeeping, transportation), and supervision. Depending on licensing, the home may provide assistance with ADLs (such as bathing and grooming), dispensing of medications, dementia care, basic nursing care, and social, recreational, and spiritual activities. Many board and care homes are unlicensed, and states may only infrequently monitor the licensed homes. As a consequence, elder abuse can be an issue.

LONG-TERM SUPPORTIVE CARE

Long-term supportive care includes the many services that support functionally impaired elders in their ADLs or IADLs to allow them to remain safely at home. Informal caregiving, the most common form of long-term care in the United States, is unpaid care in the home provided by a spouse, adult child, other relative, friend, or neighbor. These caregivers provide an estimated 80% of all home- and community-based care, and one in five U.S. households is involved in caregiving for persons aged 18 and older. Most informal caregivers are women, and approximately 30% of persons caring for elderly long-term care recipients are themselves aged 65 years or older.

Informal long-term care often demands intense effort, and affects the physical and psychological health of the caregiver. Especially stressful caregiving situations may increase the risk of caregiver abuse or neglect of care recipients. Use of caregiver support services has been shown to have positive effects,

and includes the National Family Caregiver Support Program, support groups, and respite care. Other community-based supportive services include attendant care, personal care, housekeeping and homemaking, and home-delivered meals. Senior Centers/Congregate Meal Sites provide older adults a supportive environment for socialization and recreational activities. Most senior centers and all other congregate meal sites offer a meal, and transportation to sites may be available.

THE PROGRAM OF ALL-INCLUSIVE CARE FOR THE ELDERLY

Many states have requested "waivers" to pay for normally uncovered home- and community-based services for Medicaid-eligible persons who might otherwise be institutionalized. One state option is known as the PACE[22] a capitated benefit that features a comprehensive service delivery system and integrated Medicare and Medicaid financing. In 1987, inspired by San Francisco's On Lok program, Medicare and Medicaid started a demonstration program option called PACE. In 1997, the Balanced Budget Act legislated PACE to be considered on a state-by-state basis as a permanent Medicaid waiver provider. PACE functions within the Medicare program as well.

Participants must be at least 55 years old, live in the PACE service area, and be certified as eligible for nursing home care by the appropriate state agency. While enrolled, the participant must receive Medicare and Medicaid benefits solely through the PACE organization. PACE benefits for all participants include a comprehensive package of services, such as medical care, personal care and support, meals, transportation, restorative therapies, prosthetics and other durable medical equipment, medications, laboratory tests, x-rays and other diagnostic procedures, acute inpatient care, nursing facility care, and other services determined necessary by an interdisciplinary team. PACE care is provided in adult day health centers, homes, hospitals, and nursing homes. Each PACE center must have a comprehensive interdisciplinary team that is responsible for initial and periodic assessments, care planning, and coordination of 24-hour care delivery.

THE VETERANS HEALTH ADMINISTRATION

The Veterans Health Administration (VHA) offers a spectrum of geriatric and extended care services to enrolled veterans through its 159 VHA medical centers, more than 700 ambulatory care and community-based clinics, 134 nursing homes, and 42 domiciliaries. More than 90% of the VHA medical centers provide home and community-based outpatient long-term care programs. Among the continuum of services are the Home-Based Primary Care Program, Contract Home Health Care, Adult Day Health Care, Homemaker and Home Health Aide (H/HHA), Community Residential and Domiciliary Care, Respite Care, Home Hospice Care, and Telehealth programs.

THE INDIAN HEALTH SERVICE

The Indian Health Service (IHS), an agency within the Department of Health and Human Services, is an additional resource for community-based care for American Indian and Alaska Native elders. Although comprehensive, integrated long-term care has not been a part of the total package of health care provided by the IHS, local sites and Indian Health sites, both tribal and federal, have utilized IHS appropriations to support community-based long-term care services. For example, the IHS Public Health Nursing and Community Health Representative programs provide skilled nursing visits, case management, personal care, and transportation. The IHS also provides grant funding to support the planning and implementation of community-based long-term care by tribes and communities.[23] Other community-based long-term care services are provided by tribal area agencies on aging.

Suggested Resources: Information and Referral Services; Federal government information for seniors, www.seniors.gov; Healthfinder (U.S. Department of Health and Human Services), www.healthfinder.gov/; The National Hospice and Palliative Care, www.nhpco.org.

REFERENCES

1. Center for Home Care Policy and Research. Policy Brief, No. 22. *Long-Term Care: An Overview.* 2005. Available at: http://www.vnsny.org/research/. Accessed in June 21, 2008.
2. Family Caregiver Alliance. *Selected Long-Term Care Statistics.* 2000. Available at: http://www.caregiver.org/caregiver. Accessed June 21, 2008.
3. U.S. General Accounting Office. *Aging Baby Boom Generation Will Increase Demand and Burden on Federal and State budgets* [GAO-02–544T]. 2002. Available at: www.gao.gov/. Accessed June 21, 2008.
4. American Medical Association, Council on Scientific Affairs. Home care in the 1990's. *JAMA.* 1990;263:1241–1244.
5. Levine SA, et al. Home Care. *JAMA.* 2003;290:1203–1207.
6. Ramsdell JW et al. The yield of a home visit in the assessment of geriatric patients. *J Am Geriatr Soc.* 1989;37:17–24.
7. McAlister FA, Stewart S, Ferrua S, McMurray JJ. Multidisciplinary strategies for the management of heart failure patients at high risk for admission: a systematic review of randomized trials. *J Am Coll Cardiol.* 2004;44:810–819.
8. Pearson S, et al. Prolonged effects of a home-based intervention in patients with chronic illness. *Arch Intern Med.* 2006;166:645–650.
9. Smith KL, Ornstein, K. Soriano, T, Muller D, Boal J. A multidisciplinary program for delivering primary care to the underserved urban homebound: looking back, moving forward. *J Am Geriatr Soc.* 2006;54:1283–1289.
10. Muramatsu N, Mensali E, Cornwell T. A Physician Housecall Program for the Homebound. VNA Housecalls of Greater Cleveland Home Health Care Serv Q. 2006.
11. Hughes SL, et al. Department of VA Cooperative Study Group on Home-based Primary Care. Effectiveness of team-managed home-based primary care: a randomized multicenter trial. *JAMA.* 2000;284:2877–2885.
12. Smith KL, Soriano TA, Boal J. Brief communication. National quality-of-care standards in home-based primary care. *Ann Intern Med.* 2007;146:188–192.
13. Shepperd S, Illiffe, S. Hospital-at-home versus in-patient hospital care. *Cochrane Database Syst Rev.* 2005, Issue 2 Art.
14. Leff B, Burton L, Mader SL, et al. Hospital-at-home: feasibility and outcomes of a program to provide hospital-level care at home for acutely ill older patients. *Ann Intern Med.* 2005;143:798–808.
15. Steele L, et al. The quality of life of hospice patients: patient and provider perceptions. *Am J Hospice Palliative Med.* 2005;22:95–110.
16. National Adult Day Services Association. *Adult Day Services: The Facts.* Available at: http://www.nadsa.org/. Accessed in June 21, 2008.
17. Forster A, Young J, Langhorne P, for the Day Hospital Group. Medical day hospital care for the elderly versus alternative forms of care. *Cochrane Database Syst Rev.* 1999;3:CD001730.
18. LeFaou A-L, et al. "A geriatric day care unit: a health promoting hospital initiative. *Promo Educ.* 2004;11:1–16.
19. Consumer Reports. Assisted living: how much assistance can you really count on? 2005;70:28–33.
20. Golant S. Do impaired older persons with health care needs occupy U.S. assisted living facilities? An analysis of six national studies. *J Gerontol Soc Sci.* 2004;59B:S68–S79.
21. Aud M, et al. Developing a residential care facility version of the observable indicators of nursing home care quality instrument. *J Nurs Care Qual.* 2004;19:48–57.
22. Centers for Medicare and Medicaid Services. *PACE.* Available at; http://www.cms.hhs.gov/pace/. Accessed June 21, 2008.
23. Elder Care Initiative Long Term Care Grant Program, Office of Clinical and Preventive Services, Indian Health Service, U.S. Department of Health and Human Services. *Fed Reg.* 71(73);April 17, 2006. Notices.

43

INSTITUTIONAL LONG-TERM CARE

Rebecca D. Elon, MD, MPH, Marshall B. Kapp, JD, MPH

QUALITY NURSING HOME CARE: REFORM AND UTOPIA

The American nursing facility is an important community resource, a refuge of last resort for those among us whose needs exceed the capacities of our families to provide care at home. Although often feared and reviled, the American nursing home is a dynamic microcosm, a subculture within the broader community. Nursing homes reflect the values of the communities of which they are a part. The call for "culture change" within the nursing home is really a call for an examination and evolution of the parent culture that created the nursing home in the first place.[1] If the nursing home neglects its residents, the blame in part may be placed at the feet of the community. Although a corporation may own the nursing home, it belongs to the community in a moral sense. In America today, however, we are more apt to adopt a highway than a nursing home or the nursing home resident without any family of her own.

The best nursing homes are likely to be those staffed by local men and women who take pride in their work and are respected for helping their neighbors care for family members who are infirm and disabled.[2] They are likely to be those facilities in which: families, including children, remain actively involved in the lives of their loved ones entrusted into institutional care; organizations such as faith communities, schools, and clubs are routinely present to enrich and enhance the quality of life for the residents; and frail older people can remain spiritually alive and engaged in relationships, celebrations, and community life. The best nursing homes have corporate leadership and ownership that understand and act on their responsibility, not just for shareholder profits, but also for the social fabric within the facility and their relationship to the community at large.

Although much is written about the problems and shortcomings associated with nursing facility care and calls for reform are ubiquitous, little is written that articulates a utopian vision of what ideal care should be. Yet, the concepts of reform and utopia go hand in hand. Without a clear vision of where we wish to go, efforts for reform will lead us blindly nowhere. Richard Hofstadter viewed the surge for reform as a quintessentially American phenomenon, defining much of nineteenth and twentieth century American politics. "A great part of both the strength and weakness of our national existence lies in the fact that Americans do not abide very quietly the evils of life. We are forever relentlessly pitting ourselves against them, demanding changes, improvements, remedies, but not often with sufficient sense of the limits the human condition in the end insistently imposes upon us."[3]

History may well judge the American nursing home reform movement as one of the great democratic social reform efforts of the late twentieth century. The origins of nursing home reform can be traced back to a book published in 1977 by Linda Horn and Elma Holder (nee Griesel).[4] In her introduction to this book, Gray Panther founder Maggie Kuhn stated that institutional care, in and of itself, is by its very nature a destructive force for both older and younger people alike. In her call for expanding community-based services to meet the needs of disabled persons of all ages in their own homes, she acknowledged that institutional care is unlikely to be eliminated entirely. "We cannot shrug off nursing home reform for the home health bandwagon." Horn and Holder proclaimed, "the long-term care required by the old and disabled should be one of the most tender and effective services a society provides."[4] Their book documented the failures of the nursing home industry and health professionals, including physicians, to meet the needs of the institutionalized population. Its reform agenda focused heavily on correcting the failures of government oversight, and demanded enhanced government intervention. This book was the precursor to the formation of the National Citizens Coalition for Nursing Home Reform (see www.nccnhr.org), the 1986 Institute of Medicine Report on improving nursing home care through improved regulation,[5] and the federal nursing home reform amendments of the Omnibus Budget Reconciliation

Act of 1987 with their subsequent interpretive guidelines for surveyors and enforcement regulations.[6] It is remarkable how much of Horn and Holder's citizens' action guide blueprint was indeed implemented over the ensuing 30 years, focusing on regulation and direct government intervention. It is instructive to note that Elma Holder, founder of the National Citizens Coalition for Nursing Home Reform (NCCNHR) worked for Ralph Nader early in her career. The approach to nursing home reform that she led through NCCNHR may be labeled "Naderian," in that it promulgated a command and control style of government regulatory intervention and enforcement.[7] The regulatarian approach to improving nursing home care has dominated the past 30 years of reformist intervention.

Although it is widely accepted that the nursing home reform regulations have resulted in improvements in certain aspects of care[8,9] we certainly have not yet achieved the utopian vision of nursing home care that successful reform would demand.[10,11] The Eden Alternative[12,13] founded by William Thomas, acknowledges that even nursing homes with perfect scores on the state and federal regulatory inspection surveys do not provide the kind of care that most people would want for themselves or their loved ones. Thomas identified the major problems encountered by the nursing home residents as loneliness, helplessness, and boredom. He labels these the three plagues. They are indeed existential plagues that are beyond the scope of current regulatory mechanisms. Interventions to combat the three plagues focus on companionship with children, animals, and plants, and giving the residents opportunities to participate in the community of caring. The Eden Alternative combats the regimented nature of institutional life that a focus on regulatory compliance tends to create. Thomas' introduction to the Eden Alternative quotes John Milton's *Paradise Lost*, and the summary statement calls the Eden Alternative the beginning of an epic journey.[13] In its name and its mission the Eden Alternative is utopian in scope. Although it will not likely replace regulation as the dominant force in American nursing home reform, it can certainly guide us in our search for the utopia of elder care. Even NCCNHR, the leading proponent and advocate for a tough regulatory approach to quality improvement, discovered in surveying nursing home residents that being treated with kindness was the most important factor for the residents' own perceptions of quality care.[14] The survey agency has stated it has no way of measuring kindness and no regulatory mandate that allows it to give citations for lack of kindness, unless the magnitude of its absence rises to the level of actual abuse. Therefore, from a regulatory perspective, this most important factor for residents is not on the radar screen in a substantive fashion. Nancy Foner has documented that our current system of care selects for workers who are efficient, rather than kind, and that those workers who exhibit extraordinary kindness find it interferes with efficiency. They therefore often are fired or flee the nursing home work environment.[15]

The opposite of utopia has been termed dystopia. If utopia is the place where everything is perfect, then dystopia is where everything is imperfect.[16] If striving for utopia is the mission

to create heaven on earth, then dystopia is hell on earth. For many frail elders, nursing homes still are viewed and experienced as dystopian environments, despite 30 years of efforts for reform. "We need the idea of an improvable human society, because without it we slide into dystopia. But if you try to implement a utopia in a doctrinaire, programmatic way, you are going to end up with dystopia. You have to keep the spirit of utopia alive without trying to impose it in any wholesale Pol Pot way."[16]

The remainder of this chapter will explore legal aspects and medical aspects of promoting quality care for those entrusted to our nation's nursing homes. Can law and medicine help us achieve the vision for caring for frail elders within nursing facilities that provide technically expert and compassionate care, that are freed from the three plagues, and are indeed valued as an important community resource in which residents and family members can be confident of receiving excellence in service? The answer may lie in our ability to apply our current knowledge in action within our local communities.

PROMOTING QUALITY LONG-TERM CARE IN INSTITUTIONAL SETTINGS: LEGAL CONSIDERATIONS

Legal Regulation of Nursing Homes

The Current Regulatory Environment

Nursing homes in the United States today are extensively regulated legally in a broad variety of ways. The regulatory environment, both as it actually exists and as it is perceived by regulated providers and their risk management advisors and insurers, exerts a powerful influence on the access to, and quality of, services experienced by prospective and existing nursing home residents.

First, nursing homes are subject to regulatory penalties being imposed as part of the required annual state licensure renewal and Medicare/Medicaid survey and certification processes. Applicable standards for nursing homes are contained in state licensure statutes and the federal Omnibus Budget Reconciliation Act of 1987 and its implementing administrative regulations and interpretive guidelines for state survey agencies. Sanctions for deviation from required standards may include suspension or revocation of the facility's license to operate, termination of the Medicare and/or Medicaid provider agreement that is necessary for the facility's financial survival, temporary receivership, denial of payment for all admissions or for new admissions, civil money penalties, state monitoring, transfer of residents, a directed plan of correction, or directed in-service training. In addition to being subject to mandatory federal – and state government – established standards, many nursing homes voluntarily agree to comply with the standards set by private accrediting bodies, most notably the Joint Commission on Accreditation of Healthcare Organizations (JCAHO). Even though neither JCAHO nor any other private accrediting body currently provides for nursing homes the kind of "deemed status" (making a separate government inspection unnecessary) enjoyed by JCAHO in the acute care hospital context, a number of nursing homes pursue private accreditation as a marketing tool.

Additionally, criminal prosecutions may be initiated by local prosecutors and states' Attorneys General charging nursing homes and/or individual staff members with abuse and neglect of residents and, in the case of deceased residents, even homicide.[17] Also, federal prosecutors working in collaboration with the Department of Health and Human Services' Office of the Inspector General have brought several criminal indictments against nursing homes based on the theory that a nursing home that bills the Medicare or Medicaid programs for payments when the care provided was of substandard quality is guilty of defrauding the government in violation of the False Claims Act. The submission of allegedly fraudulent claims through the mail or electronic transfers allows the government to additionally invoke the Mail and Wire Fraud Acts, which are considered predicate offenses (i.e., offenses that may create criminal liability) under the federal Racketeer Influenced and Corrupt Organizations Act. Moreover, most states have enacted their own counterparts to the federal False Claims Act, making it unlawful to fraudulently bill their respective state Medicaid programs.

Criminal prosecutions initiated against nursing homes are relatively infrequent, but extensively publicized when they do occur and carry the possibility of substantial penalties upon conviction or guilty plea. In addition to criminal penalties, conviction under the civil version of the False Claims Act exposes nursing homes to significant monetary fines. The threat of legal action being brought against a nursing home is exacerbated by the right of private individuals to act as "private Attorneys General" or "relators" and bring their own civil False Claims Act *qui tam* (whistleblower) actions against nursing homes. If the government chooses to bring a criminal prosecution based on the relator's evidence, then the relator receives between 15% and 25% of the ultimate recovery.

Historically, nursing home residents have been quite statistically underrepresented as plaintiffs in private civil lawsuits brought by or on behalf of particular residents against specific facilities and/or their staff members claiming professional malpractice. Attorneys working under contingency fee arrangements generally have not been eager to represent old, frail, unemployed individuals with short life expectancies because such individuals have a limited ability to command substantial compensatory damages under the American civil justice system. Nursing home residents whose care is paid for by Medicaid have lacked a financial incentive to sue because most of their financial recovery would ordinarily be diverted either to repay the state for providing care or to resident spend down until a new period of Medicaid eligibility became effective. Furthermore, proving that the nursing home's negligent conduct proximately or directly caused the injury often is difficult for a plaintiff who already had multiple, serious underlying medical problems. Finally, the majority of older nursing home residents just did not have the physical and mental stamina, and the availability of adequate support by family or friends, needed to initiate,

prosecute, and (literally) outlive the demands of complex civil litigation.

For a variety of reasons, including the enactment of legislation in multiple jurisdictions facilitating (and even encouraging) the filing of personal injury claims against nursing homes, the increased availability of a cadre of willing plaintiff expert witnesses, and a growing propensity of trial juries to award large judgments (often including punitive or exemplary damages) in nursing home malpractice cases, the legal picture has changed. The plaintiffs' personal injury bar has discovered and begun to cultivate this potentially lucrative sphere of practice, as widespread advertising for nursing home clients by plaintiffs' attorneys abundantly illustrates. As plaintiffs' attorneys representing allegedly injured residents and/or their families often work collaboratively with nursing home residents' advocates, long-term care ombudsmen offices, consumer groups, and government and private regulators, the volume of civil malpractice actions brought against nursing homes and staff has escalated dramatically. Most civil claims initiated against nursing homes stem factually from alleged medical care problems (such as the development of pressure ulcers and the occurrence of medication errors), falls, resident-to-resident assaults, resident abuse, elopements, and violations of residents' rights.

Nursing homes also may be subject to suit for discriminating in their provision of services. Requirements of the Americans with Disabilities Act and the Rehabilitation Act, as well as their state counterparts, regarding affirmative obligations to accommodate disabled persons apply with full force to nursing homes both as places of public accommodation and recipients of government payments. Moreover, a nursing home encounters the possibility of legal claims based on allegations that, by providing inadequate services, it violated express or implied promises made to the resident in the admission agreement.

Behavioral Manifestations of the Regulatory Environment

The current extensive regulatory and litigation climate engulfing nursing home operations in the United States creates a great deal of anxiety and apprehension among individual and institutional long-term care providers. Overwhelmingly, regulators (including plaintiffs' attorneys and the courts) are seen by providers as police officers who only review nursing homes' performance for the purpose of finding noncompliance and applying sanctions, rather than as consultants who share information with providers to help them improve practice and solve problems that might otherwise lead to legal violations. Worse yet, providers generally believe that regulators carry out their policing role in an arbitrary and capricious fashion, driven in their aggressiveness more by local political forces than by a fair and accurate factual appraisal of the circumstances. As stated in one comprehensive report:

Indeed, one of the most disconcerting aspects of government regulation of long-term care is its inconsistent application both within and across regions over time. Providers want consistency in the regulatory environment – it is difficult to play by the rules if the interpretation of the rules keeps changing or varies from one area to another.[18]

This legally induced apprehension exerts an important impact on provider behaviors in a panoply of ways. Some of these behavioral manifestations are salutary, such as paying more attention to residents' rights, more careful and constrained use of physical and chemical restraints, more complete documentation of care, and the implementation of more rigorous quality-assurance and resident safety mechanisms. Some of the kinds of behaviors inspired by providers' perceptions of a police model of external oversight ("Let's catch the bad guys and punish them") actually affect antitherapeutically the manner in which providers relate to residents.[19] The phenomenon of negative defensive practice or (at least perceived) risk management resulting from an atmosphere of shame, blame, and punishment has led many both within and outside of the nursing home industry to recommend that "[t]he relationships among regulators, providers, clinicians, quality improvement organizations and, of course, the consumer, need to be re-examined in order to realign incentives, to be 'smarter' about regulations, and to regulate more transparently."[18]

Legal anxieties influence provider behaviors, and hence residents' quality of care and quality of life, in many respects. For one thing, apprehension about exposure to negative legal (and consequently financial) consequences inhibits much needed efforts to improve the timely and honest reporting, disclosure, and dissection of errors in resident care. Admitting errors to health care consumers and their families, who generally are the de facto if not the de jure plaintiffs in malpractice lawsuits, is difficult for providers in all care delivery environments, but the problem is even more complicated in the nursing home setting. Family members, often feeling guilty and unhappy about their need to admit a loved one to a nursing home in the first place, may be antagonistic toward the nursing home and even more disposed toward pursuing legal redress for perceived shortcomings than would be families of consumers in other health care settings. Nursing home staff are reminded daily of the frequently strained rapport with families, and this surely discourages open acknowledgment of, and therefore opportunities for positive learning from, facility errors.

Moreover, providers' legal apprehensions may play out negatively in terms of encouraging behaviors that, ironically, conflict with fuller respect for residents' rights. If, for example, a nursing home is concerned about being held liable for the injuries sustained by a resident who trips and falls while carrying a tray of food back to his room where he prefers to eat, then the facility is likely to pursue the goal of resident safety in this situation even when that means adopting a policy that forbids residents from eating their meals in their own preferred locations. Overly defensive, risk-averse behavior that limits or coerces resident options is, in addition to its violation of the ethical autonomy principle, antitherapeutic because it teaches residents learned helplessness and conveys to them a lost sense of control.

When finite staff time and energy is suboptimally allocated because of perceived risk management demands, there may be a detriment to the quality of resident care. Additionally, facilities may refuse to share, or unduly encumber the sharing of, pertinent resident information out of concern about liability for claimed breaches of confidentiality, especially in light of the federal Health Insurance Portability and Accountability Act, thereby imperiling the optimal continuity of care for residents who need to go back and forth between the nursing home and hospital, rehabilitation facility, or outpatient setting.

One area in which provider behavior driven in a perverse direction by anxieties about the legal environment is especially harmful is that of medical care for residents nearing the end of life. In this context, legal anxieties may compel nursing homes to overtreat (and thereby jeopardize the comfort and dignity of) dying residents with nonbeneficial or only marginally beneficial technological interventions such as artificial feeding and hydration, respirators, antibiotics, dialysis, and cardiopulmonary resuscitation. Such disproportionately aggressive intervention not infrequently takes place despite the existence of an advance directive or do not resuscitate order instructing providers to do the opposite.

Conversely, legal worries may induce providers to insufficiently treat dying residents. Undertreatment may occur in the sense of providers refraining from, because of concern about criminal prosecution under narcotics control statutes or disciplinary action before the state medical licensing board, or skimping on adequate pain control for residents who clinically require narcotics such as opioids to alleviate their serious pain. Undertreatment also may take the form of failing to give a resident a time-limited trial of a particular potentially beneficial treatment out of a misguided, but understandable, concern that it would be difficult if not impossible to ever discontinue the intervention once it had been initiated.

Another perverse but unfortunately common behavioral manifestation of providers' felt need to avoid regulatory sanctions and malpractice litigation involves premature or unnecessary transfers of critically ill residents to hospital emergency departments when it appears (usually to a nurse who is relaying information to a physician by telephone) that the resident's survival is imminently endangered. When a resident without clear limitation orders in the medical chart "goes sour" (even when this turn of events has been anticipated), nursing homes routinely transfer the resident to the hospital to try to protect themselves from state surveyors and family members who may find fault because the resident expired within the facility. This defensive behavior is undesirable for several reasons, among them the facts that the quality of end-of-life care in hospitals often leaves much to be desired from a humane perspective and that transfer to a hospital may conflict with the resident's strong preference regarding the site of end-of-life care and the dying process and event.

Finally (although this brief list of the adverse repercussions of negative legally defensive practice does not purport to be complete), when regulation imposes extra financial costs on providers without producing a greater corresponding benefit for residents, those costs – ultimately borne by the residents – are harmful. For the resident, regulatory costs may take the form of higher monetary fees for services (for privately paying residents), decreased quality of care because of staffing cutbacks made in response to budgetary constraints, or reduced availability of valuable but legally optional activities.

Opportunities for Improvement

Despite the several useful functions it serves, the prevailing regime of negative command and control regulation coupled with private malpractice litigation is inadequate, and may actually be counterproductive, to the task of maximizing resident quality of care and quality of life in nursing homes. Positive incentives to supplement the combined regulatory bludgeon are essential.

Positive incentives may take a variety of forms. First, changing the methodology through which Medicaid and Medicare payments to nursing homes are calculated to reward facilities for performance in providing a relatively higher quality of care and life for their residents, based mainly on realistic outcome measures, could be a valuable "carrot" to encourage desirable provider conduct.

Second, facilitating the collection and dissemination of information to the public regarding quantitative indicia of quality of care and quality of life measured in particular nursing homes can empower potential residents and their families to wield meaningful clout within the competitive environment of nursing home marketing. Informed consumer choice, in turn, creates a continuous incentive for nursing homes to improve quality so as to compete successfully for customers to fill their beds.

Third, industry initiatives – whether truly voluntary or undertaken in reaction to exogenous pressures – aimed at affirmatively changing the nursing home environment should be encouraged and supported as a fundamental adjunct to regulatory strategies more narrowly (and negatively) focused on the limited goal of preventing calamities rather than making good things happen. "Smart" regulations thus will coordinate synergistically with industry efforts to facilitate a robust marketplace rather than supplant it. It is imperative "that we rationalize and integrate the precepts of quality improvement and regulatory oversight in a manner that is transparent and sends a clear message to long-term care providers."[18]

PROMOTING QUALITY LONG-TERM CARE IN INSTITUTIONAL SETTINGS: MEDICAL CONSIDERATIONS

The services offered by American nursing facilities have changed significantly since the 1980s. This is based on changes in reimbursement to hospitals and opportunities for nursing facilities to admit postacute or subacute patients with higher medical acuity, leading to higher rates of facility reimbursement. The change in nursing facility populations and programs

has necessitated a change in the organization of the medical care delivered there. Medical care delivery to nursing facility patients/residents in many settings is still playing "catch up" with the programmatic and structural changes that have already occurred in the facilities. This section focuses on the programs and populations found in nursing facilities and current approaches to medical care delivery in response to these changes.

POPULATIONS AND PROGRAMS

Short-Stay Residents/Patients in the Nursing Facility

Postacute, Subacute Care

Although the American nursing home is considered a site for "institutional long-term care," it houses many short-stay, short-term care programs. Many nursing facilities provide rehabilitation services for patients after stroke, joint replacement, fracture repair, or for reconditioning and strengthening after an acute medical illness or surgery. The duration of stay for such short-term residents/patients is generally days to weeks. Medicare Part A includes a benefit that pays 100% for the first 20 days of skilled nursing facility care, if indicated by the patient's needs and progress. This benefit is only activated if the patient has a 3-night qualifying stay in an acute care hospital prior to nursing facility admission. After the first 20 days, there is a daily copayment ($119/day in 2007) for the care provided on days 21–100. Some, but not all, Medi-gap, secondary insurance policies will pay this copayment. After 100 days total, the Medicare benefit is exhausted and the patient converts to private pay if institutional skilled care or long-term care is required.[20] People who are enrolled in Medicare managed care programs will have different rules and requirements governing their eligibility for skilled nursing facility rehabilitation and postacute/subacute services. The 3-night hospital stay is typically waived for skilled benefit eligibility. These programs must offer as a minimum benefit at least what is offered through standard Medicare benefit.

The medical needs of rehabilitation patients are quite variable. These patients often need medical visits weekly, or more often if they are experiencing medical complications or set backs in their rehabilitation progress. In general, rehabilitation patients in the nursing facility are expected to return to independent living in their own homes.

In the early 1980s, in response to escalating hospital expenditures, Medicare changed its hospital reimbursement policy from a cost-plus methodology to a prospective payment system (PPS). Hospital reimbursement became based on the patient's diagnosis (known as the "diagnostic related group" [DRG]), which was calculated in part based on the average number of hospital days required to treat the main diagnosis responsible for the hospitalization. Because the payment to the hospital was the same whether the patient stayed for the average number of days or was discharged sooner or later than average, there was a huge financial incentive to discharge patients at least by the average duration of stay, and preferably sooner. If all of the hospital's patients could be discharged sooner than the average, revenue over expenses (i.e., profit or margin) would be maximized under the DRG-PPS system. This incentivized the hospital to discharge patients more quickly, often before the acute episode had been fully treated or stabilized.

The American nursing home industry responded to this demand for quicker hospital discharges by creating postacute or subacute care programs in their community nursing facilities. Patients who were too sick to be discharged directly home from the hospital could enter the nursing facility for ongoing medical monitoring and skilled nursing interventions; intravenous therapies such as prolonged courses of antibiotics or parenteral nutrition; chronic ventilatory support with or without attempts at weaning; complex wound care; hemodialysis or peritoneal dialysis; and/or rehabilitation, as described previously. The shift in Medicare hospital payment policy to the DRG-PPS methodology was a win–win situation for both hospital and nursing facility revenue generation. Its impact on the patients themselves and the quality or outcomes of the care delivered has never been fully evaluated. The structure and quality of medical care in most nursing facilities today is still playing "catch-up" in response to the higher-acuity needs of the patients in the postacute and subacute programs. This will be discussed in more detail in the section on the organization of nursing facility medical care. The goals and focus of the postacute and subacute nursing facility units are generally medical and short-term in nature.

Respite Care Residents/Patients

Another group of people who may be short-term residents/patients of nursing facilities are those who are admitted for respite care. These people generally pay the daily rate out of pocket, unless they have a long-term care insurance policy that includes a respite care benefit. The average daily rate for non–postacute/subacute nursing home care across the United States in 2006 was $206/day, or approximately $75,000/year.[21] A typical respite care scenario would be the short-term admission of a person with dementia who requires 24-hour supervision at home, so that the family caregiver could take a trip, attend to their own personal health issues such as the need for elective surgery, or just have a rest. Respite care residents/patients are usually medically stable and are expected to return to their homes in a matter of days or weeks. Eventually many of those admitted for recurrent short-term respite care become long-stay residents.

Terminal Care/Hospice Care in the Nursing Facility

End-of-life care has become part of the scope of practice of American nursing facilities. A decade or more ago, many nursing facilities transferred back to the hospital any resident/patient who was dying, for fear that a death in the facility might lead to a charge of negligence. With greater acceptance of advance directives and advance care planning, residents and their families have greater autonomy in deciding how they want

the end of life to be approached. There are people who wish to "rage against the dying of the light"[22] and want all possible medical interventions applied that might have even a small chance of prolonging life. Others recognize that repeated hospitalizations as death approaches and attempts at cardiopulmonary resuscitation for people with end-stage conditions are rarely useful and often traumatic to the dying person. For these people, hospice-type care in the nursing facility is often desirable. Although the Medicare Hospice benefit may be applied within the nursing facility, it cannot be implemented along with the Medicare Part A skilled nursing benefit. Because the Medicare Hospice benefit does not pay for the room and board aspect of nursing home care, those who qualify for the Medicare Part A skilled nursing benefit would have an increase in their out-of-pocket expenses by signing on to Medicare Hospice. Under these circumstances, hospice-type care may be employed without invoking the Medicare Hospice benefit, per se.

Long-Stay Residents/Patients in the Nursing Facility

Typically, over half of the long-term care residents in a nursing facility suffer from dementia. Over the last decade, in response to the demand for more homelike environments, the assisted living industry has built thousands of facilities that provide care in the community for frail elders who have dementia. This trend has left the more medically complex, functionally and behaviorally impaired residents with dementia in the nursing home. It has also made lack of resources a distinguishing feature between those persons with dementia who can afford to enter the higher-amenity assisted living site versus those who cannot afford assisted living and end up admitted to the more institutional, lower-amenity, nursing facility site, with Medicaid payment. Some states have Medicaid waivers that allow persons to leave the institutional nursing home setting and have Medicaid pay for the more homelike assisted living setting, which is often lower cost than the nursing home.

Disabled younger persons often must resort to living within a nursing home, when community options are inadequate for their care needs. The social needs of younger, physically impaired persons are dramatically different from the needs of frail elders with dementia, and often the nursing home struggles with meeting those needs. Although the preadmission screening and referral process is mandated by federal law and requires nursing facilities to identify persons with developmental disabilities and mental illness to promote community placement, it is rare that the preadmission screening and referral process actually results in an alternative site of care for these specialized populations. Specialized facilities and better community options are necessary to meet the needs of younger persons with functional deficits, including those with developmental disabilities and chronic mental illness. The nursing facility often remains the community refuge of last resort. Although the 1999 United States Supreme Court Olmstead Decision requires states to create community-based alternatives to institutional long-term care in the nursing facility, the alternative options in many states have been slow to emerge.

STRUCTURE OF NURSING FACILITY MEDICAL PRACTICE

Private Practitioner, Continuity of Care Model

It is desirable from a continuity of care perspective for a primary care physician to continue to care for his or her own patients once they enter a nursing facility. The long- established doctor–patient relationship can help the nursing home staff understand the new resident within a historical context. The physician can help the patient and family adjust to the strange, new environment and serve as a patient advocate within the facility. It was not long ago that primary care physicians followed their patients across any site of care in which they found themselves. Although the initial relationship was forged through the outpatient office, the physician would appear at the emergency room to care for the patient on an urgent basis, would serve as the attending physician during acute hospital episodes and for any nursing home stay, and would come to the home when the patient was too infirm to travel to the office.

Today emergency room visits are usually managed by the board-certified emergency medicine physician. The hospital admission is increasingly managed by the hospital-based inpatient team hospitalist physician. When intensive care is required, the attending in the intensive care unit is often a board-certified intensivist physician, and when nursing home care is needed, the care is often provided by a physician devoting all or much of his or her time to the nursing facility.

The ideal of continuity of care that was taught to twentieth-century medical students as a hallmark and pillar of quality primary care has fallen victim to the demand for efficiency, productivity, and the industrialization of medical care delivery in twenty-first-century America. Physicians today are more likely to define their practice by a particular site of care, i.e., the hospital, the emergency room, the intensive care unit, the office, or the nursing home, rather than define it by wherever the physician's patient may be.

The major factors determining where a person is admitted for nursing home care are geography (proximity to family), bed availability (to speed discharge from the hospital in communities where nursing facilities have high occupancy, regardless of proximity to family or physician), or specialty programs (such as dialysis onsite or chronic ventilator capacity). This means that a physician trying to provide continuity of care could have one or two patients in a dozen or more nursing facilities. This becomes logistically challenging to impossible, both for the physician and for the facility. Continuity of care remains an important principle, and primary care physicians who are able to provide high-quality care and meet all the regulatory requirements are usually welcome onto the nursing facility staff in most community settings. Often, however, it is in the best interests of the patient, the facility, and the physician to have

the nursing home resident assigned to a physician who has a high enough number of patients in the facility to warrant at least weekly onsite visits to the facility.

Private Practitioner, Unassigned Admissions Physician

Some physicians in private practice will accept patients under their care within the nursing facility when the patients' own attending physicians do not attend there. These patients are termed "unassigned admissions," as opposed to the patients who are assigned to their community physicians who are on staff at the facility. The physicians accepting unassigned admissions typically make visits on site at the nursing home several days each week and are responsive to the nursing staff calls. Most community nursing homes have several physicians in this category. Often new physicians in a community will find it advantageous to work with the local nursing home early in their career to build a caseload while the office-based practice is growing. Once the office practice has grown and is demanding more time, the physician may take him or herself off of the unassigned admissions roster or may leave the nursing home practice entirely.

Full-Time Facility-Based Physician

Some physicians work full time within a nursing facility. Settings employing full-time nursing home physicians include: academic facilities such as those affiliated with medical schools or teaching hospitals; governmental facilities such as Veterans Administration or state-owned nursing facilities; large religious or nonsectarian not-for-profit nursing facilities; and some large for-profit nursing facility chains. Some physicians in private practice have chosen to devote their careers to serving nursing home residents. In recent years malpractice insurance coverage for a physician practicing only in a nursing facility setting has been difficult to acquire in some jurisdictions due to the legal climate described previously.

Nurse Practitioner and Physician Assistant Care of Nursing Facility Residents

Although nurse practitioner (NP) and physician assistant (PA) scope of practice and licensing requirements vary state to state, federal Medicare policy has had a major impact on their ability to function within nursing facilities. In the late 1990s, Medicare's decision to allow NPs and PAs to have their own provider numbers and bill the Medicare system as independent practitioners allowed the expansion of NPs and PAs practice within nursing facilities. Prior to that decision, they were required to bill under the physician's Medicare number, "incident to" the physician's practice, effectively requiring that the physician be on-site at the time of the NP or PA visit. The NP or PA visits are billed under the same current procedural terminology codes used by the physicians, but Medicare reimburses their work at a discounted rate relative to physician reimbursement (85% in

2006.) Authorization of prescriptive privileges for NPs and PAs that occurred in many states in the 1990s also promoted their ability to play a major role in nursing facility care.

Another impact of Medicare reimbursement policy on the role of NPs and PAs within nursing facilities is the interpretation of the original Medicare legislation that requires the physician to make the "initial visit" to the nursing home resident within 30 days of admission to the facility. Centers for Medicare and Medicaid (CMS) has determined that this physician function cannot be delegated to the NP or PA. Current medical practice within nursing facilities often requires that the first visit to the nursing home resident be made within 24–72 hours of admission. NPs and PAs are often the ones to make this "first visit" due to purely logistical considerations within a busy medical practice. NPs and PAs are able to perform an initial history-taking and physical examination of a patient in all other sites of care including within the hospital. Therefore, this restriction on their practice within nursing facilities is anachronistic. CMS has had to issue numerous clarifications regarding this discrepancy between their payment rules and current standards of community practice.[21] CMS has indicated that the "first visit" can be made by the NP or PA if it is medically necessary prior to the "initial visit," which must be made within the first 30 days by the physician. If the NP or PA does make the "first visit" prior to the "initial visit" made by the physician, it must be billed as a "subsequent visit," even if the patient is new to the practice, because legislatively only the physician can bill for the "initial visit." These complicated sorts of semantic gymnastics reflect the fact that the federal government reimbursement policy should not be dictating how medical practice occurs in the community but rather should be responsive and supportive to the delivery of quality medical care to frail elders. The current methodology often obfuscates and denies frail elders access to the care that they need and deserve.

Medicare managed care programs that rely on NPs in the nursing facility are increasingly common but still serve less than 10% of all nursing home residents nationwide. Enrollment in the managed care product is necessary to access the NP's services. The financial success of such a model is based on controlling hospital utilization. A perceived weakness of this model is that the NP acts as both the primary clinician and gatekeeper for clinical services. Although the managed care NP model can improve outcomes for nursing home residents, additional mechanisms for increasing NP and PA activity in nursing facilities are necessary that do not force residents/patients into managed care models.

Future Models: Restructuring the Care Delivery and the Financing of Medical Care

The inadequate participation of physicians, NPs, and PAs in many nursing homes indicates a need for new practice structures for medical care in this setting. The current situation is in part a direct result of inadequate reimbursement strategies and the hostile regulatory atmosphere within nursing facilities.

In the mid 1980s in response to fraudulent "Medicaid Mill" "gang visits" within nursing facilities, Medicare refused to pay for more than one visit every 30 days, even if the physician provided documentation of medical necessity in trying to manage acute problems within the nursing home setting. Although this reimbursement limitation was removed in the 1990s, the current payment only for the face-to-face visit within the nursing facility does not cover the cost of the amount of time required to provide quality care to frail elders and postacute care patients. If Medicare is interested in paying for quality performance in the nursing facility, it must acknowledge through its reimbursement policies that communication with families, nursing home staff, and various members of the interdisciplinary team is essential. Medicare reimbursement will never cover the true cost of providing care to the nursing home population until it analyses and properly compensates clinicians for the time it takes to provide quality care, including all of the nonface-to-face communication, on-call time, and paperwork that is required.

In former times, the stipend paid to the facility medical director was considered a partial reimbursement for the time required to provide proper clinical care to the nursing home residents. Because the medical director is now required under federal regulation to perform an increasingly active and scrutinized administrative role within the nursing facility, and also is less likely to be the physician caring for the majority of the nursing home residents, this form of subsidy for nursing home clinical care is no longer adequate. Physician administrative work in today's medical marketplace generally is reimbursed at a higher rate than the physician's nonprocedural, evaluation and management clinical work. In that respect, more experienced physicians may need to perform increasing amounts of administrative work reimbursed by a third party, because Medicare reimbursement is the same, whether the physician is fresh out of training or has several decades of experience. Unlike other professions, such as law, where the senior partners bill at a higher rate than the junior partners, to cover their higher salary expectations, Medicare limits what any physician may receive for his or her time, regardless of rank, experience, expertise, or market demand for a particular clinician's outstanding skills and service. Thus, Medicare's monopoly on payment for clinical care for frail elders limits their access to the most highly skilled and experienced physicians. This is just one of the many factors in the need of reevaluation in how Medicare reimburses the care of frail elders.

Anytime an order is written for a nursing home resident to receive a controlled substance, federal Drug Enforcement Administration requirements mandate that the dispensing pharmacy have an original physician prescription on file, in addition to the order received from the nursing home. This anachronistic policy is unlikely to prevent diversion of controlled substances or result in any other benefit to the patient, the facility, or the integrity of the prescribing process. Yet millions of prescriptions are sent to physicians' offices each year for signature, creating an added burden of paperwork for any physician agreeing to do nursing facility work. This Drug

Enforcement Administration requirement should be reevaluated for its effectiveness and cost/benefit ratio, and abandoned unless its worth can be demonstrated.

Many physicians refuse to work in nursing homes because of the difficulty with inappropriate and excessive number of telephone calls from the staff all throughout the day and nighttime. Dysfunctional communication patterns are often a direct result of the hostile regulatory environment. Staff members are often "written up" for failing to call the physician in a timely fashion about every detail of resident care and life. One nursing home corporation actually stated that it views it to be in their best corporate interest to require staff to call physicians in the middle of the night for non-urgent issues, rather than have the staff fail to notify the physician, for example, about a fall with no injury at 3 AM. Although the facility does not receive a regulatory deficiency citation for "over notification," it does receive citations for failure of physician notification. The hidden cost to the facility, and to all nursing home residents, is that profligate abuse of physician availability results in reasonable physicians simply refusing to participate in such a system. Successful models for nursing home practice must address communication patterns between the facility and the clinicians. The American Medical Directors Association ([AMDA] www.amda.org) has developed protocols to help facilities and physicians collaborate on productive and safe mechanisms for information transfer. Nursing facilities should be able to rely on responsive physician participation; however, the facilities must be conscientious stewards of the resource of physician availability and access. In some of the newer structures of nursing home medical practice, all nursing home calls are handled by on-call NPs. They communicate electronically with the physician for nonurgent issues, and place an urgent telephone only call when a true emergency exists that is beyond the NP's scope of clinical decision making.

QUALITY IMPROVEMENT FOR NURSING HOME MEDICAL PRACTICE

Many organizations are promulgating various clinical practice guidelines for medical care of frail elders and medical care within the nursing facility. CMS,[24] the Rand Corporation,[25] AMDA,[26] American Geriatric Society,[27] and others have published guidelines for managing specific diseases or conditions. Guidelines for appropriate prescribing for frail elders have also been developed.[28,29] Concerns have been raised about the use of such guidelines in the population of elders who have multiple, chronic conditions and whose goals of care may be more appropriately palliative than curative or even restorative.[30–32] Most of these guidelines are based on expert opinion in the absence of randomized, controlled trials for the conditions prevalent within the nursing home population. Data on the feasibility of implementing such guidelines within the current staffing levels and structure of nursing home care are limited. Also lacking are data on outcomes of implementing clinical guidelines within the institutional setting.

Clinical practice guidelines are in a sense basic recipes that should have been learned in school. They may help guide or evaluate practice but like basic recipes in the kitchen, they cannot substitute for an experienced chef. "Developing skills in the kitchen has much to do with practice, like any physical activity requiring coordination. Yet it seems more to the point to address the question of how one develops a feel for cooking or how to arrive at the point when the recipe can be put aside and instinct and confident intuition take over. Good cooking is in the very best sense a craft, involving the heart, head and hands simultaneously. It is important to know what you are doing and why you are doing it. Cooking is commonsense practice, not alchemy. Listening and watching closely while you cook will reveal a richly shaded language understood by all the senses – the degrees of a simmer, the aroma of a roast telling you it is done, the stages of elasticity of kneaded dough, the earthy scent of a vegetable just pulled from the ground – it is everything to mind these details. This is cooking. Following a recipe rigidly is a dry, mechanical exercise unless you re-create it yourself by asking questions along the way, remaining alert and responsive, and making judgments of your own."[33] It is my wish that someday our clinical practice guidelines will appear as well-worn volumes on the shelf, and we will rediscover ourselves as experienced professional chefs.[33]

The most important factor in promoting quality medical care within the nursing facility is the active presence of physicians, NPs, and PAs who are technically knowledgeable about the care of frail elders, who are passionate about their commitment to quality care, who are capable of participating as active members of the interdisciplinary team, and who can weather the storms on the rocky coast of utopia.[34]

SUMMARY

Although the focus on increasing the availability of community-based long-term care services for frail elders and disabled persons of all ages is extremely important, as most people prefer to stay at home rather than enter an institutional setting, it is doubtful that the need for nursing facility services will completely disappear. A more balanced continuum of care is certainly an important public policy goal, with institutional long-term care constituting a less lopsided component in the future.

Although the purpose of legal and regulatory interventions is to improve the quality of care and the quality of life of nursing home residents, the current approaches may have "antitherapeutic effects." Government regulatory interventions and current legal approaches need to be evaluated for their efficacy in achieving the desired outcomes and also for their burdens, costs, and unintended negative consequences relative to the provision of high-quality nursing facility care. Reform may be needed within the extant mechanisms working to reform long-term care.

Expert and attentive medical care can play a large role in improving the overall quality of care and quality of life in a nursing facility. Innovations in the way that care is delivered and reimbursed are needed to serve appropriately the needs of the residents/patients. There are many exciting possibilities for physicians, NPs, and PAs to be part of an emerging cadre of health professionals committed to providing the highest quality of care for the elders of our nation. The future possibilities may be limited only by our imagination and diligence.

REFERENCES

1. Weiner AS, Ronch JL. *Culture Change in Long-term Care*. Binghamton, NY: Haworth Press; 2003.

2. Pillemer K. *Solving the Frontline Crisis in Long-term Care: A Practical Guide to Finding and Keeping Quality Nursing Assistants*. Cambridge, MA: Frontline Publishing; 1996.

3. Hofstadter R. *The Age of Reform*. New York: Vintage Books; 1960.

4. Horn L, Griesel E. *Nursing Homes: A Citizens' Action Guide*. Boston: Beacon Press; 1977.

5. The Committee on Nursing Home Reform. *Improving the Quality of Care in Nursing Homes. Institute of Medicine Report*. Washington DC: National Academy Press; 1986.

6. Medicare and Medicaid Programs: Survey certification and enforcement of skilled nursing facilities and nursing facilities; final rule. *Fed Reg*. November 10, 1994;59:42 CFR Parts 401, 431, 435, 440, 441, 442, 447, 483, 488, 489, and 498.

7. Bok D. *The Trouble with Government*. Cambridge, MA: Harvard University Press; 2001.

8. Detmer DE, McNeil BJ. *Improving the Quality of Long-term Care. Institute of Medicine Report*. Washington DC: National Academy Press; , 2001.

9. Kapp MB. Quality of care and quality of life in nursing facilities: what's regulation got to do with it? *McGeorge Law Rev*. 2000;31:707–721.

10. Kane RL, West JC. *It Shouldn't be this Way: The failure of Long-term Care*. Nashville: Vanderbilt Press; 2005.

11. Gass T. *Nobody's Home: Candid Reflections of a Nursing Home Aide*. Ithaca, NY: Cornell University Press; 2004.

12. Thomas WH. *Life Worth Living: How Someone You Love Can Still Enjoy Life in a Nursing Home. The Eden Alternative in Action*. Acton, MA: VanderWyk & Burnham: 1996.

13. Thomas WH. *What Are Old People For? How Elders Will Save the World*. Acton, MA: VanderWyk & Burnham: 2004.

14. Burger SG, Fraser V, Hunt S, Frank B. *Nursing Homes: Getting Good Care There*. San Luis Obispo, CA: Impact Publishers; 1996.

15. Foner N. *The Caregiving Dilemma: Work in an American Nursing Home*. Berkeley: University of California Press; 1994.

16. Atwood M. An imperfect world: an interview with Margaret Atwood. *Lincoln Center Theater Rev*. 2006, Fall/Winter; No 4311–4314.

17. Long S. *Death Without Dignity: The Story of the First Nursing Home Corporation Indicted for Murder*. Austin: Texas Monthly Press; 1987.

18. Miller EA, Mor V. Out of the Shadows: Envisioning a Brighter Future for Long Term Care in America. A Brown University Report for the National Commission for Quality Long Term Care. Providence, Rhode Island; 2006.

19. Kapp MB. *The Law and Older Persons: Is Geriatric Jurisprudence Therapeutic?* Durham: Carolina Academic Press; 2003.

20. Medicare and You. http://www.cons.hhs.gov/Partnership/22_MY.asp. Accessed October 14, 2008.

21. Provider Magazine, American HealthCare Association and National Center for Assisted Living, 2006. http://www.providermagazine.com. Accessed October 14, 2008.

22. Thomas D. *Do Not Go Gentle into that Good Night. The Poems of Dylan Thomas*. New York: New Directions Books; 1952.

23. Medicare Part B News Letter No.04–043, May 28, 2004.

24. www.medicare.gov

25. Saliba D, Solomon D, Rubenstein L, et al. Quality indicators for the management of medical conditions in nursing home residents. *J Am Med Dir Assoc*. 2004;5:297–309.

26. www.AMDA.org

27. www.AGS.org

28. Beers MH, Ouslander JG, Rollinger I, et al. Explicit criteria for determining inappropriate medication use in nursing home residents. *Arch Intern Med*. 1991;151:1825–1832.

29. Fick DM, Cooper JW, Wade WE, et al. Updating the Beers criteria for potentially inappropriate medication use in older adults: results of a US consensus panel of experts. *Arch Intern Med*. 2003;163:2716–2724.

30. Tinetti ME, Bogardus ST, Agostini JV. Potential pitfalls of disease-specific guidelines for patients with multiple conditions. *NEJM*. 2004;351:2870–2874.

31. Boyd CM, Darer J, Boult C, et al. Clinical practice guidelines and quality of care for older patients with multiple comorbid diseases: Implications for pay for performance. *JAMA*. 2005;294:716–724.

32. Durso SC. Using clinical guidelines designed for older adults with diabetes mellitus and complex health status. *JAMA*. 2006;295:1935–1940.

33. Bertolli P, Waters A. *Chez Pannise Cooking*. New York: Random House; 1987.

34. Stoppard T. *The Coast of Utopia. Part I, Voyage. Part II, Shipwreck. Part III, Salvage*. New York: Grove Press; 2002.

44

CARE FOR THE ELDERLY PATIENT AT THE END OF LIFE

Seema Modi, MD, Terri Maxwell, MSN, PhD

INTRODUCTION TO PALLIATIVE CARE

Although the concept and provision of palliative care is as old as medicine itself, it is only recently that palliative care programs have increased in both visibility and numbers. Palliative care is an interdisciplinary team approach to optimizing symptom management and quality of life for those with serious or life-threatening illnesses. It is care that addresses the physical, psychosocial, and spiritual needs of the patient and family according to their preferences and cultural beliefs.[1] This differs from most allopathic care, which is directed toward the diagnosis and cure of disease. The notion and practice of palliative care continues to evolve and broaden.[2] The four main attributes of palliative care include: 1) total, active, and individualized patient care, 2) support for the family, 3) an interdisciplinary approach, and 4) effective communication.[2]

THE GROWTH OF PALLIATIVE CARE

Based on changes in the leading causes of death during the past century, a medical care system that was initially designed to focus on acute care is now becoming dominated by patients with incurable, progressive, and debilitating illnesses.[3] The current health care system excels at providing acute care for problems such as trauma and sudden illness; however, it is inadequately prepared to provide comprehensive, coordinated care for those with chronic conditions, especially for those near the end of life.[4-6] This is epitomized in the landmark study sponsored by the Robert Wood Johnson Foundation in the mid-1990s, called the Study to Understand Prognoses and Preferences for Outcomes and Risks of Treatment. This prospective study was aimed at understanding the end-of-life experiences of seriously ill hospitalized Americans and uncovered many shortcomings in the quality of care received at the end of

life, including ineffective communication between patients and providers about care preferences, lack of advanced care planning, and high prevalence of moderate-to-severe pain among dying patients.[4] Similarly, the Means to a Better End Report indicated that although more than 70% of Americans express a preference for dying at home, only approximately 25% of deaths occur at home in most states.[7] In 2001, 23% of deaths occurred in a nursing home and approximately 50% of deaths occurred in an acute care hospital.[8] Thus, a majority of patients with advanced or life-threatening illnesses continue to receive care in traditional acute care settings, necessitating diverse and innovative models of palliative and end-of-life care.

The reasons for a failure to attend to the needs of dying patients and their families are many. Some include system-related problems stemming from a lack of financial reimbursement for palliative care. Also, the health care system is guided by a well-ingrained medical model that focuses on treating disease, rather than focusing on quality of life in those with advanced illness. In addition to these system-related barriers to good palliative care, clinicians are too often unprepared to manage the complex physical and psychosocial problems experienced by patients and their families at the end of life. Few health professionals are trained in palliative care, and few medical schools and nursing programs include palliative care in their formal curricula.[9] These educational shortcomings and the lack of systematic training in palliative care contribute to inadequate care at the end of life.

Fortunately, leaders in palliative care are addressing these deficiencies and adapting new models of palliative care into acute care and community settings. Formal palliative care programs are becoming an established feature in many hospitals and academic medical centers.[10] In addition, several national initiatives were launched to improve palliative care in the hospital setting, including the Center to Advance Palliative Care project,[11] and the Joint Commission on Accreditation of Healthcare Organizations pain management standards.[12]

Annual awards are now given to medical and nursing textbooks for end-of-life content. Many medical and nursing schools are developing formal courses to better address the needs of dying patients. In 2006, the American Board of Medical Specialties voted unanimously to establish a subspecialty in palliative care. Also in 2006, the Accreditation Council for Graduate Medical Education approved the establishment of an accreditation process for hospice and palliative medicine fellowship training programs. As part of their national board and licensure examinations, medical and nursing students now encounter questions related to palliative care, and certification is available in palliative care for physicians, and for nurses at both the basic and advanced practice level.

DISTINGUISHING PALLIATIVE CARE FROM HOSPICE

Although all good hospice care is palliative, not all palliative care qualifies as hospice care. It is necessary to define both terms, as they are often used interchangeably in the literature. Palliative care spans the continuum of care and is not limited by the patient's prognosis or therapeutic plan of care. Palliative care can be initiated early in the disease process, while the patient is still receiving aggressive therapies, including radiation therapy and chemotherapy. This allows the patient to benefit from skilled symptom management and supportive services while still actively treating the underlying disease.

Hospice care entails interdisciplinary support and skilled care for persons in the final months of incurable disease, so that the dying may live as comfortably as possible. Hospice recognizes dying as a normal part of life and focuses on maintaining the quality of remaining life; it neither hastens nor prolongs death. Hospice care embraces the belief that with the appropriate care and a community sensitive to their needs, patients and their families may attain a degree of mental and spiritual preparation for a good death.[13,14]

Unlike palliative care, admission criteria for Medicare- and Medicaid-funded hospice programs require that the patient no longer be pursuing curative treatment, that a physician's written prognosis be 6 months or less based on the natural course of the illness, and that the majority of care be delivered in the home or in a long-term care setting. Hospice care is provided at the end of the palliative care spectrum and remains an appropriate option when the burden of treatment outweighs the benefit to the patient.[15] Hospice should be considered part of a seamless progression of services delivered to the patients with advanced irreversible illness.

Figure 44.1 illustrates how allopathic medicine is traditionally practiced with regard to a life-threatening illness. Figure 44.2 shows a palliative model of care, in which palliative care begins at the time of diagnosis and gradually increases until death.

In the United States, hospice care evolved as an alternative to an increasingly technological death, a death in which the dying persons' personal values and preferences were often not

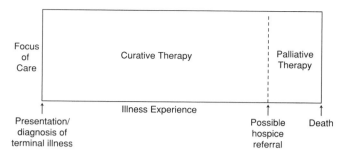

Figure 44.1. Traditional model of care at the end of life.

respected, and patients all too frequently died in pain and isolation. Pioneered in England by Dame Cicely Saunders, hospice began as a grass roots movement in the 1970s. It was initially designed for patients dying of cancer who preferred to die at home and who had available and supportive caregivers. In the 1980s, hospice programs underwent rapid expansion and continued modernization, which was largely a result of the enactment of the Medicare Hospice Benefit in 1982. This legislation transformed hospice from a cottage industry to an organized program with a payment source.

The hospice industry grew considerably after Medicare raised payment rates by 20% in 1989. There are now more than 4,500 hospice programs nationwide and much of the recent growth in the hospice industry has been seen in small freestanding for profit programs.[16] As the numbers of programs have grown, so have the numbers of patients being served by hospice. There has been a 162% increase in the number of hospice recipients in the past 10 years.[16] By 2006, hospices enrolled approximately 36% of all Americans who died.[16] In addition to growth in numbers served, the hospice industry went beyond primarily caring for those with cancer to include all patients with life-limiting illnesses, such as those with end-stage cardiac or pulmonary disease, advanced dementia, and other neurological conditions. Currently, more than half of all hospice patients have terminal diagnoses other than cancer.

Patients appropriate for hospice care have a diagnosed terminal illness with a limited life expectancy. Written certification by a physician of life expectancy of 6 months or less is a requirement for admission to Medicare and Medicaid hospice programs. The benchmark of a prognosis of 6 months or less

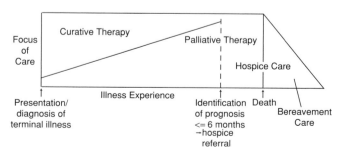

Figure 44.2. Palliative model of care (adapted from the World Health Organization).

Table 44.1. Ten Principles of Hospice Care

Patient and family are regarded as the unit of care.

Services are physician directed and nurse coordinated.

Emphasis is on control of symptoms (physical, sociological, spiritual, and psychological)

Care is provided by an interdisciplinary team.

Trained volunteers are an integral part of the team.

Services are 24 hours a day, 7 days a week, on call, with emphasis placed on availability of medical and nursing skills.

Family members receive bereavement follow-up.

Home care and inpatient care are coordinated.

Patients are accepted on the basis of health needs, not on ability to pay.

There are structured systems for staff support and communication.

Table 44.2. Questions to Consider When Recommending a Hospice Agency

■ Is the hospice agency Medicare certified and state licensed?

■ Is the medical director board certified in Hospice and Palliative Medicine?

■ Are physician consultations (preferably in the home) available for the palliative management of difficult symptoms?

■ How do they handle inpatient care and respite services for caregivers?

■ What types of therapies do they provide?

■ Will they accept patients who have no insurance? Most hospices should be willing to provide care to uninsured patients.

■ Does the hospice agency contract with long-term care facilities? How does the facility rate the care provided by this particular program? Does the long-term care facility have an exclusive contract with only one hospice agency?

came into existence in 1983 as part of the parameters established for the Medicare hospice benefit (U.S.C. Section 1965 et seq.), which served as a reimbursement model and helped to define the essential components of hospice care.

Terminal illness, however, is difficult both to define and to diagnose. Errors in prognosis are common and usually lead to overstated life expectancy, which may partially explain very short and declining durations of stay for hospice patients.[18] Prognoses of life-limiting diseases such as acquired immunodeficiency syndrome or end-stage cardiac, hepatic, pulmonary, renal, or neurological diseases are often more difficult to predict than prognoses of advanced cancers. Patients with noncancer diseases often have other known probable causes of death, such as multiple organ failure or persistent recurrent infection, in addition to their primary diagnosis. Also, a patient may have multiple medical problems, none of which may individually amount to a terminal diagnosis but when taken together, create a terminal condition.

The National Hospice Organization has published medical guidelines, currently being updated, for determining prognosis in selected noncancer diseases to aid clinicians with prognostication.[19] The prognosis of terminal illness depends on clinical judgment combined with the following: objective assessment of the natural history of the disease; treatments and response to date; performance status; thorough physical assessment, including neurological and orthopedic; and knowledge of the psychological and sociological factors of the patient, family, and physician.

Patients and families can select a hospice program by using the criteria listed in Table 44.2. At the time of admission to a hospice program, treatment decisions such as do-not-resuscitate status are explored in conjunction with the patient's values, preferences, and goals for care. Do-not-resuscitate status is not required for hospice admission. Using physician input, knowledge of the disease process, therapeutic options, and discussion

with the patient and family, an advanced care team may help to determine when the goals of care should change from life prolonging to comfort.

HOSPICE AND PALLIATIVE CARE IN THE LONG-TERM CARE SETTING

Many elderly people are dying in long-term care settings in the United States. In 2000, there were more than 1.5 million persons aged 65 and older in nursing homes[20] and almost 1 million functionally impaired older adults living in assisted living facilities.[21] As many as one-third of patients die during the year after nursing home admission.[22] One-quarter of deaths in older adults occur in nursing homes. Two-thirds of nursing home residents remain in the facility rather than being transferred to a hospital to die.[23] Assisted living facilities are increasingly serving as the location for end-of-life care; one study found a 16%–22% mortality rate for assisted living facility residents.[24]

Improving access to palliative care or hospice involvement in appropriate nursing home residents is one way to improve end-of-life care in nursing homes. Nursing home residents who died with hospice care in place had improved pain assessment and management, and lower rates of hospitalization, restraint use, and artificial nutrition and hydration.[25–27] In nursing homes with many residents enrolled in hospice, both the hospice residents and the other residents experienced lower rates of hospitalization, higher frequency of pain assessment, and higher rate of opioid use for control of pain or dyspnea, when compared with patients who died in nursing homes with limited hospice involvement.[26]

Case-controlled studies have found that families report significantly improved symptom management after adding hospice services to U.S. nursing home care, and that overall family

Table 44.3. Standardized Approach for Communicating Bad News

1) Set the scene (quiet location, turn off phones and pagers, sitting if possible.) Decide which team and family members should be present.

2) Elicit patient perceptions. "What do you understand about your situation/diagnosis?"

3) Learn patient's preferences regarding information. "How much do you want to know, details vs. big picture? If you don't want to know, whom can we talk to about decision making?"

4) Give the information. Start with a statement such as, "I wish I had better news for you." State things as simply and clearly as possible without jargon: "The cancer is worse." Pause and allow the patient time to react.

5) Respond to patient's emotions. If there is no reaction, ask what the patient is thinking or feeling at that moment.

6) Arrange for follow-up. "I have given you a lot to think about; let's meet again soon to talk more."

satisfaction with end-of-life care was higher when hospice was in place.[25–27] Palliative care teams or hospice can teach family and caregivers to care for the dying patient and can offer emotional, psychological, and spiritual support to the patient and family, as well as bereavement care and counseling to family and friends, both before and after the patient's death.

COMMUNICATION ISSUES IN PALLIATIVE CARE

Some of the most difficult situations in palliative care involve a lack of open and honest communication among patients, their families, and members of the healthcare team. Communication with patients with life-threatening illness can be facilitated by use of a standardized approach (see Table 44.3) that involves active listening, clear language, and preparing the patient and family to receive the information.[28]

If a family member requests that the bad news not be shared with the patient, the clinician may need to explore possible cultural or religious beliefs surrounding the sharing of bad news because sharing bad news is less acceptable in some cultures. Frequently, family members make this request to protect their loved one from receiving bad news. Simply asking why such a request is made, or suggesting that you ask the patient their preferences about receiving information with family present, may resolve the situation. If language barriers are present, it is important to use a skilled professional translator and not rely on family members as interpreters.

Communication about prognosis decreases uncertainty, helps the patient and family understand the implications of the diagnosis and options for treatment,[29] and helps ensure that treatment choices reflect the patient's values.[30] When communicating prognosis to patients and families, it is useful to acknowledge the uncertainty inherent in any prognosis and to

avoid giving an exact timeframe for expected death; instead, give ranges such as hours to days, days to weeks, weeks to months, or months to years. Specialty consultants can help to determine prognosis. It is also important to explain that prognosis may vary with different treatment options.

After the patient and/or decision maker has a clear understanding of the diagnosis and prognosis, the clinician should help define the goals of care. Asking questions such as the following about a patient's values can provide information to help negotiate goals of care:

"What is most important to you right now?"
"What do you enjoy most now?"
"What concerns you most about your disease?"
"What are you expecting in the coming weeks or months?"
"What have you seen in others you have known with the same disease?"

Formulating goals of care with the patient involves discussion of the relative risks, benefits, and alternatives to the various treatment options. The initial discussion of goals of care will generate an ongoing dialogue; in subsequent discussions, the patient's clinical situation and response to treatment are continually reassessed. The patient and/or decision maker has the right to refuse treatment. Carefully exploring patient's concerns about the treatment may facilitate subsequent care.

SYMPTOM MANAGEMENT

A key component of preventing suffering at the end of life is meticulous attention to symptom management. Despite almost universal agreement that pain and other symptoms should be aggressively managed, especially for those at the end of life, many patients still die with poorly managed symptoms. The following sections provide a concise review of suggested approaches for symptom evaluation and management.

PAIN

Assessment

Initial evaluation of a patient's report of pain begins with a detailed history-taking and physical examination directed to the source of the pain. The severity of pain can be rated according to a numeric scale or using visual tools (see Figure 44.3).[31] Questions should also include the pain's location, character, radiation, temporal profile, exacerbating or relieving factors, and previous response to medications. The character of the pain includes descriptors such as sharp, dull, or throbbing, which will be helpful in determining the type of pain being experienced: nociceptive, neuropathic, or mixed. Nociceptive pain is generally described as pain with both sharp and dull components, sometimes throbbing. Visceral pain is usually described as deep or dull. Neuropathic pain is described as

WHICH FACE SHOWS HOW MUCH HURT YOU HAVE RIGHT NOW?

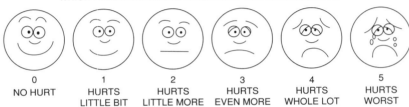

| 0 | 1 | 2 | 3 | 4 | 5 |
| NO HURT | HURTS LITTLE BIT | HURTS LITTLE MORE | HURTS EVEN MORE | HURTS WHOLE LOT | HURTS WORST |

Figure 44.3.

burning, tingling, electric, or shooting. Mixed pain is a combination of neuropathic and nociceptive. Pain can be constant, intermittent, or breakthrough. Incident pain is intermittent pain caused by a precipitating event such as movement. Breakthrough pain is a combination of constant and intermittent pain in which there is a constant baseline level of pain with intermittent episodes of more severe pain. Response to therapy provides the clinician with information about medications the patient has found effective or ineffective and any side effects they may be experiencing. A careful pain history must also include a thorough assessment of the psychological and social factors affecting the patient's expression of pain.[32–38]

Management

Pain Medication Selection

The World Health Organization (WHO) Analgesic Ladder (see Figure 44.4) was found to control pain in 90% of cancer patients and 70% of terminally ill patients.[39] The WHO Analgesic Ladder is most applicable to nociceptive or mixed pain.

Step 3, Severe Pain (7-10)
Morphine
Hydromorphone
Methadone
Fentanyl
Oxycodone
± Nonopioid
analgesics
± Adjuvants

Step 2, Moderate Pain (4-6)
APAP
Codeine
Hydrocodone
Oxycodone
Tramadol (alone or combination with APAP)
± Adjuvants

Step 1, Mild Pain (0-3)
Acetaminophen (APAP)
Nonsteroidal anti-inflammatory drugs (NSAIDs)
± Adjuvants

"Adjuvants" refers either to medications that are co-administered to manage an adverse effect of an opioid, or are added to enhance analgesia.

Figure 44.4. Adapted from the WHO Analgesic Ladder.

Scheduling and Dosing

Based on the WHO guidelines, any patient with constant or breakthrough pain requires scheduled pain medication around the clock. Immediate-release opioids such as morphine, hydromorphone, oxycodone, and hydrocodone should be dosed every 4 hours, as the half-life is approximately 4 hours, regardless of the route of administration. Because the time to maximum blood levels via the oral route is approximately 1 hour, as-needed oral doses for breakthrough pain should be given every hour. For intermittent pain, around the clock dosing is generally inappropriate; instead, immediate-release medication should be given on an as-needed basis at the onset of pain.

Choosing an appropriate dose involves starting an empiric regimen. For severe pain, a first-line medication is immediate-release morphine sulfate. In the elderly, start dosing low and adjust slowly, especially for around-the-clock medication. Most of the strong opioids are renally excreted, so dose adjustments are necessary for patients with impaired renal function.

For moderate-to-severe constant pain in an opioid-naive elderly patient, consider an initial regimen of morphine sulfate 2.5 mg orally every 4 hours around the clock and 2.5 mg orally every hour as needed for breakthrough pain. This dose is equivalent to hydrocodone/acetaminophen 2.5/325 mg (see Table 44.4). Frequent reassessment of efficacy is important. Methadone is a unique opioid that is thought to have enhanced activity in neuropathic or mixed pain states. Its pharmacokinetics can vary greatly between individuals, with a half-life of up to 72 hours. Because of its potential to accumulate over time, it should be carefully titrated and monitored in elderly patients.

Conversion

If the patient is currently taking a strong opioid or combination product and the regimen is ineffective or causing side effects, converting to a different agent may improve pain control. Table 44.4 allows direct conversion between opioids.

Additional Considerations for Management of Pain with Opioids in the Elderly

- Avoid meperidine, which has neurotoxic metabolite that can accumulate in elderly patients, is poorly absorbed orally, and has low potency.
- Avoid propoxyphene, because of poor efficacy and high potential for adverse effects.
- Use caution when starting long-acting medications such as fentanyl transdermal patches and sustained-released opioids in opioid-naïve patients.

Table 44.4. Equianalgesic Doses

Oral Dose (mg)	Analgesic	Parenteral Dose (mg)
15	Morphine	5
150	Codeine	50
10	Oxycodone	–
3	Hydromorphone	1
15	Hydrocodone	–
0.3 (transmucosal)	Fentanyl	0.05
2	Levorphanol	1
150	Meperidine	50

- Consider alternate routes: morphine and oxycodone are available in concentrated forms (20 mg/mL) that can be given sublingually. All parenteral opioids can be given subcutaneously, either intermittently or via patient-controlled analgesia.

- Approximate time to maximum blood levels for opioids is 60 minutes orally, 30 minutes subcutaneously, and 6 minutes intravenously. This should be used as a guide in determining how often to give as-needed doses.

- There is no standard or ceiling dose of opioids. Opioid dose can be slowly increased until pain is relieved or until limited by side effects.

- Always prescribe opioids with appropriate laxatives, such as senna with docusate sodium, and monitor closely for constipation and impaction.

Alternative Routes of Opioid Delivery

Although the oral route is preferred, it is occasionally necessary to consider a transdermal, sublingual, buccal, rectal, parenteral, (including portable subcutaneous or intravenous patient-controlled analgesia), inhaled, or spinal route. Advantages of and indications for topical analgesics are convenience, long-term use, confusion, difficulty swallowing, and reluctance to use injections early in the pain management regimen. Intractable neuropathic pain may necessitate consideration of intraspinal nerve blocks and epidural administration of opioids. The elderly and the dying should be evaluated carefully for benefit versus burden. In the elderly, as in other populations with chronic pain, the simplest dose schedule and least invasive modalities should be used first.

Adjuvant Agents Used for Pain Management

Adjuvant agents are those that have primary indications for other nonpain therapy but have additional utility in pain management. They play an important role in the management of neuropathic pain or in reducing opioid requirements, thereby decreasing opioid toxicity. Adjuvant agents should be considered for all patients, especially those with neuro-

pathic or bone pain. Neuropathic pain may require adjuvant medications such as the anticonvulsants pregabalin, gabapentin, carbamazepine*, valproic acid* (*requires blood level monitoring); tricyclic antidepressants including amitriptyline, desipramine, and nortriptyline; ketamine; and lidocaine. Nonsteroidal antiinflammatory drugs have been recommended for the treatment of bone pain secondary to bone metastasis because of their antiinflammatory properties. They should be used in all patients with bone metastasis, unless contraindicated. Corticosteroids and neuroleptics may also be indicated, especially if nerve root involvement is present.

Nonpharmacological Methods of Pain Control

Although not well researched in elderly populations, potentially helpful nonpharmacological methods of pain management include alternative therapies such as guided imagery, music, meditation, self-expression with art and drawing, acupressure, therapeutic touch, physical therapy, transcutaneous electrical nerve stimulation, repositioning or splinting a painful extremity, application of heat or ice, and massage. These measures can be used alone or in combination with medications.

Pain Management in Cognitively Impaired Patients

Pain is especially difficult to assess in cognitively impaired patients. Observing for behaviors such as grimacing, moaning, or crying out with turning, dressing changes, or other therapies can help anticipate and prevent unnecessary pain in cognitively impaired patients. Confused or demented patients who have difficulty communicating their pain to health professionals often receive weak opioids or nonopioids because their caregivers mistakenly believe that they cannot tolerate opioid agents.[40] If nonopioids alone are ineffective, it may be helpful to add low doses of short-acting opioids and escalate until optimal pain relief is achieved. Frequent communication with the patient, family, and caregivers is essential to monitor side effects and response to therapy.

DELIRIUM

A change in mental status is a common neurological symptom in those near the end of life. Clinicians should maintain a high index of suspicion for delirium in patients who are very ill.

Assessment

Delirium can be differentiated from pain, anxiety, depression, or dementia using the Confusion Assessment Method.[41]

1) Acute change in mental status from baseline with a fluctuating course
2) Inattention: unable to pay attention or follow a conversation
3) Disorganized thinking: rambling and incoherent, or irrelevant conversation

4) Altered level of consciousness: can be either hyperactive (hypervigilant), or hypoactive (lethargic, stuporous or comatose).

A diagnosis of delirium requires that the patient have criteria 1 and 2 and either 3 or 4.

Differential Diagnosis

The differential diagnosis of delirium in the elderly patient is covered elsewhere in this text. Delirium seen in the palliative care setting may be related to the direct effects of disease progression (such as brain metastasis), side effects to treatment, or the indirect effects of progressive disease, such as electrolyte imbalance, metabolic encephalopathy, infection, or paraneoplastic syndromes. Before undertaking an exhaustive evaluation, the following simple reversible causes should be excluded: use of medications such as tricyclic antidepressants, antihistamines, benzodiazepines, and some opioids; urinary retention; fecal impaction; infection including urinary tract infection, pneumonia, and sepsis; electrolyte imbalances; and dehydration. Assessment includes complete blood count and complete chemistry panel. Myocardial infarction and stroke can also precipitate delirium and should be considered as well.

Treatment

The treatment of delirium in patients at the end of life involves treatment of the underlying cause when possible. Often, however, a comprehensive workup is not desirable, and the cause remains elusive or is irreversible. Nonpharmacological measures should be initiated; the patient can also be started on a neuroleptic such as haloperidol in low doses (0.5–1 mg po/im/iv/sq q 12 h) repeated hourly as needed.[42] Once the total daily dose is determined, it can be given in divided doses two–three times a day. Chlorpromazine can be given when sedation is desired. Newer antipsychotics such as olanzapine[43] or risperidone[44] may be effective for treating agitation but have less evidence to support their use. Patients treated with these and all antipsychotic medications should be closely monitored for adverse effects and outcomes of therapy. They can be considered in patients with Parkinson's disease, in whom the extrapyramidal side effects of haloperidol may be problematic. Benzodiazepines, such as lorazepam, are used in alcohol or benzodiazepine withdrawal.[45]

NAUSEA AND VOMITING

Assessment

The assessment of nausea and vomiting includes a careful history-taking that includes onset, frequency, duration, bowel habits, ability to keep liquids down, recent treatments (surgery, chemotherapy, radiation etc.), exacerbating and relieving factors, and a thorough review of medications. The physical examination should be guided by the history, such as assessing papilledema in cancer patients with concern of brain metastases; abdominal examination for masses, organomegaly,

ascites; and a rectal examination to check for fecal impaction. Laboratory data can include a complete blood count to screen for infection and blood loss, and a complete metabolic panel to look for uremia, hypercalcemia, hyponatremia, hypokalemia, and liver dysfunction. Plain x-rays of the abdomen may reveal bowel obstruction, whereas electrocardiography and cardiac evaluation may identify atypical presentations of cardiac ischemia.

Management

Initial management begins with reversing underlying causes when possible, such as correcting metabolic abnormalities, treating constipation or fecal impaction, or discontinuing offending medications. Medication should be targeted to the most likely mechanism for the nausea and vomiting. A wide variety of receptor types and neurotransmitters are found in areas of the brain thought to control vomiting and each may have a role in emesis. Antagonists of the receptors for each of these transmitters have antiemetic effects. For example the 5-HT_3 antagonists are effective against chemotherapy- and radiation-induced nausea and vomiting, but do not inhibit nausea and vomiting resulting from opiate administration or motion. Drug therapy is most likely to work if started prophylactically; the oral route is preferred if there has been no vomiting.

Start with metoclopramide around the clock for nausea and vomiting caused by gastric stasis, ascites, hepatomegaly, and gastrointestinal tumor infiltration. Metoclopramide is contraindicated in Parkinson's disease and renal failure. For nausea and vomiting that is secondary to opioid therapy, uremia, or liver metastases, use haloperidol or chlorpromazine. If secondary to brain metastases, add a corticosteroid such as dexamethasone 4 mg daily. Antihistamines such as hydroxyzine, promethazine, or diphenhydramine may be added to these etiology-specific treatments if nausea and vomiting are not fully controlled. Ondansetron (Zofran®) may be added if nausea is due to moderately to severely emetic chemotherapeutic agents, such as cisplatin. Nausea and vomiting due to anxiety can also be treated with antihistamines or anticholinergics such as scopolamine. For nausea from a vestibular etiology, use a scopolamine patch or promethazine.[46]

In a meta-analysis of nonpharmacological interventions, postsurgical patients found benefit equivalent to pharmacology when using acupuncture, electroacupuncture, transcutaneous electrical nerve stimulation, acupoint stimulation, and acupressure.[47] Guided imagery and hypnosis may also be helpful.[48]

DYSPNEA

Dyspnea, the subjective sensation of difficulty breathing, is a common symptom at the end of life. It can be either an acute or chronic symptom. Objective signs, such as respiratory rate and pulse oximetry, may not match the patient's perception of dyspnea. One study of terminally ill cancer patients found a relationship between a high level of dyspnea and low will to live.[49]

Mechanisms

In patients at the end of life, dyspnea often has multiple causes. Pulmonary causes of dyspnea include pulmonary embolism; obstructive processes such as bronchospasm, tumor invasion, and chronic obstructive pulmonary disease; interstitial processes including pulmonary edema, pneumonia and pneumonitis; and restrictive processes including neuromuscular dysfunction, pneumothorax, and pleural effusions. Cardiovascular causes include heart failure, coronary artery disease, superior vena cava syndrome, and pericardial effusion or tamponade. In addition, dyspnea can be caused by deconditioning, cachexia, hypercapnea, anxiety, anemia, and acidosis.

Assessment

Detailed history-taking, appropriate physical examination, and diagnostic studies such as complete blood count, basic chemistries, arterial blood gas levels, electrocardiography, and chest x-ray may be helpful to evaluate the underlying cause of the dyspnea.

Management

Management should begin with treatment of the underlying cause of the dyspnea if possible. Simple nonpharmacological measures include the movement of air over the face via fans, guided imagery and hypnosis, and emotional support. Pharmacological approaches include bronchodilators, corticosteroids, benzodiazepines, and opioids. It is postulated that opioids decrease respiratory distress by altering the perception of breathlessness and decreasing ventilatory response to lowering oxygen and rising CO_2 levels. Opioids have been shown to improve dyspnea without causing significant deterioration in respiratory function. Quality of life in terminally ill patients experiencing dsypnea can be improved through use of low-dose opioids such as morphine sulfate immediate-release 2.5 mg by mouth every hour as need, and then every 4 hours around the clock, with the dose titrated upward until symptoms are controlled.[50]

For patients already taking opioids daily, the baseline dose can be increased by 25%–50% depending on the severity of the dyspnea. Patients requiring at least 30 mg orally daily might benefit from a long-acting opioid preparation. A breakthrough dose of approximately 10% of the total daily long-acting opioid dose should be made available. Caution should be used in patients with chronic obstructive pulmonary disease secondary to the risk of hypoventilation and hypercapnia, but opioids have been found to be effective even in those patients[51] especially when started at low doses. Nebulized opioids have been recommended in the past, but data are inconclusive about their overall efficacy.[52,53] Benzodiazepine use can be reserved for when anxiety is thought to be a strong component of the dyspnea.[54]

Supplemental oxygen is not required for patients experiencing dyspnea when the other measures outlined are effective. When oxygen is required to help relieve dyspnea, nasal prongs are preferred over oxygen masks, which tend to be isolating and can be frightening to patients.

CONTROLLED SEDATION FOR INTRACTABLE SUFFERING

Some patients at the end of life have symptoms that cannot be controlled despite maximal medical interventions. A symptom is considered refractory to treatment if it cannot be controlled adequately despite aggressive efforts to identify a tolerable therapy that does not compromise consciousness, if additional invasive and noninvasive interventions are incapable of providing adequate relief, and if the therapy directed at the symptom is associated with excessive and intolerable acute or chronic morbidity and/or is unlikely to provide relief within a tolerable time frame.[55] Controlled palliative sedation may be a treatment option for patients with intractable symptoms.

The purpose of palliative sedation is symptom relief; it should not be confused with physician-assisted suicide. If palliative sedation is being considered, it is important to communicate with the entire team caring for the patient and build consensus. While the patient is still coherent, discussion of all potential treatment options, including palliative sedation, will help the family and care team have greater comfort with the decision. When instituting palliative sedation, open conversations with the family members who are holding vigil will alleviate accusations of unethical practices.

When the decision is made to proceed, consultation is advisable with experts in either palliative medicine or anesthesia. Although opioids are often titrated to produce sedation, they are not the best choice because of development of opioid tolerance.[56] Phenobarbital, midazolam, and propofol are preferred over opioids.[57] An analysis of patients having undergone increasing sedation at end of life found no evidence for inadvertent hastening of death.[58] Ethically, palliative sedation could be viewed as equivalent to refusing/withdrawing artificial nutrition and hydration.[57]

IMPAIRED NUTRITIONAL STATUS

Although it has been well established in law, ethics, and medicine that patients have a right to refuse treatments that are invasive and unwanted, withholding artificial feedings and hydration continue to be a difficult issue for patients, families, and health care providers. Questions from family members about starvation and dehydration are common in caring for the dying. Numerous studies show that terminally ill patients generally do not get hungry, and those who do need only small amounts of food for alleviation, not artificial feeding or hydration.[59,60] Thirst and dry mouth can be relieved with ice chips, and family members can learn to provide excellent oral hygiene for comfort. Caregivers, patients, and families need to be informed that loss of appetite is to be

Table 44.5. Ten Aspects of Spiritual Pain

Abandonment	A feeling of being forgotten by God
Anger	May be directed toward God or people
Betrayal	Similar to abandonment but with an extra valance
Despair	Being without hope, having nowhere to turn
Fear, dread	What does death mean? What will it bring? Where? May be directed toward the process of dying or toward what comes afterward
Guilt	Self-recrimination, feelings of having left undone things that should have been done, or having done what should not have, a sense of death as deserved punishment
Meaninglessness	A feeling that life is without purpose, has no fundamental meaning
Regret	Sadness is associated with irreversibility, of dreams that must remain unfulfilled, of a deeper painful wish or longing for what cannot be
Self-pity	Why me? Why should I be in this condition?
Sorrow, remorse	Profound sadness, likely to be associated with impending separation from loved ones

expected in the dying and is generally thought not to contribute to suffering.

SPIRITUAL DIMENSIONS OF HOSPICE AND PALLIATIVE CARE

Theologian Dorothee Soelle, in her classic text on suffering, pointed out two very important components of suffering: perceived powerlessness and perceived meaninglessness. It is in that struggle against powerlessness, the struggle to find meaning in our lives, that so much important work is done at the end of life.[61] In this most personal and profound part of life's journey, the power of life review and the personal narrative are critical for the dying and their families. Spirituality plays an important role in the struggle to find meaning at the end of life. Spirituality does not relieve us of suffering; rather, spirituality can provide guidance and encouragement. Readings, spiritual prayers, rites, and sacraments may be helpful to some.

Much has been written about the isolation of the dying, avoidance by friends and families who do not know what to say and by health care professionals who think they no longer have anything to offer. Assisting in the spiritual work of dying requires excellent listening skills, respect for the person, reflection, and empathic awareness of the patient's situation and story. The fact that human life has spiritual dimensions becomes acutely evident as the end of life approaches and patients want to bring spiritual feelings to the forefront. A major component of pain is spiritual (Table 44.5).[62]

Table 44.6. Expected Changes When Death Is Imminent

Social

- Withdrawal; decreased responsiveness
- Increasing somnolence, confusion
- Decreased hearing and vision
- Decreased appetite and thirst

Physical

- Decreased urine output
- Mottling (bluish purple discoloration of the extremities); cyanosis; cool extremities
- Changes in breathing: Cheyne Stokes, tachypnea, rapid shallow breathing, apnea
- Tachycardia bradycardia
- Fever hypothermia
- Waxy appearing skin

The resources a hospice pastoral caregiver can bring to the patient and family depend, of course, on the spiritual dynamics that motivate a particular person. Every religious value system has corresponding sources of spiritual strength. In the Christian context some of these sources of spiritual strength are forgiveness, God, hope, prayer, rites, and trust.[63] Many persons must face spiritual issues if death is to occur with any kind of acceptance.

EXPECTED PHYSICAL CHANGES AS A PATIENT NEARS DEATH

Patients and families are vulnerable and often fearful about the impending death. They turn to their health care practitioners for information and reassurance. Health care providers play an important role in helping patients and families to feel comfortable with the dying process by providing information about it. Unfortunately, very few physicians and midlevel providers have received adequate training in the changes associated with the dying process or have witnessed the natural death of a patient.

There are anticipated changes at the end of life, as listed in Table 44.6. Some patients will exhibit all of these changes; a few patients will not exhibit any. Many of the changes wax and wane, and changes often do not proceed in a stepwise fashion. The social changes generally precede the physical changes.

ANTICIPATING FAMILY CONCERNS

Some questions frequently asked by families at the end of life:
Are you sure we are doing the right thing?
Reassurance may be helpful. Consider responding, "Why do you ask?" This may help unearth ambivalence or the need

for reassurance. Making sure the goals of care are established ahead of time can make this a much easier question to answer.

Do you think she is suffering?

Again, often reassurance is all that is needed. Explain that a useful proxy for distress in a nonverbal patient is looking at the area between the eyebrows: if it is relaxed, the patient is likely not in distress; if it is wrinkled, the patient may be experiencing discomfort. Again, consider asking an open-ended question like "What are you seeing that concerns you she may be suffering?"

How long does he have?

Avoid giving a specific number of hours or days. If the patient is manifesting several of the signs seen in Table 44.4, it is appropriate to give a range "hours to days."

Why is she not on an IV?

Reassurance to the family that the patient is dying from their underlying disease process can be very helpful, especially in the patient in whom death appears imminent. A recent, small study of terminal cancer patients showed a modest improvement in symptoms with low-volume hydration.[64] At worst, fluids run at a maintenance rate will increase secretions and potentially lead to anasarca and pulmonary edema. Intravenous access may be very difficult obtain or maintain in patients at the end of life. Parenteral fluids should only be initiated or continued if such use is consistent with the goals of care and clinical condition. If there is increasing edema or the development of terminal secretions, discontinuation of intravenous fluid is appropriate. Ongoing communication with the family is the key to all changes in the plan of care.

SUMMARY

Death is an anticipated outcome for any clinician providing care for the elderly. Comprehensive care for the elderly includes excellent care for the dying. Attention to the principles of palliative care and appropriate symptom management ensure that elderly persons at the end of life endure a minimum of suffering and experience a good death. Hospice referral for patients with an expected prognosis of 6 months or less can provide an interdisciplinary team approach to end-of-life care. Prognostication can be difficult for many clinicians; providing a range of expected lifespan can help convey the uncertainty inherent in any prognosis. High-quality palliative care can be provided to all elderly patients with chronic disease by focusing on comfort rather than exclusively on disease management and life prolongation.

REFERENCES

1. Hauptman PJ, Havranek EP. Integrating palliative care into heart failure care. *Arch Intern Med.* 2005;165:374–378.
2. Meghani SH. A concept analysis of palliative care in the United States. *JAdv Nurs Sci.* 2004;46:152–161.
3. Lynn J, Adamson DM. Living well at the end of life: adapting health care to serious chronic illness in old age. Rand White Paper. Santa Monica: Rand; 2003. Available at http://www.rand.org/pubs/white_papers/WP137/.Accessed June 22, 2008.
4. SUPPORT Principle Investigators. A controlled trial to improve care for seriously ill hospitalized patients: the study to understand prognosis and preferences for outcomes and risks for treatment. *JAMA.* 1995;274:1591–1598.
5. Bodheimer T, Wagner EH, Grumbach K. Improving primary care for patients with chronic illness. *JAMA.* 2002;288:1775–1779.
6. Foley KM, Gelband H, eds. *Improving Palliative Care for Cancer.* Washington, DC: National Academy Press; 2001.
7. Means to a Better End: a report on dying in America today. Robert Wood Johnson Foundation, 2002. Available at: http://www.rwjf.org/files/publications/other/meansbetterend.pdf. on Accessed June 22, 2008.
8. Facts on Dying: policy relevant data on care at the end of life. Available at: http://www.chcr.brown.edu/dying. Accessed June 22, 2008.
9. Field MJ, Cassel CK, eds. *Approaching Death: Improving Care at the End of Life.* Executive Summary. Committee on Care at the End of Life. Institute of Medicine. Washington, DC: National Academy Press; 1997.
10. Pan CX, Morrison RS, Meier DE, et al. How prevalent are hospital-based palliative care programs? Status report and future directions. *J Palliat Med.* 2001;4:307–308.
11. Center to Advance Palliative Care. Available at: http://www.capc.org. Accessed June 22, 2008.
12. Joint Commission on Accreditation of Healthcare Organizations (JCAHO). Pain management standards (standards RI 2–8 and PE 1.4). In: *Comprehensive Accreditation Manual for Hospitals.* Washington, DC: JACHO; 2001.
13. Veteran Administration's Hospice and Palliative Care Initiative. Available at: http://www1.va.gov/geriatricsshg/page.cfm?pg = 65. Accessed June 22, 2008.
14. *Standards of a Hospice Program of Care.* Arlington, VA: National Hospice Organization; 1993.
15. Conant L, Lowney A. The role of hospice philosophy of care in nonhospice settings. *J Law Med Ethics.* 1996;24:365–368.
16. National Hospice and Palliative Care Organization (NHPCO) Facts and Figures: Hospice Care in America, November 2007 Edition.
17. National Hospice and Palliative Care Organization (NHPCO) Facts and Figures, 2004.
18. *Hospice fact sheet.* Arlington, VA: National Hospice Organization, July 1996.
19. National Hospice Organization. *Medical Guidelines for Determining Prognosis in Selected Non-cancer Diseases.* Arlington, VA: National Hospice Organization; 1995.
20. Hetzel L, Smith A. The 65 Years and over Population 2000: Census Brief. U.S. Census Bureau 2000. Available at http://www.census.gov/main/www/cen2000.html. Accessed June 22, 2008.
21. Golant SM. Do impaired older persons with health care needs occupy U.S. assisted living facilities? An analysis of six national studies. *J Gerontol B Psychol Sci Soc Sci.* 2004;59B:S68–S79.
22. Hanson LC, Henderson M, Rogman E. Where will we die? A national study of nursing home death. *J Am Geriatr Soc.* 1997;47:9.
23. Kiely DK, Flacker JM. The protective effect of social engagement on 1-year mortality in a long-stay nursing home population. *J Clin Epidemiol.* 2003;56:472–478.
24. Zimmerman S, Sloane PD, Eckert K. *Assisted Living: Needs, Practices, and Policies in Residential Care for the Elderly.* Baltimore: Johns Hopkins Press; 2001.

25. Miller S, Gozalo P, Mor V. Outcomes and utilization for hospice and non-hospice nursing home decedents. 2002. Available at: http://aspe.hhs.gov/daltcp/reports/oututil.htm. Accessed June 22,2008.

26. Miller S, Gozalo P, Mor V. Hospice enrollment and hospitalization of dying nursing home patients. *Am J Med.* 2001;111:38–44.

27. Baer WM, Hanson LC. Families' perception of the added value of hospice in the nursing home. *J Am Geriatr Soc.* 2000;48:879–882.

28. Buckman R, Kason Y. *How to Break ad News – A Practical Protocol for Healthcare Professionals.* Toronto: University of Toronto Press; 1992.

29. Christakis NA. *Death Foretold: Prophecy and Prognosis in Medical Care.* Chicago: University of Chicago Press; 1999.

30. Weeks JC, Cook EF, O'Day SJ, et al. Relationship between cancer patients' predictions of prognosis and their treatment preferences. *JAMA.* 1998;279:1709–1714.

31. Wong DL, Baker CM. Pain in children: comparison of assessment scales. *Pediatr Nurs.* 1988;14:9–17.

32. Rousseau P. Hospice and palliative care. *Dis Mon.* 1995;41:779–842.

33. Doyle D, Hanks G, McDonald N, eds. *Oxford Book of Palliative Medicine.* Oxford: Oxford University Press; 1993.

34. Enck RE. A review of pain management. *Am J Hosp Palliat Care.* 1992;8:6–9.

35. Cleeland CS, Gonin R, Hatfield AK, et al. Pain and its treatment in outpatients with metastatic cancer. *NEJM.* 1994;330:592–596.

36. Kaiko RF. Age and morphine analgesia in cancer patients with post-operative pain. *Clin Pharmocother.* 1980;28:823–826.

37. Agency for Health Care Policy and Research. Management of Cancer Pain. Clinical Practice Guideline 9 (AHCPR 94–0592 Rockville, MD: US Department of Health and Human Services, Public Health Service, Agency for Health Care Policy and Research; 1994.

38. Portenoy RK. Chronic opioid therapy in nonmalignant pain. *J Pain Symptom Manage.* 1990;5:S46–S62.

39. Cancer Pain Relief and Palliative Care. Technical Report Series 804. Geneva: World Health Organization; 1990.

40. Agency for Health Care Policy and Research. Management of Cancer Pain. Clinical Practice Guideline 9 (AHCPR 94–0592 Rockville, MD: US Department of Health and Human Services, Public Health Service, Agency for Health Care Policy and Research; 1994.

41. Inouye SK, van Dyck CH, Alessi CA, Balkin S, Siegal AP, Horwitz RI. Clarifying confusion: the confusion assessment method. A new method for detection of delirium. *Ann Intern Med.* 1990;113:941–948.

42. Breitbart W, Marotta R, Platt MM, et al. A double-blind trial of haloperidol, chlorpromazine, and lorazepam in the treatment of delirium in hospitalized AIDS patients. *Am J Psychol.* 1996;153:231–237.

43. Skrobik YK, Bergeron N, Dumont M, Gottfried SB. Olanzapine vs haloperidol: treating delirium in a critical care setting. *Intens Care Med.* 2004;30:444–449.

44. Han CS, Kim YK. A double-blind trial of risperidone and haloperidol for the treatment of delirium. *Psychosomatics.* 2004;45:297–301.

45. Mayo-Smith MF. Pharmacological management of alcohol withdrawal. A meta-analysis and evidence-based practice guideline. American Society of Addiction Medicine Working Group on Pharmacological Management of Alcohol Withdrawal. *JAMA.* 997;278:144–151.

46. Weissman D. Fast Fact and Concepts #05: Treatment of Nausea and Vomiting. 2000. End-of-Life Physician Education Resource Center. Available at: http://www.eperc.mcw.edu. Accessed June 22, 2008.

47. Lee A, Done ML. The use of nonpharmacologic techniques to prevent postoperative nausea and vomiting: a meta-analysis. *Anesth Analg.* 1999;88:1362–1369.

48. Burish TG, Tope DM. Psychological techniques for controlling the adverse side effects of cancer chemotherapy: findings from a decade of research. *J Pain Symptom Manage.* 1992;7:287–301.

49. Tataryn D, Chochinov HM. Predicting the trajectory of will to live in terminally ill patients. *Psychosomatics.* 2002;43:370–377.

50. Jennings AL, Davies AN, Higgins JP, Gibbs JS, Broadley KE. A systematic review of the use of opioids in the management of dyspnoea. *Thorax.* 2002;57:939–944.

51. Light RW, Muro JR, Sato RI, Stansbury DW, Fischer CE, Brown SE. Effects of oral morphine on breathlessness and exercise tolerance in patients with chronic obstructive pulmonary disease. *Am Rev Respir Dis.* 1989;139:126–133.

52. Harris-Eze AO, Sridhar G, Clemens RE, Zintel TA, Gallagher CG, Marciniuk DD. Low-dose nebulized morphine does not improve exercise in interstitial lung disease. *Am J Respir Crit Care Med.* 1995;152:1940–1945.

53. Noseda A, Carpiaux JP, Markstein C, Meyvaert A, de Maertelaer V. Disabling dyspnoea in patients with advanced disease: lack of effect of nebulized morphine. *Eur Respir J.* 1997;10:1079–1083.

54. Smoller JW, Pollack MH, Otto MW, Rosenbaum JF, Kradin RL. Panic anxiety, dyspnea, and respiratory disease. Theoretical and clinical considerations. *Am J Respir Crit Care Med.* 1996;154:6–17.

55. Cherny NI, Portenoy RK. The management of cancer pain. *CA Cancer J Clin.* 1994;44:263–303.

56. Storey P, Knight CF, Schonwetter RG. *Pocket Guide to Hospice/ Palliative Medicine.* American Academy of Hospice and Palliative Care. Glenview, IL: Haworth Medical Press; 2003.

57. Quill TE, Byock IR. Responding to intractable terminal suffering: the role of terminal sedation and voluntary refusal of food and fluids. ACP-ASIM End-of-Life Care Consensus Panel. American College of Physicians–American Society of Internal Medicine. *Ann Intern Med.* 2000;132:408–414.

58. Sykes N, Thorns A. Sedative use in the last week of life and the implications for end-of-life decision making. *Arch Intern Med.* 2003;163:341–344.

59. Easson A, Hinshaw D, Johnson D. The role of tube feeding and total parenteral nutrition in advanced illness. *J Am Coll Surg.* 2002;194:225–228.

60. Shragge JE, Wismer WV, Olson KL, Baracos VE. The management of anorexia by patients with advanced cancer: a critical review of the literature. *Palliative Med.* 2006;20:623–629.

61. Cassell EJ. Recognizing suffering. *Hastings Cent Rep.* 1991;21:24–31.

62. Abbott JW. *Hospice Resource Manual for Local Churches. Spiritual Pain and Spiritual Growth: Ten Aspects of Spiritual Pain.* New York: Pilgrim Press; 1987:21.

63. Abbott JW, ed. *Hospice Resource Manual for Local Churches.* Pilgrim, OH: Pilgrim Press; 1988.

64. Bruera E, Sala R, Rico MA, et al. Effects of parenteral hydration in terminally ill cancer patients: a preliminary study. *J Clin Oncol.* 2005;23:2366–2371.

45

ASSESSMENT OF DECISION-MAKING CAPACITY

Jeffrey Philip Spike, PhD

Case 1: Mr. Allen. Mr. Allen is an 80-year-old widower living alone in an unheated rural shack. His family says he is an alcoholic of 20 years and a loner. He is successfully treated for pneumonia in the hospital, but the antibiotic leaves him with a life-threatening coagulopathy. He insists on going home but does not seem to appreciate the seriousness of his condition, and there is concern he will not take the pills he needs to remain alive. The social worker wonders if this would be a safe discharge or whether he should be discharged to a nursing home.

Case 2: Mrs. Benson. Mrs. Benson is a 75-year-old widow with advanced vascular dementia and end-stage congestive heart failure. She listens to a description of the benefits and burdens of having a do-not-resuscitation (DNR) directive, and when her physician recommends it, she agrees. The next day she has no memory of the discussion, so her physician repeats the consent process, and she again agrees. Her physician wonders if she could have capacity when her memory is so compromised.

CAPACITY AND COMPETENCE

Capacity and competence are among the most important ethical and legal issues in geriatrics. Although the terms are often used interchangeably in conversation, it is advisable to keep capacity and competence as two distinct concepts, with capacity as a *clinical* concept and competence as a *legal* concept. It is not that the two words have different meanings in our everyday discourse, but that it is best to remind ourselves that sometimes we are talking about legal conflicts that can only be resolved in court whereas other times we are talking about clinical decisions that are best made without any legal complications (or costs).

Capacity and competence are presumed for all adults in the United States. Hence capacity and competence do not require

any sort of test. Lack of capacity can be determined by any clinician and does not require any court action. Incompetence, in contrast, must be determined by a court, and thus typically involves the use of expert witnesses for both the plaintiff and defendant.

Capacity is also something that can vary from day to day or according to the task at hand. Just as a person might be able to play checkers but not chess, a person might be able to make simple medical decisions, but not ones requiring processing complex statistics. In contrast competence is generally seen as global, and once a person is judged to be incompetent, a guardian or conservator is usually appointed to make decisions for the person, and the specific types of decisions removed from the person are defined (often including financial issues, such as selling of property, giving of gifts, and estate planning as well as medical decisions).

To help keep the distinction clear, it is increasingly common to refer to the clinical concept as *decision-making capacity*. Decision-making capacity deliberately links the concept of capacity to the concept of informed consent. The bulk of this chapter will focus on decision-making capacity because cases that go to court to determine competence are removed from the primary care arena into the legal world of expert witnesses. It is important, however, to know what goes on in court, if only to appreciate the value of avoiding that option when possible; therefore, competence will be covered briefly in the final section of the chapter.

DEFINING CAPACITY: CAPACITY AS A FUNCTIONAL CONCEPT

There are various definitions of decision-making capacity but all share some basic tenets. Some definitions propose additional elements, making them more stringent. It is best to begin with the basic elements on which all definitions agree.

To assess capacity, the clinician needs to determine that the patient:

1) *Understands* the nature of her illness and all of the reasonable treatment options
2) *Appreciates* the benefits and burdens (risks and benefits) of each of the reasonable options
3) Makes a *voluntary* choice (free from coercion)
4) *Communicates* her choice.

The basic concept is often distilled to this: the patient must *understand and appreciate* the relevant medical information and then make an authentic choice, that is, one that reflects the patient's values.

Each of these elements can benefit from some clarification. The conjunction "understand *and* appreciate" is a reminder that this is not just a matter of cognition or comprehension of information but an appreciation of the impact of the decision on the person's life. It is a common mistake to think that the patient does not understand enough because of an assumption based on an imaginary ideal patient's comprehension. An elderly patient or a patient from a different culture may well have never understood modern Western medicine, and this alone cannot mean they lose the right to make their own decisions. It simply means the clinician must work a little harder at translating or interpreting what the patient needs to know. The most important information the patient must comprehend is not the medical details (such as the treatment process or its probabilities of success), but the expected physical and emotional consequences of the decision he or she has made. Hence that should be the focus of the assessment. The patient need not have any higher degree of comprehension of the medical or surgical option itself than is required for the appreciation of its *consequences*.

The patient probably ought to understand the organ system that is the source of the problem, whether the illness is life threatening, and the difficulty of the recovery period for each of the alternative interventions. Thus, for surgical interventions, they should understand the rehabilitation required, including the duration and the location of the rehabilitation. They do not need to know any of the details of the procedure, any more than they need to understand the chemical pathways of a medication.

Informed consent requires that *all reasonable options* should be presented, not just the one that most people might choose. It also requires that the option to refuse medical treatment be included. The benefits and burdens of each option must be explained in terms the patient can understand. Thus, if the patient refuses a life-saving surgery, the clinician should explain that the patient will most likely die as a result. This should not be done in a threatening tone, as if to coerce intervention. It may be that the patient is prepared to die and prefers a sooner death to a difficult or painful recovery period or a long period of inevitable decline. One should also mention that refusing all the options for curative treatment does not in any way preclude either hospice or palliative care. No patient should ever be made to fear dying alone or in pain.

Patients may choose any of the reasonable options, but this does not mean patients may choose any option. They may not choose options that are considered unreasonable, unproven, or physiologically futile, for example. Neither may they choose illegal options. *Most importantly*, they must appreciate the consequences of the option they choose. If they can say, "I know I will die, but I have been prepared for that for many years now," then there is no need to try to talk them out of it or to consider them suicidal (as they have not attempted suicide during those years).[1,2]

Sometimes there is a question of whether a patient is making a free and voluntary choice or is being coerced by either her doctor or her family. There is much the clinician can do to prevent the former, and there is a little the clinician can do to prevent the latter.

Some physicians express skepticism about the value of informed consent, saying that all their patients take their recommendations. Implicit in this claim may be an assumption that the doctor always recommends what is best, and any patient who refused the recommendation would be making a bad choice. It is rarely the case that there is only one good choice that is best for everybody. Furthermore, any physician who considers a patient's choice contrary to the doctor's recommendation as a personal rejection is at risk for becoming coercive.

Of course patients go to a doctor for advice, and generally hold doctors' recommendations in high regard. So it is reasonable to expect patients to accept physicians' recommendations most of the time. If more than one reasonable option is available, then it is sensible to expect some variation in the choices patients make, which reflect their personal value systems. Hence if all of a physician's patients make the same choice this is a prima facie warning sign of a coercive informed consent process.

Patients will often ask a health care provider what the provider would do in his or her situation. It is important to answer patient's questions, but it is also important to encourage patients to make their own decisions. Thus it is good to begin by replying, "Well, you have to understand that I am a __ (e.g. a 45-year-old Indian woman, and not a Christian), and so I may have very different values than you. And it is very hard for me to know what I would do unless I was in your situation. As a clinician I do know the medical facts, but you're the person who is going to reap the benefits or suffer the consequences of the treatment, not me. I can make a recommendation, but you must make the final decision."

If pressed for an answer, or faced with a patient who cannot make a decision without some external prompting, clinicians must be very careful not to impose their views. Many physicians have a natural bias toward medical treatment, which they must try to counterbalance. One might respond: "I know it would be a very difficult decision, and I might decide it was better to __ (e.g., go back to my family one last time) rather than go right into the hospital for treatment. You may be different from me, and I want you to think about what is best for you." This reminds them that there are at least two choices and that they do not need to agree with you, and even invites them to differ with you by giving them your reason for your choice so they can see if they share the same values.

It is harder to guarantee that family members are not influencing a patient's decision. Some degree of influence from loved ones is to be expected and is often welcomed by the patient. The clinician need not try to prevent all family input. The general principle of respect for persons requires that clinicians have at least one initial private conversation with their patient, without other family members present. At that meeting emphasize that this is the patient's decision, and it is up to the patient how much information she wishes to share with the family and how much of their advice to follow. Reassure the patient that if she ever feels pressured or coerced by her family she can request another private meeting and that you will respect her wishes. At the same time you can explain that it will be the patient's family who will make decisions for the patient if the patient loses capacity, unless the patient explicitly names an agent on an advance directive.[3]

It is also important to remember that patients may communicate their choice in many ways and not just by talking. Written notes, American Sign Language, hand squeezes, blinking, eye movements, and word, letter, and signboards are all useful tools in enabling nonverbal patients to communicate.

CAPACITY AND CONSISTENCY OVER TIME: THE ROLE OF THE FAMILY AND THE PRIMARY CARE PHYSICIAN IN ASSESSMENT

The basic concept of capacity has been described in the previous section, but there are some additional conditions that are debated as part of the concept. One, the concept that a decision be "rational," has been widely rejected, whereas the other, consistency, is sometimes a useful additional condition but must be applied with care.

The condition that the patient's decision must be rational before the patient is judged to have capacity has been rejected in ethics and law as outcome based, that is, according to what decision he makes. This falsely assumes there is only one rational choice, and that all patients with capacity must be rational. Rationality is at best an abstract ideal; it could well exclude 90% of humanity as everyone harbors some beliefs that are not well founded or based on scientific evidence. Religious beliefs, for example, can be defined as based on faith rather than reason, but we accept that patients can make decisions based on their religious beliefs if they choose.

Some definitions of capacity use the ambiguous term "reasoned choice." It can be interpreted as either the patient "gives a reason" for her choice or the patient makes a choice that is considered to be reasonable by her physician. Because of the etymological tie between "reason" and "rational," all such definitions invite a paternalistic restriction upon patients based on thinking physicians have a more reasoned understanding of medicine than do their patients. So long as the options being considered are all reasonable options, then there is no need for this additional condition.

If one wants to raise the standard for having capacity so the standard is restricted to persons who can give some justification for their choice, it is better to ask that patients be able to *explain* their choice rather than require they make a reasoned choice. Idiosyncratic or culturally determined explanations (e.g., based on folk medicine) are less likely to be rejected using this language as we are accustomed to appreciating the importance of respect for cultural diversity. (See the chapter on ethnic diversity.)

A more useful addition to the definition of capacity is that the patient makes a decision *consistent with their past choices*. This is a way to test for authenticity of belief, representing the ethical goal of having a patient make autonomous choices or choices that represent his core values or deeply held beliefs.

The idea of consistency over time as a way to judge whether a patient is making an authentic choice has some advantages: 1) it helps to identify decisions made in a state of panic or anxiety that the patient may later regret, and 2) it emphasizes the link between the concepts of decision-making capacity and surrogate decision-making, because surrogates of incapacitated patients are expected to make decisions that are consistent with those the patient made when capacitated.

Adding the condition of consistency over time also comports with an ethical methodology that has garnered much interest in the past decade: narrative ethics. Narrative ethics holds that a human life is best seen as a story: it has a beginning, middle, and end, with each stage growing naturally out of earlier stages, and with some sort of identifiable thread woven through it that is held together by the consistency over time of the subject's personality, memories, values, goals, and social network. Judging someone to have capacity is then saying that they are still in charge of their life-story and have the right to decide its ending.

The case of Mrs. Benson (case 2 described previously) demonstrates the potential importance of consistency over time. When physicians discovered that she had no memory of agreeing to be DNR the day before, they wisely repeated the entire informed consent process. When she agreed once again to the DNR directive they realized that her consistency sufficed for them to be comfortable that her choice represented her core values, even though she could not remember any conversation from one day to the next.

There is another interesting consequence of adding consistency to the criteria for capacity and that is that the experts about consistency would be the persons who have best known the patient over time. Thus a capacity assessment would have to include a family member, friend, or long-term care provider who has known the patient well for an extended period of time (e.g., when the patient clearly had decision-making capacity).

There is a drawback to adding consistency over time as an additional criterion: it could dissuade us from thinking that people who change their minds have capacity. Often a person who has stated a certain opinion for years when healthy may feel differently once confronting a serious illness. Thus the best practice is to not require consistency over time unless the patient has some confusion, depression, or memory impairment. In those cases consistency with past choices can be used to extend the range of cases in which patients remain in control of their medical care, thus maximizing patient self-determination.

EVALUATING CAPACITY: ASSESSMENT, TESTING, AND CONVERSATION

There is no single widely used and validated test for lack of capacity. This is not so much the fault of the tests as a consequence of the concept: the objective testing of subjective states is inherently limited. Nevertheless, any clinician should be able to assess whether her patient lacks capacity, it simply does not require a test or other objective assessment tool.

One point cannot be stressed enough: the commonly used Folstein Mini-Mental State Examination (MMSE) does not assess capacity, and using it for that purpose is a mistake.[4] The MMSE is designed to assess dementia and is validated for that purpose. It was never intended for assessing capacity. Indeed, any reference to an MMSE score in a psychiatry note responding to a request for a capacity evaluation is more of an indicator of confusion on the part of the consultant than the patient. Mrs. Benson would probably score less than a 15/30 on the MMSE, but still was rightly judged to have the capacity to agree to a DNR order. Interestingly, a patient can also score a perfect 30 on the MMSE and lack capacity. The point is the same: the MMSE simply does not test for capacity.

Similarly, tests for depression, although simple and potentially beneficial, do not test for capacity. A patient may have mild-to-moderate depression, as well as mild-to-moderate dementia and still be capable of informed decision making. If either dementia or depression is suspected the clinically relevant question is whether it is affecting patients' decisions or whether they are making the same decision they would make regardless of the diagnosis.

There are other more recent tests designed specifically to assess capacity such as the Aid to Capacity Evaluation[5] and the MacArthur Competence Assessment Tool-Treatment.[6] These tools are especially useful in research settings where one must be careful to be consistent in how one enters all the study subjects, especially when there is doubt about whether the study will have any medical benefit for the patient. They offer no advantage over a well-documented half hour conversation with a patient about his illness and all of the reasonable treatment options. Following such a discussion, if the patient understands his options, makes a choice, and understands the consequences, then the patient has capacity. A note documenting those facts in the chart is adequate legally to justify orders that are intended to achieve the patient's goals. It is not necessary for the note to review the entire medical history, although doing so is acceptable. It will be helpful if the note quotes *verbatim* a few of the questions asked of the patient and his or her replies. These can prove enormously helpful to the staff and the family later in the hospitalization, should the patient lose capacity.

There may be some concern that this time is not reimbursed; however one can be reimbursed for talking about advance directives, and short visits can always be billed for short conversations. This time can also be part and parcel of the informed consent process. "Informed consent" is not a form and it is not accomplished by obtaining a patient's signature, it is an informational process whose goal is patient self-determination. If it is given short shrift, then considering it as a simultaneous capacity assessment might encourage a more careful and complete process.

There is normally no need for a psychiatric consult to assess capacity. Recognizing this is important, given the shortage of psychiatrists, especially geriatric psychiatrists. The exceptions are when a patient already has a diagnosis that might benefit from a specialist, especially to determine if a condition that is interfering with capacity might be reversible. Thus a psychiatric consult can be justified for patients with refractory psychosis or delirium; just as a neurology consult or neuroimaging can be justified for stroke and dementia patients. It is typically the case that the geriatrician can assess capacity better than the specialist; thus the purpose of any consult must be made clear and not invite 'turfing' decisions better made by the doctor who has known the patient over time and knows the patient best.

There is another reason why capacity is best assessed by the patient's geriatrician or primary care physician as part of the consent process, rather than by a consulting psychiatrist. It is not uncommon for patients to resent being asked to talk to a psychiatrist for fear of being found to lack capacity and forced into a nursing home. As a result, patients sometimes refuse to meet with a psychiatrist. This can cause delays and frustration, but it is important to avoid interpreting a patient's refusal to meet with a psychiatrist to be evidence of a lack of capacity. If anything, it could be argued that refusing to talk to a psychiatrist is a sign of insight insofar as it shows an understanding of what the psychiatrist is there to evaluate and its possible consequences.

For hospitalized patients there may be another useful resource in cases where capacity is doubted or disputed: the *ethics consultation service*. These are available at most teaching hospitals in the United States and Canada, and their consultants (who are usually doctors, nurses, or philosophers with hospital-based training) will often have experience with other similar cases in the same hospital and will be familiar with local laws and policies.

DIMINISHED AND FLUCTUATING CAPACITY

Capacity is not all or nothing; some patients have it at some times of day and not at others. Some patients have capacity while medicated but not when the medications wear off, whereas others have it when the medications wear off but not when medicated. Yet other patients have capacity to make some decisions but not other decisions. Because of potential contingencies such as time of day and medication side effect, the clinician should always be careful in a chart note to say of a patient who lacks capacity that this may not be a chronic or irreversible condition and that one will return to reassess at a different time of day or after a change in medication or a wash-out period.

There is no need to worry that a patient with fluctuating capacity and resulting apparent "changes of mind" somehow cancels out the validity of her choices. The clinician in this case must clearly chart what the patient said during her lucid phases and make clear that occasional contrary statements were made during times of incapacity.

In addition, different levels of cognitive complexity are required for decisions choosing between medical interventions and choosing a durable power of attorney for health care (also known as a health care proxy in some states such as New York and New Jersey, and a health care surrogate in Florida). If a patient should be found to lack capacity to make some complex decisions, she may still have capacity to choose a loved one trusted to represent her wishes. This can be a critical last chance to maintain some control over the remainder of her life.

Helping patients make medical decisions and fill out advance directives is an absolutely essential task for geriatricians. A general discussion about attitudes about aggressive treatment, intensive care, feeding tubes, and nursing homes should be subtly woven into the last 10 minutes of every annual exam. Information garnered should be included in the chart for future reference. Advance directives, including naming a durable power of attorney for health care, should be suggested to every patient and help given in filling out the forms and putting them in the chart and having them implemented. Helping the patient select the friend or family member best able to handle the common pressures presented by the health care system (and avoid choosing someone who "cannot live without them") is also very important. This should not be seen as merely or routinely identifying the "next of kin."

It is never too late to address these issues. If clinicians offer to discuss them with a particular patient annually but are repeatedly rebuffed, that does not mean the patient will not want to address the issues after being hospitalized with a life-threatening illness. A visit to a patient in the hospital will never be forgotten by the patient or his family, and a documentation of capacity by the patient's private attending may allow a patient to maintain control over his life in the midst of a hospital chart filled by notes of numerous experts who are strangers to the patient.

PLACEMENT OR DISPLACEMENT? WHEN SAFETY AND FREEDOM CONFLICT

Mr. Allen's case (case 1 described previously) probably exemplifies the most common problem that triggers a capacity assessment, namely a patient who refuses beneficial treatment or who is making a decision that is considered dangerous.[7] Such decisions and the capacity assessments they trigger are usually made in the hospital, but the consequences often extend beyond the period of hospitalization.

For Mr. Allen and many other patients, the determination regarding capacity will decide whether he is allowed to return home or be discharged to a nursing home over his objections. His children were convinced that he would not take the medicine he needed to survive, but they also agreed that his refusal was consistent with his life-long values and actions. They were certain that living in a nursing home would be unacceptable to him, and he would try every way to escape, even if it risked death. Most importantly, his family did not feel like they had the right to make decisions for him, as they felt he could make his own decisions. This was a good example of the use of the optional fifth condition for capacity, consistency over time, and especially the important role of family in judging whether a patient meets that criterion. Mr. Allen did indeed go home, surviving for about a month (thanks to subtle surveillance by his family and his family physician). During that time he was very happy to have won this final battle, bragging to friends about how he outsmarted all of his doctors.

Thus, another issue raised by the case is when *involuntary placement* in a nursing home can be justified. In general, if a patient with capacity refuses placement, that wish must be respected. If discharge to home is not felt to be safe, that does not automatically justify nursing home placement. Safety is not an absolute value, but one value that must be balanced with others. Freedom to live where you want and especially freedom to live in your own home is an important liberty we enjoy in our society.

In situations where safety and freedom collide, the weighing of each must be done with meticulous attention to detail: Can the home be modified to enhance safety, such as switching a gas stove to an electric stove? Can a cleaning service be engaged to shovel out years of hoarded newspapers and clean and disinfect the kitchen and bathrooms? If so, then the value of respecting the decisions of patients with capacity clearly prevails. Or, on the other hand, can the nursing home be interviewed in advance for its willingness to allow eccentric individuals to maintain their lifestyle, such as sleeping late every day, or drinking or smoking in their room? Can a nursing home be located with a dominant ethnic group that will make the patient feel more at home than he would feel isolated at home, such as one with many Asian or Hispanic residents? If so, then perhaps the patient can be persuaded to change his mind and give it a try.[8–10]

Giving these controversies their due attention, including a capacity assessment, is very important. In the long run, the worst outcomes could result from well meaning but one-sided safety concerns: elderly patients might prefer not to call 9-1-1 if they think every hospitalization carries with it the risk of an involuntary placement (or as it might more accurately be called, "displacement"). Documentation of a patient's decision that he or she understands and appreciates the risks will keep the responsibility for the consequences with the patient who knowingly chooses independence over safety and will minimize any legal risk to the physician.

PATIENTS WHO LACK CAPACITY: WHEN RESPECT FOR PERSONS REPLACES AUTONOMY

The emphasis so far has been on cases in which the patient was assessed to have capacity, despite initial doubts. What about cases in which the patient does not have capacity? There is often a misperception that determining a "difficult patient" lacks capacity will make decision-making easier; however, this is seldom the case. Someone will still have to make the decisions, and it is rarely the doctor who will be empowered to do that. So a finding of incapacity sets in motion a search for a suitable surrogate, and then the informed consent process must begin again with the surrogate.

It is not necessarily easier to deal with a healthy adult child of an elderly patient. There may be great emotional difficulties in making decisions to stop life-sustaining treatment, for example, especially in cases in which there are no advance directives. There may be differences of culture and location: You may have to wait for someone to travel 3,000 miles and then find that they are less trusting of your advice than was your patient.

When a patient lacks capacity there is no choice but to begin this process of family decision making. Most states have laws with an ordinal list of surrogates, starting with the spouse followed by adult children, then siblings, and ending with close friends. It should be kept in mind, however, that one is really seeking those who can best represent the patient's preferences, and that anyone on the list of surrogates can defer to someone else lower on the list if they feel that other person can do a better job. Then the goal of the informed consent process becomes a collaborative effort between the clinician and the surrogate(s) to decide what the patient would have wanted in the circumstances. This is called *substituted judgment*.[11,12]

In the situation in which the patient lacks capacity and there is no family member who is able to help with substituted judgment (due to lack of family members or unwillingness of family members to make decisions), then clinicians are counseled to do what is best for the patient. This is commonly known as *the best interest standard*. This judgment should include both the benefits and the burdens of all the treatment options, so as to weigh quality of life as well as duration of life. This should not be taken to mean "do everything" or "always err on the side of life." Clinicians must still obey the Hippocratic advice to "At least, Do No Harm," that is, do not pursue interventions that are likely to make things worse or prolong suffering. If the decision to withhold or withdraw some life-sustaining treatment is to be made, it is be advisable to request a review by the ethics consultation service. Their role, however, is not to make the decision but to confirm its reasonableness in the given circumstances.

Once any medical decisions are arrived at using either substituted judgment or the best interest standard, it is important that someone inform the patient. If the patient objects, then one must carefully review the reasons it was felt she lacked capacity, and consider whether the patient's objection is worthy of reassessing the evaluation. Sometimes it will become evident on reassessment that the patient does understand and appreciate her situation, in which case the family will often accept the patient's decision (and feel relieved of the burden of deciding).[13]

Generally speaking, courts do not like to hear cases that are "just" about medical decisions, especially end-of-life decisions. Furthermore, going to court will usually take more than a month (even expedited hearings usually take at least 2 weeks), and means engaging in a system that is by definition adversarial. There are fees for the court, for the lawyers, and for the expert witnesses. One can never predict the outcome of a hearing or all of its long-term consequences. Often a guardian will be appointed who is unfamiliar with the patient. Hence it might only be advisable to go to court to determine whether the patient can be declared incompetent when 1) a patient is determined to lack capacity, *and* 2) there is reason to think this condition will not be reversible, *and* 3) there are no friends or family available to help make decisions for the patient, *and* 4) there are likely to be a number of important decisions to be made for the patient (such as involuntary placement and selling of property and other financial issues).[14]

To paraphrase one of the great judges in American history: "Hell is filled with lawyers paying more attention to due process than to achieving justice." Hence courts should generally be seen as a last resort, and an indication that issues were not properly addressed by the patient and primary care doctor when they should have been. Before beginning down that road, it is always advisable to ask oneself if there is any way to improve your patient's understanding and appreciation of the situation by improving one's communication skills. It has been said that half the problem with noncompliant patients is doctors who do not give adequate time to patient education, and it might also be true that half the problem with incapacitated patients is doctors who do not take the time to listen.

REFERENCES

1. Lane v. Candura, 6 Mass. App. 377,376 N.E. 2nd 1232 (1978).
2. Meisel A, Cerminara KL. *The Right to Die*. 3rd ed. New York: Aspen Publishing; 2004.
3. Lo B, Steinbrook RL. Resuscitating advance directives. *Arch Intern Med*. 2004;164:1501–1506.
4. Folstein MF, Folstein SE, McHugh PR. Mini-mental state: a practical method for grading the cognitive state of patients for the clinician. *J Psychiatr Res*. 1975;12:189.
5. Aid to Capacity Evaluation (ACE) was developed at the University of Toronto Center for Bioethics. Available at: http://www.jointcentreforbioethics.ca/tools/ace.shtml. Accessed June 22, 2008.
6. Grisso T, Appelbaum P. *Assessing Competence to Consent to Treatment: A Guide for Physicians and Other Health Professionals*. Oxford: Oxford University Press; 1998.
7. Spike JP, Greenlaw J. Ethics consultation: refusal of beneficial treatment by a surrogate decision maker. *J Law Med Ethics*. 1995;23:202–204.

8. Kane RA and Caplan AL. *Everyday Ethics: Resolving Dilemmas in Nursing Home Life*. New York: Springer;1990.

9. Spike JP. Personhood and a paradox about capacity. In: Thomasma D, Weisstaub D, eds. *Personhood in Healthcare*. New York: Kluwer Academic Publishers; 2001.

10. Spike JP. Capacity is not in your head. In: Thomasma D, Weisstaub D, eds. *Variables of Moral Capacity*. New York: Kluwer Academic Publishers; 2004.

11. Singer PA, Martin DK, Lavery JV, et al. Reconceptualizing advance care planning from the patient's perspective. *Arch Intern Med*. 1998;158;879–884.

12. Arnold RM, Kellum J. Moral Justifications for surrogate decision making in the ICU. *Crit Care Med*. 2003;31:S347–S353.

13. Spike JP. Narrative unity and the unraveling of personal identity: dialysis, dementia, stroke, and advance directives. *J Clin Ethics*. 2000;11:367–372.

14. In re Jobes, 529 A 2nd 434 (N.J. 1987).

46

INJURIES IN OLDER ADULTS

Amy R. Ehrlich, MD, Keiko Kimura, MD, Jody Rogers, MD

Injuries are an important cause of morbidity and mortality in the elderly and are the ninth leading cause of death in the United States for all persons aged 65 years and older.[1] The contemporary model of injury prevention and control is based on the concept that the event leading to the injury is distinct from the injury itself. Injuries can be prevented by altering the precipitating event, changing the impact of the event on the individual, or modifying the environment.[2] Passive injury prevention strategies, such as modifications in the environment or product design, are generally the most successful. Active injury prevention strategies that require an individual to change their behavior are more prone to failure.[2,3]

The leading causes of injuries in the elderly are a diverse group of events including falls, motor vehicle accidents (see Chapter 48), fires and burns, poisoning, choking, and environmental exposures. Falls are the most frequent cause of injuries in older adults accounting for 61% of nonfatal injuries and 40% of fatalities. Motor vehicle accidents are the second most common cause for injury and death outside the home in the elderly.[4] Most nonvehicular injuries occur within the home environment. Rates of home injury–related death increase with advancing age, rising from 7 per 100,000 in those aged 60–69 years to 48 per 100,000 in those aged 80 years and older. Fire- and burn-related injuries are the second most common cause of death in the home, followed by poisoning and choking.[5,6] Heat and cold exposure injuries also pose a significant threat in older adults.

Injuries in the geriatric population can be conceptualized as a "geriatric syndrome," arising from a complex interplay of predisposing risk factors including advancing age, and functional, sensory, and cognitive impairment.[7] Extrapolating from the extensive literature on falls, additional risk factors contributing to injuries are likely to include the use of multiple medications and specifically the use of psychotropic medications.[8] The role of dementia, with its accompanying deficits in memory and judgment, as a contributing factor to household injuries has

not been fully elucidated. Dementia is present in up to 50% of community-dwelling persons older than the age of 85 years. Dementia is frequently not recognized by the treating physician, with up to two-thirds of patients with moderate dementia not correctly identified by physicians in the office setting or the emergency department.[9,10] It is, however, reasonable to postulate that a frail older adult with cognitive as well as functional and sensory deficits who is at increased risk for falls is also at risk for other household injuries. Experts recommend a multifactorial intervention strategy for patients who have fallen or are thought to be at high risk for falling and a similar approach should be considered to prevent other injuries in older adults.[11]

The U.S. Preventive Services Task Force recommends counseling adults to prevent household accidents; however, there are no trials on the outcome of including counseling as a part of the routine office-based health care of elderly patients.[11] A referral to a home care agency, for a home safety assessment, may be warranted for patients at high risk for a household injury. A home safety evaluation by allied health professionals can explore potential risks for common injuries that exist in the home environment. Multiple home safety assessment tools are available to aid health professionals in reviewing safety risk during a home visit, although no tools have been used in large trials and no outcome data exist to evaluate individual tools (Table 46.1).[12,13]

FIRES AND BURNS

The risk of injury and death in a residential fire increases with advancing age. Adults aged 85 years and older have a relative risk of death by fire that is 4.6 times higher than the national average. The highest fire fatality rates are seen in males and within the African American community, reflecting both the increased poverty rates and increased burden of medical illness.

Table 46.1. Home Safety Checklist

General Housing
- Smoke detectors
  - Present and in working order
  - Location: on every floor, away from air vents, near bedrooms, on ceiling or 6–12 in below ceiling
- Carbon monoxide detector present
- Telephones
  - Emergency numbers next to phone
  - Phones accessible
- Medications
  - Properly stored and clearly labeled
  - No expired medications
- Hazardous materials stored properly
- Adequate heating and cooling
  - Space heaters/wood burning stoves
    - Located away from flammable materials
    - Appear properly installed and maintained
- Emergency exit plan in place

All Rooms/Hallways
- Passageways
  - Free from objects and clutter
- Cords
  - Out of the flow of traffic. Not under rugs
- Lighting adequate
- Floor coverings
  - No unsecured throw rugs/runners; carpets lie flat

Specific Rooms/Areas
- Kitchen
  - Flammable and combustible objects stored away from burners and ovens
  - Cooking supplies stored away from burners
  - Frequently used supplies within easy reach
  - Sturdy step stool available
  - Refrigerator free of spoiled food
- Bathroom
  - Nonslip surface or nonskid mats on bathroom floor
  - Nonskid surface (mat or abrasive strips) in bath/tub
  - Grab bars for bath/tub
  - Hot water temperature <120°F
  - *Patients with fall risk*
    - *Raised toilet seat*
    - *grab bars by toilet*
    - *Bath bench/shower seat*
    - *Handheld shower device*
- Bedrooms
  - Phone accessible from bed
  - Lamp/light accessible from bed
  - Adequate light from bed to toilet
- Stairs
  - Handrail secure
  - Steps and coverings in good repair
  - Light switches at top and bottom of stairs
  - Lighting adequate to visualize each step

African American males aged 85 years and older have a relative risk of death in a residential fire that is 21.5 times higher than the overall population.[14] The mortality rate for older adults admitted to burn centers also rises with age, although advances in contemporary burn care have improved survival rates in the oldest of the old.[15,16] Common causes of residential fires involving the elderly include cigarette smoking, cooking, and heating equipment.[14]

Alcohol and Benzodiazepines

Alcohol is the single most important independent risk factor for death in all residential fires.[17] In autopsy series, up to three-quarters of middle-aged adults are reported to have a positive alcohol level at the time of fire death. The association is less significant in elderly fire victims, nonetheless up to 30% of decedents aged 60 years and older have a positive alcohol level.[18,19] Similarly, positive alcohol levels are found in 9%–21% of elderly patients admitted with a major burn.[20,21]

Benzodiazepines, which are associated with multiple increased adverse drug events (ADEs) including an increased risk of falls, are commonly prescribed for community-dwelling elderly.[22] In one retrospective study, almost one-third of elderly patients admitted with a major burn had a positive toxicology screen for benzodiazepines, cocaine, or marijuana.[21] Although these data have not been replicated in other trials, they are consistent with the finding of increased ADEs with the use of benzodiazepines. Elderly persons with dementia and functional disabilities are at increased risk for both major burns and fire death.[19] In one retrospective chart review of elderly patients admitted to a burn unit, up to 30% were found to have dementia.[23] A similar study found that two-thirds of patients with a diagnosis of dementia were unsupervised at the time of their burn injury; these accidents occurred when the patients were bathing or cooking.[24]

Cigarettes

Cigarettes are the leading cause of fire fatalities in the elderly. The high morbidity and mortality rates from cigarette smoking are related to the ignition of bedding or clothing, with subsequent severe burns and smoke inhalation. The majority of older adults who die in a fire are sleeping or bedridden.[25] Strategies to aid the elderly in smoking cessation are similar to those used for the rest of the adult population. High-risk activities, such as smoking in bed, should be specifically addressed.[26] Patients with cognitive deficits who continue to smoke pose a complex management problem for families and physicians. Every attempt should be made to encourage such patients to participate in smoking cessation; however, families and other caregivers may need to be instructed by the physician to stop providing the homebound, demented patient access to cigarettes, as these patients represent an unacceptably high risk for accidental injury to self or others.

Cooking

For older adults, accidents while cooking are the single most important cause of burns and a leading cause of death in residential fires. Cooking burns account for up to 40% of major burns and 70% of emergency department visits for minor burns in elderly adults.[27,28] The most common cause of major cooking burns is the "granny-gown" burn: the ignition of loose fitting clothing while reaching across a stove.[29,30] Strategies to limit cooking burns include patient and family education regarding safe cooking techniques, and environmental modifications such as the use of stoves with side mounted controls, and the removal of cooking supplies from the back of the stove.

There are few data to guide the physician in evaluating an elderly patient's risk in cooking. Warning signs of unsafe behavior may include a history of minor burns, reports of burned food or utensils, or leaving on the gas. The use of timers may be a useful adjunct for patients with mild cognitive impairment who have insight into their deficit. Patients with significant cognitive deficit, unless directly supervised, need to discontinue cooking. If necessary, caregivers may need to be instructed to remove the knobs from the stove and disconnect kitchen appliances to prevent cooking while unsupervised.

Bath and Shower Burns

Scald burns from hot tap water are associated with a high morbidity and mortality. Over half of fatal tap water burns in the United States occur in patients aged 75 years and older.[31] The causes of bathtub burns include inappropriate handling of the hot water taps, falls, seizures, and syncope.[32] In one series of elderly patients admitted with major bathtub-related scald burns, two-thirds were found to be demented.[23]

To reduce injury, the recommended maximum temperature for residential hot water heaters is 120°F; estimates are that it takes 5 minutes to develop a full thickness burn at this temperature.[33] The majority of adults in the United States do not know the setting of their hot water heater, and studies that have directly measured residential hot water temperatures have found a significant prevalence of dangerously high water temperatures.[34] Basic safety equipment is frequently not present in the homes of community-dwelling elderly. Bath and shower safety equipment has been studied in relationship to patients with bathing disability. In one large trial, up to 50% of community-dwelling elderly who were functionally at risk for falls lack basic safety equipment such as grab bars and shower seats.[35,36] A successful public health initiative to prevent household injuries including falls, burns, and scalds emphasized lowering hot water thermostats and installing grab bars and nonskid strips.[37] Physicians should review the presence of both adequate supervision and bathroom safety equipment for patients with cognitive deficits and those at high risk for falls or burns. In addition to testing and maintaining hot water temperature at less than 120°F, recommendations to prevent hot tap water injuries include filling bathtubs with cold water first.

Medical Equipment Associated with Burns

Heating Pads

Heating pads result in 1,600 emergency room visits annually in the United States, with the elderly accounting for almost half of heating pad–related burns. Heating pads may also lead to major burns requiring admission to a burn center. Patients with sensory deficits or cognitive deficits are at increased risk for burns from these devices. High-risk behaviors include sitting or lying on a heating pad or use while sleeping.[27,38,39] Recommendations for the use of heating pads in any elderly patient need to be carefully weighed against the potential for misuse resulting in a burn.

Home Oxygen

More than 90% of burns or fires caused by home oxygen occur in patients who smoke; other causes include lighting a family member's cigarette or a pilot light on a furnace.[40] In elderly patients receiving home care services, factors contributing to burns or fire include cognitive impairment, nonfunctional smoke detectors, and living alone. Poor communication among the multiple health care providers involved with the homebound patient (primary care physician, home care team, and medical supply company) also plays a role in these accidents. Recommendations to reduce risk associated with home oxygen include ensuring that systems are in place for training and education of caregivers, notifying the physician if a patient resumes smoking, and testing for a functional smoke detector.[41]

Vaporizers

Vaporizers that are used for the treatment of respiratory infections may lead to scald burns.[42] In frail patients, with cognitive and sensory deficits, who are at increased danger from a home injury, the potential benefits of a vaporizer need to be weighed against the risk a burn.

Common Consumer Products and Environmental Hazards

A wide range of consumer products is associated with burns in the elderly. Hair care products, including curling irons and hair dryers, are a frequent cause of ocular burns requiring emergency department visits in the pediatric population and have also been reported in the elderly.[43] Contact burns from heating radiators or hot pipes have also been responsible for burns in vulnerable adults and can be prevented with a variety of structural modifications.[27,44]

Minor Burns

Of the approximately 1.1 million annual burn injuries in the United States that come to medical attention, only 5% are estimated to require admission to the hospital. The remaining 95% are minor burns that can be safely managed in the outpatient setting.[45] It is not known if minor burns are a marker for patients who are at increased risk for a life-threatening burn. There are no clinical trials evaluating interventions for elderly patients presenting for treatment of minor burns, nor are there studies describing the long-term outcome for such patients. A retrospective study found that elderly patients with minor burns and multiple chronic medical problems, who were treated and discharged from an emergency department, were rarely referred to a home care agency for further evaluation.[28] Physicians should consider referral to a home care agency for patients who present with a minor burn. The patient must have a skilled need, in the field of nursing, physical therapy or social work, for the referral to be part of a Medicare covered benefit. In this setting, a home safety evaluation by allied health professionals can explore potential risks for recurrent burns that exist in the home environment.

Physicians caring for a patient with a minor burn should consider the possibility of cognitive impairment as a contributing factor in the accident. Additionally, a medication history should be reviewed for use of benzodiazepines and other psychotropic medications, as well as the use of cigarettes and alcohol. High-risk activities should be targeted in patients found to have cognitive deficits, including smoking, cooking, bathing, and use of consumer products associated with burns.

Smoke Alarms

The presence of a functioning smoke alarm reduces mortality from residential fires by up to 60%.[19] Although the number of homes with smoke alarms has continued to rise, up to one-quarter of smoke alarms in United States households are estimated to be nonfunctional. On average, 70% of fire deaths occur in the United States in homes with no functional smoke alarm.[46] In one study, smoke alarms were found to be protective in the homes of vulnerable elderly with either physical or cognitive disabilities.[19] Special smoke alarms are made for the deaf or hard of hearing, which use strobe lights or vibrating devices. Other safety recommendations for residential homes include having a fire extinguisher and a preplanned fire escape route, although there are few data available to support these practices.[34] Hospital-based home care nurses, during the assessment of new referrals, have been effective at screening the apartments or houses of homebound patients for the presence of a functional smoke detector, and assisting in the installation of smoke detectors in the homes of this high-risk population.[47] During a home visit, a review of smoke detectors, fire extinguishers, and knowledge of fire exits should be part of the home safety evaluation.[12]

POISONINGS AND OVERDOSES

Drug overdose and poisoning, either intentional or unintentional, are major causes of injuries in the home for older adults. Adults aged 65 years and older comprise approximately 12% of the total U.S. population but are responsible for 30% of the total prescription drug use and 40% of the over-the-counter-drug purchases.[48,49] ADEs include allergic reactions, undesirable pharmacological effects or toxic effects, secondary side effects such as falls, but exclude intentional overdoses and poisonings.[50] The frequency of ADEs and potential for drug toxicity both rise with the increasing numbers of medications used per patient.[51] ADEs in the outpatient setting increase dramatically with advancing age and lead to a higher

hospitalization rate in the elderly.[50] The distinction between ADEs and poisoning may be less clear than in a younger population.[52] Older adults are at greater risk of death from both intentional and unintentional overdose than younger adults. In 2004, just over 2.4 million exposures were reported to U.S. poison centers. Although persons aged 60 years and older represented only 5% of these exposures, they accounted for 15% of poisoning-related deaths and the fatality rate was highest among those aged 80 years and older.[53]

Unintentional accidental exposures are the most common cause of poisonings in the elderly.[54,55] Intentional drug overdose remains the most common method for suicide attempts, although firearms account for the greatest number of successful suicides in the elderly.[56] Age-related changes in pharmacokinetics and pharmacodynamics make the elderly more susceptible to poisoning.[57,58] Older patients often have comorbid conditions, resulting in decreased physiological reserve when confronted with poisoning. Recommendations to reduce unintentional poisoning and overdoses in the elderly include counseling patients and their families regarding proper storage and labeling of all toxic substances and medications. Patients with cognitive deficits also require adequate supervision of their medication management and administration.

Presentation

Overdoses in the elderly may be difficult to diagnose for multiple reasons. First, they frequently present with nonspecific signs and symptoms, such as altered sensorium, changes in sleep patterns, or cognitive dysfunction. Second, toxicity is frequently due to chronic or subacute exposure, so a clear history of excessive drug ingestion may be nonexistent or difficult to obtain.[52] Third, the presenting signs and symptoms may mimic other disease processes. For example, the diagnosis of chronic salicylate toxicity is often delayed in the elderly because the clinical presentation is similar to other disease states such as infection or delirium.[59] A high level of suspicion must be maintained for an atypical or subtle presentation of drug toxicity and overdose in an elderly person presenting with unexplained symptoms or change in functional status.

Diagnosis

The approach to the poisoned patient requires using multiple diagnostic tools. A detailed history of medication use and toxic exposures must be obtained. The physical examination may help elucidate an etiology by suggesting a toxidrome: the various signs and symptoms that are referable to one toxic substance or class of substance. There are several common toxidromes including anticholinergic, opioid, cholinergic, and sympathomimetic (Table 46.2). Recognition of the anticholinergic toxidrome is of particular importance in the elderly, as they may be more susceptible to these effects and have signs of toxicity even at therapeutic dosing. Anticholinergic toxicity is commonly seen with ingestion of tricyclic antidepressants, first generation antihistamines, antipsychotic, and antiparkinsonian medications. Laboratory studies that should be obtained

Table 46.2. Common Toxidromes

Anticholinergic Toxidrome:
Delirium with psychomotor agitation or somnolence, tachycardia, mydriasis, hypertension, hyperthermia, dry mucous membranes, dry flushed skin, absent bowel sounds, urinary retention

Opioid Toxidrome:
Central nervous depression, respiratory depression, miosis, bradycardia, hypothermia, gastrointestinal stasis

Cholinergic Toxidrome:
Muscarinic Effects: salivation, lacrimation, urination, defecation, vomiting, bradycardia, bronchorrhea, miosis

Nicotinic Effects: muscle weakness, fasciculations, paralysis, diaphoresis, mydriasis, tachycardia, hypertension

Sympathomimetic Toxidrome:
Hypertension, tachycardia, hyperthermia, agitation, diaphoresis, mydriasis.[52]

in every acute suicidal overdose or unknown ingestion include electrolytes, glucose, blood urea nitrogen, and creatinine to screen for acidosis and renal failure. Aspirin and acetaminophen levels should be part of every initial evaluation because these are common, potentially fatal toxins for which early intervention can be life saving. Additional laboratory studies to consider during potential overdose cases include arterial blood gas levels, prothrombin time and partial thromboplastin time, liver function tests, blood ethanol levels, carboxyhemoglobin, and specific individual drug levels.[52] Because chronic drug toxicity is of particular concern in the elderly, individual drug levels may be helpful in the diagnosis of chronic aspirin, digoxin, theophylline, and lithium toxicity. The results of an electrocardiogram may be suggestive of toxicity from several drugs including digoxin, calcium channel blockers, β-blockers, and tricyclic antidepressants and can also reveal cardiac ischemia from carbon monoxide or stimulants. Routine urine drug screening has never been shown to contribute to the immediate clinical management of the overdose patient although urine drug screens have a role in patients with delirium, tachycardia, or unexplained seizures.[60]

The management of overdoses in the elderly, although similar to that of younger patients, is often complicated by the presence of comorbid medical conditions and threshold for admission to an intensive care unit should remain low. Management may require a multidisciplinary approach including consultation with a local poison center or toxicologist, and transfer to a tertiary hospital.

Choking

Inhalation of food or other objects into the respiratory tract, leading to choking and suffocation, is an important cause of mortality for older adults in the home.[5] The literature, however, is almost entirely limited to aspiration-related syndromes in the hospital and nursing home.[61,62] Age-related impairment of swallowing reflex may be exacerbated by comorbid medical conditions, cognitive impairment, neurological illness such as stroke, Parkinson's disease, medications, and alcohol use, placing many older persons at risk for aspiration. The most common aspirated material is organic matter, followed by dental appliances; aspiration of foreign bodies comprise approximately 0.2% of bronchoscopies performed in all adults and peak incidence is in the sixth decade.[63–65] Sudden onset of choking with intractable coughing as well as chronic cough are common presenting symptoms of foreign body aspiration; occult foreign body aspiration is rarely seen.

Recommendations for the prevention of aspiration-related injuries in the community can only be extrapolated from data on prevention in institutionalized older adults. For patients at risk, it would be reasonable to recommend evaluation by a speech pathologist, adequate supervision during eating, with appropriate modifications in food texture and feeding and swallowing techniques.[61] Several early trials demonstrate potential benefits from medications in the treatment of swallowing dysfunction in older persons but have not been repeated in larger trials.[66,67]

HYPOTHERMIA AND HYPERTHERMIA

Aging is associated with lower metabolic rate and impaired thermoregulation. In response to cold, older persons have decreased ability to generate heat, along with decreased ability to vasoconstrict appropriately, resulting in increased heat loss. They are less able to maintain core temperature during a cold challenge, have reduced cutaneous thermal sensitivity, and may need a colder stimulus to initiate protective actions to shield themselves from the cold.[68] Older persons also have decreased heat tolerance, that is, reduced sweating response in hot, dry environments.[69] Blunted thirst response is common and many elderly are unable to achieve adequate hydration. Although accidental deaths from hypothermia and hyperthermia are relatively uncommon, older adults people are disproportionately affected. There is an increased rate of accidental deaths due to hypothermia or hyperthermia with advancing age, and many of these fatalities are preventable.[70,71]

Hypothermia is defined as a decline in the core temperature to less than 95°F or 35°C and is classified according to measured core temperature as mild (35–32°C), moderate (<32–28°C), and severe (<28°C).[72] Deaths from hypothermia often result from both excessive heat loss through environmental exposure and inadequate heat protection. Immersion in water results in more rapid onset of hypothermia because water has greater thermal conductivity compared with air and promotes heat loss. Symptoms of mild hypothermia are vigorous shivering, tachycardia, and cold white skin. With moderate hypothermia, there is amnesia, apathy, and loss of coordination. In severe cases, loss of consciousness and reduced cardiac and respiratory rate are seen, along with fixed dilated pupils and areflexia, mimicking death.

Deaths from hypothermia are probably underreported. In the U.S. there are approximately 700 deaths per year due to hypothermia, and over half are in persons aged 65 years and older.[73] The risk factors for accidental deaths from hypothermia identified by the Centers for Disease Control and Prevention include age older than 65 years old, mental impairment, and substance abuse, most commonly alcohol.

Hyperthermia is defined as core body temperature above 103°F or 39.4°C, resulting from environmental exposure or strenuous exercise.[74] Heat exhaustion is a milder condition, characterized by cool and sweaty skin, fatigue, muscle cramps, dizziness, nausea and vomiting. Progression to heat stroke is almost always fatal and is accompanied by dry, red, hot skin and confusion leading to loss of consciousness.

Heat-related deaths increase with advancing age, rising from 2 deaths per 1 million population to 6 deaths per 1 million in those aged 65 and older. Advanced age and inability for care for oneself were identified as two major risk factors for heat-related deaths by the Centers for Disease Control and Prevention.[71,75]

Many of the heat-related deaths take place during heat waves, most notably in the July 1995 heat wave in Chicago that resulted in 739 deaths. Summer heat waves are defined by the National Weather Service as 3 or more consecutive days of air temperature *higher than* 90°F. The strongest risk factors for death during the 1995 heat wave in Chicago were being confined to bed and living alone.[76] In addition, a higher mortality rate was observed among frail elderly, defined as those receiving home care services such as visiting nurse, home care aides, housekeepers and Meals-on-Wheels, compared with those who did not require such services. Protective factors were having a working air conditioner and having access to transportation. Decreased risk of death was also seen with social worker visits prior to the heat wave.

Comorbid health problems such as cardiac and respiratory diseases are exacerbated with extremes of temperature. The presence of comorbid medical problems and use of multiple medications may contribute to development of hypo- and hyperthermia. Common clinical conditions in the elderly include cerebrovascular accident, impairing central thermoregulation, and dementia, leading to poor judgment. Medications such a narcotics and benzodiazepines may affect cognition. Diuretics and anticholinergics interfere with salt and water balance and neuroleptics interfere with thermoregulation. Additionally, excessive alcohol and use of multiple medications may contribute to the development of hypo- or hyperthermia. These factors, along with decreased ability to care for oneself, financial stresses that lead to parsimony with energy expenditures, and lack of social support make older persons vulnerable to cold- and heat-related deaths.

In recent years, public awareness of the vulnerability of the elderly to heat and cold has grown and local emergency response plans have been implemented. During times of extreme weather, health warnings are televised, emphasizing extra attention to those who are frail and elderly. Recommended preventive measures are to monitor the elderly living alone, and encourage them to have a working cooling or heating source. In some cities, local officials have developed and implemented emergency response plans when extreme weather is forecast. Chicago increased the number of daily contacts with the elderly during the 1999 heat wave, reducing the death toll.[71] Additional public health strategies such as opening cooling centers during heat waves and warm shelters during extreme winters may help to minimize weather-related deaths.

REFERENCES

1. National Vital Statistics Reports: Deaths: Leading Causes for 2002, 53:17. 2005. Center for Disease Control and Prevention. Available at: www.cdc.gov/nchs/data/nvsr/nvsr53_17.pdf. Accessed July 2008.
2. Rivara FP, Grossman DC, Cummings P. Injury prevention. First of two parts. *NEJM*. 1997;337:543–548.
3. Robertson L. *Injuries: Causes, Control Strategies, and Public Policy*. Lexington, MA: Lexington Books; 1983.
4. National Center for Injury Prevention and Control. Web-based Injury Statistics Query and Reporting System (WISQARS), 2003. Centers for Disease Control and Prevention. Available at: www.cdc.gov/ncipc/wisqars. Accessed June 22, 2008.
5. Runyan CW, Perkis D, Marshall SW, et al. Unintentional injuries in the home in the United States Part I: mortality. *Am J Prev Med*. 2005;28:73–79.
6. Injury Facts, 2004. National Safety Council. Available at http://www2.nsc.org/library/facts.htm (7/13/08).
7. Tinetti ME, Inouye SK, Gill TM, Doucette JT. Shared risk factors for falls, incontinence, and functional dependence. Unifying the approach to geriatric syndromes. *JAMA*. 1995;273:1348–1353.
8. Tinetti ME. Clinical practice. Preventing falls in elderly persons. *NEJM*. 2003;348:42–49.
9. Hustey FM, Meldon SW, Smith MD, Lex CK. The effect of mental status screening on the care of elderly emergency department patients. *Ann Emerg Med*. 2003;41:678–684.
10. Callahan CM, Hendrie HC, Tierney WM. Documentation and evaluation of cognitive impairment in elderly primary care patients. *Ann Intern Med*. 1995;122:422–429.
11. Health Services/Technology Assessment Text: Guide to Clinical Preventive Services, 3rd ed. Agency for Health Care Research and Quality. Available at: http://www.ahrq.gov. Accessed June 22, 2008.
12. Tanner EK. Assessing home safety in homebound older adults. *Geriatr Nurs*. 2003;24:250–254, 256.
13. Safety for Older Consumers Home Safety Checklist. Consumer Product Safety Commission. Document #701.on. Available at: www.cpsc.gov/CPSCPUB/PUBS/705.pdf. Accessed July 2008.
14. Fire and the Older Adult. U.S. Fire Administration/National Fire Data Center. 2006. Homeland Security. Available at: http://www.usfa.dhs.gov/downloads/pdf/publications/fa-300.pdf. Accessed June 22, 2008.
15. Pomahac B, Matros E, Semel M, et al. Predictors of survival and length of stay in burn patients older than 80 years of age: does age really matter? *J Burn Care Res*. 2006;27:265–269.
16. Lionelli GT, Pickus EJ, Beckum OK, DeCoursey RL, Korentager RA, et al. A three decade analysis of factors affecting burn mortality in the elderly. *Burns*. 2005;31:958–963.
17. Runyan CW, Bangdiwala SI, Linzer MA, Sacks JJ, Butts J. Risk factors for fatal residential fires. *NEJM*. 1992;327:859–863.

18. McGwin Jr. G, Chapman V, Curtis J, Rousculp M. Fire fatalities in older people. *J Am Geriatr Soc.* 1999;47:1307–1311.

19. Marshall SW, Runyan CW, Bangdiwala SI, et al. Fatal residential fires: who dies and who survives? *JAMA.* 1998;279(20):1633–1637.

20. Hunt JL, Purdue GF. The elderly burn patient. *Am J Surg.* 1992;164:472–476.

21. McGill V, Kowal-Vern A, Gamelli RL. Outcome for older burn patients. *Arch Surg.* 2000;135(3):320–325.

22. Leipzig RM, Cumming RG, Tinetti ME. Drugs and falls in older people: a systematic review and meta-analysis: I. Psychotropic drugs. *J Am Geriatr Soc.* 1999;47:30–39.

23. Hill AJ, Germa F, Boyle JC. Burns in older people–outcomes and risk factors. *J Am Geriatr Soc.* 2002;50:1912–1913.

24. Alden NE, Rabbitts A, Yurt RW. Burn injury in patients with dementia: an impetus for prevention. *J Burn Care Rehabil.* 2005;26(3):267–271.

25. The Fire Risk to Older Adults, in Topical Fire Research Series. 2004. Available at: http://www.usfa.dhs.gov/Accessed June 22, 2008.

26. *Guide to Clinical Preventive Services: Report of the U.S. Preventive Services Task Force.* 2nd ed. Baltimore: Williams & Wilkins; 1996.

27. Rossignol AM, Locke JA, Boyle CM, Burke JF. Consumer products and hospitalized burn injuries among elderly Massachusetts residents. *J Am Geriatr Soc.* 1985;33:768–772.

28. Ehrlich AR, Kathpalia S, Boyarsky Y, Schechter A, Bijur P. Elderly patients discharged home from the emergency department with minor burns. *Burns.* 2005;31(6): 717–720.

29. Turner DG, Leman CJ, Jordan MH. Cooking-related burn injuries in the elderly preventing the "granny gown" burn. *J Burn Care Rehabil.* 1989;10:356–359.

30. Ryan CM, Thorpe W, Mullin P, et al. A persistent fire hazard for older adults: cooking-related clothing ignition. *J Am Geriatr Soc.* 1997;45:1283–1285.

31. Walker AR. Fatal tapwater scald burns in the USA, 1979–86. *Burns.* 1990;16:49–52.

32. Cerovac S, Roberts AH. Burns sustained by hot bath and shower water. *Burns.* 2000;26:251–259.

33. Tap Water Scalds. U.S. Consumer Product Safety Commission. 2004. Available at: http://www.cpsc.gov/CPSCPUB/PUBS/5098.html. Accessed June 22, 2008.

34. Runyan CW, Johnson RM, Yang J, et al. Risk and protective factors for fires, burns, and carbon monoxide poisoning in U.S. households. *Am J Prev Med.* 2005. 28:102–108.

35. Naik AD, Gill TM. Underutilization of environmental adaptations for bathing in community-living older persons. *J Am Geriatr Soc.* 2005;53:1497–1503.

36. Gill TM, Robison JT, Williams CS, Tinetti ME. Mismatches between the home environment and physical capabilities among community-living older persons. *J Am Geriatr Soc.* 1999;47:88–92.

37. Plautz B, Beck DE, Selmar C, Radetsky M. Modifying the environment: a community-based injury-reduction program for elderly residents. *Am J Prev Med.* 1996;12(4 Suppl):33–38.

38. Federal Drug Administration, C.P.S.C., Hazards Associated with the use of Electric Heating Pads. 1995. Available at www.fda.gov/CDRH/heatpad.pdf. Access July 2008.

39. Bill TJ, Edlich RF, Himel HN. Electric heating pad burns. *J Emerg Med.* 1994;12:819–824.

40. Robb BW, Hungness ES, Hershko DD, Warder GD, Kagan RJ. Home oxygen therapy: adjunct or risk factor? *J Burn Care Rehabil.* 2003;24:403–406; discussion 402.

41. Sentinel Event Alert. Lessons Learned: Fires in the Home Care Setting. Joint Commission on Accreditation of Healthcare Organizations. 2001. Available at: http://www.jointcommission.org/SentinelEvents/SentinelEventAlert/sea_17.htm Accessed June 22, 2008.

42. Barillo DJ, Coffey EC, Shirani KZ, Goodwin CW. Burns caused by medical therapy. *J Burn Care Rehabil.* 2000;21(3):269–73; discussion 268.

43. Qazi K, Gerson LW, Christopher NC, Kessler E, Ida N. Curling iron-related injuries presenting to U.S. emergency departments. *Acad Emerg Med.* 2001;8:395–397.

44. Harper RD, Dickson WA. Domestic central heating radiators: a cause for concern in all age groups. *Burns.* 1996;22:217–220.

45. Brigham PA, McLoughlin E. Burn incidence and medical care use in the United States: estimates, trends, and data sources. *J Burn Care Rehabil.* 1996;17:95–107.

46. Ahrens M. *U.S. Experience with Smoke Alarms and Other Fire Detection/Alarm Equipment.* Quincy, MA: National Fire Protection Association; 2004.

47. Schmeer S, Stern N, Monafo WW. An outreach burn prevention program for home care patients. *J Burn Care Rehabil.* 1988;9:645–647.

48. Hohl CM, Dankoff J, Colacone A, Afilalo M. Polypharmacy, adverse drug-related events, and potential adverse drug interactions in elderly patients presenting to an emergency department. *Ann Emerg Med.* 2001;38:666–671.

49. Wan H, Sengupta M, Velkoff MA, DeBarros KA. US Census Bureau, Current Population Reports, P23-209, 65+ in the United States: 2005, US Government Printing Office, Washington, DC, 2005.

50. Budnitz DS, et al. National surveillance of emergency department visits for outpatient adverse drug events. *JAMA.* 2006;296:1858–1866.

51. Chutka DS, Evans JM, Fleming KC, Mikkelson KG. Symposium on geriatrics – Part I: Drug prescribing for elderly patients. *Mayo Clin Proc.* 1995;70:685–693.

52. Goldfrank LR. *Goldfrank's Toxicologic Emergencies.* 8th ed. New York: McGraw-Hill; 2006.

53. Watson WA, Litovitz TL, Rodgers Jr GC, et al. 2004 Annual report of the American Association of Poison Control Centers Toxic Exposure Surveillance System. *Am J Emerg Med.* 2005;23:589–666.

54. Haselberger MB, Kroner BA. Drug poisoning in older patients. Preventative and management strategies. *Drugs Aging.* 1995; 7:292–297.

55. Kroner BA, Scott RB, Waring ER, Zanga JR. Poisoning in the elderly: characterization of exposures reported to a poison control center. *J Am Geriatr Soc.* 1993;41:842–846.

56. Frierson RL. Suicide attempts by the old and the very old. *Arch Intern Med.* 1991;151:141–144.

57. Schmucker DL. Liver function and phase I drug metabolism in the elderly: a paradox. *Drugs Aging.* 2001;18:837–851.

58. Lindeman RD, Tobin J, Shock NW. Longitudinal studies on the rate of decline in renal function with age. *J Am Geriatr Soc.* 1985;33:278–285.

59. Durnas C, Cusack BJ. Salicylate intoxication in the elderly. Recognition and recommendations on how to prevent it. *Drugs Aging.* 1992;2:20–34.

60. Montague RE, Grace RF, Lewis JH, Shenfield GM. Urine drug screens in overdose patients do not contribute to immediate clinical management. *Ther Drug Monit.* 2001;23: 47–50.

61. Oh E, Weintraub N, Dhanani S. Can we prevent aspiration pneumonia in the nursing home? *J Am Med Dir Assoc.* 2005;6(3 Suppl):S76–S80.

62. Marik PE. Aspiration pneumonitis and aspiration pneumonia. *NEJM.* 2001;344:665–671.

63. Limper AH, Prakash UB. Tracheobronchial foreign bodies in adults. *Ann Intern Med.* 1990;112:604–609.

64. Baharloo F, Veyckemans F, Francis C, Biettlot M-P, Rodenstein DO. Tracheobronchial foreign bodies: presentation and management in children and adults. *Chest.* 1999;115:1357–1362.

65. Chen C-H, Lai C-L, Tsai T-T, Lee Y-C, Perng R-P. Foreign body aspiration into the lower airway in Chinese adults. *Chest.* 1997;112:129–133.

66. Ebihara T, Takahashi H, Ebihara S, et al. Capsaicin troche for swallowing dysfunction in older people. *J Am Geriatr Soc.* 2005;53:824–828.

67. Ebihara T, Ebihara S, Okazaki T, et al. Theophylline-improved swallowing reflex in elderly nursing home patients. *J Am Geriatr Soc.* 2004;52:1787–1788.

68. Smolander J. Effect of cold exposure on older humans. *Int J Sports Med.* 2002;23:86–92.

69. Kenney WL, Hodgson JL. Heat tolerance, thermoregulation and ageing. *Sports Med.* 1987;4:446–456.

70. Hypothermia-Related Deaths – Suffolk County, New York, January 1999–March 2000 and United States, 1979–1998. Centers for Disease Control and Prevention. 2001. Available at: http://www.cdc.gov/mmwr/preview/mmwrhtml/mm5004a1.htm. Accessed June 22, 2008.

71. Heat-Related Deaths – Chicago, Illinois, 1996–2001, and United States, 1979–1999. Centers for Disease Control and Prevention. 2003. Available at: http://www.cdc.gov/MMWR/preview/mmwrhtml/mm5226a2.htm. Accessed June 22, 2008.

72. Mallet ML. Pathophysiology of accidental hypothermia. *QJM.* 2002;95:775–785.

73. Hypothermia-Related Deaths – United States, 2003–2004. Centers for Disease Control and Prevention. 2005. Available at: http://www.cdc.gov/MMWR/preview/mmwrhtml/mm5407a4.htm. Accessed June 22, 2008.

74. Bouchama A, Knochel JP. Heat stroke. *NEJM.* 2002;346:1978–1988.

75. Heat-related illnesses and deaths – Missouri,1998 and United States 1979–1996. Centers for Disease Control and Prevention. 1999. Available at: http://www.cdc.gov/mmwr/preview/mmwrhtml/mm4822a2.htm. Accessed June 22, 2008.

76. Semenza JC, Rubin CH, Falter KH, et al. Heat-related deaths during the July 1995 heat wave in Chicago. *NEJM.* 1996;335:84–90.

47

The Mistreatment of Older Adults

James G. O'Brien, MD

INTRODUCTION

Mistreatment of older adults is not a new phenomenon; it has been a feature of society since antiquity. Among nomadic tribes, older adults who could no longer contribute to the welfare of the tribe were often abandoned when the tribe moved on. King Lear is an example of severe abuse during Shakespeare's era. In the agrarian society of the latter 1800s and early 1900s, when multiple generations lived together, there were many instances of abuse documented in court records and sermons of that time. Sometimes maintaining an elderly parent in the home had more to do with ensuring the transfer of an inheritance than borne out of love or a sense of responsibility.

The 1960s was the decade for the recognition of child abuse followed by spouse abuse in the 1970s. In the 1980s some preliminary studies and hearings confirmed the presence of elder abuse. From the initial evidence it appeared elder abuse was widespread and crossed all social, racial, and economic barriers. Various types of abuse such as physical, psychological, material, and violation of rights occurred. The most common type was neglect, with family members being the most common perpetrators. Most states then rushed to develop legislation to combat abuse, but fewer states provided the necessary services to deal adequately with the problem.

The mistreatment of older adults includes several types of abuse. Physical abuse includes direct physical assaults, from slapping to homicide. This also includes sexual assaults, which some authorities place in a separate category. Physical neglect is the failure to provide a dependent older adult with the necessities of life, such as food, clothing, medicine, a safe living environment, and assistive devices. Psychological abuse and neglect include verbal abuse; threats, a common one being the threat to place the elder in a nursing home; or isolating the person from social contact. Exploitation, or financial abuse, includes actions taken against an older adult's property or other items and forcing an older adult to make decisions against his or her will, such as forcing a change in residence or a will or preventing a marriage or divorce.

These categories are often interrelated. Most cases of victimization involve more than one type, and the less severe types, such as psychological abuse or neglect and exploitation, are often precursors of the more life-threatening physical abuse and neglect. The perpetrator is most frequently a family member.[1] Most laws focus on mistreatment at the hands of others, and typically exclude self-neglect, which is being reported with increasing frequency in most states and can be particularly challenging to deal with.

It is difficult to obtain accurate data on the prevalence of elder mistreatment because victims and their families are prone to hide such behavior. Official statistics fail to include large numbers of cases, and studies tend to use small, biased samples. Estimates of the frequency of elder abuse range from 2%–10% based on various sampling definitions and survey methods.[2] The problem appears to be increasing as noted in the 2004 Survey of Adult Protective Services that showed a 19.7% increase in reported cases from the 2000 survey. Self-neglect (26.7%) was the most frequent type of case encountered followed by caregiver neglect (23.7%).[3]

Because this survey excluded some types of elder mistreatment, this figure should be considered to be a minimum. Recent attempts by the National Center on Elder Abuse to access other data sets including FBI crime data, Medicare Discharge Data and Centers for Disease Control and Prevention data revealed that abuse and neglect are rarely documented or occur so infrequently, that they lack mention.[4]

Mistreatment can occur in the older adult's own home, the homes of relatives, and in institutional facilities. Not all elder mistreatment is a deliberate action taken to injure the victim. Families often face serious dilemmas in caring for an aged member. For example, older adults often fail to recognize their failing capacities and may insist on living alone when they no longer are capable of caring for themselves. Their children must either violate their rights by forcing them to move or worry that they may later be charged with neglect if the older adult should fall or otherwise be injured.

Primary Care Practitioners

Primary care practitioners (PCP) have a unique opportunity to detect abuse and neglect. Most PCPs see elderly patients on a regular basis and frequently provide care in ambulatory, hospital, and nursing home settings and occasionally in the home, which provides unique access and opportunity for detection. Therefore they are in a position to identify many cases of mistreatment that would not otherwise come to public attention. Older adults also trust physicians and other practitioners and are likely to confide in them. In many instances, practitioners have contact with the older adult's family and may understand the factors surrounding the mistreatment. They also have access to critical tests needed by other professionals to verify abuse.

LEGAL REQUIREMENTS

As a means to deal with mistreatment of older adults, as of 1990 all states had passed legislation requiring reporting of this problem. These laws vary somewhat from state to state. All are designed to protect "vulnerable" adults, which includes adults who because of advanced age and/or physical or mental disability are not able to protect themselves. In such instances, the state intervenes on their behalf. Mandatory reporting laws require health and social service professionals to report suspected cases of elder mistreatment to an adult protective services agency. Practitioners are usually among those required to report and should determine the specific reporting requirements for their particular state and county. State laws generally provide protection for reporters, keeping the identity of the reporter confidential and guaranteeing immunity from litigation to those who report. Some state laws overemphasize the vulnerability and dependency of elder victims as independent elderly may also be victimized.

Adult protective service workers investigate the reports, usually within a specified time and document whether mistreatment has indeed occurred, and provide assistance. This may include referral to police or other authorities to protect the victim from the abuser. Laws also require that the autonomy of mentally competent elders be protected and that their decision not to receive services will be respected, which is frequently the dilemma encountered in cases of self-neglect in which services and assistance are refused.

WHO IS AT RISK?

Mistreatment of older adults can occur among all social, economic, ethnic, and religious groups. Because most older adults are women, most victims of elder mistreatment are also women.

Practitioners should never assume that any segment of their patient population is free from risk. At particularly high risk, however, are patients who are isolated; are highly dependent on others for their care; have been dependent for an extended period; have dementia, depression, or other psychiatric problems; or engage in behaviors, such as wandering or aggressiveness, that make caregiving difficult.

Certain characteristics of the family and caregiver are also associated with a high risk of abuse, such as elders in families with a history of poor relationships, especially those involving conflict, abuse, or violence. If the caregiver or other family members have mental or psychological problems or are substance abusers, the older adult is at greater risk. Many older adults are alone; they are often at the mercy of caregivers, neighbors, or scam artists.

Even in families with a high level of cohesion and resourcefulness, long-term care of an older adult can stretch tolerance and resources to the breaking point. Care of an aged adult is highly disruptive of normal family status and power relationships. A parent who is dependent on an adult son or daughter may attempt to maintain his or her former authority, resulting in tension, conflict, and possible violence. A well-meaning caregiver may be overwhelmed from multiple demands from a parent, children, and work and may lack the knowledge and ability to meet the needs of an elderly parent resulting in neglect or abuse. This situation lacks intentionality.

CLINICAL IDENTIFICATION OF MISTREATMENT

Because physicians and other primary care practitioners are more likely to observe the older adult than any other professional, they are likely to be better able to identify persons at risk or actually victims of mistreatment.[5] Because mistreatment frequently escalates over time, early identification may allow intervention to prevent the more life-threatening types that may occur later. Warning signs as depicted in Table 47.1 profile victims who may be at increased risk.

A protocol for interviewing potential victims is outlined in Table 47.2.

When injury from abuse or neglect has occurred, families are likely to take the victim to different medical facilities, particularly emergency centers, in the hope that health care providers will not see a pattern and recognize the mistreatment. Other indicators include a sudden decline in function, failure to thrive, frequent use of medical facilities, noncompliance with medical advice, failure to appear for appointments, and delay in seeking treatment. In addition, specific indicators can be delineated for each type of mistreatment.

Physical abuse can be identified by observing repeated or unusually placed injuries. For example, physical examinations or radiographs may indicate previous injuries that have been neglected.

Bruises should be carefully examined for special patterns. These may include bruises that take the pattern of the object inflicting them, such as a belt, electric cord, hanger, or the

Table 47.1. Warning Signs of Possible Elder Mistreatment[5,6,7,8,9]

History

Pattern of "physician hopping"

Unexplained delay in seeking treatment

Previous unexplained injuries or injuries inconsistent with medical findings

Previous reports of injuries similar to the current ones

Conflicting accounts between patient and potential abuser

Physical findings

Fractures, falls, dislocations

Evidence of physical restraint

Bruises, hematomas, welts, lacerations, abrasions, punctures

Burns of unusual shape or in unusual locations

Injuries that are bilateral, clustered, or in various stages of healing

Evidence of overmedication or undermedication

Unexplained sexually transmitted disease or genital infection

Pain, itching, bruising, or bleeding in genital area

Signs of poor personal hygiene, decubitus ulcers, dehydration, malnutrition

Inadequate or inappropriate clothing

Absence of needed eyeglasses, hearing aids, dentures, prostheses

Poor walking indicating hidden injuries or sexual assault

Evidence of substance abuse in patient or caregiver

Clinical observations

Signs of withdrawal, depression, agitation, low self-esteem, infantile behavior

Mental status changes from previous examination

Evidence of sleep disorder or deprivation

Ambivalence, resignation, fearfulness toward caregiver or family members

Substandard care despite adequate financial resources

Confusion over or lack of knowledge of financial situation

Sudden transfer of assets to a family member

Sudden inability to meet financial needs

Caregiver refusing to let patient see physician alone

Unusual behavior patterns between patient and caregiver

Adapted from AMA Department of Mental Health. Diagnostic and Treatment Guidelines on Elder Abuse and Neglect. Chicago, 1992. Available at: www.ama-assn.org/ama1/pub/upload/mm/386/elderabuse.pdf; The Mount Sinai/Victim Services Agency Elder Abuse Project. Elder mistreatment guidelines for health care professionals: Detection, assessment and intervention. New York, 1988; The Harborview Medical Center Department of Social Work. Protocol for Identification and Assessment of Elder Mistreatment. Seattle, 1992; Beth Israel Hospital Elder Abuse/Neglect Protocol. Boston, 1991; and Bloom JS, Ansell P, Bloom MN. Detecting elder abuse: a guide for physicians. *Geriatrics.* 1969;44:40–56.

Table 47.2. Guidelines for Interviewing Victims[10]

Ensure privacy

Separate victims from caregivers

Ensure confidentiality

Allow adequate time for response

Progress from general (screening) to specific (direct) questions

Keep questions simple and appropriate for educational level

Respect cultural and ethnic differences

Do not blame victims

Do not blame or confront perpetrators

Do not show frustration

Acknowledge that this process may require multiple interviews

Determine whether cognitive impairment is present

Use other people, such as office or emergency room nurses to conduct the interview if this is less threatening to victims

Reprinted with permission from O'Brien JG. A primary care clinician's perspective. In: Baumhover LA, Beall SC, eds. *Abuse, Neglect, and Exploitation of Older Persons.* Baltimore: Health Professions Press; 1996:51–64.

fingers of the human hand. It is difficult to determine the age of bruises as color changes are not always predictable.

A thorough history-taking and physical examination are essential, so the patient should be undressed and gowned. Careful attention should be paid to any injuries that do not match the patient's history. Particular attention should be paid to injuries in the breast or perineal areas, which may indicate that sexual abuse has occurred. The feet need to be examined for injuries to the soles or extreme neglect of toenails that otherwise might avoid detection. Overmedicating and symptoms of alcohol or drug overdose may also be signs that a caregiver is using these as methods of control.

Physical neglect may be present if the patient exhibits a lack of any necessities. Unexplained weight loss, not following prescribed medical protocols, or lack of such aids as dentures, eyeglasses, or hearing aids may indicate that a dependent patient is not receiving proper care.

Psychological abuse and neglect are more difficult to identify. Depression, withdrawal, fear of the caregiver, or isolation from others may be indicators. Observing exchanges between patient and caregiver may indicate problems. Office staff can be trained to notice these interactions, which otherwise may be hidden from the physician.

Exploitation can be observed in the medical setting by noting whether a mentally competent older adult is in control of his or her health care and finances. If a caregiver or others try to prevent a patient from consulting a physician alone or make decisions for him or her, this may be evidence of mistreatment. If a patient is unable to pay for treatment or prescribed medications, especially if this is a change from an earlier pattern, the patient's funds may have been misappropriated. Identification

Table 47.3. Suggested Questions from the Hwalek–Sengstock Elder Abuse Screening Test[11,12]

Items indicating violation of personal rights or direct abuse

4. Who makes decisions about your life, like how or where you should live?

9. Does someone in your family make you stay in bed or tell you you're sick when you know you're not?

10. Has anyone forced you to do things you didn't want to do?

11. Has anyone taken things that belong to you without your permission?

15. Has anyone close to you threatened to hurt you or harm you recently?

Items indicating characteristics of vulnerability

1. Do you have anyone who spends time with you, taking you shopping or to the doctor?

3. Are you sad or lonely often?

6. Can you take your own medication and get around by yourself?

Items indicating a potentially abusive situation

2. Are you helping to support someone?

5. Do you feel uncomfortable with anyone in your family?

7. Do you feel that nobody wants you around?

8. Does anyone in your family drink a lot?

12. Do you trust most of the people in your family?

13. Does anyone tell you that you give them too much trouble?

14. Do you have enough privacy at home?

Adapted from Hwalek MA, Sengstock MC. *The Elder Abuse Screening Test ("EAST")*. Detroit: SPEC Associates, 1986; Neale VA, Hwalek MA, Scott RO, et al. Validation of the Hwalek–Sengstock Elder Abuse Screening Test. *J Appl Gerontol.* 1991;10:40–418.

of the problem at this point may prevent an escalation at a later time. Medical facilities sometimes facilitate exploitation, by inviting family members to provide information or make decisions, rather than allowing older adults to do these things for themselves.

INTERVIEWING VICTIMS AND POSSIBLE PERPETRATORS

As has been noted, a critical component of identifying elder mistreatment is obtaining an accurate case history. A number of techniques may help to accomplish this, as noted in Table 47.3. First, it is essential that the older adult be interviewed apart from the suspected abuser or any other family member; during this period another staff member may interview family members to obtain additional information. Both should be interviewed in a quiet, private, nonthreatening setting. Both should be assured of confidentiality: without telling the family what

the older adult has said or vice versa. In both instances, the interviewer should make an effort at the outset to develop rapport. It is challenging to accomplish this in the setting of a busy office but an extended Medicare visit will help defer the cost.

The interviewer can assist the interview by judicious questioning. Questions should proceed from the general to the specific. In this private setting, do not be afraid to ask the older adult directly if he or she has been injured or threatened. Ask the respondent to describe a typical day. Both the older adult and the family members are likely to describe stresses and problems, as well as defenses. Statements need to be recorded verbatim. The abuser and even the victim may defend the abuser's behavior; interviewers should allow them to maintain these defenses. It is not the practitioners' responsibility to prove abuse or neglect but to describe objectively observations and findings and then report to the appropriate authority.

As indicated, a thorough physical examination of the older adult is also critical; the physician should explain the need for this and ask the patient's permission. All findings in both history and physical examination should be clearly documented in the event of a later investigation. Bruising or other visible injuries should be photographed after permission is provided. Photos should be dated and a reference such as a coin or easily recognized item may be useful to demonstrate the size of a bruise or wound. It is important at this point to determine the degree of danger or urgency of the situation. Patients whose lives may be in danger must be handled differently from those to whom the threat is less serious or immediate; this may require calling police, or a temporary hospital admission for observation.

In interviewing the alleged abuser or other family members, attempt to determine both stresses and possible supports. What caregiving problems exist? What other personal or family problems are present? Are there resources in the family that can be called upon for support?

A number of approaches should be avoided in these interviews. Avoid blaming the victim for his or her situation. Also avoid confronting the suspected abuser with his or her actions. In most instances confrontation is not useful, and in any event, this is the role of protective services or legal authorities, not the physician. If a report is mandatory, avoid using it as a threat. Rather present it as a means of protection and assistance, but do not suggest that protective services can solve all problems. Good data from a thorough history-taking and physical examination can have considerable value to protective services in any further action on the case.

CASE MANAGEMENT

A protocol developed by the American Medical Association.[5] suggests a sequence (see Figure 47.1) that can be utilized in most settings. Assistance to older patients who have suffered mistreatment is a long-term process.

There are short- and long-term management goals. *Short-term management* includes actions that must occur within the 24- or 48-hour period immediately following the discovery

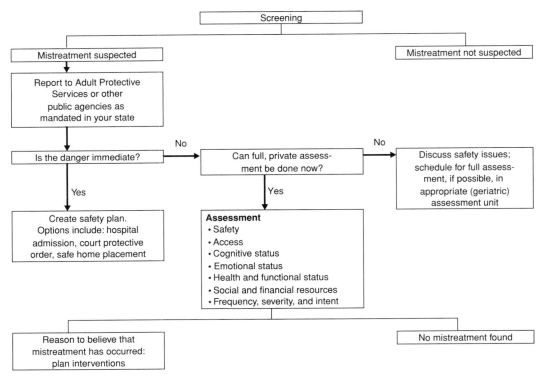

Figure 47.1. Screening and assessment for elder abuse and neglect should be based on an algorithm such as this one, developed and recommended by the American Medical Association. (Adapted from American Medical Association Department of Mental Health. *Diagnostic and Treatment Guidelines on Elder Abuse and Neglect.* Chicago: American Medical Association, 1992.)

of mistreatment. During this period it is critical to assess the degree of danger to the older adult. If physical abuse has already occurred or is threatened and the alleged abuser still has access to the patient, immediate separation of victim and abuser is imperative. Experts have determined that risk is particularly high if there are guns or other weapons in the home, if drug or alcohol abuse is present, or if there has been previous serious injury or threats of homicide or suicide.[13]

Ideally the abuser, rather than the victim, should be removed from the home. Often this is not possible, and placement of the older adult in other living arrangements may be necessary for his or her own protection. Sometimes another relative or friend is available or the patient may be placed in foster care or a nursing home or a senior shelter that may be available in some communities. Temporary hospitalization under the abuse-related, diagnosis-related groups may be an option, particularly if there are other diagnoses that justify the admission. For example, a vulnerable demented victim could be admitted to a geropsychiatry unit, if available. Consultation with your hospital's utilization review department can be useful.

Financial abuse may also require speedy action. If a person's assets are being misappropriated, a great deal of harm can result in only a few hours. Legal action may be required to change a guardian or conservator, eliminate a power of attorney, and so on. Referring the patient to an attorney or legal services agency may assist with these problems. When the patient or his or her assets do not appear to be in immediate danger, the physician,

staff, and protective services agency can take somewhat longer to develop a plan of action.

Long-term *case management* is necessary in all cases of elder mistreatment because these situations involve ongoing family patterns that are rarely resolved in a short time. Patients who suffer from mistreatment generally require a great many services, not only for the older adult, but also for the family, to prevent further mistreatment. These services are rarely within the scope of any single professional and often require interdisciplinary involvement. The practitioner's role in these cases varies with the relationship with the patient. An emergency physician's role differs from that of a physician who has an ongoing relationship with the patient and family.

When the patient or families are continuing patients, the practitioner should continue to be involved in case management. The involvement of a case manager who identifies and locates needed services and coordinates their implementation has been found to be critically important in these cases. When no single person is in charge, the older adult is likely to become confused or discouraged and terminate services. Some practitioners prefer to retain this role in their own office or clinic. Another option is to refer the case management role to a formal case management agency.

The types of services that should be involved vary with a wide variety of factors, including, among others, the degree of dependence of the patient, health insurance, financial resources, the supports available in the family, and the intention of the alleged abuser. For example, a fully functioning older adult who is being mistreated may alter the situation by means of a change of residence or social contacts, while a dependent patient may require extensive help in changing caregiving arrangements.

The intention of the suspected abuser is a critical factor in determining services. Where the mistreatment appears to be an intentional act, separation of the victim and the abuser is usually necessary, and may require criminal prosecution or civil action to force the abuser to avoid the patient.

In many instances, however, the mistreatment is not a deliberate act. It may result from lack of knowledge of proper care techniques on the part of the caregiver or from extreme stress. In such instances, providing services to alleviate these stresses may resolve the situation. Visiting nurses, respite care, or home health aids, for example, may provide needed caregiving information or help a caregiver cope. A family coping with marital or unemployment problems may be more effective in caregiving once these difficulties have been alleviated. Some caregivers have physical or mental impairments that render them incapable of providing proper care. The knowledgeable case manager can identify these situations and make appropriate referrals.

ELDER ABUSE IN THE NURSING HOME

Abuse and neglect in nursing homes is common and a major problem in the United States. Ombudsman programs nationally investigated more than 20,000 complaints of abuse and neglect and discovered physical abuse was most common.[14] In Georgia, a study of problem homes revealed that 38% of residents reported abuse with 45% reporting that they had been treated roughly.[15] When one matches the most vulnerable, those with cognitive impairment, dependence, frailty, and lacking resources with a workforce that is frequently undertrained, overworked, underpaid with rapid turnover, no one should be surprised that abuse and neglect occurs in institutions. Practitioners who care for institutionalized elderly need to monitor carefully for signs of abuse and neglect as previously described but particularly for malnutrition, weight loss, polypharmacy, and use of restraints. Reporting suspected abuse and neglect typically comes under the purview of the Ombudsman and not Adult Protective Services.

CONCLUSION

It is disappointing after almost three decades since gaining public recognition that so little progress has occurred. We are still unsure as to the prevalence and outcome data. We have an inconsistency of state laws and definitions and have an absence of federal legislation. More importantly, however, we lack adequate resources and treatment options when abuse and neglect are identified. Mistreatment of an elder, at a minimum, compromises quality of life during the remaining years and may in fact result in his or her premature death. As such, it should be a matter of concern to physicians and other health care providers. Considering the physician's unique opportunities in terms of knowledge of patient and family, access to diagnostic and management strategies, and general influence, intervention in such cases may achieve an outcome that rivals the successful treatment of a medical condition.

Furthermore, an interdisciplinary style of practice, with the incorporation of other providers such as nurses, nurse practitioners, home health nurses, social workers, and case managers, provides an ideal setting for efficient management of abuse cases. Great societies should be judged by how they treat their most vulnerable citizens, the very young and the very old. We are not earning a passing grade.

REFERENCES

1. Sengstock MC, Barrett SA. Abuse and neglect of the elderly in family settings. In: Campbell J, Humphreys J, eds. *Nursing Care of Survivors of Family Violence*. St. Louis: Mosby; 1993:173–208.
2. Lachs M, Pillemer K. Elder abuse. *Lancet*. 2004;364:1192–1263.
3. Teaster PB, Dugar TA, Mendiondo MS, Abner EL, Cecil KA. The 2004 Survey of State Adult Protective Services: Abuse of Adults 60 Years of Age and Older. The National Center on Elder Abuse, Washington, D.C. February, 2006.
4. Wood EF. The Availability and Utility of Interdisciplinary Data on Elder Abuse: A White Paper for the National Center on Elder Abuse. The National Center on Elder Abuse, Washington, D.C. May, 2006.
5. American Medical Association Department of Mental Health. *Diagnostic and Treatment Guidelines on Elder Abuse and Neglect*. Chicago: American Medical Association; 1992.
6. The Mount Sinai/Victim Services Agency Elder Abuse Project. *Elder Mistreatment Guidelines for Health Care Professionals: Detection, Assessment and Intervention*. New York, 1988.
7. The Harborview Medical Center Department of Social Work. Protocol for Identification and Assessment of Elder Mistreatment. Seattle, 1992.
8. Beth Israel Hospital Elder Abuse/Neglect Protocol. Boston, 1991.
9. Bloom JS, Ansell P, Bloom MN. Detecting elder abuse: a guide for physicians. *Geriatrics*. 1969;44:40–56.
10. O'Brien JG. A Primary care clinician's perspective. In: Baumhover LA, Beall SC, eds. *Abuse, Neglect, and Exploitation of Older Persons*. Baltimore: Health Professions Press; 1996:51–64.
11. Hwalek MA, Sengstock MC. *The Elder Abuse Screening Test ("EAST")*. Detroit: SPEC Associates; 1986.
12. Neale VA, Hwalek MA, Scott RO, et al. Validation of the Hwalek-Sengstock Elder Abuse Screening Test. *J Appl Gerontol*. 1991;10:40–418.
13. Campbell JC. Prediction of homicide of and by battered women. In: Campbell JC, ed. *Assessing Dangerousness*. Thousand Oaks, CA: Sage; 1995:96–113.
14. National Ombudsman Reporting System Data Tables. 2003. Washington, DC: U.S. Administration on Aging.
15. Hawes C. Elder abuse in residential long-term care facilities: what is known about prevalence, causes, and prevention. Testimony before the U.S. Senate Committee on Finance. June 18, 2002. Available at: http://finance.senate.gov/hearings/testimony/061802chtest.pdf. Accessed June 22, 2008.

48

DRIVING AND THE OLDER ADULT

Alice K. Pomidor, MD, MPH, Joanne Schwartzberg, MD

"It's getting very hard for me to drive at night. I don't like to go out because I don't think it's safe. Is there something you can do to help me?"

"You have to talk to Dad about his driving when you go in. He almost hit someone the other day, and I don't feel like he can take the children out anymore."

"My neck is so sore from that fender-bender. The emergency room said that I had to come in and see you if the pain didn't go away after a few days."

INTRODUCTION

Almost every health care practitioner who cares for older adults has heard a variation on one of these statements. Driving is an essential instrumental activity of daily living for young and old alike in this highly mobile society, but it becomes increasingly difficult to maintain with normal aging changes and potential comorbid medical conditions. Prevention, detection, and treatment of impaired driving ability is challenging in most health care settings for many reasons, including symptoms that do not fit typical medical paradigms, lack of familiarity with effective assessment techniques, and time constraints. Concerns about significant legal and ethical questions may also deter the health care provider from addressing the issue of driving. Early intervention is important, however, to prevent injury, unnecessary disability, and the potential loss of driving skills/privileges, with ensuing adverse effects on quality of life. With the rapid increase in the population of older adults, it is estimated that 25% of drivers will be older than age 65 by the year 2030.[1] It is essential to help older adults drive safely for as long as possible and, when necessary, devise satisfactory alternative means of transportation.

DRIVING CHARACTERISTICS AND HABITS

In 2005, 191,000 older individuals were injured in traffic crashes. Although this figure accounted for only 7% of all people injured in traffic crashes during the year, older adults comprised 15% of all traffic fatalities, 14% of all vehicle occupant fatalities, and 20% of all pedestrian fatalities.[2] This disproportionate risk of injury and death compared with younger individuals may result from older adults' fragility from limited physiological reserves and greater susceptibility to impact. The consequences of this increased risk are further magnified by the fact that recent generations of older adults are more mobile compared with previous cohorts. Total miles traveled per person per day by those age 65 years and older increased by more than 50% during 1995–2001.[3]

Even though many older persons self-restrict their driving to help compensate for changes in vision and to reduce the perceived risk of an accident,[4,5] crash rates per mile traveled start increasing for drivers 75 and older and increase markedly after age 80. Elevated crash rates for older drivers when measured per mile traveled may be somewhat inflated because of the type of driving, because much of their mileage involves city driving, which generally has higher crash rates per mile than freeway driving.[6] Most traffic fatalities involving older drivers in 2005 occurred during the daytime (79%), on weekdays (73%), and involved other vehicles (73%). In two-vehicle fatal crashes involving an older driver and a younger driver, the vehicle driven by the older person was nearly twice as likely to be the one that was struck (60% and 33%, respectively). In 25% of these crashes, however, the older driver was turning left five times as often as the younger driver.[2]

Drivers age 75 years and older are at modestly increased risk of involvement in two-vehicle collisions in which occupants of other vehicles receive nonfatal injuries. With the exception of deaths among their passengers, older drivers were not

Table 48.1. Pharmacological Risk Factors for Driving

Alcohol

Angiotensin-converting enzyme inhibitors

Antidepressants

Benzodiazepines

Nonsteroidal anti-inflammatory drugs

Opioid analgesics

Table 48.2. Medical Risk Factors for Driving

Arthritis

Coronary artery disease

Dementia

Depression

Falls

Foot reaction time slowing

Orthostatic hypotension

Parkinson's disease

Renal disease

Stroke or transient ischemic attack

Visual field loss

overrepresented in crashes in which other road users were killed. Older drivers experience the most serious consequences of their collisions: two-thirds of deaths in crashes involving drivers 75 and older were the drivers themselves.[7]

AGING CHANGES AND MEDICAL RISK FACTORS

Several essential functional abilities for driving may decline due to normal changes of aging physiology, the increased likelihood of comorbid illness with age, or a combination of both.[8] Impairments in vision, neuromuscular strength and speed, cognitive function, and select medical conditions have been linked to actual crash risk for older adults.

Normal losses in visual acuity and contrast sensitivity, with increased glare sensitivity, combined with ocular diseases such as cataract formation, glaucoma, and age-related maculopathy are the most prevalent findings in older adults. These impairments can affect the Useful Field of View (UFOV), which is the visual field over which information can be acquired in a brief glance without eye or head movements. Computerized UFOV testing measures the ability to identify objects and pay attention to them, as opposed to simple confrontational visual field testing. UFOV impairment appears to be much more accurate than static visual acuity in predicting crash risk: a 40% decline more than doubles the likelihood of a crash.[9,10]

Neuromuscular factors such as reduced neck rotation, slowed foot reaction time, a greater orthostatic drop in blood pressure, and the history of a fall in the past year have all been shown to increase crash risk, particularly in women.[11–13] Medical illnesses and treatments that may be linked to driving difficulty in self-report, case-control, and retrospective population studies include a history of falls, coronary artery disease, stroke or transient ischemic attack, kidney disease, and – in women – arthritis.[14–16] Use of certain medications is also linked to increased risk, including angiotensin-converting enzyme inhibitors, benzodiazepines, opioid analgesics, alcohol, and nonsteroidal antiinflammatory drugs. Depression and the use of antidepressant medications may also impair driving performance in both younger and older populations (Table 48.1).[15,17–19]

Cognitive function and conditions such as dementia that affect mental status in older adults have been the subject of extensive study. Normal changes of aging such as decreased reaction time and longer recall time generally are compensated for in actual driving scenarios by increased experience and have not been shown to impair driving ability in most older adults. Diseases such as Alzheimer's and Parkinson's, however, have been linked to decreased driving performance and heightened crash risk because of their adverse impact on cognitive skills, including memory, visuospatial skills, attention, reaction time, processing speed, and executive function, as demonstrated on neuropsychological testing (Table 48.2).[8,20–22] Although there is no gold standard test for assessing the driving ability of patients with dementia or Parkinson's disease, the consensus among several professional organizations is that persons with moderate-to-severe disease should stop driving.[23,24] There is no reliable office assessment tool for identifying driving impairment among patients with mild dementia, and additional driving simulator or on-the-road assessments are likely to be needed.[25–27]

DRIVING ASSESSMENT

The health care clinician involved in assessing the individual older adult's ability to drive rarely has the opportunity, time, or expertise to observe the patient's driving skills directly. Office-based assessment relies on obtaining a driving history in addition to the traditional medical history from both the patient and caregiver, a physical examination targeted at abilities needed for driving in addition to typical medical conditions, and the use of simple neuropsychological tests that may provide proxy information about the cognitive skills used in everyday driving. A health care provider may wish to initiate an assessment with a patient because of concerns about another clinical condition, such as diabetes or dementia. In other likely situations, the provider may be reacting to an injury or concern presented by the patient or caregiver, or responding to a request from a motor vehicle bureau, workplace, or insurance

Table 48.3. Driving History Red Flags

Acute or unstable medical events: acute myocardial infarction, angina, hypoglycemia, stroke or transient ischemic attack, traumatic brain injury, syncope, vertigo, seizure, surgery, delirium, sleep apnea

Any expression of concern: about driving safety, from patient or caregiver

Medications: any psychoactive, cardiovascular, neurological or potentially sedating agents

Chronic medical conditions:

Vision – field cuts, cataracts, glaucoma, macular degeneration, hypertensive or diabetic retinopathy, retinitis pigmentosa

Cardiovascular disease – unstable angina, arrhythmia, valvular disease, congestive heart failure

Neurological disease – dementia, Parkinson's disease, multiple sclerosis, peripheral neuropathy, stroke

Psychiatric disease – depression, anxiety, psychosis, alcohol or substance abuse

Musculoskeletal disability – arthritis, foot abnormalities, previous fractures, cervical disease

Respiratory disease – obstructive sleep apnea, chronic obstructive pulmonary disease, asthma, disease requiring oxygen supplementation on a daily basis

Metabolic disease – diabetes, renal failure, thyroid disease

Table 48.4. Patient Driving History Questions

1. Do you now drive a car?
2. How many days did you drive this past week?
3. Have you noticed any change in your driving habits in the past year? Please check all that apply.

   Do not drive at night

   Do not drive on freeways

   Do not drive in rain/snow, bad weather

   Do not drive during rush hour

   Do not drive as far

   Only drive when I absolutely must

   Prefer for others to drive

   Have cut back because of being too sick/tired
4. In the past year, have you had any of the following events? Please check all that apply.

   Accidents

   Fender-benders

   Near-misses

   Tickets

   Discussions/warnings
5. Have you ever forgotten where you were going?
6. Do others honk at you or act irritated?
7. Have you ever gotten lost while driving?
8. Have others said they are worried about your driving, criticized you or refused to ride with you?

---

company for information on fitness to drive. The American Medical Association (AMA), in collaboration with the National Highway Safety Transportation Administration, created an advisory panel, which developed the *Physicians' Guide to Assessing and Counseling Older Drivers,* released in September 2003.[28] This contains one approach to assessment and advising based on expert consensus opinion of literature review and has the stated purpose of helping older drivers stay on the road safely to preserve their mobility and independence, as opposed to primarily detecting and removing unsafe drivers.[29] Other countries such as Canada and individual expert authors have since also released recommendations and protocols for evaluation that are similar in scope and content but vary according to whether one is targeting a high-yield population, responding to a clinical need, or doing population screening.[30–32]

History

As in a traditional medical examination, the first step of a medical assessment for driving ability is a targeted history-taking. Be alert for acute and chronic medical conditions, medications or symptoms that may impair driving skills when taking the patient's history (Table 48.3). These "red flags" deserve further evaluation and follow-up.[28]

A general driving history should include questions such as those noted in Tables 48.4 and 48.5, which give the patient and caregiver the opportunity to express concerns that might otherwise be too embarrassing to discuss or that might be

Table 48.5. Caregiver Driving History Questions

1. Does the patient drive?
2. Have you noticed any unsafe driving?
3. Do you feel uncomfortable riding with the patient?
4. Has the patient gotten lost?
5. Does the patient rely on a copilot?
6. Does the patient rely on passengers?
7. Do others worry about the patient's driving?
8. Does the patient forget where they are going?
9. Do others have to drive defensively?
10. Have others refused to ride with the patient?
11. Has the patient changed their driving habits?
12. In the past year, has the patient had any of the following? Please check all that apply.

    Accidents

    Fender-benders

    Near-misses

    Tickets

    Discussions/warnings

forgotten.[32] Some providers may wish to provide these questions or the AMA's "Am I a Safe Driver?" as a written handout for self-evaluation prior to initiating an assessment.[28]

Targeted Physical Examination

In addition to the general physical examination maneuvers needed to investigate any positive history items found above, the AMA guide recommends special items recorded on their Assessment of Driving-Related Skills ([ADReS] Figure 48.1), which evaluates vision, motor function, and cognition. Far acuity should be assessed with the traditional Snellen E chart and visual fields by confrontation testing. Although the UFOV test has better correlation with crash risk, it is not yet widely available. Testing is currently under way in pilot state departments of motor vehicles, aimed at evaluating the practicality of UFOV tests in field settings.[33] Motor function is gauged through assessments of walking, range of motion, and strength. The rapid-pace walk is based on the time (in seconds) it takes the patient to walk a 10-ft path, turn around and return. Range of motion testing consists of observing neck rotation to the right and left, having the patient make a fist with each hand, pretending the patient is holding a steering wheel to make a wide right turn and then a wide left turn, and dorsiflexing and plantarflexing both ankles. Motor strength testing is done for bilateral shoulder adduction, abduction, and flexion; wrist flexion and extension; handgrip strength; hip flexion and extension; and ankle dorsiflexion and plantarflexion, each rated on a traditional 0–5 of 5 scale.

Cognitive screening is performed using the Clock Drawing Test, in which the patient is verbally instructed to draw the face of a clock and to place the hands at 10 minutes after 11 using a blank sheet of paper and a pencil. Memory, visual spatial skills, attention, and executive skills are all used during the clock drawing task. Scoring is found on the ADReS, with greater than two errors correlating with unsafe driving behaviors on driving simulation testing.[34] The Trails-Making B test (see Figure 48.2) is also recommended, with a time for performance more than 180 seconds considered abnormal and meriting intervention. Patients are asked to connect dots in a path in sequence that alternates between numbers and letters, such as "1-A-2-B." Poor performance has been prospectively linked to crash risk in two studies in which evaluation has been tracked during license renewals.[22,33] The Trails-Making B form and directions for its use are available for free in the AMA guide, which may be obtained through National Highway Safety Transportation Administration or online through the AMA.[28]

Although not recommended as part of the AMA's driving assessment, many clinicians also perform the Folstein Mini-Mental State Examination, which has been widely used as a clinical tool to assist in the diagnosis of dementia; a score of 20/30 or lower has also been found to correlate with poor driving performance.[31] Although a low score appears to be reasonably specific for driving impairment, a higher score does not necessarily exclude driving impairment. Patients with higher scores can often have poor driving performances, and the Mini-Mental State Examination is not considered sufficient cognitive screening when used alone. Clinicians should remember that these tests are used to screen for multiple potential cognitive impairments that may lead to unsafe behaviors and do not, in and of themselves, diagnose dementia or determine the safety of persons with dementia who drive.

After completing the initial driving assessment, health care practitioners will need to assure accurate diagnosis and

---

Patient's Name: _____ **Date:** _____

1. **Visual fields:** Shade in any areas of deficit.

Patient's R   **L**

2. **Visual acuity:** _____ OU
Was the patient wearing corrective lenses? If yes, please specify:
_____

3. **Rapid pace walk:** _____seconds
Was this performed with a walker or cane? If yes, please specify:
_____

4. **Range of motion:** Specify 'Within Normal Limits' or 'Not WNL.' If not WNL, describe.

	Right	Left
Neck rotation		
Finger curl		
Shoulder and elbow flexion		
Ankle plantar flexion		
Ankle dorsiflexion		

5. **Motor strength:** Provide a score on a scale of 0-5.

	Right	Left
Shoulder adduction		
Shoulder abduction		
Shoulder flexion		
Wrist flexion		
Wrist extension		
Hand grip		
Hip flexion		
Hip extension		
Ankle dorsiflexion		
Ankle plantar flexion		

6. **Trail-Making Test, Part B:** _____ seconds

7. **Clock drawing test:** Please check 'yes' or 'no' to the following criteria.

	Yes	No
All 12 hours are placed in correct numeric order, starting with 12 at the top		
Only the numbers 1-12 are included (no duplicates, omissions, or foreign marks)		
The numbers are drawn inside the clock circle		
The numbers are spaced equally or nearly equally from each other		
The numbers are spaced equally or nearly equally from the edge of the circle		
One clock hand correctly points to two o'clock		
The other hand correctly points to eleven o'clock		
There are only two clock hands		

Figure 48.1. Assessment of Driving-Related Skills (ADReS).

Trail-Making Test, Part B
Patient's Name: _____ Date _____

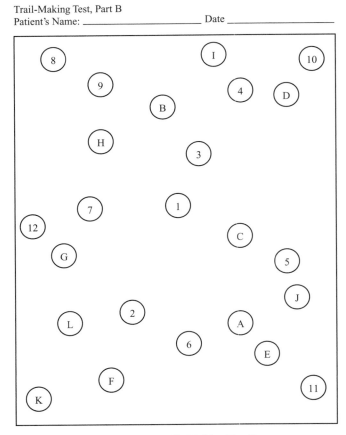

Figure 48.2. Trails-Making Test B.

treatment of any medical impairments that have been discovered. Referral for expert evaluation of visual impairment, neuropsychological deficits, and musculoskeletal disorders may be especially useful. If, however, the patient's deficits cannot be medically corrected and do not have further potential for improvement with medical intervention, referral to a driver rehabilitation specialist (DRS) may be necessary. A DRS is often an occupational therapist who undergoes additional training in driver rehabilitation. Other professionals may also receive DRS certification. A DRS is able to do either simulator and/or on-road testing to determine more specifically the patient's level of driving safety and help correct the patient's functional impairments, if possible, through adaptive techniques or devices. A list of certified DRSs can be obtained from the Association for Driver Rehabilitation Specialists.[35] Patients and health care providers need to be aware, however, that DRS services are often not covered by health insurance other than state Workers Compensation and Vocational Rehabilitation programs. Medicare and Medicaid coverage is highly variable and private insurance typically mirrors the actions of the local Medicare intermediary.[28,35]

Also, DRSs are often hard to locate outside of urban areas, which may impede referral. Local driving school referral is not equivalent to a medical DRS evaluation but may be helpful in the absence of other resources.

INTERVENTIONS

Actual or potential loss of driving ability should be viewed through the same perspective as other typical health maintenance practices for older adults: primary, secondary, and tertiary prevention of driving ability loss. *Primary* prevention identifies medical problems that may lead to impairment and optimizes the driving patient's medical condition to prevent the loss of driving ability. More than 40% of patients who have stopped driving identify medical problems as the primary reason, with changes of aging second at almost 20%, and concerns over licensure or accidents third.[4,36] Reversible or partially treatable conditions must be optimized to give the patient the best possible chance of continuing to drive without impairment. Medical interventions should also minimize the adverse effects of unavoidable medical conditions on driving ability, particularly medication side effects. These may at times be dependent on the driving situation. If a medication cannot be changed or discontinued, for example, health care providers may counsel patients not to drive when under the influence of the medication – just as they would advise patients not to drive under the influence of alcohol. Conversely, patients with significant pulmonary disease may need reinforcement to use their oxygen while driving, and patients with Parkinson's disease should be advised to drive only when their symptoms are adequately controlled and when they are well rested. Patients with visual difficulties can be counseled to minimize nighttime, high-speed, and dense traffic situations where their functional limitations put them at risk for impaired driving.[37]

Health care providers can also recommend enhancement and active maintenance of driving skills through refresher courses, self-assessment, and self-education, such as the Automobile Association of America's Senior Driver program.[38] or the American Association of Retired Persons Driver Safety Program.[39] Both programs encourage self-evaluation and recognition of potential problems, with courses intended to help improve driving skills. A recent feature of the Automobile Association of America program published in 2004 is the *Roadwise Review*, a CD-ROM computer-based home assessment program that includes assessment of leg strength and general mobility, head/neck flexibility, high- and low-contrast visual acuity, working memory, visualization of missing information, visual search, and UFOV). Currently under development, the *Driving Decisions Workbook*, a new self-assessment instrument designed to include medical content, has been compared with road test outcomes. The authors also recommend using it to facilitate conversations with family members.[40]

Secondary prevention looks at an existing problem of driving impairment in a patient and tries to minimize or compensate for the impairment, so that the patient may continue to drive safely. Vehicle and environmental adaptation strategies may be helpful, such as hand-controls that compensate for strength or range of motion impairment, use of well-maintained roads with bright and easily visible lighting and signage, and newer vehicles with better safety devices such as two-stage airbags that minimize the force of patient contact.

Seat belt use should always be encouraged. Evaluation of driving impairment with tailored compensation strategies may be available through local driving school instruction or DRS treatment programs.[41] Patients also do frequently self-restrict their driving activities when aware of driving impairment and may need their health care provider's assistance in determining when they should do so.[4,5,42] In these circumstances, health care providers may be called on to document and verify the presence of driving impairment to help obtain access and financial support for adaptive equipment, driving rehabilitation, or restricted driving privileges.

Tertiary prevention limits the adverse consequences for the patient if loss of the ability to drive cannot be prevented, and the patient must stop driving entirely – a circumstance termed driving retirement or cessation. Helping the patient to plan in advance by discussing the eventual need for driving retirement, similarly to work retirement, can minimize negative effects and facilitate a smooth transition. The multiple adverse consequences of driving cessation for older adults are well documented and include depression, dependency, caregiver strain, social withdrawal, increased risk of entry into long-term care facilities, and restricted mobility.[43–47] According to the 2001 National Household Travel Survey, approximately 90% of daily and long-distance travel is conducted in a personal vehicle. Social and recreational trips, such as visiting friends, accounted for the largest percentage of older adults' trips at 19%, with larger percentages of trips also used for shopping, medical reasons, and religious reasons compared with younger adults.[48] Driving life-expectancy rates and the duration of time for which older persons will be dependent on alternative sources of transportation were projected using data from a large, longitudinal study of community-based elderly. Male drivers aged 70–74 years at baseline would have a driving life expectancy of approximately 11 years, and approximately 7 years of transportation dependency, and women would have a similar driving life expectancy but longer life expectancy, leading to transportation dependency for approximately 10 years.[49]

The health care provider's recommendation for driving retirement should emphasize concern for the patient's safety and the safety of others as the primary reason for giving up driving. Even so, many patients are understandably upset or angry on receiving the recommendation, and in the case of cognitive impairment, some may lack the insight necessary to understand the consequences. It may be helpful to reinforce the recommendation by asking the patient to repeat back to you the reasons for driving retirement, to provide a prescription on which "Do Not Drive" is written, and to help the patient create a plan for alternative transportation. Some patients may also benefit from identifying peer driver behaviors that they consider to be unsafe and using those examples to set their own threshold for when they would consider themselves unsafe to drive. Identifying a trusted friend or family member whose opinion is honored by the impaired driver may also help to support the recommendation. Keep in mind that a spouse who depends on the patient for transportation may find it difficult to support a recommendation for driving retirement. At no time should a "copilot" be recommended to unsafe drivers as a means to continue driving, as this merely places both persons in addition to other road users at risk. There is often insufficient time in many traffic situations for the copilot to detect a hazard and alert the driver to respond quickly enough to avoid a crash, and use of a copilot also raises the issue of whether the patient is fit to drive. A follow-up letter documenting the recommendation for driving retirement should be sent to the patient, and – if the patient consents – to involved family members. A copy should also be kept in the chart for documentation.

Clinicians should attempt to see their patients for whom driving is no longer possible soon after driving retirement, both to monitor for compliance with the recommendation to stop driving and also to check for signs and symptoms of depression and failure-to-thrive. Extra care should be taken to assure that travel can be arranged for those who may have difficulty obtaining food and medications, or going for necessary medical care. Twenty-four percent of older adults report having a medical condition that potentially limits their travel outside the home, and of these, 85% report that it has decreased their travel by half.[48] Finding alternative means of transportation is difficult for older adults, particularly in rural areas and metropolitan settings that lack well-developed systems of mass transportation. Even where such transportation is available, 60% of this cohort of adults reports that they have not used public transportation on a regular basis before,[45] and only 12% have used special-needs transportation such as dial-a-ride.[48] The burden of meeting transportation needs will mostly likely fall on family, friends, and neighbors, some of whom may also suffer from undiagnosed driving impairment. Social agency and volunteer organization referrals for meeting transportation needs are an important part of the patient care plan for driving retirement, often beginning with the Area Agency on Aging.[28]

For patients who lack capacity and insight, it is essential for the appointed guardian or caregiver to help the patient comply with the recommendation to stop driving. Many strategies have been used with varying degrees of success to circumvent persistent attempts to drive, including placing reminder signage on doors or inside the windshield on the driver's side, informing the patient of cancelled insurance, providing alternative picture identification, attempting to collect and remove all sets of keys, grinding down ignition keys, disabling the vehicle by removal of parts or fluids, and removing the vehicle. A guardian may forfeit the patient's license and car on the patient's behalf if absolutely necessary as a last resort.

LEGAL AND ETHICAL ISSUES

The AMA's official ethical opinion E-2.24 regarding Impaired Drivers and their Physicians (Figure 48.3) as issued in June of 2000 lists many of the issues faced by health care providers who find themselves caring for older adult drivers. In particular, clinicians often find themselves in an ethical conflict between

The purpose of this report is to articulate physicians' responsibility to recognize impairments in patients' driving ability that pose a strong threat to public safety and which ultimately may need to be reported to the Department of Motor Vehicles. It does not address the reporting of medical information for the purpose of punishment or criminal prosecution.

(1) Physicians should assess patients' physical or mental impairments that might adversely affect driving abilities. Each case must be evaluated individually since not all impairments may give rise to an obligation on the part of the physician. Nor may all physicians be in a position to evaluate the extent or the effect of an impairment (e.g., physicians who treat patients on a short-term basis). In making evaluations, physicians should consider the following factors: (a) the physician must be able to identify and document physical or mental impairments that clearly relate to the ability to drive; and (b) the driver must pose a clear risk to public safety.

(2) Before reporting, there are a number of initial steps physicians should take. A tactful but candid discussion with the patient and family about the risks of driving is of primary importance. Depending on the patient's medical condition, the physician may suggest to the patient that he or she seek further treatment, such as substance abuse treatment or occupational therapy. Physicians also may encourage the patient and the family to decide on a restricted driving schedule, such as shorter and fewer trips, driving during non-rush-hour traffic, daytime driving, and/or driving on slower roadways if these mechanisms would alleviate the danger posed. Efforts made by physicians to inform patients and their families, advise them of their options, and negotiate a workable plan may render reporting unnecessary.

(3) Physicians should use their best judgment when determining when to report impairments that could limit a patient's ability to drive safely. In situations where clear evidence of substantial driving impairment implies a strong threat to patient and public safety, and where the physician's advice to discontinue driving privileges is ignored, it is desirable and ethical to notify the Department of Motor Vehicles.

(4) The physician's role is to report medical conditions that would impair safe driving as dictated by his or her state's mandatory reporting laws and standards of medical practice. The determination of the inability to drive safely should be made by the state's Department of Motor Vehicles. Physicians should disclose and explain to their patients this responsibility to report.

(5) Physicians should disclose and explain to their patients this responsibility to report.

(6) Physicians should protect patient confidentiality by ensuring that only the minimal amount of information is reported and that reasonable security measures are used in handling that information.

(7) Physicians should work with their state medical societies to create statutes that uphold the best interests of patients and community, and that safeguard physicians from liability when reporting in good faith. (I, III, IV, VII)

Issued June 2000 based on the report "Impaired Drivers and Their Physicians," adopted December 1999.

Figure 48.3. American Medical Association Ethical Opinion E-2.24 Impaired Drivers and Their Physicians.

the standard of patient confidentiality and the duty to safeguard public safety. Many primary care providers may also be reluctant to report impaired drivers to their local drivers licensing authority for fear of jeopardizing their relationship with the patient. These concerns, however, must be weighed against state requirements for reporting unsafe drivers. It is essential for providers to know and comply with their state's reporting laws and to document all activities in the patient's chart. All conversations and efforts to communicate with the patient and caregiver, recommendations, referrals for further testing, direct observations, counseling, formal assessment, medical interventions, patient education handouts, and referral reports related to your recommendations regarding driving should be clearly documented, and copies should be kept in the patient's chart for future reference and possible protection in the event of third-party litigation. It is important to keep in mind that the health care provider cannot suspend or remove the right to drive. Only the state Department of Motor Vehicles has the authority to perform a legal action regarding licensure. Chapter 8 of the AMA Guide provides a directory of state licensing requirements and reporting laws current as of September 2003.[28]

LOOKING TO THE FUTURE

In Western societies driving remains a critical function for instrumental activities of daily living, and the federal government is beginning to recognize the need to improve standards for assessment and licensure across the states. The National Highway Transportation Safety Administration and American Association of Motor Vehicle Administrators are working together to fund efforts to improve specific protocols at the local licensing agency level. Pilot assessment studies are ongoing in California, Florida, and Maryland at motor vehicle administration field sites to evaluate performance-based measures such as the Gross Impairment Screening Battery. The entire protocol is designed as an 11-minute assessment, combined with a subtest of the UFOV, and, either a Mobility or Driving Habits questionnaire, for a total assessment time of approximately 20 minutes.[33,50] The Gross Impairment Screening Battery consists of a rapid-pace walk, foot tap, arm reach, head/neck rotation, cued and delayed recall, symbol scan, visual perception test, and the Trails-Making A and B tests. Older drivers presenting for license renewal were followed prospectively for subsequent motor vehicle crashes; participants 78 years of age and older who demonstrated impairment on one of several components had double the risk of involvement in an at-fault motor vehicle crash.[33] This type of functional screen may significantly improve the effectiveness of driver screening for impairment at the level of licensure, and enhance the detection and referral of impaired drivers for rehabilitation and medical assessment.

Social support and transportation infrastructures have not been well planned or prepared either at the individual driver or governmental level. Florida, often considered the vanguard of the aging population, has determined that the following elements are needed to address the needs of mature drivers: 1) continued research into assessment methods and transportation alternatives, 2) development and implementation of widespread public information and education, materials, and programs, 3) focused training for law enforcement, social service, and health care providers, 4) expansion of services for assessment, remediation, and transportation alternatives, 5) funding initiatives to support development of community-based programs, 6) establishment and extension of community-based services, and 7) creation of an action plan.[51]

For the health care provider, the detection, prevention, and treatment of driving impairment captures the classic problem of the needs and priorities of the individual versus the needs and priorities of society. The clinician must help to negotiate a delicate balance between the two.

REFERENCES

1. Lyman S, Ferguson SA, Braver ER, Williams, AF. Older driver involvements in police reported crashes and fatal crashes: trends and projections. *Inj Prev.* 2002;8:116–120.

2. National Highway Transportation Safety Administration. Traffic Safety Facts 2005 data. Older Population DOT HS 810 622: 1–6.

3. Austin RA, Faigin BM. Effect of vehicle and crash factors on older occupants. *J Safety Res.* 2003;34:441–452.

4. Ball K, Owsley C, Stalvey B, et al. Driving avoidance and functional impairment in older drivers. *Accid Anal Prev.* 1998;30:312–322.

5. Ragland DR, Satariano WA, MacLeod KE. Reasons given by older people for limitation or avoidance of driving. *Gerontologist.* 2004;44:237–244.

6. Institute for Highway Safety. Q &A: Older People, 2006. Available at: http://www.iihs.org/research/qanda/older_people.html#2. Accessed June 22, 2008.

7. Braver ER, Trempel RE. Are older adults actually at greater risk of involvement in collisions resulting in deaths or non-fatal injuries among their passengers and other road users? *Inj Prev.* 2004;10:27–32.

8. Anstey KJ, Wood J, Lord S, Walker JG. Cognitive, sensory and physical factors enabling driving safety in older adults. *Clin Psych Rev.* 2005;25:45–65.

9. Owsley C, Ball K, McGwin G, et al. Visual processing impairment and risk of motor vehicle crash among older adults. *JAMA.* 1998;279:1083–1088.

10. Clay OJ, Wadley VG, Edwards JD, Roth DL, Roenker DL, Ball, KK. Cumulative meta-analysis of the relationship between useful field of view and driving: current and future implications. *Optom Vis Sci.* 2005;82:724–731.

11. Marottoli RA, Richardson ED, Stowe MH, et al. Development of a test battery to identify older drivers at risk for self-reported adverse driving events. *J Am Geriatr Soc.* 1998;26:562–568.

12. Margolis KM, Erani RP, McGovern P, et al. Risk factors for motor vehicle crashes in older women. *J Gerontol Med Sci.* 2002;57A:M186–M191.

13. Isler RB, Paronson BS, Hansson GJ. Age related effects of restricted head movements on the useful field of view of drivers. *Accid Anal Prev.* 1997;29:793–801.

14. Lyman JM, McGwin G, Sims RV. Factors related to driving difficulty and habits in older drivers. *Accid Anal Prev.* 2001;33:413–421.

15. Sims RV, McGwin G, Allman RM, Ball K, Owsley C. Exploratory study of incident vehicle crashes among older drivers. *J Gerontol Med Sci.* 2000;55A:M22–M27.

16. McGwin G, Sims RV, Pulley LV, Roseman JM. Relations among chronic medical conditions, medications and automobile crashes in the elderly: a population-based case-control study. *Am J Epidemiol.* 2000;152:424–31.

17. Ray WA, Fought RL, Decker MD. Psychoactive drugs and the risk of injurious motor vehicle crashes in elderly drivers. *Am J Epidemiol.* 1992;136:873–883.

18. Edwards JG. Depression, antidepressants and accidents. *BMJ.* 1995;311:887–888.

19. Brunnauer A, Laux G, Geiger E, Soyka M, Moller HJ. Antidepressants and driving ability:results from a clinical study. *J Clin Psychiatry.* 2006;67:1776–1781.

20. Uc EY, Rizzo M, Anderson SW, Sparks JD, Rodnitzky RL, Dawson JD. Impaired visual search in drivers with Parkinson's Disease. *Ann Neurol.* 2006;60:407–413.

21. Grace J, Amick MM, D'Abreu A, Festa EK, Heindel WC, Ott BR. Neuropsychological deficits associated with driving performance in Parkinson's and Alzheimer's disease. *JINS.* 2005;11:766–775.

22. Stutts JC, Stewart JR, Martell C. Cognitive test performance and crash risk in an older driver population. *Accid Anal Prev.* 30;1998:335–346.

23. Brown LB, Ott BR. Driving and dementia; a review of the literature. *J Geriatr Psychiatry Neurol.* 2004;17:232–240.

24. Adler G, Rotunda S, Dysken M. The older driver with dementia; an updated literature review. *J Safety Res.* 2005;36:399–407.

25. Brown LB, Ott BR, Papandonatos GD, Sui Y, Ready RE, Morris JC. Prediction of on-road driving performance in patients with early Alzheimer's disease. *J Am Geriatr Soc.* 2005;53:94–98.

26. Ott BR, Anthony D, Papandonatos GD, et al. Clinician assessment of the driving competence of patients with dementia. *J Am Geriatr Soc.* 2005;53:829–833.

27. Molnar, FJ, Patel A, Marshall SC, Man-Son-Hing M, Wilson KG. Clinical utility of office-based cognitive predictors of fitness to drive in persons with dementia; a systematic review. *J Am Geriatr Soc.* 2006;54:1809–1824.

28. Wang CC, Kosinski CJ, Schwartzberg JG, Shanklin AV. Physician's guide to assessing and counseling older drivers. Washington, DC: National Highway Traffic Safety Administration; 2003. Available at: http://www.ama-assn.org/go/olderdrivers. Accessed June 22, 2008.

29. Wang CC, Carr DB. Older driver safety: a report from the older drivers project. *J Am Geriatr Soc.* 2004;52:143–149.

30. Molnar FJ, Byszewski AM, Marshall SC, Man-Son-Hing M. In-office evaluation of medical fitness to drive: practical approaches for assessing older people. *Can Fam Physician.* 2005;51:372–379.

31. Murden RA, Unroe K. Assessing older drivers: a primary care protocol to evaluate driving safety risk. *Geriatrics.* 2005;60:20–24.

32. Odenheimer GL. Driver safety in older adults: the physician's role in assessing driving skills of older patients. *Geriatrics.* 2006;61:14–21.

33. Ball KK, Roenker DL, Wadley VG, et al. Can high-risk older drivers be identified through performance-based measures in a department of motor vehicles setting? *J Am Geriatr Soc.* 2006;54:77–84.

34. Freund B, Gravenstein S, Ferris R, Burke BL, Shaheen E. Drawing clocks and driving cars. *J Gen Intern Med.* 2005;20:240–244.

35. Association for Drivers Rehabilitation Specialists. (Accessed January 28, 2007 at http://www.driver-ed.org)

36. Dellinger AM, Sehgal M, Sleet DA, Barrett-Connor E. Driving cessation: what older former drivers tell us. *J Am Geriatr Soc.* 2001;49:431–435.

37. Freeman EE, Munoz B, Turano KA, West SK. Measures of visual function and their association with driving modification in older adults. *Invest Ophthalmol Vis Sci.* 2006;47:514–520.

38. American Automobile Association. Senior Drivers Tools/Resources. Available at: http://www.aaaexchange.com. Accessed June 22, 2008.

39. AARP Driver Safety. Available at: http://www.aarp.org/families/driver_safety. Accessed June 22, 2008.

40. Eby DW, Molnar LJ, Shope JT, Vivoda JM, Fordyce TA. Improving older driver knowledge and self-awareness through self-assessment: the driving decisions workbook. *J Safety Res.* 2003;34:371–381.

41. Stutts JC, Wilkins JW. On-road driving evaluations: a potential tool for helping older adults drive safely longer. *J Safety Res.* 2003;34:431–439.

42. Stutts JC. Do older drivers with visual and cognitive impairments drive less? *J Am Geriatr Soc.* 1998;46:854–861.

43. Ragland DR, Satariano WA, MacLeod KE. Driving cessation and increased depressive symptoms. *J Gerontol Med Sci.* 2005;60A:399–403.

44. Marottoli RA, Mendes de Leon CF, Glass TA, Williams CS, Cooney LM, Berkman LF. Consequences of driving cessation: decreased out-of-home activity levels. *J Gerontol Soc Sci.* 2000;55B:S334–S340.

45. Kostyniuk LP, Shope JT. Driving and alternatives: older drivers in Michigan. *J Safety Res.* 2003;34:407–414.

46. Freeman EE, Gange SJ, Munoz B, West SK. Diving status and risk of entry into long-term care in older adults. *Am J Public Health.* 2006;96:1254–1259.

47. Taylor BD, Tripodes S. The effects of driving cessation on the elderly with dementia on their caregivers. *Accid Anal Prev.* 2001;33:519–528.

48. Collia DV, Harp J, Giesbrecht L. The 2001 national household travel survey: a look into the travel patterns of older Americans. *J Safety Res.* 2003;34:461–470.

49. Foley DJ, Heimovitz HK, Guralnik JM, Brock DB. Driving life expectancy of persons aged 70 and older in the united states. *Am J Public Health.* 2002;92:1284–1289.

50. Vance DE, Roenker DL, Cissell GM, Edwards JD, Wadley VG, Ball KK. Predictors of driving exposure and avoidance in a field study of older drivers from the state of Maryland. *Accid Anal Prev.* 2006;38:823–831.

51. Florida At Risk Driver Council. The effects of aging on driving ability report. Florida Department of Highway Safety and Motor Vehicles; 2004.

49

INTEGRATIVE MEDICINE IN THE CARE OF THE ELDERLY

Joel S. Edman, DSc, FACN, Bettina Herbert, MD

INTRODUCTION AND BACKGROUND

The emergence of Integrative Medicine or Complementary and Alternative Medicine (CAM) was first recognized in 1993 with a report of a survey in the *New England Journal of Medicine* that found that one in three respondents had had a CAM treatment within the last year.[1] These visits were mostly for chronic disorders, sought without physician referrals, and in more than 70%, the respondents did not inform their physician. Integrative medicine is defined by the Consortium of Academic Health Centers for Integrative Medicine as "the practice of medicine that reaffirms the importance of the relationship between practitioner and patient, focuses on the whole person, is informed by evidence, and makes use of all appropriate therapeutic approaches, healthcare professionals and disciplines to achieve optimal health and healing."

Table 49.1 outlines a classification for integrative medicine practice although there may be overlap between categories. Many integrative medicine practices provide a range of these therapies with the ability to integrate them with allopathic medical approaches and practitioners. These integrative therapies, when carefully applied, are safe and have the potential for bringing greater well-being to all patients.

Currently, the older-than-65 years age group has the lowest integrative medicine/CAM use of any age group;[3] however, the demographic bubble of the baby boomers is starting to move into the 60 plus part of the population and will soon enlarge the 'elderly' stratum of U.S. society. Although at least 30% of the elderly have used integrative medicine, the boomers' use is at least 50% and increasing. Therefore more and more elderly will routinely be using these therapies. Predictors of integrative medicine use include poorer health (more chronic conditions), higher education, chronic conditions not responsive to conventional care, and increased age.[3,4]

An important challenge for integrative medicine is to establish its efficacy. This is not an easy task given the multifactorial nature of chronic diseases, and the combination of modalities that are often recommended. Although there is ongoing classic research to examine individual therapy influences on specific diseases and symptoms, true integrative medical clinical practice and research applies and attempts to quantify benefits derived from dietary guidelines, nutritional supplements, stretching/exercise/yoga, stress management techniques, therapeutic touch, and/or other approaches followed at the same time. There are no simple research models that can do this; so new approaches are being developed, although significant resources and time are needed.

With an increasing elderly population in the United States, with increasing amounts of chronic diseases that often are a challenge to manage, integrative medical therapies can give patients individual attention from a variety of practitioners, a practitioners touch, an ability to participate in their care, and a range of natural approaches that can be helpful. Our focus will be on illustrating how integrative medicine is applied as well as describing core approaches such as nutrition, physical fitness and falls prevention, pain management, stress management, and mind–body medicine.

NUTRITION

Good nutrition is an important foundation for optimal aging and for an integrative medicine approach to symptoms and disorders common in the elderly. This includes both the use of specific dietary guidelines and targeted nutritional supplementation.

It is well established that older individuals are at significant risk for malnutrition, and clinical or subclinical nutritional

Table 49.1. Classification of Integrative Medicine/Complementary and Alternative Medicine Practices with Examples

Dietary, Nutritional Supplement, Herbal and Other Biological Therapies

Use of diet and supplementation for therapeutic and preventive purposes

Therapeutic diets	Intravenous therapies
Vitamins, minerals, fatty acids, etc.	Aromatherapy
Herbs	Detoxification

Manual Healing Methods

Systems that are based on manipulation and/or movement of the body

Osteopathic manipulative therapy	Pressure point therapies
Chiropractic	Postural/Movement reeducation therapies
Massage therapy	Bioenergetic systems

Mind–Body Interventions

Behavioral, psychological, social, and spiritual approaches to health.

Biofeedback	Mindfulness-based stress reduction (MBSR)
Meditation	Hypnosis and imagery
Yoga	Prayer and mental healing
Tai chi and Chi gong	Art and music therapy

Alternative Medical Systems

Complete systems of theory and practice that have been developed mostly outside of the Western biomedical model.

Traditional oriental medicine	Naturopathic medicine
Acupuncture	Homeopathic medicine
Ayurvedic medicine	Environmental medicine
Energy medicine	

Source: Adapted from Monti DA, Stoner M. Complementary and Alternative Medicine. In *Textbook of Women's Mental Health.*[2]

deficiencies. Many common factors may contribute to nutritional inadequacy including poor appetite, depression, isolation, and disability, although there are many other influences that can have important effects in individual circumstances. Rates of nutritional deficiency range from 10%–50%,[5,6] with the most common nutrient deficiencies found for folate, vitamin D, calcium, zinc and magnesium.[5-8]

There are a few key differences between medical nutrition therapy practiced in an integrative or CAM clinic in comparison to a dietetics setting. One primary difference is that integrative nutritionists or dietitians are much more likely to recommend therapeutic diets (e.g., vegetarian, rotation/elimination, sugar-free, or lower carbohydrate), at least for a specific period of time, because they can be an important part of an integrative program. Another important distinction is that nutritionists and integrative medical practitioners are much more likely to prescribe nutritional supplements to go along with therapeutic diets, whereas most dieticians are often not trained in the use

of nutritional supplements and have little experience with their therapeutic potential.

Dietary Guidelines

Many dietary guidelines and considerations that are presented and recommended in the earlier nutrition chapter are in agreement with integrative medicine and nutrition. Research supports these guidelines in the prevention and adjuvant treatment of heart disease, cancer, and neurocognitive decline.[9-11]

Three primary dietary approaches that are frequently addressed in integrative medicine are: a) antiinflammatory diets; b) elimination or rotation diets for food intolerance or food allergy; and c) balance of macronutrients and other factor-specific guidelines for hypoglycemia, abnormal glucose tolerance and insulin resistance. Depending upon the symptom or disorder, various levels of dietary guidelines could be

Table 49.2. Healthy Dietary Fat

Omega 3 Fatty Acids	Monounsaturated Fatty Acid
Fish – salmon, mackerel, sardines, others	Olive oil and olives
Ground flax seeds or flax oil	Nuts and seeds
Soy products	Avocado
Nuts and seeds	
Dark green leafy vegetables	

recommended and/or a combination of these approaches as described below.

Recent research and commentary suggests that aging may be an inflammatory process.[12] Although most research suggests that omega 3 fatty acids have the most significant anti-inflammatory effects, there is also some evidence to support the effects of monounsaturated fat, antioxidants, phytonutrients and possibly other factors.[13] These guidelines can be encouraged by recommending omega 3 fats and monounsaturated fats listed in Table 49.2.

Rotation and elimination diet can be useful for stomach and intestinal disorders (IBS, IBD and GERD), migraines, autoimmune disorders, chronic inflammatory or pain disorders, skin conditions, allergies or others. These diets can be applied in 3 primary ways, including: a) a rotation diet (1–2 times per week of foods in Level 1 or Level 2); b) a "Level 1" elimination diet – avoid sugars, dairy, wheat, alcohol and caffeine; and c) "level 2" elimination diet – avoid foods from Level 1 plus other potentially offending foods such as peanuts, soy, other gluten grains (rye, barley and oats), corn, citrus, eggs, and any other foods that may be suspected. The patient's ability and willingness to comply even for a short time is important to consider.

It is possible that abnormal glucose tolerance in underweight people (hypoglycemia) and insulin resistance in overweight or obese individuals reflect a continuum that can be addressed in similar ways. This includes: limiting or avoiding sugars and refined carbohydrates; balancing meals for protein, healthy fat and complex carbohydrate; limiting caffeine; eating smaller, more frequent meals and snacks, regular stretching and exercise; and possibly specific nutrients such as magnesium and/or chromium.

The challenge to nutritionists is to target the optimal diet and supplement program that can produce results yet are not so difficult that compliance is sacrificed. Therefore this requires dialogue and understanding, as well as informational and practical support. Finally, the guidelines should be recommended for a finite period of time such as 2–8 weeks to see if results are achieved. An example recommendation could be to avoid or rotate sugar, wheat, dairy and alcohol for four weeks and see what results are produced.

Sometimes by just applying therapeutic diets for a short time it can be determined if this will be beneficial. Although there may be many patients who cannot follow strict guidelines, there are many who can and are encouraged to follow through, especially if they can feel better or see the changes they are looking for.

Nutritional Supplementation

Supplement sales have increased to more than $23 billion per year.[14] Although taking supplements can have significant preventive and therapeutic effects, it is also important for practitioners to know what patients are taking and if there are significant nutrient–drug interactions.

The consideration for the use of nutritional supplements in clinical practice is to a certain degree a question of philosophy and practice orientation. For integrative or CAM practitioners, supplements are a part of the framework of natural approaches that include diet, exercise, stress management, and other modalities such as acupuncture or massage. For allopathic physicians where insurance and time constraints often limit the degree to which other health-related issues can be addressed, it is an important question to ask whether supplements should be included. This is particularly true because the supportive clinical research is often weak, especially when compared with pharmaceutical research – this is largely due to the lack of financial incentives to conduct this research and significant methodological problems. Geriatric practice, however, could be particularly responsive to targeting key supplements to avoid adding to the number of other medications that may already be being taken and potential adverse effects or interactions.

The primary legislation that regulates all aspects of supplements, including manufacturing, quality control, labeling, and marketing is The Dietary Supplement Health and Education Act passed by Congress in 1994. There is a large range of supplements that practitioners may recommend or that patients may try on their own. These categories of supplements include vitamins, minerals, fatty acids, amino acids, antioxidants, probiotics and prebiotics, herbs and botanicals, enzymes, hormones, glandulars, functional foods and food concentrates, homeopathic remedies, and others.

There are many reasons to suggest why supplements may benefit a patient, including poor dietary choices, variations in soil nutritional content, micronutrient losses from food processing and cooking, and genetic polymorphisms or variations in individual nutrient requirements.[15] To understand how supplements can benefit the patient population, it is possible to use several models, including nutritional deficiency, subclinical nutritional deficiency, biological response modifiers, and mass action effects.[16] The overt nutritional deficiency is well defined and most often utilized in medical and nutritional practice. Classic examples are iron and vitamin B_{12} deficiencies that produce clinical symptoms, can be identified through laboratory analyses, and supplemented and monitored for symptom and assay changes.

More challenging is the evaluation of the other three research models in which there may be varying levels of supportive evidence from in vitro, animal, and clinical research.

For example, a subclinical magnesium deficiency is the reason many integrative medicine practitioners recommend magnesium despite normal serum or red blood cell magnesium levels.[17] Magnesium is a cofactor for over 300 enzymes and is a calcium channel blocker. Research supports magnesium's influence in hypertension, diabetes and glucose tolerance, migraines, allergies, muscle cramps, constipation, neurocognitive function, and possibly other disorders.[18,19] Because magnesium is often inadequate in the diet and can be depleted by chronic disease, it is often prescribed by primary health care providers to help address a range of symptoms.

Omega-3 fatty acids or fish oil supplements are a good example of supplements that have biological response–modifier effects. Supplements can enhance dietary influences, as described in the previous dietary section, and can effectively alter the synthesis of proinflammatory versus antiinflammatory eicosanoids. Omega-3 fatty acids are potentially beneficial in a range of disorders due to their antiinflammatory effects and impact on cellular membrane fluidity and function because of their effects on membrane fatty acid composition.[20] There is no established nutritional status measure, although some studies have quantified blood levels of specific omega-3 fatty acids or omega-3/omega-6 fatty acid ratios.[21] These are two good examples (among many) in which there are no accurate nutritional status measures available. This lack of effective assessment measures and data makes it much more difficult to conduct research that can quantify supplement recommendation effects and lead to valid clinical protocols.

With regard to 'mass action' effects, Ames and colleagues have written an excellent review of the biochemical influences of high-dose vitamins on enzyme binding and activity.[16] As many as 50 genetic diseases and many genetic polymorphisms have shown improvement through a range of nutritional supplementation, with other polymorphism effects to be determined as their identification and clinical effects are more thoroughly understood.

Despite the challenges presented, supplements can be effectively utilized in patient care, especially in the elderly, once a reliable source of products is identified. Table 49.3 describes an effective framework from which supplements can be recommended.

There are some dietary or nutritional supplements that can be safely recommended and may be beneficial. Table 49.4[22] presents some of the most important and useful supplements (the first three could be considered a foundation approach).

Intravenous Nutrients

Many integrative medicine/CAM practitioners recommend intravenous (IV) nutrients and chelation therapy for cardiovascular disease;[34] IV vitamin C and other nutrients for cancer;[35] and IV nutritional protocols for a variety of other disorders. This can also be considered for elderly patients who may have poor nutritional status resulting from malabsorption and/or a range of other contributing factors including metabolic consequences of chronic disease.[36]

Table 49.3. Framework for Recommending Supplements

Healthy diet as a foundation

Evidence base that includes a sound rationale and mechanism

Positive benefit/risk ratio

Defined dose and timeframe to assess effects

Targeted populations to treat such as: patients with adverse or inadequate responses to medication; patients or families who would like to try nutrition and/or natural therapies before taking pharmaceuticals; or elderly patients who are already taking many medications

Herbal Medicine

Herbal medicine or the use of plant-based products to influence symptoms or disorders is often included with the use of nutritional supplements as part of a nutritional supplement/herbal regimen. Herbs may also be recommended, however, as part of traditional medical approaches such as Ayurveda, traditional Chinese medicine, and Tibetan medicine or east Asian medicine that have been practiced for thousands of years. Significant research, largely supported by the National Center for Complementary and Alternative Medicine (NCCAM) and the Office of Dietary Supplements, is now being conducted to examine the effects of herbal therapies. NCCAM has also established a Botanical Research Center Program that supports university-based research centers that are investigating age-related diseases, metabolic syndrome, women's health, immunomodulators, botanical lipids, and phytomedicine. In Europe and Australia herbal products are regulated by government agencies to assure product quality. An ongoing debate compares the use of standardized herbal products indexed to specifically identified and quantified active ingredients versus the use of whole herbs (leaves and/or stems) that may have multiple active ingredients.

An example of a commonly used herb is saw palmetto (Serenoa repens) for benign prostatic hypertrophy. The active ingredients have been identified as β sitosterol, campesterol and stigmasterol. Research suggests that its influence in benign prostate hypertrophy is derived from an inhibition of 5α-reductase and 3-ketosteroid reductase, as well as blocking the binding of dihydrotestosterone to prostate cells.[37]

St. John's Wort (Hypericum peforatum) is another example of an herb, frequently recommended, for mild-to-moderate depression. Although not as well known, St. John's Wort may also be helpful for wound healing and antiviral effects. Although research suggests that this herb can be beneficial, it is not well understood which of the mechanisms are most important including: inhibition of reuptake of norepinephrine, serotonin, dopamine, and γ-aminobutyric acid; upregulation of serotonergic receptors; inhibition of catechol-o-methyltransferase; inhibition of monoamine oxidase-A and monoamine oxidase-B activities; and/or others. It is also a good example of an herbal product that can significantly influence the

Table 49.4. Important and Useful Dietary Supplements

Supplement	Rationale
Multivitamin and mineral	Despite some conflicting results, research has suggested that multivitamin and mineral supplements may reduce the risk for heart attacks and certain types of cancer, as well as reduce C-reactive protein, and infection rates in diabetics and the elderly.[23–27] Taking a multivitamin and mineral every day can reinforce healthy behaviors that contribute to a healthy lifestyle.
Omega-3 fatty acids or fish oil	Health benefits of fish were described earlier in this chapter. It should also be noted that fish oil is now endorsed by the American Heart Association for the prevention of cardiovascular disease. There are at least six mechanisms by which omega-3 fatty acids reduce cardiovascular disease risk including: 1) anti-inflammatory; 2) hypolipidemic; 3) anti-thrombotic; 4) cytokine inhibition; (5) antiarrhythmic; and 6) endothelial-derived nitric oxide stimulation.[28]
Calcium, magnesium, and vitamin D	Important for bone health and the many important aspects of magnesium influence that were listed earlier. Also, there is some recent provocative research suggesting that vitamin D may be involved in immune function and cancer, autoimmune disorders, insulin resistance, and possibly other disorders, especially in the elderly.[29]
Probiotics	Have been shown to be helpful for symptoms such as constipation and diarrhea, and they are very safe.[30] They may also be helpful for irritable bowel syndrome, inflammatory bowel disease, atopic disease and *Clostridium difficile* infections with a yeast supplement, *Saccharomyces boulardii.*[31]
Glucosamine sulfate and chondroitin sulfate	Good research suggests that glucosamine and chondroitin sulfate can help reduce stiffness and pain in osteoarthritis.[32]
Coenzyme Q10	CoQ10, or ubiquinone, is an important part of the oxidative phosphorylation chain leading to mitochondrial ATP synthesis. 3-hydroxy-3-methyl-glutaryl–coenzyme A reductase inhibitors or statins lower circulating levels of CoQ10, but the consequences are not well understood. Perhaps the most common symptom would be muscle cramps. Supplementation may be warranted especially in susceptible populations such as those >65 years of age or those with congestive heart failure.[33]

circulating levels and/or effectiveness of pharmaceuticals. This results because St. John's Wort induces cytochrome P450 enzymes, particularly CYP 3A4, which can lower plasma levels of alprazolam, amitriptyline, cyclosporine, digoxin, indinavir, methadone, simvastatin, theophylline, warfarin, oral contraceptives, and other medications.[38]

It is beyond the scope of this chapter to provide a detailed list and description of the use of herbs in the elderly but this is described elsewhere,[39] and there are resources listed at the end of this chapter. Herbal products can be useful, although more caution is necessary because there are more common interactions between some herbs and pharmaceuticals.

Homeopathy

Homeopathy is an approach to health and healing that is based on the principle of *similia similibus curantur* or like heals like. The founder and primary developer of Homeopathy was the German physician Samuel Hahnemann (1755–1843). He spent most of his life testing and documenting remedy effects and recording them in the Organon of Medical Art. For most of the nineteenth century and early twentieth century homeopathy was the mainstream medicine practiced in the United States.

Homeopathy specifically challenges the biological system or physiology of an individual by exposing it to a remedy that causes the symptoms that an individual is reporting. In so doing, the body's own healing mechanisms are stimulated to respond, thus promoting homeostasis or healing to occur. Although controversial, there is an emerging body of medical literature and research that shows benefits of homeopathic approaches for fibromyalgia syndrome, respiratory symptoms, postoperative swelling and pain, and other disorders.[40–42] Homeopathic remedies are easy to take because the delivery mechanism is small sugar pellets. They generally do not cause side effects, are nonhabit forming, and are regulated by the Food and Drug Administration as over- the-counter medications. Instead of building up a tolerance and requiring more of the medicine, patients generally need less and less over time because of the healing effect of the medicines.[43]

The two main approaches to the practice of homeopathy are classic homeopathy and the use of combination remedies. Classic homeopathy involves the recommendation of an individualized single remedy based on a thorough and comprehensive interview with a patient. This would include the totality of symptoms and any other characteristics that may be considered important or relevant. In contrast, combination or complex remedies are in essence manufactured by homeopathic companies for a range of disorders or symptoms such as colds, cough, allergies, headaches, diarrhea, and so forth. Although these remedies are available in most health food or supplement stores and can be effective, classic homeopathy is considered to be more specific and individualized for a patient, and a truer form of homeopathy. Classic homeopathy also requires considerable experience to work effectively with patients.

In treating the elderly, homeopathy is an important approach to consider because it can be helpful and does not interfere with other modalities. This may be particularly helpful in elderly patients who may already be taking many medications. Much more information is available through the resource listed at the end of the chapter.

PHYSICAL MEDICINE

Fitness

At any age, for almost any condition, some form of movement is beneficial. It is best to find something that gives a patient pleasure. For a lifelong athlete, continuing in a chosen sport is ideal; levels of training are often naturally modified. For others, just getting started will help with affect, cardiovascular disease, sleep, immune function, musculoskeletal complaints, and overall strength, balance, and endurance.

For the completely deconditioned, "TV exercises" are a good start. Patients can perform ankle circles, leg lifts, or arm strengthening with 2-lb weights (even soup cans) during commercials. Keeping the upper extremities as strong as possible is key to using any assistive device such as a walker or cane. Of course, care must be exercised not to injure shoulders or other vulnerable joints. Sometimes a short course with a skilled physical or occupational therapist is a wise start. A fitness class will often provide incentive as well as social interaction.

Fall Prevention

Because 5-year survival after hip fractures in the elderly is very low, preventing falls is essential. Several strategies, best if combined, can reduce falls: patient education, home safety evaluations, specific exercise methods, and assistive devices.

Educating patients about home safety is key; they should be encouraged to secure area rugs, tuck away cords, put nonskid surfaces on slippery stairs and install bars in the shower and toilet. A one-time home evaluation by an occupational therapist may be very useful.

Patients may also be encouraged to forego vanity and use an assistive device when out of the house for both balance and reassurance. For the more active, walking sticks (modified ski poles) are a welcome suggestion. They imply activity rather than infirmity and can be used both indoors and outdoors.

Paradoxically, fear of falling can increase the risk of falling, because it leads to tight muscles that reduce balance recovery. In winter, walking sticks or canes with carbide tips (found in outdoor stores and catalogues) and slip-on gripper soles for shoes are very useful for negotiating icy surfaces.

Movement Therapies

Gait is a predictor of balance. A number of interventions have been shown to improve gait; they include many safe and effective movement therapies that can be practiced in groups or alone and can be modified to meet individual needs.

Some of the best ways to restore or maintain fitness, balance, and strength are through the mind–body practices, such as Tai Chi, Qi Gong and yoga. A large multicenter study by Emory University found that Tai Chi – done for an hour twice weekly – is the single most effective intervention widely available, reducing falls by 47.5% in people older than 70.[44] More recently they studied the "transition to frailty" elderly who had fallen at least once, and even they experienced a 40% reduction in falls by the 4th month.[45]

Both Tai Chi and Qi Gong are gentle martial arts practices that have been used for centuries in China. In addition to creating better balance with slow, fluid exercises, they reduce stress, as evidenced by α and τ brain wave increases, increases in β endorphin levels and drops in adrenocorticotropic hormone levels.[46]

Yoga is an ancient practice developed in India that addresses the physical, mental, and spiritual aspects of the individual. There are many different forms of yoga, each emphasizing different skills, goals and philosophies. Hatha yoga, the physical practice of integral yoga, is the best-known approach in the United States and is used here mainly as a form of exercise and stress management. It is easily adaptable to patients with physical limitations.

TREATMENT OF CHRONIC PAIN

Pain is one of the most common reasons people turn to integrative medicine. A growing body of evidence also suggests that a multidisciplinary treatment approach to pain – one that addresses its physical, emotional, functional and social aspects – offers the best chance of long-term success. Hence, integrative medicine may be especially appropriate for, as well as attractive to, patients with chronic pain. Conventional treatments can be thoughtfully combined with nutritional support, plant-based remedies as well as manual, movement, and mind–body therapies.

Perhaps the most common cause of pain in the elderly is osteoarthritis (OA). Back, neck, and joint pain are prevalent. With the declining use of the COX2 inhibitors, many patients are turning to other therapies to minimize pain and increase function, put off joint replacement, and stay as active as possible. Several modalities have research to support their use in OA.

ACUPUNCTURE

Acupuncture, part of traditional Chinese medicine, an ancient healing modality, is one of the more widely studied therapies. There is increasing evidence that it is safe and efficacious for pain of OA both as an adjunct (complementary) treatment and as an alternative.[47–49] Acupuncture has also been shown to be valuable in stroke rehabilitation, migraine and tension headaches, tennis elbow, fibromyalgia, myofascial pain, low-back pain, and carpal tunnel syndrome.[50–56] The World Health Organization lists over 40 common conditions for which acupuncture should be considered as treatment.

An acupuncturist inserts very thin needles into specific points to normalize and maintain energy (Qi) flow in the body. Although that is a different paradigm from the allopathic model, there has been some success in studying acupuncture. Data suggest that several mechanisms of action lead to decreases in pain. Needle stimulation may affect pain transmission locally through release of spinal dynorphins, centrally via central nervous system endorphin and neurotransmitter release (mood and pain perception) and systemically via adrenocorticotropic hormone–activated endogenous corticosteroids.[57–60] Decreasing use of pain medications has been reported.[61]

Adverse events such as needle pain are common but minor and, overall, acupuncture is well tolerated by even the frailest patients.[62] The author has often referred patients to experienced acupuncturists after critical illness or surgery to increase vitality.

Manual Therapies

Osteopathic Manipulative Medicine (Osteopathic Manipulative Treatment)

A physician who is managing an older patient with multiple chronic neuromusculoskeletal conditions (such as OA, cervicalgia, osteoporosis, low back pain, or neurodegenerative disease) may find it useful to consult an osteopathic physician well trained in osteopathic manipulative medicine (OMM). In the United States, but not in Canada or Great Britain, osteopaths (DOs) have exactly the same medical education as allopaths (MDs). They have an additional perspective: that a body's structure affects its function and, given proper alignment, the body will heal itself as much as possible. Osteopaths use manual therapies to restore good body biomechanics to decrease myofascial strain and restore blood and lymph circulation.

"Cracking," or high velocity low amplitude is perhaps the best-known OMM direct technique. Although other direct approaches such as muscle energy and myofascial release are well tolerated by most, there are other gentle, comforting techniques that are effective and safe even for frail patients. These 'indirect' osteopathic techniques work on soft tissue and effect changes that may be deep and long lasting, without running the risk of damaging osteoporotic bones or calcified tendons. Often, manipulation is delivered in the "direction of ease," rather than pushing against the restriction, and gradually the body (joint, muscle, bone, organ, and spine) releases its tension. Some of the most frequently used indirect techniques include the following

- Strain/counterstrain and its offshoot, positional release – use positions of comfort to decrease painful tender points and decrease pain overall

- Cranial osteopathy also known as craniosacral therapy – the gentle manipulation of tissues surrounding the central nervous system (including the dura mater attachments at the skull and sacrum) to free restrictions of a subtle fluid respiratory rhythm
- Functional technique (one of the gentlest) – treatment only in position of ease
- Visceral manipulation: a technique developed in France for releasing restrictions and adhesions in fascia suspending specific organs.

In addition to reducing pain, data suggest many additional benefits of OMM. They include acutely increasing gait length in Parkinson's disease, utilizing the viscerosomatic reflexes to diagnose and treat same-spinal-cord-level-related somatic and visceral structures, and improving posture, gait, and balance to improve quality of life in neurodegenerative disease.[63–69]

Chiropractic

Chiropractors have training focused on disorders of the musculoskeletal and nervous systems, spinal manipulation, biomechanics, and palpation skills. Their course of study, especially clinical training, is usually significantly shorter than those of allopathic and osteopathic physicians. Because they comprise the largest group of alternative practitioners, chiropractic is the most studied of manipulative therapies. These studies have provided useful data.

The most common technique, spinal manipulation (to restore joint mobility), alone has been shown to be as effective as other common approaches to low back pain such as analgesics, back school, and so forth.[70] It has also proven effective as conservative management of neck pain.[69] There is growing evidence that manipulation/mobilization plus exercise is more effective in reducing pain than either one alone.[71,72] Most of the studies, however, have been performed using a younger population.

It would be inadvisable to subject elderly patients with potential osteoporosis and atherosclerosis to direct thrust or high velocity–low amplitude techniques ("cracking"). If anything, only soft tissue techniques, known as "chiropractic mobilization," should be applied to this at-risk population.

Therapeutic Massage

Massage is the use of manually applied pressure on soft tissues. It has many benefits, including the relief of pain in the low back, tight muscles. and arthritic joints. It softens hard musculature and increases blood flow, promotes restful sleep, releases endorphins, and increases levels of serotonin and dopamine.[73–76] It is even more effective for pain relief when combined with exercise or physical therapy.[77] For the elderly, who often live alone, it also provides that much-needed kind human touch.

In an older population, massage strokes should be slower, gentler, and take into account a patient's frailties, including osteopenia and warfarin use. Contraindications for massage include deep vein thrombosis, burns, skin infections, eczema, open wounds, bone fractures, and advanced osteoporosis.[78]

POSTURAL/MOVEMENT REEDUCATION THERAPIES

Yoga is also useful in pain management. Studies have demonstrated decreases in serum cortisol levels, increases in brain α and τ waves, reduced pain of OA and carpal tunnel syndrome, stress reduction, and mood elevation.[79,80] Certain asanas ("postures that bring steadiness and comfort") have been shown to decrease blood pressure.[81] The combination of yoga and meditation is an integral and successful part of the well-known Stress Reduction and Relaxation Program at the University of Massachusetts, founded by Jon Kabat-Zinn, PhD, to treat patients who have chronic pain.[82–85]

Tai Chi and Qi Gong, when combined with education and relaxation training, have been shown to be effective for several pain syndromes, including complex regional pain syndrome, fibromyalgia, and chronic low back pain.[86–88]

Western movement approaches are also often utilized by patients with chronic pain. A few of the more commonly used ones will be discussed here.

The Feldenkrais Method consists of a large variety of very gentle, simple exercises to develop graceful, efficient movement patterns that are pain free. The work consists of two parts: group movement lessons and individual, hands-on sessions. Studies of the Feldenkrais Method suggest that it may be useful for anxiety, neck and shoulder pain, and both disability and anxiety in multiple sclerosis patients.[89–92] Data also suggest it is useful for stroke recovery.[93] It is a key component in some multidisciplinary pain programs.

The Alexander Technique, often used for chronic back and neck pain, uses verbal instructions and light touch to guide the patient to improve postural habits. Clinical trials are promising and suggest that this technique is useful in reducing disability from Parkinson's disease and in improving back pain.[94–96] Small studies have also suggested benefits for reduction of both stress and chronic pain, enhanced relaxation, improved balance in older women, and enhanced respiratory function.[94,97,98]

The Trager Approach also combines table work and simple movement practices to release accumulated tension and help the patient learn ways to move freely. Table work consists of gentle movements to release restrictive holding patterns that create pain. Patients are taught to recreate the feelings of relaxation that they felt during the sessions. A recent study combining the Trager Approach and acupuncture found that the treatment was effective in reducing shoulder pain in spinal cord injury patients.[98] It may also be effective in other musculoskeletal problems.[100]

Mind–Body Approaches to Pain Management

Advanced brain imaging has shown that pain simultaneously activates several regions of the brain, including somatosensory representations of the body along with frontal structures such as the anterior cingulate and prefrontal cortex.[101–105] Because the latter are involved in affect, mind–body techniques such as meditation, relaxation, and biofeedback are useful in treating patients with chronic pain. Biofeedback, for example, is useful for tension headaches.[106] Generally, these techniques are beneficial in any condition in which stress exacerbates symptoms. Many of the movement therapies, such as yoga and Tai Chi, are in actuality mind–body approaches.

ENERGY THERAPY

The NCCAM, part of the National Institutes of Health, divides energy work into two types. Biofield therapy manipulates the human life force or energy field. Forms of energy work that use hands on or off the body include Reiki, a traditional Japanese system of energy work and stress reduction; therapeutic touch, healing touch, and Qi Gong. Although the actual energy field has not yet been successfully measured, there is evidence of beneficial effects. For example, Reiki treatments may lower stress hormones, heart rate, and blood pressure.[107] These are also low-risk interventions that may prove helpful to many patients.

The second type of energy therapy, pulsed electromagnetic therapy, has been used for many years to aid healing in fractures. Recent data suggest it may reduce pain in several chronic conditions including knee and cervical OA, rheumatoid arthritis, fibromyalgia, and lumbar radiculopathy.[108–111]

EMOTIONAL AND SPIRITUAL WELL-BEING AND STRESS MANAGEMENT

This last section is in many ways the heart of integrative medicine and describes an important goal of integrative medicine practice. Disease is thought to be significantly influenced by stresses, thought processes and emotional factors, as well as one's spiritual life. Healing therefore is most likely to occur when a practitioner not only examines the physical body, but also considers mental and emotional characteristics, stresses that may be present, as well as influences of spiritual beliefs and practices. Although some of these issues may not be unique to most geriatric practices or centers, the integrated and interrelated concept of mind, body, and spirit often is.

There are so many ways to evaluate and encourage emotional and spiritual well-being that only an overview can be presented within this chapter. What is important to recognize is that illnesses and stresses with aging and end of life can lead to considerable suffering or discomfort that can often be affected by attention to emotional and spiritual factors, as well as a variety of stress management techniques. These techniques range from various psychological or talk therapies to bodywork, exercise or yoga, to enjoyable and therapeutic activities, hobbies and social networking.

Within integrative medicine, a technique that has been embraced and well researched is MBSR, developed by Jon Kabat-Zinn.[112] Based on a Zen Buddhism tradition, it is a good illustration of the mind, body, and spirit concept by encouraging the experience of life and living with an observer's perspective or mind, to be present to stress-related physical sensations, thoughts and feelings as well as any other related issues. Accumulating evidence supports the beneficial effects of MBSR for stress levels, mood, sleep, and/or quality of life in a variety of disorders including depression and anxiety, fibromyalgia, cancer, chronic pain, menopausal hot flashes, organ transplants, and other populations.[113–117]

Attitude is also of prime importance. George Vaillant, director of the Harvard Study of Adult Development, succinctly lists several attributes on the "aging gracefully scale."[118] These include staying open to new ideas, retaining a sense of humor as well as a capacity for joy and play. Maintaining or regaining initiative, trust, and social utility are key in the mind–body arena.

It is by now well documented that many symptoms and diseases have a 'mind–body' connection. Ongoing research is now attempting to clarify mechanisms and identify biological markers and valid characteristics or scales that can be useful. This research is examining functional disorders such as irritable bowel syndrome, fibromyalgia and chronic fatigue, headaches and migraines, immune deficiency and auto-immune disorders, heart attacks, and many others.

Another piece within integrative medicine is that the concepts and practice of spirituality and/or religion are considered very important to well-being and strongly supported. Evidence suggests that this is an important aspect of American life and is associated with good health.[119] Significant research has also examined the potential healing benefit of various types of prayer.[120]

There are many ways that emotional, psychological, and spiritual factors can influence health and disease, and this has been effectively illustrated by Rachel Naomi Remen in her lectures and books.[121] Dr. Remen encourages practitioners to be present and listen effectively so that a caring environment can allow patients the opportunity to share and to uncover the stories that shape all lives.

Although it is beyond the scope of this chapter to discuss thoroughly psychological and spiritual aspects of aging and illness, it is important to recognize that aging and end-of-life experiences will often reflect the influences of a life's events and moments that may or may not have occurred as one had hoped or dreamed. It may also have included significant traumas or stresses that may need to be acknowledged or dealt with before they can be let go of and allow for healing to occur.

SUMMARY AND CONCLUSION

Integrative medicine is a developing approach to health care that is increasing in demand and in many ways seeks to return to a system that is personal, supportive, as noninvasive as possible, and holistic. This is especially important and useful in a geriatric population. Although there are many areas that require significantly more research and development, many of the techniques can be safely and effectively used.

An important consideration for the use of integrative medicine is how to find qualified practitioners who can effectively contribute to a patient's care and participate in a health care team. Because credentialing will vary according to the specialty being considered, potential practitioners could be identified from academic or hospital settings, colleague recommendations, from patients who have had good experiences, and/or other sources. In addition, although physician visits are often covered (especially as an out of network consultation), acupuncture, chiropractic treatments, nutritional counseling, and massage are usually only covered in some cases. Some modalities, however, such as yoga, Feldenkrais, Tai Chi, Qi Gong and others, may be accessed through group classes, books, tapes, and videos.

Integrative medicine approaches can be beneficial for wellness and preventive care, as well as for integrative or adjuvant treatment for chronic disorders. Unfortunately, many come only when they have exhausted conventional treatments and they may have unrealistic expectations for dramatic results when integrative medicine approaches often have a longer timeframe or produce more gradual benefits. Hopefully, as more preventive and lifestyle approaches are incorporated into health care, there will also be more discussion by physicians with their patients about some of these integrative medicine treatment options and current patient lifestyle characteristics. This should help to encourage two important tenets of integrative medicine: self-care and responsibility.

Future developments will significantly influence how broadly and effectively integrative medicine modalities will be utilized. Therefore, many resources and references are included herein to explore, understand, and monitor the progress of integrative medicine.

WEBSITES AND RESOURCES

American Academy of Medical Acupuncture (AAMA) and Medical Acupuncture Research Foundation, 5820 Wilshire Boulevard, Suite 500, Los Angeles, CA 90036; (323) 937–5514; www.medicalacupuncture.org.

American Association of Acupuncture and Oriental Medicine, 433 Front Street, Catasauqua, PA 18032; (610) 266–1433; www.aaom.org.

American Association of Naturopathic Physicians, 4435 Wisconsin Avenue, NW, Suite 403, Washington, DC 20016; (866) 538–2267; www.naturopathic.org.

American Botanical Council, 6200 Manor Road, Austin, TX 78723;(512) 926–4900; http://www.herbalgram.org.

American Chiropractic Association, 1701 Clarendon Boulevard, Arlington, VA, 22209; (703) 276–8800; www.amerchiro.org.

American Holistic Medical Association, PO Box 2016, Edmonds, WA, 98020; (425) 967–0737; www.holisticmedicine.org.

American Institute of Homeopathy, 801 N. Fairfax Street, Suite 306, Alexandria, VA 22314; (888) 445–9988; www.homeopathyusa.org.

American Massage Therapy Association; www.amta.org; Foundation research database – www.amtafoundation.org.

American Osteopathic Association, 142 E. Ontario Street, Chicago, IL, 60611; (800) 621–1773; www.osteopathic.org.

Association for Applied Psychophysiology and Biofeedback, 10200 W. 44th Avenue, #304, Wheat Ridge, CO, 80033; (303) 422–8436; www.aapb.org

Bravewell Collaborative, 1818 Oliver Avenue South, Minneapolis, MN 55405; www.bravewell.org.

Consortium of Academic Health Centers for Integrative Medicine; www.imconsortium.org.

Duke University's Center for the Study of Religion, Spirituality and Health; www.dukespiritualityandhealth.org.

Institute for Functional Medicine, 4411 Pt. Fosdick Drive NW, Suite 305, P.O. Box 1697, Gig Harbor, WA 98335; (800) 228–0622, Fax: (253)853–6766; http://www.functionalmedicine.org/.

National Center for Complementary and Alternative Medicine (NCCAM), National Institutes of Health (NIH); 6707 Democracy Boulevard, Suite 401, Bethesda, MD, 20892; (888) 644–6226; http://nccam.nih.gov.

Natural Medicines Comprehensive Database (subscription required) http://www.naturaldatabase.com.

Office of Dietary Supplements, NIH, 6100 Executive Boulevard, Room 3B01, MSC 7517, Bethesda, MD, 20892; (301) 435–2920; http://ods.od.nih.gov.

REFERENCES

1. Eisenberg DM, Davis RB, Ettner SL, et al. Trends in alternative medicine use in the United States, 1990–1997: results of a follow-up national survey. *JAMA.* 1998; 280:1569–1575.
2. Monti DA, Stoner M. Complementary and alternative medicine. In: Kornstein SG, Clayton AH, eds. *Textbook of Women's Mental Health.* New York: Guilford Publications; 2002:344–355.
3. Herman CJ, Allen P, Hunt WC, Prasad A, Brady TJ. Use of complementary therapies among primary care clinic patients with arthritis. *Prev Chronic Dis.* 2004; 1:A12.
4. Ai AL, Bolling SF. The use of complementary and alternative therapies among middle-aged and older cardiac patients. *Am J Med Qual.* 2002; 17:21–27.
5. Guigoz Y. The Mini Nutritional Assessment (MNA) review of the literature – What does it tell us? *J Nutr Health Aging.* 2006;10:466–485; discussion 485–487.
6. Biesalski HK, Brummer RJ, Konig J, et al. Micronutrient deficiencies. Hohenheim Consensus Conference. *Eur J Nutr.* 2003;42:353–363.
7. Chandra RK. Nutrition and the immune system from birth to old age. *Eur J Clin Nutr.* 2002; 56 Suppl 3:S73–S76.
8. Ames BN. Low micronutrient intake may accelerate the degenerative diseases of aging through allocation of scarce micronutrients by triage. *Proc Natl Acad Sci USA.* 2006; 103:17589–17594.
9. Hu FB, Willett WC. Optimal diets for prevention of coronary heart disease. *JAMA.* 2002; 288:2569–2578.
10. Kushi LH, Byers T, Doyle C, et al. American Cancer Society Guidelines on Nutrition and Physical Activity for cancer prevention: reducing the risk of cancer with healthy food choices and physical activity. *CA Cancer J Clin.* 2006;56:254–281.
11. Van Dyk K, Sano M. The impact of nutrition on cognition in the elderly. *Neurochem Res.* 2007;32:893–904.
12. Sarkar D, Lebedeva IV, Emdad L, Kang DC, Baldwin AS Jr, Fisher PB. Human polynucleotide phosphorylase (hPNPaseold-35):

13. a potential link between aging and inflammation. *Cancer Res.* 2004;64:7473–7478.
13. Kontogianni MD, Zampelas A, Tsigos C. Nutrition and inflammatory load. *Ann NY Acad Sci.* 2006;1083:214–238.
14. National Institutes of Health State-of-the-science conference statement: multivitamin/mineral supplements and chronic disease prevention. *Ann Intern Med.* 2006;145:364–371.
15. Oakley GP Jr. Eat right and take a multivitamin. *NEJM.* 1998;338:1060–1061.
16. Ames BN, Elson-Schwab I, Silver EA. High-dose vitamin therapy stimulates variant enzymes with decreased coenzyme binding affinity (increased K(m)): relevance to genetic disease and polymorphisms. *Am J Clin Nutr.* 2002;75:616–658.
17. Olerich MA, Rude RK. Should we supplement magnesium in critically ill patients? *New Horiz.* 1994;2:186–192.
18. Ueshima K. Magnesium and ischemic heart disease: a review of epidemiological, experimental, and clinical evidences. *Magnes Res.* 2005;18:275–284.
19. Swain R, Kaplan-Machlis B. Magnesium for the next millennium. *South Med J.* 1999;92:1040–1047.
20. Yehuda S, Rabinovitz S, Mostofsky DI. Essential fatty acids and the brain: from infancy to aging. *Neurobiol Aging.* 2005; 26 Suppl 1:98–102.
21. Tiemeier H, van Tuijl HR, Hofman A, Kiliaan AJ, Breteler MM. Plasma fatty acid composition and depression are associated in the elderly: the Rotterdam Study. *Am J Clin Nutr.* 2003;78:40–46.
22. Edman JS, Horvitz E. Dietary and nutritional supplements. In: Deen D, Hark LA, eds. *The Complete Guide to Nutrition in Primary Care.* London: Wiley Publishing; 2007.
23. Holmquist C, Larsson S, Wolk A, de Faire U. Multivitamin supplements are inversely associated with risk of myocardial infarction in men and women–Stockholm Heart Epidemiology Program (SHEEP). *J Nutr.* 2003;133:2650–2654.
24. Fuchs CS, Willett WC, Colditz GA, et al. The influence of folate and multivitamin use on the familial risk of colon cancer in women. *Cancer Epidemiol Biomarkers Prev.* 2002;11:227–234.
25. Barringer TA, Kirk JK, Santaniello AC, Foley KL, Michielutte R. Effect of a multivitamin and mineral supplement on infection and quality of life. A randomized, double-blind, placebo-controlled trial. *Ann Intern Med.* 2003;138:365–371.
26. Church TS, Earnest CP, Wood KA, Kampert JB. Reduction of C-reactive protein levels through use of a multivitamin. *Am J Med.* 2003;115:702–707.
27. El-Kadiki A, Sutton AJ. Role of multivitamins and mineral supplements in preventing infections in elderly people: systematic review and meta-analysis of randomised controlled trials. *BMJ.* 2005;330:871.
28. Holub DJ, Holub BJ. Omega-3 fatty acids from fish oils and cardiovascular disease. *Mol Cell Biochem.* 2004;263:217–225.
29. Holick MF. Vitamin D: Its role in cancer prevention and treatment. *Prog Biophys Mol Biol.* 2006;92:49–59.
30. Boyle RJ, Robins-Browne RM, Tang ML. Probiotic use in clinical practice: what are the risks? *Am J Clin Nutr.* 2006;83:1256–1264; quiz 1446–1447.
31. Katz JA. Probiotics for the prevention of antibiotic-associated diarrhea and Clostridium difficile diarrhea. *J Clin Gastroenterol.* 2006;40:249–255.
32. Richy F, Bruyere O, Ethgen O, Cucherat M, Henrotin Y, Reginster JY. Structural and symptomatic efficacy of glucosamine and chondroitin in knee osteoarthritis: a comprehensive meta-analysis. *Arch Intern Med.* 2003;163:1514–1522.

33. Witte KK, Nikitin NP, Parker AC, et al. The effect of micronutrient supplementation on quality-of-life and left ventricular function in elderly patients with chronic heart failure. *Eur Heart J.* 2005;26:2238–2244.

34. Villarruz MV, Dans A, Tan F. Chelation therapy for atherosclerotic cardiovascular disease. *Cochrane Database Syst Rev.* 2002: CD002785.

35. Padayatty SJ, Riordan HD, Hewitt SM, Katz A, Hoffer LJ, Levine M. Intravenously administered vitamin C as cancer therapy: three cases. *CMAJ.* 2006;174:937–942.

36. Thomas DR, Zdrodowski CD, Wilson MM, Conright KC, Diebold M, Morley JE. A prospective, randomized clinical study of adjunctive peripheral parenteral nutrition in adult subacute care patients. *J Nutr Health Aging.* 2005;9:321–325.

37. Buck AC. Is there a scientific basis for the therapeutic effects of Serenoa repens in benign prostatic hyperplasia? Mechanisms of action. *J Urol.* 2004;172:1792–1799.

38. Izzo AA. Drug interactions with St. John's Wort (Hypericum perforatum): a review of the clinical evidence. *Int J Clin Pharmacol Ther.* 2004;42:139–148.

39. DerMarderosian A, Briggs M. Supplements and herbs. In: Mackenzie ER, Rakel B, eds. *Complementary and Alternative Medicine for Older Adults: A Guide to Holistic Approaches to Healthy Aging.* New York: Springer; 2006:31–78.

40. Bell IR, Lewis DA 2nd, Brooks AJ, et al. Improved clinical status in fibromyalgia patients treated with individualized homeopathic remedies versus placebo. *Rheumatology.* 2004;43:577–582.

41. Brinkhaus B, Wilkens JM, Ludtke R, Hunger J, Witt CM, Willich SN. Homeopathic arnica therapy in patients receiving knee surgery: results of three randomised double-blind trials. *Complement Ther Med.* 2006;14:237–246.

42. Haidvogl M, Riley DS, Heger M, et al. Homeopathic and conventional treatment for acute respiratory and ear complaints: a comparative study on outcome in the primary care setting. *BMC Complement Altern Med.* 2007;7:7.

43. Riedlinger J, Lennihan B. Homeopathic medicine. In: *Handbook of Non-Prescription Drugs.* Washington, DC: American Pharmacists Association; 2002.

44. Wolf SL, Barnhart HX, Kutner NG, McNeely E, Coogler C, Xu T. Reducing frailty and falls in older persons: an investigation of Tai Chi and computerized balance training. Atlanta FICSIT Group. Frailty and Injuries: Cooperative Studies of Intervention Techniques. *J Am Geriatr Soc.* 1996;44:489–497.

45. Wolf SL, Sattin RW, Kutner M, O'Grady M, Greenspan AI, Gregor RJ. Intense tai chi exercise training and fall occurrences in older, transitionally frail adults: a randomized, controlled trial. *J Am Geriatr Soc.* 2003;51:1693–1701.

46. Ryu H, Lee HS, Shin YS, et al. Acute effect of qigong training on stress hormonal levels in man. *Am J Chin Med.* 1996;24:193–198.

47. Berman BM, Lao L, Langenberg P, Lee WL, Gilpin AM, Hochberg MC. Effectiveness of acupuncture as adjunctive therapy in osteoarthritis of the knee: a randomized, controlled trial. *Ann Intern Med.* 2004;141:901–910.

48. Witt CM, Jena S, Brinkhaus B, Liecker B, Wegscheider K, Willich SN. Acupuncture in patients with osteoarthritis of the knee or hip: a randomized, controlled trial with an additional nonrandomized arm. *Arthritis Rheum.* 2006;54:3485–3493.

49. White A, Foster NE, Cummings M, Barlas P. Acupuncture treatment for chronic knee pain: a systematic review. *Rheumatology.* 2007;46:384–390.

50. Hsieh RL, Wang LY, Lee WC. Additional therapeutic effects of electroacupuncture in conjunction with conventional rehabilitation for patients with first-ever ischaemic stroke. *J Rehabil Med.* 2007;39:205–211.

51. Vickers AJ, Rees RW, Zollman CE, et al. Acupuncture of chronic headache disorders in primary care: randomised controlled trial and economic analysis. *Health Technol Assess.* 2004;8:1–35.

52. Melchart D, Weidenhammer W, Streng A, Hoppe A, Pfaffenrath V, Linde K. Acupuncture for chronic headaches–an epidemiological study. *Headache.* 2006;46:632–641.

53. Trinh KV, Phillips SD, Ho E, Damsma K. Acupuncture for the alleviation of lateral epicondyle pain: a systematic review. *Rheumatology.* 2004;43:1085–1090.

54. Martin DP, Sletten CD, Williams BA, Berger IH. Improvement in fibromyalgia symptoms with acupuncture: results of a randomized controlled trial. *Mayo Clin Proc.* 2006;81:749–757.

55. Audette JF, Blinder RA. Acupuncture in the management of myofascial pain and headache. *Curr Pain Headache Rep.* 2003;7:395–401.

56. Weidenhammer W, Linde K, Streng A, Hoppe A, Melchart D. Acupuncture for chronic low back pain in routine care: a multicenter observational study. *Clin J Pain.* 2007;23:128–135.

57. Napadow V, Kettner N, Liu J, et al. Hypothalamus and amygdala response to acupuncture stimuli in carpal tunnel syndrome. *Pain.* 2007. 130(3):254–266.

58. Han JS. Acupuncture and endorphins. *Neurosci Lett.* 2004; 361:258–261.

59. Ulett GA, Han S, Han JS. Electroacupuncture: mechanisms and clinical application. *Biol Psychiatry.* 1998;44:129–138.

60. Wu MT, Hsieh JC, Xiong J, et al. Central nervous pathway for acupuncture stimulation: localization of processing with functional MR imaging of the brain – preliminary experience. *Radiology.* 1999;212:133–141.

61. Carlsson CP, Sjolund BH. Acupuncture for chronic low back pain: a randomized placebo-controlled study with long-term follow-up. *Clin J Pain.* 2001;17:296–305.

62. White A, Hayhoe S, Hart A, Ernst E. Survey of adverse events following acupuncture (SAFA): a prospective study of 32,000 consultations. *Acupunct Med.* 2001;19:84–92.

63. Lesho EP. An overview of osteopathic medicine. *Arch Fam Med.* 1999;8:477–484.

64. Andersson GB, Lucente T, Davis AM, Kappler RE, Lipton JA, Leurgans S. A comparison of osteopathic spinal manipulation with standard care for patients with low back pain. *NEJM.* 1999; 341:1426–1431.

65. Licciardone JC, Brimhall AK, King LN. Osteopathic manipulative treatment for low back pain: a systematic review and meta-analysis of randomized controlled trials. *BMC Musculoskelet Disord.* 2005;6:43.

66. Wells MR, Giantinoto S, D'Agate D, et al. Standard osteopathic manipulative treatment acutely improves gait performance in patients with Parkinson's disease. *J Am Osteopath Assoc.* 1999;99:92–98.

67. Nicholas AS, DeBias DA, Ehrenfeuchter W, et al. A somatic component to myocardial infarction. *BMJ.* (Clin Res Ed) 1985;291:13–17.

68. Johnston WL, Kelso AF. Changes in presence of a segmental dysfunction pattern associated with hypertension: Part 2. A long-term longitudinal study. *J Am Osteopath Assoc.* 1995;95:315–318.

69. Yates HA, Vardy TC, Kuchera ML, Ripley BD, Johnson JC. Effects of osteopathic manipulative treatment and concentric and eccentric maximal-effort exercise on women with multiple sclerosis: a pilot study. *J Am Osteopath Assoc.* 2002;102:267–275.

70. Bronfort G, Haas M, Evans RL, Bouter LM. Efficacy of spinal manipulation and mobilization for low back pain and neck pain: a systematic review and best evidence synthesis. *Spine J.* 2004;4:335–356.

71. Aure OF, Nilsen JH, Vasseljen O. Manual therapy and exercise therapy in patients with chronic low back pain: a randomized, controlled trial with 1-year follow-up. *Spine.* 2003;28:525–531, discussion 531–532.

72. Evans R, Bronfort G, Nelson B, Goldsmith CH. Two-year follow-up of a randomized clinical trial of spinal manipulation and two types of exercise for patients with chronic neck pain. *Spine.* 2002;27:2383–2389.

73. Cherkin DC, Sherman KJ, Deyo RA, Shekelle PG. A review of the evidence for the effectiveness, safety, and cost of acupuncture, massage therapy, and spinal manipulation for back pain. *Ann Intern Med.* 2003;138:898–906.

74. Field T. Massage therapy. *Med Clin North Am.* 2002;86:163–171.

75. Field T, Hernandez-Reif M, Diego M, Schanberg S, Kuhn C. Cortisol decreases and serotonin and dopamine increase following massage therapy. *Int J Neurosci.* 2005;115:1397–1413.

76. Kennedy E, Chapman C. Massage therapy and older adults. In: Mackenzie ER, Rakel B, eds. *Complementary and Alternative Medicine for Older Adults: A guide to holistic approaches to Aging.* New York: Springer; 2002:135–148.

77. Furlan AD, Brosseau L, Imamura M, Irvin E. Massage for low-back pain: a systematic review within the framework of the Cochrane Collaboration Back Review Group. *Spine.* 2002; 27:1896–1910.

78. Tan JC. Massage as a form of complementary and alternative healing modality for physical manipulation. In: Wainapel SF, Fast A, eds. *Alternative Medicine and Rehabilitation: A Guide for Practitioners.* New York: Demos Medical Publishing; 2003:90–91.

79. Garfinkel M, Schumacher HR Jr. Yoga. *Rheum Dis Clin North Am.* 2000;26:125–132, x.

80. Kamei T, Toriumi Y, Kimura H, Ohno S, Kumano H, Kimura K. Decrease in serum cortisol during yoga exercise is correlated with alpha wave activation. *Percept Mot Skills.* 2000;90:1027–1032.

81. Fishman L. Yoga in medicine. In: Wainapel SF, Fast A, eds. *Alternative Medicine and Rehabilitation: A Guide for Practitioners.* New York: Demos Medical Publishing; 2003:151–158.

82. Kabat-Zinn J, Lipworth L, Burney R. The clinical use of mindfulness meditation for the self-regulation of chronic pain. *J Behav Med.* 1985;8:163–190.

83. Aftanas LI, Golocheikine SA. Human anterior and frontal midline theta and lower alpha reflect emotionally positive state and internalized attention: high-resolution EEG investigation of meditation. *Neurosci Lett.* 2001;310:57–60.

84. Kjaer TW, Bertelsen C, Piccini P, Brooks D, Alving J, Lou HC. Increased dopamine tone during meditation-induced change of consciousness. *Brain Res Cogn Brain Res.* 2002;13:255–259.

85. Davidson RJ, Kabat-Zinn J, Schumacher J, et al. Alterations in brain and immune function produced by mindfulness meditation. *Psychosom Med.* 2003;65:564–570.

86. Wu WH, Bandilla E, Ciccone DS, et al. Effects of qigong on late-stage complex regional pain syndrome. *Altern Ther Health Med.* 1999;5:45–54.

87. Taggart HM, Arslanian CL, Bae S, Singh K. Effects of T'ai Chi exercise on fibromyalgia symptoms and health-related quality of life. *Orthop Nurs.* 2003;22:353–360.

88. Creamer P, Singh BB, Hochberg MC, Berman BM. Sustained improvement produced by nonpharmacologic intervention in fibromyalgia: results of a pilot study. *Arthritis Care Res.* 2000;13:198–204.

89. Malmgren-Olsson EB, Branholm IB. A comparison between three physiotherapy approaches with regard to health-related factors in patients with non-specific musculoskeletal disorders. *Disabil Rehabil.* 2002;24:308–317.

90. Johnson SK, Frederick J, Kaufman M, Mountjoy B. A controlled investigation of bodywork in multiple sclerosis. *J Altern Complement Med.* 1999;5:237–243.

91. Huntley A, Ernst E. Complementary and alternative therapies for treating multiple sclerosis symptoms: a systematic review. *Complement Ther Med.* 2000;8:97–105.

92. Lundblad I, Elert J, Gerdle B. Randomized controlled trial of physiotherapy and Feldenkrais interventions in female workers with neck-shoulder complaints. *Jocc Rehabil.* 1999;9:179–194.

93. Batson G, Deutsch JE. Effects of Feldenkrais awareness through movement on balance in adults with chronic neurological deficits following stroke: a preliminary study. *Complement Health Practice Rev.* 2005;10:203–210.

94. Ernst E, Canter PH. The Alexander technique: a systematic review of controlled clinical trials. *Forsch Komplementarmed Klass Naturheilkd.* 2003;10:325–329.

95. Elkayam O, Ben Itzhak S, Avrahami E, et al. Multidisciplinary approach to chronic back pain: prognostic elements of the outcome. *Clin Exp Rheumatol.* 1996;14:281–288.

96. Stallibrass C, Sissons P, Chalmers C. Randomized controlled trial of the Alexander technique for idiopathic Parkinson's disease. *Clin Rehabil.* 2002;16:695–708.

97. Dennis RJ. Functional reach improvement in normal older women after Alexander Technique instruction. *J Gerontol A Biol Sci Med Sci.* 1999;54:M8–M11.

98. Austin JH, Ausubel P. Enhanced respiratory muscular function in normal adults after lessons in proprioceptive musculoskeletal education without exercises. *Chest.* 1992;102:486–490.

99. Dyson-Hudson TA, Shiflett SC, Kirshblum SC, Bowen JE, Druin EL. Acupuncture and Trager psychophysical integration in the treatment of wheelchair user's shoulder pain in individuals with spinal cord injury. *Arch Phys Med Rehabil.* 2001;82:1038–1046.

100. Foster KA, Liskin J, Cen S, et al. The Trager approach in the treatment of chronic headache: a pilot study. *Altern Ther Health Med.* 2004;10:40–6.

101. Treede RD, Kenshalo DR, Gracely RH, Jones AK. The cortical representation of pain. *Pain.* 1999;79:105–111.

102. Morone NE, Greco CM, Weiner DK. Mindfulness meditation for the treatment of chronic low back pain in older adults: a randomized controlled pilot study. *Pain.* 2007;134(3):310–319.

103. Jensen IB, Bergstrom G, Ljungquist T, Bodin L. A 3-year follow-up of a multidisciplinary rehabilitation programme for back and neck pain. *Pain.* 2005;115:273–283.

104. Carson JW, Keefe FJ, Lynch TR, et al. Loving-kindness meditation for chronic low back pain: results from a pilot trial. *J Holist Nurs.* 2005;23:287–304.

105. Astin JA. Mind-body therapies for the management of pain. *Clin J Pain.* 2004;20:27–32.

106. Arena JG, Hannah SL, Bruno GM, Meador KJ. Electromyographic biofeedback training for tension headache in the elderly: a prospective study. *Biofeedback Self Regul.* 1991; 16:379–390.

107. Mackay N, Hansen S, McFarlane O. Autonomic nervous system changes during Reiki treatment: a preliminary study. *J Altern Complement Med.* 2004;10:1077–1081.

108. Hulme J, Robinson V, DeBie R, Wells G, Judd M, Tugwell P. Electromagnetic fields for the treatment of osteoarthritis. *Cochrane Database Syst Rev.* 2002:CD003523.

109. Sutbeyaz ST, Sezer N, Koseoglu BF. The effect of pulsed electromagnetic fields in the treatment of cervical osteoarthritis: a randomized, double-blind, sham-controlled trial. *Rheumatol Int.* 2006;26:320–324.

110. Shupak NM, McKay JC, Nielson WR, Rollman GB, Prato FS, Thomas AW. Exposure to a specific pulsed low-frequency magnetic field: a double-blind placebo-controlled study of effects on pain ratings in rheumatoid arthritis and fibromyalgia patients. *Pain Res Manage.* 2006;11:85–90.

111. Thuile C, Walzl M. Evaluation of electromagnetic fields in the treatment of pain in patients with lumbar radiculopathy or the whiplash syndrome. *NeuroRehabilitation.* 2002;17:63–67.

112. Kabat-Zinn J. *Full Catastrophe Living: Using the Wisdom of Your Body and Mind to Face Stress, Pain and Illness.* New York: Dell Publishing; 1990:467.

113. Reibel DK, Greeson JM, Brainard GC, Rosenzweig S. Mindfulness-based stress reduction and health-related quality of life in a heterogeneous patient population. *Gen Hosp Psychiatry.* 2001;23:183–192.

114. Plews-Ogan M, Owens JE, Goodman M, Wolfe P, Schorling J. A pilot study evaluating mindfulness-based stress reduction and massage for the management of chronic pain. *J Gen Intern Med.* 2005;20:1136–1138.

115. Kreitzer MJ, Gross CR, Ye X, Russas V, Treesak C. Longitudinal impact of mindfulness meditation on illness burden in solid-organ transplant recipients. *Prog Transplant.* 2005;15:166–172.

116. Carlson LE, Garland SN. Impact of mindfulness-based stress reduction (MBSR) on sleep, mood, stress and fatigue symptoms in cancer outpatients. *Int J Behav Med.* 2005;12:278–285.

117. Carmody J, Crawford S, Churchill L. A pilot study of mindfulness-based stress reduction for hot flashes. *Menopause.* 2006;13:760–769.

118. Vaillant GE, Mukamal K. Successful aging. *Am J Psychiatry.* 2001;158:839–847.

119. Park CL. Religiousness/spirituality and health: a meaning systems perspective. *J Behav Med.* 2007;30(4):319–328.

120. Jantos M, Kiat H. Prayer as medicine: how much have we learned? *Med J Aust.* 2007;186:S51–S53.

121. Remen RN. Kitchen Table Wisdom. New York: The Berkley Publishing Group; 1996.

50

SUCCESSFUL AGING: OPTIMIZING STRATEGIES FOR PRIMARY CARE GERIATRICS

Thomas L. Edmondson, MD, CMD, AGSF, William Dean Charmak, PhD

INTRODUCTION

Since publication of the article *Geriatrics* by I. L. Nascher, M.D., almost a century ago in *The New York Medical Journal*, the field continues to evolve in its view of the concept of aging.[1] In 1909, Dr. Nascher coined the word geriatrics from the Greek words *geras*, old age, and *iatrikos*, relating to the physician. The field of geriatrics has since explored aging, successful aging, healthy aging, productive aging, usual aging, homeostenosis (the depletion of physiological reserves resulting from aging), frailty, and senescence. For the purposes of this chapter, we will use the word 'successful' interchangeably with optimal and healthy. As individuals age, how can the process of aging occur in a manner viewed as successful or healthy continues to be a topic of interest to individuals and cultures alike. The concept of successful aging implies that some age successfully whereas others do not. How one defines successful aging varies greatly by person, physician, and researcher. As Thomas Glass notes, we know little about how older people define successful aging and what they value in the quality of their life and death.[2] Review of the literature on successful aging reveals no clear consensus as to the definition of successful aging. Although different types of aging are denoted, one finds all three descriptors used widely in the literature to represent similar ideas. Now 100 years after Dr. Nascher wrote his article, geriatricians researching this topic typically present a philosophical discussion about the interplay of aging, disease, pathology, and senescence. When changes in function or a characteristic/variable are noted, do the changes represent the passage of time, "wear and tear," disease due to either lifestyle or genetics or both, or rather homeostenosis and/or senescence? Thus, when reviewing the literature on successful aging, which adjective is most appropriate to describe the aging process depends much on the models' underlying premises regarding the methods applied to examine the aforementioned changes.

To date, there is a lack of consensus on the required components of successful aging. Proposed models include the following approaches: biomedical, psychosocial, cognitive, and multicriteria models.[3] Also lacking consensus, is whether successful aging should be defined objectively by others or subjectively by elders themselves and about which components are necessary and/or sufficient.[3,4] The most frequently discussed model is promulgated by Rowe and Kahn, in which they describe successful aging as involving freedom from disability along with high cognitive, physical, and social function;[5] this model identifies successful agers objectively.[3] Other definitions examine the degree to which elderly individuals adapt to age-associated changes, view themselves as successfully aging, or avoid morbidity until the latest time point before death.[4,6–9]

The aforementioned models may not be helpful to a clinician whose patients' health status improves or declines over time, and research is lacking to help address the other following practical issues. Should successful aging be defined arbitrarily as those individuals with attributes measured within the upper tertile or even quintile of the variable of interest? At what age does one become a candidate to be thought of as aging or even aging successfully? Can a senior citizen be judged in one model as aging successfully but not by the criteria of another model? Over time, if judged to be an unsuccessful ager, can one change to then later be categorized as a successful ager? Or, can a successful ager subsequently lose the characteristics that made her successful? Can a person aging successfully free of morbidity in his 20s suffer the accidental loss of a limb and later have the required characteristics to be judged as a successful ager if he reaches age 95, or was the individual eliminated from the possibility of aging successfully due to the accidental loss of a limb? Last, should a highly educated person (such as a physician) in his 30s with hypertension and obesity be viewed as not aging successfully? This chapter will explore definitions, the prevailing models of optimal aging, and suggest strategies for primary care geriatrics practice.

DEFINITIONS

What is successful aging? To date, there is no consensus on what constitutes 'successful' aging and a definition likely entails more factors than the minimization or avoidance of frailty. In a comprehensive review of larger quantitative studies regarding definitions of successful aging, Depp and Jeste identified 28 studies with 29 different definitions.[4] The mean reported proportion of successful agers was 35.8%. Twenty-six of 29 definitions included disability and/or physical function usually measured by self-reported activities of daily living and less often by instrumental activities of daily living and objective performance. They note that the most frequent significant correlates of the various definitions of successful aging were age (young-old), nonsmoking, and absence of disability, arthritis, and diabetes. Moderate support was found for greater physical activity, more social contacts, better self-rated health, absence of depression and cognitive impairment, and fewer medical conditions. Gender, income, education and marital status generally did not relate to successful aging in this review. Depp and Jeste note that the majority of definitions were based on the absence of disability with lesser inclusion of psychosocial variables. In the next section, we will examine in more detail biological models and models that use psychosocial, cognitive, or multiple criteria in defining successful aging.

The biological model of successful aging is based on two main concepts: longevity and the compression of morbidity. Data on the oldest old are difficult to validate and vary based on the database and criteria used to substantiate age. The oldest individual ever confirmed and recorded was Jeanne Calment, who died at the age of 122 years.[10] Data on the numbers of supercentenarians (people aged 110 and older) are noted in a paper by Schoenhofen et al. in which the number of supercentenarians living in the United States is estimated by the Gerontology Research Group to be approximately 60–70 and worldwide, approximately 250–300.[10] The determinants of maximum lifespan are thought to be partially from genetic factors although environmental, attitudinal, or lifestyle factors have not been excluded as playing roles.[3]

The concept of compression of morbidity may be described as avoidance of morbidity until the latest time point before death. A useful measurement may be the index of health expectancy at birth. In 2000, the World Health Organization created an index of health expectancy at birth, which calculates the number of years an individual is expected to live without major disease.[3] In the United States, the average healthy active life expectancy in 2000 was 67 years of age for males and 71 years of age for females. Data since 1982 show a decline of approximately 2% per year in disability trends in contrast with a decline in mortality rates of approximately 1% per year, thereby documenting compression of morbidity in the United States at the population level.[11] Fries notes that persons with few behavioral health risks have only one-quarter the disability of those who have more risk factors, and the onset of disability is postponed from 7 to 12 years. He also notes that randomized, controlled trials of health enhancement programs in elderly populations show reduction in health risks, improved health status, and decreased medical care utilization.[11]

A recent study of supercentenarians supports the finding that the incidence of disease peaks and then declines. In a descriptive study of 32 supercentenarians, data showed that only 41% required minimal assistance or were independent and that they markedly delayed and even escaped clinical expression of vascular disease toward the end of their lives.[10] In this study, rates of vascular-related disease were relatively rare: myocardial infarction, 6%; stroke, 13%; and hypertension, 22%.

In a study by Karlamangla et al. using data from the MacArthur Successful Aging cohort of high-functioning adults aged 70–79, the researchers developed a scoring system based on continuous values of risk factors to measure the total dysregulation across multiple physiological systems.[12] The internal physiological milieu adapts to environmental demands, a phenomenon referred to as allostasis. When adaptation efforts are excessive, the body gradually loses the ability to maintain system parameters within normal operating ranges. Frequent or chronic arousal has been associated with ultimate dysregulation of major physiological systems, including the hypothalamic-pituitary-adrenal axis, the sympathetic nervous system, and the immune system.[12] Allostatic load is the total accumulation of such dysregulation across physiological systems and was hypothesized to mediate the effects of stress on health risks. Ten biological markers were used to create allostatic load scores for the cohort followed over 7 years. Results showed that compared with participants whose allostatic load score decreased between 1988 and 1991, individuals whose allostatic load score increased had higher all-cause mortality between 1991 and 1995 (15% versus 5%). Karlamangla et al. conclude that even in older ages, risk factor changes are associated with mortality risk and that risk assessment can be enhanced by following changes in composite risk scores such as allostatic load.

Psychosocial models of successful aging feature social interaction, life satisfaction, and well-being as major determinants of successful aging.[3] Lower mortality risks and better mental and physical health outcomes are associated with older adults who report a greater number of social ties, social integration, and social support. Social integration and support are also linked to protection against physical and mental health conditions such as cardiovascular diseases, hypertension and depression, each of which is related to cognitive decline.[3] Moreover, two studies have found social engagement and greater reported social networking to be protective against cognitive impairment and the onset of dementia, respectively.[13,14]

Personality traits early in life have been shown to be potent predictors of psychological well-being.[3,15] McCrae found that positive affect was associated with extraversion and high well-being, whereas negative affect was associated with neuroticism and low levels of well-being. These results suggest that well-being, as a marker of successful aging, might be highly dependent on certain personality traits, which develop very early in life. Lupien and Wan note that this supports the idea that the pathways to successful aging are determined very early in life.[3]

Cognitive models of successful aging are based on the measurement of individuals' performance in comparison with other groups. Using this methodology, a given individual could be defined as a successful ager by using one type of comparison, and as a normal or pathological ager by using another type of comparison.[3] Bias also exists due to older individuals who volunteer for a study are generally more educated, have a higher income, and are in better physical shape than those who do not readily volunteer.[3] An inherent problem using comparison with the mean of an aged population is that some view this as leading to an elitist definition of successful aging.[3] As cognitive function is positively related to education level, it is highly likely that those defined as successful agers will be those who were successful during their entire life (high education and high income).

Each of these models helps to further delineate components of what may be described as successful aging; yet each model fails to account for the other models' components and strengths. Development of more comprehensive models has been promulgated by two recent approaches. The first model by Rowe and Kahn provides for an objective identification of individuals who have high cognitive, physical, and social function.[16] Two critiques of this model cite potential bias in the study population and over-reliance on objective measurements. The second model proposed by Baltes and Baltes in 1990 views successful aging as a process of continuous adaptation to late-life changes.[2,3]

Rowe and Kahn's paper on usual and successful aging described three components of successful aging: avoidance of disease and disability, maintenance of cognitive capacity, and active engagement.[16] In the MacArthur Studies of Successful Aging, successful aging was defined as performance in the top third of functional ability in both physical and cognitive function. Significant results included elevated baseline plasma level of interleukin-6 as a significant predictor of cognitive decline 2.5 years later; certain measures of learning, memory, and low emotional support at baseline were strong predictors of cognitive decline measured 7 years later. Additionally, a low number of social ties at the time of entry into the study predicted cognitive decline 7 years later.[3]

To be categorized as a successful ager, this model recognizes heterogeneity in aging among a cohort and deems those successful who were measured to be in the top 30% of the population in terms of cognitive factors. Because education level and socioeconomic income are positively related to cognitive function, choosing to define a successful ager as one in the top 30% of cognitive function reflects those individuals who were successful during their entire life. As such, Lupien and Wan question the usefulness of generalizing the findings from the MacArthur studies to the general population.[3] A second critique is a lack of inclusion of self-rated reports on successful aging and well-being. In one study of participants aged 65–99 years, the percentage of those rating themselves as aging successfully was 50.3% compared with 18.8% classified according to Rowe and Kahn's criteria.[17] Many participants with chronic conditions and with functional difficulties still rated themselves as aging successfully whereas none were so classified according to Rowe and Kahn's criteria.

The second model using multiple criteria also accounts for heterogeneity of the aging process by defining successful aging as a process of continuous adaptation.[3] In Baltes and Baltes' model of selective optimization with compensation (SOC), they describe a strategy of successful aging designed to serve as a guideline for an individual's thoughts and actions and for social policy.[2,18] The model emphasizes the need to maintain a sense of control over one's environment in the face of the dynamic interplay between gains and losses in late life[2] and explains how individuals make adaptations when faced with changes brought about by the aging process.[3]

The first element, selection, refers to the conscious restriction of the range of functional activities in response to age-related losses of capacity and reserve. Selection implies that individuals adjust their expectations to allow the subjective experience of satisfaction and personal control.[3,18] The second, optimization, is the strategy of engaging in actions and behaviors that enhance or augment remaining strengths and capacities. People engage in behaviors that assist them in reaching higher and more desirable levels of functioning to achieve their individual goals in the face of simultaneous losses.[3] The third element, compensation, involves the use of psychological strategies or compensatory technology to replace lost functional abilities.[2] The process of compensation occurs when an individual's behavioral capacities are lost or reduced below a level necessary for adequate functioning. Compensatory strategies include the use of mnemonic devices when internal memory strategies are inadequate[3,18] or compensatory technology such as hearing aids to replace lost functional abilities.[2]

Two critiques of this model are a lack of inclusion of biological or cognitive criteria and the reliance on the individual as the source of successful aging.[3] As Lupien and Wan point out, the Israeli Kibbutz communities have shown the impact of social arrangements and social support as strong predictors of successful aging. When faced with structural changes, the Kibbutz' society adapts to the needs of its members, which in turn leads them to age successfully. This is in contrast to the SOC models' theory that successful aging is the successful adaptation of the individual to changes during the course of aging.[3] Although the SOC model may have these weaknesses, the model has been found to predict several measures of well-being independent of other predictors of successful aging as found in the Berlin Aging Study.[19]

PSYCHOSOCIAL CONSIDERATIONS AND SUCCESSFUL AGING

Western culture's paradoxical model of successful aging continually encourages the population older than 40 to deter what is perceived as inevitable decline. The ever-blurring boundary between media and medicine, synergistically and continually perpetrates the manifest message that healthy living is achieved by placing a moratorium on aging. Deterring the effects of aging has long become synonymous with avoiding the life crises of demise of physical well-being, the loss of and reduced ability to accrue income, access to myriad opportunities afforded to the young to include beginning new endeavors and finding a life partner. It is this latter premise of loneliness and isolation that most of the aging populous fears.

In many respects, societal thinking continues to value youth over age, while youth becomes equated with beauty and beauty with goodness.[20] Generally, these factors are considered crises by health providers who in turn seek to ameliorate suffering, which accompanies the loss of physical and at times mental prowess. This pathologized view of the aging process has prompted many to engage in prevarication about their age, deny associations with past events (revealing one's age), and deny that one is one's chronological age. Approbation for looking or behaving younger than one's stated age is coveted especially when such compliments in American culture are paid not on the basis that one has successfully made it to a given age, but defied the very process itself.

The Western concept of aging follows a curvilinear format; the rewards of maturity, which may include access and privilege, peak and inevitably decline. Loss by its very definition describes a state of impermanence and struggle. Kubler-Ross, whose model of grief and loss describes its passages, avers that in its final stage, acceptance is not synonymous with happiness but simply an ability to coexist with what once was. Loss, too, is synonymous with oppression; relegation to a social and/or distinct class who by its devalued status is forced into an encapsulated existence by the holders of privilege.[21] Goldenberg aptly denotes that "the process of accommodating oneself to a life essentially devoid of possibilities is not easy. It is not simple to learn to accept one's impotence in a world supposedly replete with surging energy and ever-increasing mastery."[22] He postulates that reattainment of access is modeled via traversing the narrow tube of an hourglass, separating the holders of privilege from those who lost or never had it. Cultural cognizance of the disenfranchisement, which accompanies age, calls clinicians to advocate against this process as well as secure the privileges that should not be lost with age. Obviously, decline in physical and mental abilities concomitant with age may signify an end to occupational capability, independent living, and athletic activity. Yet, the pronounced proclivity to equate these changes with growing older has become biased and automatic. It is just as critical to point out the spurious notion that the aforementioned age curve is necessarily reflective of later stage human development.

Creativity as a variable is less related to age than time spent in occupation.[23] The plethora of research, which supports ultimate decline after attaining some defined pinnacle of achievement, is predicated on biased research. Friedan continues to point out that when creativity is plotted along *individual* life curves, the predicted declines are inconsequential.

Undoubtedly, successful aging is associated with good health, longevity, and life satisfaction.[24] The lack of operational terms in this definition, however, easily lends itself to misinterpretation, even by well-meaning clinicians. As with the preponderance of tomes outlining recommended or good palliative care, the medical community is again led to a potentially biased understanding of what the elderly need or desire. Experienced clinicians understand that their patients can increase internal locus of control (self-efficacy) by taking an active role in both their care and treatment.

It is logical to assume that the process of choosing to participate in an activity is, in itself, both empowering and control enhancing (given that the decision to risk involvement is made through an individual's own volition).[25] Many health providers are tempted to assume that rote, prescriptive approaches should improve both quality and outlook on life for the aging patient. It has been demonstrated on countless occasions that the most effective understanding of behavior is ultimately gained from the internal frame of reference of the individual himself.[26]

Most important, the equation of aging with death must be handled with utmost objectivity. As Viorst astutely observes, although the fear of death may not be universal, it is nonetheless a thought, which many of us cannot abide – especially when one perceives that loneliness and isolation precede death.[27] Clark also succinctly describes the dying process as going alone and/or the dread of parting.[28] We therefore eschew the idea of death, avoid painful consequences typically associated with loss, and inanely resist its inevitability.

A paucity of medical training programs address death as a topic of study, almost suggesting that the developmental process of old age perseverates along an imaginary continuum, or gradually dissolves into nonexistence. Although death is a consequence of age, it need not be the reward for painful decline. To the disbelief of many scholars and practitioners, in 1970, gerontologist Bernice Neugarten postulated that anticipated life events (crises) include menopause, retirement from work, and loss of a spouse, lacked the distressing qualities thought to be associated with these developmental hallmarks.[29] That is, the acceptance of these passages as expected occurrences made them acceptable as life events. Perhaps then, it can be postulated that practitioners may at times be culpable of unwittingly projecting their own uncertainties of death onto the patient: it is well known that health care professionals frequently avoid working with the terminally ill as they fear that bonding with patients will heighten their own experiences of loss.[30]

Clearly, the perception of aging both as cultural and intrinsic processes demands reconceptualization not from the standpoint of biased professionals but from the geriatric population itself. Continuance and resonance of the myth of age as decline is not what the aged are promulgating. Friedan via her own experience found aging near the end of her own life to be likened with adventure along with the realization that exploration of a new agenda is merely heightened by wisdom acquired through life experience.[23] It is one intent of this chapter to promote dissolution of the culturally promulgated myth, which views youth as Mecca.

STRATEGIES FOR PRIMARY CARE

Patients, physicians, and geriatricians all would like to understand and implement strategies that would lead to optimal aging, and the literature may, or may not depending on one's understanding of successful aging, point toward useful strategies. Findings from research on successful aging have yet to be translated into evidenced-based, practical strategies for clinicians. Although the definition of successful aging is still controversial, the various models of successful aging fail to synthesize the strengths of other models and fail to overcome the disadvantages inherent to that model's assumptions. Furthermore, research is lacking on older individuals' values and understanding of what it means to age successfully.[2] Until studies are completed, clinicians may best optimize strategies for their patients based on individualized interviews and assessments of their patients' values, goals, and skills. Indeed, primary care providers may choose to refer to different models of successful aging for different patients depending on the individual patients' values, belief system and physical, mental, and biopsychosocial health. Whereas one model of optimal aging may be applicable for one patient, that same version of successful aging may not be generalizable to all patients.

Research in both the biological and psychological models is beginning to yield some promising results, however. Data obtained from the Atherosclerosis Risk in Communities Study show that newly adopting a healthy lifestyle (as defined by a diet of at least five daily servings of fruits and vegetables, exercise, maintaining a healthy weight, and not smoking) results in a substantial reduction in all-cause mortality and cardiovascular disease events, 40% and 35% respectively, over the subsequent 4 years.[31] Of the two age groups studied, the older group aged 55–64 was statistically significantly more likely to adopt a healthy lifestyle than those aged 45–54.

Research on the perception of age and aging stereotypes has shown that well-being and a positive view of aging are major protective factors against the effects of age.[3] In a study on the effects of negative and positive attitudes toward aging, introducing positive views of aging reduced cardiovascular stress in the sample being studied.[32] In an observational study, those who expressed a more positive self-perception of aging compared with those holding more negative perceptions had a 7.5-year mean survival advantage.[3,33] Regarding memory performance, older adults exposed to negative age stereotypes tend to worsen their memory performance, self-efficacy, and judgments of other elderly people.[3,34] In earlier work, older adults

who perceived their age as younger than others of the same age had more internal control, which has been related to more positive functioning and enhanced life satisfaction.[3,35] Positive attitudes toward aging have been shown to have positive influences on memory performance, longevity, health, well-being, life satisfaction, will to live, and other physiological and psychological function.[3]

REFERENCES

1. Nascher IL. Geriatrics. *NY Med J.* 1909;358–359.
2. Glass, TA. Assessing the success of successful aging. *Ann Intern Med.* 2003;139:382–383.
3. Lupien SJ, Wan N. Successful ageing: from cell to self. *Phil Trans R Soc Lond B.* 2004;359:1413–1426.
4. Depp CA, Jeste DV. Definitions and predictors of successful aging: a comprehensive review of larger quantitative studies. *Am J Geriatr Psychiatry.* 2006;14:6–20.
5. Rowe JW, Kahn RL. Human aging: usual and successful. *Science.* 1987;237:143–149.
6. Baltes PB. On the incomplete architecture of human ontogeny. *Am Psychol.* 1997;52:366–380.
7. Schulz R, Heckhausen J. A life span model of successful aging. *Am Psychol.* 1996;51:702–714.
8. von Faberm, Bootsma-van der Wiel A, Van Excel D, et al. Successful aging in the oldest old: who can be characterized as successfully aged? *Arch Intern Med.* 2001;161:2694–2700.
9. Fries JF. Successful aging – an emerging paradigm of gerontology. *Clin Geriatr Med.* 2002;18:371–382.
10. Schoenhofen EA, Wyszynski DF, Andersen S, et al. Characteristics of 32 supercentenarians. *J Am Geriatr Soc.* 2006;54:1237–1240.
11. Fries JF. Measuring and Monitoring Success in Compressing Morbidity. *Ann Intern Med.* 2003;139:455–459.
12. Karlamangla AS, Singer BH, Seeman TE. Reduction in allostatic load in older adults is associated with lower all-cause mortality risk: MacArthur Studies of Successful Aging. *Psychosom Med.* 2006;68:500–507.
13. Bassuk SS, Glass TA, Berkman LF. Social disengagement and incident cognitive decline in community-dwelling elderly persons. *Ann Intern Med.* 1999;131:165–173
14. Fratiglioni L, Wang HX, Ericsoon K, Maytan M, Winblad B. Influence of social network on occurrence of dementia: a community-based longitudinal study. *Lancet.* 2000;355:1315–1319.
15. McCrae RR. The maturation of personality psychology: adult personality development and psychological well-being. *J Res Personal.* 2002;36:307–317.
16. Rowe JW, Kahn RL. Human aging: usual and successful aging. *Science.* 1987;237:143–149.
17. Strawbridge WJ, Wallhagen MI, Cohen RD. Successful aging and well-being: self-rated compared with Rowe and Kahn. *Gerontologist.* 2002;42:727–733.
18. Baltes PB, Baltes MM. Psychological perspectives on successful aging: the model of selective optimization with compensation. In: Baltes PB, Baltes MM, eds. *Successful Aging: Perspectives from the Behavioral Sciences.* New York: Cambridge University Press; 1990:1–34.
19. Freund AM, Baltes PB. Selection, optimization, and compensation as strategies of life management: correlations with subjective indicators of successful aging. *Psychol Aging.* 1998;13:531–543.

20. Dion KK, Berscheid E, Walster E. What is beautiful is good. *J Personal Soc Psychol.* 1972;24:285–290.

21. Kubler-Ross E. *On Death and Dying.* London: Collier-Macmillan Limited; 1969.

22. Goldenberg II. *Oppression and Social Intervention: Essays on the Human Condition and the Problems of Change.* Chicago: Nelson Hall; 1978:73.

23. Friedan B. *The Fountain of Age.* New York: Touchstone; 1993:637–638.

24. Palmore EB. Successful aging. In Maddy GD, ed. *Encyclopedia of Aging: A Comprehensive Resource in Gerontology and Geriatrics.* 2nd ed. New York: Springer; 1995:914–915.

25. Charmak WD. The Effects of a Psychosocial Intervention Program on Sense of Control in Cancer Patients. Anne Arbor, MI: UMI Dissertation Information Service; 1988.

26. Rogers CR. *Client Centered Therapy: Its Current Practices, Implications And Theory.* Boston: Houghton Mifflin; 1951:494.

27. Viorst J. *Necessary Losses.* New York: Random House; 1986:342–343.

28. Clark C. *How to Face Death: What Happens When We Die – and Afterwards.* London: The Faith Press Limited; 1958:15.

29. Neugarten B. Dynamics of transition of middle age to old age. *J Geriatr Psychiatry.* 1970;4:77–80 and In Friedan B. *The Fountain of Age.* New York: Touchstone; 1993:120.

30. Kalish RA, ed. *Death Grief and Caring Relationships.* 2nd ed. Monterey, CA: Books/Cole; 1985 and In Kalichman SC. *Understanding AIDS: A Guide for Mental Health Professionals.* Washington, DC: American Psychological Association; 1995: 199.

31. King DE, Mainous AG, Geesey ME. Turning back the clock: adopting a healthy lifestyle in middle age. *Am J Med.* 2007; 120:598–603.

32. Levy B, Hausdorff J, Hencke R, Wie J. Reducing cardiovascular stress with positive self-stereotypes of aging. *J Gerontol Psychol Sci.* 2000;55B:205–213.

33. Levy B, Slade M, Kundel S, Kasl S. Longevity increased by positive self-perceptions of aging. *J Personal Soc Psychol.* 2002;83:261–270.

34. Levy B. Improving memory in old age through implicit self-stereotyping. *J Personal Soc Psychol.* 1996;71:1092–1107.

35. Linn MW, Hunter K. Perceptions of age in the elderly. *J Gerontol.* 1979;34:45–52.

51

CELL BIOLOGY AND PHYSIOLOGY OF AGING

Richard Falvo, PhD

"Our culture's compulsive spinning of old age into gold can inflict psychospiritual harm when it lures people into expecting a perpetually gilded existence, with an infomercial alchemist available at every rough and turbulent bend in the road to provide correctives that keep our lives shiny. Without more prevalently honest cultural representations of aging to inform our sensibilities, many of us approach the prospect of becoming old as though it were an option, and we view any failure to grab the gold as an anomaly, a personal flaw, the result of a doctor's incompetence, an HMO's stinginess with resources, or some great cosmic unfairness".[1]

Human aging can be defined as that time in postreproductive development when systematic deterioration begins at various rates and severity in multiple organ systems and results in random physiological disorder, which ultimately precedes death.

Although there may be some legitimacy that basic aging research appears to overlook the potential translation of findings to patient care, overall the intention has been to keep an "eye on the prize," that is, to "understand" the complex phenomenon known as aging. It is only through work on yeast, worms, flies, mice, monkeys, and humans will an understanding be reached of this long-pondered puzzle of nature. This inquiry, to most investigators, is neither to view aging as a disease nor to extend the human life span[2] but rather to understand the basic biology of aging and to translate these findings to help promote "successful aging." The term "functional longevity,"[3] which implies a facilitation of sensory, cognitive, and physical stability enabling elderly individuals to enjoy fully their ever-increasing golden years, would appear to be a most desirable description of successful aging.

A value-added aspect of aging research is the accumulation of further insights and correlations between normal processes related to homeostatic controls and how these processes become "unstable" and lead to age-related diseases (e.g., Alzheimer's disease [AD], diabetes mellitus, cardiovascular disease).

If asked by a patient how he/she could ensure a long and healthy life, the answer given by most health care providers would include, among nonrisk taking behaviors, maintenance of both mental and social activities; attainment of an ideal weight that would promote good insulin sensitivity; maintenance of a normal blood pressure; a promotion of high high-density lipoprotein (HDL)/low-density lipoprotein (LDL) ratio via a sensible diet including fish and vegetables (possibly with the use of a cholesterol lowering drug); low alcohol intake; no nicotine use; moderate exercise (e.g., strength enhancement and aerobics) and possibly some supplements and pharmacological interventions, such as vitamins and antioxidants.

Therefore, are there any data gleaned from aging research that imply following such a regimen or life style improves one's chances for increased longevity (attribute of being long-lived)? Are there additional interventions that an individual could take to ensure functional longevity? Or is it all based on genetics? Below is a short review of *some* of the major theories of aging. A discussion of calorie restriction and its implication for humans will be followed by a short review of the human lifespan, centenarians, and a conclusion describing how some of these data help us understand aging and what potential this research has for translation to patient care.

AGING THEORIES

Although it has been suggested there are as many theories of aging as researchers in the field, this is untrue. However, most investigators divide aging theories into random alterations (stochastic) (i.e., somatic mutation, error catastrophe, protein alterations and oxidative stress) and genetic–physiological

536

Table 51.1. Definitions of Acronyms and Terms Used in the Chapter

Antagonistic pleiotropy (theory stating that during aging, processes are expressed that although beneficial early in life have unintended deleterious effects during aging).

Antioxidants (chemicals that slow down oxidation and help remove free radicals [atoms or groups of atoms with an odd or unpaired number of electrons]. Examples are peroxidases, catalases, and superoxide dismutase).

Apoptosis (programmed cell death).

Cytokines (secreted signaling molecules).

Genomics (systematic use of genome information).

GH (growth hormone – an anterior pituitary gland hormone).

IGF-1 (insulin-like growth factor-1; one of many growth factors secreted normally by the liver in response to growth hormone stimulation).

Interleukins e.g., IL-1, IL-6, etc. (a group of secreted signaling molecules that are a major functioning aspect of the immune system).

Lifespan (maximum known duration of life of an organism).

Longevity (attribute of being long-lived).

PARP-1 (enzyme poly[ADP-ribose] polymerase 1) (a nuclear repair enzyme).

Mimetics (e.g., drugs that can mimic calorie restriction).

NSAIDS (nonsteroidal antiinflammatory drugs).

Nutraceutical (supplement with beneficial effects on human health).

p53 (tumor suppressor protein).

PPAR (peroxisome proliferator-activated receptor, e.g., thiazolidinediones) (PPAR agonists that act to increase insulin sensitivity).

Proteomics (study of protein structure and function as associated with genomics).

Resveratrol (polyphenolic component of red wine and peanuts).

Senescence (e.g., cellular, cells become arrested and do not proliferate).

Sirtuins (silent information regulators [a family of protein deacetylases] – these enzymes removed N-acetyl groups from amino side chains to permit gene transcription).

Stochastic (randomness).

Telomeres (repeating base pairs located on the ends of chromosomes that protect the chromosomes from degradation).

Transcription factor (protein that binds DNA at a specific site [promoter or enhancer] where it regulates gene transcription).

(genetics, cellular senescence/death, neuroendocrine, immunological, and inflammation). The treatment and organization of these theories varies and what follows is one approach. For clarification, the definition of certain acronyms and terms used in the chapter are listed in Table 51.1.

Somatic Mutation

This theory implies damage to sensitive cellular and genetic components over time by environmental "hits" (insults). As these hits (which can be genetic or epigenetic) continue, damage occurs in various tissues. As risk factors increase or tolerance is exceeded, age-associated diseases occur. To counter this, DNA repair occurs using, for example, the enzyme PARP-1. PARP-1 is one important factor among other repair systems and the

level of activity of this factor has been shown to be related to longevity.[4]

Error Catastrophe

Briefly, this theory states that over time the cellular machinery of the cell breaks down (becomes erratic) and as a result errors occur in protein formation and metabolic pathway control and the cells become dysfunctional or die.[5]

Protein Alteration

Some investigators have described this phenomenon as analogous to the "browning of a turkey." Over time proteins become overly glycated (sugar coated), leading to disruption of cell function. Proteins also are oxidized, and cross-linking occurs leading to stiffness, inflammation, and other problems that can lead to age-related diseases.[6]

Neuroendocrine

The nervous–endocrine system interaction has profound influences on the body. It is an exquisitely fine-tuned system, which starts functioning long before birth, triggers puberty, and controls reproduction and function of major endocrine glands in the body. It has control over water balance, electrolyte balance, and countless other homeostatic systems. During aging both neuronal and hormonal attenuation occurs and this can have an enormous impact on every organ system in the body (e.g., loss of muscle strength and bone density, which presents a fundamental problem causing frailty in the aged.[7] In addition, there are the well-known aspects of reproductive changes in aging organisms.

Immunological Aging

Aging reduces the ability to resist infection, and this deficiency increases with a concomitant greater incidence and morbidity associated with infectious diseases. In addition vaccine efficiency declines.[8] Because the T-lymphocytes, specifically helper T cells, play a major role in both humoral and cellular immune responses, their age-associated dysfunctions have a major impact on aging.

Genetics

Aging is a multilevel phenomenon with biochemical, cellular, and regulatory alterations in different tissues and organs systems at different times and at different rates. How genes are involved in aging is not easy to appreciate because selection pressures would tend to be over once postreproductive years have been reached. Basically there are probably no genes "for aging."[9] According to our current understanding of "the genetics of aging," genes not under the pressures of natural selection have survived and express themselves during aging in an environment totally novel from which they arose. Hence aging phenotypes exist because the younger organism has evolved processes for cellular maintenance, reproductive fitness, and genetic viability, which incur various "costs" in terms of aging and longevity (see later). Thus during aging, processes are expressed that although beneficial early in life have unintended deleterious effects during old age – this is what is known as antagonistic pleiotropy.[9]

Despite this viewpoint, genetic manipulation in animals as diverse as yeast, nematode worms, fruit flies, and mice[10] can increase longevity as much as sixfold by slowing down the aging process. What is fascinating is that many of these manipulations appear to influence a highly conserved metabolic pathway, that is, the insulin/IGF1-like pathway. In mice, either natural or induced mutations that interfere with

GH production, GH receptor binding, or production of IGF lead to extended longevity (see Table 51.1 for explanation of GH in this pathway).[11] All of these gene manipulations appear to somehow reduce the susceptibility to stress (see later).

Cellular Senescence/Apoptosis (Cancer and Aging – Parallel Changes)

There are a few observations that help give deeper insights into the complexity of cellular aging. During development, certain cells divide continually, and unlike their postmitotic or nondividing siblings, are more prone to cancers, which typically are more likely to occur as the organism ages. The protection that young organisms possess that old ones do not is an extensive tumor suppressive network. In humans, following stress, such as DNA damage, hypoxia, and cell cycle disruption, one major and critical tumor suppressor protein that responds to protect the genome is p53.[12,13]

Organisms protect themselves from cancer by shielding the genome from potential damage by either elimination (apoptosis) or arrest (cellular senescence) of cells, which are or can become neoplastic.

Apoptosis is programmed cell death (not necrosis) and ensures the timely removal of cellular products and debris and thus insulates the surrounding cells from potentially harmful products (enzymes, etc.). Apoptosis is also essential for normal embryological development. Along with these useful properties, unfortunately, any alteration in the normal apoptotic response can result in disease. Cancer cells, in the absence of appropriate apoptotic signals, find themselves in a proliferative environment, which is permissive to their destructive properties.

Cellular senescence occurs in cells that are not terminally differentiated and hence still retain the capacity to undergo cell division. When appropriately stimulated, such cells can respond by undergoing neoplastic transformations. Although apoptosis eliminates cells, cellular senescence describes a situation in which cells are arrested and do not proliferate, that is, do not self-renew. This is critical, because such cells will not become malignant, but they do remain viable for extended periods of time.[14] Cellular senescence apparently occurs due to replicative senescence–repeated cell division.[12] The cause of replicative senescence is thought to be related to telomere shortening over time.

Telomeres protect chromosomes from degradation. After each division, telomeres shorten (this is not true for cancer cells or reproductive tissue that have the telomerase enzyme that restores them). Following multiple divisions, the original "telomere theory" of aging[15] [and updated to the present[16]] suggests that this repeated genomic instability could make further division impossible. In response to this instability, following multiple divisions, cells either undergo apoptosis or cellular senescence. Certain progeroid syndromes, disorders that mimic physiological aging at an accelerated rate (e.g., Werner syndrome), do show shortened telomeres.[17]

The parallel changes of aging and cancer are another excellent example of antagonistic pleiotropy – although both apoptosis and cellular senescence are beneficial in the young organism, they may have unselected deleterious effects later in life, contributing both to aging and susceptibility to diseases. For example, apoptosis eliminates unwanted cells (beneficial) but can potentially deplete cells and/or stem cell lines (harmful). Senescence prevents proliferation of unwanted cells (beneficial) but can change the metabolic behavior of remaining cells, which can lead to production and secretion of unwanted molecules (e.g., cytokines, growth factors, and destructive enzymes), which can destroy homeostasis and potentially lead to age-related pathologies. Hence the cells have a choice to protect against cancer or postpone aging. Indeed humans with genetic variability (polymorphisms) of p53, which promotes the best cancer protection (apoptosis and cell senescence), also show signs of decreased longevity. Another downside is that senescent cells that remain in check may renew their cell cycle activity and give rise to common cancers later in life.[14] On a similar theme is a description of the link between cellular aging and tumor suppression. A gene has been identified that prevents cancer cells from dividing but during aging, as its activity increases, stem cell renewal is reduced. In mice, if the activity of this gene were attenuated, islet cells could continue to proliferate like in young animals. If the activity was overexpressed, the stem cells aged prematurely and stopped dividing. These results, albeit limited but supported by others, clearly show antagonistic pleiotropy in action.[18]

Oxidative Stress

The oxidative stress theory (formerly called the free radical theory) is thought to be one of the major causes of aging, although not all investigators are convinced.[19]

Mammalian cells are continually insulted by reactive species (RS) such as reactive oxygen species, nitrogen-derived reactive species, and others. This hostile environment during aging, coupled with a reduced defense system (antioxidants) is considered one component responsible for the pathology observed in inflammation, age-related degeneration, tumor formation, diabetes mellitus, and other diseases.[20] The targets of RS are DNA, proteins, lipids, and cellular organelles. The sources of RS include cellular metabolism, ischemia, ionizing radiation, injury and resulting inflammation, air pollution, and cigarette smoke. Without proper scavenging by antioxidants, the levels of the RS build up and subsequent damage (aging) occurs. The human organism possesses defense mechanisms that suppress generation of RS. Antioxidant vitamins (C and E) scavenge RS. There are also repair enzymes that attempt to reconstitute damaged structures and molecules. Supported by a vast array of animal experimentation, oxidative stress and the resulting damage appear to have an impact on lifespan. For example, alteration of antioxidant gene expression can extend lifespan; that is, more than 20% in mice.[21]

Molecular Inflammation

Emerging evidence shows that age-related human diseases (e.g., atherosclerosis, arthritis, dementia, osteoporosis, and cardiovascular diseases) all have an inflammatory basis.[22] This so-called "molecular inflammation theory" proposes a possible link between aging and age-related diseases. The basis of this theory states that activation of very sensitive reduction-oxidation sensitive transcription factors coupled with age-related disruption of gene expression via oxidative stress is the underlying cause. Well known specific molecular inflammatory markers, for example the interleukins, have been implicated. Indeed it has been recently reported that the decline in mortality in certain countries can be attributed to a life-long reduction of infection and inflammatory burden.[23]

CALORIE RESTRICTION

The only known intervention to consistently increase longevity in all species in which it has been tried is caloric restriction (CR) (usually a 30%–40% reduction of calories] along with maintenance of proper nutritional requirements. This is true in well-documented cases in, among others, yeast, worms, flies, and rodents.[24]

Most pertinent to humans is the study of CR (30% reduction) in rhesus monkeys,[24] which is a National Institute on Aging–supported project at five primate research centers in the United States. The rhesus monkey shows many of the aging characteristics of its more famous relative such as presbyopia, presbycusis, and declines in motor activity, learning and memory, metabolic rate, body temperature, cardiovascular function, and appetite. Rhesus also shows some neural pathology similar to AD and show changes in hormone levels and reproductive decline. Approximately 15 years into the study many parameters/categories, which change in response to CR in these monkeys, are similar to those observed in long-lived humans not practicing CR. For example, monkeys under a CR regimen show the expected decreases in body weight, fat deposition, metabolic rate, and body temperature. They have increased insulin sensitivity, decreased fasting blood glucose, and decreased IGF-1. Their blood pressure, heart rate, triglyceride, LDL, and certain interleukins are reduced. They also show a decrease in oxidative stress in muscle; however, their time to sexual maturity is lengthened. These monkeys have been reported to outlive their non-CR restricted controls.[25]

A potential consensus is emerging that CR reduces oxidative stress; induces reduction in the insulin–IGF pathway; increases insulin sensitivity; decreases blood glucose; delays immune senescence; and reduces inflammation. As a result of the decreased energy intake, there is also less hyperplasia and hence less chance of tumor initiation and growth.[26]

Additionally sirtuins have been implicated as key components of aging.[27] These proteins sit in an advantageous position to monitor energy supply by encoding a nuclear protein deacetylase. These deacetylases have profound impacts on gene expression. The homologs of these mammalian proteins in yeast and worms, when overexpressed, promote longevity. Sirtuins are being described as a link among CR, cancer, and aging.

Human Implications of CR

CR or at least calorie reduction has potential health benefits for humans. Humans practicing CR have a decreased body weight and fat stores along with the expected increased insulin sensitivity and decreased fasting glucose. Likewise their triglyceride levels and HDL/LDL profiles are ideal. Their blood pressures and heart rates are lower and the incidence for vascular disease is less. They are less susceptible to diabetes mellitus and metabolic syndrome. Some of these effects, in addition to weight reduction may be due to the corresponding decreases in insulin, glucose, and IGF-1/GH levels in the blood. They tend to have a lower risk of cancer and vascular diseases and an overall decreased mortality from cancer and other age-related diseases.[28]

CR, which lowers oxidative damage, lowers the incidence of AD. A comparison of countries with reduced fat and caloric intake (e.g.,China, Japan, and Nigeria] compared with the United States and western Europe with an opposite type of diet, shows a lower incidence of AD by up to 50%.[26,29] Dietary modification, for example a Mediterranean diet, appears to be neuroprotective and this may be due to the high antioxidant activity, low fat content, and reduced caloric intake associated with this diet.[30,31] Dietary intake of several exogenous antioxidants and nonsteroidal antiinflammatory drugs may also be associated with a lower risk for AD.[32,33]

Although not conclusively proven, resveratrol, a polyphenolic component of red wine and peanuts, activates the sirtuin pathway (as noted previously)and extends life in both yeast and worms. Although the connection of resveratrol to longevity in humans is at best speculative, it is interesting to note the link between resveratrol and the known benefit of red wine drinking that accompanies the supposed life-prolonging effects of the Mediterranean diet.[34]

Downside of CR

When human CR is practiced (restricted ~40%, although this varies) individuals do have the expected loss of weight and adipose tissue. They may also show cardiovascular (hypotension), reproductive (menstrual irregularities, loss of libido, infertility), skeletal (bone thinning and osteoporosis) and psychological (depression, subdued affect and irritability) problems. They are cold sensitive, have loss of muscle strength/stamina and wound-healing takes longer.[35] On the other hand, many practitioners report excellent health, ideal mental attitude, and maintain productive lifestyles.[36]

Alterative Interventions to CR

Research is underway to develop drugs which would have the same biological effects as CR without the reduction of caloric intake. Such drugs are known as CR mimetics and can include nutraceutical, pharmaceutical, and hormonal preparations.[37] In addition to novel chemicals, a well-known drug in the treatment of diabetes (metformin), which produces a reduction in hepatic glucose production and heightened insulin sensitivity, is being tested as a CR mimetic.[38] Furthermore drugs that inhibit glycolysis, agonists of peroxisome proliferator-activating factor (thiazolidinediones) and IGF-1 signaling inhibitors are being tested.[37] All of these interventions are based on some of the aging theories and their biological bases, which were explained previously.

THE HUMAN LIFESPAN

The maximum human lifespan (maximum observed lifespan of the human species) is now approximately 122 years of age.[39] The major influence on longevity is not determined by genetic influences but by environmental conditions.[40] Indeed, there is an increasing body of data accumulating that indicate nurture does have a positive impact on the attenuation of certain diseases that are typically considered age related.[30,31]

Furthermore, those who live to old age have only a rare genetic advantage, which although having a significant impact on individual longevity has minimal impact on the average human lifespan. The genetic differences between those who die prematurely (early aging syndromes]) and those who live to attain old age (centenarians) is probably quite small.[41] Due to the fact that more individuals are surviving childhood illness due to improved living conditions, nutrition, improved health care, and so forth, these "centenarian" genes may become more prevalent in our population and provide some added genetic advantage to their descendents (recall antagonistic pleiotropy).

CENTENARIANS

Achieving centenarian status occurs in 1/10,000 individuals in the United States.[42] They appear to age successfully, pass on their survival advantage to offspring, and provide a fascinating human model for longevity studies. They reach this age through a complex interaction of genes, lifestyles, and environment. Third generation offspring of centenarians have a lower incidence of or a delay in the onset of age-related diseases. These individuals have larger HDL levels and particle size and low LDL levels.[43]

Although centenarians have a complex genotypic and phenotypic background and other unique characteristics, a few of these attributes can be more compelling, based on both experimental results and current aging theories. For example, although cancer does occur in centenarians the disease appears to occur 20 years later and in a milder form. They have excellent glucose tolerance, low IGF-1/GH, and a low incidence of diabetes mellitus, metabolic syndrome, and hypertension. Although many are taking antihypertensive medications, they still display a reduced incidence of vascular problems (stroke and myocardial infarctions) possibly due to their known natural protection against inflammation. They also have a lower incidence of age-related dementia (AD) and Parkinson's disease. Furthermore, centenarians appear to have protection against RS and heightened abilities to generate antioxidant defense mechanisms.[42–44] Interestingly, these centenarians who are being studied today survived pandemics during the early part of the last century and seem to have an exceptional resistance to disease. Once again, not everyone is in agreement.[45] It must also be pointed out that despite all of these findings, centenarians are not necessarily disease free.[46]

SUMMARY

Aging is determined by a complex interaction between genes, the environment, and randomness.[47] Furthermore, the "typical" person is probably genetically "programmed" to live to be approximately 85–90 years of age (depending on other nonbiological factors as described at the end of this chapter). This is true if they are fortunate enough not to have a certain genetic constituency that harbors age-related/cancer-inducing conditions. To become a centenarian (adding $\sim$ 10–15 years) appears to be a genetic rarity.[48] Therefore what advice can a physician give patients who wish to help ensure their own functional longevity? Much of the "theoretical" data or basic research on aging speak directly to this in a very profound manner. If a patient would begin with an honest attempt to maintain a healthy weight or to shed extra pounds via modest CR (8%–25% or every other day feeding; -[EODF]),[49] this coupled with exercise could lead to an increase in insulin sensitivity and reduced glucose levels. In addition there can be added benefits of increased HDL and reduced LDL levels along with a decrease in blood pressure. There is even a suggestion that fasting itself, that is, EODF, rather than the calories themselves may slow the aging process.[35]

These interventions apparently may reduce oxidative stress, inflammation, and lower the risks for all types of age-related diseases (e.g., arthritis, diabetes mellitus II, atherosclerosis, cardiovascular, AD).[49]

In addition the potential of functional longevity benefits offered by both the nutritional supplementation (vitamins, antioxidants, etc.] and pharmaceutical (nonsteroidal antiinflammatory drugs, cholesterol lowering drugs, etc.) industries, although somewhat speculative at this point, do show some promise in RS and inflammatory attenuation. Data, although scattered and obtained from those following the Mediterranean diet and other long-term dietary modifications, along with modest alcohol consumption, olive oil use and so forth, show clear evidence that reducing energy production and increasing naturally occurring antioxidants may aid in the achievement of functional longevity.

For the present, until future research on genomics, proteomics, and mimetics yields additional information about the secrets of longevity, this is the best message to relay to patients.

In addition, none of these recommendations are considered harmful to the average person.

FINAL COMMENT

Although the thrust of this chapter has been very biologically oriented, some recent findings are sobering. C-reactive protein (CRP) is produced by the immune system in response to acute infection or injury and is part of the inflammatory response. Low socioeconomic status (SES) is a major risk factor for a host of diseases (age related and not) and recently low SES has been shown to be correlated with elevated CRP levels, especially in the elderly.[50] Likewise disturbing data outlining health disparities due to race, income, and location in the United States have recently been reported in the *New York Times*.[51] Of specific interest to the topic of this chapter, women in a particular county in New Jersey typically reach 91 years of age whereas Native American men in parts of South Dakota die at approximately 58 years of age. In addition, Asian-American women have a life expectancy 13 years longer compared with low-income African-American women in the rural south. Finally, millions of the lowest income Americans have life expectancies similar to those observed in developing countries. Many factors contribute to these differences including health care opportunities. Aging research opens many interesting scientific pathways to aid the human condition, but it must be linked to proper and equitable medical care. All parties in a position of influence should carefully evaluate dispensing expectations regarding longevity enhancement that are neither attainable nor desirable.

REFERENCES

1. Scannell K. An aging un-American. *NEJM*. 2006;355:1415–1417,
2. Marshall J. Life extension research: an analysis of contemporary biological theories and ethical issues. *Med Health Care Phil.* 2006;9:87–96.
3. Yu BP. Why caloric restriction would work for human longevity. *Biogerontology.* 2006;7:179–182.
4. Bürkle A, Beneke S, Muira M-L. Poly[ADP]-ribosylation and aging. *Exp Gerontol.* 2004;39:1599–1602.
5. Semsei I. On the nature of aging. *Mech Ageing Dev.* 2000;117:93–98.
6. Furber JD. Extracellular glycation crosslinks: prospects for removal. *Rejuv Res.* 2006;9:274–278.
7. Lamberts SWJ, van den Beld AW, van der Lely A-J. The endocrinology of aging. *Science.* 1997;278:419–424.
8. Kovaiou RD, Grubeck-Loebenstein B. Age-associated changes within CD4+T cells. *Immunol Lett.* 2006;107:8–14.
9. Kirkwood TBL. Genes that shape the course of ageing. *Trends Endocrinol Metab.* 2003;14:345–347.
10. Partidge L, Gems D. Beyond the evolutionary theory of ageing, from functional genomics to evo-gero. *Trend Ecol Evol.* 2006;21:334–340.
11. Bartke A. Minireview: role of the growth hormone/insulin-like growth factor system in mammalian aging. *Endocrinology.* 2005;146:3718–3723.

12. Campisi J. Cellular senescence and apoptosis: how cellular responses might influence aging genotypes. *Exp Gerontol.* 2003;38:5–11.

13. Van Dyke T. p53 and tumor suppression. *NEJM.* 2007;356:79–81.

14. Mooi WJ, Peeper DS. Oncogene-induced cell senescence-halting on the road to cancer. *NEJM.* 2006;355:1037–1046.

15. Hayflick L. How and why we age. *Exp Gerontol.* 1998;33:639–654.

16. Patil CK, Mian ID, Campisi J. The thorny path linking cellular senescence to organismal aging. *Mech Ageing Dev.* 2005;126:1040–1045.

17. Eller MS, Liao X, Liu S, et al. A role for WRN in telomere-based DNA damage responses. *Proc Natl Acad Sci USA.* 2006;10:15073–15078.

18. Janzen V, Forkert R, Fleming HE, et al. Stem-cell ageing modified by the cycling-dependent kinase inhibitor p16[INK4a]. *Nature.* 2006;443:421–426.

19. Kregel KC, Zhang HJ. An integrated view of oxidative stress in aging: basic mechanisms, functional effects and pathological considerations. *Am J Physiol Integr Comp Physiol.* 2007;292:R18–R36.

20. Cooke MS, Evans MD. Reactive oxygen species: from DNA damage to disease. *Sci Med.* 2005;10:98–111.

21. Schriner SE, Linford NJ Martin GM, et al. Extension of murine life span by overexpression of catalase targeted to mitochondria. *Science.* 2005;308:1909–1911.

22. Chung HY, Sung B, Jung KJ, et al. The molecular inflammatory process in aging. *Antiox Redox Signal.* 2006;8:572–581.

23. Crimmins EM, Finch CE. Infection, inflammation, height, and longevity. *Proc Natl Acad Sci USA.* 2006;103:498–503.

24. Roth G, Mattison J, Ottinger MA, et al. Aging in Rhesus monkeys: relevance to human health interventions. *Science.* 2004;305:1423–1426.

25. Hansen BC, Bodkin LH, Ortmeyer HK. Calorie restriction in nonhuman primates: mechanisms of reduced morbidity and mortality. *Toxicol Sci.* 1999;52(2 Suppl):56–60.

26. Martin B, Mattson MP, Maudsley S. Caloric restriction and intermittent fasting: two potential diets for successful brain aging. *Ageing Res Rev.* 2006;5:332–353.

27. Longo VD, Kennedy BK. Sirtuins in aging and age-related diseases. *Cell.* 2006;126:257–268.

28. Hursting SD, Lavigne J, Berrigan D, et al. Calorie restriction, aging and cancer prevention: mechanisms of action and applicability to humans. *Ann Rev Med.* 2003;54:131–152.

29. Grant W. Dietary links to Alzheimer's disease: 1999 Update. *Alzheimers Dis.* 1999;1:197–201.

30. Solfrizzi V, Capurso C, Panza E. Adherence to a Mediterranean dietary pattern and risk of Alzheimer's disease. *Ann Neurol.* 2006;59:912–921.

31. Steele M, Stuchbury G, Münch G. The molecular basis of the prevention of Alzheimer's disease through healthy nutrition. *Exp Gerontol.* 2007;42(1/2):28–36.

32. McGeer PL, Rogers J, McGeer EG. Inflammation, antiinflammatory agents and Alzheimer's disease: the last 12 years. *J Alzheimers Dis.* 2006;9(3 Suppl):271–276.

33. Rutten BP, Steinbusch HW, Korr H, et al. Antioxidants and Alzheimer's disease: from bench to bedside (and back again). *Curr Opin Clin Nutr Metab Care.* 2002;5:645–651.

34. Baur JA, Sinclair DA. Therapeutic potential of resveratrol: the in vivo evidence. *Nature Rev Drug Discov.* 2006;5:493–506.

35. Dirks AJ, Leeuwenburgh C. Caloric restriction in humans: potential pitfalls and health concerns. *Mech Ageing Dev.* 2006;127:1–7.

36. Mason M. One for the ages: a prescription that may extend life. *New York Times.* October 31, 2006.

37. Ingram DK, Zhu M, Mamczarz J, et al. Calorie restriction mimetics: an emerging research field. *Aging Cell.* 2006;5:515–524.

38. Kirpichnikov D, McFarlane SI, Sowers JR. Metformin: an update. *Ann Intern Med.* 2002;137:25–33.

39. Vijg J, Suh Y. Genetics and longevity and aging. *Ann Rev Med.* 2005;56:193–212.

40. Herskind AM, McGue M, Holm NV, et al. The heritability of human longevity: a population-based study of 2872 Danish twin pairs born 1870–1900. *Hum Genet.* 1996;97:319–323.

41. Cutler RG. Evolution of human longevity and the genetic complexity governing aging rate. *Proc Natl Acad Sci USA.* 1975;72:4664–4668.

42. Perls TT. The different paths to 100. *J Clin Nutr.* 2006;83:484S–487S.

43. Atzmon G, Rincon M, Rabizadeh, Barzilai N. Biological evidence for inheritance of exceptional longevity. *Mech Ageing Dev.* 2006;126:341–345.

44. Schoenhofen EA, Wyszynski DF, Andersen S, et al. Characteristics of 32 supercentenarians. *J Am Geriatr Soc.* 2006;54:1237–1240.

45. Adachi T, Wang J, Wang XL. Age-related change of plasma extracellular-superoxide dismutase. *Clin Chim Acta.* 2000;290:169–178.

46. Andersen-Ranberg HR, Jeune B, Nybo H et al. Low activity of superoxide dismutase and high activity of glutathione reductase in erythrocytes from centenarians. *Age–Ageing.* 1998;5:643–648.

47. Martin GM. Keynote, mechanisms of senescence: complicationists versus simplifications. *Mech Ageing Dev.* 2002;123:65–69.

48. Perls T, Terry D. Genetics of exceptional longevity. *Exp Gerontol.* 2003;38:725–730.

49. Fontana L, Meyer TE, Klein S, et al. Long-term calorie restriction is highly effective in reducing the risk for atherosclerosis in humans. *Proc Natl Acad Sci USA.* 2004;101:6659–6663.

50. Alley DE, Seeman TE, Ki Kim J. Socioeconomic status and C-reactive protein levels in the US population: NHANES IV. *Brain Behav Immun.* 2006;20:498–504.

51. Perez-Pena R. Bergen county N.J. is long in longevity. *New York Times.* September 12, 2006.

52

IMPLICATIONS OF AN AGING SOCIETY

Daniel Swagerty, MD, MPH, Jonathan Evans, MD, MPH

INTRODUCTION

Understanding the changing demography of the growing older adult population is essential to providing quality medical care to older adults. With the growing numbers of adults older than age 65 years, almost every medical specialty will be impacted by this phenomenon. The fastest growing population cohort in the United States are adults older than age 85. Understanding the differences in older adult care for the young-old and old-old provides an important basis for the study of geriatrics. In fact, individual variation is more pronounced in the older adult population than in any other age group. The chapter aims to explain the urgent and growing need for health professionals to be skilled in the care of older adults.

Over the last century the world has dramatically aged. Life expectancy has steadily increased, particularly in the developed world. There are many reasons for this significant increase in life expectancy including improvements in hygiene, sanitation, and medical advances. At the same time, birth rates have declined. The net effect on society as a whole is an older population.[1]

This aging of our society is expected to have many far-reaching consequences on the U.S. and world culture, economy, social relationships, health care delivery, and governmental responsibilities. An aging population will have an impact on everyone in society regardless of age. Moreover, population aging is occurring around the world, most notably in developed countries, but also to a significant extent in the developing world. It is difficult to predict all of the ways in which our nation and the world will be challenged in the next several decades as a result of the aging population. Many of the effects are already evident, such as increased health care costs and demand for health care and social services. Nevertheless, there is still a great deal of uncertainty because this phenomenon has not previously occurred to this extent. Our historical experience will be

a very limited guide as we confront unprecedented acceleration in the growth and complexity of an aging population.[1-3]

The impact of aging on individual seniors must be considered in the context of the aging population. An individual's needs, preferences, goals, resources, and abilities change throughout the lifespan. As one grows, matures, and ages, there is a change in one's living situation, finances, functional independence, and self-reliance. Of particular concern to most everyone is how much we must rely on others (such as family members, friends, the local community, and government) for our instrumental and basic activities of daily living. As the age of an entire society increases, more people reach advanced age without a proportional increase in the number of younger people to care for them. This shift in population demographics will likely cause fundamental changes in the nation's economy, labor force, the role of government, and the ability of government to provide needed services. There is also a fundamental shift in the ability, and perhaps willingness, of the younger members of society to provide for the needs of older generations.[4-9]

As described in other chapters in this book, it is well known what happens to the human body with normal aging. It is therefore possible to anticipate and extrapolate those changes to groups of individuals; however, a society is more than the sum of all of the individual members. Some of the consequences of an aging society will be obvious and predictable whereas others will be more obscure and unpredictable. The following sections will explore how the effects of individual aging can be extrapolated to predictable social impacts and how such impacts can also be difficult to predict for many reasons.

This chapter will discuss the impact of an aging society on health care delivery, government, the economy, and on family relationships. It will explore some of the difficulties of anticipating future changes and needs, as well as some of the dilemmas that our and other aging societies face now and in the future. Population aging will be examined in an effort to understand

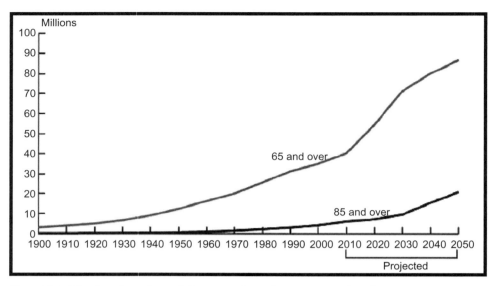

Figure 52.1. Number of people aged 65 years and over, by age group, selected years 1900–2000. *Note:* Data for 2010–2050 are projections of the population. *Reference population:* These data refer to the resident population. *Source:* U.S. Census Bureau, Decennial Census and Projections. See color plates.

better what the implications are for both older adults and the rest of society.

CURRENT AND PROJECTED SIZE OF THE U.S. OLDER ADULT POPULATION

The post–World War II baby boom generation in the United States is fast approaching age 65 and older. There are more people 65 years of age or older alive today in the United States, as well as the world, than have ever reached that age throughout our history. In the United States alone, the population age 65 years and older is currently 36 million or 13% of the overall population. Figure 52.1 shows how as the baby boom generation ages, those older than 65 years will double in number by the year 2050 to 90 million or 20% of the U.S. population. Particularly rapid growth is anticipated in the older-than-85 age group. The elderly population is also expected to become more ethnically diverse. Consequently, we are entering a completely new era, with little in our past to guide our future.[1,2]

Life Expectancy

In the United States, improvements in health have resulted in increased life expectancy and contributed to the growth of the older population over the past century. As shown in Figure 52.2,

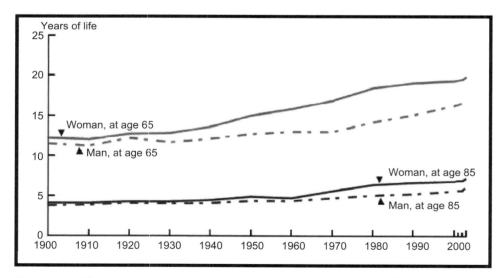

Figure 52.2. Life expectancy at ages 65 and 85 years, by sex, selected years 1900–2003. *Reference population:* These data refer to the resident population. *Source:* Centers for Disease Control and Prevention, National Center for Health Statistics, National Vital Statistics System. See color plates.

Americans are living longer than ever before. Life expectancies at both age 65 and 85 years have increased. Current life expectancy is approximately 86 years for women and 78 years for men. Under current mortality conditions, men who survive to age 65 can expect to live an average of 17 years and for women, the life expectancy at 65 is currently 20 years. The life expectancy of people who survive to age 85 today is 6 years for men and 7.2 years for women. The further one progresses beyond age 65 years, the longer one is expected to live. Although life expectancies have improved dramatically over the last decade in the United States, individual life expectancies vary based on existing comorbidities, quality of life, race, and socioeconomic status.[10,11]

Life expectancy at age 65 in the United States is lower than that of many other industrialized nations. The longest life expectancies are for Japanese women. Within the United States, the longest life expectancies are in Hawaii. Life expectancy also varies by race but the differences change with age. In the United States, life expectancy at birth and at age 65 is higher for white people than for black people. At older ages, however, the life expectancy among black people is slightly higher than among white people. This has been attributed to a "healthy survivor" effect, more social support, and other factors. Not surprisingly, differences in life conditions of older persons with inadequate income and those above the median income in the United States have led to the conclusion that there is a major discrepancy of 1–2.5 years in active life expectancy between the poor and the nonpoor.[10,11]

Active Life Expectancy

The concept of active life expectancy is useful in thinking about functional status and independence in older adulthood. In life expectancy, the end point is death. In active life expectancy we are also concerned with the loss of independence or the need to rely on others for assistance with daily activities. Simplistically put, the remaining years of life for a group of persons can be "active" or "dependent," or some combination thereof. Active life expectancy answers the question: "Of the remaining years of life for this cohort of persons, what proportion is expected to be spent disability free?" The answer has implications for individuals, families, and societies. As Abraham Lincoln once said, *"And in the end, it's not the years in your life that count. It's the life in your years."*

THE IMPACT OF DEATH RATE ON SOCIETY

The impact of an aging population on death rates and the subsequent broad social impact illustrate the complex consequences of an aging society. Currently, three-fourths of all deaths in the United States occur among those 65 years of age and older. Consequently, the overall number of deaths per year is expected to increase as the population increases in age. A predictable consequence will be an increased demand across the spectrum of health care services for the quality and quantity of end-of-life care. It can also be expected that the new demand

for end-of-life care services will require increases in specific health care education for multiple disciplines, the number of individual and organizational providers, and the financing of this health care service. The broader social impact is less predictable. More deaths may increase demand for the number and types of funeral services. Growth in funeral services will require a commensurate growth in the mortuary sciences as well as an increased demand for land for cemeteries. An additional social impact could be in greater tension over land use and zoning in certain municipalities and neighborhoods. This is just one instance in which the effects of an aging society will have broad, and not always predictable, effects on our local, regional, national, and global communities.[2–4,6–8,12–18]

CROSSING THE STREET

Among the myriad changes of normal aging are a decrease in stride length and a consequent reduction in gait speed. That is, older pedestrians walk slower. Studies of ambulatory community-dwelling elderly individuals have found that the time allotted at a crossing signal (i.e., how long the "Walk" sign remains illuminated) is inadequate to allow many older adult pedestrians to cross the street before traffic resumes, thus creating a potentially serious safety hazard. The obvious solution to accommodate an increasingly older populace and promote functional independence is to change the timing of the traffic lights to allow more time for crossing the street. Changing the timing of traffic lights, however, has an obvious slowing effect on traffic flow. Any change in traffic flow also has a significant effect on safety, as well as the economy. In fact, controlling and linking traffic signals across large metropolitan areas has been a primary means by which an increase in cars has been accommodated over several decades without building new roads. In some areas, even changing a single traffic signal can have a major effect. Thus, a number of difficult choices confront society in the coming years as the older adult population grows. The unintended social consequences of one decision to accommodate the needs of an increasing number of older adults may not be as obvious as changing a stoplight.[19–21]

CONSUMER SPENDING, WORK, AND THE ECONOMY

Our economy has undergone tremendous change over the last few decades for a multitude of reasons such as new technology, globalization, and a shift from manufacturing to service sector jobs. Although these changes have little to do with population aging, the increasing age of a population has dramatic effects on the economy. As the population ages, the labor market changes: It becomes older and decreases in size. It is likely that the retirement age will increase for many people, particularly professionals. Similarly, it is likely that the service sector will continue to grow, particularly in health care, financial services, travel, and generally in the professions. The kind of work that

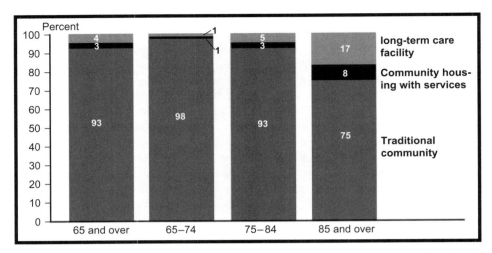

Figure 52.3. Percentage of Medicare enrollees aged 65 years and over residing in selected residential settings, by age group, 2003. *Note:* Community housing with services applies to respondents who reported they lived in retirement communities or apartments, senior citizen housing, continuing care retirement facilities, assisted living facilities, staged living communities, board and care facilities/homes, and other similar situations, AND who reported they had access to one or more of the following services through their place of residence: meal preparation, cleaning or housekeeping services, laundry services, help with medications. Respondents were asked about access to these services but not whether they actually used the services. A residence is considered a long-term care facility if it is certified by Medicare or Medicaid; or has 3 or more beds and is licensed as a nursing home or other long-term care facility and provides at least one personal care service, or provides 24-hour, 7-day-a-week supervision by a caregiver. *Reference population:* These data refer to Medicare enrollees. *Source:* Centers for Medicare & Medicaid Services. Medicare Current Beneficiary Survey. See color plates.

older workers desire and are able to do, particularly those who remain in the workforce beyond retirement age, is different from the kind of work done by young people just entering the work force. This shift in the available workforce will have a tremendous economic impact.[3,8,17,22]

Consumer spending is also largely dependent on the age of consumers. The demand for goods and services will change as the needs and preferences of consumer's change with age. A shift in consumer spending may have far-reaching economic impacts. For example, trade deficits with other nations may continue to rise as a result of our shifting national economy. There will also be relative shortages in the number and expertise of our labor pool. Labor shortages of this nature will result in upward wage pressure and outsourcing. Additionally, government spending on health care and retirement benefits will significantly affect government priorities, tax policy, the federal debt burden, and the government's ability to impact the economy through public policy. It is quite possible that the size of the overall economy could shrink, if the numbers and types of workers decrease without significant increases in individual productivity.[1–3,5,8,13,22–25]

HOUSING

The housing needs and preferences of seniors are different from younger homeowners. After retirement, many people opt to downsize to a smaller home or apartment to access home equity, to reduce the time and expense of housekeeping and maintenance, to accommodate disabling medical conditions, or to relocate to another community. If a large number of people in a particular real estate market were to make similar decisions at the same time, real estate prices would be expected to change. Regardless of such an abrupt market change, it is likely that demand will change significantly over a long period of time, resulting in changing prices and supply. Increasingly, newer homes are built incorporating the principles of "universal design," or architectural features to accommodate lifelong aging as well as the occurrence of disability. In that retrofitting (involving redesign and construction on) older homes is expensive, this has been a welcome change in home design; however, affordable housing is currently in short supply in many communities, regardless of age. Affordable housing that is also accessible for adults with disabilities is in even shorter supply. Moreover, affordable housing coupled with assistance for activities of daily living (i.e., assisted living facilities) for low-income older adults is nonexistent in many communities.

The default for many poor older adults who require even limited assistance with activities of daily living is long-term nursing facility placement because Medicaid pays for it. Figure 52.3 shows the increasing reliance on long-term care facilities to provide a residence for older adults who require assistance with their activities of daily living. Although only

1.5% of all individuals aged 65–74 years live in long-term care, this rises to nearly 25% for those older than 85. The numbers living in long-term care facilities are declining slowly but the level of disability of residents is significantly increasing. These older adults often enter long-term care facilities on a short-term basis following acute care hospitalization. They cannot, however, be discharged to the community, despite clinical improvement, because their care needs cannot be affordably met elsewhere. To avoid the demand for significant increases in nursing facility construction in the future, there must be much greater availability of affordable housing with services for older adults who require assistance with their activities of daily living. This will likely require the concerted cooperation between government at all levels and the private sector.[2–9]

GOVERNMENTAL CHANGE

If government does indeed serve the people, then the role, size, scope, and priorities of government will surely change as an aging society's needs change.

Just as older consumers have different preferences and needs, so do older voters, and the adult children who serve as caregivers for older family members. Attitudes toward taxation and spending priorities vary by age. As already evidenced in our society, an older voter on a fixed income may be both particularly concerned about paying increasing taxes and about any threatened cuts to government programs from which they benefit. Younger voters may likewise be concerned about shouldering an even bigger burden of higher taxes to support retirement programs, particularly if they do not trust that those same programs will be available for them in the future. Additionally, funding for schools and roads compete with funding for health care and housing for older adults. To the extent that families have become smaller and geographically separated, many more older adults need to rely on all levels of government to meet their basic needs of health, nutrition, safety, and security.[3–5,9,23,25–27]

FEDERAL AND STATE ENTITLEMENT PROGRAMS

A large and growing proportion of federal government spending goes to the large-scale entitlement programs that provide a variety of essential benefits to older adults – namely Social Security, Medicare, and Medicaid. As the number of Americans age 65 and older increases, the cost of each of these programs also increases. Meanwhile, the proportion of younger Americans age 65 and younger contributing to these three programs through payroll taxes is decreasing. Additionally, the amount of money paid out in benefits has grown faster than overall tax revenues or the economy has grown. Consequently, these programs represent an increasing percentage of the federal budget, and an increasing percentage of the national Gross Domestic Product. Each of these 3 programs will be discussed in greater detail below.

Social Security

When the Social Security program was developed in the 1930s, the population of the United States was much younger and life expectancy was much shorter. Relatively few people were expected to live long enough to collect any retirement benefits, and even fewer retirees would live to collect benefits for many years. In addition, for every one person collecting retirement benefits, there were more than 20 younger, working Americans paying into the system through payroll taxes. Subsequently, life expectancy has increased by more than 15 years, and the number of retirees has dramatically increased. By 1960, there were only five workers paying Social Security taxes for every Social Security beneficiary. Currently there are a little more than three workers for every beneficiary. By 2020, the number will be reduced to fewer than three workers and by 2040 to just two workers. In the next half century, barring any changes to taxes or benefits, the Social Security Trust Fund will be depleted.[2,3,8]

To prevent or forestall future insolvency of the Social Security program, a variety of proposals to raise the minimum retirement age, reduce benefits, and/or raise payroll taxes have been debated. Others have proposed partially or completely privatizing Social Security. It should be noted, however, that Social Security income represents a large proportion of overall income for most retirees. Consequently, any reduction in benefits or any threat to the stability of the program is expected to have a major and broad societal impact.[2,3,6,8,22]

Medicare

Medicare is "the" health care insurance program for Americans aged 65 and older and for the disabled. The Medicare program was developed to provide insurance coverage for seniors in response to what many economists termed a "market failure." That is, prior to Medicare's inception in the 1960s, many older Americans with chronic illnesses found themselves 'uninsurable' in the private insurance market, despite their ability to pay insurance premiums. Consequently, Medicare was developed as a program for all older adults, regardless of income or wealth. Despite concerns about the inefficiency of the large bureaucracy of the federal government, Medicare is very efficiently run compared with most private insurance companies, virtually all of which spend a substantially larger proportion of premiums on overhead compared with Medicare. In addition, Medicare has controlled costs better than the private sector. Consequently, the rate of increase in health care inflation has been much lower over the last two decades within the Medicare program when compared with the private sector. Because Medicare is very effective in controlling costs, projections about large increases in overall program costs (with the exception of Medicare Part D drug coverage) have been related more to the growth in the size of the number of beneficiaries resulting from population aging rather than to runaway health care costs. One way in which Medicare has effectively controlled spending has been to reduce and limit payments to hospitals, physicians, and other health care providers. In recent years, however, many private insurers reduced payments or eligibility for covered services even further, such that hospitals generally regard Medicare as a reliable, if not preferred payer.[13,24,25,28,29]

Changes implemented by Medicare since the late 1980s, such as the Diagnosis-related Group Prospective Payment System for hospitals have fundamentally changed health care delivery in this country, resulting in reduced hospital duration-of-stay patterns, a shift of care away from hospital settings, and tremendous growth in home health care and skilled nursing facility utilization. How much Medicare pays for a given service in a given site of care affects access to care, the location where care is provided, and even health care quality. Moreover, although Medicare has sometimes taken its lead from the private sector, such as in offering Managed Care coverage, private insurance coverage for patients of all ages is also affected by coverage decisions made by Medicare. In many respects, Medicare has served as a model that private insurers have subsequently followed. Medicare also pays to train resident physicians at teaching hospitals throughout the nation. As a result, any changes made to Medicare have the potential to affect health care delivery for everyone. As the largest of the federal entitlement programs, and with significant programmatic cost increases projected, an increase in revenues through taxation, premium increases, co-payment increases, or a reduction in benefits is inevitable.[25,28–30]

The Medicare Part D drug coverage program has extended prescription drug coverage to many and has partially privatized the Medicare program for others. The federal laws that created this program also restricted the ability of Medicare administrators to control costs by specifically prohibiting price controls on prescription drugs. Due to these restrictions, there is little doubt that the cost of the Medicare program will increase dramatically in the coming decades. The impact and fate of the Medicare Part D prescription drug program in the future are more uncertain. Some sources predict that the Medicare Part D prescription drug program will threaten the integrity of the entire Medicare program.[25,28–30]

In addition to the impact of population aging on Medicare, the future of this program will also be affected substantially if coverage is extended to younger Americans. Extending Medicare eligibility or offering 'Medicare-style' benefits to the working uninsured is one of many ideas that has been suggested by legislators, policy makers, business leaders, and others to deal with the dual crises of uninsurance affecting more than 47 million Americans, most of whom work, as well as a crisis in the current employee-sponsored insurance system, which is insufficient to provide coverage to tens of millions of uninsured working Americans. The employee-sponsored insurance system is expensive and burdensome to employers, adds to the cost of goods and services produced in this country, and is consequently seen as a threat to economic competitiveness in the global marketplace. American producers are competing with producers from other nations, virtually all of which have some sort of government-sponsored universal health care coverage.[23,24,28,31]

Medicaid

Medicaid is funded jointly by the federal and state governments. Each state has its own Medicaid program, with slightly different eligibility criteria and covered services. Medicaid pays for health services for the poor of all ages. Currently approximately 10% of older adults live in poverty with the remainder equally divided among "high," "middle," and "low" incomes. Rates of poverty vary considerably by education level, race, and sex. Approximately half of all elderly black women who live alone are poor. The projected financial status of "baby boomers" in old age is highly controversial and likely to show a wide range of financial status.[10]

Although Medicare is intended entirely for the aged and/or the disabled, Medicaid provides health care benefits to eligible Americans of all ages, and disability is not an eligibility requirement for younger beneficiaries. Medicaid programs and services for children are among the most celebrated successes since Medicaid's inception 40 years ago. Like Medicare, Medicaid programs have been very effective in controlling costs per beneficiary. Medicaid also pays for long-term nursing facility care for poor older adults. Considering that nursing facility care may cost 200 dollars per day or more, it does not take long for most Americans to become impoverished as a result of nursing facility placement. As a consequence, Medicaid has effectively become Long-Term Nursing Facility insurance for many, if not most Americans. Therefore, it is not surprising that over the last decade as the population has aged, the fastest-growing segment of Medicaid expenditures in every state is long-term facility care for older adults. As the postwar baby boom generation ages and develops diseases or impairments over the coming decades, the need for long-term nursing facility placement is expected to increase further. Medicaid spending is therefore expected to increase, affecting government spending in all 50 states as well as the federal government, unless benefits are reduced or eligibility is limited. Without a substantial increase in Medicaid spending, and perhaps even with such an increase in funding, there is the real possibility of erosion in the quality of care to nursing facility Medicaid recipients. The quality of care would suffer due to the increased number of residents and complexity of care presenting to nursing facilities, which would also have increasing limitations in the number of available staff, adequately trained staff, and financial resources.

Moreover, many expect that there will be a significant increase in the number of poor older adults with inadequate housing, care, and assistance in the community, who are unable to find or afford residential long-term care. Within the Medicaid program itself, providing long-term care to a growing older adult population will affect the provision of services to younger beneficiaries, unless overall spending increases. To continue the same Medicaid benefits for a growing older adult population will likely require increased taxation at the state and federal level or a reduction in government spending elsewhere.[3,8,23,28,32]

CAREGIVER SHORTAGES

Not only are Americans living longer, they are also healthier overall and are generally living longer before disabling medical illness occurs. Increases in health have a modifying effect on the need for assistance with daily activities as well as on hospital utilization and other aspects of health care delivery. Improvements in health and a reduction in disability rates are not of sufficient magnitude to counter the overall effects of population aging on the need for health care services or the need for paid caregivers to assist with activities of daily living such as bathing, dressing, grooming, toileting, and ambulation.[2,3,13,33]

At present, there is an overall national shortage of both nurses and physicians. There is even a greater shortage of nurses and physicians who have been specifically trained to serve the needs of older adults. There are wide geographical variations as well as more acute shortages in some communities compared with others in the same area. Likewise, the shortages are greatest among some medical specialties compared with others. In general, primary care specialties are in shortest supply, and these shortages are expected to be exacerbated substantially in the future as society ages.

It is estimated that 36,000 geriatricians will be needed in the United States by 2030. There are currently 7,128 certified geriatricians and 1,596 certified geriatric psychiatrists. The current training output of geriatricians is inadequate to reach the goal of 36,000 geriatricians by 2030. Family medicine, internal medicine, and general psychiatry are the sources of applicants for geriatric fellowship programs. Since 2003, the number of U.S. medical school graduates selecting these careers has declined. With an insufficient number of geriatricians and geriatric psychiatrists to provide direct care to all older adults, it is generally agreed that the future role of these providers will be to train other physicians and health care providers. Given the recent decline in the primary specialties providing geriatrics fellowship applicants, it is unlikely that there will be enough geriatric specialists to fulfill the training role. Because of the expense involved in training health care professionals as well as a shortage of all health care faculty, especially those teaching the care of older adults, schools of nursing and medicine are not expected to expand enough in the future to reduce disparities in health care delivery to older adults below current levels.[34-39]

Access to care is particularly problematic for older adult patients with cognitive or functional impairment who have difficulty seeking care. This population is increasing so rapidly that our current system of 'complaint'-based health care with an emphasis on the provision of care in ambulatory clinics is expected to be even more inadequate for a growing number of older adult patients who are unable to ambulate, recognize medical concerns, and/or communicate their 'complaints' to an appropriate health care provider.[13-16]

Notwithstanding society's ability or willingness to pay for more physicians, nurses, and other caregivers such as nursing assistants, it is unlikely that there will be enough professional care providers to meet the needs of all older adults who require care. This creates a number of difficult issues for society. Given the limited availability of paid caregivers, the quality of care will suffer as care providers are increasingly burdened by workload. Avoiding this degradation in health care quality will be very difficult under such circumstances. Many have asked who should be responsible for addressing this pressing societal issue. Some have suggested that immigration laws should be relaxed to allow an influx of relatively low skilled foreign workers to fill entry-level jobs as nursing assistants. It is difficult to imagine in the current political climate that immigration laws will be substantially changed in this manner. Moreover, as the shortage of paid caregivers worsens, raising or merely attempting to maintain standards through regulation, such as minimum staffing requirements for long-term care facilities will likely mean raising the quality of care for a relatively few, while limiting access to care for many others. Also there will be a shifting of the burden away from the public sector onto individuals and families, irrespective of their ability to provide or to pay for care. Placing additional burdens on families will mean that some family members will have to leave the workforce, and the productivity of others will suffer as family members miss work for caregiving emergencies. There will be a substantial effect on the economy as a whole.[3-7,9,13]

HEALTH CARE DELIVERY

Health care needs are changing, and these changes will be amplified as the population continues to age. Aging is associated with an increase in the prevalence of chronic conditions. In addition, modern medicine has succeeded in transforming what were once fatal illnesses (such as human immunodeficiency virus) into chronic diseases. The societal effect has been a significant increase in health care costs due to greater prescription drug use and costs, healthcare utilization, the complexity of medical care, and an expansion of the health care continuum. A health care system built around a model of acute management of single illnesses in isolation, either in the ambulatory or hospital setting, is now obsolete. Most acute care hospitalizations and deaths are now caused by acute exacerbations or complications of chronic disease. Much more health care is needed and must be provided in settings other than the ambulatory and hospital care settings. It is increasingly rare for the care of a single episode of illness to take place in only one site of care. Newer sites of care have been developed, such as the unfortunately named "Long-Term Acute Care Hospital." Consequently, care and communication is increasingly fragmented across multiple sites and multiple providers, creating new and greater challenges for care delivery. Hospital care is shifting toward more invasive, expensive, high-technology care in an increasingly more intensive care setting. The traditional services of the general hospital are increasingly provided in sites outside of the hospital. In the future, these services may not be provided in the hospital at all. Acute care hospitals may effectively become towers of intensive care units and complex surgery centers. Thus, the shifting of sites of care will continue. Hospital care will be deemphasized for all but the most critically ill patients.

As the nursing shortage becomes more critical, the trend toward task segmentation and 'off-loading' of historically nursing responsibilities will continue to shift toward lower skilled and lower paid employees. Likewise, the growing number of midlevel care providers is expected to increase as the physician shortage increases; however, increasing the number of nurse practitioners will decrease the number of nurses. Similarly, adding more medical schools or increasing medical school class size in an effort to increase the number of physicians will likely decease the number of prospective nurses, physical therapists, and other health care providers. One example of the impact of health care provider supply on society is found in the significant shortage of pharmacists. The shortage of pharmacists has been made especially acute in recent years due to the relative explosion in prescription drug use, a trend which is expected to continue for the foreseeable future. Substituting pharmacy technicians and technological solutions, such as robots, to ease the burden on pharmacists has played an increasingly important role in delivering more pharmacy care with a limited number of trained professionals. Legitimate concerns about patient safety exist, however, as the role of the best-trained health care provider (pharmacist) changes and their ability to provide direct oversight of care is potentially compromised.[2,3,13–16,18,30,31,33]

FAMILY RELATIONSHIPS

It has often been said that as a result of population aging, the 'family tree' is getting 'taller,' not 'wider.' That is to say that more and more children now and in the future will have the experience of knowing their grandparents as well as their great grandparents but will have fewer siblings and cousins than in past generations. The opportunity to share the collective wisdom of generations, the experience of having healthy, older relatives as role models, and the added attention that a child might experience as a result of having more older relatives and fewer age peers to compete with for their attention are all potentially positive aspects of aging families. On the other hand, the relationships within families change as individuals age and the demands on younger family members increase as their numbers decrease.[2–4,9,13]

More than 65% of those aged 65–74 live with their spouse. Single and widowed individuals also overwhelmingly live in the community. Families and others provide a tremendous amount of support to the elderly. Role reversals occur when adult children become caregivers for aging parents, particularly those with Alzheimer's disease and other conditions resulting in cognitive impairment. Significant emotional and financial stress related to care giving or financially supporting older relatives will take a heavy toll on many. Moreover, the necessity of attending to medical emergencies or other health-related crises for older family members will affect attendance at work for younger family members, which could negatively affect productivity as well as job security. Although intergenerational family groups living together in one home will likely become more common, this will increasingly require some family members to move great distances from their home or work, causing significant stress, the loss of social support, and/or income disruption, because many parents do not currently live in the same community as their adult children.

More and more adult children will experience the stress and/or joy of watching widowed parents or grandparents remarrying or entering into significant personal relationships with others, causing the perception of one's own family to change as well. Thus there is the potential for richer family relationships, strengthened family bonds, a greater respect for older generations, and a more fulfilling life through family interaction. There will, however, also be excruciatingly painful decisions for many, related to caregiving, finances, and threats to one's ego and identity as roles, relationships, needs, and abilities change throughout life.

SUMMARY

The aging of America, as well as the entire world, will have wide-ranging consequences on our society, economy, government, and our own lives, irrespective of our age. Everyone will be affected in some way by this demographic change. Untold opportunities and challenges will present themselves. A shortage of clinicians and paid caregivers will put greater strain on a health care system that many feel is already broken. Ensuring the health and welfare of our nation, including those who are most vulnerable, will require a reassessment of personal and governmental priorities. It is likely that more of the caregiver burden will be shifted to families and informal care giving networks and more of the financial burden for long-term care will shift away from government onto the private sector. Necessary increases in government spending on Social Security, Medicare, and Medicaid, even if individual benefits decrease, will result in decreased discretionary spending by state and federal governments. There will also be a greater burden on local governments and communities to meet the needs of a growing number of older adults. Cultural attitudes toward the aged will likely change – hopefully for the better but not necessarily so. Nevertheless, the opportunity for many to live longer, better lives is a real possibility. People will continue to enjoy the company of loved ones, to learn from elders, and impart that wisdom to younger generations. This is an invaluable gift which many more of us will experience and benefit from in the years to come.

REFERENCES

1. Kinsella K, Velkoff VA. An Aging World: 2001. November 2001. Washington, DC: Department of Health and Human Services; P95/01–1.
2. Gist YJ, Hetzel LI. We the People: Aging in the United States. Washington, DC: United States Census Bureau; December 2004 CENSR-19.
3. Reznik GL, Shoffner D, Weaver DA. Coping with the demographic challenge: fewer children and living longer. *Soc Secur Bull.* 2005–2006;66:37–45.
4. Eckert JK. Morgan LA. Swamy N. Preferences for receipt of care among community-dwelling adults. *J Aging Soc Policy.* 2004;16:49–65.
5. Golant SM. Political and organizational barriers to satisfying low-income U.S. seniors' need for affordable rental housing with supportive services. *J Aging Soc Policy.* 2003;15:21–48.
6. Newman S. The living conditions of elderly Americans. *Gerontologist.* 2003;43:99–109.
7. Oswald F, Wahl HW. Housing and health in later life. *Rev Environ Health.* 2004;19:223–252.
8. Burham K. Expenditures of the aged. *Soc Secur Bull.* 2007;67:45–51.
9. Kelman HR, Thomas C, Tanaka JS. Longitudinal patterns of formal and informal social support in an urban elderly population. *Soc Sci Med.* 1994;38:905–914.
10. General Interagency Forum on Aging-related Statistics. *Older American Update 2006: Key Indicators of Well-Being. Federal Interagency Forum on Aging-Related Statistics.* Washington, DC: US Government Printing Office; 2006.
11. Health Status. Available at: http://www.agingstats.gov/agingstatsdotnet/Main_Site/Data/2006_Documents/Health_Status.pdf. Accessed June 27, 2008.
12. Murphy SL. Deaths: final Data for 1998. *Natl Vital Stat Rep.* 2001;48.
13. Fleming KC, Evans JM, Chutka DS. Caregiver and clinician shortages in an aging Nation. *Mayo Clin Proc.* 2003;78:1026–1040.
14. Reuben DB, Zwanziger J, Bradley TB, et al. How many physicians will be needed to provide medical care for older persons? Physician manpower needs for the twenty-first century. *J Am Geriatr Soc.* 1993;41:444–453.
15. Cooper RA, Getzen TE, McKee HZJ, Laud P. Economic and demographic trends signal an impending physician shortage. *Health Affil.* 2002;21:140–151.
16. Chiang L. The geriatrics imperative: meeting the need for physicians trained in geriatric medicine. *JAMA.* 1998;279:1036–1037.
17. Stewart SD. Effect of changing mortality on the working life of American men and women, 1970–1990. *Soc Biol.* 1997;44:153–158.
18. Smith DW. Changing causes of death of elderly people in the United States, 1950–1990. *Gerontology.* 1998;44:331–335.
19. Hoxie RE, Rubenstein LZ. Are older pedestrians allowed enough time to cross intersections safely? *J Am Geriatr Soc.* 1994;42:241–244.
20. Langlois JA, Keyl PM, Guralnik JM, Foley DJ, Marottoli RA, Wallace RB. Characteristics of older pedestrians who have difficulty crossing the street. *Am J Public Health.* 1997;87:393–397.
21. Koepsell T, McCloskey L, Wolf M, et al. Crosswalk markings and the risk of pedestrian-motor vehicle collisions in older pedestrians. *JAMA.* 2002;288:2136–2143.
22. Ozawa MN, Yeo YH. The effect of disability on the net worth of elderly people. *J Aging Soc Policy.* 2007;19:21–38.
23. Rowland D. Medicaid: implications for the health safety net. *NEJM.* 2005;353:1439–1441.
24. Foster RS, Clemens MK. Medicare financial status, budget impact, and sustainability – which concept is which? *Health Care Financ Rev.* 2005–2006;27:127–140.
25. Davis K, Collins SR. Medicare at forty. *Health Care Financ Rev.* 2005–2006;27:53–62.
26. Turner MJ, Shields TG, Sharp D. Changes and continuities in the determinants of older adults' voter turnout 1952–1996. *Gerontologist.* 2001;41:805–818.
27. Binstock RH. Older voters and the 2004 election. *Gerontologist.* 2006;46:382–384..
28. Iglehart JK. The Centers for Medicare and Medicaid Services. *NEJM.* 2001;345:1920–1924.
29. Newhouse JP. Financing Medicare in the next administration. *NEJM.* 2004;351:1714–1716.
30. Lichtenberg FR. Sun SX. The impact of Medicare Part D on prescription drug use by the elderly. *Health Affairs.* 2007;26:1735–1744.
31. Anonymous. By the numbers. Vital statistics. *Mod Healthcare.* 2007;Suppl:78–79.
32. MetLife Mature Market Institute. The MetLife Market Survey of Nursing Home and Home Care Costs, September 2006. Available at: http://www.metlife.com/WPSAssets/21052872211163445734V1F2006 NHHCMarketSurvey.pdf. Accessed June 27, 2008.
33. National Center for Health Statistics. *Health, United States, 2007. Chartbook on Trends in the Health of Americans.* Available at: http://www.cdc.gov/nchs/hus.htm. Accessed June 27, 2008.
34. Association of Directors of Geriatric Academic Programs (ADGAP). The Status of Geriatrics Workforce Study. Fellows in Geriatric Medicine and Geriatric Psychiatry Programs. *Training and Practice Update.* 2007;5:3–5.
35. Alliance for Aging Research. *Ten Reasons Why America is Not Ready for the Coming Age Boom.* Washington, DC: Alliance for Aging Research; 2002.
36. Association of Directors of Geriatric Academic Programs (ADGAP). Status of Geriatrics Workforce Study. Figures 1.4 and 1.8. Available at: http://www.ADGAPstudy.uc.edu. Accessed June 27, 2008.
37. Graduate medical education tables. *JAMA.* 2003;290:1234–1248.
38. Graduate medical education tables. *JAMA.* 2006;296:1154–1169.
39. Graduate medical education tables. *JAMA.* 2007;298:1081–1096.

53

ETHNOGERIATRICS

Fred Kobylarz, MD, MPH, Gwen Yeo, PhD

ETHNIC, RACIAL, AND CULTURAL ASPECTS OF HEALTH CARE FOR OLDER ADULTS

Introduction and Demographics

Because effective geriatric care is heavily influenced by cultural beliefs and practices of elders and their family members and the differential health risks of specific populations, any comprehensive discussion of geriatrics needs to include the recognition of the growing ethnic and racial diversity* of America's older population. One measure of the growing diversity is the projection that elders from populations described as ethnic and racial minorities will grow from 18% to 39% of all older Americans by mid-century.

Table 53.1 summarizes the projected increases in ethnic and racial minorities of older adults aged 65 years and older by race and Hispanic origin. These projections, however, drastically understate the cultural diversity that geriatric providers will increasingly face because within each of these categories there is great heterogeneity, for example, the rapidly increasing population of Asian American elders include immigrants from more than 30 countries with very different cultures, and the non-Hispanic white category includes elders from the diverse Middle Eastern and eastern European countries as well as those from western European ancestry. Then within each of the ethnic and racial populations, there are vast differences in acculturation levels to the mainstream society, English language proficiency, educational and occupational backgrounds, income, religion, and family structure; all of which effect their interactions and expectations with health care providers.

So, how can geriatric team members attempt to work effectively in the face of such growing diversity? Part of the solution is knowing as much as possible about the background of the elders

and their families the providers are likely to see, which may be challenging in very diverse regions. In addition, knowing some basic techniques to establish trust and to elicit the information needed for appropriate care and methods of adapting clinical behavior to meet the patients' needs increases the probability of a positive therapeutic relationship. This chapter will attempt to provide some resources for both efforts.

As background for providers, Table 53.2 summarizes some of the clinically relevant characteristics of elders from the larger ethnic populations. Of note are groups with high proportions of less educated elders, which would make their risk of low health literacy greater and their ability to use written health promotion materials, even in their native language, less. These individuals include those from Vietnamese, Chinese, and Mexican backgrounds; in fact in one large population-based study of older Mexican Americans in 1998–1999, 22% of those whose primary language was Spanish had zero years of school.[1] Among older Korean Americans, women are particularly educationally disadvantaged; their proportion with less than nine years of school is three times that of older men.

Noting the populations with large percentages who speak little or no English allows providers to be aware of the need to have professionally trained interpreters available for appointments with patients from those groups. Limited English proficiency is frequently associated with elders who are not highly acculturated to the mainstream American society and probably American health care as well, and they may be more accustomed to nonwestern medical practices common in their countries of origin. More than 80% of elders in all the Asian subgroups except Japanese Americans were born outside the United States.[2]

A particularly economically disadvantaged group is older Black women living alone, 40% of whom have incomes below poverty.[3] Among those patients, transportation and other access issues may be barriers to adequate care.

---

* In this chapter, the term race is used to mean the socially constructed categories commonly used in the United States and not to imply that there are significant biological differences between population groups.

Table 53.1. U.S. Population Aged 65 Years and Older by Race and Hispanic Origin, 2004 and Projected 2050

Race and Hispanic Origin	2003 Estimates		2050 Projections	
	No.	Percent	No.	Percent
Total older population	36,293,985		86,705,637	
Nonhispanic White alone	29,732,252	81.9	53,259,961	61.3
Black/African American alone	3,046,896	8.4	10,401,575	12.0
Asian alone	1,048,030	2.9	6,776,033	7.8
All other races alone or in combination	429,464	1.2	2,326,390	2.7
Hispanic/Latino (of any race)	2,164,987	6.0	15,178,025	17.5

Source: U.S. Census Bureau, Population Estimates and Projections 2004; Federal Interagency Forum on Aging Related Statistics.

Table 53.2. Selected Demographic and Background Characteristics of the Larger Populations of Elders (65+ Years) from Diverse Ethnic Populations in the U.S.: U.S. Census, 2000 and 2004[a]

Demographic	Percent in Poverty	Living Alone %Men/%Women	Education ≤9 yr/ ≥High School	%Speak Little or No English[b]
Total population	9.8	18.8/39.7	*16.8/73.1*	*4.0*
Nonhispanic White[c]	7.5	18.7/41.1	*12.9/78.0*	*1.2*
Black/African American[c]	23.9	26.6/41.4	*30.6/52.5*	*1.2*
Hispanic/Latino	18.7	15.7/24.8	*51.1/37.6*	*38.4*
Mexican		*19.1/12.0*	*59.0/25.1*	*35.1*
Asian[c]	13.6	9.9/26.7	*30.9/64.8*	*40.0*
Chinese	*16.2*	*8.7/18.9*	*40.0/49.9*	*60.0*
Filipino	*8.4*	*4.4/8.6*	*29.5/60.5*	*22.6*
Japanese	*5.6*	*13.8/26.0*	*11.3/75.9*	*10.7*
Korean	*22.1*	*8.8/26.2*	*31.7/55.0*	*63.9*
Asian Indian	*9.1*	*6.0/6.9*	*31.6/54.1*	*35.4*
Vietnamese	*16.0*	*6.7/8.0*	*47.2/32.4*	*73.5*
American Indian/Alaska Native	23.5	19.4/28.4	*36.6/41.9*	*11.2*

[a] Figures in *italics* were compiled by the author (GY) from U.S. Census, 2000, Summary Files 1, 2, and 4; others are from 2004 based on Current Population Survey, Annual Social and Economic Supplement, 2005 as reported in the Older Americans Update, 2006.
[b] From responses reported as "Speak English not well" and "Speak English not at all."
[c] Alone (as opposed to in combination with other races) particularly educationally disadvantaged; their proportion with less than 9 years of school is three times that of the older men.

Causes of Death

Overall, older Black Americans experience much poorer health than Whites. According to Cohen, for Black Americans, age-adjusted death rates are 33% higher than for Whites. In contrast, for other ethnic and racial groups, age-adjusted death rates are lower than the comparable rates for Whites. For Hispanics, age-adjusted death rates are 22% lower than for non-Hispanic Whites. For American Indian/Alaskan Native and Asian and Pacific Islander groups, age-adjusted death rates are also lower than for non-Hispanic Whites.[4]

Table 53.3 summarizes the top five leading causes of death for those aged 65 and older in the four major ethnic and racial categories for the past two decades.[5] Of note, leading causes of death are heart disease and cancer in all groups.

According to National Center for Health Statistics data, among the youngest age group, 65–74 years of age, cancer is as common as heart disease; however, it decreases in importance with age, ranking third among women 85 years of age and older. The third leading cause of death is stroke for most groups except American Indians for whom diabetes is in third place.

Table 53.3. Leading Causes of Death for Persons 65 Years of Age and Older

White	Black/African Americans	American Indian	Asian or Pacific Islander	Hispanics
Heart disease	Heart disease	Heart disease	Heart disease	Heart disease
Cancer	Cancer	Cancer	Cancer	Cancer
Stroke	Stroke	Diabetes	Stroke	Stroke
COPD	Diabetes	Stroke	Pneumonia/influenza	COPD
Pneumonia/Influenza	Pneumonia/influenza	COPD	COPD	Pneumonia/influenza

Source: Trends in causes of death among the elderly. Aging Trends; No.1. Hyattsville, Maryland: National Center for Health Statistics. 2001.

Among White men and women 65–74 years of age, the third leading cause of death is chronic obstructive pulmonary disease (COPD) and other chronic respiratory disease.

Alzheimer's disease and renal disease have gained importance as causes of death among the elderly in the past two decades. Alzheimer's disease is now among the 10 leading causes of death for older White persons but not for other ethnic and racial groups. Renal disease ranks between the 6th and 10th leading cause of death and is more common in Blacks than Whites. Pneumonia and influenza also remain among the top five causes of death and has increased in recent years for all age, race, and -sex groups.

Significant trends worth noting in death rates among ethnic and racial groups have also occurred over the past two decades.[6] Heart disease decreased at a slower rate for Blacks than for Whites (20% vs. 37% for ages 65–74 years; 16% vs. 32% for ages 75–84 years; and 8% vs. 18% for ages 85+ years). Stroke followed a similar pattern with the decrease more moderate for the Black population. Hypertension death rates declined among older White men (75–84 and 85+ years) but dramatically increased among older Black men. Similarly, death from hypertension increased among older White women; however, the increase was much greater among older Black women.

Other trends worth noting include rates of cancer death. Over the past 10 years, there has been an overall downward trend among White men 65–74 (3%) and 75–84 years of age (6%) and among Black men 65–74 (9%) and 75–84 years of age (2%). This trend varied by type of cancer. For example, lung cancer has decreased in White men 65–84 years of age; however, it increased among Black men, the oldest old, and all women. Breast cancer has increased in the oldest group of both White and Black women older than 75 years of age. Prostate cancer rates remain higher in Black than White groups.[7]

Pharmacotherapy

Literature from the 1990s suggests that there may be population-based differences in response to some medications. Thiazide diuretics and calcium channel blockers were found to be more effective in treating hypertension in African Americans than were β-blockers.[8,9] Regarding heart disease, BiDiL®, a combination of isosorbide and hydralazine provoked controversy in 2005 as the first drug approved for a single-race group (Black/African Americans) in the treatment of congestive heart failure.[10]

National Institute of Mental Health-funded Research Center on the Psychobiology of Ethnicity reviews of research on ethnic differences in response to specific types of drugs report that among Chinese, Japanese, Korean, and Vietnamese patients, smaller doses of tricyclic antidepressants than usually used to treat depression in Caucasian patients may be effective. Mean dosage levels of benzodiazepines for Asian patients were one half to two thirds that of their Caucasian counterparts in a survey of American and Canadian clinicians. Studies of haloperidol showed 40%–50% higher plasma concentrations for Chinese than non-Chinese patients with similar doses. Some studies have attributed the differences to slower metabolism among some Asian patients.[11] This suggests the increased importance of the geriatric pharmacotherapy adage "start low and go slow" among Asian populations.

Complimentary and alternative medicine therapies are increasingly used in older American populations in general and are especially likely to be used by elders less acculturated to the U.S. health care system from countries with long traditions of herbal medication use.[12–14] The most common practice reported is use of both Western biomedical pharmaceuticals and culture-specific alternative medicines, which are not reported unless specifically queried by the provider.[13] In a recent survey of older adults, Asian elders have significantly greater odds than other racial and ethnic groups of using any complimentary and alternative medicine.[15]

Select Diseases

It is beyond the scope of this chapter to discuss the differential prevalence of individual diseases among different racial and ethnic populations in detail. As an example, the short summary below focuses on dementia.

Dementia

No national data sets on the prevalence of dementia in the United States are available. Rather, much of what we know about the prevalence of dementia in racial and ethnic groups in the United States is based on population studies in specific communities. Analysis of these data are difficult because of lack

Table 53.4. Components of the ETHNICS Mnemonic

E: Explanation	Why do you think you have this (use patient's phrase for his or her) symptom/illness/condition?
T: Treatment	What have you tried for this (use patient's phrase for his or her) symptom/illness/condition?
H: Healers	Who else have you sought help from for this (use patient's phrase for his or her) symptom/illness/condition?
N: Negotiate	How best do you think I can help you?
I: Intervention	This is what I think needs to be done now.
C: Collaborate	How can we work together on this and who else should be included?
S: Spirituality	What role does faith/religion/spirituality play in helping you with this (use patient's phrase for his or her) symptom/ illness/ condition?

Adapted from Kobylarz FA, Heath JM, Like RC. The ETHNICS Mnemonic: A clinical tool for ethnogeriatric education. *J Am Geriatr Soc.* 2002;50:1582–1589.[20]

Table 53.5. Components of the SPEAK Mnemonic

S: Speech	How will the health care provider's speech be received by the patient and/or caregiver?
P: Perception	How will the patient and/or caregiver perceive both the verbal and written content during the communication with the health care provider?
E: Education	What is the education level of the patient and/or caregiver?
A: Access	How will the clinical encounter provide for a respectful and safe environment?
K: Knowledge	How will assessment of health literacy be carried out, and what tools will be used?

Adapted from Kobylarz, FA, Pomidor A, Heath JM. SPEAK Mnemonic: A Clinical Tool for Health Literacy in Geriatric Clinical Encounters. *Geriatrics.* 2006;61:20–27.[26]

of comparability, eligibility criteria, and different measures of dementia. Some populations have many available data sets, whereas Asian subpopulations other than Japanese and American Indian subgroups in the United States are completely devoid of data on dementia prevalence.

According to Yeo, most, but not all, of the available studies have found that Blacks have higher dementia rates than whites. Significantly higher rates of vascular dementia were found among Black populations. Among the Hispanic/Latino populations, Dominican and Puerto Rican elders had higher rates of Alzheimer's disease than non-Hispanic Whites. Among Mexican Americans, rates of dementia were reported to be similar to those for non-Latino Whites. Among Japanese Americans, rates of Alzheimer's disease were found to be the same as studies of Whites, but rates of vascular dementia were much higher in Hawaii. Other studies in Japan and some Asian countries also found higher rates of vascular dementia.[16]

Cross-Cultural Communication

Cultural and linguistic competence is an essential component of providing health care to older adult patients. Once cultural differences are recognized by geriatric providers and the need to elicit additional information is determined, explanatory model frameworks can be utilized to facilitate communication.[17–19] Table 53.4 provides an example of a useful and practical cross-cultural interviewing tool in the form of questions for geriatric providers, the mnemonic ETHNICS (explanation, treatment, healers, negotiate, intervention, collaborate, and spirituality).[20] Other considerations include health literacy issues such as education level, overcoming sensory impairments in either vision or hearing that impact communication, and sensitivity to nonverbal communication techniques that

can greatly influence cultural perceptions of touch, eye contact, facial expression, and vocal tone between patient and health care provider. Simple technologies such as the use of an assistive listening device for hearing-impaired individuals without their own hearing aides and the availability of the mental status assessments, geriatric depression scale, and other common geriatric "tools" in languages other than English (and preferably validated on the population being cared for) can also add to the effective cross-cultural communication. Simple but effective strategies such as addressing elders by their last name in a formal and polite manner will also show respect and help to establish a trusting relationship, and even more effective is using culturally specific strategies to show respect, especially because respecting elders is an important value in many cultures.[21,22]

Health Literacy

The Institute of Medicine report, Health Literacy: A Prescription to End Confusion, defines health literacy as the degree to which individuals have the capacity to obtain, process, and understand basic health information and services needed to make appropriate decisions.[23] This definition encompasses components beyond the immediate communication elements of speaking, reading, and writing to include educational attainment, culture of origin and acculturation, and health care systems level institutional issues, which are often less likely to be considered during patient care. Low health literacy is a significant barrier to achieving effective care and most adversely affects the elderly and racial and ethnic minorities seeking health care.[24] Consequences may include less health knowledge, poorer health status, high rates of health services use and costs, and decreased patient safety, including errors in self-administration of medications.[25]

Geriatric providers can enhance the effectiveness and efficiency of the care they provide by recognizing their patient's health literacy. Table 53.5 provides a useful tool in the form of questions that health care providers can ask themselves to improve the care of elders they suspect have limited health literacy.[26] In addition, the American Medical Association, National Institute on Aging, and American College of Physicians Foundation have developed initial communication and health literacy materials.[27–29] It should be recognized that the assessment of the level of health literacy is especially difficult when providers and patients do not speak the same language and when the expectations of the clinical encounter may differ because of different cultural perceptions.

INTERPRETERS

Studies on the use of professional interpreters have shown positive benefits on communication (errors and comprehension), utilization, clinical outcomes, and satisfaction with care.[30] Geriatric providers caring for older adults from diverse racial and ethnic populations should be aware of language barriers among patients and their caregivers during clinical encounters and seek to remove them if possible. In 2000, the United States Census Bureau report revealed that approximately 7% of persons 65 years or older did not speak English, and in some ethnic populations, more than 70% of elders speak little or no English (Table 53.2).[31,32]

In caring for non-English proficient or limited-English proficient patients, geriatric providers should be aware of recent federal requirements regarding appropriate language assistance options and interpreters, which should be accessed during clinical encounters. The National Standards on Culturally and Linguistically Appropriate Services in Health Care guidelines state, "health care organizations must offer and provide language assistance services, including bilingual staff and interpreter services, at no cost to each patient/consumer with limited English proficiency at all points of contact, in a timely manner during all hours of operation."[33] The Office for Civil Rights policy discusses acceptable language assistance options that can be used when caring for limited-English proficient patients.[34] With respect to interpreters, providers should be aware of the recent guidelines for The National Standards of Practice for Healthcare Interpreters and the American Geriatrics Society.[35,36] In cases in which there can be no trained interpreters available in person for a specific language, health care organizations are encouraged to provide clinicians technology allowing remote access, such as telephonic language banks, video interpreting, or remote simultaneous interpreting.[37] Although the practice of using younger family members to interpret for monolingual non-English speaking elders is very common in geriatric care, the practice can result in censored or inaccurate information. Serious clinical omissions or mistakes can result from incomplete or inaccurate translations due to the family member's insufficient vocabulary in one of the languages or to censoring of personally uncomfortable or culturally inappropriate material. This is especially likely to occur in cases of potential elder abuse or when cultural norms of modesty discourage the discussion of issues such as genitourinary problems in the

Table 53.6. Components of the TRANSLATE Mnemonic

T: Trust	How will trust be developed in the patient-clinician-interpreter triadic relationship? In relationships with the patient's family and other health care professionals?
R: Roles	What role(s) will the interpreter play in the clinical care process (e.g., language translator, culture broker/informant, culture broker/interpreter of biomedical culture, advocate)?
A: Advocacy	How will advocacy and support for patient- and family-centered care occur? How will power and loyalty issues be handled?
N: Nonjudgmental Attitude	How can a nonjudgmental attitude be maintained during health care encounters? How will personal beliefs, values, opinions, biases, and stereotypes be dealt with?
S: Setting	Where and how will medical interpretation occur during health care encounters (e.g., use of salaried interpreters, contract interpreters, volunteers, or telephonic interpreter services)?
L: Language	What methods of communication will be used? How will linguistic appropriateness and competence be assessed?
A: Accuracy	How will knowledge and information be exchanged in an accurate, thorough, and complete manner during health care encounters?
T: Time	How will time be appropriately managed during health care encounters?
E: Ethical Issues	How will potential ethical conflicts be handled during health care encounters? How will confidentiality of clinical information be maintained?

Adapted from Levin SJ, Like RC, Gottlieb JE. 2000. "Appendix: Useful Clinical Interviewing Mnemonics." Patient Care Special Issue, "Caring for Diverse Populations: Breaking Down Barriers," May 15, 2000, p. 189.[38]

presence of certain family members. Use of minor children as health interpreters can be especially traumatic and is highly discouraged. Table 53.6 provides a useful tool for working with medical interpreters.[38]

End of Life

Caring for terminally ill older patients entails encountering diverse beliefs from many cultures held by family members about what constitutes a "good death," under what circumstances an elder should be allowed to die, and whether or not to prolong life.[39] In some cases, historical experience of severe discrimination in health care (e.g., among African Americans, especially related to the Tuskegee experiment) or attempted annihilation (e.g., American Indians) has resulted in distrust of providers' decision making around treatment at the end of life.

Family decision making is the norm in many Asian and Latino families so this becomes critical in end-of-life situations.[40,41] In some cases, a certain member of the family is culturally designated as the decision maker related to treatment of the older patient, but that member may live in another city or even in another country. It might include, for example, the oldest son, the oldest male relative, an extended family leader, or a clan or religious leader. If at all possible, before older adults become severely ill, it is very helpful to have private conversations with them in which they can express their preferences for decisions and decision makers. In some cases, however (e.g., Chinese and Navajo), the cultural norms do not favor the direct discussion of death itself, so indirect references need to be used.[42,43]

It is not uncommon for health care providers to encounter pleas from family members, especially those from some Asian backgrounds, not to tell their parents that they are terminally ill or that they have cancer because it might lead to their giving up hope. Providers then feel conflicted between these requests to honor the filial respect of the family members and their obligation to the autonomy of their older patients. Prior conversations asking elders how much they would like to know if they have a serious condition would be helpful in resolving these dilemmas.

In end-of-life issues, geriatric health care providers need to make every effort to recognize the uniqueness of both the individuals they care for and their cultural backgrounds,[44] although this frequently involves considerable clinical complexity. In managing that complexity of cross-cultural end-of-life care, a major support for health care providers can be cultural guides or cultural brokers. Locating religious or cultural leaders from their patients' background who are bilingual and understand both the patients' and the providers' health care cultures can be invaluable resources in critical times when patients are facing death.

REFERENCES

1. Haan MN, Mungas DM, Gonzalez HM, et al. Prevalence of dementia in older Latinos: the influence of type 2 diabetes mellitus, stroke, and genetic factors. *J Ame Geriatr Soc.* 2003;51:169–177.

2. Yeo G, Hikoyeda N. Asian and pacific island elders. In: Schulz R, Noelker LS, Rockwood K, Sprott R, eds. *Encyclopedia of Aging.* 4th ed. New York: Springer; 2006.

3. Federal Interagency Forum on Aging Related Statistics. Older Americans Update 2006: Key Indicators of Well-Being. Available at http://www.agingstats.gov/Agingstatsdotnet/Main_Site/Data/2006_Documents/OA_2006.pdf. Accessed July 2008.

4. Cohen B. Introduction. In Anderson BN, Bulatao RA, Cohen B, eds. *Critical Perspectives on Racial and Ethnic Differences in Health in Later Life.* Washington, DC: National Academic Press; 2004:1–22.

5. Heron MP, Smith BL. Deaths: Leading causes for 2003. National vital statistics reports. Hyattsville, MD. National Center for Health Statistics. Available at: http://www.cdc.gov/nchs/products/pubs/pubd/hestats/leadingdeaths03/leadingdeaths03.htm#ref1. Accessed June 27, 2008.

6. Sahyoun RN, Lentzner H, Hoyert D, Robinson KN. Trends in Causes of Death Among Elderly. Aging Trends No. 1 Center For Disease Control and Prevention. March 2001. Available at www.cdc.gov/nchs/data/ahcd/agingtrends/01death.pdf. Accessed July 2008.

7. Peters N, Armstrong K. Racial differences in prostate cancer treatment outcomes: a systematic review. *Cancer Nurs.* 2005;28:108–118.

8. Francis CK. Hypertension and cardiac disease in minorities. *Am J Med.* 1990;88:3B–3S.

9. Moser M. Hypertension treatment results in minority patients. *Am J Med.* 1990;88:24S–31S.

10. Brody H, Hunt LM. BiDil: Assessing a race-based pharmaceutical. *Ann Fam Med.* 2006;4:556–560.

11. Lin K-M, Poland RE, Nakasaki, G, eds. *Psychopharmacology and Psychobiology of Ethnicity.* Washington, DC: American Psychiatry Press, 1993.

12. Sternberg SA, Chandran A, Sikka, M. Alternative therapy use by elderly African americans attending a community clinic. *J Am Geriatr Soc.* 2003;51:1768–1772.

13. McBride MR, Morioka-Douglas N. Yeo G. *Aging and Health: Asian and Pacific Islander American Elders.* 2nd ed. SGEC Working Paper Series 3. Stanford, CA: Stanford Geriatric Education Center; 1996.

14. National Center for Complementary and Alternative Medicine. Complementary and Alternative Medicine Usage in the United States. Available at: http://nccam.nih.gov/news/camsurvey_fs1.htm. Accessed July 2008.

15. Arcury TA, Suerken CK, Grwacz JG, et al. Complementary and alternative medicine use among older adults: ethnic variation. *Ethn Dis.* 2006;16:723–731.

16. Yeo G. Prevalence of dementia among ethnic populations. In: Yeo G, Gallagher-Thompson D, eds. *Ethnicity and the Dementias.* 2nd ed. New York: Taylor and Francis; 2006:3–9.

17. Kleinman A, Eisenberg L, Good B. Culture, illness and care: clinical lessons from anthropologic and cross-cultural research. *Ann Intern Med.* 1978;88:251–258.

18. Berlin EA, Fowkes WC. A teaching framework for cross-cultural health care. *West J Med.* 1982;139:934–938.

19. Stuart MR, Lieberman JA III. *The Fifteen-Minute Hour: Applied Psychotherapy for the Primary Care Physician.* 2nd ed. New York: Praeger; 1993.

20. Kobylarz FA, Heath JM, Like RC. The ETHNICS mnemonic: a clinical tool for ethnogeriatric education. *J Am Geriatr Soc.* 2002;50:1582–1589.

21. Adler RN, Kamel HK, eds. *Doorway Thoughts: Cross-Cultural Health Care for Older Adults.* American Geriatrics Society, Vol. 1. Sudbury MA: Jones and Bartlett Publishers; 2004.

22. Adler RN, ed. *Doorway Thoughts: Cross-Cultural Health Care for Older Adults.* American Geriatrics Society, Vol. 2. Sudbury MA: Jones and Bartlett Publishers; 2006.

23. Institute of Medicine. *Health Literacy: A Prescription to End Confusion.* Washington, DC: National Academic Press; 2004.

24. Berkman ND, DeWalt DA, Pignone MP, et al. *Literacy and Health Outcomes. Evidence Report/Technology Assessment No. 87.* (Prepared by RTI International. University of North Carolina Evidence-based Practice Center under Contract No. 290-02- 0016). AHRQ Publication No. 04-E007–2. Rockville, MD: Agency for Healthcare Research and Quality; 2004.

25. Weiss BD. Epidemiology of low literacy. In: Schwartzberg JG, VanGeest, JB, Wang CC, eds. *Understanding Health Literacy: Implications for Medicine and Public Health.* Chicago, IL: American Medical Association Press; 2004:17–42.

26. Kobylarz FA, Pomidor A, Heath JM. SPEAK mnemonic: a clinical tool for health literacy in geriatric clinical encounters. *Geriatrics.* 2006;61: 20–27.

27. Weiss BD. Health literacy: A manual for clinicians. In: *Health Literacy: Help your Patients Understand.* A multimedia program for health professionals. Chicago, IL: American Medical Association Foundation and AMA; 2003.

28. National Institute on Aging. A Guide for Older People: Talking with Your Doctor. Available at: http://www.niapublications. org/pubs/talking/index.asp. Accessed June 27, 2008.

29. American College of Physicians Health Literacy Solutions. Available at: http://foundation.acponline.org/health_lit.htm. Accessed June 27, 2008.

30. Karliner LS, Jacobs EA, Chen AH, Mutha S. Do professional interpreters improve clinical care for patients with limited English proficiency? A Systematic Review of the Literature. Health Research and Educational Trust. *Health Serv Res.* 2007 Apr;42(2): 727–754.

31. Census Report Language Use and English-Speaking Ability: Census 2000 Brief C2KBR-29. 2003. Available at: http://www. census.gov/prod/2003pubs/c2kbr-29.pdf. Accessed June 27, 2008.

32. U.S. Census Bureau, Census 2000 Summary File 4. Available at http://www.census.gov/Press-Release/www/2003/SF4.html.

33. *Federal Register. National Standards on Culturally and Linguistically Appropriate Services in Health Care.* Washington, DC; Office of Minority Health. 2000;65:80865–80879. Available at: http://www.omhrc.gov/clas. Accessed June 27, 2008.

34. Federal Register. Policy Guidance: Title VI Prohibition Against National Origin Discrimination as it Affects Persons with Limited English Proficiency. Washington, DC: Office of Civil Rights. 2000;65:52762. Available at: http://www.hhs.gov/ocr/lep/ guide.html. Accessed June 27, 2008.

35. National Standards of Practice for Health Care Interpreters September 2005. Available at http://www.ncihc.org/mc/page. do?sitePageId=57768&orgId=ncihc.

36. American Geriatrics Society. Use of Interpreters During Clinical Encounters Position Paper. Available at: http://www. americangeriatrics.org/products/positionpapers/interpreter_ 022307.shtml. Accessed June 27, 2008.

37. Roat CE. Addressing Language Access Issues in Your Practice: A Toolkit for Physicians and their Staff Members. California Academy of Family Physicians and CAFP Foundation. 2005. Available at: http://www.familydocs.org/news-media/toolkits. php.

38. Levin SJ, Like RC, Gottlieb JE. 2000. "Appendix: useful clinical interviewing mnemonics." *Patient Care.* 2000;34:188–189.

39. Braun KL, Pietsch JH, Blanchette PL, eds. *Cultural Issues in End-of-Life Decision Making.* Thousand Oaks, CA: Sage Publications;2000.

40. Mouton C. Cultural and religious issues for African Americans. In: Braun KL, Pietsch JH, Blanchette PL, eds. *Cultural Issues in End-of-Life Decision Making.* Thousand Oaks, CA: Sage Publications; 2000:71–82.

41. Talmantes MA, Gomez C, Braun KL. Advance directives and end-of-life care: the Hispanic perspective. In: Braun KL, Pietsch JH, Blanchette PL, eds. *Cultural Issues in End-of-Life Decision Making.* Thousand Oaks, CA: Sage Publications; 2000:83–100.

42. Yeo G, Hikoyeda N. Cultural issues in end-of-life decision Mmaking among Asians and Pacific Islanders in the United States. In: Braun KL, Pietsch JH, Blanchette PL, eds. *Cultural Issues in End-of-Life Decision Making.* Thousand Oaks, CA: Sage Publications; 2000:101–125.

43. Westlake Van Winkle. N. End-of-life decision making in American Indian and Alaska Native cultures. In: Braun KL, Pietsch JH, Blanchette PL, eds. *Cultural Issues in End-of-Life Decision Making.* Thousand Oaks, CA: Sage Publications; 2000:127–144.

44. Searight RH, Gafford J. Cultural diversity at the end of life: issues and guidelines for family physicians. *Am Fam Physician.* 2005;71:515–22.

ETHNOGERIATRICS – SELECTED RESOURCES

Articles and Books

Adler RN, Kamel HK, eds. *Doorway Thoughts: Cross-Cultural Health Care for Older Adults.* American Geriatrics Society, Vol. 1. Sudbury MA: Jones and Bartlett Publishers; 2004.Adler RN, ed. *Doorway Thoughts: Cross-Cultural Health Care for Older Adults.* American Geriatrics Society, Vol. 2. Sudbury MA: Jones and Bartlett Publishers; 2006.Curry L, Jackson J. *The Science of Inclusion: Recruiting and Retaining Racial and Ethnic Elders in Health Research.* Washington, DC: Gerontological Society of America; 2003.

Duffy SA, Jackson FC, Schim SM, Ronis DL, Fowler KE. Racial/ethnic preferences, sex preferences, and perceived discrimination related to end-of-life are. *J Am Geriatr Soc.* 2006;54:150–157.

Ferris M. Racial disparities in health care for elderly. *Geriatr Times.* 2000; I. Available at: http://www.geriatrictimes.com/ g001209.html.

Gallagher-Thompson D. Development and implementation of intervention strategies for culturally diverse caregiving populations. In: Schulz R, ed. *Handbook on Dementia Caregiving.* New York: Springer; 2000:151–183.

Gornick ME, Eggers PW, Reilly TW, et al. Effects of race and income on mortality and use of services among medicare beneficiaries. *NEJM.* 1996;335:791–799.

Hallenback J, Goldstein M, Mebane EW. Cultural considerations of death and dying in the United States. *Clin Geriatr Med.* 1996;12:393–406.

Hayes-Bautista D, Hsu P, Perez A, Gamboa C. The 'browning' of the graying of America: diversity in the elderly population and policy implications. *Generations.* 2002;26:15–24.

Kagawa-Singer M, Blackhall LJ. Negotiating cross-cultural issues at the end of life. 'You've got to go where he lives.' *JAMA.* 2001;286:2993–3001.

Kobylarz FA, Heath JM, Like RC. The ETHNICS mnemonic: a clinical tool for ethnogeriatric education. *J Am Geriatr Soc.* 2002;50:1582–1589.

Kobylarz FA, Pomidor A, Heath JM. SPEAK mnemonic: a clinical tool for health literacy in geriatric clinical encounters. *Geriatrics.* 2006;61:20–27.

McBride M, Lewis, I. African American and Asian American elders: an ethnogeriatric perspective. *Ann Rev Nurs Res.* 2004;22:161–214.

Miles T. Ethnogeriatrics comes of age. *J Am Geriatr Soc.* 2001;49:995.

Moldm F, Fitzpatrick J, Roberts J. Minority ethnic elders in care homes: a review of the literature. *Age Ageing.* 2005;34:107–113.

Stahl S, Vasquez L. Approaches to improving recruitment and retention of minority elders participating in research. *J Aging Health.* 2004;16(Suppl5):9S–17S.

Takeshita J, Ahmed I. (2004). Culture and geriatric psychiatry. In: Tseng WS, Streltzer J, eds. *Cultural Competence in Clinical*

Psychiatry Washington, DC: American Psychiatric Association; 2004:147–161.

Smedley BD, Stith AY, Nelson AR. Institute of Medicine, Committee on Understanding and Eliminating Racial and Ethnic Disparities in Health Care. *Unequal Treatment: Confronting Racial and Ethnic Disparities in Health Care.* Washington, DC: National Academy Press; 2003.

Xakellis G, Brangman S, Hinton WL, et al. Curricular framework: core Ccompetencies in multicultural geriatric care. *J Am Geriatr Soc.* 2004;52:137–142.

Valle R. Culturally attuned recruitment, retention, and adherence in Alzheimer disease and associated disorders: a best practices working model. *Alzheimer Dis Assoc Dis.* 2005;19:261–266.

Valle R. *Caregiving Across Cultures with Dementia Illness and Ethnically Diverse Populations.* Washington, DC: Taylor & Francis; 1996.

Yeo G, Gallagher-Thompson D. *Ethnicity and the Dementias.* Washington, DC: Taylor and Francis 1996

Yeo G, Gallagher-Thompson D. *Ethnicity and the Dementias.* 2nd ed. Washington, DC: Taylor & Francis; 2006.

Websites

Alzheimer's Association's Diversity Toolbox
www.alz.org/alzheimers_disease_caring_for_diverse_populations.asp.

American Geriatrics Society – Position Statement on Ethnogeriatrics, Prepared by the Ethnogeriatrics Committee
www.americangeriatrics.org/staging/products/positionpapers/ethno_committee.shtml.

American Geriatrics Society – Position Statement on Interpreters, Prepared by the Ethnogeriatrics Committee
www.americangeriatrics.org/products/positionpapers/interpreter_022307.shtml.

American Academy of Hospice and Palliative Medicine
www.aahpm.org/cgi-bin/wkcgi/browse?category=article&section=CC.

Administration on Aging – Addressing Diversity
www.aoa.gov/prof/adddiv/adddiv.asp.

BIBLIOGRAPHY IN ETHNOGERONTOLOGY

culturedmed.sunyit.edu/bib/ethnogerontology/index.html

Core Curriculum in Ethnogeriatrics. Gwen Yeo, PhD, et al. Developed by the Members of the Collaborative on Ethnogeriatric Education, Supported by the Bureau of Health Professions, Health Resources and Services Administration, USDHHS, October 2000
www.stanford.edu/dept/medfm/ebooks/intro.pdf.

Cultural Competency for Health Professionals in Geriatric Care

Western Reserve Geriatric Education Center

www.nethealthinc.com/cultural/index.asp.

Culture & End-of-Life Care (Phase I e-learning course), Talaria Inc.
elearning.talariainc.com/pageview.asp?pagekey = 4052.

Cross-Cultural Resources. Focus: Death and Dying. Cross-Cultural Health Care Program, Seattle, Washington
ethnomed.org/clin_topics/cchcp/CCRHFeb2003_rev.pdf.

Ethnic Elders Care

www.ethnicelderscare.net/.

GeroNurseOnline.org

Select topic: Ethnogeriatrics and Cultural Competence
www.geronurseonline.org/.

National Asian Pacific Center on Aging
www.napca.org.

National Caucus and Center on Black Aged
www.ncba-aged.org/.

National Hispanic Council on Aging, Inc.
www.nhcoa.org.

National Indian Council on Aging
www.nicoa.org.

54

RETIREMENT

Gordon F. Streib, PhD

The word retirement has three major meanings: an event, a process, and a social institution, and all three meanings have implications for the person who comes to a health professional for diagnosis and treatment.

Retirement is generally an event in the later life course. Employment is terminated and when paid work stops, major changes occur in a person's roles, source of income, activities, and life rhythms.[1] Retirement is also a process because it has continuity and goes on through time. As a social institution, retirement involves governmental and private organizations, pension plans, age requirements, and the customs, practices, and behaviors that revolve around the process of stopping work in later life.[2]

CONTEXT: GOVERNMENT AND MARKET FACTORS

The larger social and cultural context established by social policies and market forces deserves consideration for they define and establish significant parameters of retirement living. A fundamental program that shapes context is Social Security that was established more than 70 years ago.[3] In May 2006 almost 49 million persons were beneficiaries. Primary benefits are based on indexed monthly earnings. Eighty-six percent of beneficiaries were older than 65 years of age, and 14% were younger than 65. Among the 65 years and older beneficiaries, 82% were retired workers, and 18% were survivors and dependents. In December 2005 the average benefit for all retirees was $1,002 per month. Currently, a person must be 65 to receive full benefits or age 62 for reduced benefits. Beginning in 2000 the age of entitlement will gradually rise from 65 to 67 years of age.[4] Social Security was enlarged in 1966 to include Medicare, the health insurance program that provides hospital and medical care benefits for persons who are 65 years old.

Market forces are also a major part of the retirement context. For example, many cities in the northeast and midwest have been adversely changed by declining markets, new technologies, and the transfer of industries to other regions or overseas. These large, contextual market shifts have brought about the early retirement of some current cohorts of retirees.

Retirement was a transition experienced mainly by men for the first half of the twentieth century. During the last 50 years retirement also became a disengaging process from work for women. Single women, women of color, and some lower income women have had an involvement in the labor market over the years and are now eligible for various kinds of benefits.[5]

Retirement evolved within a specific time and national frame. There are many commonalities of pensions, benefits, health insurance, and so forth in other industrialized nations that are similar to the United States, but the United States is the focus in this chapter.

VULNERABILITY AND RETIREMENT

"Vulnerability science" has been utilized in research studies related to disasters in both the west and the developing world.[6] The vulnerability concept provides leverage in understanding retirement when we consider the meaning of the word: susceptible to negative results.

Retirement and vulnerability may begin with the person and the choices that have been made over a lifetime. Those decisions that increased one's vulnerability may be related to hereditary factors over which the person may have only limited control. Vulnerability may also be increased by social factors that originate in the family and then are enhanced or decreased by one's immediate environment, the neighborhood, job experience, and so forth.

The larger social world may increase one's vulnerability in retirement. Retirees were undoubtedly more vulnerable in retirement before the initiation of social programs: Social

Security and Medicare. Those programs do provide a basic safety net reducing one's economic and health vulnerability. The role of chance in one's vulnerability should not be forgotten. Working in a hazardous occupation: coal mining or chemical work may increase the probability of being hurt or penalized in some form. Chance may also affect one's economic vulnerability in retirement because one's employer goes bankrupt resulting from fraud, market conditions, or foolish decisions by executives. In short, economic and health vulnerability in retirement is probably the result of life-long processes that may have resulted from a single factor or combination of personal, familial, economic, and social factors.

One can divide retirement roughly into three stages of increasing vulnerability. Newly retired persons (perhaps 65–74 years) are often healthy and active and continue functioning as they did in their middle years. They usually continue to live in their own homes, and some may face moderate health decline. The next cohort (roughly 75–84 years) is starting to experience health decrements or declining energy and may start to look for supportive services and more health providers. The last segment – those older than 85 years – is increasingly vulnerable, due to failing health, loss of a spouse or loss of friends, and neighbors who have died or moved away. They are most likely to need supportive services or family caregivers. They may no longer be able to drive. An increasing number each year are relocating to retirement communities.

In summary, vulnerability is a linking concept between the person and the environment. Retirement is associated with aging processes and they increase vulnerability. The resilience, adaptability, and coping style of the individual are also the result of life course behaviors and experiences. The great variation in the resilience of humans to stress and change is a remarkable social phenomenon, and it is involved in the success or failure of the diagnosis and treatment offered by health care providers.

CONTEXT: THE RETIREE'S LIVING ARRANGEMENTS

Context is a broad concept that involves many aspects of the retiree's life and his/her ability to adapt to the changes that occur in this phase of life. Context includes several important but differing environments in which persons live: their homes and neighborhoods and the larger community. The context of home is significant because retirees generally spend more time there than they did while working. Whether the retiree lives alone or with others certainly influences the course of retirement living and may be a factor the health professional should consider. A major characteristic of U.S. housing is the high percentage of homeowners. About three-fourths of the retired population own their own homes, and the majority are usually free of mortgage debt. Repairs and upkeep become an increasing burden, however.

Retired persons who are renters often face problems in finding affordable, safe housing. Subsidized public housing for older persons and the disabled has been operating for more than a half a century, but in recent years there has been marked decline in the number and quality of such projects. Some public housing has been eliminated because of health and safety requirements.

The housing market in the United States is dominated by private enterprise. The growth of the market, as well as many improvements and innovations in planning, constructing, and financing have been largely due to the activities of real estate, builders, and financial organizations.

CONTEXT: RETIREMENT AND THE FAMILY

Health providers need to consider the relationship between retirement and the family. The family in the United States comes in many shapes and varieties. One major family factor that affects retired person's health and adjustment is the mobility of family and the separation of the generations. As the retirees become less functional, support in various forms becomes a necessary reality. Among the millions of persons who need long-term care, most live at home or in community settings *not* in nursing homes.[7] Approximately three-quarters of retirees who receive long-term care at home get that care from unpaid family and friends, mostly wives and adult daughters. For those retirees without family or whose family members are scattered and live far apart, the problem of finding long-term care is complicated and often frustrating.

In addition, more women are in the workplace, and this causes a juggling process, as they seek to cover their parents' or spouses' needs. Finding a satisfactory substitute for a family caregiver can be frustrating. There is often frequent turnover, and it is difficult to predict caregiver outcomes. Assessment is difficult to handle and cultural barriers may be involved. The older housebound retiree faces a difficult situation. There are a few technological advances that may be of help, but in the final analysis, a human caregiver seems to be a requirement.

Retirement affects not only the retiree but also other members of the retiree's family. Available research shows there are few role realignments.[8] Retired husbands may "help" their wives more than before retirement, but the division of labor in the home generally remains traditional. The most difficult aspect of retirement that couples may face is the serious illness or death of a spouse. The generations may not have kept intimate ties over time because they require some cultivation and nurturing. There is the possibility that retired parents may become overly dependent on adult children. This can become burdensome to the children who are involved. Unexpected family responsibilities may also occur and change the positive opportunities in retirement. The individual should plan retirement priorities carefully but be prepared for possible changes.

RETIREMENT COMMUNITIES

Health professionals need to have an awareness of the various kinds of contexts in which retirees live.[9] Most older

Americans tend to live in traditional homes or apartments. There is a growing segment of the retired population, however, who are living in various kinds of retirement communities that address many of their vulnerabilities. These can be sorted into three general categories.

The first type is called the Naturally Occurring Retirement Community (NORC). These are age-dense places: neighborhoods and subdivisions that result from the fact that many people age in place and do not consider a move. NORCs also result from demographic concentrations of the old residents remaining and young people departing. NORCs have some positive outcomes for retirees, for many prefer to live near familiar places or landmarks: stores, churches, professional services. Age-dense neighborhoods do enhance social contacts among the residents and are more likely to provide helping networks than do more heterogeneous age neighborhoods.

A second kind of retirement community is the Leisure-oriented Retirement Community. These are usually located in the sunbelt states, but the housing industry has found a growing niche for building leisure-oriented retirement communities in the suburbs of northern cities. These communities provide many more opportunities for supportive neighbors and friends, exercise and social and intellectual activities. The new opportunities for physical and mental activity are life enhancing, and some retirees are stimulated by the presence of retired neighbors as role models and the proximity of facilities.

A third, and growing kind of retirement community, is the Continuing Care Retirement Community (CCRC). These communities are organized around the idea of a continuum of living arrangements. Most residents live independently in apartments or villas. A smaller number of apartments are called assisted living units and a third level is the skilled nursing unit. The distribution of the number of these types of housing units is based on careful actuarial studies that have steadily improved as the database has increased and the record keeping has been carefully noted.

The continuum is predicted on the fact that older persons may periodically experience health or mobility problems that make it difficult to live independently. The person who has had a fall, an operation, or some other health problem may move temporarily to the assisted living apartments or to the skilled unit, where support and therapies are provided on site. The person may move back to her own apartment or villa for continued independent living. As the population ages, there is an increasing number of residents who move to assisted living or the skilled nursing unit.

CCRCs are a form of long-term care insurance because the financial arrangements are carefully organized and estimated in terms of actuarial assumptions that are based on average lifetime health needs and life expectancies. A substantial upfront payment is required to cover the possible housing and health care needs for the lifetime of the residents. Most CCRCs have a broad program of social, cultural, intellectual, and physical activities. The richness and variety will depend on the residents' initiatives and tastes. Many older Americans have the financial resources to live in a CCRC, but only a small percentage may move to one.

With the mobility and separation of family members, CCRCs provide security for the retirees and some assurance for family members that the exigencies of late life may be dealt with responsibly and professionally. Living in a CCRC may provide single and widowed persons an opportunity for psychological security and social support that is unique in an individualistic, mobile society.

All these types of age-dense communities, whether planned or naturally occurring, have positive consequences that are related to the fact that neighbors, friends, and even acquaintances share information about health conditions, health care, and the complex processes of assessing the care system and learning about the insurance or payment system.

Living around large numbers of older persons may increase awareness that the end of life is a natural process. It has been noted that because neighbors and friends die periodically, survivors are commonly very helpful to one another during the bereavement process.

COORDINATION OF SERVICE AND TEAMWORK

Focusing on retirement housing and living arrangements opens a broad window on the importance of teamwork in providing appropriate care of retirees. Most private health care providers will not have a range of health and social service providers. This discussion may increase awareness among health providers and perhaps alert patients to possible vulnerabilities when returning home from a hospital stay. There are referral agencies, area agencies on aging, senior centers, and other agencies and groups – both private and governmental – that may help the retired patient.

One advantage of living in a retirement community is that it increases knowledge of community services. Retirement communities have lectures, discussion groups, and postings that increase health awareness, and some communities have organized "buddy systems" that function in many informative and supportive ways to enhance information. Maintaining health and enhancing recovery is more than an individual matter for many.

SOCIAL SCIENCE RESEARCH FINDINGS

A major finding of recent retirement research is that this last phase of life is not a uniform, simple model of sudden changes. Many workers do retire in one sudden step but others seek and find bridging jobs. The dynamics of changes in the economy, in technology, and in the workplace have interrupted work for many persons for short periods before retirement. Before that final move to a retirement role, there are a variety of paths that people follow as a result of choices, opportunities, or fate. It is pertinent to note, "The experience of being an ex- of one kind or another is common to most people in modern society."[10]

The dynamics of role change continue as one grows older in retirement. For some persons who retire healthy and active, the path in retirement may be long and fulfilling. For others, retirement is marked by the decline of an active retiree role to that of the disabled or chronically ill. Some retirees may face intermittent or continued health problems and practitioners or clinicians will find retirees requiring the full panoply of diagnosis and treatment.

The Health and Retirement Study is a nationally representative sample of the older U.S. population who have been reinterviewed several times.[11] The 2000 survey asked people how satisfied they were with retirement and 60% said it was very satisfying, 32% considered it moderately satisfying, and less than 8% said not at all satisfying.

These broad positive answers about retirement reflect the confirming data of most researchers. They contradict the expectations of early gerontologists, who thought that retirement would have a great number of negative effects. These early gerontologists thought that negative outcomes were related to the loss of identity that had been defined by one's occupation; however, for many people, daily work was something that could be given up without much psychic damage. There is a minority of persons for whom work is the major way they have an identity, and retirement is definitely a negative situation for them.

Many retirees define and experience retirement as differential disengagement. One might view differential disengagement as a kind of universal social process, because most of life is marked by changing roles, many of which are "forced" and others chosen.[12] Thus, disengaging from work is just another shift in a series of role changes. Because work does occupy a central demand on time and energy, its loss may be traumatic for some. It must also be pointed out that many jobs are boring, overdemanding, and unpleasant, so giving up the work role is a welcome end to this phase of life. Differential disengagement also means that other roles may continue or expand and fill the role space brought about by retirement. Differential engagement also occurs when new roles that are interesting and attractive are taken on. These may involve travel, volunteer work, family, or opportunity to spend more time at hobbies or athletics.

Retirement may also have a salutary effect on some retiree's health for the daily demands and stresses of work stop.

Retirement researchers have also found that people who have a more satisfactory retirement experience have generally better health, higher income, and adaptive personality and a strong social network. All of these factors foster a positive adjustment to retirement and are supportive at all stages of life. Retiree dissatisfaction is more apt to occur when retirement occurs suddenly. Retirees who have anticipated and accepted retirement in advance of its happening tend to cope better. Formal retirement preparation programs, however, are limited. There are many popular and available sources about retirement

and its financial implications for persons who are "planners." Generally, those who anticipate this new phase seek information and talk to others about the personal experience of a retiree and have a sharper definition of the retiree role and an easier adjustment.

THE FUTURE OF RETIREMENT

Health professionals treating retirees will observe that they have continuity of personality and coping styles that have been followed for a half century. The social science findings about adaptation to retirement summarized here can offer the practitioner insight and some reassurance that an unadjusted retiree is probably not the typical case.

Retirement has become institutionalized in American society and accepted quite widely. The dynamic social and economic contexts are undergoing changes for many Americans however. Retirement income security is worrisome for many and the changing and controversial health insurance milieu is one that may be confusing and threatening to many older Americans. The way in which prescription drugs are obtained and paid for is another challenge that faces retirees and the providers of health care.

Retirement now and for the foreseeable future will involve increasingly diverse patterns. A major pattern is the increasing inequalities in income and pensions.[13] Health insurance may or may not be carried over from one's employment. Differing age and sex patterns will also be involved, and finally there will be different meanings attached to retirement as a social institution.

Future retirees will probably face a more uncertain situation.[14] A major issue will be whether retirement will be as sustainable economically and politically as it has been in the past. The worldwide shifts labeled globalization have had major political and economic outcomes. Pension coverage has shifted in the United States. The contribution arrangement has been realigned and plans have moved from defined benefits to defined contributions presenting the individual with more choices and probably increased personal financial risks.[15]

When Social Security was created the retirement base was portrayed as a three-legged stool: Social Security, a pension from one's employer, and private savings. For many in the future there will be only a one-legged stool: Social Security benefits.

As our society matures, it is hoped that health professionals will have an understanding of the changing context in which the retirees live and which is part of their thinking and behavior as they move through the health care process.

REFERENCES

1. Atchley RC. Retirement. In: Birren JE, ed. *Encyclopedia of Gerontology.* Vol. 2. San Diego, CA: Academic Press; 1996:437–449.

2. Monk A. *The Retirement Handbook*. New York: Columbia University Press; 1994.

3. Quadagno J. *The Transformation of Old Age Security: Class and Politics in the American Welfare State*. Chicago: The University of Chicago Press; 1988.

4. *The World Almanac and Book of Facts*. New York: World Almanac Book; 2007:381–383.

5. Eckerdt D, Dennis H. (guest eds.) Retirement: new chapters in American life. *Generations*. 2002;26:6–89.

6. A symposium on natural disasters. *Contemp Sociol*. 2006;207–227.

7. Family Caregiver Alliance. *Caregiver Assessment: Principles, Guidelines and Strategies for Change. Report from a National Consensus Development Conference*. Vol. I. San Francisco: 2006.

8. Dorfman LT. Retirement and family relationships: an opportunity in later life. *Generations*. 2002;26:74–79.

9. Streib GF, (guest ed). Retirement communities. *Res Aging*. 2002;24(1):3–164.

10. Ebaugh HRF. *Becoming an Ex: The Process of Role Exit*. Chicago: University of Chicago Press; 1988.

11. Bender KA, Jivan NA. What makes retirees happy? Issue in Brief – Center for Retirement Research. Boston: Center for Retirement Research, Boston College. 2005;28:1–11.

12. Streib GF, Schneider CJ. *Retirement in American Society: Impact and Process*. Ithaca, NY: Cornell University Press; 1971.

13. O'Rand AM, Henretta JC. *Age and Inequality: Diverse Pathways Through Later Life*. Boulder, CO: Westview Press; 1999.

14. Magnusson P. Why so many Americans may be working when they retire. *AARP Bull*. 2006;(July-August):22–23.

15. Lowenstein R. We regret to inform you that you may no longer have a pension. *New York Times Magazine*. Oct. 30, 2005/Section 6:56–63,70,82,90.

55

GERIATRIC SEXUALITY

Lisa Granville, MD, Karen Myers, ARNP

INTRODUCTION

Sexuality is an important part of health and quality of life and thus is an important area for health care providers to address. Although much has been written about sexuality in adolescence and adults, relatively little information regarding sexuality in older populations is available. With the aging of the baby boom generation, different attitudes and mores regarding sexuality are coming forward as a result of growing up in the "free love" generation. In time, discussion of sexuality with older adults is anticipated to be more direct, open, and often initiated by well-informed patients.

At this time a number of fallacies regarding sexuality later in life prevail. Many prefer to believe that sexuality in older adults simply does not exist. Brogran notes, "there is a general societal belief that old people are, or should be, asexual and a false assumption exists that physical attractiveness depends on youth and beauty."[1] Alternatively, sexuality in older adults is considered a laughing matter. Comical cards and ones on old age often give messages about physical weakness and failures in sexual performance.[2] Sexuality in older adults is sometimes seen as something distasteful or disgusting with references to "dirty old men" and "lecherous old women." Although often these fallacies of sexuality are held by youthful members of society, perhaps just as often they are believed by older adults themselves.[3] It becomes apparent that the health care providers' involvement in promoting health and well-being of older adults through discussions of sexuality is often hindered by misinformation and misperceptions.

SEXUAL ACTIVITY

The sexual behaviors of older adults are not well studied. There are both physical and emotional aspects to sexuality and the desire for intimacy continues throughout life.[4] Physical close-ness can be expressed in many ways including holding hands, hugging, kissing, mutual stroking, masturbating, oral sex, and intercourse. Studies have shown that for older adults current level of activity correlates with past sexual frequency and most older adults desire more activity than what they have.[5] Lack of partners and lack of privacy are significant obstacles for sexual expression. Adults living in age-segregated environments, such as retirement communities, express more interest in sexual activity and engage in sexual activity more often than their cohorts who are not age segregated.[6] Adults with partners are much more likely than those without partners to engage in interpersonal sexual activities such as kissing, hugging, oral sex, and intercourse.[6,7] Adults with partners express more emphasis on having a satisfying sexual relationship, more frequent sexual activity, and more sexual satisfaction overall.[4,7] Some older adults report that sex became more pleasurable and of greater importance with age.[4]

Avis examined the impact of age and sex on sexual function and found that older women reported a cessation of sexual relations due to a death of a spouse (36%), illness of a spouse (20%), or a spouse's inability to perform sexually (18%). Only 10% of the older women reported a cessation of sexual activity because of their own illness, loss of interest, or inability to perform.[8] Szwabo noted that as roles change within a relationship, so can the sexual behaviors of the couple. If the wife has assumed the caregiver "nursing" role, it may make sexual feelings and expressions less intense as the spouse may be seen as a patient rather than a sexual partner.[9]

Adults without partners appear to adjust their sexual expectations and priorities. In one study it was noted that most people reporting no importance of sex were found to have no current partner and no anticipation of a partner in their lifetime.[4] Women aged 75 years and older are much less likely than older men to have a partner (58% vs. 21%).[7] In 1999, the American Association of Retired Persons surveyed 1,382 people 45 years and older. In this study, across all age groups, sexuality was more important to men than women. Men had more frequent sexual thoughts, feelings of sexual desire, and engaged in self-stimulation more often than women. Contrary to popular stereotypes, men's satisfaction with their sex lives was related to the romantic qualities of their partner and whether or not their partner was perceived as sensitive to their moods and needs. Women's satisfaction was more related to their feelings that their partner was imaginative about sex and exciting.[7]

BARRIERS TO TREATMENT

Several barriers to seeking treatment for sexual problems were revealed in an interview study of 45 adults aged 50–92 years old.[10] Patients expressed a preference to consult a general practitioner of similar age and sex with the goal of minimizing embarrassment through discussing concerns with someone likely to have had similar experiences themselves. It was also noted that patient perceptions of providers' attitudes toward sexuality in later life may be a hindrance if perceptions exist that older people are or should be asexual or access to treatments included age-based rationing. In this study 97% said they would discuss sexuality if the provider brought it up and 80% stated a willingness to return for a designated sexual concerns appointment.

Reasons for health care providers' reluctance to initiate discussions about sexual concerns in the older population have been noted.[10] These include believing the myths and stereotypes regarding the lack of sexuality in the older population, fear that patients may be offended, and lack of confidence in the ability to approach and discuss sexual issues. In a recent study by Nusbaum, 68% of older women interviewed stated that the topic of sexuality was never approached during office visits.[15] The older women stated that they brought up the topic 22% of the time, and only 10% of the time the physician initiated the subject. Of those who discussed sexual issues, 94% reported that the discussions were helpful. Nearly all older women in the study, 97%, said that they would have discussed the topic had the physician asked about any sexual concerns.

Both providers and patients may mistakenly attribute sexual problems to "normal aging" and both may lack knowledge about services and resources. As with many potentially sensitive issues it appears that patients are waiting for their health care providers to raise the topic. Providers can take measures to help reduce the potential discomfort in dealing with sexual concerns. These include maintaining a professional demeanor, displaying comfort with the topic, and remaining kind, empathic, and understanding.[15]

INSTITUTIONALIZED ELDERLY

The institutionalized elderly face many additional obstacles in meeting their sexual needs. Nursing homes are by design open, public spaces. Lack of privacy is a significant barrier to sexual expression. Lack of a partner is also very common and

solitary sexual expression may become a necessity. Although nursing home residents are frail and functionally dependent, sexual desire persists and the importance of noncoital sexuality is increased. Sexual behaviors are often viewed by staff as problems and an asexual environment is promoted. Patients with dementia raise additional concerns among staff and family such as sexually disinhibited behavior and capability for consensual sexual activity.[16]

SEXUAL RESPONSE CYCLE AND COMMON DISORDERS

The sexual response cycle has four phases. The first phase, desire, involves the brain and one's interest in or urge for sexual activity. The second phase, arousal, involves the vascular system and the body's response to stimulation. In men this is primarily recognized by penile erection, and in women by vaginal lubrication and genital engorgement. The peak of arousal is referred to as plateau. The third phase, orgasm, involves the spinal cord and perineal musculature. In this phase the body experiences involuntary contractions of the pelvic muscles and reproductive organs and men experience ejaculation of seminal fluid. In the fourth phase, resolution, the body recovers from orgasm with a physiological rest period.[11]

In 1966, Masters and Johnson's landmark study of older persons' sexuality noted that natural aging leads to a need for more time to engage in sexual activities. Advancing age is associated with delayed arousal and a greater need for genital stimulation, reduced penile rigidity and vaginal lubrication, loss of the sensation of ejaculatory inevitability, and increasing anorgasmia.[12]

Tables 55.1 and 55.2 outline sex-specific sexual response cycle markers, changes with aging, and common disorders for men and women. Whereas women experience menopause and its impact on sexuality over a relatively short period of time, men's physiological changes are thought to occur over a longer period of time with less awareness as change is occurring. The physiological changes with age alone are insufficient cause to cease sexual activity and for some these changes are felt to enhance their sexual activity.

MISCONCEPTIONS REGARDING SEXUALLY TRANSMITTED INFECTIONS

Age does not protect against sexually transmitted infections. Sexually transmitted infections, including human immunodeficiency virus/acquired immunodeficiency syndrome (HIV/AIDS), are indeed transmitted in the elderly population. HIV/AIDS infection affects 65,000 Americans older than the age of 50 years.[13] Almost 27% of the overall HIV population in the United States is older than the age of 50 years.[14] Sexual contact is the leading mode of transmission and accounts for more than 60% of the diagnosed elderly cases of HIV. According to the Centers for Disease Control and Prevention, AIDS cases among

Table 55.1. Men

Sexual Response Cycle: Men	Markers	Changes with Aging	Disorders
Desire: brain	Desire/urge for sexual activity	Testosterone decrease at 55+ years may affect libido	Affected by illness, performance anxiety, relationship problems

Arousal: vascular system	Penile erection
	Genital engorgement
	   Testes
	   Scrotum
		Longer time for arousal (often need physical stimulation), erections less firm, sperm production declines	Erectile dysfunction (most common male dysfunction)

Plateau: (peak of arousal)	Full penile erection Testicular elevation and swelling Pre-ejaculatory fluid		Premature ejaculation
Orgasmic: spinal cord and perineal musculature	Involuntary rhythmic contractions of the pelvic muscles, reproductive organs Ejaculation of seminal fluid	Ejaculatory control improves, fewer contractions per orgasm, volume of ejaculate decreased	Orgasmic disorder
Resolution:	Subjective sense of relaxation "Refractory period"	Physiologically extended refractory period	

Table 55.2. Women

Sexual Response Cycle: Women	Markers	Changes with Aging	Disorders
Desire: brain	Desire/urge for sexual activity	Unclear: theory of low estrogen causing decreased libido is being reconsidered	Affected by illness, performance anxiety, relationship problems Hypoactive Sexual Desire disorder

Arousal: vascular system	Vaginal lubrication
	Clitoral erection
	Genital engorgement
	   Vulva
	   Vagina
	   Uterus
	Breast changes
		Less increase in breast size, reduced elasticity of vaginal walls, decreased vaginal lubrication, less muscle tension	Female sexual arousal disorder (lack of lubrication/lack of pleasure despite adequate stimulation)
			Note: often related to estrogen deficiency

Plateau: (peak of arousal)	Vasocongestion of outer third of uterus, vagina Elevation of uterus		
Orgasmic: spinal cord and perineal musculature	Involuntary rhythmic contractions of the pelvic muscles, reproductive organs	Fewer contractions per orgasm, ability for multiple orgasms may decrease	Orgasmic disorder (more common in women than men)
Resolution:	Subjective sense of relaxation	May have refractory period	

people older than 50 years have increased 22% since 1991, making heterosexuals 50 years and older the most rapidly growing AIDS population.[15] Postmenopausal women are more susceptible to the transmission of HIV because of atrophic changes in the vaginal mucosa.[13]

Unfortunately, there are misunderstandings concerning safer sex practices in the older population. HIV/AIDS is often not acknowledged in the aging community because of the common misconception that older adults are not at risk, either because they are in stable relationships or because they are no longer sexually active. Nusbaum found that significantly few women older than 65 years had concerns regarding safer sex, sexually transmitted diseases, or HIV/AIDS.[15] This correlates with the misconception that the elderly are not an at-risk population. Some physicians do not perceive the older adult as being at risk for HIV and are less likely to test for the virus.[14]

Many older adults have been in long-term sexually monogamous relationships and may be unsure or unaware of the risks of sexually transmitted diseases including HIV. With the loss of a partner, the survivor may begin dating for the first time in years and become at risk for exposure to HIV. Condom use for other than protection from pregnancy is not the norm. According to the National Association on HIV Over Fifty (NAHOF), HIV prevention programs are needed that encourage older adults to take steps to protect themselves from HIV.[17] In recognition of the increasing prevalence of HIV, the Centers for Disease Control and Prevention issued a new guideline September 2006 advocating "in all health-care settings, screening for HIV infection should be performed routinely for all patients aged 13–64 years."[18] According to Medicare guidelines, testing for HIV is a covered benefit only if there is a documented risk of exposure. In the absence of a documented AIDS-defining or HIV-associated disease, sign or symptom, or documented exposure to a known HIV-infected source, Medicare considers HIV testing a screening activity and does not cover it as a benefit.[19]

COMMON MEDICAL CONDITIONS AND SURGICAL PROCEDURES

A number of medical conditions contribute to sexual dysfunction and raise patient concerns regarding health consequences of sexual activity. Medical conditions and their treatments may negatively alter one's perception of body image, create preoccupation with concern of exacerbation of symptoms, reduce exercise tolerance, and limit flexibility and positions of comfort. Tables 55.3 and 55.4 outline patient advice for common medical conditions and common surgical procedures.[19,20]

SEX-SPECIFIC CONDITIONS

Erectile dysfunction (ED) is the most common disorder of men's sexual health. ED is defined as the recurrent inability to attain or maintain a penile erection sufficient for sexual perfor-

mance. The prevalence of ED increases with age. In the Massachusetts Male Aging Study of 1,290 men aged 40–70 years, the probability of severe ED tripled from 5.1% to 15%; the probability of moderate ED doubled from 17% to 34%, and the probability of mild ED remained constant at 17%.[22] Many medical conditions and their treatments contribute to the development of ED. Common etiologies include diabetes mellitus, hypertension, cardiac disease, depression, and prostate cancer.[23] Treatment options are varied and include medications, penile implants, and vacuum devices. For most men oral agents are the first-line treatment option for ED. Phosphodiesterase type 5 inhibitors, such as sildenafil citrate, are the most commonly used, and they normalize erectile function in approximately 40% of men with severe ED and 79% of men with mild ED.[24] Side effects of these medications include headache (17%), flushing (13%), and dyspepsia (8%), and they should not be used by men taking nitrates.[23] Intracavernosal injection of vasoactive agents, such as papaverine hydrochlorate and prostaglandin E_1, are also effective. The most commonly reported side effect is penile pain (24%); some men are averse to needle use. Intracavernosal therapy has a success rate of 60%–70%.[25] Intraurethral insertion of vasoactive agents is an alternative. This approach is termed medicated urethral system for erection and is successful approximately 44% of the time.[26] Side effects include urethral irritation in patients and some partners. Vacuum pump with constrictive bands is a common alternative to medications. This method often achieves an erection; however, patient satisfaction varies between 27% and 74%.[26] The vacuum pump requires some skill and an understanding partner. Men receiving adequate training report better satisfaction.[23] Penile implants are generally reserved for those in whom alternatives were unsuccessful. The operation requires destruction of the corpus cavernosus, thus eliminating any future pharmacological treatments.[23]

SEX TOYS

Health care providers should develop a general awareness of the types of sex toys that are commonly used and related health care considerations. There are several reasons why a patient may develop an interest in toys including lack of a partner, reentering the dating scene, and interest in adding variety. The patient may look to the health care provider for guidance in how to use toys, validation that toy use is an acceptable practice, and health risk education. In addition to these roles the physician may need to assist with retrieval of misplaced or out of reach equipment.

The following guidelines facilitate the safe use of toys. When putting something in a body opening be aware that sharp, breakable, and hard to hold on to objects can be problematic and are discouraged from use. One should listen to his/her body; pain is a good indicator to slow down, pull out, or explore other options. Toys should be cleansed thoroughly between use with soap and water and allowed to dry completely. When cleaning porous materials (silicone, latex) a little bleach can be

Table 55.3. Common Medical Conditions

Condition	Advice and Information
Myocardial infarction	■ Abstinence often advised for 8–14 weeks although there is limited data to support this practice
	■ Duration of abstinence depends primarily on patient desire, general fitness, conditioning
	■ Ability to climb 1–2 flights of stairs is generally considered adequate fitness for sexual activity
Angina	■ Late morning activity after a full night's rest
	■ Use of supine position to reduce exertion level
	■ Creation of a relaxed atmosphere for sexual encounters
Heart failure exacerbation with pulmonary edema	■ Abstain from sexual activity 2–3 weeks or until ability to climb 1–2 flights of stairs is restored
Hypertension	■ No need to limit sexual activity
	■ Be aware that antihypertensive medication and untreated hypertension lead to erectile dysfunction in men; effects in women not well studied
Stroke	■ Sexual function may be impaired, desire is usually unaffected
	■ If loss of desire is present, screen for depression
	■ Physical stimulation can be focused on the unaffected side of the body
	■ Pillows and headboards can be used for support
Emphysema and other causes of shortness of breath	■ Use intervals of rest
	■ Select positions requiring limited exertion
	■ Use oxygen as needed
Arthritis	■ Use general pain reduction approaches: exercise, rest, warm baths, analgesics prior to exertion
	■ Try different sexual positions to minimize joint pain
	■ Use time of day when pain and stiffness are least severe
Diabetes mellitus	■ Sexual desire is unaffected
	■ Male erectile dysfunction (ED) is 2–5 times more common than in general population
	■ For some men establishing good control of diabetes reestablishes potency
	■ If diabetes is already well controlled, ED is likely irreversible, consider ED management approaches
Depression	■ Sexual desire is affected
	■ Treatment of depression restores sexual interest

added. Battery or electronically operated equipment should not be completely submerged. A condom can be used on many toys and will significantly facilitate cleanliness. Condoms should always be changed between partners and when moving from anus to vagina. Using a toy with only one individual, termed dedicated use, is another effective strategy for safer sex toy use.

LUBRICANTS

There are many different lubricants available. Lubricants are used with condoms, with toys, for masturbation, for anal sex, and frequently in postmenopausal women for vaginal dryness. When selecting a lubricant there are three main considerations: the ingredients; the purpose; and reactions between the chemicals and the person, toys, and safer sex supplies. The three main types of lubricants are: water based, silicone based and oil based. Water-based lubricants are very popular because they are safe to use with latex condoms and rubber toys. Advantages include ease of cleaning, stain free unless color has been added, nongreasy feel, and reactivation with water or saliva. Silicone-based lubricants last a long time, do not dry out, and small amounts are very effective. Limitations include difficulty in cleaning, damage to silicone toys, and vaginal irritations and

Table 55.4. Common Surgical Procedures

Condition	Advice and Information
Hysterectomy	▪ Abstinence advised 6–8 weeks to allow adequate wound healing
	▪ Women sensitive to cervical and uterine contractions during orgasm may notice the loss of these sensations
	▪ Depression is common and may impair desire
Oophorectomy	▪ Effects of decreased androgen, estrogen, progesterone not well studied
	▪ Sexual frequency is sometimes increased with removed fear of pregnancy
Mastectomy	▪ Loss of desire occurs with embarrassment, perceived loss of femininity, fear of being unattractive
	▪ Periodic depression common for 1–2 years post procedure
	▪ Rehabilitation programs encouraged for patients and partners to deal with physical/psychological concerns and enhanced communication
Prostatectomy	▪ Abstinence advised for 6 weeks to allow wound healing
	▪ Transurethral resection of prostate, used for benign prostatic hypertrophy, leads to retrograde ejaculation and erectile dysfunction
	▪ Complete prostatectomy, used for prostate cancer, leads to erectile dysfunction in 60% or more
Orchiectomy	▪ Psychological impact substantial; physical impairment of function limited
	▪ Counseling before and after surgery is highly advocated

infections. Oil-based lubricants are most often used for male masturbation. Limitations include difficulty in cleaning, not recommended for vaginal use, and damage to rubber toys and latex condoms. Lubricants may have additives. Anal lubricants may contain benzocaine as a desensitizing agent. Although this may assist initiation of anal sex, caution is advised that decreased sensation may increase injuries. Additives may also include flavors and scents. Plain lubes taste mildly chemical and slightly bitter. Edible lubricants are water based and often contain glycerin. Patients should be advised that in warm, moist environments such as the vagina, sugar promotes yeast and bacterial infections. Lubricants also vary in consistency from light liquids to heavy gels. Heavier lubricants are recommended for anal sex. Patients are encouraged to test a small quantity of lubricant for adverse reactions, especially if using for vaginal intercourse.

COITAL POSITIONS

With advancing age, a number of factors may influence a patient's preference for coital positions. Considerations include limited exercise tolerance, pain aggravated by certain positions, and embarrassment related to medical devices (ostomy pouch) or procedures (mastectomy, orchiectomy). The man on top (missionary) position facilitates intimacy including talking, hugging, kissing, eye contact, and close body contact. Touching by the man is limited because he must hold himself up and prolonged activity may be physically challenging. Women may find

this position uncomfortable if the man is heavy. The woman on top position facilitates intimacy for similar reasons. With the woman in control of depth, speed, and rhythm of penetration, a woman's orgasm may be facilitated and pain with penetration can be minimized. This position works well for partners of different heights. Prolonged activity may be physically challenging for the woman. The sitting/kneeling position may be a desired alternative for patients with abdominal bloating, discomfort, or medical devices. Although some consider lack of eye contact impersonal, this may be an advantage for those embarrassed by altered body image. If this position is hard on the knees, use of a chair may facilitate comfort. The rear entry (doggie-style) position also facilitates touching, is easy on the muscles, and requires less energy than those positions previously mentioned. This position facilitates deep penile penetration and has limited eye contact. The side-by-side (spoons) position requires the least amount of energy and is therefore useful for patients with limited mobility or stamina. This position facilitates touching, close body contact, and slower encounters. With increased time and less deep penile penetration, this position is useful for patients with premature ejaculation.

Patients of all ages have concerns about sexuality; however, many providers may not feel comfortable in talking about sexual issues or even taking a sexual history, especially in their older patient population. As the number of older adults continues to increase, the health care providers' responsibility to this segment of the population grows. Sexual activity is an important component of quality of life, and sexually transmitted disease is an important threat to health and well-being in all ages. It is imperative that the health care provider gain knowledge and skill in discussing sexual issues and routinely provide the initiative for conversations on these topics. The health care provider at ease with handling sexuality issues allows older patients to be more comfortable and open in their discussions.

REFERENCES

1. Brogan M. The sexual needs of elderly people: addressing the issue. *Nurs Stand.* 1996;10:42–45.
2. Bytheway B. *Ageism.* Buckingham, UK: Open University Press; 1995.
3. Kessel B. Sexuality in the older person. *Age Ageing.* 2001;30:121–124.
4. Gott M, Hinchcliff S. How important is sex in later life? The views of older people. *Soc Sci Med.* 2003;56:1617–1628.
5. Ginsberg TB, Pomerantz SC, Kramer-Feeley V. Sexuality in older adults: behaviours and preferences. *Age Ageing.* 2005;34:475–480.
6. Weinstein S, Rosen E. Senior adult sexuality in age segregated and age integrated communities. *Int J Aging Hum Dev.* 1988;27:261–270.
7. AARP/Modern Maturity Sexuality Survey. *Mod Maturity.* 1999; Sept/Oct: 57–69.
8. Avis NE. Sexual functioning and aging in men and women: community and population-based studies. *J Gender-Specif Med.* 2000;2:37–41.
9. Szwabo P. Counseling about sexuality in the older person. *Clin Geriatr Med.* 2003;19:595–604.
10. Gott M, Hinchcliff S. Barriers to seeking treatment for sexual problems in primary care: a qualitative study with older people. *Fam Pract.* 2003;20:690–695.
11. McKenzie LJ, Carson SA. Human sexuality and female sexual dysfunction. In: Scott JR, Gibbs RS, Karlan BY, Haney AF, eds. *Danforth's Obstetrics and Gynecology.* 9th ed. Lippincott Williams & Wilkins; 2003.
12. Masters WH, Johnson VE. *Human Sexual Response.* Boston: Little, Brown and Co; 1966.
13. Wilson MM. Sexually transmitted diseases. *Clin Geriatr Med.* 2003;19:637–655.
14. Karpiak SE, Shipley RA, Cantor MH. *Research on older adults with HIV.* New York: AIDS Community Research of America; 2006.
15. Nusbaum MR, Singh AR, Pyles AA. Sexual healthcare needs of women age 65 and older. *J Am Geriatr Soc.* 2004;52:117–122.
16. Hajjar RR, Kamel HK. Sexuality in the nursing home. Part 1: attitudes and barriers to sexual expression. *J Am Med Dir Assoc.* 2003;4:152–156.
17. National Association on HIV over fifty. Available at http://www.hivoverfifty.org. Accessed October 21, 2007.
18. Branson BM, Handsfield HH, Lampe MA, et al. Revised Recommendations for HIV Testing of Adults, Adolescents, and Pregnant Women in Health-Care Settings. *MMWR.* 2006;55(RR14):1–17.
19. NCD for Human Immunodeficiency Virus (HIV) Testing (Diagnosis). Available at http://www.viahealth.org/documents/laboratory%20forms/manual0708HIVdiagnosis.pdf.
20. "Chapter 114 Sexuality" In: Beers MH, Berkow R, eds. *Merck Manual of Geriatrics.* 3rd ed. New Jersey: Merck Laboratories; 2000.
21. Morley JE, Tariq SH. Sexuality and disease. *Clin Geriatr Med.* 2003;19:563–573.
22. Johannes CB, Araujo AB, Feldman HA, et al. Incidence of erectile dysfunction in men 40 to 69 years old: longitudinal results from the Massachusetts Male Aging Study. *J Urol.* 2000;163:460–463.
23. Morales A. Erectile dysfunction: an overview. *Clin Geriatr Med.* 2003;19:529–538.
24. Seftel A. From aspiration to achievement: assessment and non-invasive treatment of erectile dysfunction in aging men. *J Am Geriatr Soc.* 2005;53:119–130.
25. Tariq SH, Hallem U, Omran ML, et al. Erectile dysfunction: etiology and treatment in young and old patients. *Clin Geriatr Med.* 2003;19:539–551.
26. Mulligan T, Reddy S, Gulur PV, et al. Disorders of male sexual function. *Clin Geriatr Med.* 2003;19:473–481.

56

THE ELDERLY, THEIR FAMILIES, AND THEIR CAREGIVERS

Susan Mockus Parks, MD, Laraine Winter, PhD

The extraordinary projected growth in the elderly population has prompted concern both about their care and about the impact the provision of that care will have on society. In 1900 only 4.1% of the population was 65 and older and only 0.2% was 85 and older. By 2050 an estimated 20.7% will be at least 65 years old and 5.0% at least 85.[1] Thus, the population aged 65 or older increased from approximately 3 million in 1900 to nearly 35 million in 2000 and is projected to reach nearly 90 million in the year 2060.[2]

Families are the most important providers of care for elderly people, with primary caregivers most likely to be immediate family.[3] In fact, 78% of adults receiving care at home rely exclusively on care from family members.[4] It is estimated that 9.4 million people in the United States are providing care to a relative or friend with a chronic health problem.[4] The importance of the family support system on the well-being of patients has been recognized for almost 4 decades. The families who provide such care have been called one of society's great assets.[5]

Seventy three percent of caregivers are spouses or children.[2] Adult daughters make up 29% of caregivers and wives another 23%.[2] Thus, the overwhelming majority of family caregivers are women. Because most elderly men are married and most elderly women are not, men tend to have a spouse for assistance whereas women do not. Thus, husbands constitute only 13% of caregivers.[1]

Despite concerns about the continuing availability of family caregivers in the future, the demographic trend described by Himes' 1992 study is reassuring, at least for the next two decades.[6] The cohort now in old age or entering it consists of parents of the baby boom generation. This is a group for whom childbearing was extremely common, and most families had more than one child. Decreases in child mortality have also contributed to the availability of caregivers for this cohort. Thus, the majority of the elderly consists of people with adult children, and the great majority will have a child available for support in 2010.[6]

Future cohorts of elderly people, however, may have a different experience, based on trends in the structure of the American family. In 2002, only 7% of U.S. households fit the definition of the traditional family, with the husband working in the labor force and the wife at home. Household structure has been altered especially by trends in marriage and fertility. Divorce is a particular concern because of its potential to undermine affective bonds between parents and children, especially fathers and children.[7] Future cohorts of older adults may therefore be less able to rely on spouses and children.[2]

Chronic conditions increase the risk of functional limitations that threaten independence and increase dependence on family caregivers. In 2000, more than 100 million Americans had a chronic condition, with that number expected to increase to 158 million by 2040. Chronic conditions are more disabling for the elderly than for younger adults. Nearly 45% of older adults are functionally limited as a result of chronic conditions, the most common being arthritis, hypertension, hearing loss, heart disease, and cataracts.[2]

Trends in disability are encouraging, however. Surveys have consistently documented declines in disability and improvements in instrumental activities of daily living and function in the elderly population.[8] Lower rates of disability portend a better quality of life, greater independence for elders, and lower demands on families and government programs.

CAREGIVING AND CAREGIVER BURDEN

Nevertheless, even in the best-case scenarios of improving health, decreasing disability, and available family caregivers, the projected increase in the older adult population will inevitably place demands on both American families and government programs for the elderly.[2] The cohort of family caregivers – defined as people who live with and care for a relative with physical or cognitive limitations – in the United States will continue to increase. A wide variety of physical and cognitive disabilities affecting the elderly can require the assistance of a caregiver, including dementias, advanced cancers, and end-stage congestive heart failure.

The term "caregiver burden" was coined in the early 1980s. It has been defined as the "physical, emotional, social, and financial toll of providing care,"[9] or the extent to which caregivers perceive their emotional or physical health, social life, and financial status as suffering as a result of caring for their relative.[10] The term is used in both the medical and lay communities to describe the stress felt by those in the caregiving role.

Despite the abundant literature on caregiver burden, some authors think that the term caregiver burden is too broad in trying to encapsulate the stresses associated with this role. In addition, the degree of physical and emotional stress associated with caregiving is very individualized. Thus, we will outline individual components of health and well-being that are affected by caregiving.

IMPACT OF CAREGIVING

Family caregiving and its effects on health and well-being have been topics of a large body of research since the term was introduced. Some caregivers report high satisfaction with their role. Work by Donelan found that 89% of caregivers feel appreciated by their care recipient and 71% report that the relationship between them and their care recipient has improved.[11]

Nevertheless, caregiving has well-documented negative effects on mortality, morbidity, and emotional and financial well-being. Higher caregiver burden has been associated with multiple ill effects on the caregiver, the care recipient, and the family as a whole.

Becoming a caregiver can have a significant economic and lifestyle impact.[12] Many caregivers are forced to leave their jobs to provide adequate care for their relative. This can have far-reaching effects on caregivers' financial status and sense of worth. Likewise, many caregivers feel a sense of isolation as their new role does not allow them the time to participate in social or self-care activities. Marital and family conflict may also emerge from the stress of providing care.[13]

The health impact of caregiving has been well studied and widely reported. A landmark study by Shultz and Beach[5] documented increased mortality, especially in spousal caregivers. In this study, spousal caregivers who experienced burden had a 63% higher mortality rate compared with caregivers who did not experience burden during a 4-year study period.[5] More recent work has determined that mortality rates after the hospitalization of a spouse varied according to the diagnosis requiring admission.[14] The highest mortality rates among both men and women spousal caregivers occurred when hospitalization was for psychiatric disease or dementia.[14]

Many caregivers experience symptoms of depression and anxiety. Studies have found that the incidence of depression among caregivers ranges from 31% to 46%.[15–17] A large epidemiological study in Ontario, California revealed an increase in any psychiatric diagnosis among caregivers compared with noncaregivers, 20.6% compared with 14.9%.[18] Specifically for anxiety disorders, the increase among caregivers was 17.5% compared with 10.9% for noncaregivers.[18] The only category not higher among caregivers was substance abuse.[18] Two other studies showed equal or less alcohol use among caregivers.[15,19]

Caregiving burden is also associated with increased risk of institutionalization of the care recipient.[20] Institutional placement is more closely associated with family support system collapse rather with the patient's own health deterioration.[21] Also, increased use of formal in-home services is seen in cases of high caregiver burden.[20]

Because caregiving is often a protracted experience and the health conditions that afflict relatives have changing trajectories, caregiving has been conceptualized as a career.[12] Some researcher have investigated psychological trajectories in the caregiving career, documenting decreasing sense of mastery and competence among many family caregivers.[22,23]

IDENTIFYING FAMILY CAREGIVERS AND ASSESSING BURDEN

Family caregivers have long been recognized as "hidden patients."[25] Therefore, assessment of their physical and mental health status represents an emerging topic in the health care literature. It has been suggested that primary care physicians are in the unique position to discover patients who may be in the caregiving role by asking about caregiving during a social history.[26] Caregivers, however, have multiple other entry points into the health care community, such as when applying for social services. The best time and place for caregiver assessment has been debated; however, it is universally agreed on that some form of caregiver assessment is a good practice. An expert panel on caregiving, the National Consensus Development Conference for Caregiver Assessment: Translating Research into Policy and Procedure, was assembled in 2005 and developed a consensus report on caregiver assessment. Their recommendations were extensive but included identification, assessment of stressors, and current and needed resources.[28] One author described some of the outcomes of caregiver assessment as maintaining caregivers' health and well-being, preventing social isolation of caregivers, and providing appropriate support to caregivers.[27]

Researchers have developed several instruments with which to describe and quantify the degree of burden felt by caregivers. One such instrument, the Zarit Burden Interview, has become widely used by researchers studying caregivers.[29] Although this questionnaire was developed for research purposes, primary care providers should screen their patients for the overall degree

Table 56.1. Screening Questions for Health Care Providers to Assess Degree of Caregiver Burden

Are you taking care of a relative at home?

Do you feel that you are currently under a lot of stress because of your caregiving responsibilities?

Are there family or friends who help you care for your loved one?

Do you have time to take care of yourself on a daily basis?

of burden perceived by their patients who are caring for a relative.

Health care providers should screen patients for depression if they are providing care to a relative. The 15-item Geriatric Depression Scale is a useful clinical tool for elderly caregivers;[24] however, simply asking, "are you often sad or blue?" is also an effective screening question.

Table 56.1 gives health care providers sample screening questions to quickly identify caregivers and assess for burden in their patients.

SUPPORT FOR FAMILY CAREGIVERS

A variety of support services are available to assist caregivers, including information and assistance services, technology (including assistive devices and home modifications), education and training, support groups and counseling, respite care, and financial support.[4] There is evidence that support groups can improve the psychological well-being of caregivers.[30] Some evidence suggests that support groups can be most beneficial when they have an educational focus, such as helping with behavior management issues for those caring for a loved one with dementia.[31] Other benefits of support groups include sharing difficult issues, sharing coping strategies, and lessening the feelings of isolation.[4] Respite services provide family caregivers with much needed rest from their caring responsibilities. Respite can be provided either inside or outside the home. Adult day care programs are considered a form of respite care. Such care has been shown to have a varied effect on caregiver burden.[32–34]

Financial support may have a profound effect on those in the full-time caregiving role. Currently, the state of California offers a caregiver support program.[4] On the federal level, the National Family Caregiver Support Program (NFCSP) exists under the Older Americans Act Programs administered by the Administration on Aging and the state and local aging agencies. The NFCSP had its first year of funding in 2001. This program is earmarked for caregivers of those 70 years and older to provide information about existing services, assistance to access these services, counseling, support groups and training around issues of problem solving, respite care, and other services such as home modification.[4] In 2002, the NFCSP provided information on services to 4 million people, counseling to 182,000 people, and respite services to 76,000 people.[35] Table 56.2 details national resources for caregivers.

CROSS-CULTURAL PERSPECTIVES

Caregiving experiences vary across different countries and cultures. Recent work by Belle et al. has shown that a

Table 56.2. Caregiver Resources

Name	Phone No.	Web Address	Description
Family Caregiver Alliance	800–445-8106	www.caregiver.org	National caregiver support organization. On-line support groups available.
National Area Agencies on Aging (AAA)	Eldercare locator 800–677-1116	www.eldercare.gov	Links to local AAAs. Assist with insurance issues, legal issues, etc
Alzheimer's Association	800–272-3900	www.alz.org	Information specific to caring for people with dementia.
Meals-on-Wheels Association of America	703–548-5558	www.mowaa.org	Links people to their local Meals-on-Wheels and other nutritional support programs.
Medicare	800–633-4227	www.medicare.gov	Assistance with insurance coverage issues, Medicare D programs, etc.
American Association for Retired Persons (AARP)	888–687-2277	www.aarp.org	Section on Web site on caregiver health, legal issues, and long-distance caregiving
National Family Caregiver Support Program of the Administration on Aging	Links by Eldercare locator 800–677-1116 or through Family Caregiver Alliance at 800–445-8106	www.aoa.gov	Information for caregivers including individual counseling, training, and respite options usually managed through AAAs

multicomponent intervention improves quality of life and depression among caregivers across different ethnic and racial groups within the United States.[36] Outside the United States, some cultures consider family caregiving as a key component of their long-term care. Germany, Australia, and the United Kingdom are examples of countries where caregivers are considered integral to the functioning of their long-term care systems. Legislation has dictated this. In other cultures, however, caregiving is considered the cultural norm. The provision of care by families is expected, not considered the exception. In those societies, nursing homes are few and families provide care to their elder relatives in the home setting.

As our country faces an enormous increase in the number of older Americans, the role of family caregivers will become increasingly important. It is the role of many health care professionals, especially primary care physicians, to identify people in the caregiving role and to screen for caregiving stress or burden. It is likewise important to screen for health effects including depression, anxiety, and substance abuse. It is also key to link caregivers to local resources. These include the area agencies on aging, the Alzheimer's Association, support groups, individual counseling, respite services, and adult day services. Occupational and physical therapy may also be useful services for family caregivers of frail or demented elders. Caregivers should also be assisted in applying for services through available financial resources, especially through the NFCSP or other organizations that exist in most communities.

REFERENCES

1. Agency on Aging. 2006. Available at: http://www.aoa.gov/prof/ Statistics/online_stat_data.
2. Wilmoth JM, Longino CF. Demographic trends that will shape U. S. policy in the twenty-first century. *Res Aging.* 2006;28:269–288.
3. Stone R., Cafferata GL, Sangl J. Caregivers of the frail elderly: A national profile. *Gerontologist.* 1987;27:616–626.
4. Thompson L. Long-term care: support for family caregivers. Georgetown University Long-term Financing Project. 2004. Available at: http://ltc.georgetown.edu. Accessed June 28, 2008.
5. Shultz R, Beach SR. Caregiving as a risk factor for mortality. The Caregiver Health Effects Study. *JAMA.* 1999;282:2215–2219.
6. Himes CL. Future caregivers: projected family structures of older persons. *J Gerontol Soc Sci.* 1992;47:S17–S26.
7. Amato P, Booth A. A prospective study of divorce and parent-child relationships. *J Marriage Fam.* 1996;58:356–365.
8. Freedman VA, Martin LG, Schoeni RF. Recent trends in disability and functioning among older adults in the United States: a systematic review. *JAMA.* 2002;288:3137–3146.
9. George LK, Gwyther LP. Caregiver well-being: a multidimensional examination of family caregivers of demented adults. *Gerontologist.* 1986;26:253–259.
10. Zarit, SH, Todd PA, Zarit JM. Subjective burden of husbands and wives as caregivers: a longitudinal study. *Gerontologist.* 1986;26:260–266.
11. Donelan K, Hill CA, Hoffman C, et al. Challenged to care: informal caregivers in a changing health system. *Health Aff.* 2002;21:222–231.
12. Aneshensel C, Pearlin L, Mullan J, et al. *Profiles in Caregiving: The Unexpected Career.* New York: Academic Press; 1995.
13. Semple SJ. Conflict in Alzheimer's caregiving families: its dimensions and consequences. *Gerontologist.* 1992;32:648–655.
14. Christakis NA, Allison PD. Mortality after the hospitalization of a spouse. *NEJM.* 2006;354:719–730.
15. Baumgarten M, Hanley JA, Infante-Rivard C, et al. Health of family members caring for elderly persons with dementia. *Ann Intern Med.* 1994;120:126–132.
16. Rosenthal CJ, Sulman J, Marshall VW. Depressive symptoms in family caregivers of long-stay patients. *Gerontologist.* 1993;33:249–256.
17. Williamson GM, Schultz R. Coping with specific stressors in Alzheimer's disease caregiving. *Gerontologist.* 1993;33:747–755.
18. Cochrane JJ, Goering PN, Rogers JM. The mental health of informal caregivers in Ontario: an epidemiologic survey. *Am J Pub Health.* 1997;87:202–207.
19. Kiecolt-Glaser JK, Dura JR, Speicher CE, et al. Spousal caregivers of dementia victims: longitudinal changes in immunity and health. *Psychosoc Med.* 1991;53:345–362.
20. Brown LJ, Potter JF, Foster BG. Caregiver burden should be evaluated during geriatric assessment. *J Am Geriatr Soc.* 1990;38:455–460.
21. Lowenthal MF, Berkman P. *Aging and Mental Disorders in San Francisco.* San Francisco: Jossey-Bass; 1967.
22. Lawton MP, Moss M, Hoffman C, et al. Two transitions in daughters' caregiving careers. *Gerontologist.* 2000;40:437–448.
23. Skaff M, Pearllin LI, Mullan JT. Transition in the caregiving career: effects on sense of mastery. *Psychol Aging.* 1966;11:247–257.
24. Yesavage JA, Brink TL, Rose TL, et al. Development and validation of a geriatric depression screening scale: a preliminary report. *J Psych Res.* 1982–1983;17:37–49.
25. Andolsek KM, Clapp-Channing NE, Gehlbach SH, et al. Caregivers and elderly relatives: the prevalence of caregiving in a family practice. *Arch Intern Med.* 1988;148:2177–2180.
26. Parks SM, Novielli KD. A practical guide to caring for caregivers. *Am Fam Physician.* 2000;62:2613–2620.
27. Nicholas E. An outcomes focus in carer assessment and review: value and challenge. *Br J Soc Work.* 2003;33:31–47.
28. National Consensus Report on Caregiver Assessment. Vols. I and II. Available at: http://www.caregiver.org/caregiver/jsp/content_node.jsp?nodeid=1630. Accessed June 28, 2008.
29. Zarit SH, Reever KE, Bach-Peterson J. Relatives of the impaired elderly: correlates of feelings of burden. *Gerontologist.* 1980;20:649–655.
30. Mittleman M, Ferris SH, Shulman E, et al. A comprehensive support program: effect on depression in spouse-caregiver of AD patients. *Gerontologist.* 1995;35:792–802.
31. Haley WE. The family caregiver's role in Alzheimer's disease. *Neurology.* 1997;48:S25–29.
32. Lawton MP, Brody EM, Saperstein AR. A controlled study of respite service for caregivers of Alzheimer's patients. *Gerontologist.* 1989;29:8–16.
33. Forde OT, Pearlman S. Breakaway: a social supplement to caregiver's support groups. *Am J Alz Dis.* 1999;14:120–124.

34. Feinberg LF, Whitlach C. *Family Caregivers and Consumer Choice.* San Fransico: Family Caregiver Alliance; 1996.

35. Administration on Aging. The Older Americans Act: National Family Caregivers Support Program (Title III-E and Title VI-C): Compassion in Action. Washington, DC: US Department of Health and Human Services, Administration on Aging; 2004.

36. Belle SH, Burgio L, Burns R, et al. Enhancing the quality of life of dementia caregivers from different ethnic or racial groups. *Ann Intern Med.* 2006;145:727.

57

SYSTEMATIC APPROACHES TO PREVENTING ERRORS
IN THE CARE OF THE ELDERLY

Jeanette Koran, BS, RN, Amy Talati, PharmD, Albert G. Crawford, PhD, MBA, MSIS

INTRODUCTION

According to estimates from the Institute of Medicine, 44,000–98,000 patients die in U.S. hospitals annually because of injuries sustained because of errors. Unsafe and inadequate care in other settings such as physician offices, emergency departments, and nursing homes compounds the problem. This chapter will review three systematic approaches to preventing errors in the care of the elderly:

1. Improving coordination of care, especially during transitions of care
2. Reducing medication errors through improved guidelines and practices for prescribers, nurses, and pharmacists, and systems for tracking and reporting medication errors
3. Health information technology (IT), including computerized alerts and reminders and decision support systems, and electronic health records (EHRs).

COORDINATION DURING TRANSITIONS OF CARE

Problem

The Joint Commission on Accreditation of Healthcare Organizations (November 1999 Institute of Medicine [IOM] Report) reports that communication issues were the root cause of approximately 65% of the 2,966 sentinel events identified from 1995 to 2004,[1] and approximately 64% of the 3,548 sentinel events reported by 2005.[2]

"Hand-offs," or transfers of patient care, are inevitable in health care. Home to facility, facility to facility, shift to shift, caregiver to caregiver intensive care and emergency department transfers or procedure back to floor and visa versa, and facility to home and/or home care are some examples of occasions when effective communication is critical or crucial to ensure that safe care is rendered. The potential for error then because of missed communication is multiplied when dealing with a geriatric population struggling with the complexities of comorbid disease conditions and health care treatments, confusing medical jargon, and the fear that can be associated with unfamiliar surroundings.

Changes in how medical care is delivered impact continuity and coordination of care. For instance, the recent mandate by the Accreditation Council of Graduate Medical Education of an 80-hour work week for residents necessitates more frequent sign-off of patients from one caregiver to another. The shortage of nurses and the use of temporary staff are other factors that may result in increased hand-offs to individuals who are unfamiliar with particular patients. Care fragmentation and the complexity of care pose a challenge for the medical community. This challenge is being addressed by governmental and regulatory agencies and is being met by the physicians, nurses, and organizations that provide care to patients.

Organizational Response – Progress Toward a Solution

The National Patient Safety Goals required by The Joint Commission on Accreditation of Healthcare Organizations in 2006 introduced a new element under the requirements for Goal 2: Improve the effectiveness of communication among caregivers – 2e: Implement a standardized approach to "hand-off" communications, including an opportunity to ask and respond to questions.[3] In terms of Implementation Expectations: The following are attributes of effective 'hand off' communications.

- Hand offs are interactive communications allowing the opportunity for questioning between the giver and receiver of patient/client/resident information.
- Hand offs include up-to-date information regarding the patient's/client's/resident's care, treatment and services, condition and any recent or anticipated changes.

- Interruptions during hand offs are limited to minimize the possibility that information would fail to be conveyed or would be forgotten.
- Hand offs require a process for verification of the received information, including repeat-back or read-back, as appropriate.
- The receiver of the hand off information has an opportunity to review relevant patient/client/resident historical data, which may include previous care, treatment and services.[4]

These basically address the who, what, where, and when of patient communication.

On July 20, 2006, the Center for Medicare and Medicaid Services (CMS) issued a response to the IOM report about identifying and preventing medication errors. Among the standards introduced by CMS was "working with local Quality Improvement Organizations (QIOs) to use medication reconciliation and focus on the reliability of transfers and hand-offs from one care setting to another."[5] Broad standards such as this provide an atlas rather than a road map for organizations to reach the quality destination or desired outcome. Organizational leadership must encourage collaborations with QIOs, local organizations struggling with the same issues, and national programs publishing possible "solutions."

The National Committee for Quality Assurance (NCQA) provider evaluation program, Physician Practice Connections, recognizes and rewards physician practices that use information systematically to enhance the quality of patient care.[6] Theoretically an interoperable EHR would provide a transparent and comprehensive view of a patient's health record/history. NCQA realizes the importance of communication to facilitate continuous, coordinated care across the health care continuum. NCQA evaluates standards that cover:

- Enabling patients to communicate with and access the practice easily
- Using systems to track patients, their treatments, and conditions
- Managing patients' care proactively over time
- Supporting patients' self-management of their health
- Using electronic prescribing tools
- Tracking and following up laboratory and imaging tests
- Tracking and following up referrals
- Measuring performance and working to improve care
- Updating to interoperable electronic systems.

Programs that reward health care providers for providing safe care such as the Bridges to Excellence Coalition utilize Physician Practice Connections as a performance assessment measure.[6]

So, what is being done at the organizational level? How can these standards/recommendations be put into practice? Can we measure effectiveness? Finally, can we motivate patients to be active participants in their care? The University Health-System Consortium, an organization composed of representatives from academic medical centers across the country, pools data and addresses quality and safety issues that medical centers are facing nationwide. Organizations such as this strive to provide road maps for implementation that can be adopted at the facility level. The University HealthSystem Consortium develops best practice recommendations that can be reviewed and adopted by members of the consortium. In addition, organizations have published information that chronicles the implementation of various methods to improve communication. Standardized, electronic, and team oriented are adjectives used to describe techniques aimed at standardizing communication.

What are the elements necessary to provide the framework for an effective transfer of patient care? Information shared must be accurate and timely delivered in an atmosphere with minimal distractions and an opportunity for questions. There is no easy answer, but by utilizing data from the electronic medical record for demographics and laboratory and test results supplemented by an interactive piece for sign-out notes and augmented with face-to-face time is a reasonable place to start.

One communication technique, Situation-Background-Assessment-Recommendation or SBAR provides a framework for communication between members of the health care team about a patient's condition. The acronym is an easy-to-remember, concrete mechanism useful for framing any conversation, especially critical ones, requiring a clinician's immediate attention and action. This technique was developed by Michael Leonard, physician leader for patient safety, along with colleagues Doug Bonacum and Suzanne Graham at Kaiser Permanente of Colorado. It can be downloaded from the Institute for Healthcare Improvement website, which provides resources for the improvement of health care.[7]

Several hospitals are addressing this issue and have published studies documenting their experience. At the University of Washington, a group of 28 residents, representing eight services, participated in the design of a computerized resident sign-out system. "Accuracy, flexibility, and portability were identified as key elements by the design team."[8] In February 2003, at the Jacobi Medical Center (Bronx, NY) internal medicine residents began using a computerized sign-out program that had been incorporated into the computerized medical record. It was recognized by physicians and nurses on a medicine ward that communication between nurses and house staff was getting in the way of patient care. The hospital started a pilot study to explore the potential benefits of offering inpatient nurses access to the sign-out program. Nurses were able to print out the sign out sheet to utilize this information in planning care and at the end of shift report. The nurses reported increased job satisfaction and an increased ability to care for patients secondary to increased understanding of the rationale for admissions and increased communication among house staff.[9] The Veterans Affairs Medical Center in Massachusetts published a study that evaluated the impact of a computerized sign-out program after a 4-month implementation period. They concluded that house staff are willing participants in efforts to measure and improve the quality of health care and the intervention may have reduced the risk for medical injury associated with discontinuity of inpatient care.[10]

A recent report by the IOM[11] addresses the need for systems for rewarding quality measurement and public reporting of quality measures by providers. Additionally, the IOM recommendations focus on the critical importance of two quality improvement approaches emphasized in this chapter. First, the significance of care coordination is addressed in an IOM recommendation: "Recommendation 8: CMS should design the Medicare pay-for-performance program to include components that promote, recognize, and reward improved coordination of care across providers and through entire episodes of illness. Thus, CMS should 1) encourage beneficiaries and providers to identify providers who would be considered their principal responsible source of care, and 2) pay for and reward successful care coordination that meets specified standards for providers who take on that role."

Exercise

Have someone read the following paragraph to you in a crowded cafeteria or restaurant without the opportunity to ask questions

An 84-year-old female patient, A.P., transferred from an extended care facility s/p fall with complaints of dizziness. Co-morbidities include: non-insulin dependent diabetes mellitus, hypertension, hypercholesterolemia, osteoporosis, early senile dementia. Current medications include: Glucophage 850 mg tid, hydrochlorothiazide 25 mg bid, Captopril 25 mg qday, Simvastatin 10 mg qday, Raloxifene 60 mg qday, and ASA 81 mg qday. Fall not witnessed by staff. No fractures per x-ray, bruising on lower spine. Cat scan negative for bleed. Most recently, a GI virus had been diagnosed in approximately 40% of the residents at the extended care facility although patient did not present with signs and symptoms of GI distress. Prior to this incident patient required minimal assistance with ADLs including encouragement to po feed. Mrs. P's Glucophage had recently been increased to tid dosing from 500 mg bid and her roommate of 2 years had transferred to a facility in another state 2 days prior to the fall.

Several hours later confer with your notes and look at the following questions:

1. Do you have all of the information recorded?
2. Theoretically, is all the information you need to care for this patient provided in this blurb?
3. What questions does this generate?
4. Could you organize this into a template?

PREVENTING MEDICATION ERRORS

Introduction

Due to advancements in health care and technology, people in the United States are remaining healthier and living longer. Currently, the approximately 36 million individuals aged 65 years or older represent 15% of the total U.S. population.[12] Because the frequency of acute and chronic illness increases with age, the elderly receive disproportionate amounts of medications compared with the general public, consuming nearly 33% of all prescription medications and 40% of over-the-counter medications.[12] In 2003, approximately 50% of all seniors and 70% of those with *more than three* chronic conditions were consuming *more than five* prescription medications a day.[13]

According to a report published by the IOM[14] in July 2006, 1.5 million U.S. patients are harmed or killed each year because of medication errors. The report states that a) on average, a patient hospitalized in the United States will experience at least one medication error per day, and b) each year, medication errors cause at least 400,000 preventable injuries and deaths in hospitals, more than 800,000 in nursing homes and long-term care facilities, and more than 530,000 among Medicare beneficiaries treated in outpatient settings.[14]

Medications are unquestionably a vital and cost-effective component of the health management of seniors. They play an essential role in improving an older adult's health status and overall quality of life. Given the elderly's large consumption of medications, decline in physiological function due to aging and various comorbidities, it is not surprising that they are at greater risk for experiencing an adverse drug event (ADE) or medication error.

Medication Errors: Definition

According to the National Coordinating Council for Medication Error Reporting and Prevention ([NCCMERP] www.nccmerp.org/aboutMedErrors.html) a medication error can be defined as follows:

> A medication error is any preventable event that may cause or lead to inappropriate medication use or patient harm while the medication is in the control of the health care professional, patient, or consumer. Such events may be related to professional practice, health care products, procedures, and systems, including prescribing; order communication; product labeling, packaging, and nomenclature; compounding; dispensing; distribution; administration; education; monitoring; and use.

Medication errors are the result of multidisciplinary and multifactorial sources. Errors result from lack of knowledge, poor performance, or system failure. The Institute for Safe Medication Practices (ISMP) identifies the following areas as potential causes of medication errors (ISMP Website, www.ISMP.org. Accessed October 26, 2006; Jackson MA, Reines WG. A Systematic Approach to Preventing Medication Errors. Available at: www.uspharmacist.com. Accessed September 29, 2006):

- Failed communication
- Poor drug distribution practices
- Complex or poorly designed technology
- Access to drugs by nonpharmacy personnel

Table 57.1. Types of Medication Errors[a]

Type	Definition
Prescribing error	Incorrect drug selection (based on indications, contraindications, known allergies, existing drug therapy, and other factors), dose, dosage form, quantity, route, concentration, rate of administration, or instructions for use of a drug product ordered or authorized by physician (or other legitimate prescriber); illegible prescriptions or medication orders that lead to errors that reach the patient.
Omission error[b]	The failure to administer an ordered dose to a patient before the next scheduled dose, if any.
Wrong time error	Administration of medication outside predefined time interval from its scheduled administration time (this interval should be established by each individual health care facility).
Unauthorized drug error[c]	Administration to the patient of medication not authorized by a legitimate prescriber for the patient.
Improper dose error[d]	Administration to the patient of a dose that is greater than or less than the amount ordered by the prescriber or administration of duplicate doses to the patient.
Wrong dosage-form error[e]	Administration to the patient of a drug product in a different dosage form that ordered by the prescriber.
Wrong drug-preparation error[f]	Drug product incorrectly formulated or manipulated before administration.
Wrong administration-technique error[g]	Inappropriate procedure or improper technique in the administration of a drug.
Deteriorated drug error[h]	Administration of a drug that has expired or for which the physical or chemical dosage-form integrity has been compromised.
Monitoring error	Failure to review a prescribed regimen for appropriateness and detection of problems, or failure to use appropriate clinical or laboratory data for adequate assessment of patient response to prescribed therapy.
Compliance error	Inappropriate patient behavior regarding adherence to a prescribed medication regimen.
Other medication error	Any medication error that does not fall into one of the previously predefined categories.

[a] The categories may not be mutually exclusive because of the multidisciplinary and multifactorial nature of medication errors.

[b] Assumes no prescribing error. Excluded would be 1) a patient's refusal to take the medication or 2) a decision not to administer the dose because of recognized contraindications. If an explanation for the omission is apparent, that reason should be documented in the appropriate records.

[c] This would include, for example, a wrong drug, a dose given to the wrong patient, unordered drugs, and doses given outside a stated set of clinical guidelines or protocols.

[d] Excluded would be 1) allowable deviations based on preset ranges established by individual health care organizations in consideration of measuring devices routinely provided to those who administer drugs to patients or other factors such as conversion of doses expressed in the apothecary system to the metric system and 2) topical dosage forms for which medication orders are not expressed quantitatively.

[e] Excluded would be accepted protocols that authorize pharmacists to dispense alternate dosage forms for patients with special needs as allowed by state regulators.

[f] This would include, for example, incorrect dilution or reconstitution, mixing drugs that are physically or chemically incompatible, and inadequate product packaging.

[g] This would include doses administered 1) via the wrong route (different from the route prescribed), 2) via the correct route but at the wrong site, and 3) at the wrong rate of administration.

[h] This would include, for example, administration of expired drugs and improperly stored drugs.

- Workplace environmental problems that lead to increased job stress
- Dose miscalculations
- Lack of patient information
- Lack of patients' understanding of their therapy

Medication errors may be committed by any members of the health care team, including pharmacists, physicians, nurses, supportive personnel, students, clerical staff, pharmaceutical manufacturers, patients and their caregivers, and others. Although the outcomes of many errors may be minimal, some result in serious morbidity or mortality (ASHP Guidelines on Preventing Medication Errors in Hospitals. Available at: www.ashp.org/bestpractices/MedMis/MedMis_Gdl_Hosp.pdf. Accessed September 29, 2006).

Table 57.1, adapted from the ASHP Guidelines on Preventing Medication Errors in Hospitals, highlights various types of medication errors including prescribing errors, dispensing errors, and medication administration errors. Although this list has been compiled to apply to an inpatient hospital setting, many of the errors are applicable to other practice settings.

Table 57.2. Recommendation to Enhance Accuracy of Prescription Writing: Dangerous Abbreviations

Abbreviation	Intended Meaning	Common Error
U	Units	Mistaken as a zero or a four (4) resulting in overdose. Also mistaken for "cc" (cubic centimeters) when poorly written.
μg	Micrograms	Mistaken for "mg" (milligrams) resulting in an overdose.
Q.D.	Latin abbreviation for every day	The period after the "Q" has sometimes been mistaken for an "I" and the drug has been given "QID" (four times daily) rather than daily.
Q.O.D	Latin abbreviation for every other day	Misinterpreted as "QD" (daily) or "QID" (four times daily). If the "O" is poorly written, it looks like a period or "I."
SC or SQ	Subcutaneous	Mistaken as "L" (sublingual) when poorly written.
TIW	Three times a week	Misinterpreted as "three times a day" or "twice a week."
D/C	Discharge; also discontinue	Patient's medications have been prematurely discontinued when D/C, (intended to mean "discharge") was misinterpreted as "discontinue," because it was followed by a list of drugs.
HS	Half strength	Misinterpreted as the Latin abbreviation "HS" (hours of sleep).
cc	Cubic centimeters	Mistaken as "U" (units) when poorly written.
AU, AS, AD	Latin abbreviation for both ears; left ear; right ear	Misinterpreted as the Latin abbreviation "OU" (both eyes); "OS" (left eye); "OD" (right eye)
IU	International Unit	Mistaken as IV (intravenous) or 10 (ten)

See the full Council Recommendation, Recommendations to Enhance Accuracy of Prescription Writing © 1998–2006 National Coordinating Council for Medication Error Reporting and Prevention. All Rights Reserved. Used with permission.

Beers Criteria

Inappropriate prescribing has been reported as the most prominent cause of ADEs.[15] One study reported that 17% of all hospital admissions by elderly patients were the result of ADEs.[15] Beers and colleagues published an explicit list of criteria in 1991 in an attempt to create structure regarding appropriate prescribing for the elderly. This list defines and identifies medications and classes of medications that should be avoided and has become the most widely used consensus criteria for appropriate medication use in the elderly.[16] This list of medications was established by an expert consensus panel and has been updated twice (1997 and 2003) since its inception.[16,17] According to the Beers criteria, potentially inappropriate medications are defined as drugs that are ineffective, pose unnecessarily high risks for patients, or are available in safer alternative forms.[17–19]

At the point of prescribing, it is important to avoid using medications that may be inappropriate in the elderly. Reliance on the Beers criteria can help guide use of medications associated with the least risk for an older adult. Chapter 5, Appropriate Use of Medications in the Elderly, addresses the Beers criteria in more detail.

Recommendations for Preventing Medication Errors

Various national organizations such as the IOM, the ISMP, the ASHP, and the Food and Drug Administration (FDA) have each published guidelines and recommendations for the prevention of medication errors. All of these guidelines include strategies for preventing errors at an individual and organizational level and also discuss methods of managing errors once they have occurred. This chapter focuses solely on approaches that a health care provider (prescriber, nurse, and pharmacist) can utilize in their daily practice. Strategies for incorporating safety measures into organizational systems such as computerized physician order entry (CPOE) systems, electronic prescribing, and bar coding are beyond the scope of this chapter. The following recommendations for prescribers, nurses, and pharmacists

Table 57.3. Official "Do Not Use" List[a]

Do Not Use	Potential Problems	Use Instead
U (unit)	Mistaken for "0" (zero), the number "4" (four) or "cc"	Write "unit"
IU (international unit)	Mistaken for IV (intravenous) or the number 10 (ten)	Write "international unit"
Q.D., QD, q.d., dq (daily)	Mistaken for each other	Write "daily"
Q.O.D., QOD, q.o.d., qod (every other day)	Period after the Q mistaken for "I" and the "O" mistaken for "I"	Write "every other day"
Trailing zero (X.0 mg)[b]	Decimal point is missed	Write X mg
Lack of leading zero (.X mg)		Write 0.X mg
MS	Can mean morphine sulfate or magnesium sulfate	Write "morphine sulfate"
MSO$_4$ and MgSO$_4$	Confused for one another	Write "magnesium sulfate"

[a] Applies to all orders and all medication-related documentation that is handwritten (including free-text computer entry) or on preprinted forms.

[b] Exception: A "trailing zero" may be used only where required to demonstrate the level of precision of the value being reported, such as for laboratory results, imaging studies that report size of lesions, or catheter/tube sizes. It may not be used in medication orders or other medication-related documentation. www.ismp.org.

have been adapted from the ASHP Guidelines on Preventing Medication Errors in Hospitals.

Prescribers

Because many medication errors arise when medications are being prescribed, ASHP recommends the following for physicians and other prescribers.

1. To determine appropriate drug therapy, stay abreast of the current state of knowledge through literature review, consultation with pharmacists and other physicians, participation in continuing education programs, and other means.
2. Evaluate the patient's total status and review all existing drug therapy before prescribing new or additional medications.
3. In hospitals, be familiar with the medication ordering system.
4. Drug orders should be complete and include patient name, generic drug name, trademarked name, route and site of administration, dosage form, strength, quantity, frequency of administration, and prescriber's name. Prescribers should review all drug orders for accuracy and legibility immediately after they have prescribed them.
5. Care should be taken to ensure that the intent of medication orders is clear and unambiguous. Tables 57.2 and 57.3 highlight dangerous abbreviations that should be avoided.
6. Written drug or prescription orders should be legible.
7. Verbal drug or prescription orders should be reserved only for those situations in which it is impossible or impractical

for the prescriber to write the order or enter it in the computer. A written copy of the verbal order should be placed in the patient's medical record.
8. When possible, drugs should be prescribed for administration by the oral route rather than by injection.
9. When possible, talk with the patient or caregiver to explain the medication prescribed and any special precautions or observations that might be indicated, including any allergic or hypersensitivity reactions that might occur.
10. Follow up and periodically evaluate the need for continued drug therapy for individual patients.
11. Instructions with respect to "hold" orders for medications should be clear.

Nurses

Due to their constant interaction with patients, nurses are in an excellent position to detect and report medication errors. In an inpatient setting, nurses often serve as the final point in the checks-and-balances triad for the medication use process and thus they play a crucial role in error reduction. The following recommendations are made:

1. Be familiar with the medication ordering and use system.
2. Review patients' medications with respect to desired patient outcomes, therapeutic duplications, and possible drug interactions.
3. All drug orders should be verified before medication administration.
4. Patient identity should be verified before the administration of each prescribed dose.

5. All doses should be administered at scheduled times unless there are questions or problems to be resolved.

6. When standard drug concentrations or dosage charts are not available, dosage calculations, flow rates, and other mathematical calculations should be checked by a second individual.

7. The drug distribution system should not be circumvented by "borrowing" medications from one patient to give to a different patient or by stockpiling unused medications.

8. If there are questions when a large volume or number of dosage units is needed for a single patient dose, the medication order should be verified.

9. All personnel using medication administration devices should understand their operation and the opportunities for error that might occur with the use of such devices.

10. Talk with patients or caregivers to ascertain that they understand the use of their medications and any special precautions or observations that might be indicated.

11. When a patient objects to or questions whether a particular drug should be administered, the nurse should listen, answer questions, and (if appropriate) double check the medication order and product dispensed before administering it to ensure that no preventable error is made. If a patient refuses to take a prescribed medication, that decision should be documented in the appropriate patient records.

Pharmacists

The pharmacist plays a vital role in preventing medication misuse. As drug experts, pharmacists should be involved in assessment, management, and surveillance of drug regimens. They can advise providers on elements of appropriate drug use for the elderly, while also serving as a liaison between the patient and provider in an effort to maintain communication and prevent medication errors. It is also important that the pharmacist devote careful attention to dispensing processes to ensure that errors are not introduced at that point in the process. The following recommendations are suggested for pharmacists.

1. Participate in drug therapy monitoring and DUE activities to help achieve safe, effective, and rational use of drugs.

2. To recommend and recognize appropriate drug therapy, stay abreast of the current state of knowledge.

3. Make themselves available to prescribers and nurses to offer information and advice about therapeutic drug regimens and the correct use of medications.

4. Be familiar with the medication ordering system and drug distribution policies and procedures.

5. Never assume or guess the intent of confusing medication orders.

6. When preparing drugs, maintain orderliness and cleanliness in the work area and perform one procedure at a time with as few interruptions as possible.

7. Before dispensing a medication in nonemergency situations, review an original copy of the written medication order.

8. Dispense medications in ready-to-administer dosage forms whenever possible.

9. Review the use of auxiliary labels and use the labels prudently when it is clear that such use may prevent errors.

10. Ensure that medications are delivered to the patient care area in a timely fashion after receipt of orders.

11. Observe how medications are actually being used in patient care areas to ensure that dispensing and storage procedures are followed and to assist nursing in optimizing patient safety.

12. Pharmacy staff should review medications that are returned to the department.

13. When dispensing medications to ambulatory patients, counsel patients or caregivers and verify that they understand why a medication was prescribed and dispensed, its intended use, any special precautions that might be observed, and other needed information.

14. Maintain records sufficient to enable identification of patients receiving an erroneous product.

Tracking and Reporting Medication Errors

If a medication error has occurred, it is important to document its cause and then study it to improve systems as an effort to minimize recurrences. It is important to classify the potential seriousness and clinical significance of the detected error. This classification should be based on predefined criteria established within the organization. Use of a classification system allows for better management and follow-up activities upon error detection.

The NCCMERP adopted a *Medication Error Index* that classifies an error according to the severity of the outcome. The NCCMERP hopes that this index will help practitioners and institutions track errors in a consistent, systematic manner. The index considers factors such as whether the error reached the patient and, if the patient was harmed, to what degree. A copy of the *Medication Error Index* is available at www.nccmerp.org/medErrorCatIndex.html.

The following organizations accept medication error reports from consumers and health professionals. If a medication error has occurred at your institution, a report should be submitted to the most applicable organization listed below.

The Food and Drug Administration

The FDA accepts reports from consumers and health professionals about products regulated by the FDA, including drugs and medical devices, through MedWatch, the FDA's safety information and adverse event reporting program.

Phone: 1–800–332–1088

www.fda.gov/medwatch/how.htm

Institute for Safe Medication Practices

The ISMP accepts reports from consumers and health professionals related to medication. They also publish *Safe Medicine*, a consumer newsletter on medication errors.

Phone: 215–947-7797

www.ismp.org/pages/consumer.html

U.S. Pharmacopeia

The U.S. Pharmacopei runs MedMARX, an anonymous medication error-reporting program used by hospitals.

Phone: 1–800-822–8772

www.medmarx.com or www.usp.org

HEALTH INFORMATION TECHNOLOGY

Health IT that can play a key role in preventing errors in the care of the elderly includes: computerized alerts, reminders, and decision support tools, and EHRs.

Computerized Alerts, Reminders, and Decision Support Tools

There is an emerging understanding that humans are inherently fallible and that part of the solution to the problems of inadequate quality and safety of care lies in redesigning systems of care to reduce the likelihood of errors. Health IT can play a key role in facilitating clinicians' memory, information processing, and decision making, in applications ranging from automated alerts and reminders to computerized decision support. For example, a randomized controlled trial (RCT) found that computerized reminders to physicians about when to repeat tests reduce unnecessary testing.[20] Similarly, another RCT found that automated alerts including critical laboratory test results reduce time to appropriate treatment, compared with conventional hospital pages.[21] A related application of health IT is standardized protocols; for example, one study of patients in intensive care units with severe respiratory disease found that computerized treatment protocols resulted in a fourfold increase in the survival rate.[22] Similarly, a systematic review of assessments of the effects of computerized decision support systems in 1998 found beneficial effects on physician performance in 43 of 65 studies, and beneficial effects on patient outcomes in 6 of 14 studies.[23]

Several studies demonstrate benefits for patient safety in particular:

- A computerized decision support system combined with CPOE reduced the incidence of ADEs during antibiotic administration by 75% and also reduced orders for drugs where there were patient reports of allergies or antibiotic-related ADEs.[24,25]
- Automated reminders were found to increase orders for recommended services from 22% to 46%.[26]
- A CPOE/decision support system increased use of appropriate medications in high-risk situations, e.g., use of subcutaneous heparin to prevent venous thromboembolism,

from 24% to 47% and decreased medication errors by 19%–84%.[27,28]

Electronic Health Records

Introduction

EHRs have long been promoted as central to the solution of the problems of high cost, inefficiency, and inadequate quality and safety in the U.S. health care system; however, at present, only approximately 24% of physician office practices have adopted ambulatory EHRs.[29] Nevertheless, we may now be witnessing a turning point in the adoption process, with a number of developments combining to promote widespread implementation of ambulatory EHRs. Such recent developments include President Bush' 2004 goal that all Americans should have access to EHRs within 10 years, his administration's creation that year of the Office of the National Coordinator for Health Information Technology (ONCHIT), the increasing focus by all parties on quality and safety, and improved incentives for adoption offered by payers. Specifically, many payers have been motivated by the increasingly popular idea that widespread EHR adoption can generate huge cost savings and have developed pay-for-performance (P4P) initiatives to promote value in health care purchasing. P4P systems can promote adoption of ambulatory EHRs in two ways:

1. *Directly*, as in the case of the Leapfrog Group's statement on safety practices, that is, "Research shows that if the first three leaps (CPOE, Intensive Care Unit Physician Staffing, and Evidence-based Hospital Referral) were implemented in all urban hospitals in the United States we could save up to 65,341 lives, prevent as many as 907,600 serious medication errors each year, and save $41.5 billion."[30]
2. *Indirectly*, by rewarding high-quality care, given that a prerequisite for quality, and quality improvement, is an ambulatory EHR that allows quality measurement.

Medicare and Medicaid are, of course, the largest payers in the United States, and the IOM has recently recommended that the CMS promote the use of health IT as follows: Recommendation 9: Because electronic health information technology will increase the probability of a successful pay-for-performance program, the Secretary of DHHS should explore a variety of approaches for assisting providers in the implementation of electronic data collection and reporting systems to strengthen the use of consistent performance measures.[11]

How to Evaluate and Select Ambulatory EHR Systems

The most valuable guide in selecting an ambulatory EHR system is whether it been certified by the Certification Commission for Healthcare Information Technology (CCHIT), a federally supported private testing organization.[31] CCHIT designed its voluntary certification program to clarify the confusing HIT market and to promote EHR adoption. Some 38 products met the 2006 ambulatory certification criteria; an up-to-date list can be found at: www.cchit.org/certified/products.htm.

Useful Websites

National Patient Safety Goals	www.jointcommission.org/PatientSafety/NationalPatientSafetyGoals/06_npsgs.htm
National Committee for Quality Assurance, Physician Practice Connections	www.ncqa.org/ppc/
Institute of Healthcare Improvement	www.ihi.org
National Coordinating Council for Medication Error Reporting and Prevention	www.nccmerp.org/aboutMedErrors.html
The Institute for Safe Medication Practices	www.ismp.org
ASHP Guidelines on Preventing Medication Errors in Hospitals	www.ashp.org/bestpractices/MedMis/MedMis_Gdl_Hosp.pdf
Beers Criteria	archinte.ama-assn.org/cgi/reprint/163/22/2716/pdf
NCCMERP Medication Error Index	www.nccmerp.org/medErrorCatIndex.html
The Food and Drug Administration MedWatch program	www.fda.gov.medwatch/how.htm
ISMP's *Safe Medicine*, consumer newsletter on medication errors	www.ismp.org/pages/consumer.htm
U.S. Pharmacopeia MedMARX program	www.medmarx.com
Certification Commission for Healthcare Information Technology (CCHIT) Ambulatory Certification Criteria	www.cchit.org/certified/products.htm

Support in Implementing and Maintaining an EHR System

A recent CMS initiative promoting health IT is its Doctor's Office Quality-Information Technology (DOQ-IT) program, implemented through the national network of regional QIOs. The main goals of the DOQ-IT program are to provide:

- Help in evaluating practice needs and capabilities.
- Education on features, functionality, and options for purchasing EHRs.
- Objective information and assistance with vendor selection.
- Advice on refining processes and office workflow to improve efficiencies and patient care.
- Enhanced knowledge of available technology from an objective and reliable source.
- Understanding of how to achieve optimal use of technology.
- Access to the latest innovations in health information technology.

CONCLUSION

This chapter has reviewed three systematic approaches to preventing errors in the care of the elderly:

1. Improving coordination of care, especially during transitions of care.
2. Reducing medication errors through improved guidelines and practices for prescribers, nurses, and pharmacists, and systems for tracking and reporting medication errors.

3. Health IT, including computerized alerts, reminders, and decision support systems, and EHRs.

The authors hope that the reviews of these systematic approaches will aid clinicians in their efforts to promote high-quality, safe care of the elderly.

REFERENCES

1. Gmah L. Hand offs – a link to improving patient safety. *AORN J.* 2006;83:227–230.
2. The Joint Commission's Annual Report on Quality and Safety 2007. Improving American's Hospitals. Available at: http://www.jointcommissionreport.org/performanceresults/sentinel.aspx. Accessed 8/10/2008.
3. The Joint Commission. National Patient Safety Goals (effective January 1, 2006). Available at: http://www.jointcommission.org/PatientSafety/NationalPatientSafetyGoals/06_npsgs.htm. Accessed June 29, 2008.
4. The Joint Commission. 2008 National Patient Safety Goals Disease-Specific Care. Available at: http://www.jointcommission.org/PatientSafety/NationalPatientSafetyGoals/. Accessed 8/10/2008.
5. U.S. Department of Health and Human Services. CMS administrator speaks to Institute of Medicine report. *CMS News.* 2006;9/28/2006.
6. Physician Practice Connections. NCQA acknowledging outstanding performance. *Physician Pract Connect.* 7/24/2006.
7. Institute for Healthcare Improvement. Patient safety tools. Available at: http://www.ihi.org/IHI/Topics/PatientSafety/SafetyGeneral/Tools/SBARTechniqueforCommunicationASituationalBriefingModel.htm, Accessed 8/8/2008.

8. Van Eaton EG, Horvath KD, Lober WB, Pellegrini CA. Organizing the transfer of patient care information: the development of a computerized resident sign-out system. *Surgery*. 2004;136:5–13.

9. Sidlow R, Katz-Sidlow RJ. Using a computerized sign-out system to improve physician-nurse communication. *Jt Comm J Qual Patient Saf*. 2006;32:32–36.

10. Petersen LA, Orav EJ, Teich JM, O'Neil AC, Brennan TA. Using a computerized sign-out program to improve continuity of inpatient care and prevent adverse events. *Jt Comm J Qual Improv*. 1998;24:77–87.

11. Institute of Medicine Committee on Redesigning Health Insurance Performance Measures, Payment, and Performance Improvement Programs. *Rewarding Provider Performance: Aligning Incentives in medicare (Pathways to Quality Health Care Series)*. The National Academies Press, Washington, DC. 2007. Available at: http://books.nap.edu/catalog.php?record_id=11723, Accessed 8/8/2008.

12. Arnet RH III, Blank LA, Brown AP, et al. National health expenditures. *Health Care Financ Rev*. 1998;11:1–41.

13. The Henry J Kaiser Family Foundation. *Medicare Chartbook*. 3rd ed. Available at: http://www.kff.org/medicare/upload/Medicare-chart-book-3rd-edition-summer-2005-report.pdf. Accessed June 28, 2008.

14. Institute of Medicine. Preventing medication errors. Available at: http://www.iom.edu/Object.File/Master/35/943/medication%20errors%20new.pdf. Accessed June 29, 2008.

15. Beard K. Adverse reactions as a cause of hospital admission in the aged. *Drugs Aging*. 1992;2:356–367.

16. Beers MH, Ouslander JG, Rollingher I, et al. Explicit criteria for determining inappropriate medication use in nursing home residents. *Arch Intern Med*. 1991;151:1825–1832.

17. Fick DM, Cooper JW, Wade WE, Waller JL, MacLean JR, Beers MH. Updating the Beers criteria for potentially inappropriate medication use in older adults: results of a US consensus panel of experts. *Arch Intern Med*. 2003;163:2716–2724.

18. Beers MH. Explicit criteria for determining potentially inappropriate medication use by the elderly. an update. *Arch Intern Med*. 1997;157:1531–1536.

19. Gurwitz JH, Rochon P, Food and Drug Administration (U.S.). Improving the quality of medication use in elderly patients: a not-so-simple prescription. *Arch Intern Med*. 2002;162:1670–1672.

20. Bates DW, Kuperman GJ, Rittenberg E, et al. A randomized trial of a computer-based intervention to reduce utilization of redundant laboratory tests. *Am J Med*. 1999;106:144–150.

21. Kuperman GJ, Teich JM, Tanasijevic MJ, et al. Improving response to critical laboratory results with automation: results of a randomized controlled trial. *J Am Med Inform Assoc*. 1999;6:512–522.

22. Morris AH. Protocol management of adult respiratory distress. *New Horizons*. 1993;1:593–602.

23. Hunt DL, Haynes RB, Hanna SE, Smith K. Effects of computer-based clinical decision support systems on physician performance and patient outcomes. *JAMA*. 1998;280:1339–1345.

24. Evans RS, Classen DC, Pestotnik SL, Clemmer TP, Weaver LK, Burke JP. A decision support tool for antibiotic therapy. *Proceedings from the Nineteenth Annual Symposium on Computer Applications in Medical Care*. 1995;19:651–655.

25. Evans RS, Pestotnik SL, Classen DC, et al. A computer-assisted management program for antibiotics and other antiinfective agents. *NEJM*. 1998;338:232–238.

26. Overhage JM, Tierney WM, Zhou XH, McDonald CJ. A randomized trial of "corollary orders" to prevent errors of omission. *J Am Med Inform Assoc*. 1997;4:364–375.

27. Bates DW, Leape LL, Cullen DJ, et al. Effect of computerized physician order entry and a team intervention on prevention of serious medication errors. *JAMA*. 1998;280:1311–1316.

28. Teich JM, Merchia PR, Schmiz JL, Kuperman GJ, Spurr CD, Bates DW. Effects of computerized physician order entry on prescribing practices. *Arch Intern Med*. 2000;160:2741–2747.

29. Burt CW, Hing E, Woodwell D. Electronic medical record use by office-based physicians: United States, 2005. Available at: http://www.cdc.gov/nchs/products/pubs/pubd/hestats/electronic/electronic.htm. Accessed June 29, 2008.

30. Birkmeyer JD, Dimick JB. Potential benefits of the new leapfrog standards: effect of process and outcomes measures. *Surgery*. 2004;135:569–575.

31. Certification Commission for Healthcare Information Technology. CCHIT certified products by product. Available at: http://www.cchit.org/ , Accessed on 8/8/2008.

58

HEALTH CARE ORGANIZATION AND FINANCING

Peter Hollmann, MD

An understanding of the organization of the health care system enables the clinician to better navigate the system on behalf of the patient. It provides important insights that improve the ability of health care professionals to continue to operate in their chosen profession, increasing the likelihood of succeeding and surviving financially. The United States health care system is frequently described as "broken." To understand how it can be improved, it is useful to have an appreciation of how it presently is configured and how it evolved. The purpose of this chapter is to provide an overview of fundamental principles of financing health care and insurance. The most relevant programs for the elderly, Medicare and Medicaid, are addressed. There are multiple complex and interacting segments that comprise the health care delivery and financing system. Where the money comes from, where it goes, and why so much is spent will be examined. Possible responses to a system under stress that is facing the challenges of changing demographics and relentless cost trends are presented.

THE HEALTH CARE "SYSTEM"

It is useful to remember that the care of the elderly patient occurs in a system that is complex and provides and finances for care for well children, disabled adults, the uninsured, that is, the entire population. The many elements of the financing and delivery system are interdependent. Cross-subsidization occurs. This results in all elements being relevant to the elderly patient. It is Medicare, however, that has come to symbolize the health care system for the geriatric patient. Medicare is far more complex than a governmental insurance company paying claims for persons older than 65 years of age. Medicare also pays for care provided to the disabled and those on dialysis; it contracts with private health plans and drug plans to provide required and supplemental benefits to beneficiaries. It has a major role in financing medical education, researching

the impact of system change through demonstration projects, and shaping the delivery system. Private insurance often mimics Medicare payment and benefits policies; however, Medicare is a financing system, not the delivery system. Health care is delivered by providers such as doctors and hospitals. There are suppliers such as drug and device manufacturers who not only provide important tools for improving health and preventing disease, but also significantly impact the cost and politics of health care. The system includes private and governmental payers other than Medicare. These payers ostensibly act on behalf of and respond to demands of employers and the voting populace and finance a greater dollar volume of health care than does Medicare. Their impact on the system is substantial. Private insurance is important for the elderly, as most have some form of coverage beyond traditional Medicare, whether it is employee or retiree coverage, a Medicare Advantage plan, or "gap" coverage. Medicaid is critical for low-income seniors and those in long-term care institutions. The Veterans Administration plays an important role in funding and delivery of care. The most important parts of the health care system are the patients and their families. The elderly, although just a population subset, are patients of great diversity in employment status, cultural, behavioral, financial, educational, health, and functional attributes.

There is general popular agreement that our system is seriously flawed. It is often stated that aligning incentives will improve the likelihood that the system will better serve the needs of society. A common goal of achieving a healthy population is agreed on (assuming providers of goods and services believe they will still be needed), but the uniformity of viewpoints stops there. Complex systems also have great inertia because any change in one part of the system tends to affect another. The ripple from any change may be predictable, based on study of the past, such as service volume increasing in response to price reduction, or dauntingly unknown, such as the use of services by a baby boom cohort that may be of improved health status, yet accustomed to aggressive consumption of new technologies. The health care system also exists within a social milieu in which health care consumes resources that might otherwise be used for education or housing. Health care professionals may not naturally operate on an assumption that the growth rate of the economy is as relevant to health care organization and financing, and therefore their practice of medicine, as is the latest treatment innovation for a condition of interest. Furthermore, the financing and delivery system often seems to be no system at all with conflicting interests, as hospitals compete with doctors for fee updates and payers seek to avoid any updates in the face of increased utilization of services. Yet clinicians impact the system one patient at a time and have a unique potential to lead system change: a potential that comes with the experience of operating daily at the interfaces of finance, delivery, and caring for our patients.

Insurance Basics

Health insurance serves two fundamental goals: prepay predictable expenses and provide financial protection against the cost of infrequent but very costly events. It is well established that the uninsured and underinsured do not receive recommended and necessary services. Traditionally, health insurance allowed the individual to obtain treatment for an acute illness that could otherwise not be purchased due to limitations of personal financial resources. The reason to prepay predictable expenses is a newer insurance phenomenon related to payment for prevention. It is intended to encourage appropriate use of services that will prevent disease, disability, and future medical expenses. It is also a mechanism to provide services at a contracted amount as compared with charges and with fund care for persons with essentially no resources, such as those with poverty-level incomes. Increasingly, insurance finances health care for chronic illness. Insurance also finances the delivery system infrastructure.

Insurance is foremost a pooling or spreading of risk across a large population. It works by everyone paying a little into a pool that few will use. Those few who use it will exhaust the pool, less administrative costs and some reserves for unexpected variation. The reserves, besides being a cushion, produce investment income, lowering the amount needed to be collected from each person, known as the premium. In this manner, health insurance is no different than automobile, homeowners, or professional liability insurance. In 2002, 12% of all Medicare beneficiaries accounted for 69% of Medicare spending, but approximately one in three beneficiaries did not even see a physician (Kaiser Family Foundation). In younger populations where the prevalence of chronic illness is lower, the contrast between the few who spend a great deal and those who use little to no services is more stark. The high-use population is composed of different types of people. Some have one-time high-cost events, such as those who survive major trauma without disability or those who die after an expensive course of care. Others have chronic illness punctuated with rare high-cost events such as coronary artery disease with bypass surgery or chronic illness

with recurrent costly events such as congestive heart failure and recurrent inpatient care. In 2001, the 23% of Medicare beneficiaries with five or more chronic conditions accounted for 68% of the program expenditures.

The effect of spreading risk works best when it is spread over the largest possible population. Any segmentation creates the potential for the effects of what is known as "adverse selection." The United States does not have a system in which the entire population is enrolled in one insurance program. Many provider groups receive payment that is at least partially based on some form of prepayment per person or "capitation," and therefore the provider assumes some insurance function or risk. Therefore, adverse selection is very relevant. Consider two health plans: Plan A has 5% of its members with a serious chronic illness; Plan B has 6% of its members with the same condition. The difference at first appears trivial; however, because the 5% account for 50% of all expenses in Plan A, that means that each 1% change in the sick population will result in a 10% difference in total expenses. If Plan B is to make ends meet, it will raise its premiums to cover its greater costs. This may lead people who do not use services and thus see less value in health insurance to leave to a lower premium plan, which then only decreases the pool of healthier people over which to spread the risk. Plan B spirals into insolvency. Risk or case mix–adjusted premiums might work, but the high-risk people may not be able to afford the higher premium. Adjusting premiums to risk also defeats the principle of pooling risk, unless the risk level is under the control of the insured, for example by using tobacco or not. It also is the case that the risk adjustors account for a relatively limited amount of the per person variance because there remains a significant degree of unpredictability in expenses. Most insurance today has some form of risk adjustment. Large employer groups may be rated (have their premiums priced) by historical use experience. Small groups may be rated by age or sex adjustments. Medicare risk adjusts payments to Medicare Advantage plans based on factors such as diagnoses and whether the person is institutionalized. One of the largest challenges in a voluntary health insurance system is setting premiums for well young adults at a level at which they will purchase coverage. They are indeed low risk and often see little value in insurance that they perceive as inadequately risk adjusted.

Benefits are what insurance covers or pays for. Benefit design is a critical element in understanding health care financing, as it defines what is being financed through insurance. If hospital care is covered by insurance, then the price and volume of hospital services must be calculated and spread over the population paying premiums. If long-term nursing home care is not covered, then its cost and volume is irrelevant. Because insurance is a legal contract between the insurer and the insured, careful definition is critical. Certain services may be essential to the health of the patient, but that fact does not make them covered. Until Medicare created a prescription drug plan, there was no coverage for medications, yet medications were more important than many covered services to the health of most Medicare patients. Medicare does not cover long-term care in a nursing facility yet it is necessary for many. Benefit design may create or minimize adverse selection risk. Presume our example Plan B was different from Plan A not by random chance but because Plan B had slightly different benefits that made it much more attractive to people with chronic illness. Perhaps coverage for a certain drug important to a person with the illness was slightly better. By providing better benefits Plan B created its problem. Provider network may also create selection risk for a health plan. This same type of issue can affect physicians or physicians groups who accept some of the risk by becoming paid by capitation. Group A has no geriatricians and has a typical complexity patient panel mix. Group B has geriatricians who attract complex patients. If the two groups are paid the same amount per patient, Group B will have to do a far superior management job. There is a great deal of unexplained variation or waste in health care services utilization, but the disease burden of the patient, not the management skill of the clinicians, will dictate most of the cost of caring for the patient. It is unlikely that Group B will succeed financially.

Long-term care provides a good example for two other important points: calculating cost-offsets or "savings" and behavior change. Insurance coverage of a service will make it more accessible. This will expand its use and create a market for providers who will seek to expand it further. If home care is paid fully out of pocket, some will utilize it. If it is insured, the use will grow. Behavior changes with coverage. It is almost certain that some nursing home residents can be cared for more cost effectively at home with home care services supporting other caregivers. If $50 per day on home care would prevent $150 per day of nursing home care, it would seem a good buy. It is a gross miscalculation, however, to base savings on the experience expected for one person. Insurance covers populations. In structuring the home care benefit to cover that nursing home patient who could be cared for at home, it might be that five people at home who need home care, but are presently paying out of pocket, now become eligible for insurance to pay. The $150 per day "saved" results in $300 per day of home care for six patients, not $50 per day for one. Perhaps five caregivers missed less work, saving their employer costs and boosting productivity and society was better off. The health care insurance costs were not reduced however.

This brings us to the point of total costs, insurance costs, cost shifting, and returns on investment. Whether the insurance is provided by a for-profit company or the government, there is a budget of sorts. One way to control the budget is to shift costs to the patient by limiting the benefit. Medicare Part D drug coverage has beneficiary cost sharing so that it could be affordable to society (at least to the degree that Congress determined). States and the federal government have different programs that have unique budgets, but a single patient may be a beneficiary of both programs. Ideally, such shifting and fragmentation does not create unintended or harmful gaps or increase total costs, but this is not always the case. It frequently creates administrative processes and added expense. More significantly, one payer may take actions to save a little for itself, even if it results in higher total costs or higher cost to the other payer and patient. Costs may also be shifted over time periods by

making an investment. A diabetes program that delays diabetic morbidity may save an employer-sponsored private insurance company money if an upfront investment in the member's care can be amortized over years of membership premiums and the most costly episodes are prevented or deferred to an age of Medicare eligibility and thus shifted to the Medicare program. The insurance company will see a return on the investment assuming the member remains with them long enough. One of the consequences of Medicare programs helping a person survive to another year is that there will be another year of Medicare expenses. If Medicare is to have a return on investment, it must reduce lifetime expenditures, which is very difficult to accomplish. For Medicare, a smaller population is less costly. Private insurance has a per member premium. Reducing membership reduces income and is not financially desirable.

An insurance company can control costs in limited ways. It can reduce the price of a service or it can reduce the frequency of a service: pay less or buy less. One way to reduce the price is to shift some cost to the member or to not cover the service at all. Price reductions may stimulate providers to increase volume to make up for lost income. Price reductions may make a service unavailable due to provider drop out. If the reduction is achieved by shifting the cost to the member, the member may forego the service. If the service was particularly cost effective this would be deleterious. The price change could result in substitution with a more costly service or result in disease progression to more costly stages due to lack of the service. If the service was not cost effective, the frequency reduction achieved is positive. Attempting to reduce frequency by means other than price can have the same risk/benefit calculus. Administrative costs may be incurred implementing programs designed to reduce volume of services. Seemingly simple actions can have complex unanticipated results.

Financial Principles

In a system in which there are issues such as cost shifting and adverse selection, it may appear that standard business principles do not apply; however, the delivery system is a business and fundamentals generally do apply. The financing system may contribute to confusion over fundamentals. For example, payments may be based on historical charges and not based on current true costs. Every business has income and expenses. It has a product that it provides and makes money per some unit of product. It can have loss leaders or provide charitable services, but it cannot lose money on every service and survive.

A solo practitioner running his or her office must have a good sense of these realities. There is the rent, the utilities, the employees and their benefits, professional liability insurance, and supplies. Then there is income that is typically fee for service. Each patient is a little different, but overall there is a predictable gross income per unit of patient service. Income must exceed expenses. There are also variable and fixed costs to consider. One more patient on the schedule will not change the rent or staffing, which are the fixed costs. That patient may use another paper gown as a variable cost, but mostly the patient is pure net income. At some number of additional patients, more staff will need to be added or another doctor asked to join the practice. At that point there might need to be a subsidy of the new doctor's salary. The practice founder will assess the value of the investment in the new doctor by estimating the cost today as compared with what a similar investment would generate over time and decide whether to bring on the associate or to purchase mutual fund shares for a better return on investment. Of course, there are also estimates of intangibles such as reduced on-call schedule, ability to better manage unexpected surges in patient demand, and other nonfinancial calculations that will occur.

The same principles apply for health care systems. A hospital-employed geriatrician may directly produce income that exceeds his expenses and salary plus benefits. In such a case, that single unit is profitable. The geriatrician might be using only variable costs, if the clinic space and staffing is fixed anyway, but it is likely that fixed costs would be proportionally allocated to all users of facility and staff. The geriatrician may be a feeder of patients to the specialists and hospital. Hospitals have huge fixed costs. A few extra admissions incur few variable costs and are usually highly desirable. If the hospital believes that the geriatrician's patients would not have been at the hospital were it not for his employment, this might be recognized as his contribution to another cost or profit center. The geriatrician's patients may also give generously to the hospital capital campaigns. On the other hand, if the hospital concludes that the geriatrician's patients always incur costs of care exceeding the reimbursement the hospital receives, the hospital may wish to no longer employ the doctor even if he earns his salary based on the office/clinic income. A geriatrician may work for a nursing facility–based special needs health plan that employs physicians and receives Medicare capitation payments. The plan may determine that a skilled geriatrician results in markedly fewer transfers to the hospital, better drug and laboratory usage, more appropriate specialty care, and lower costs. The number of patients seen per day is only relevant to the extent that it results in better, more cost-effective care; payment generated per nursing home visit is not relevant. The bottom line is that regardless of the setting, there is a calculation of productivity or income by some measure. There is a calculation of costs or resources used. There is either profit and sustainability, or loss and eventual demise. These calculations may be complex and involve assumptions that are controversial or flawed. If profit margins of a larger organization are good, the effect of a small unit may not be calculated or be worth the attention, but ultimately real income and real expense exist in any endeavor and are likely to be a factor.

Other basics warrant mention. The most salient is that in the financing and delivery dyad, costs to one party is income to another. Any cost reductions for payers result in income loss for the providers in the aggregate, although not necessarily for an individual provider. The tension is obvious. Efficient provider units lower health care costs without losing profitability of the unit. They can maintain the same profit margin by reducing expenses while lowering the price of their services.

This is the typical economic paradigm in competitive markets; however, health care markets are distorted by many factors. A cost-effective provider is not the same as an efficient provider as described previously. Cost-effective providers could reduce their income because fewer services are used or increase their incomes because they shared in the cost savings, or because the more cost-effective services were the more profitable services for them. Another important point concerns growth rates and compounding. In a mortgage a lower principle will save great sums when interest is applied over time, but the interest rate can be more significant. Baseline expenditures and the growth trend are principle and interest in another setting. An extremely high trend in a service that accounts for a minute portion of total expenditures has an insignificant effect compared with modest growth in services that are responsible of a high proportion of total costs. Sustained high growth rate can, however, make a service that was once an inconsequential expense become very significant. An example of this in health care is the projected costs of high-cost "specialty" drugs such as the biological agents.

MEDICARE

Medicare was established in July 1966 by Title XVIII of the Social Security Act for people 65 and older regardless of income or health status. It has played a major role in reducing poverty rates among the aged and increasing access to care. It has funded infrastructure development, education and training, and been a major part of the social transformation of changing health care from a service paid by cash or barter to one paid by insurance. It actually accounts for less than 1 in 5 dollars spent on health care in America. It only pays for 45% of the health care expenditures of the Medicare beneficiary (calculated in 2002, prior to Part D) and has recently been surpassed by Medicaid as the biggest governmental program by enrollment. Nonetheless, the impact of Medicare on the health care system and the lives of the elderly would be difficult to overstate. Medicare is an "entitlement" program, contrasted to Medicaid, which is "welfare" or a needs-based program. Medicare benefits and costs were historically the same regardless of beneficiary income or wealth. In 2007 Medicare introduced a variable premium for Part B services based on income. Part D, the pharmacy benefit, which originated in 2006, is supported by income-adjusted beneficiary premiums.

There are four parts to Medicare and each has different funding and benefits. They are: Part A (hospital insurance); Part B (medical insurance); Part C (Medicare Advantage); and Part D (prescription drug plan). In 1972, Medicare added eligibility for the disabled. People with end-stage renal disease (ESRD) are also eligible. People are entitled to Medicare if they or a spouse are eligible for Social Security, Railroad Retirement, or equivalent federal benefits due to age, or they are eligible due to disability (i.e., receive Social Security Disability Income (SSDI)), or if they have ESRD. The aged are eligible the first day of the month of their 65th birthday. SSDI recipients are eligible after 2 years of social security eligibility. ESRD and people with amyotrophic lateral sclerosis are eligible at the time of initiating dialysis or Social Security payment eligibility, respectively. There are approximately 43 million people covered by Medicare. Seven million are also eligible for Medicaid and 47% of Medicare beneficiaries have incomes below 200% of the Federal Poverty Level. The Congressional Budget Office estimated 2006 spending to be $374 billion and 14% of the federal budget:36% of the beneficiaries have three or more chronic conditions; 14% have three to six limitations in activities of daily living; 12% are older than age 85 and 15% are younger than age 65. Medicare has benefits that have deductibles, copayments (set dollar amounts), and coinsurance (percent dollar amounts), that is, the beneficiary pays part of the bill or cost shares for any specific service. Some benefits have limits so that the beneficiary pays for all the service at some point. Parts B and D of Medicare have premiums, that is, the beneficiary must pay to enroll in that part of Medicare, whereas this is generally not the case for Part A. The "payment gap" created by deductibles, coinsurance, and benefit limits is often covered by "gap" insurance. Many beneficiaries purchase "gap" coverage offered by private insurers. Those eligible for Medicaid have coverage for this liability from Medicaid. The benefits structure for private insurance gap coverage is regulated by Medicare, but there are variations allowed.

Medicare Part A

Part A is hospital insurance but it also covers skilled nursing care and hospice. It covers home health care following an inpatient stay. Part A accounts for 41% of benefit spending (2006). Hospitals receive 34% of Medicare funds. Part A is mostly funded by a payroll tax of 2.9% of earned income, with additional income from interest on savings in the trust fund and taxes on high-income earners' Social Security checks. The funds are held in the Hospital Insurance Trust Fund and may not be used for other purposes. Expenses are anticipated to outstrip income and savings so that around 2018 the Hospital Insurance Trust will be insolvent. The trust fund has frequent calculations of solvency and has had adjustments made in taxes and other income sources. Like Social Security, it is payroll based at present and therefore meeting the burden of rising expenditures falls to working people. Part A has benefits and deductibles in a given benefit period. The benefit period is defined by a 60-day continuous break without hospital or skilled nursing care. In 2008, there is a $1,024 deductible per benefit period for a hospital stay. There are copayments of $256 per day for hospital days 61–90 and $512 for days 91–150. Days over 150 are paid by the beneficiary. There is a $128 per day copayment for days 21–100 of a skilled nursing facility (SNF) stay. There is no copayment for SNF days 1–20 and days over 100 are entirely the responsibility of the beneficiary. Hospice covers those with a terminal illness who are expected to live 6 months or less. It provides drugs, medical care, and support for those enrolled in an approved program. It accounts for 2% of Medicare expenditures, has seen a growing use, and serves over 1 million beneficiaries annually. Many think it is underused

due to misconceptions such as being limited to care for terminal cancer, when actually less than half of the hospice enrollees have this condition. It covers and has eligibility criteria for conditions such as Alzheimer's disease, pulmonary disease, heart disease, and general debility. It covers services typically not covered by Medicare such as respite and grief counseling. Care in the home has no beneficiary cost sharing.

Part B

Part B covers medically necessary services furnished by physicians in settings such as the hospital, office, or ambulatory surgery center. Home health (not following an inpatient stay), ambulance, durable medical equipment and surgical supplies, clinical laboratory and diagnostic services, and services by certain practitioners (e.g., nurse practitioners, clinical psychologists, and physical therapists) are paid by Part B. It covers the facility and professional components of outpatient services as well as drugs and biologicals that are not self-administered or otherwise part of Part D. It accounted for 35% of Medicare expenditures in 2006. Physicians and suppliers received 25% of Medicare expenditures with facilities receiving 10%. Part B is funded mostly by the general treasury, with premiums from beneficiaries accounting for 25% of program support. Premium payments in 2008 are $96.40 per month. Premiums are adjusted annually. Premiums vary for higher-income individuals. (In 2008, monthly premiums are $122.20 for single persons with income of $82,000 or couple with income of $164,000. The highest-income beneficiaries have premiums of $238.40 per month). Funding for Part B is through the Supplemental Medical InsuranceTrust Fund. The Supplemental Medical Insurance Trust has a Part B and a Part D fund within it. Part B services have an annual deductible ($135 in 2008) and a coinsurance of 20% of the allowance. This means the beneficiary is responsible to pay 20% of the allowed charge (Medicare's fee for a provider). For mental health services, the coinsurance is 50%. Note that the allowed charge is made up of the amount that Medicare pays and the amount that the beneficiary (or the gap insurance) pays. It is a common misconception that the fee is reduced for mental health services. In fact, a physician is expected to charge and collect in total the same amount for an office visit whether the visit is for arthritis or depression.

Part C

Part C is the Medicare Advantage (MA) program. These are private health plans that receive Medicare payments to provide actuarially equivalent benefits. The Part A and Part B benefits are both provided and the deductible, copayments, and coinsurance are typically covered by a premium charged by the MA plan. In addition, the beneficiary must continue to pay their Part B premium. Although MA plans cover the Medicare deductibles, copayments, and coinsurance, they typically have their own forms of cost sharing, such as office visit copayments, which can be substantial in the aggregate for high utilizers. Most MA plans include Part D. Therefore, these plans are typically

A, B, D, and gap coverage all rolled up into one product. Covered benefits must include all services covered by Medicare, but typically additional services such as more extensive preventive care are added. Part C accounted for 14% of Medicare spending in 2006. MA and the predecessor Medicare + Choice (M+C) plans have had variable membership and regional distribution over the years, in part affected by profitability based on federal payment schedules. Some regions have had a strong and durable presence of MA or M+C plans, whereas other areas have seen plans leave the market. With the advent of Part D and other factors, plans have grown and approximately 16% of the Medicare population is in an MA plan. Beneficiary choice has been an objective of the Centers for Medicare and Medicaid Services ([CMS], the federal agency that administers the two programs). The Medicare Payment Advisory Commission (an advisory body to Congress) estimates that MA plans receive 110% of what Medicare would have paid for such services outside of Part C. For some high service use beneficiaries, out-of-pocket costs may be higher than traditional Medicare in these plans. Because MA plans represent a subset of the population, adverse selection or the converse "cherry picking" becomes a concern. This is worsened if beneficiaries can move freely back and forth between plans and traditional Medicare. If the MA plan is restrictive but less costly, patients may move into the traditional program when they become ill and the loss of premium savings is outweighed by ease of service use found in traditional Medicare. For this reason, CMS has created lock-in provisions restricting movement.

Part D

Part D is the prescription drug benefit. It is funded with premiums (averaging $25–$30/month, varying by plan selected), general revenues, and state revenues that previously were used for Medicaid prescription drug coverage. Part D coverage is provided by private insurers approved by CMS. There is a low-income subsidy for premiums. Part D was not optional for Medicaid enrollees who are also Medicare beneficiaries (the dual eligibles). The standard plan for 2008 has a $275 deductible and 25% coinsurance for the first $2,510 after the deductible. For the next $3,216 of true out-of-pocket expenses for the year, the beneficiary pays 100%. This is commonly labeled the "donut hole." Beneficiaries may receive help on the out-of-pocket expenses from family or state assistance programs, but not the Part D plan. After $5,726 of total drugs costs ($4,050 out of pocket) there is a 5% coinsurance. Only 12% of 2008 plans use this standard design. Most have no deductible and use tiered copayments but retain the coverage gap. Those plans that provide coverage in the gap typically just cover generic drugs. Part D plans have formularies with preferred drugs having different coverage than other drugs or noncoverage for some drugs. CMS requires certain drugs to be on all formularies and designated classes must have a representative drug. Some drugs are excluded from Part D plan coverage by law, such as benzodiazepines. Physician-administered drugs remain on Part B. It is estimated that 7% of beneficiaries have

out-of-pocket drug expenses over $3,600. Sixty percent will have out-of-pocket expenses of $750 or less. The program is projected to be costly, $50 billion in 2007 and $932 billion for 2008 through 2016. Cost to Medicare means that beneficiaries will consume more medications or save money or both. Part D provides some drug coverage to nearly 24 million Medicare beneficiaries. Other Medicare enrollees have coverage through plans such as retiree or employee benefits so that more than 90% of Medicare beneficiaries now have drug coverage.

What Medicare Does Not Cover

Medicare does not cover acupuncture, routine vision care and eyeglasses, dental services, hearing examinations and aids, and long-term custodial care. Care outside the United States is generally not covered. It does not cover all preventive care, specifically an annual examination for preventive purposes other than one for new enrollees. Claiming a routine preventive examination as a condition-related medically necessary visit is prohibited. In recent years, however, Congress has added selective preventive services to the benefits and each service is specified in law, that is, there is no categorical coverage for all preventive services, such as all those advised by the U.S. Public Health Service. Because Medicare covers skilled nursing care and skilled home care, the greatest misconception of the public regarding coverage relates to these services. Many beneficiaries believe long-term nonskilled or "custodial" nursing home care is covered. That is incorrect. Benefits are set by statute. This means Congress defines the coverage, not CMS. CMS may provide greater detail but is not able to add benefits outside an existing category of covered service. Medicare covers only 45% of Medicare beneficiary health care costs because of services that are excluded from coverage and because of cost sharing. The other costs are out of pocket (or indirectly out of pocket through the purchase of gap coverage) or paid by other programs such as Medicaid, the Veterans Administration, or employment-related coverage.

MEDICAID

Medicaid was begun in 1965 as a state and federal shared program to help the poor with medical expenses. It is Title XIX of the Social Security Act. The program was established so that it would be funded by state funds with federal matching monies. States could determine eligibility (with some restrictions set by the federal government) and select the covered services, payment rates, and administer the program. It is "needs based" with eligibility determined by income and assets limits, that is, it is a welfare program. Over time, the program has changed and the federal government has placed some further requirements on the states for them to receive matching funds, but fundamentally it remains state specific. Therefore, eligibility and benefits do vary and a beneficiary who moves from one state to another may be at risk for losing coverage. Medicaid covers poor women and their children, the blind or disabled, the medically needy, and funds the Programs for All Inclusive Care of the Elderly along with Medicare. The medically needy elder is typically a nursing home resident who was always poor or who has exhausted her savings and "spent down" to eligibility. The Programs for All Inclusive Care of the Elderly participants receive all their services through the program, require a nursing facility level of care, but are managed in an alternative setting by using flexible benefits not typically provided by Medicare. Medicaid funds 40% of all nursing home care. It provides gap coverage for deductibles, copayments, and coinsurance for Medicare benefits, and prior to 2006, paid for prescription drugs. Because of the high per person costs for the elderly nursing home resident and the disabled, these aged and disabled comprise only 25% of the Medicaid population, yet account for 75% of Medicaid spending.

DELIVERY SYSTEM FINANCING AND ORGANIZATION

There are multiple components of the delivery system, but we will describe only a few key provider types.

Hospitals

There are approximately 5,000 hospitals in the United States. In the past decade the duration of inpatient stays has dropped slightly and leveled off. The number of admissions fell until the mid-1990s and since then has slowly risen. Therefore, the number of inpatient days has remained fairly stable. Over the past decade outpatient hospital services growth has been strong. Hospitals have also consolidated, giving them much greater market power in negotiating rates with private payers. This has been useful as they have seen their profit margins from Medicare decline. Since the 1980s hospital inpatient services have been paid by Medicare with a prospective payment system called Diagnosis-Related Groups (DRG). A hospital receives a single payment for an inpatient admission based on the diagnosis that caused the admission. Procedures and complications affect the DRG selection and there are special allowances for extreme outlier stays. The goal of such a system is to create incentives for the hospital to improve efficiency. Hospitals also receive payment updates based on a willingness to report quality performance measures. Private payer inpatient payment methodologies vary by payer and hospital.

Physicians

Physician supply has steadily increased; however, most of the increase has been in nonprimary care specialties. The growth in larger group practices that could support infrastructure investments such as electronic health records is slower in primary care compared with specialist groups. The physician workforce is changing: women now outnumber men in medical schools and more physicians are employees than in the past. Physicians are paid by Medicare on a modified fee for service or

"piece-work" basis. The modification consists of surgical procedures being paid with one fee for all related services within a "global" time period and for reductions when multiple surgical procedures are performed on the same day. Related services in the global period include the office visit services called "evaluation and management." These are the history, examination, assessment, and plan "cognitive" services. In general, the physician payment methodology by CMS has a financial incentive to perform more services. Since 1992, all Medicare fees are determined by a conversion factor and relative value units (RVUs). This is called the Resource-Based Relative Value System (RBRVS). Services of all types (procedural and evaluation and management) are ranked in a relative manner based on physician work. Work is determined by time, technical skill and effort, mental effort and judgment required, and stress due to risk to the patient. RVUs are assigned using a previously valued service as the reference or comparator. Valuation based on relativity to a reference service is the origin of the term "relative value." Practice expenses are then calculated based on the expenses incurred for clinical staff, supplies, and other costs associated with a specific procedure, and converted to RVUs by using a mathematical formula. Finally, professional liability costs related to a specific procedure are estimated and given a RVU amount. The three components of the RVUs are added up and converted to dollars by using a conversion factor (CF). For example, five RVUS with a CF of $30 would result in an allowance of $150. Practice expenses vary by whether a procedure is done in a facility, whereby the facility incurs the expense, or whether the service was nonfacility, that is, in the doctor's office.

A committee of physicians representing multiple specialties (including primary care–oriented specialties) is convened by the American Medical Association to oversee the valuation process and make recommendations for RVUs to CMS. CMS can accept the recommendations or not, but the acceptance rate is over 90%. The RBRVS methodology replaced a physician charge-based system and was intended to rationalize payment and reduce a disparity favoring procedure-oriented specialties. Congress defined the basics and CMS determines significant details. The ultimate valuations are based on work, practice expense, and liability costs, which is the basis for it being called "resource based." It is noteworthy, and a source of some criticism, that the current methodology does not create payment based on concepts such as cost effectiveness, quality, value to society, or the need to support a primary care infrastructure. Other payers do not necessarily use the Medicare payment methodology, but the majority uses some variant.

The highest volume and highest total cost service in medicine is the office visit. The cost per service is relatively low, but the volume is staggering. RBRVS values office visits and other evaluation and management services based on different levels defined by the amount of history, examination, and medical decision making required. Included in the valuation is some amount of work before the face-to-face service, such as reviewing a record sent in advance, and some amount of work after the service, such as dictating a consult note or following up on a laboratory result with the patient. There is a growing sentiment and evidence base that the valuations inadequately recognize the work and practice expense of care coordination required for the medically complex, chronically ill patient.

The process by which a physician is paid starts with the reporting of that service to a payer by using a Current Procedural Terminology (CPT) code. CPT is the nomenclature system maintained by the American Medical Association (AMA). Payers (in Medicare, CMS) assign each code a coverage determination (covered, not covered, or included in the payment of another service) and a fee. The claim a physician submits will be processed through an electronic claims system that may look for or have "edits" based on multiple factors such as diagnoses to indicate whether the service is medically necessary or covered. There are typically edits to be sure that one service may be paid with another service on the same day, or not because reporting both is incorrect. The rules for correct procedure code selection, knowing what Medicare covers and payment processing steps can be confusing and require education.

CMS assigns an allowance for every procedure. Physicians who participate in Medicare (i.e., agree to the Medicare fee as payment) are paid the allowance, less coinsurance and deductibles, directly by Medicare. Physicians who do not participate in Medicare may bill the patient, but only up to 109.25% of the allowance and then the physician must collect from the patient who is the recipient of the Medicare payment. Physicians may "opt-out" of Medicare. In this case the physician privately contracts with the patient, is not bound by any allowance, and neither the patient nor the doctor may receive Medicare funds for the doctor's service. The physician who opts out is completely out of Medicare. The patient who sees such a physician may still receive services paid by Medicare from other providers. Medicare physician participation rates and rates of physicians willing to see new Medicare patients remain high and steady despite Medicare physician fee updates not keeping up with practice cost inflation. Whether Congress interprets this as professionalism or sufficient satisfaction with the program is uncertain.

Nursing Facilities

Approximately 5% of all Medicare payments were for skilled nursing facility (SNF) care. SNF reimbursement is based on a variation of the DRG. Facilities receive a global per diem payment that covers all services such as nursing, therapies, room and board, and medications. The payment is based on a Resource Utilization Group that is determined from information provided as part of the Multidisciplinary Resident Assessment process.

PERSPECTIVES ON HEALTH CARE COSTS

Health care costs have outpaced inflation and the growth of the economy so that an increasing percentage of the Gross Domestic Product (GDP) is devoted to health care. If the GDP

pie grows sufficiently, the nonhealth care portion or slice in absolute size may be larger in successive years, even if it is a smaller portion of the pie. Consumption of health care does correlate with wealth, in international comparisons and by socioeconomic class in America. All of the GDP will be used for something, why not health care? Increased life years, including when adjusted for quality of life (function), have resulted from the health care system and almost certainly not just from other effects such as secular dietary changes and no smoking policies. A part of the reason for increased volume of services is that more meaningful care can be provided for an expanding group of patients. We now do better controlling diabetes and hypertension and detecting breast cancer in early stages. Costly drugs really do help people with rheumatoid arthritis. The cost of health care insurance, however, is rising at a rate that is suppressing wages and leading employers to discontinue or reduce coverage. Many elderly are using a growing portion of their income for health care. The federal budget is strained by cost trends that are independent of demographic change, which itself will further stress the budget. Health is determined by more than health care. Spending on housing, education, and nutrition may be much more effective in promoting the next advance in function or longevity than spending on, for example, a new drug to treat advanced malignancy. Studies on regional variation on spending in health care indicate that higher expenditures are inversely correlated with measurable quality. Concerns about quality, value, and sustainability indicate that the cost trend warrants critical review.

Many have examined costs in America. Although there may not be unanimity of opinion, there are some summary conclusions that can be reasonably made. It is useful to note that there are likely many factors and an improvement in any one area should not be cast away as irrelevant. No magic bullet is likely. Demographics account for a relatively small aspect of the trend. Care at the end of life does consume a large percentage of total expenditures, but this is true at all ages. The costs are growing at the same rate as other services and the costs for the very old are not due to futile intensive care unit days, but due to long-term and palliative care. Competition has had mixed effects. When payers with market clout forced hospitals and others to compete for patients by price, there was a period of trend reduction. Typically competition has resulted in one facility trying to outdo the other in technology arms races that fuel the fire of cost growth. Price is a factor with drugs and devices costing more than in other international systems that negotiate better with industry. Physicians earn more relative to the rest of the population when compared with western European countries. Our employer-based insurance system that became the model for our governmental programs was created by providers, presumably for providers, although that seems a distant memory to those battling with these payers today. Administrative costs are significant, typically described as the low single digits for Medicare and 10%–15% for commercial insurance. This has been fairly stable, is not the bulk of costs, and may include investments in technology and services that will improve efficiency and quality. There is still an opportunity to create savings from better administrative efficiency and reduced marketing costs. Disease frequency, some of which is preventable by lifestyle interventions, may account for significant differences in per capita spending in international comparisons. Most agree that the biggest factor is the use and rapid diffusion of new technology, typically without a strong evidence base of utility established at the time of diffusion. Cost effectiveness is rarely assessed.

Attempts to reign in costs have had mixed effects. Fraud, although rare, exists and must be rooted out continuously. Fraud reduction programs generally more than pay for themselves. Payer-created price reductions often resulted in cost shifting to other payers or increased volume of services to maintain gross income. Copayments or deductibles designed to moderate patient demand obviously shift cost to the patient, but the sickest patients account for most of the costs. Their services are typically the least discretionary, so savings from reduced utilization may not result. Removing some cost insulation may lead to consumers being more aware of and engaged in solving a national social problem. A forceful control on technology diffusion does forestall costs for awhile but requires a political will that is currently lacking. Systems that operate within a budget such as an integrated delivery system that also provides financing or assumes financial risk do best in cost control. In our pluralistic payment system budgets are not like those of single-payer systems in other countries and accordingly are harder to enforce. Furthermore, the delivery system is not a system organized with the capacity, authority, and information systems necessary to control expenditures within a national or regional budget. A primary care focus has had success, although restrictions by "gatekeepers" have not.

It is hoped that costs can be controlled by reducing duplication of care, errors, and other waste through use of an electronic health record and other delivery system changes. The same information systems can facilitate more effective use of evidence-based medicine. In an example of misaligned incentives, the cost of the system changes may be borne by a provider, but the benefit may accrue to the financing system. Changing payment from one that favors new procedures and volume of services to one that supports chronic disease care using teams, nonface-to-face interventions, and community resources (the Chronic Care Model of Wagner) may be effective, if not in saving money, in improving care. Disease management programs that properly target the most at risk and use effective interventions do save money by reducing hospitalization and, ergo, serious morbidity. Identification of at risk persons who are about to cross the threshold from average utilizer to high-cost utilizer may be possible. There needs to be a substantial investment into better understanding comparative cost effectiveness of medical interventions. Only now, after years of resistance, are we developing ways to measure quality and efficiency and make them transparent and actionable for the provider and consumer alike. There will be stumbling along the way as this process matures. The financing and payment system must support a transformation in health care, but there is legitimate concern about the predictability of the result of many interventions. There will be those who are adversely affected by change and will oppose it. Ultimately, all these efforts to improve our system will still require a social calculation of value. It seems likely that such a transformational process will only occur under duress.

REFERENCE

1. Anderson GF. Medicare reform. *NEJM*. 2001;345(24):1780–1781.

59

ADVANCE CARE PLANNING: VALUES AND FAMILIES IN END-OF-LIFE CARE

David J. Doukas, MD, Laurence B. McCullough, PhD, Stephen S. Hanson, PhD

After the protracted 15-year Florida legal case of Terri Schiavo concluded in 2005 (discussed in this chapter's fourth section), most Americans have heard about advance directives (i.e., living wills and durable powers of attorney for health care), and most (hopefully) now have also learned the valuable lesson that an oral expression for future care may not lead to the intended consequence.[1] This chapter focuses the reader's attention on using *written* preventive ethics tools in geriatric practice in planning for end-of-life care. This chapter first examines the legal development and ethical significance of the living will and durable powers of attorney for health care, then examines some of the ethical conflicts that can be associated with the use of written advance directives, and considers a stepwise preventive ethics approach to these advance directives in clinical practice.

THE BEGINNINGS OF ADVANCE DIRECTIVES

Although the concept of living wills began in the 1960s, the legal beginnings of what we now call "advance directives" arose from a grassroots response to *In Re* Quinlan, decided by the New Jersey Supreme Court in 1976.[2] Ms. Quinlan, a 21-year-old woman, suffered two prolonged anoxic episodes of unknown origin, was resuscitated by a rescue team, hospitalized, and subsequently was in a persistent vegetative state (PVS). Her father petitioned the court for guardianship of her person for the purpose of requesting that respirator support be discontinued, with the understanding that the higher probability was that his daughter would die. His request was eventually granted by the Supreme Court of New Jersey. One legal root of the *Quinlan* decision has its support of patient decision making from the 1914 New York State Appeals Court decision, *Schloendorff v. Society of New York Hospital,* which stated "Every person of adult years and sound mind has the right to determine what shall be done to his body, and a surgeon who performs an operation without the patient's consent commits an assault."[3] All competent, adult patients have the right to control what is done or not done for him or her.

Quinlan also has roots in the United States Supreme Court decision on abortion in 1973, *Roe v. Wade.*[4] *Roe* and cases that preceded it established that there is a constitutional protection of privacy and that this constitutional protection extends to the physician–patient relationship. Privacy creates a zone of noninterference around the physician–patient relationship into which the state may not intrude without sufficiently compelling reason. The courts recognize the compelling interest of the state in protecting life; however, when the Supreme Court of New Jersey decided *Quinlan,* the court argued that the rights of legal self-determination and privacy could override that compelling interest.

Portions of that Court's reasoning are crucial for the reader to understand. The Court determined that Ms. Quinlan's prior statements were not specific enough to count as advance informed refusal and instead turned to the constitutional right of privacy, reasoning that "the individual's right to privacy grows as the degree of bodily invasion increases and the prognosis dims. Ultimately there comes a point at which the individual's rights overcome the State interest in preserving life."[2] Ms. Quinlan could not exercise her rights for herself, and they would have to be exercised for her. Mr. Quinlan could play this role because he had shown himself convincingly to be a suitable guardian. Each of us retains privacy rights, even into and despite loss of the capacity to make our own decisions, including irreversible loss of such capacity. The Quinlan case thereby establishes the legal background to: 1) allow patients to make written or oral advance declarations regarding their own end-of-life treatment (i.e., the living will); 2) allow patients to appoint proxy decision makers (i.e., the durable power of attorney for health care); and 3) emphasize the meaningful discourse on values and the place of other important family and loved ones in future end-of-life treatment (relevant later in the concepts of the *Values History* and the *family covenant*).

THE LIVING WILL

After *Quinlan,* many states codified the right to refuse medical treatment, in advance of a time when one was no longer competent and terminally ill (and in most states, also if in a PVS), termed the "living will." California first enacted such legislation in 1976, and all but three states (Massachusetts, Michigan and, New York) currently have such a statute. Even in these three states, living will documents are used by health care providers as evidence of a patient's preferences to assist in guiding medical care for those incompetent to make their own medical decisions.[5,6]

Self-determination is exercised by an individual through his making, and then projecting into the future, the refusal of medical interventions. This refusal is binding on physicians and institutions. Numerous aspects of many states' living will, natural death, or advance directive acts, as they are variously known, seek to balance this right and the right to privacy with the state's interest in the preservation of life. For example, many states suspend the implementation of living wills for women while they are pregnant. Furthermore, while only competent adult patients may execute a living will, statutes generally make no provision requiring competency in revoking a living will. This makes sense only on the assumption that the statute expresses the legislature's interest in preserving life when in doubt. Living will laws also provide for criminal and civil immunity for physicians and institutions that carry out the instructions contained in a valid living will in which no malpractice occurs. There are no reported cases challenging this protection anywhere, indicating a very wide acceptance of living wills.

The living will, then, is an expression of informed refusal in advance of the time in which the patient is terminally ill (or persistently vegetative depending on the relevant statute) and has lost decision-making capacity. The latter is a clinical judgment, to be made according to prevailing standards of reasonable clinical judgment. States vary according to whether the patient's declaration or living will must be written. In addition, states vary on whether a written or oral declaration must take a particular form. In addition, many states allow surrogate decision makers to exercise the rights to refuse for patients without living wills, usually family members in a rank ordering determined state by state. The reader should familiarize himself with the details in relevant statutes for the reader's jurisdiction. The federal government recognizes the living will as well, for example, in Veterans Affairs institutions. One important note, some persons who wish not to have treatments discontinued have resorted to executing a so-called "affirmation of life." If a therapy is not beneficial (i.e., per evidence-based medicine criteria or credible physiologic reasoning), however, it may still be morally acceptable for a physician or health care facility to refuse to provide it.

THE DURABLE POWER OF ATTORNEY FOR HEALTH CARE

As experience was gained with living wills, a concern arose that the scope of advance informed refusal in living wills was not broad enough. There were clinical situations in which the patient was not necessarily terminally ill or persistently vegetative, but was not competent, and it was questioned whether aggressive management of the patient is what the patient would have wanted. In such cases, patient's wishes would best be represented by family members or other loved ones.

For many years common and statutory law have allowed for a durable power of attorney. A *power of attorney* is the assignment of certain legal powers to others, for example, to dispose of property in the physical absence of the owner. A simple power of attorney is not *durable*; that is, it does not persist beyond that individual's loss of decision-making capacity. The *durable* power of attorney was developed precisely to permit the conveyance of one's legal powers to another upon one's loss of capacity to make decisions. The durable power of attorney for health care (DPAHC), also called a health care proxy, permits a named other (termed variously in different states, the "agent," "health care surrogate," or "proxy") to make one's health care decisions upon one's loss of decision-making capacity of any type. As with living wills, the loss of decision-making capacity is a clinical judgment, to be made in accordance with prevailing standards of reasonable medical judgment, without the need for formal evaluation by the court. The onus is on the physician to show that the patient lacks capacity, although with difficult or ambiguous cases, psychiatric consultation may be needed.

As with living wills, there is no reported case of legal challenge, especially for wrongful death, against a physician or hospital that has let a patient die subsequent to the decision by an agent holding a legally valid DPAHC. An important distinction between the DPAHC and the living will is that the latter typically requires terminal illness, whereas the former takes effect with any form of a loss of decision-making capacity. Also, although the former can be used to request or to refuse *any* intervention, the latter typically applies only to life-prolonging interventions. Many states stipulate the form that the DPAHC must take, so that the reader should familiarize himself with applicable statutes.

THE PATIENT SELF-DETERMINATION ACT

A major shift occurred soon after the Nancy Cruzan case in 1990.[7,8] Nancy Cruzan, 23, lost control of her car on the night of 11 January 1983. Paramedics in Jasper County, Missouri discovered her lying face down in a ditch and without detectable pulse or respiration – apparently anoxic for approximately 12–14 minutes. After resuscitation, Cruzan entered a PVS, sustained by gastrostomy tube feedings. After several years, her parents requested that her artificial feeding be discontinued to allow her death. Informal wishes expressed to her parents and roommate were rejected by the Missouri Supreme Court (to whom this case had been appealed) as insufficient for a "clear and convincing" standard of evidence. This court added that nutrition and hydration should be viewed as basic life support and not as medical therapy. The U.S. Supreme Court, in June 1990, affirmed the Missouri Supreme Court decision, but did not concur with all of its reasoning. The Court stated that patients with capacity have a right under the U.S. Constitution to refuse medical therapy (and further stated that artificial nutrition and hydration were indistinguishable from other forms of medical therapy that could be refused). The Court stated that although a state has an interest in preserving life, the constitutional right to refuse therapy takes precedence over the state's interest. The state of Missouri, however, was allowed to exercise its interest in preserving life for the incompetent patient by requiring a standard of evidence that a proxy must meet before being allowed to refuse life-prolonging treatment on the patient's behalf. Justice O'Connor (in a separate opinion) noted that few patients have advance directives and that "clear and convincing" evidence may not exist. Her opinion is a clarion call to the U.S. public to use both living wills and durable powers of attorney for health care to strive toward that standard of evidence.

A major federal legal development after *Cruzan* was the Patient Self-Determination Act (PSDA) of 1990, which took effect in December of 1991. A parallel policy for Veterans Affairs institutions took effect in 1992. The PSDA aims to reduce the number of situations in which patients do not have written advance directives by requiring institutions that receive federal funds and HMOs to notify their patients on admission (or enrollment in the case of HMOs) about their relevant rights under relevant state law to execute an advance directive. In addition, patients are to be notified about their rights of informed consent generally. Finally, among other provisions, the law also requires hospitals to have policies on these matters, to notify patients that there are such policies, and provide information to patients about these policies.

Although the PSDA has increased patient awareness of advance health care planning, the reader should not assume that the PSDA solves the problem of patients not having advance directives.[9,10] Regrettably, the PSDA often does not get carried out by health care professionals, but instead is usually a single query to the patient or family by admissions personnel or is in a raft of documents mailed to a new patient joining an HMO. It takes time, discussion, and patient education to effect an increased usage of advance directives.[11,12] The reader should assume that he or she bears significant responsibility for discussing advance directives with patients in the outpatient setting and for anticipating and seeking to prevent ethical conflicts that can arise in association with advance directives.

ETHICAL CHALLENGES WITH ADVANCE DIRECTIVES

There are currently two advance directive instruments, and even a federal law on requesting about their use. Just as these advances were being put forward, the Terri Schiavo case unfolded.[13] In February 1990, Theresa (Terri) Marie Schiavo, 27 years old, suffered a cardiac arrest with resultant severe brain damage (PVS). Terri Schiavo had no living will or durable power of attorney for health care. She remained in a PVS for 15 years, maintained on artificial nutrition and hydration. Michael Schiavo, her husband, attempted to discontinue the feeding tube when he realized over several years that her remaining in a PVS was counter to her wishes. Several witnessed discussions in which she had stated these wishes were put forward as best representing her autonomous preferences. Terri's parents, the Schindlers, opposed the removal due to a belief that she was not in a PVS and could somehow be rehabilitated with therapy, and based on their desire to keep Terri alive. Over several years of media-inflamed coverage and posturing in both the Florida legislature and U.S. Congress, the U.S. Supreme Court declined *five times* to review the case. Michael Schiavo's request to withdraw the feeding tube was ultimately allowed and Terri Schiavo died March 31, 2005. The autopsy on Terri Schiavo demonstrated that at her death, she had a brain weight half that of normal. Her autopsy revealed massive damage to her brain, and the coroner opined that she was "irrecoverable and no amount of treatment or rehabilitation could have reversed" her condition.

The Schiavo case helps to point out that there are ethical challenges with advance directives, many of which are best addressed before they become problems. First, patients may not realize that having an advance directive is important to their own future.[14] In their absence, decisions may be made contrary to those the patient might make. Decisions might also be made by others than those the patient would prefer or would want to trust with such decisions. Second, in some states a standard living will lacks detail. Typically, statutes refer to the withdrawal of mechanical or other artificial means of sustaining life. Some states, however, are explicit that all life-sustaining treatment (which is defined in the statute) should be withheld or discontinued. These states may also allow patients to choose which categories of treatment they wish continued and which withheld.

Third, a patient may fail to provide future health instructions to his proxy. This lapse may occur because the patient trusts the agent named to make decisions and believes that trust is sufficient, or because the patient has not been provided the opportunity to make such decisions. Patients may also write instructions or make oral statements in association with a living will or durable power of attorney for health care that strike the physician as unreasonable (e.g., "Do everything – he's a fighter"), or as vague (e.g., "Don't keep me alive if I'm a vegetable"). These may be requests either for treatment or against treatment. Aggressive management does not make sense in all cases any more than nonaggressive management makes sense in all cases. Unreasonable instructions by patients need to be identified when they are made and discussed with the patient, *before* they lead (usually late at night) to ethical conflict.

Fourth, patients or their families can sometimes overestimate what their religious traditions require of them in resisting death. Religious advisers can sometimes influence patients or families, even if the adviser is not well informed about the patient's condition and its prospects. Patients sometimes misinterpret what their religion "requires" of them in fighting illness, and their religious advisor can rectify these erroneous beliefs.[15] Fifth, one's professional colleagues may have difficulty with some strategies for permitting patients to die, the withdrawal of nutritional therapy in particular. Some take the view that withdrawal of nutritional therapy is tantamount to starvation and suicide. As mentioned previously in the *Cruzan* case, the U.S. Supreme Court examined this matter and held that nutritional therapy is the same as any other medical intervention and that its withdrawal is like that of a ventilator, not a killing. Some state statutes also make this clear.

Sixth, the patient's family members and loved ones may have objections to the patient's decisions as expressed in advance directives. Family members may disagree about how or when to implement a living will based on differing views of "hope." The worst time for conflicts about such matters is *after* the patient has lost decision-making capacity. It is far better to help the patient identify and deal with potential problems within his family in advance of the loss of capacity.

An advance directive is not a physician's order. Advance directives do need to be translated directly into physician's orders upon entry into the health care system. These orders should be explicit, comprehensive, and timely. No professional caring for the patient should have any doubt about just what is and is not to be done when life-threatening events occur. The physician's obligations do not end with writing orders for nonaggressive management. There are substantive ethical obligations to the dying and their families. The patient is owed appropriate palliative management of pain and suffering and threats to dignity. The family is owed assurance and support that the patient's wishes are being carried out and that, therefore, everything that ought to have been done was indeed done.

A RESPONSE TO THESE ETHICAL CHALLENGES: THE VALUES HISTORY

These ethical challenges of advance directives led investigators to develop an explicitly value based advance directive instrument called the Values History to address prospectively these challenges.[13,16–18] The term "values history" has its roots in Dr. Edmund Pellegrino's description in the 1980s of the interactive discussion and narrative of values that can and should take place between patient and physician.[19] The patient's values and beliefs serve as an important basis for further understanding why these advance directives were executed by the patient. The Values History promotes patient autonomy by eliciting value-based discourse that can then be utilized in unanticipated future medical scenarios that cannot readily be addressed by means of a standard advance directive.

Documenting the patient's values helps to contextualize these preferences for future use (in the absence of a known illness). The values in the Values History have been empirically evaluated and significant correlations have been found between patient values and the medical therapies that patients would wish to forgo if they were terminally ill. Specifically, individuals often wish to forego end-of-life treatment that will be financially, emotionally, or physically burdensome to their family.[20–22] These findings support the claim that patient values can help the patient and the patient's family and physician better understand how to invoke the patient's specific directive preferences in future, unforeseen medical circumstances. This approach allows for greater flexibility in the physician's response to the patient's future incapacity by heightening awareness of why patients would prefer or not prefer treatment modalities. These values can then assist the family and physician in writing orders when the need for them later arises. Almost all jurisdictions and Department of Veterans Affairs policy allow specific directive statements to be added to a living will as well as the DPAHC, when their intent is in concordance with the advance directive (the reader is directed to review the advance directive from their own jurisdiction: State Links at www.press.jhu.edu/books/supplemental/9306_4.html and VA Link: www.ethics.va.gov/ETHICS/activities/policy.asp

The Values History contains two parts: 1) an identification of values (Values Section), and 2) preference statements based on the patient's values (Directives Section). The Values Section elicits from the patient her values regarding end-of-life care. The patient is first asked to evaluate her future life in the context of duration of life versus quality of life. The patient is then asked to identify the end-of-life values that are most important to her. The reader is encouraged to discuss the patient's values at length to allow for their elaboration or for the addition of other values that more completely reflect the individual's concerns or beliefs about end-of-life treatment. The Directives Section invites the patient to select specific treatment directives in light of those values and beliefs. The goal of this two-part approach is to encourage patient–physician discussion on the use of medical treatments at the end of life, which may assist the patient to understand better and articulate his values. In turn, the physician can better respect the patient's autonomy by helping remove constraints that could potentially hinder the informed consent process.[23]

The Values History's Directives Section list of treatment preferences is *intended* to be exhaustive, as it is an ideal to strive for, while focusing first on those that are most likely to be used for the patient, given their current medical problems. The Directives Section begins with treatment preferences in acute care situations: consent for or refusal of cardiopulmonary resuscitation, ventilator use, and endotracheal tube use. Preferences regarding chronic care modalities follow, including those for use of intravenous fluids, enteral feeding tubes, and total parenteral nutrition, medication, and dialysis. During this part of the Values History process the physician explains the treatment modalities, their beneficial effects, short-term and long-term consequences, and possible harms in the contexts of terminal illness, irreversible coma, and PVS. During conversations on discontinuing treatment, the patient should be reassured that the administration of medications for symptom relief (including treatment for pain, nausea, and shortness of breath) would not be withheld if required for comfort care, even if such therapy may involve an incremental increase of the risk of mortality.

The Values History is different from the living will and DPAHC in that "trials of intervention" can be more easily articulated for specific treatments.[24] This concept of trials of intervention is important in critical care, replacing the "all or nothing" approach.[25] The clinical reality is that aggressive management is often undertaken in a trial to see if it will benefit the patient. Trials of intervention also create the possibility of finding common ground between the patient's values and the physician's values.

For all of the above directives (except cardiopulmonary resuscitation), the patient may choose intervention, a trial of intervention (limited by time or medical judgment), or non-intervention. The patient may decide that after a set time trial attempting an intervention, if no benefit of the therapy were apparent, the intervention should be discontinued. The patient can instead decide to have a treatment continued so long as it benefits the patient, in the physician's best medical judgment. Benefit-based trials require a significant level of trust among the patient, the proxy, and the physician. The task for the physician is to allow adequate time for a therapy to benefit the patient before considering stopping it. The parameters the physician will use should be discussed with the patient. Benefit-based trials more accurately convey how the DPAHC agent may approach intervention in an unforeseen future medical condition. Trials thereby allow for assignment of treatment as a trial with subsequent decisions made on the basis of benefit (or lack of it), time, or a later decision by the patient's proxy. Identifying common ground of values is the core strategy of preventive ethics.

The Values History also offers several unique directives: refusal of intensive care treatment, autopsy, a "Proxy Negation" directive to exclude a specific potential decision maker (due to differing values) and "Do not call 911" for patients in long-term care facilities or home care.[16] The end of the Directive section allows the patient to add consent, refusal, or trials of intervention to other specific directives not otherwise addressed (e.g., specific types of surgery).

THE FAMILY COVENANT IN ADVANCE CARE PLANNING

In a series of recent publications, the *family covenant* has been put forward as a means to negotiate the place of family and significant others in the patient's health decisions. The family covenant is a health care agreement that can facilitate proactive

discourse on advance care planning. The family covenant articulates the roles of the patient, family or loved ones, and physician, as they define them in an interactive conversation. An initial health care agreement delineates boundaries of information sharing and proxy consent, with the physician serving as facilitator in potential future times of conflict.[26,27] This process- (rather than form-) based approach is intended to provide a richer context of values and preferences through interactive discussion, as voiced by the participants.

The family covenant, then, is an open health care agreement predicated on a promise among the patient, physician, and those loved ones designated by the patients who agree to participate (including the patient's health care surrogate/proxy). The initial promise is then reinforced by time and trust in the ongoing bond between the parties, with the physician serving as facilitator if conflict arises. The family covenant's construct then determines the level and scope of persons who have informational access to the patient's future health affairs, both when able and incapacitated, and designates which loved ones may participate in future decision making on behalf of the incapacitated patient. The family covenant helps to clarify the values of each participant at its outset by articulating parameters concerning information sharing and surrogate decision making in end-of-life care. These parameters are defined by those participating in the covenant. It promotes communication, collaboration, and transparency while being pragmatic in understanding that loved ones sometimes can benefit from the facilitative assistance of the patient's physician.

The family covenant adds an important aspect to advance care planning – articulating the role of loved ones, and the discourse among them in forging an ongoing health agreement. This advance directive model can therefore help with the difficulties of health care proxies when a loved one is not sure what the patient would want done and turns to other family members for assistance.[28] It also would help when a living will's original premises are found to be so vague as to be uninformative in medical decision making, and information from others knowledgeable about the incapacitated patient is required for their care. Very importantly, it explicitly identifies those loved ones who are *included* in the covenant – such that those outside of the covenant do not have standing in the sharing of information or decision making for the patient. The family covenant may have avoided the moral problems of proxy consent that were evident between the husband and parents in the PVS case of Terri Schiavo.[1,29]

A PREVENTIVE ETHICS STRATEGY FOR ADVANCE DIRECTIVES

The ethical challenges discussed previously usually occur because the physician waits too long to involve the patient (and his loved ones) in decision making in the outpatient setting, well in advance of hospitalization or admission to a nursing home. Regular discussion of advance directives with all geriatric patients should be regarded as the ethical standard of care. These discussions should take place at hospital admissions – and the response of the reader's institutions to the PSDA should not be presumed to be sufficient – but should also take place in other potentially less stressful settings.

Advance directives should be discussed in the outpatient setting.[30] Discharge planning should also be utilized as an additional setting in which decision-making discussions can be initiated, in anticipation of readmission. Too many ethical conflicts continue to occur because physicians are not initiating timely conversations with geriatric patients about advance directives. The primary clinical task, therefore, is to prevent such conflicts, particularly those discussed in the previous section.

The authors believe that, when possible, a patient should complete advance care planning over several visits. Such a methodology has two advantages over precipitous consent to an advance directive.[31,32] The process is intended to be a reflective process by the patient, so that decisions are made thoughtfully. With discussion occurring over time, the physician can distribute the time required for these discussions over several medical visits.

The family and other loved ones can be part of this process when the patient consents to their involvement. The patient's loved ones, and specifically the DPAHC agent, should receive a copy of the completed living will, DPAHC, Values History, and family covenant. Any misunderstandings should be clarified at the meeting of family members, agent, patient ,and physician. The authors urge that all advance directives be reviewed with the patient periodically (every 6–12 months), especially if there is a significant deterioration in the patient's health status or change in family dynamics. This way, changes in values or preferences that may occur over time can be documented, as well as discussed. Orders could then be updated as necessary.

The authors propose the following eight steps as a preventive ethics strategy for advance directives. Although these steps take time, they will be cost beneficial in the time, stress, and ethical conflicts that they can prevent for the reader, for patients, for patients' families and loved ones, for institutions, and for society.

First, explain that there are two forms of advance directives and that they serve different purposes and take effect under different conditions. The living will can be used by the patient only to refuse (or request) certain types of treatment in advance of the time that the patient is both terminally ill (as defined in relevant state or federal statute) and found in reasonable clinical judgment to have lost the capacity for making his own decisions. The reader should be clear with the patient about whether the applicable law permits an advance directive to be implemented only when a person is terminally ill or if it may also be implemented when a person is in a PVS. If the state law narrowly restricts the types of situations in which a living will may be implemented, the patient is well advised to consider executing a durable power of attorney for health care that can be implemented in a broader range of health circumstances.[33] The DPAHC can be used to assign to someone else the power to make decisions for the patient when in reasonable clinical

judgment the patient has lost the capacity to make his own decisions. The patient need not also be terminally ill, as is the case for living wills. If relevant statutes exclude from the agent's authority the right to authorize certain types of treatment (e.g., electroshock therapy), these exclusions should be made clear to the patient.

Patients' instructions on their DPAHC document should be reviewed. If the patient's instructions could in some circumstances be reliably judged to be unreasonable or difficult to implement, this should be explained to the patient, so that the patient can clarify his intent and preferences. For example, a request that everything be done may not make sense for a patient who is irreversibly dying despite aggressive management that results, on balance, only in unnecessary pain and suffering. Such an outcome is justifiably regarded as unreasonable in beneficence-based clinical ethical judgment, and this should be explained to the patient. All alternatives should be reviewed so that potential conflicts between the patient's preferences and beneficence-based clinical ethical judgment are understood and satisfactorily addressed.

For patients who have executed both documents, the living will and DPAHC should be reviewed for potential areas of conflict. These should be pointed out to the patient and the patient's preference for the management of such conflict elicited. The patient should be asked to make note of such preference in the documents and the reader should record such preferences in the patient's record.

Second, the patient should be provided with a frank description of the kinds of interventions that are employed in aggressive management of life-threatening events, especially critical care interventions. The patient should be provided a brief but accurate description of such interventions as intubation and support by mechanical ventilation, cardiopulmonary resuscitation, admission to the critical care unit, the administration of medication, fluid, and nutrition by peripheral and central lines, etc.[34] Both the short- and the long-term consequences should be discussed, including reliable estimates of the probability of successfully implementing the patient's preferences given the patient's present and future expected health status.[35] Patients with chronic diseases need to appreciate that life-threatening events usually accelerate the process of decline, and aggressive management followed by survival usually leaves the patient with a lower baseline than before the event.

It is especially important that the concept of trial of intervention be discussed with the patient.[36] A trial may be (and is often) stopped when it is no longer benefiting the patient. In particular, the patient should understand that in contemporary critical care, an admission to the intensive care unit is also a trial of intervention. This trial usually is undertaken to know whether it will benefit the patient, because it is still quite difficult to reliably predict which patients will and which patients will not benefit from intensive care admission. This trial, too, can be ended if the intended effect is not forthcoming – and the patient should articulate what such an endpoint would be.

Third, many patients make health care decisions on the basis of their religious beliefs, traditions, and convictions.

Patients often turn to religious advisers for help in making decisions about advance directives. When they do, the religious adviser should not be offering advice in a vacuum. With the patient's permission, therefore, the religious adviser should be provided with the information described in the previous two steps. In addition, the reader should be aware that most faith communities do not make it obligatory to resist death at all costs. Rather, moral theological views tend to recognize limits to what medicine can accomplish.[37] As noted previously, patients sometimes may not be aware of this and so may overestimate what their faith requires of them. If a patient or a religious adviser insists that the patient's faith requires that everything be done, this should be discussed with the patient and advisor in a frank way, apprising them of the prospects of success and the resulting cost in unnecessary morbidity, pain, and suffering. It may be appropriate to ask them to reconsider.

Fourth, the patient should be asked whether the patient anticipates whether anyone in the patient's family may have concerns, problems, or objections to the patient's decisions in her advance directives. For example, a patient may prefer to name an adult child as agent with DPAHC, rather than her spouse. The patient's spouse may be unaware of this preference. Offer the patient the opportunity to meet with family members, so that the patient's preferences and decisions can be explained. Family members have an ethical obligation to respect the patient's choices. Adult children, especially, need to be made aware of role reversal, taking over decision making as if the patient were now a child and the adult children were now parents of the patient. Family members, especially those named as a DPAHC, should be included in discussions about the patient's health care preferences, when possible.

Fifth, beware of ever using the language of withdrawing or withholding "care." Treatments may be withheld or withdrawn, while *caring* for patients never stops. Caring for patients also includes diligent attention to, and palliative management of, pain and suffering and protection of the patient's dignity.

Sixth, ask the patient where the patient keeps originals of his advance directives and who has copies. The reader should be sure that there are copies of the patient's directives in the patient's office records, the hospital records, and the nursing home's records. In particular, the reader should be certain that the emergency department of the patient's hospital has copies of the patient's directives. The patient's DPAHC agent, if one is named, should also have copies.

Seventh, ask yourself and ask your colleagues – especially nursing colleagues, as well as trainees – if any of them have concerns, problems, or objections to the patient's advance directives. When possible, you should plan for these contingencies. For example, some individuals may object to withdrawal or withholding of nutrition as a form of killing by starvation. Two responses to this can be considered. The first is, if the patient is being supported by other interventions, for example, a ventilator, or antibiotics, or pressor drugs, one or more of these could be discontinued to allow the patient to die comfortably. For patients on multiple life supports, this may provide a resolution acceptable to all.

The second response applies when nutritional therapy is the main or sole intervention that is preventing the patient's death. This is frequently the case for patients in a PVS. Not everyone accepts the explanation that death subsequent to discontinuation of nutritional support is caused by gastrointestinal tract and immune system failure secondary to irreversible central nervous system injury or disease. In 1990, Justice Antonin Scalia argued against this in his concurring opinion in Cruzan v. Director, Missouri Department of Health.[7] It is arguably a right in conscience for health care professionals who agree with Justice Scalia to withdraw from the care of the patient from whom nutritional support will be withheld or withdrawn provided sound transfer of medical care to another physician is facilitated. The reader's practice and institutional policy where the reader practices should recognize and respect such a right and the conscientious views that lead to its exercise. There is no conclusive ethical argument that Justice Scalia and those who share his views are mistaken. This view must therefore be regarded as reasonable and respected. Nevertheless, this view cannot be allowed to stand in the way of implementing an advance directive, because there is also no conclusive argument that withdrawal or withholding of nutrition must be regarded as killing by starvation in all cases. As professionals, individuals who share Justice Scalia's views must respect the patient's preference as also being reasonable and in conscience they are free to withdraw from the patient's case after ensuring that the patient will not suffer any loss of care by their withdrawal.

Eighth, having undertaken the previous seven steps, the reader is in a position to write an order that implements the patient's advance directive(s). The reader's orders should be comprehensive and clear. The goal is the following: no professional with responsibility for the patient, upon reading the orders, should be unclear or uncertain in any way about what should and should not be done in the case of a life-threatening event. These orders should be readily accessible in the patient's chart, that is, as a face sheet.

As noted previously, there are serious beneficence-based and autonomy-based obligations to dying patients. Chief among these obligations are adequate pain and suffering control and maintenance of dignity. Seriously ill patients can tolerate high doses of analgesics, if the level is titrated appropriately. This approach minimizes the risk of mortality from aggressive pain and suffering management. Because the patient's death can be acceptable in both beneficence-based and autonomy-based clinical judgment, an increased risk of mortality for the sake of adequate pain and suffering control does not violate beneficence-based clinical ethical judgment. Quality assurance mechanisms should be extended to cover review of pain and suffering management for dying patents, so that these matters can be addressed openly and with institutional sanction.

SPECIAL CONSIDERATIONS

Implementing advance directive orders for patients in nursing homes, for patients electing to die at home, and for surgery involves special considerations. For nursing home patients, the order written in step eight, in addition to pain and suffering control, might simply be "Do Not Call 911." This strategy avoids all forms of aggressive management in nursing homes without resuscitation equipment and personnel trained in its appropriate use.

This strategy may meet some institutional resistance, given the present regulatory environment of nursing homes in the United States. Some managers of nursing homes want to avoid any mortality in the nursing home and so may resist the "Do Not Call 911" order. There have been no reported cases against physicians or hospitals that have implemented valid advance directives in accordance with the patient's wishes. Nursing homes can develop policies that respect and implement living wills, a process that will be self-educating for the institution's personnel and leadership.

For patients at home, there are now several states that allow "Do Not Call 911" orders by statute.[38] There are several problems with this strategy. First, orders are usually written not for family members but for professional colleagues and trainees. The physician does not stand in a hierarchical relationship of power with respect to family members. Second, family members may justifiably place limits in their spousal and filial obligations, including the obligation to care for a loved one dying at home.[39] Some family members may reasonably judge the care burdens of doing so to be beyond their capacities, physical, emotional, or financial. A patient does not have an unlimited, autonomy-based positive right to impose unreasonable care burdens on family members. To prevent future ethical conflict, the writing of a "Do Not Call 911" order should be conducted with a frank and mutually respectful discussion of the sense of family members' obligations and an articulation of their limits.

Conflicts in this area can be prevented in several ways. Family members need to be informed honestly about the care burdens involved and also about home services, such as hospice, that could reduce those burdens to a reasonable level. Family members also need to know that ambulance crews usually employ full resuscitation protocols for all rescues in response to 911 calls. Families can avoid this outcome by bringing the patient to the hospital before an emergency or perceived emergency. Some states have laws allowing an out-of-hospital do-not-resuscitate (DNR) order that do permit emergency palliative therapies to be provided without being required to provide cardiopulmonary resuscitation. How these laws operate, and the familiarity that health care facilities and providers have with them, vary widely.[40,41] The reader should evaluate local laws before writing or guiding patients to create out-of-hospital DNR orders. In addition, the reader can write orders that will address how the patient is to be managed once the patient reaches the emergency department of the hospital. The reader should work with colleagues in the emergency department and hospital administration on policies that will sanction such orders.

Patients for whom orders have been written to implement their advance directive(s) may require surgery to reduce the patient's pain and suffering. The patient may be a reasonable,

Table 59.1. Advance Care Planning from Documents to Families

1. After patient execution of either or both, the living will and DPAHC (as part of well elder care), the physician asks the patient which loved ones he would want as part of their own family covenant to share information, as well as to help the proxy (or clarify the living will) in future circumstances of incapacity. The members of this family covenant then meet (in person or by phone) to determine the boundaries that the patient and each member hold as a promise to each other.

2. The physician discusses with the patient values regarding quality of life versus duration of life, as part of the values history.

3. The physician reviews the patient's quality-of-life values with the patient and requests that the patient select those most important to her, while exploring other alternative patient values as well.

4. Using the patient's values as a framework, the patient and physician discuss the various therapeutic options in the directive section, especially examining "why" a therapy is accepted or refused.

5. The physician facilitates the consent process:

   a. By framing the process in relation to known patient values.

   b. By exploring other values that may emerge in the process.

   c. By clarifying for the patient inconsistencies between values and directives in a nonpaternalistic fashion, by removing reversible constraints to consent.

   d. By framing treatment options in terms of known patient conditions and diseases as well as high-risk activities and genetic propensities.

6. Other specific advance directive preferences concerning surgery, and calling 911 from home or the nursing home should be discussed.

7. The directives individually should be initialed and dated. The patient signs, dates, and has witnessed the completed values history, with copies placed in the medical chart (i.e., doctor's office, hospice, and/or extended care facility). The original should be placed in a readily available place in the patient's home (known to family and friends). The family covenant members should be participants in reviewing these values and preferences (as consented to in the covenant).

8. Periodically, these values and preferences should be reviewed among physician, patient, and family covenant members.

albeit high, risk for surgical intervention. From a surgical point of view, the problem with DNR orders remaining in effect during surgery is that administration of anesthesia or intraoperative technique can result in life-threatening events, from which the patient has a reasonable probability of recovering and then going on to enjoy the benefits of the surgery. It makes little or no sense in beneficence-based clinical ethical surgical judgment to let the patient die from reversible iatrogenic events when the patient is reliably expected to benefit from surgery. This line of reasoning is sound beneficence-based clinical ethical judgment and explains surgeons and anesthesiologists who reverse DNR orders during surgery, despite autonomy-based arguments to the contrary.[42]

Maintaining DNR orders during surgery could result in some patients' pain and suffering being unnecessarily worse than it has to be. The preventive ethics strategy here is not surprising: negotiation with the surgical team. The reader should be prepared to present a clear statement of the patient's problem and why surgery is reliably expected to be effective in addressing that problem. The reader and the surgical team should undertake a frank appraisal of the patient's surgical risk. The reader should also negotiate with the surgical team when the reader's orders for nonaggressive management of life-threatening events will again take effect (i.e., essentially a postoperative trial of intervention). The reader needs to be aware of surgeons' understandable sensitivities about mortality rates. The reader and surgical colleagues should work with their institutions and payers to ensure that death subsequent to surgery and reinstatement of the reader's orders for nonaggressive management of life-threatening events is an acceptable form of postoperative mortality.

To summarize an optimal means to address advance care planning, Table 59.1 depicts this process in brief. The family can be part of this process when the patient consents to their involvement. At its completion, the patient's loved ones, and specifically the DPAHC agent, should receive a copy of the completed living will, DPAHC, Values History, and family covenant.

CONCLUSION

As one can understand from the Schiavo case, the moral weight of future treatment refusal should not be left to oral statements. The legally recognized written advance directives, the living will, and the DPAHC are essential tools in advance care planning. The Values History and family covenant are powerful supplementary documents that can add clarity and meaning to these advance directives by facilitating patient conversation on end-of-life care with family and physicians. Taken together, these advance directives allow the physician to respect patient autonomy and to understand better his patient's values and preferences regarding end-of-life care.

My Advance Directive for Future Medical Treatment

Patient's name:

_____

I currently have signed
[] Living Will
Date signed: _____
Location: _____
Discussed with
[] My doctor:
Name _____ Date _____
[] My Proxy/Health Surrogate
Name _____ Date _____
[] My other family members
Name _____ Date _____

Name _____ Date _____
Name _____ Date _____
Name _____ Date _____
Name _____ Date _____
[] My Durable Power of Attorney for Health Care:
Proxy Name: _____
Address: _____ Phone _____
Date signed: _____
Location: _____
Discussed with
[] My doctor:
Name _____ Date _____
[] My Proxy/Health Surrogate
Name _____ Date _____
[] My other family members
Name _____ Date _____
Name _____ Date _____
Name _____ Date _____
Name _____ Date _____
Name _____ Date _____
[] My Organ Donation Card:
Date signed: _____
Location: _____
Discussed with
[] My doctor:
Name _____ Date _____
[] My Proxy/Health Surrogate
Name _____ Date _____
[] My other family members
Name _____ Date _____
Name _____ Date _____
Name _____ Date _____
Name _____ Date _____
Name _____ Date _____

My Family Covenant

I have entered a family covenant with my doctor _____ and the following family members and friends:
Name _____
Name _____
Name _____
Name _____
Name _____

(Reprinted with permission from Johns Hopkins University Press, Doukas, DJ, Reichel, W. *Planning for Uncertainty.* 2nd ed. Baltimore: Johns Hopkins University Press, 2006.)

If other family members or friends are not included above, they are not to be consulted about my health, given medical information without my consent or that of my proxy, and they are not to be part of any medical decision making on my behalf.

My family covenant directs members to carry out my autonomous values and preferences in the following way, in conjunction with my living will and/or durable power of attorney for health care:

[Potential Areas for consideration:]

[] Who Has Access to My Health Care Information (Confidentiality)

[] Who Else May Participate in My Health Care Decisions

[] Who Is My Proxy and Whom Else Should He or She Consult (or Not)

Describe here:

_____
_____
_____
_____

Signature: _____ Date: _____
Witness/Address: _____
Witness Signature: _____ Date: _____
Witness/Address: _____
Witness Signature: _____ Date: _____

The Values History

Patient's name: _____

This Values History serves as a set of my specific value-based directives for various medical interventions. It is to be used in health care circumstances when I may be unable to voice my preferences. These directives shall be made a part of the medical record and shall be used as supplements to my living will and/or durable power of attorney for health care if I am terminally ill and unable to communicate, if I am in an irreversible coma or persistent vegetative state, or if I am in end-stage dementia and unable to communicate.

I. Values Section

There are several values important in decisions about end-of-life treatment and care. This section of the Values History invites you to identify your most important values.

A. Basic Life Values

Perhaps the most basic values in this context concern length of life versus quality of life. Which of the following two statements most accurately reflects your feelings and wishes? Write your initials and the date next to the number you choose.

_____ 1. I want to live as long as possible, regardless of the quality of life that I experience.

_____ 2. I want to preserve a good quality of life, even if this means that I may not live as long.

B. Quality-of-Life Values

There are many values that help us to define for ourselves the quality of life that we want to live. The following values appear to be those most frequently used to define quality of life. Review this list and circle the values that are most important to

your definition of quality of life. Feel free to elaborate on any of the items in the list, and to add to the list any other values that are important to you.

1. I want to maintain my capacity to think clearly.
2. I want to feel safe and secure.
3. I want to avoid unnecessary pain and suffering.
4. I want to be treated with respect.
5. I want to be treated with dignity when I can no longer speak for myself.
6. I do not want to be an unnecessary burden on my family.
7. I want to be able to make my own decisions.
8. I want to experience a comfortable dying process.
9. I want to be with my loved ones before I die.
10. I want to leave good memories of me for my loved ones.
11. I want to be treated in accord with my religious beliefs and traditions.
12. I want respect shown for my body after I die.
13. I want to help others by making a contribution to medical education and research.
14. Other values or clarification of values above:

II. Directives Section

The following directives are intended to clarify what you want and do not want if one day you are terminally ill and unable to communicate, you are in an irreversible coma or persistent vegetative state, or you are in end-stage dementia and unable to communicate. Some directives involve a simple yes or no decision. Others provide for the choice of a trial of intervention. Write your initials and the date next to the number for each directive you complete.

Initials/Date

_____ 1. I want to undergo cardiopulmonary resuscitation.

_____ YES

_____ NO

Why?

_____ 2. I want to be placed on a ventilator.

_____ YES

_____ TRIAL for the TIME PERIOD OF _____.

_____ TRIAL to determine effectiveness using reasonable medical judgment.

_____ NO

Why?

_____ 3. I want to have an endotracheal tube used in order to perform items 1 and 2.

_____ YES

_____ TRIAL for the TIME PERIOD OF _____.

_____ TRIAL to determine effectiveness using reasonable medical judgment.

_____ NO

Why?

_____ 4. I want to have total parenteral nutrition administered for my nutrition.

_____ YES

_____ TRIAL for the TIME PERIOD OF _____.

_____ TRIAL to determine effectiveness using reasonable medical judgment.

_____ NO

Why?

_____ 5. I want to have intravenous medication and hydration administered. Regardless of my decision, I understand that intravenous hydration to alleviate discomfort or pain medication will not be withheld from me if I so request them.

_____ YES

_____ TRIAL for the TIME PERIOD OF _____.

_____ TRIAL to determine effectiveness using reasonable medical judgment.

_____ NO

Why?

_____ 6. I want to have all medications used for the treatment of my illness continued. Regardless of my decision, I understand that pain medication will continue to be administered including narcotic medications.

_____ YES

_____ TRIAL for the TIME PERIOD OF _____.

_____ TRIAL to determine effectiveness using reasonable medical judgment.

_____ NO

Why?

_____ 7. I want to have nasogastric, gastrostomy, or other enteral feeding tubes introduced and administered for my nutrition.

_____ YES

_____ TRIAL for the TIME PERIOD OF _____.

_____ TRIAL to determine effectiveness using reasonable medical judgment.

_____ NO

Why?

_____ 8. I want to be placed on a dialysis machine.

_____ YES

_____ TRIAL for the TIME PERIOD OF _____.

_____ TRIAL to determine effectiveness using reasonable medical judgment.

_____ NO

Why?

_____ 9. I want to have an autopsy done to determine the cause(s) of my death.

_____ YES

_____ NO

Why?

_____ 10. I want to be admitted to the Intensive Care Unit.

_____ YES

_____ NO

Why?

_____ 11. *For a patient in a long-term care facility or for a patient receiving care at home who experiences a life threatening change in health status:* I want 911 called in case of a medical emergency.

_____ YES

_____ NO

Why?

_____ 12. Other directives:

I consent to these directives after receiving honest disclosure of their implications, risks, and benefits from my physician, being free of constraints, and being of sound mind.

Signature: _____ Date: _____

Witness/Address: _____

Witness/Address: _____

13. Proxy Negation: I request that the following persons NOT be allowed to make decisions on my behalf in the event of my disability or incapacity:

Name _____ Date _____

Name _____ Date _____

Reprinted by permission of Appleton & Lange, Inc. Adapted from Doukas D, McCullough L. The values history: the evaluation of the patient's values and advance directives. *J Fam Pract.* 1991;32:145–153.

REFERENCES

1. *Schiavo v. Schiavo*, No. 8:05-CV-530-T-27TBM (M.D. Fla. Mar. 22, 2005), aff'd, No. 05–11556 (11th Cir. Mar. 23, 2005).
2. *In Re Quinlan*, 70 N.J. 10, 355 A.2d 647 (1976).
3. *Schloendorff v. Society of New York Hospital*, 211 N.Y. 125, 105 N.E. 92 (NY Ct. App., 1914).
4. *Roe v. Wade*, 410 U.S. 113 (1973).
5. http://www.oag.state.ny.us/health/EOLGUIDE012605.pdf. Accessed July 10, 2006.
6. http://bhs.msu.edu/mnp.htm. Accessed July 10, 2006.
7. *Cruzan v. Director, Missouri Department of Health*, 497 U.S. 261 (1990).
8. *Omnibus Budget Reconciliation Act of 1990.* Pub L. No. 101–508.
9. Robinson M, Dehaven M, Koch K. Effects of the patient self-determination act on patient knowledge and behavior. *J Fam Pract.* 1993;37:363–368.
10. Silverman H, Tuma P, Schaeffer M, Singh B. Implementation of the patient self-determination act in a hospital setting: an initial evaluation. *Arch Intern Med.* 1995;155:502–510.
11. Bailly D, and DePoy E. Older people's responses to education about advance directives. *Health Soc Work.* 1995;20:223–228.
12. Hoffman LJ, Gill B. Beginning with the end in mind. *Am J Nurs.*2000;Suppl:38–41.
13. Doukas DJ, Reichel W. *Planning for Uncertainty: Living Wills and Other Advance Directives for You and Your Family.* 2nd ed Baltimore: John Hopkins University Press; 2007.
14. Sulmasy DP, Terry PB, Weisman CS, et al. The accuracy of substituted judgments in patients with terminal diagnoses. *Ann Intern Med.* 1998;128:621–629.
15. Brett AS. "Inappropriate" treatment near the end of life: conflict between religious convictions and clinical judgment. *Arch Intern Med.* 2003;163:1645–1649.
16. Doukas DJ, McCullough LB. The values history: the evaluation of the patient's values and advance directives. *J Fam Pract.* 1991;32:145–153.
17. Doukas DJ, McCullough LB. Assessing the values history of the aged patient regarding critical and chronic care. In: Gallo JJ, Reichel W, Andersen L, eds. *Handbook of Geriatric Assessment.* 1st ed. Rockville, MD: Aspen Publishers, Inc.; 1988:111–124.

18. Doukas DJ, Lipson S, McCullough LB. Value history. In: *Clinical Aspects of Aging*. 3rd ed. Baltimore: Williams & Wilkins; 1989:615–616.
19. Pellegrino ED. Personal communication, 1981.
20. Doukas DJ, Gorenflo DW. Analyzing the values history: an evaluation of patient medical values and advance directives. *J Clin Ethics*. 1993;4:41–45.
21. Doukas DJ, Antonucci TA, Gorenflo DW. A multigenerational assessment of values and advance directives. *Ethics Behav*. 1992;2:51–59.
22. Doukas DJ, Gorenflo DW, Venkateswaran R. Understanding patients' values. *J Clin Ethics*. 1993;4:199–200.
23. Ackerman T. Why doctors should intervene. *Hastings Center Rep*. 1982;12:14–17.
24. Wear S. Anticipatory ethical decision-making: the role of the primary care physician. *HMO Pract*. 1989;3:31–46.
25. Civetta J, Taylor R, Kirby R, eds. *Critical Care*. Philadelphia:J. B. Lippincott; 1988.
26. Doukas DJ. Autonomy and beneficence in the family: describing the family covenant. *J Clin Ethics*. 1991;2:145–148.
27. Doukas DJ, Hardwig J. Using the family covenant in planning end-of-life care: obligations and promises of patients, families, and physicians. *J Am Geriatr Soc*. 2003;51:1155–1158.
28. Upadya A, Muralidharan V, Amoateng-Adjepong Y, Manthous CA. Patient, physician, and family member understanding of living wills. *Am J Respir Cri Care Med*. 2002;166:1430–1435.
29. Doukas DJ. Currents in contemporary ethics–family in advance care planning: the family covenant in the wake of Terri Schiavo. *J Law Med Ethics*. 2005;33:372–374.
30. Emanuel LL, Barry MJ, Stoeckle JD, et al. Advance directives for medical care – a case for greater use. *NEJM*. 1991;324:889–895.
31. Scissors K. Advance directives for medical care. *NEJM*. 1991; 325:1255.
32. Forrow L, Gogel E, Thomas E. Advance directives for medical care. *NEJM*. 1991;325:1255.
33. Emanuel LL, Danis M, Pearlman RA, et al. Advance care planning as a process: structuring discussions in practice. *J Am Geriatr Soc*. 1995;43:40–46.
34. Moore KA, Danks JH, Ditto PH, et al. Elderly outpatients' understanding of a physician-initiated advance directive discussion. *Arch Fam Med*. 1994;3:1057–1063.
35. Uhlmann RF, Pearlman RA. Perceived quality of life and preferences for life-sustaining treatment in older adults. *Arch Intern Med*. 1991;151:495–497.
36. Reilly R, Teasdale T, McCullough LB. Option of trial in advance directives. *Gerontologist*. 1992;32:69.
37. Grodin MA. Religious advance directives: the convergence of law, religion, medicine, and public health. *Am J Public Health*. 1993;83:899–903.
38. Stollerman G. Decisions to leave home. *J Am Geriatr Soc*. 1988;36:375–376.
39. Jecker NS. The role of intimate others in medical decision making. *Gerontologist*. 1990;30:65–71.
40. Sabatino CP. Survey of state EMS-DNR laws and protocols. *J Law, Med Ethics*. 1999;27:297–315.
41. Feder S, Matheny RL, Loveless RS Jr, Rea TD. Withholding resuscitation: a new approach to prehospital end-of-life decisions. *Ann Intern Med*. 2006;144:634–640.
42. Cohen CB, Cohen PJ. Required reconsideration of "do-not-resuscitate" orders in the operating room and certain other treatment settings. *Law Med Health Care*. 1992;20:354–363.

60

ETHICAL DECISION MAKING IN GERIATRIC MEDICINE

Brooke E. Salzman, MD, Danielle Snyderman, MD, Robert Perkel, MD

INTRODUCTION

Ethical decision making is essential in the practice of medicine. The foundation of the provider–patient relationship rests on moral principles expressed in professional oaths that serve to protect and promote the interests and welfare of patients. Even the most mundane medical interactions usually involve weighing competing values and priorities to arrive at a management plan that is sound both from medical and moral vantage points. Health care providers, like most people, derive moral guidance from multiple sources including their personal upbringing and experiences, education, cultural traditions, and religious beliefs. Nevertheless, providers may not be adequately prepared to carry out their unique, professional ethical obligations and to facilitate resolutions of ethical dilemmas in a clinical setting. Knowledge of and skills pertaining to ethics in clinical practice and in training have been shown to be highly variable and frequently deficient.[1–3] Therefore, increasing efforts to educate health care providers in clinical ethics are important.

New ethical considerations in clinical practice will continually emerge along with advances in medical technology and life-sustaining therapies. Such advances have already raised fundamental ethical questions in areas pertaining to issues of life and death, and one's right to consent to, request, or refuse treatment, for example. Providers who care for geriatric patients may be more likely to confront ethical issues that concern end-of-life care and quality-of-life questions. The role of ethical analysis in medicine will become even more critical as the aging population expands along with increasing technological advances.

This chapter describes several case scenarios that raise ethical dilemmas commonly confronted in the care of elderly patients. In clinical medical ethics, there are few, if any, absolutes and generally no single correct answer. Our goal is *not* to provide readers with answers to difficult ethical disputes, but rather to offer some helpful approaches to analyzing and resolving ethical conflicts in medical practice.

CURRENT APPROACHES TO CLINICAL MEDICAL ETHICS

The terms "morality" and "ethics" are often used interchangeably but deserve distinction. Morality refers to beliefs about right and wrong in relation to human behavior. Ethics refers to the discipline that studies principles that govern good and bad behavior. Medical ethics or bioethics is a subset of the discipline that pertains to examining ethics within the context of medicine or science. More specifically, clinical ethics involves "the systemic identification, analysis and resolution of ethical problems" in the clinical practice of medicine.[4] A systematic approach to clinical ethics not only assists clinicians in ethical decision making, but also protects the rights and interests of patients, and supports collaborative relationships among patients and those close to patients, clinicians, and health care institutions.[4] Clinical ethics may be differentiated from the larger framework of medical ethics or bioethics in that it focuses more on being practice oriented and therefore, applicable in a clinical setting. Bioethics is broader in scope and encompasses more theoretical discussions of ethics in medicine and science.

One important approach to clinical ethics is termed *principlism*, which outlines a set of moral principles that can function as a template or framework for ethical analysis and decision making. Such principles are not moral absolutes and often come into conflict with one another in the clinical context. These principles can, however, serve as a useful framework for analyzing challenging ethical cases. The four key categories of moral principles include: 1) respect for autonomy, 2) nonmaleficence, 3) beneficence, and 4) justice.[5]

The principle of respect for autonomy asserts that competent adult patients have the right to make decisions about basic personal matters, such as their health care. The concept of autonomy encompasses notions of self-determination, independence, and freedom. This principle obliges health care providers to facilitate patient involvement in treatment decisions. Furthermore, the principle of respect for patient autonomy establishes the basis for several other standard clinical practices including informed consent, truth telling, confidentiality, and advance care planning.[3] The principle of beneficence represents the fundamental duty of medical professionals to do good for patients, to help patients who are in need, and to promote their well-being. The principle of nonmaleficence stems from the obligation of physicians to do no harm to patients. This principle underscores the importance of considering the negative consequences and burdens of medical treatments. Furthermore, it compels health care providers to weigh such outcomes against the possible benefits to determine the best course of action. Nonmaleficence may be particularly relevant when considering end-of-life care, precisely because some medical interventions may cause suffering with minimal benefit for the patient's duration or quality of life. Finally, the principle of justice concerns the notion of being fair and treating patients equally. Specifically, given our current medical and societal paradigms, distributive justice relates to the allocation of limited medical resources in an equitable fashion.

Although principlism is a useful, practical, and popular methodology for examining clinical ethics, it has been criticized for its limitations and inadequacies. Alternative approaches have been developed that offer additional insights for resolving ethical dilemmas. For instance, casuistry, or case-based ethics, emphasizes the importance of examining the particular features of a specific case and then comparing that case to other cases to achieve moral understanding. Supporters of this approach argue that a case-based approach is more practical than trying to apply abstract principles to real-life situations.[6]

Feminist approaches to clinical ethics challenge essential assumptions that shape moral principles that possibly perpetuate patriarchal notions of the human experience. For instance, respect for autonomy gives precedence to individualism and self-determination, whereas a care-based approach upholds the underlying concepts of connection and relationships, and emphasizes ideals of caring and justice.[7] Other ethical perspectives arising from disadvantaged or marginalized groups favor morals derived from personal experience over abstract moral principles. Such theorists value narratives by people in their own voices and focus on the moral perceptions expressed in those narratives.[8,9] Finally, virtue theory describes an approach to clinical ethics that underscores core qualities and attributes of the physician, rather than examining how a physician's actions support certain ethical principles. According to this theory, the virtues of a good physician should include characteristics such as compassion, integrity, respect, loyalty, altruism, honesty, impartiality, and self-effacement.[10]

An approach to clinical ethics need not align itself with one particular methodology but can utilize relevant aspects of various methods. It is certainly both reasonable and practical to blend different models for ethical decision making.

Furthermore, several other sources of moral guidance such as law, public policy, and spirituality may aid in analyzing ethical issues. We will review several ethical dilemmas and approaches to resolving such dilemmas in the cases that follow.

PRACTICAL CONSIDERATIONS IN APPROACHING ETHICAL DILEMMAS

Whether addressing an ethical dilemma as a formal consultation or not, it is imperative for the clinician to gather all pertinent information about the patient and the "ethics case." A thorough collection of such information will frame the relevant details necessary for case analysis. Initially, when faced with an ethical question, the clinician needs to identify the patient's diagnosis, prognosis, options for care, and the benefits and risks of alternative treatments.[11] It is necessary to assess patients' goals and objectives, their understanding of the situation, their decision-making capacity, and in some cases, whether there is a written advance directive or proxy medical decision maker. It is also critical for the clinician to investigate the key people and relationships involved in the particular case. For example, who is the primary decision maker? What is the relationship among the patient, family members, and other significant persons? Who are the key providers for this patient (including primary care and/or specialist health care providers as well as personal, emotional, financial, and fiduciary providers)?

To facilitate a resolution to an ethical issue, it is crucial to explore and understand the attitudes, beliefs, and interests of the patient and of the other relevant individuals involved.[12,13] Such attitudes and beliefs can be influenced by multiple factors including but not limited to religion, culture, education, age, and economic status. Clarifying the views of the health care team is also critically important.

The clinician needs to name and clarify the ethical dilemma at issue. Sometimes this is not as easy or automatic as might be surmised. An ethical conflict exists precisely because there are competing moral considerations or differing views about what is right or wrong. The reasons supporting each opposing potential course of action should be elucidated. It also behooves the clinician to investigate pragmatic issues that may be influencing the case such as interpersonal conflicts among family members, poor communication with the hospital team, time or financial pressures, hospital policy, or insurance coverage.[11,12]

In addition to evaluating the patient, it is usually helpful if not crucial to meet with the family or key persons involved in the care of the patient. Team meetings can be instrumental in facilitating communication among the patient, family members, and the health care team. Facilitating such meetings may involve acknowledging or validating different perspectives and explicitly discussing emotions, beliefs, and attitudes as well as interpersonal conflicts. In some cases, it is necessary to seek further assistance to resolve an ethical dilemma. This may entail asking for a hospital or institutional ethics committee consultation and/or involving an ombudsman or legal counsel.

Case Number 1 (The Right to Drive)

A widowed, 85-year-old man comes into your office for a routine physical examination. He is active, lives alone, and drives regularly. He has a medical history of hypertension, diabetes, and prostate cancer. During your visit, you notice that the patient has trouble telling you the names of the medications he takes and how he takes them. On a Mini-Mental Status Examination, he loses points for attention, calculation, recall, and visuospatial tasks. His total score is 21 of 30, likely placing him in the mild dementia category. His blood pressure in the office is elevated at 165/85 mm Hg. Otherwise, his physical examination, including vision and neurological examinations, is normal. He denies being involved in any recent motor vehicle accidents. He admits to getting lost one night while driving home from visiting family but attributes this incident to forgetting his glasses. You recommend to the patient that he obtain a driver's evaluation, but he refuses and responds, "What for? I haven't had any problems. Besides, without a car, I'd die. I wouldn't be able do anything."

Later that day, you get a phone call from this patient's son asking you to tell his father not to drive anymore. He tells you that his father's driving skills have significantly declined and that he frequently gets lost while driving, even when he is only a few miles from his house.

DISCUSSION

The number of older drivers is progressively increasing in parallel with the growing elderly population. By 2030 people age 65 years and older are expected to represent 25% of the driving population and 25% of fatal crash involvements.[14] Increasingly, older patients and their families will turn to their physicians for guidance in assessing the ability to drive and with concerns about safe driving. Patients may be reticent to raise concerns to their physician about driving because they do not want the privilege revoked. To many older adults, driving represents a critical cornerstone of independence and self-reliance. People frequently need to drive to perform basic activities of daily living and to provide social contact. Relinquishing the privilege of driving may be perceived as tantamount to becoming dependent, lonely, and vulnerable. Such fears may render patients unwilling to recognize the decline in their driving abilities. Moreover, some patients, due to their underlying medical conditions, may be unable to perceive deficiencies in their driving abilities. Therefore, it is incumbent upon the physician to inquire about whether her patients drive, if they have experienced difficulties driving, and to assess medical conditions that may affect driving abilities.

Numerous medical conditions may cause impaired driving abilities including but not limited to epilepsy, Alzheimer's disease and other etiologies of cognitive deficit, syncope, cerebrovascular disease, macular degeneration, glaucoma, Parkinson's disease, osteoarthritis, and alcoholism.[15] Advanced age alone has been associated with an increase in motor vehicle crashes and fatal car accidents.[14] Nevertheless, the ability to drive should not be solely based on having a particular diagnosis or on being a certain age.[16] Older patients and patients with various medical conditions represent a tremendously diverse population and therefore should be considered and evaluated on a case-by-case basis.

One of the major ethical conflicts represented in this case is weighing an individual's right to confidentiality (and the physician's duty to provide confidentiality) versus the physician's moral obligation to override that confidentiality to prevent potential harm to third parties. The principle of regard for patient autonomy may suggest respecting the patient's continuing decision to drive and the physician's need to maintain confidentiality, particularly in relation to the son's intervention. The principles of justice and nonmaleficence, however, may require the physician to breach confidentiality to protect the safety of others, let alone the safety of her patient. The legal case of *Tarasoff v. Regents of the University of California* recognized inherent limitations to patient–physician confidentiality and the physician's duty to reveal protected information in certain circumstances. "A physician may not reveal the confidence entrusted to him in the course of medical attendance . . . unless he is required to do so by law or unless it becomes necessary in order to protect the welfare of the individual or of the community."[17]

Regarding the specific issue of driving, clinicians need to be aware of their specific state's laws and regulations. Policies for obtaining, renewing, and restricting drivers' licenses vary from state to state. For example, some jurisdictions require additional driving tests or documentation for all people in older age groups. All 50 states have regulations supporting voluntary reporting of unsafe drivers by physicians, especially when the patient does not comply with requests to be tested or stop driving. Several states mandate physicians to report certain medical conditions to state authorities. Many physicians are unaware of state reporting requirements. Two particularly helpful resources include the *Physician's Guide to Assessing and Counseling Older Drivers*[18] from the American Medical Association, which details reporting regulations for each state, and the Insurance Institute for Highway Safety.[14] Importantly, whether or not one's driver's license is limited or revoked based on reported information represents a determination of the state department of motor vehicles and lies not within the authority of the patient's physician.

Physicians are obliged to advise and counsel their patients regarding their medical conditions and possible medication side effects that may impair their ability to drive safely. Case law illustrates that failure to advise the patient about such issues is considered negligent behavior.[18] In fact, physicians have been held liable for their patients' car accidents and for third-party injuries caused by their patients because physicians failed to advise patients about medical conditions and medication side effects that impaired driving performance.[18] In most states, when reporting unsafe drivers to state authorities, physicians are generally protected from liability if the report is made in good faith and without malice. Physicians in some states may be liable for reporting a patient with questionable driving abilities for violating patient–physician confidentiality.[18]

Physicians often fear that reporting patients will adversely impact the provider–patient relationship and this fear may serve as a barrier to discussing driving with patients.[19] However, patients prefer to hear about driving concerns from their doctors rather than other sources.[20] Furthermore, older adults may be more willing to follow recommendations to stop driving from their well meaning and trusted physician rather than from family members.[21] The ethical dilemma of whether or not to report someone to state authorities may be preempted altogether by a thorough and sensitive discussion with the patient about recommendations regarding driving retirement.[22] In particular, educating patients and family members about community resources and alternatives to driving may alleviate some of the concerns about dependence and social isolation. If a patient who is clearly impaired refuses to stop driving despite the provider's best efforts and advice, it may be necessary to breach patient confidentiality and report the patient to the Department of Motor Vehicles. Health care providers are encouraged to review applicable driving laws with their patients and to discuss and clearly document their medical recommendations to their patients.

Case Number 2 (Disclosing Diagnosis)

An 82-year-old woman is brought into your office by her daughter. The daughter tells you about her mother's memory loss, which has gradually worsened over the past few years, and that she is becoming more and more forgetful. In addition, the patient has expressed paranoid thoughts that her daughter wants to put her in a nursing home and that people are stealing her possessions. The patient lives alone but nearby her daughter. The patient is adamant about continuing to live on her own and has expressed that living in a nursing home is a fate worse than death. She currently dresses and bathes herself. The daughter conducts most of her mother's finances, arranges and administers her medications, and also does her shopping. There have been no significant accidents or incidents in which the mother is wandering or is lost. After a thorough evaluation, you feel this patient most likely has dementia caused by Alzheimer's disease. When you express this to the patient's daughter, she requests that you not tell her mother as it would only anger, depress, or worry her. The daughter would like you to start a medication for dementia but asks you not to tell the patient the real purpose of the medication.

DISCUSSION

The physician's primary obligation is to her patient. A clinician is required to disclose to the patient all reasonable information relevant to her condition and treatment options so that the patient can make an appropriate, autonomous decision about her own health care. The principle of respect for an individual's autonomy underscores the patient's right to be informed about her condition and her right to participate in her own treatment plan. The fact that the information regarding early dementia may be upsetting to the patient does not in and of itself provide adequate justification to withhold that information from the patient. With skillful and sensitive physician questioning, the patient may then communicate with her doctor how much or what type of information about her condition she would like to have.

The right to be told the truth has evolved over time along with changing attitudes of physicians regarding the doctor–patient relationship. Prior to the 1970s, it was common for physicians not to disclose a diagnosis such as cancer to a patient.[23] Assertions of nonmaleficence were invoked to justify paternalism. By the mid-1970s, however, mirroring the consumer rights revolution in the United States, a significant shift occurred in attitudes supporting patients' rights and autonomy. The majority of health care providers began to affirm the patient's right to full disclosure of diagnosis and prognosis and thereby empower patients to make informed treatment decisions.[23]

A family member's assertion that a patient would be unable to handle upsetting information is generally not a sufficient reason to deny the patient information. The physician must gently inform a well-meaning family member that the health care professional's duty is to assess whether or not a patient wishes to be informed about her condition even if it may be distressing. Dialogue with the patient and family is critical in these situations. Of note, there is little evidence to support the notion that patients wish to be shielded from distressing information. In fact, evidence from pubic opinion polls suggests that most people want to hear the details of their condition, even if the information is burdensome or devastating.[24,25]

There are, however, limited circumstances in which a physician may be excused from disclosing information to a patient. Such circumstances arise when there is ample evidence that the patient is not psychologically or emotionally equipped to consider the information or that the disclosure of information itself would pose serious and immediate harm to the patient. This is known legally as the therapeutic exception to informed consent; however, this exception should be invoked in only a few, highly selected situations.

In some situations, a patient's cultural or ethnic background may have some bearing on her preferences for disclosing information. A patient may wish to delegate authority regarding her health care to someone else. For instance, a patient may want a certain family member to be the primary decision maker. Such a delegation of authority should be clearly stated by the patient and thoroughly documented in medical records. Moreover, the clinician needs to address these issues with the patient and not make assumptions based on cultural or ethnic identity.

Family members and/or clinicians may erroneously presume that an elderly patient lacks decision-making capacity merely because of her age, physical frailty, or cognitive decline.[4] This may lead caregivers and/or clinicians to circumvent inquiring about and fulfilling the patient's preferences and wishes. Furthermore, clinicians may assume that family members should be informed about the patient's situation without seeking the patient's permission first. Such assumptions should be avoided, and patient information should be discussed with family members only after a patient gives permission to do so.

This case clearly illustrates the importance of dialogue with a patient while she still possesses decision-making capacity. Discussing patient preferences, goals, and priorities early on gives the patient the opportunity to consider her situation and contribute to the management plan. Such communication helps guide future medical decisions as the disease progresses to the point when the patient may lack decision-making capacity.

Case Number 3 (Substituted Judgment and Medical Futility)

An 89-year-old African American woman has a history of diabetes, hypertension, congestive heart failure, chronic obstructive pulmonary disease, and advanced dementia. She has been a resident in a nursing home for the last 5 years. You meet this patient and her family when she is hospitalized for a hip fracture. Soon after her hip repair, the patient develops pneumonia. She requires oxygen therapy to maintain appropriate oxygen saturation; however, the patient has become delirious and frequently takes off the oxygen. The house staff orders restraints to keep the oxygen therapy in place. Furthermore, the patient's intake of fluids and nutrition has substantially decreased during this admission. She develops acute renal failure associated with dehydration. An intravenous catheter is placed to administer fluids that, despite her restraints, is quickly torn out by the patient. Further attempts to place an intravenous catheter are unsuccessful.

You meet with the family to discuss this patient's complicated hospital course, her prognosis, and the goals of care for this patient. You ask the family about the patient's wishes regarding resuscitation and the use of other life-sustaining medical therapies. The patient has not executed an advance directive or living will. One daughter says that the patient did not previously express treatment wishes but she believes that her mother would want everything done to keep her alive and would not want a do-not-resuscitate order. She requests that the patient be transferred to the intensive care unit for aggressive management.

DISCUSSION

This commonplace ethical dilemma in hospital practice illustrates selected core ethical issues. In this case, the clinician has no precise, unequivocal statement of the patient's prior autonomous wishes. The clinician has asked for the daughter's recall of her mother's previously expressed desires regarding treatment. One potential difficulty with this approach lies in the assumption that the daughter may, in fact, accurately be able to represent the true autonomous wishes of her mother.

Multiple studies reviewed by Shalowitz et al., however, demonstrate that patient-designated and next-of-kin surrogates incorrectly predict patients' end-of-life treatment preferences in at least one-third of cases.[26] Furthermore, data suggest that surrogates' own personal treatment preferences significantly influence their predictions of patients' preferences.[27] Therefore, one important distinction the clinician must address with family members in cases such as this is that of substituted judgment or clarification of what the *patient's* wishes would be were she magically able to sit up and in a competent and lucid manner tell us what she would desire. Too often, what clinicians receive from well-meaning but distraught family members is what they, the *family members*, would want (either for themselves in such a situation or for their loved one) rather than a statement of what the family members can best estimate their loved-one would want in this situation.

This case involving a patient with advanced dementia and the question of what level of aggressiveness of care to use also highlight the need for discussion with family concerning the issue of medical futility. Although considerable controversy exists about how "medical futility" should be defined, it generally expresses the concept that a medical intervention will not be successful, in that the intervention will not help restore the physical function(s) it is attempting to restore, it will not result in a meaningful benefit, and/or it will not fulfill the patient's goals.[28] For example, performing a medical intervention on a patient with a terminal illness may have no beneficial effect on her underlying medical condition or impact her duration or quality of life. The intervention may even adversely affect her quality of life by causing pain, suffering, or worsening disability.

When considering cases of medical futility, defining a terminal state may not always be straightforward and easy. The debate regarding medical futility stems less from medical uncertainty than from the value judgments (of the physician, patient, and/or family) inherent in making determinations about quality of life, goals of care, and what constitutes a terminal state and a meaningful benefit. Therefore, the patient's best interests and the deliberation over medical futility should be explored with an open discussion with key persons involved, making sure to address the different values and perceptions that inform the decision to pursue or not pursue medical intervention(s).

To recognize a case of medical futility, the health care team must, of course, understand the disease process and establish as accurate a prognosis as possible based on available medical literature. Equipped with these data, a sensitive discussion with family may often allow the invocation of futility to make a decision for less intervention with less aggressive intent. Rather than simply offer the entire menu of treatment choices in cases of true futility, the thoughtful clinician may invoke some degree of beneficence (paternalism) to guide a family toward a more gentle model of palliative and supportive care.

In cases in which there are multiple family members involved with no one designated health care proxy, it can be helpful if the family can appoint one representative who can speak for the family on behalf of the patient. This may allow better communication between health care team and family and obviate the all too common dilemma of different family members hearing different (and sometimes seemingly competing) messages at different times.

Although providers and families can differ in opinion regarding cases of medical futility, providers are usually more comfortable with and respectful of surrogates who attempt to assert the patient's right to refuse care than with surrogates who demand a level of treatment that is more aggressive than the provider's best notion of appropriate care.

In fact, clinicians are not obliged to provide medical treatment they believe is futile and outside of the accepted standard of care. Nevertheless, it is essential that clinicians clearly communicate to family members their medical perspective regarding the patient's condition, prognosis, treatment options, and rationale for their recommendations. It is worthwhile if not critical to take the time to explore respectfully the reasons behind requests for futile medical treatment with the patient and/or family. If, despite numerous efforts to communicate about the patient's poor prognosis, the patient and/or family still demand seemingly futile treatment, then it may be sensible to offer a trial of treatment with a mutually agreed on end point.[28]

This case also illustrates one of the most common scenarios in which a hospital or institutional ethics committee consultation may be of value. Family and health care team should be jointly invited to such a meeting during which a careful explication of issues stated previously can be addressed with the involved parties. Everyone's best intentions and well meaning can be explicitly stated with the same information flowing to all interested parties so then an acceptable solution may be reached in difficult cases near or at the end of life.

We would be remiss if we did not include a brief discussion of the need to think through allocation of resource issues and consideration of culture in matters of futility. Our current medical environment all too often seems to embrace the notion of doing "everything that can be done." This represents neither good nor thoughtful medical practice. Knowing when to say no to technological interventions is as important as knowing when to say yes. Sometimes it simply seems easier to use the technology because it is available. The time to invoke resource utilization and, therefore, social justice arguments, may not necessarily be at the bedside of the individual patient in question. Thoughtful clinicians must help set institutional policy so that some of these matters may be decided with a degree of anticipatory guidance.

Lastly, the issue of culture and race should not be underestimated. Due to a long history of abuse and oppression, documented health disparities, as well as specific important historical considerations (Tuskegee, Willowbrook, the acquired immunodeficiency syndrome genocidal theory), a certain level of mistrust exists among racial and ethnic groups for the larger medical culture. Without getting into a discussion of the propriety of these fears, we simply need to acknowledge their existence so that we may deal openly and honestly with any existing fear and mistrust among our patients and their families.

Case Number 4 (Feeding Tube)

A 77-year-old man with end-stage Alzheimer and multiinfarct dementia is admitted to a geriatric psychiatric ward for worsening aggressive behavior after physically attacking his wife. He lives at home with his wife with the live-in help of nursing assistants. The patient's intake by mouth has substantially decreased and he has lost approximately 15 lb in the past 3 months. On admission, the patient's laboratory values reflect dehydration and malnutrition. You consider placing an intravenous catheter in this patient to administer fluids. A nutrition consultation asserts that the patient requires a feeding tube to address his malnutrition. On meeting with the patient's wife, she asks you not to give her husband intravenous fluids or a feeding tube. "What good would it do in the end? Can't we just let him go?" she asks you.

DISCUSSION

This case highlights a common clinical scenario in both inpatient and long-term care settings that providers caring for patients with dementia can expect to encounter. It is anticipated that all patients with dementia who live long enough will experience difficulty with eating. As dementia worsens, patients will express less interest in eating and develop physical difficulty with chewing, swallowing, and other aspects of motor coordination involved with eating. Patients with dementia will frequently pocket their food (store food in the side compartments of the mouth) and subsequently are considered to be at greater risk of choking. The natural disease trajectory of dementia includes eventual nutritional deficiencies, weight loss, and, ultimately, terminal dehydration. Once a patient stops chewing and swallowing completely, the average life expectancy is 2 weeks.

When patients are unable to feed themselves successfully, the two main therapeutic approaches include artificial feeding by tube or careful feeding by hand. The decision for health care providers and families is often difficult due to misperceptions of the specific disease process as well as the added emotional, social, and cultural traditions and comforts involved with eating. A careful review of the indication for a feeding tube as well as the evidence supporting it can be invaluable to both providers and families when approaching a complex decision involving a patient's care.

There are four clinical scenarios in which tube feeding is deemed beneficial for patients including: head and neck cancers, neuromuscular dystrophy syndromes (specifically, amyotrophic lateral sclerosis), gastric decompression in certain gynecological or abdominal malignancies, and persistent dysphagia 30 days after a cerebrovascular accident.[29] In the latter, evidence supports that the optimal timing for placement of a percutaneous endoscopic gastrostomy (PEG) tube for dysphagia following a stroke is not until 30 days after the event.[20] This allows time to see if the dysphagia will resolve without aggressive intervention and also permits providers and families to take time to make an important decision.

Despite the evidence supporting the aforementioned indications for PEG tube placement, the most common diagnosis for patients receiving tube feeding is dementia. Additionally, patients most likely to receive PEG tubes are patients who are younger, of nonwhite race, and those who lack advance directives. There are multiple assumed benefits of placing PEG tubes in patients with dementia but little evidence to support these benefits. The belief that PEG tubes are associated with less risk of aspiration has not been proven. In fact, tube feeding is considered a risk factor for aspiration, which remains the most common cause of death in patients with PEG tubes. Additionally, there are no data to support that jejunostomy tubes are associated with a decreased risk of aspiration.[31] Although many patients, families, and/or providers may intuitively think that enteral feeding would improve nutritional status, studies have shown that, in fact, weight loss increased as the duration of tube feeding increased, lending support to the frail body's inability to utilize or absorb the extra nutrition.[32] It is also important to note that the use of enteral feeding to prevent or treat pressure sores has also not been proven. Finally, mortality data have not shown a survival benefit for patients with severe dementia receiving tube feeding.[33]

Many family members understandably fear that withholding nutrition is associated with starvation and deprivation of one of the most comforting aspects of life. Although it is difficult to assess the level of discomfort in patients with severe dementia and poor oral intake, we can extrapolate from studies of patients with terminal illnesses including cancer. Although patients often have awareness of hunger and thirst at the end of life, 84% of such patients reported that minimal interventions such as swabbing the mouth and eating small amounts of food satisfied the feelings of hunger and thirst.[34] An additional consideration in quality-of-life data includes the fact that the use of PEG tubes in severe dementia leads to increased use of restraints.[35] Lastly, a cross national survey of family members of cognitively impaired patients who received PEG tubes in nursing home settings revealed a majority of family members regretted making the decision to have a PEG tube placed in their relative.[36]

Epidemiological trends showed a doubling of the use of PEG tubes in Medicare patients at the end of the 20th century with a concomitant increase in use for nonevidenced-based indications.[37] Medicare reimbursements for tube-fed patients in long-term care settings are higher, suggesting that financial incentive may play a role in this trend. The major challenge regarding the appropriate provision (or withholding) of artificial nutrition in patients with terminal illnesses remains educational in nature. In a study addressing physicians' attitudes in decisions regarding PEG tube placement, 90% felt starting tube feeding was the correct decision if family members were in agreement but only 50% still believed it to be the right decision if family members were not in agreement.[38] It remains the health care provider's responsibility to find the balance between beneficence (promoting medical interventions that can help the patient) and nonmaleficence (not recommending interventions that are not helpful and may even be harmful to patients). Patients with end-stage dementia often rely on surrogate decision makers to determine if a feeding tube should be placed. Substituted judgment may be particularly difficult in these scenarios because they often involve beliefs and attitudes deeply rooted in cultural and religious practices. This difficulty highlights the importance of encouraging discussion of advance directives early on in the disease process. In the setting of dementia, anticipatory guidance regarding the natural history of the disease and the nutritional issues that will arise may help patients make decisions when they still possess decisional-making capacity.

CONCLUSION

Ethical decision making is an essential component of appropriate, sound, caring, and compassionate medical practice. Practitioners of geriatric medicine may be more likely to confront ethical dilemmas in clinical practice involving end-of-life care and quality-of-life issues. Particularly as the aging population expands and technology advances, ethical decision making in medicine will assume even more importance. Understanding a variety of approaches to clinical ethics, ranging from the practical to the theoretical, will undoubtedly facilitate analysis and resolution of ethical dilemmas in the clinical setting. Ultimately, both the medical care we provide and the welfare of our patients will benefit from improving our knowledge of and skills pertaining to clinical ethics.

REFERENCES

1. SUPPORT Principal Investigators. A controlled trial to improve care for seriously ill hospitalized patients: the Study to Understand Prognoses and Preferences for Outcomes and Risks of Treatments (SUPPORT). *JAMA.* 1995;274:1591–1598.
2. Wayne DB, Muir JC, DaRosa DA. Developing an ethics curriculum for an internal medicine residency program: use of a needs assessment. *Teach Learn Med.* 2004;16:197–201.
3. Carrese JA, Sugarman J. The inescapable relevance of bioethics for the practicing clinician. *Chest.* 2006;130(6):1864–1872.
4. Ahronheim JC, Moreno JD, Zuckerman C. *Ethics in Clinical Practice.* 2nd ed. Boston: Jones and Bartlett Publishers; 2005.
5. Beauchamp TL, Childress JF. *Principles of Biomedical Ethics.* 5th ed. New York: Oxford University Press; 2001.
6. Jonsen AR, Siegler M, Winslade WJ. *Clinical Ethics.* 3rd ed. New York: McGraw-Hill, 1992.
7. Gilligan C. Moral orientation and moral development. In: Kittay EF, Meyers DT, eds. *Women and Moral Theory.* Totowa, NJ: Rowman and Littlefield; 1987.
8. Dula A, Williams S. When race matters. *Clin Geriatr Med.* 2005;21(1):239–253.
9. Dula A. The life and death of Miss Mildred: an elderly black woman. *Clin Geriatr Med.* 1994;10:419–430.

10. Pellegrino ED, Thomasma DC. *The Virtues in Medical Practice.* New York: Oxford University Press; 1993.

11. Perlin TM. *Clinical Medical Ethics: Cases in Practice.* Boston: Little, Brown and Company; 1992.

12. La Puma J, Schiedermayer D,. *Ethics Consultation: A Practical Guide.* Boston: Jones and Bartlett Publishers; 1994.

13. Lo B. *Resolving Ethical Dilemmas: A Guide for Clinicians.* 2nd ed. Philadelphia: Lippincott Williams & Wilkins; 2000.

14. Insurance Information Institute. Older Drivers. 2008. Available at: http://www.iii.org/media/hottopics/insurance/olderdrivers. Accessed July 7, 2008.

15. Lantz MS. The impaired older adult driver: when is it time to stop? *Clin Geriatri.* 2007;15:17–20.

16. Dubinsky RM, Stein AC, Lyons K. Practice parameter: risk of driving and Alzheimer's disease (an evidence-based review): report of the quality standards subcommittee of the American Academy of Neurology. *Neurology.* 2000;54(12):2205–2211.

17. Beauchamp TL, Walters L. *Contemporary Issues in Bioethics.* 6th ed. Belmont, CA: Wadsworth-Thomson Learning. 2003.

18. American Medical Association. *Assessing and Counseling Older Drivers.* Available at: http://www.nhtsa.dot.gov/People/injury/olddrive/OlderDriversBook/pages/Contents.html. Accessed on July 7, 2008.

19. Bogner HR, Straton JB, Gallo JJ, Rebok GW, Keyl PM. The role of physicians in assessing older drivers; barriers, opportunities, and strategies. *J Am Board Fam Pract.* 2004;17:38–43.

20. Adler G, Kuskowski M. Driving cessation in older men with dementia. *Alzheimer Dis Assoc Disord.* 2003;17:68–71.

21. Persson D. The elderly driver: deciding when to stop. *Gerontologist.* 1993;33:88–91.

22. MacLean K, Berg-Weger M, Meuser TM, Carr D. Driving retirement: help with counseling older patients. *Fam Pract Recertif.* 2007;29:33–43.

23. Novack DH, Plumber R, Smith RL, Ochitill H, Morrow GR, Bennett JM. Changes in physicians' attitudes toward telling the cancer patient. *JAMA.* 1979;241:897–900.

24. Schattner A, Tal M. Truth telling and patient autonomy: the patient's point of view. *Am J Med.* 2002;113:66–69.

25. Jenkins V. Information needs of patients with cancer: results from a large study in UK cancer centres. *Br J Cancer.* 2001;84:48–51.

26. Shalowitz DI, Garrett-Mayer E, Wendler D. The accuracy of surrogate decision makers: a systemic review. *Arch Intern Med.* 2006;166:493–497.

27. Fagerlin A, Ditto PH, Danks JH, Houts RM, Smucker WD. Projection in surrogate decisions about life-sustaining medical treatments. *Health Psychol.* 2001;20:166–175.

28. Moseley KL, Silveira MJ, Dorr Goold S. Futility in evolution. *Clin Geriatr Med.* 2005;21:211–222.

29. Niv Y, Abuksis V. Indications for percutaneous endoscopic gastrostomy insertion: ethical aspects. *Digest Dis.* 2002;20:253–256.

30. Dennis MS, Lewis SC, Warlow C; FOOD Trial Collaboration. Effect of timing and method of enteral tube feeding for dysphagic stroke patients (FOOD): a multicentre randomised controlled trial. *Lancet.* 2005;365:764–772.

31. Lazarus BA, Murphy JB, Culpepper L. Aspiration associated with long-term gastric versus jejunal feeding: a critical analysis of the literature. *Arch Phys Med Rehab.* 1990;71:46–53.

32. Ciocon JO, Silverstone FA, Graver LM, Foley CJ. Tube feedings in elderly patients. Indications, benefits, and complications. *Arch Intern Med.* 1988;148:429–433.

33. Mitchell SL, Kiely DK, Lipsitz LA. The risk factors and impact on survival of feeding tube placement in nursing home residents with severe cognitive impairment. *Arch Intern Med.* 1997;157:327–332.

34. McCann RM, Hall WJ, Groth-Juncker A. Comfort care for terminally ill patients. The appropriate use of nutrition and hydration. *JAMA.* 1994;272:1263–1266.

35. Peck A, Cohen CE, Mulvihill MN. Long-term enteral feeding of aged demented nursing home patients. *J Am Geriatr Soc.* 1990;38:1195–1198.

36. Mitchell SL, Berkowitz RE, Lawson FM, Lipsitz LA. A cross-national survey of tube-feeding decisions in cognitively impaired older persons. *J Am Geriatr Soc.* 2000;48:391–397.

37. James SE, Price CS, Khan S. Percutaneous endoscopic gastrostomy: mortality, trends, and risk factors. *J Postgrad Med.* 2005;51:23–29.

38. Von Preyss-Friedman SM. Physicians' attitudes toward tube feeding chronically ill nursing home patients. *J Gen Intern Med.* 1992;7:46.

INDEX

973
BOO

Boorstin, Daniel J.

The Landmark history
of the American
people

$11.99

DATE			

© THE BAKER & TAYLOR CO.

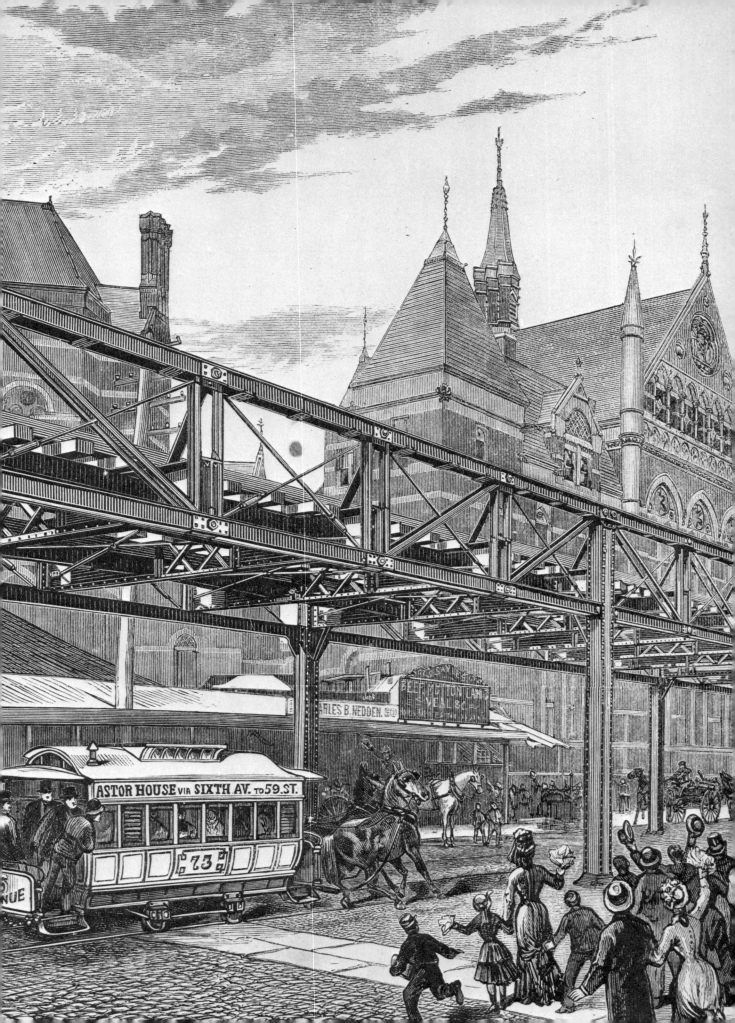

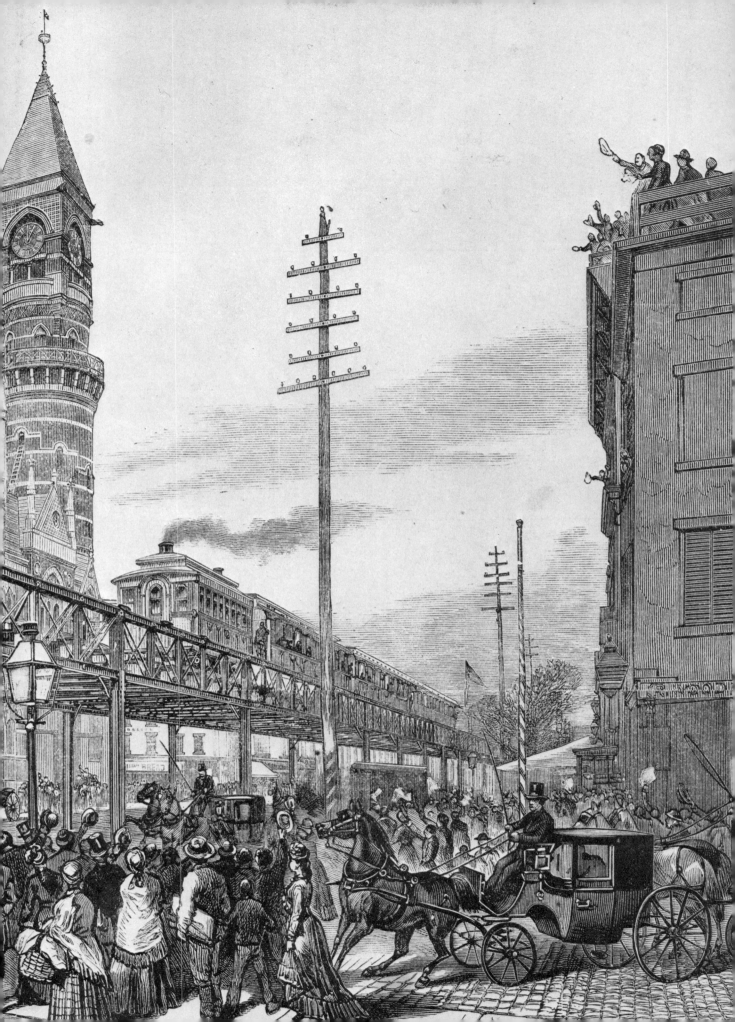

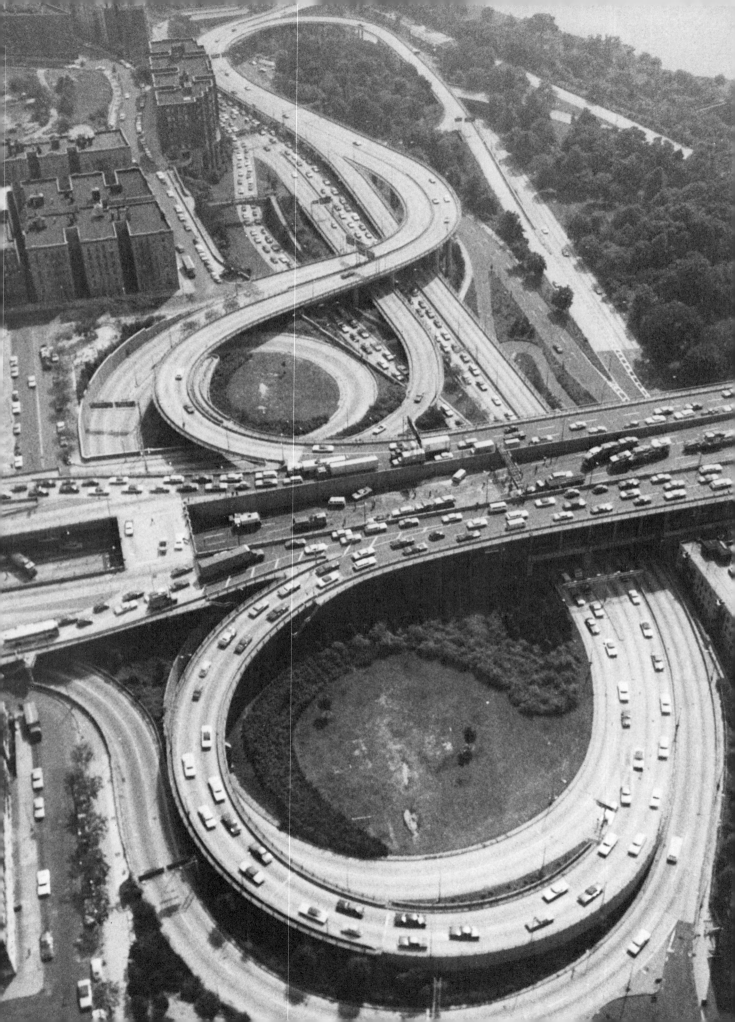

THE LANDMARK HISTORY OF THE
AMERICAN
PEOPLE

THE LANDMARK HISTORY OF THE
AMERICAN
PEOPLE

VOLUME 2
From Appomattox to the Moon
NEWLY REVISED AND UPDATED

BY DANIEL J. BOORSTIN
With Ruth F. Boorstin

Illustrated with prints and photographs

RANDOM HOUSE 🏠 NEW YORK

Author's Acknowledgments

This book has benefited from the suggestions of many friends and fellow historians, especially those at the University of Chicago and the Smithsonian Institution. At Random House, Janet Finnie proposed the book to me and helped shape it; Karen Tobias helped find and select the illustrations. Janet Schulman of Random House suggested the new edition and with the assistance of Kate Banks helped guide the updating and revisions.

Copyright © 1970, 1987 by Daniel J. Boorstin.
All rights reserved under International and Pan-American Copyright Conventions.
Published in the United States by Random House, Inc., New York, and simultaneously in Canada by Random House of Canada Limited, Toronto.

Library of Congress Cataloging-in-Publication Data:
Boorstin, Daniel J. (Daniel Joseph), 1914—   .
  The landmark history of the American people.
  Includes bibliographies and indexes.
  Contents: v. 1. From Plymouth to Appomattox—
v. 2. From Appomattox to the moon.
  1. United States—History—Juvenile literature.
[1. United States—History]   I. Boorstin, Ruth Frankel.
II. Title.
E178.1.B717   1987 973 87-9603
ISBN: 0-394-89120-1 (set);
   0-394-99118-4 (lib. bdg. : v. 1);
   0-394-99119-2 (lib. bdg. : v. 2)

Manufactured in the United States of America 1 2 3 4 5 6 7 8 9 0

*Dedicated with love
to our grandchildren,
Julia, Eric, Adam, and Ariel*

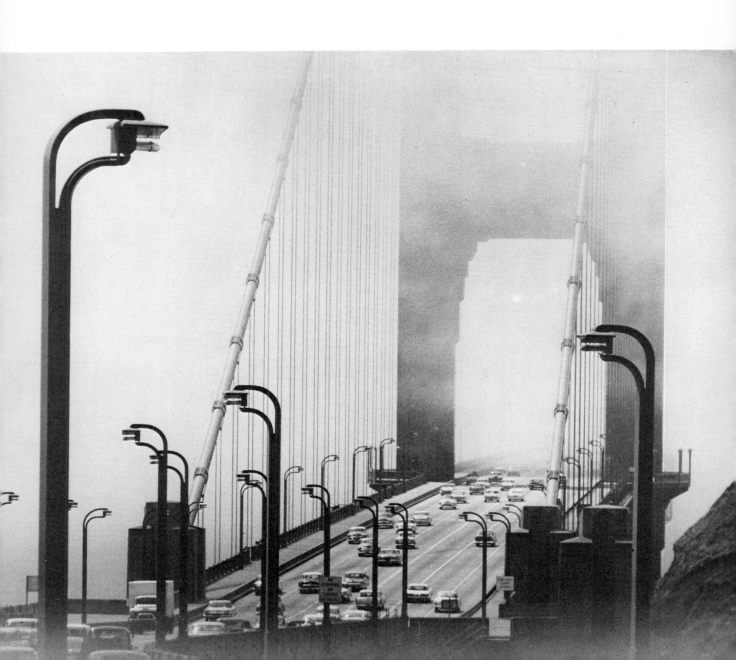

CONTENTS

Prologue: A World Transformed

Part One: The Go-Getters

Part Two: People on the Move

Part Three: Bringing People Together

Part Four: Champions for the People

Part Five: To This Whole World—and Beyond

PROLOGUE
A World Transformed

For the American people, everyday life changed in the century following the Civil War more than the life of earthlings had changed in the thousand years before.

As millions from everywhere became Americans, they invented a new Way of Life. And they gave a new meaning to almost everything.

Americans, for example, changed the meaning of day-and-night. Indoors, after sundown, could now be brighter than during the day.

Americans changed the meaning of the seasons. Wherever they lived, with central heating and air conditioning, they could be warm in winter and cool in summer. Foods of all seasons could be eaten any time. The United States became the land of strawberries in winter.

Americans changed the meaning of country-and-city. Every day the farmer, like the city man, could read his city newspaper. He wore city-made clothes and he bought city-made furniture in the latest styles—delivered right to his door.

Americans changed the meaning of distance. Faraway events were heard and seen in everybody's living room. Now millions could afford to go out by jet plane to Paris or Rome or Tokyo and see the world for themselves.

Americans even changed the meaning of the earth. Ever since the beginning of history this had been a lonely planet. The heavens were where living men could never go. Now, once again, Americans accomplished the "impossible." They walked on the moon and planned trips to Mars and beyond.

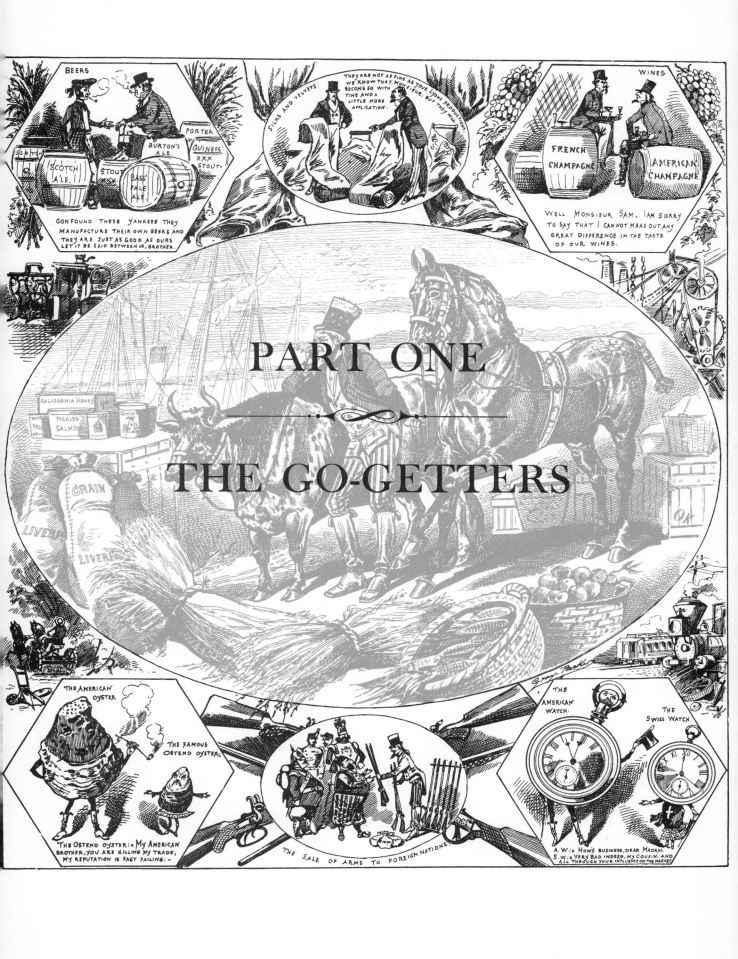

PART ONE

THE GO-GETTERS

THE GO-GETTERS

By the time of the Civil War, Americans had only begun to discover America. The land was still half-explored. The highest mountains were still unclimbed and the swiftest rivers still unmapped. Nobody had yet reached the top of Long's Peak or Mount Whitney. The Colorado River, which began somewhere high in the Rockies, had not been traced in its dangerous meanders. The shores of the Great Lakes were still a mystery. The bayous of Louisiana and the everglades of Florida seemed dark and threatening.

The Gold Rush to California in 1849 was only a first finding of the treasures in mountain streams and deep under the earth. America was full of secret resources.

A new kind of American, the Go-Getter, helped discover these treasures. Just as the nation was founded by people with assorted dreams and hopes, so a new American Way of Life was invented by a wide assortment of Go-Getters.

Some were outdoor men riding the range, leading thousands of cattle on new trails. Some were adventuring miners, risking fortunes to drill deep in search of mysterious new minerals. Some were businessmen—new-style storekeepers finding ways to make the whole nation their customers. Some were engineers and inventors, anxious to build bigger engines than the world had

ever seen, and machines which could turn out things by the millions.

E Pluribus Unum was the Latin motto of the young nation. It meant "one made from many." The Go-Getters were experts at bringing people together. Just as earlier Americans had organized thirteen new colonies and a new nation, so now the Go-Getters brought later Americans together in their cattle-trains and oil companies and department stores, and in thousands of other new enterprises. The new American Way of Life was designed for everybody.

America would be not merely a democracy of people but also a democracy of things. It would be a long time —maybe forever—before no one was poor. But after the Civil War it became easier for more and more Americans to share the good things of life. The Go-Getters, without even intending it, were bringing the whole nation together.

Some of the Go-Getters were more honest than others. Some made their fortunes by new ideas, by hard work, by being clever. Some were simply lucky. All prospered from the continent's hidden wealth.

The Go-Getters were not satisfied with the slow pace of the Old World. They wanted to see things happen fast. And by the early years of the twentieth century they had helped transform American life.

CHAPTER 1

Cattlemen and Cowboys

About the time of the Civil War, the Western cattle trade became big business. The men who made money from it were as different as possible from the European peasant who kept his few cattle at night in the room where he slept. The peasant could keep only a few because his house was small, and he had to feed his animals by hand in winter.

The Western cattleman numbered his stock by the thousands. He did not have to give them a roof, for Western cattle were tough enough to look after themselves on the range. And on the great Western plains there grew "buffalo grass" which survived drought and provided free food right on the ground throughout the winter.

Western cattlemen were bold and adventurous, willing to take big risks in a wild country. In the Old World, the expression "Man on Horseback" meant a military man, a commander of troops which he might use to take over the government. But in the American West the "Man on Horseback" was a cowboy. And the Western cattleman was a Go-Getter on horseback.

One of the first and most energetic of these was John Wesley Iliff. His father, an Ohio farmer, had offered him $7,500 if he would settle nearby on a respectable Ohio farm. But in 1856 he heard of the fortunes farther west. Young Iliff, who wanted adventure, told his father he would be satisfied with $500 if he could use it to make his start out there.

A cowboy and his horse, working together, could rescue a Longhorn from the mud. In the days before the camera could take action pictures, the artist Frederic Remington became famous for his drawings and sculptures of men and horses in action.

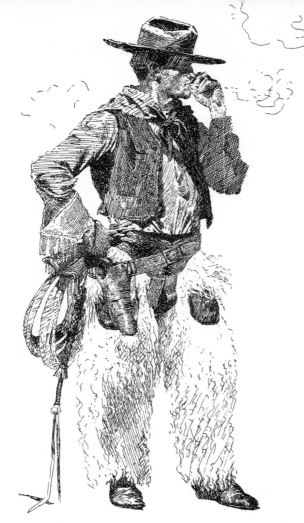

A cowboy in his "uniform," fully equipped with lariat and six-shooter. A drawing by C. M. Russell, who was born in St. Louis and went to Montana as a cowboy at the age of sixteen.

Iliff did not find gold in the Colorado mountain streams. But he did find it in the cattle that came there with Americans pushing westward.

During the Colorado Gold Rush the thousands of covered wagons that arrived near Denver—just before the climb into the mountains—wanted to lighten their load. They shed most of their belongings, so they could go ahead on foot or with a few pack mules. They were glad to sell to Iliff the footsore oxen that had pulled their wagons across the plains.

He fed these cattle free on the open range that belonged to everybody. He began breeding a herd. When the animals were fattened, Iliff sold them either to butchers in the mining camps or to travelers returning east who needed oxen to pull their wagons.

Of course there were risks, especially from winter weather and from Indian attack. Iliff became friendly with a man named Gerry, a pioneer fur trader who had married the twin daughters of Chief Swift Bird of the Oglalas. Using the information from his wives, Gerry warned Iliff whenever the Indians were about to attack, so that Iliff's cattle could be moved to a safe place.

For a Go-Getter like Iliff, even the Indians became a source of profit. He made a small fortune supplying meat to the remote western outposts where troops had been sent to fight the Indians. At the same time he sold beef to government officials so they could feed the Indians on reservations.

When railroads—promoted by Eastern Go-Getters—pushed West, they opened another new market. Now Western beef could be shipped to the growing Eastern cities. At the same time, hard-working crews building the railroads had to be well fed, and what they most wanted was meat. Iliff agreed to deliver cattle by the thousands to the Union Pacific Railroad construction gangs and to the troops guarding them against the Indians.

This was easier said than done. He had to find more beef than anyone had ever yet seen in one place. And he had to bring it to the middle of nowhere, where railroads were still to be built.

Iliff was helped by still another brand of Go-Getter, the Western Trailblazer.

One of the oldest of them was a remarkable man with the unlikely name of Charles Goodnight. His family had taken him to Texas when he was a boy of nine. In 1868 Goodnight agreed to deliver to Iliff's camp near Cheyenne, Wyoming, forty thousand dollars worth of cattle from Texas.

When Americans had come to Texas in the 1830's thousands of Longhorn cattle were running wild. These were the great-great-grandchildren of a few animals brought over by Spanish explorers in the sixteenth century. To get your herd all you had to do was to hunt and capture. Hunting wild cattle became a prosperous business. But it was not child's play. For the wild cattle of Texas, one hunter reported, were "fifty times more dangerous than the fiercest buffalo." Armed with sharp horns that they were not afraid to use, these bold beasts could not be managed by men on foot. They made the Texas cowboy get onto his horse, and they kept him there.

It was a thousand miles from the cattle country of central Texas to Goodnight's promised delivery point in southeastern Wyoming. You had to cross some of the driest, most unfriendly land in the whole continent—what maps before the Civil War called the "Great American Desert." In all that country there was no town worthy of the name. There was not even any trail. To deliver his cattle, Goodnight had to find his own way.

It would be a risky business. But it seemed worth trying, when a steer bought for four dollars in Texas sold for forty dollars in Wyoming. Multiply that by three thousand (the number of cattle Goodnight hoped to take on each

trip) and it added up to a handsome profit.

The Texas Longhorns were well equipped for long trips. Their sense of smell, the cowboys said, was as much superior to that of an ordinary Eastern cow as the bloodhound's was to that of a parlor poodle. Where water was hard to find, the Longhorn's nose for water could make the difference between life and death. Cowboys who let the leading steer act as guide sometimes found remote lakes they had never seen before.

The real problem was how to keep all those three thousand cattle together and moving at just the right speed. If they were allowed to stop or dawdle, they might never reach their goal. But if they were allowed to trot they might get out of control or exercise off the weight that was worth money in Wyoming.

Stationed at the front, or "point," of the herd were two of the most experienced men, called "pointers." They navigated for the whole herd, following the course set ahead by the foreman. Bringing up the rear were three steady cowboys whose job it was to look out for the weaker cattle—the "drags." To prevent the herd from straggling out for miles, the whole party moved no faster than the weakest "drags" at the rear. The rest of the cowboy crew were stationed along the sides to keep the herd compact and all the same width.

Every herd of cattle on the trail needed its own herd of horses to give the cowboys fresh mounts for their tricky jobs. To feed the men you needed a chuck wagon which the cook would drive fast ahead of everybody else. His job was to have food ready as soon as the weary cowboys arrived.

Communication between the front and rear of the herd was difficult. The rumbling of hoofs smothered words. The cowboys, then, borrowed a clever system of hand signals from the Plains Indians.

Apart from Indians, the greatest peril was a stampede. Suddenly at night the three thousand cattle, which a moment before had been quietly dozing, might rouse into a thundering mass. To stop a stampede, experienced cowboys made a circle to keep the animals churning and circling, always round to the right. Then by tightening their circle they squeezed the stampeding cattle tighter and tighter together till they had no place to run. The milling herd was forced to halt.

If the encircling tactic failed, all was lost. The stampede would get out of control. Then the cattle would fly out like sparks into the night, and they might never be seen again.

The cowboys had their own trail-tested ways of preventing stampedes by soothing the jumpy Longhorns. At night the men guarding the herd would sing and whistle while they made their rounds. The purpose of this "serenading," the veteran cowboy Andy Adams explained, was "so that the sleeping herd may know that a friend and not an enemy is keeping vigil over their dreams."

The cowboys called these songs "hymns" because they were sung to tunes which the cowboys remembered from their mothers' songs in childhood or from church services. But the words the cowboys sang usually were not church-words. What they sang might have shocked or startled the cattle if they could have understood. For these cowboy songs told the exploits of famous horse races and notorious criminals, or they repeated advertising texts from coffee cans or whiskey bottles, or they recited profanity sprinkled between nonsense syllables.

At the end of the Long Drive came the "Cow Town," which was as American as the cowboy. It was simply another smaller kind of "instant city" like those already dotted over the West. The Cow Town was where cowboys delivered their herd to the cattle dealers and the railroads. There, after long lonely weeks on the trail, cowboys enjoyed the company of strangers, bought liquor, and gambled away their money.

Go-Getting cattlemen made these instant towns prosper. One cattleman, Joseph G. McCoy, picked a place along the Kansas Pacific Railroad. In 1867, when he first made his plans for Abilene, it was (as he later recalled) "a very small, dead place, consisting of about one dozen log huts, low, small rude affairs, four-fifths of which were covered with turf roofing; indeed, but one shingle roof could be seen in the whole city. The business of the burg was conducted in two small rooms, mere log huts, and of course the inevitable saloon, also in a log hut, was to be found."

Within sixty days the place was transformed. As if by magic, Abilene had a shipping yard for three thousand head of cattle, besides a large pair of Fairbanks Scales to weigh the cattle on, a big barn and office, and of course "a good three-story hotel." The idea was to ship out thousands of cattle from Abilene to Chicago and other big cities.

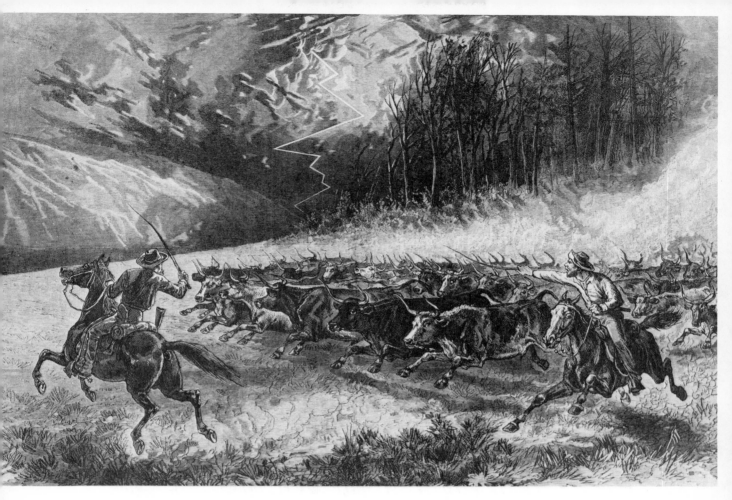

Texas cowboys trying to end a stampede of Longhorns frightened by thunder (1881). In the margin of this and the facing page are cattle brands.

On September 5, 1867, when the first shipment (twenty carloads of cattle) left Abilene, the Chicago stockmen had come there to celebrate. In tents specially erected for the occasion, they feasted, drank wine, sang, and listened to bombastic speeches. Before the end of that year Abilene shipped out 35,000 head of cattle.

The Go-Getting McCoy had paid only $2,400 for the whole Abilene townsite. Before long he was offered more than that for a single city lot. He received from the Kansas Pacific Railroad a commission of one-eighth of the freight charges on every carload of cattle. Before the end of the second year,

the railroad company owed McCoy a quarter of a million dollars.

Soon there were other prospering Cow Towns sprinkled all over the West: Schuyler and Fort Kearney and North Platte and Ogallala and Sydney in Nebraska, Pine Bluffs and Rock River and Rock Creek and Laramie and Hillsdale and Cheyenne in Wyoming, Miles City and Glendive and Helena in Montana.

The Cow Towns did not suffer from modesty. More than one boasted that she was the "Queen of Cow Towns." But Dodge City, in Kansas, and others competed for the title of the "Wickedest Little City in America."

While town-building was profitable

and exciting, prosperous cattlemen still fondly remembered their days on the trail. "All in all, my years on the Trail," Charles Goodnight remembered on his ninety-third birthday, "were the happiest I ever lived. There were many hardships and dangers, of course, that called on all a man had of endurance and bravery; but when all went well there was no other life so pleasant. Most of the time we were solitary adventurers in a great land as fresh and new as a spring morning, and were free and full of the zest of darers."

Western cattlemen and cowboys were among the first and bravest of the Go-Getters. They tried the impossible and succeeded in making something from nothing. They captured wild cattle that belonged to nobody. Then they fed the cattle on buffalo grass that nobody even imagined could be food, and grazed them on range that belonged to everybody and nobody. And they finally transported the cattle on their very own feet for thousands of miles to places where they could become beef.

Who could have imagined that the "Great American Desert" would become the greatest beef factory in the world?

CHAPTER 2

Rock Oil to Light up the World ⌘

The Indians had taught the early settlers how to raise new crops like corn and tobacco, and how to find new medicines in the forests and underground. One of these medicines was a curious black oily substance that the Seneca Indians of upstate New York saw floating on ponds. They laid their blankets on top of ponds where the oil was floating, until the blankets had soaked up the oil. Then they wrung the oil out of the blankets into a bowl. They treasured the oil as an ointment, which they thought would cure all sorts of ills.

Before the end of the eighteenth century, the American colonists had learned to use this oily medicine, and it became an item of trade with the Indians. It was called "Seneca Oil" after the Indians who sold it.

Down in Kentucky in the 1830's, when a salt well was ruined by the oil which bubbled into it, the owners discovered that the black stuff was really Seneca Oil. They stopped selling salt, and instead went into the medicine business. They put the stuff in bottles, called it "Rock Oil" or "American Oil," and sold it as a remedy for rheumatism and nearly everything else. They sold these bottles by the hundreds of thousands.

Other salt manufacturers, who found this black stuff ruining their salt wells, also went into the medicine business. One of them, Samuel Kier, put out leaflets boasting of his Rock Oil's "wonderful curative powers" for rheumatism, chronic cough, ague, toothache, corns, neuralgia, piles, indigestion, and liver ailments. He printed advertisements in

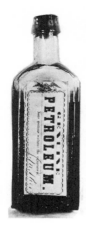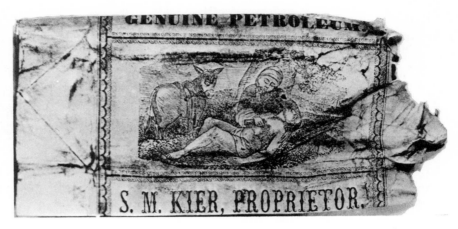

A bottle and wrapper for Kier's "Genuine Petroleum" which he sold as medicine. The scene from the Biblical story of the Good Samaritan (who helped his suffering fellowmen) was supposed to show what Kier's Genuine Petroleum could do for you.

the shape and size of paper money. These featured the number 400—the number of feet below the earth's surface from which the oil was drawn—as if every drop of the oil was worth its weight in gold.

To attract customers, Kier sent salesmen out over the countryside in circus wagons. They played music, sang songs, displayed animal freaks, and used every possible means to attract attention and sell their magic fluid. Within a few years, Kier had disposed of a quarter-million half-pints of his wonderful Rock Oil at a dollar a bottle.

But Kier's wells gushed out even more than his clever salesmen could sell. What could be done with the rest?

About the same time that Kier and other salt manufacturers found themselves flooded with Rock Oil, there was a growing need for some inexpensive kind of lighting. In those days before electric lights, home lighting came from tallow candles and oil lamps, not much different from the ones used in ancient Rome. A wick made from a twisted rag burned in a dish of fish oil or animal oil or vegetable oil. That weak flickering light of burning oil was all that people had to read and play and work by after sundown.

But oil was expensive. So most homes were usually not lit at night. And people went to bed when the sun set.

In the years before the Civil War, American cities were growing. Homes built close together lacked sunlight. At the same time city people wanted to get together more in the evenings. New factories and railroads also required more and better artificial light. As early as 1830, gas (manufactured from coal) was used to light a few streets and public buildings in Baltimore, Boston, and New York. But gas was not yet used in houses.

Some help came when Isaiah Jennings invented a new lamp oil, which he called "camphene." He used American turpentine—the yellowish sticky fluid that seeped out of holes made in certain pine trees. When this sticky stuff was heated and the product was mixed with alcohol, it made an excellent lighting fluid. It was much cheaper than the other lighting oils, and when it burned it gave a brighter, whiter light. But it had an unpleasant smell and it gave off explosive gases.

Nearly everybody agreed that American homes would not be bright at night until there was a safer inexpensive lamp oil. Where could it be found?

A hint of the great new source came when a clever Canadian doctor, Abraham Gesner, in 1850 found a way to make lighting oil from coal. He called his new product "kerosene" (from *keros,* the Greek word for wax). It had an unpleasant odor, but it could be used without danger of explosion. Doctors who had warned against the "horrors of burning fluid" now urged people to fill their lamps with the safe new "coal oil." Before the end of 1859 nearly two million coal-oil lamps had been sold. But since there were about thirty million people in the United States, the country was still a long way from the goal of "a lamp in every room."

Dr. Gesner had showed that lamp oil could be made not only from plants and animals but also from coal, which was a *mineral.* Was it possible that the new mineral product, Rock Oil, could also be used for lighting?

About this time a New Haven businessman, George H. Bissell, formed the Pennsylvania Rock Oil Company to buy lands in western Pennsylvania, where Rock Oil was found floating on ponds. He hired a famous Yale professor of chemistry, Benjamin Silliman, Jr., and agreed to pay him $500 to find out what the Rock Oil was good for.

Professor Silliman's report opened a new age for Rock Oil. He discovered that Rock Oil—by now also called "petroleum" from *petrus,* Latin for rock, and *oleum* for oil—would make an excellent oil for lamps. His process was cheap. He simply distilled the Rock Oil —that is, heated it and collected the gas that came off. When the gas cooled down into a liquid, it was lamp oil. This, he discovered, was a new way to make kerosene that was just as good as kerosene made from coal. Kerosene made from Rock Oil also gave a bright, white light, with almost no smoke, and would not explode.

The Rock Oil itself also had wonderful lubricating powers. It would keep the wheels and gears of machines from wearing out and would make them run quiet and smooth.

Rock Oil, with these valuable uses, could surely be sold in large quantities. But until then the only known way to collect it was to find it on the surface or accidentally in a salt well. Sometimes people would dig a shallow ditch to increase the flow where it was already bubbling up.

Then one day, the story goes, Bissell saw one of Kier's advertisements. It was the sheet printed to look like paper money that featured the numeral 400. "A.D. 1848," it read. "Discovered in *boring* for salt water . . . about FOUR HUNDRED FEET below the Earth's surface." Boring! If oil could be obtained when you bored for salt water, why not simply bore for the oil?

"Oil coming out of the ground!" exclaimed a friend. "Pumping oil out of the earth the way you pump water? Nonsense! You're crazy."

But Bissell and the other Go-Getting businessmen in the Pennsylvania Rock Oil Company decided to try. From New Haven they sent Edwin L. Drake out to the oil fields. One reason they picked him was that since he had been a railroad conductor, he still had a free pass on the railroads. He could go out to western Pennsylvania without it costing anybody anything.

When Drake reached Titusville, the town closest to the biggest finds of surface oil, he decided to drill for oil. But at first he could not find a driller willing to do the job. The drillers all thought that boring for oil was silly.

Then, luckily, he found an old salt driller, "Uncle Billy" Smith, who was also a skilled blacksmith and knew how to make drilling tools. Uncle Billy began drilling in June 1859. But after he reached bedrock thirty-two feet down, Uncle Billy could drill no more than three feet each day. Drake thought that to find oil they might have to drill a thousand feet.

On Saturday, August 29, 1859, the hole still reached down less than seventy feet. When Drake and Smith came back on Monday morning the hole was full of oily black stuff.

"What's that?" Drake asked.

Uncle Billy replied, "That's your fortune!"

Soon there was an oil mania. Everybody wanted to get rich from oil. The map of northwestern Pennsylvania was

---

The first oil well, Titusville, Pennsylvania. The pointed wooden structure held a derrick for pulling up the drilling tools.

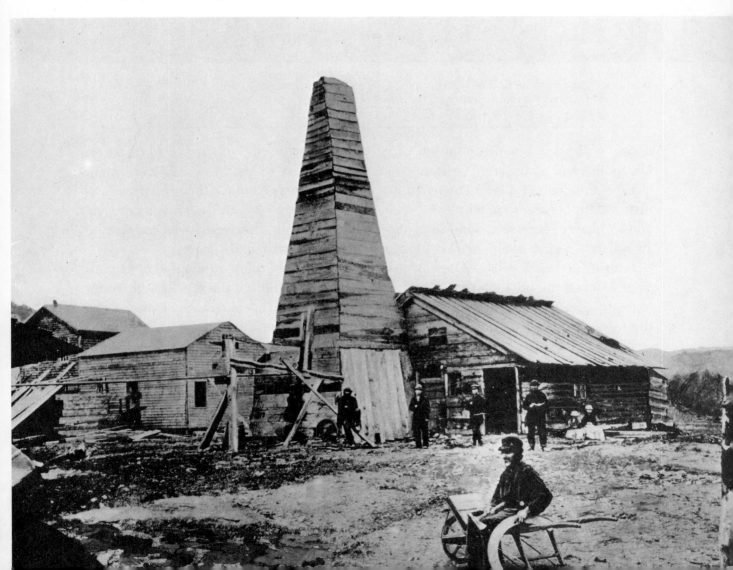

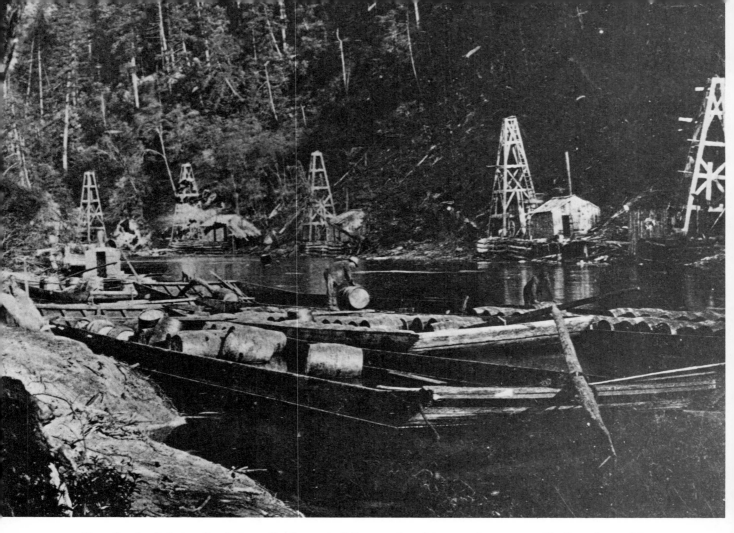

Barrels of oil being loaded on flat-bottomed barges for shipment by water. Shallow boats like these had to navigate the torrents of the Pond Freshet.

dotted with such new names as Oil City, Oleopolis, and Petroleum Center.

Like the instant Cow Towns, these instant Oil Towns boomed. They were good places for salesmen and for swindlers. Some well drillers began "doctoring" their wells. They would pour buckets of oil into their holes at night to trick buyers who came to look the next morning.

When Drake's first well began to gush oil, the oil was put into old whisky barrels, washtubs, and any other container in sight. But since the oil was inflammable, it was dangerous to store in the open. The oil was usually sealed in barrels before being loaded on wagons to

be hauled to the railroad or to docks on the nearest rivers. As roads were poor, the best way to move the oil barrels was on flatboats. But in the streams nearest the oil wells the water was too low to float the loaded flatboats.

The clever oilmen then invented their own way of filling the creeks with water to float their oil barrels to market. The name for their system was the "Pond Freshet" ("freshet" meant a sudden flood of water). For example, on Oil Creek, each oilman made his own artificial pond held back by a dam. Then, at a signal, each quickly opened the dam of his own artificial pond. This suddenly flooded the creek.

Only a few minutes before, the creek was much too shallow for the big flatboats. Now this man-made wave floated down the stream. All the flatboats along the way were alert and ready. At just the right moment, each oilman pushed his loaded boats into the flood, which carried them quickly down to the railroad center.

Just after a successful Pond Freshet, as an oilman recalled, the Oil Town was very much like a Cow Town after the arrival of a large Texas herd.

Shippers are busy paying off the boatmen, the citizens of the creek are laying in a stock of the necessaries of life, and all is bustle and business. You see men dripping with the oleaginous product. Our hotels are filled to repletion with these greasy men who are supplying light for the world. Oil is the only topic of conversation, and the air is redolent with its sweet perfumery.

The great success in oil—one of the most spectacular of all American Go-Getters—was John D. Rockefeller. He was not an inventor or an explorer. He was an organizer. His talent was like that of Charles Goodnight, who had collected thousands of cattle for the Long Drive.

Young Rockefeller went to school in Cleveland, but he never went to college. His father, who traveled through the West selling patent medicines, left young John in charge of the family long before he was grown. John D. Rockefeller was ambitious. "I did not guess what it would be," he recalled. "But I was after something big."

Even as a boy he was systematic and

well organized. While still struggling to make his way, he gave one-tenth of his income to the Baptist Church and to charities. But when it came to organizing his oil business, he did not always use Sunday School methods.

Cleveland was a good place to organize "something big" in the oil business. At the receiving end of two railroads which came from the western Pennsylvania oil fields, Cleveland was also on a lake big enough for large ships. Rockefeller determined to make Cleveland the center of the oil business, and from there to command the biggest oil company in the world. Beginning with a small sum he had made in a grain-trading business, in 1865 he bought his first Cleveland refinery. There crude oil from the fields was made into kerosene for lighting and oil for lubricating. Then he bought up the smaller refineries in Cleveland and many oil wells in western Pennsylvania.

As other oilmen went out of business, the railroads needed Rockefeller's freight more than ever. He was clever at making the two Cleveland railroads compete for his business. He bargained with one railroad by threatening to give all his business to the other. And he finally forced them to charge him lower prices than they charged anybody else. He did this by secret arrangements so other customers of the railroad could not know for sure what was happening. He pretended to pay the same prices the railroad charged everybody else. Then the railroads secretly gave him back a "rebate"—a refund on each barrel of his oil that they had hauled.

After he perfected these tactics he went to the small refiners in other parts of the country and asked them to sell to him. "If you don't sell your property," he would say, "it will be valueless, because we have advantages with the railroads."

"But we don't want to sell," they would say.

"You can never make money," Rockefeller would reply. "You can't compete with the Standard Oil Company. We have all the large refineries now. If you refuse to sell, it will end in your being crushed."

He would then offer a price far below what the owners thought their refineries were worth. But they usually sold because they realized that Rockefeller could drive them out of business.

When it became cheaper to pump oil through pipelines instead of carrying it in barrels, Rockefeller organized his own pipeline. Then, when a different kind of oil was found in Ohio, Rockefeller hired chemical engineers to invent new kinds of refineries.

Rockefeller's Go-Getting business reached around the world. To the Chinese, his Standard Oil Company sold inexpensive lamps by the millions—and then sold the oil to fill them. Before long, people on all continents were

A magazine cartoon published two years after Drake's first oil strike. Whales (whose blubber had been an important source of lamp oil) had good reason to celebrate the discovery of "mineral oil." As the new oil industry prospered, the whaling industry declined.

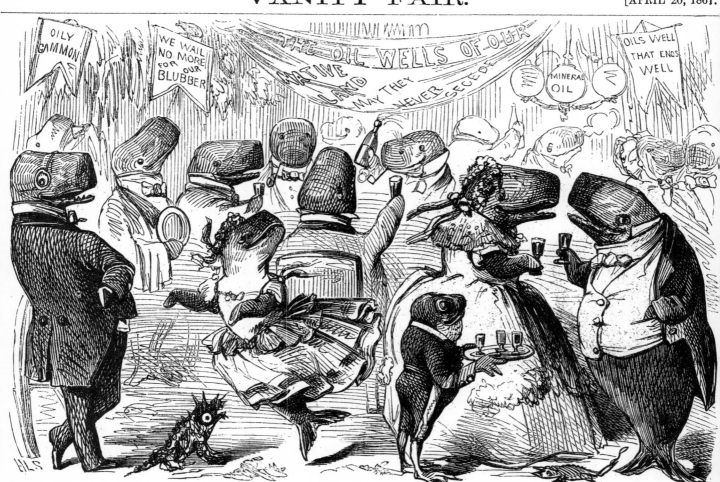

GRAND BALL GIVEN BY THE WHALES IN HONOR OF THE DISCOVERY OF THE OIL WELLS IN PENNSYLVANIA.

using lamp oil from American wells. Between the Civil War and 1900 over half the American output went abroad. In those years the giant Go-Getter, John D. Rockefeller, helped light up the world. Now Americans could afford a lamp in every room.

In the twentieth century, Rockefeller's business would grow in ways even he had never imagined. After the automobile was invented, petroleum was refined into gasoline—and Rock Oil made it possible for a whole nation to move on wheels.

CHAPTER 3

City Goods for Country Customers

During the colonial years, an American farmer made for himself almost everything he needed. He built his own house (with the help of a few neighbors) and he made his own furniture. His wife and daughters spun the thread, wove the cloth, and then made the family's clothes. The pots and pans and metal tools which he could not make for himself he would buy from a peddler. But he bought very few things. There were not many ready-made things for him to buy.

Then, in the years before the Civil War, American know-how built on ideas from Europe's Industrial Revolution to develop a new kind of manufacturing. Lots of new things were produced in vast new quantities. The new American System of Manufacture, which Eli Whitney and Samuel Colt had organized to make guns and revolvers, also turned out clocks and locks, and countless other items—both better and cheaper. Now farmers could afford to buy them.

But when a farmer wanted any of these things he had to go to the nearest village and visit the general store.

Children loved the place because it was where you could buy candy and toys. Since the storekeeper kept a good fire in his stove, the store was where you could stay warm in winter. Year round it was where you could meet friends and exchange ideas.

But it was no place for bargains. The country storekeeper, who bought only a little bit of everything, could not command the best wholesale prices from the big-city manufacturers. Each item had to be hauled by wagon over bumpy backwoods roads. Things would get dusty and out-of-date before they could be sold.

Soon after the Civil War an energetic young salesman, who had covered the West selling goods to the owners of general stores, began to think of a new plan. His name was A. Montgomery Ward. He had done all sorts of things, from working in a barrel factory and in a brickyard to selling drygoods. Often in his travels he had heard farmers complain about the small choice of goods and the high prices.

Young Ward's idea was to sell goods

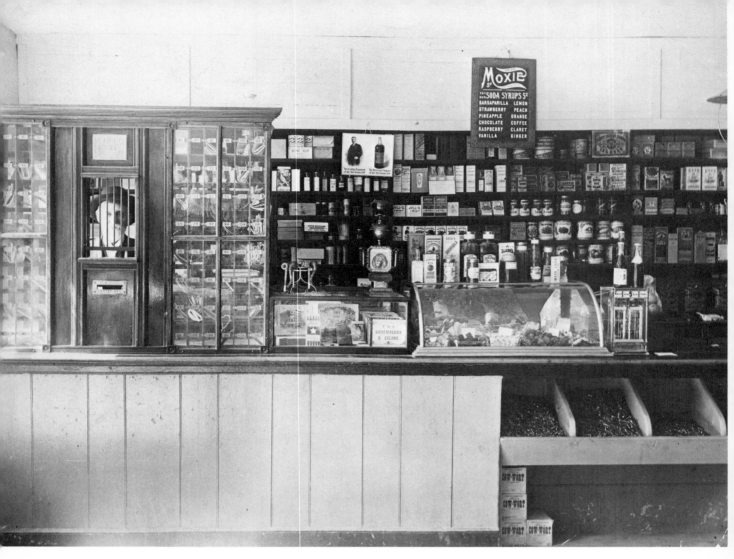

An old general store with the village post office. The storekeeper often doubled as postmaster.

in an entirely new way. Instead of the old general store which stocked only a few of each item, Ward imagined a mail-order store. The storekeeper would stay in the big city where it was easier to collect a large stock of all sorts of goods. He would send out to farmers lists of his goods with descriptions and pictures. The farmer would not need to come to the store because the store—in the form of a catalog—would go to the farmer. And the farmer would order by mail, picking out whatever he wanted from the catalog. Then the storekeeper would mail the farmer his goods.

If this new scheme worked, the store-keeper would be selling not only to the few customers in one particular village. He could sell to farmers all over America—to anyone within reach of a mail-box.

The possible customers of this new kind of store would not be just a few hundred, they might be millions! And then Ward could buy his goods from the manufacturer by the hundreds and thousands. The manufacturer could afford to give him a lower price.

For the customer, too, there were advantages. He had a much wider selection of goods. And he paid a lower price since the mail-order storekeeper, with so many more customers, could take a smaller profit on each item and yet would make more money in the long run.

Young Montgomery Ward had lost nearly all his savings in the Chicago fire of 1871, but in the very next year he managed to scrape together enough to make a start with his new idea. He put in $1,600 and a partner added $800. They rented a small room over a stable, and started modestly. Their single price-sheet listed the items for sale and told how to order. Within two years Ward was issuing a 72-page catalog with illustrations. By 1884 the catalog numbered 240 pages and listed nearly ten thousand items. Within another thirty years it was over a thousand pages and included every conceivable object for animals or men.

One way Ward rounded up customers was to get himself appointed the official supplier for the "Grange." This was one name for a large farmers' club, the Patrons of Husbandry, founded just after the Civil War. By 1875 its members numbered 750,000 and all these were likely customers. Ward offered Grange members a special discount. He stocked the official Granger hat and in his catalog printed recommendations from Grange officers. This encouraged other farmers to trust Ward's.

Trust was the most important thing for a mail-order store. If you bought in a general store you were buying from a storekeeper you knew. You could see the goods and handle them to satisfy yourself. But when you bought from a mail-order store you had to trust somebody you had never seen. You had to believe that the storekeeper would really send you the exact thing described in the catalog.

Ward was a spectacular success. The first secret of his success was not a secret at all, but simply to be honest, give good value, and always let the customer be the judge. On everything Ward's gave an ironclad guarantee. "Satisfaction or your money back!" If a customer did not like the goods when they arrived, he could always return them. If something arrived damaged, he could send it back to Ward's to be replaced. The company paid the postage both ways.

Of course there had to be trust on the company's side, too. The company had to be willing to cash the customer's checks, to believe his complaints, and to replace damaged goods without a lot of investigating. Ward was willing to do this, and to take the risks.

The catalog showed pictures of Ward himself, of the other executives, and of the men in charge of the different departments. This was to convince the customer that he was dealing with real people. Some customers wrote in to say how pleased they were to deal with such "fine looking men." Some even named babies after Ward, and said he would be an inspiration to their children.

Ward saw that their letters were promptly answered—even if they were not ordering goods but only asking advice. One customer asked how to find a baby to adopt. Others tried to sell Ward their secondhand furniture or their livestock. Parents asked help in finding boys who had run away from home. They wanted to know how to handle disobedient children. Some wrote him simply because they were lonely and had nobody else to write to.

SHOPPING by CATALOG

From the Montgomery Ward catalog, 1895. At that time both wages and prices were much lower than today. A typical workingman earned about $500 a year.

Children's Suits.

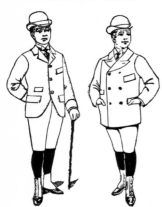

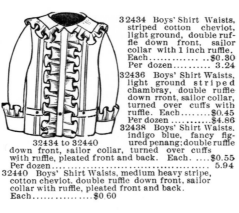

32434 Boys' Shirt Waists, striped cotton cheviot, light ground, double ruffle down front, sailor collar with 1 inch ruffle. Each................ $0.30
Per dozen......... 3.24

32436 Boys' Shirt Waists, light ground striped chambray, double ruffle down rront, sailor collar, turned over cuffs with ruffle. Each........ $0.45
Per dozen.......... $4.86

32438 Boys' Shirt Waists, indigo blue, fancy figured penang; double ruffle down front, sailor collar, turned over cuffs with ruffle, pleated front and back. Each.... $0.55
Per dozen............................. 5.94

32434 to 32440

32440 Boys' Shirt Waists, medium heavy stripe, cotton cheviot, double ruffle down front, sailor collar with ruffle, pleated front and back. Each................ $0.60

Spinning Wheels.

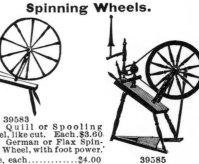

39583
39583 Quill or Spooling Wheel, like cut. Each. $3.60
39585 German or Flax Spinning Wheel, with foot power. Price, each............ $4.00

39585

Bathing Suits.

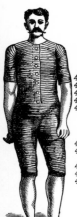

ONE-PIECE SUITS.

Knit goods, very elastic, not cloth goods. Button well down to the front, making them easy to get on or off. Extra, by mail, 5 to 10 cents. Give chest measure.

Each.
49150 Cotton, striped........ $0.75
49151 Cotton, navy blue....... 1.50
49152 Cotton, fast black....... 1.50
49153 Cotton, navy with stripes 1.25
49154 Worsted, navy blue.... 2.90

TWO-PIECE SUITS.

Consisting of quarter sleeve shirts and knee pants. Per Suit.
49155 Cotton, striped........ $1.00
49156 Cotton, navy, with stripes................ 1.50
49157 Worsted, navy blue..... 2.40
49158 Worsted, black........ 2.40
49160 Best Worsted, striped. 5.25
Extra, by mail, 15 to 20 cents.

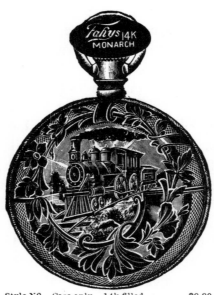

Style N2. Case only. 14k filled $8.80

36570 Child's Lawn Hat, extra shirred brim. Colors: Cardinal, white, pink or light blue. Each.. .... $0.45
Per dozen..... 5.00
36571 Child's Shirred Hat, made of Swiss embroidery shirred brim, trimmed all round with embroidered edging Each.......... $0.50
Per dozen..... 5.50

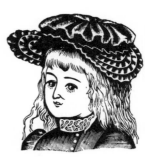

5704 Ladies' Newport Suit, same style as 5700, made of heavy all-wool storm serge, trimmed with two rows of folded satin rhadame on collar, cuffs and bottom of skirt. Colors: Black or navy blue only. A stylish and splendid wearing suit. Per suit................. $5.95

5705 Ladies' Newport Suit, same style as 5700, made of heavy English whip cord, trimmed in narrow folds of satin. Navy blue or black only. Very serviceable and elegant. Per suit. $7.50

5708 Ladies' Newport Suit, same style as 5700, made of fine all wool broadcloth, high finished; collar, cuffs and bottom of skirt trimmed with narrow fold of moire silk, very elegant. Colors: Black, brown, light or dark navy blue. Per suit... ..$8.50

5709 Ladies' Newport Suit, made of all wool cheviot serge in navy blue; new organ pipe skirt, double breasted jacket, double stitching around skirt and jacket, immense sleeves, made in first-class style. Persuit $8.75

5711 Ladies' Newport Suit, made of stylish tweed suiting, in light brown and white mixture. Very neat and serviceable, will not show dust or wear. Same style as 5709. Per suit.. ....$9.00

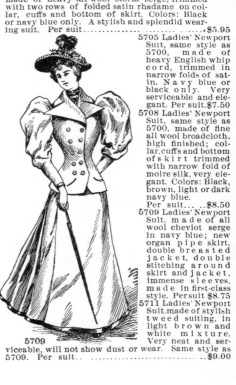

5709

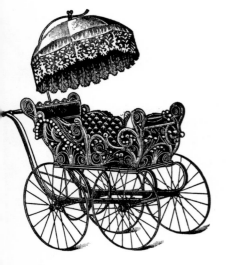

The Razor Toe.

Weight 15 ounces.

52034 This style shoe is becoming very popular on account of the long narrow toe, and patent tip, which has a tendency of giving the foot a very graceful appearance. The stock is a very soft dongola, with light flexible soles and medium but slightly concave; for a neat stylish dress boot, it has no equal and for the quality, compares favorably with many of the three dollar and a half grades now on the market. Sizes, 2½ to 7 widths, C, D, E and EE. Per pair.................... $2.50

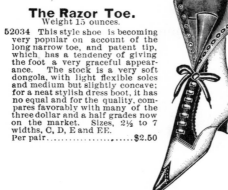

Just as the colonial tobacco planter might ask his London agent to send him whatever he needed, now the lonely farmer asked Ward's. One customer wrote:

Please send me a good wife. She must be a good housekeeper and able to do all household duty. She must be 5 feet 6 inches in height. Weight 150 lbs. Black hair and brown eyes, either fair or dark. I am 45 years old, six feet, am considered a good looking man. I have black hair and blue eyes. I own quite a lot of stock and land. I am tired of living a bachelor life and wish to lead a better life and more favorable.

Please write and let me know what you can do for me.

Ward's answered that it was not a good idea to select a wife by mail. "After you get the wife and you find that she needs some wearing apparel or household goods," Ward's added, "we feel sure we could serve both you and her to good advantage."

Some felt that Ward's would be disappointed at not hearing from them.

I suppose you wonder why we haven't ordered anything from you since the Fall. Well, the cow kicked my arm and broke it, and besides my wife was sick, and there was the doctor bill. But now, thank God, that is paid, and we are all well again, and we have a fine new baby boy, and please send plush bonnet number 29d-8077.

This friendly customer received a friendly reply. Ward's said they were sorry about his arm, glad that his wife was better, and sent congratulations on the son with hopes he would grow up to be a fine man. The order for the bonnet was acknowledged. Then, finally, Ward's asked whether the customer had noticed that there was an anti-cow-kicker for sale in the catalog.

It is not surprising that the mail-order store was a roaring success. Of course, in an age of Go-Getters, Ward was not the only man who tried his hand at building a mail-order store. One of the cleverest of these others was a young railroad station agent, Richard Sears. When a stray package of watches arrived at his station in North Redwood, Minnesota, the Chicago watch company offered to sell them to Sears at $12 apiece. Sears bought the watches and then sold them by mail to other agents along the line for $14 apiece.

Sears was in business. By selling watches to other station agents, Sears made five thousand dollars in six months, gave up his railroad job, moved to Chicago, and began selling other jewelry by mail. He found a partner in Alvah Curtis Roebuck, a watchmaker who ran a print shop where they could turn out their catalogs.

Sears was a clever man, and a near-genius at selling by mail. One of his schemes was a club plan for selling watches. He persuaded men to form a "Watch Club" of thirty-eight members. Every week each member would pay the Club one dollar. And every week when the members drew lots, one of them would win a watch. At the end of thirty-eight weeks, every club member had a watch. And they had bought all thirty-eight watches from Sears!

Of course, Sears could not have succeeded for long in the mail-order business unless he, like Ward, had been honest. He too gave good value for the money, and let customers return any goods they did not like.

But Sears was not afraid of a good joke. He knew that lonely farm families were glad to be entertained. In a rural weekly newspaper in 1889 he made an "Astonishing Offer." It was illustrated by a drawing of a sofa and two chairs, all of "fine, lustrous metal frames beautifully finished and decorated, and upholstered in the finest manner with beautiful plush." Sears offered to ship all this furniture "as an advertisement only" and "for a limited time only" for the ridiculously low price of ninety-five cents.

The customers who sent in their money really were astonished. They received a set of doll's furniture, made exactly according to the description. They had not noticed in the first line of the advertisement, in tiny print, the word "miniature."

There were lots of stories about how clever Sears was. One of his advertisements offered a "sewing machine" for a dollar. When the customer sent in his dollar, he promptly received by return mail a needle and thread. But Sears used such stunts only to attract attention.

Like Ward, Sears actually built his business on trust and on the personal touch. After the typewriter first came into general use, about 1900, some farmers still preferred to get a letter written by hand. Sears still went to the trouble of hiring people to write out handwritten letters for the company. Then farmers would not have their feelings hurt by receiving a letter that was "machine-made."

Sears knew that his catalog was both his shopwindow and his salesman. And he invented schemes for getting his catalogs around. He would send them in batches of twenty-four to people who had agreed to distribute them. But how could he be sure that the distributors would give their catalogs to the people most likely to be good customers? Sears kept a record of purchases by the new customers to whom each distributor had given his catalogs. The distributor then received a prize in proportion to the amount of money spent by his new customers. When, for example, total orders from his new customers amounted to $100, the distributor was awarded a bicycle, a sewing machine, or a stove.

Sears was constantly improving his catalog. He developed a new quick-drying ink, new systems of color printing, and thinner paper that would take color but was cheaper to mail. He found, for example, that four pages of

A four-passenger surrey advertised in 1897 by Sears Roebuck for $44. The buyer also needed a horse.

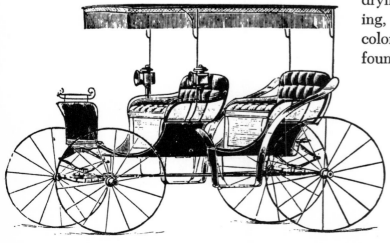

advertisements in color would sell as much of the same goods as twelve pages in black and white. His improvements were widely copied by other advertisers and by publishers of newspapers and magazines.

As Sears's catalog grew bigger and bigger it also reached more and more customers. He sent out two big catalogs a year, one in the spring and one in the fall. By 1904 each of these had a circulation of over one million. By the 1920's the figure was seven million. And it kept on rising.

As the mail-order catalog reached more and more people on remote farms, it became more and more important in their daily lives. While the farmer kept his Bible in the living room, he kept his Sears or Ward catalog in the kitchen. That was where he really lived.

There were all sorts of stories about how much faith people put in this big book. When one little boy was asked by his Sunday School teacher where the Ten Commandments came from, he said he supposed they came from Sears.

Just as Puritan boys and girls in colonial times had studied the New England Primer with its stories about God and the Devil, now Americans on farms studied the Sears catalog. In country schoolhouses, where there were few textbooks, teachers made good use of the catalog. They used it to teach reading and spelling. For arithmetic, pupils filled out orders and added up items. And they learned geography from the catalog's postal-zone maps.

In a school that had no other encyclopedia, pupils used a Ward or Sears catalog. It had a good index, it was

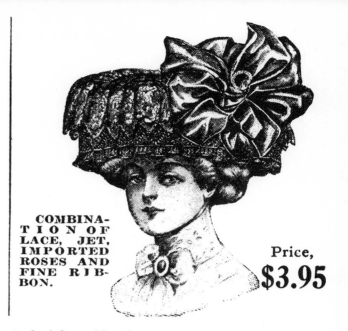

COMBINA-TION OF LACE, JET, IMPORTED ROSES AND FINE RIB-BON.

Price, $3.95

Ladies' hats, like this one advertised in the Sears catalog of 1910, offered the latest fashions for the farmer's wife—and for his daughter's paper dolls.

illustrated, it told you what things were good for, what they were made of, how long they would last, and even what they would cost. Mothers gave the catalogs to children to keep them occupied. When a new catalog arrived, the old one would be given to the girls, who cut it up for paper dolls.

Nothing did more than the new mail-order stores to change life on the farm —and to make life in America something new. Before the twentieth century most Americans still lived on the farm. Now that the American farmer could order from Ward's or Sears, his life became increasingly different from that of a European peasant. His view of the good things in the world was no longer confined to the shelves of the little village store. The up-to-date catalogs brought news of all kinds of new machines, new gadgets, and new fashions. Now American farmers could buy big-city goods at prices they could afford and from someone they could trust.

CHAPTER 4

One Price for Everybody!

Meanwhile other Go-Getters were inventing ways to attract the new millions of city customers. The big stores which now grew up in American cities were as different from the little shops in London's West End as the grand new American hotels were different from the modest Old World inns.

The new American hotels were People's Palaces. Anybody could meet his friends in the elegant lobby or, if he had the money, could entertain in a dining room with a crystal chandelier. The new department stores were Buyers' Palaces. And they, too, were democratic.

In London, nobody was admitted to the elegant shops unless he looked like a "gentleman" or a "lady." Unless the shopkeeper knew who you were, he would not let you in. You had to be a "person of quality" (as the upper classes were called) to see "goods of quality."

Department stores changed all this. Suddenly there were vast Buyers' Palaces, some large enough to fill a whole city block—specially designed to display goods of every shape, price, and description. Anybody could walk in. Now everybody could have a close look at elegant jewelry, clothing, and furniture of the kind once reserved for rich men's eyes.

Like many other American achieve-ments, this happened quickly. English ways of selling had not changed much in five hundred years. But this department-store revolution, which began shortly before the Civil War, changed the lives of American customers within a few decades.

Stewart's Cast Iron Palace, completed in 1862 in New York City, was one of the first big department stores. It was the product of two different kinds of Go-Getters—a businessman and an inventor.

A. T. Stewart, the merchant who built up the business, came to the United States from Ireland at the age of seventeen. He started by selling the Irish laces he had brought with him. But he soon branched out into all kinds of goods. He was a bold, ambitious businessman. And he decided to spend a fortune on an enormous building in an entirely new style. When Stewart decided to build his grand new store he picked an inventing genius who was sure to try something new.

James Bogardus, the man Stewart chose, had started as a watchmaker's apprentice in upstate New York. He first became famous by his new design for an eight-day clock. Then he invented all kinds of new machines—for making cotton thread, for mixing lead paint, for grinding sugar, for metering gas, and for engraving postage stamps. He patented a metal-cased pencil with a lead that was "forever pointed."

His most important new idea was to construct buildings of cast iron. Bogardus' own five-story factory, built in 1850, was probably the first cast-iron building in America. The building Bogardus built for Stewart overwhelmed everybody at the time by its height—eight stories. It quickly became famous as the biggest store in the world.

Bogardus used cast iron to make an impressive Buyers' Palace. The outside looked palatial and dignified. Graceful columns which held up thin beams made a neat repeating pattern like that found in Old World palaces. The molded iron panels between columns were painted to resemble stone. Fancy cast-iron shapes decorated the window frames.

On the ground floor the outside walls no longer needed to be thick—as they had to be when a tall building was made of stone. Now there could be larger windows on every floor. Slender iron columns held up the high ceiling of display rooms a city-block wide. The ground floor was made even more palatial by a grand central staircase and a great rotunda reaching up the full height of the building, topped by a glass roof down which the sunlight streamed. You could enjoy long indoor vistas of appealing merchandise—gloves, umbrellas, suitcases, coats, furniture, all kinds of things in all shapes and sizes and colors. All the people busy looking, buying, and admiring helped make a splendid spectacle.

Naturally the Go-Getting department-storekeepers wanted to display their

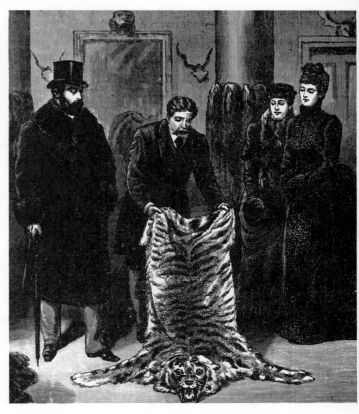

A London furrier giving personal attention to upper-class customers. Only select "gentlemen" and "ladies" would be shown the elegant stock.

goods to everybody who walked down the street. The thin cast-iron building frames made this easier, but it would not have been possible without a new kind of window. Before the age of the department store, glass was expensive. Windows had to be small. They were made to admit a little daylight or to look *out of*.

Then, not long before the Civil War, an Englishman invented an inexpensive way of rolling out glass in large sheets. These large sheets of glass now at last made possible the "show window." Americans invented this new expression for the new kind of window that was made to look *into*. Now the goods could advertise themselves.

In a store where thousands of customers were buying and hundreds of people were selling, other things had to

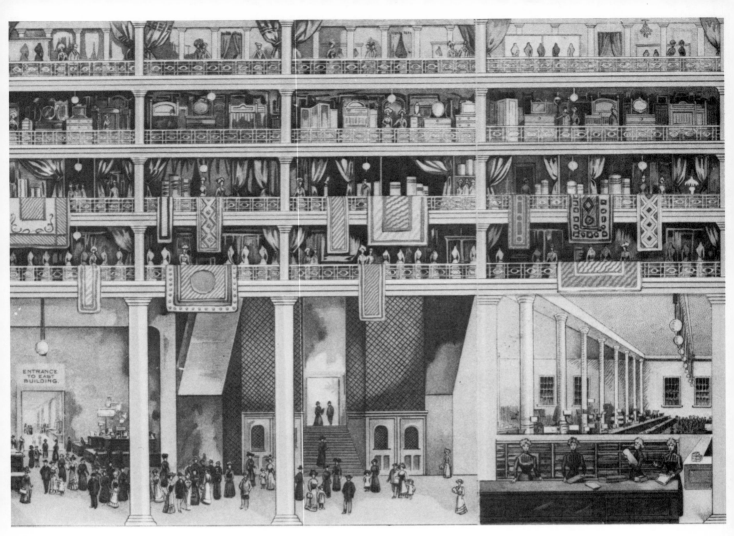

"Buyers' Palaces"—open to all—were soon found in the larger American cities. A cutaway view of Abraham & Straus department store in Brooklyn about 1892.

change. The old way of selling goods was for the storekeeper to bargain with each customer separately. He did not mark a price on the goods. Instead he asked from each customer the highest price he thought he could get. This price depended upon how rich he thought the customer was, on how much he thought the customer wanted the goods, and on how anxious he was to make a sale at that time. You could never be sure in advance how much you would have to pay. If you were a good bargainer, you could always get it for less. But bargaining took time. It did not suit Americans in a hurry.

The big department store brought the age of the "fixed price." A. T. Stewart's Cast Iron Palace employed two thousand people. Stewart himself could not know all his salesmen. How could he let them bargain for him? At Stewart's, then, everything carried a price tag. Everybody could see the price, and it was the same price for all.

When you went shopping now, you could no longer get your fun from bargaining. But you got better value, and there were new experiences to enjoy— like looking at all the elegant things you could not afford. The department store was a new, very American, and very democratic kind of entertainment where the admission was always free.

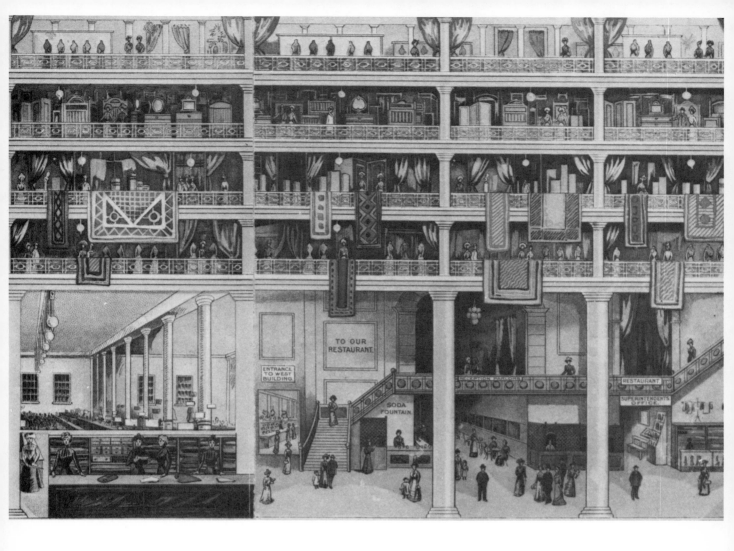

CHAPTER 5

A Democracy of Clothing

At the outbreak of the Civil War in 1861 the government had to provide hundreds of thousands of uniforms for men in the army. This was the first time in American history that so much clothing had been required all at once. During the American Revolution the colonial army had been relatively small, and most soldiers brought along their own clothing. In the later wars too—the War of 1812 and the Mexican War—

the armies were only a few thousand strong.

So in 1861 there was no large ready-made clothing industry. The simple explanation was that it had always been the custom for each family to make its own clothes. Just as the meals that American families eat today are usually made at home, so it used to be with coats, suits, socks, and nearly everything else a person wore. Only the rich few, who could afford to look elegant, would hire a skilled tailor.

In New England in the early nineteenth century there were a few shops that sold ready-made clothing. But these offered only the cheapest grades. In New Bedford, Massachusetts, for example, sailors who had just returned from a three-year whaling voyage needed new clothing quickly. Other sailors who had just signed on for a new voyage hastily had to collect supplies for their months at sea. The stores that sold them their clothing were called "slop-shops" because the clothing they sold was sailors' "slops." ("Slop" was an Old Norse word for the sailors' wide-bottomed trousers.) What sailors bought there they put on board ship in their "slopchests." Slopshop clothing was of poor quality, and the customer did not expect a good fit.

In the South, too, some plantation owners bought cheap ready-made clothing for their slaves. In Western mining towns the men who had quickly joined the Gold Rush had usually left their families behind. There were too few women to provide homemade clothing, and not enough rich people to support a tailor. Miners had to go to a store. "Store-boughten" clothing was better than nothing.

People took it for granted that if you bought ready-made clothing from a store, it could not possibly fit you well. They believed that everybody was a quite different size. Therefore, they said, the only way to make clothing fit was to have it made specially (either at home or by a tailor) to your very own measurements. How could a manufacturer possibly turn out thousands of suits, each a different size, for thousands of different people? A suit you bought in a store would surely be too loose in some places and too tight in others. Manufacturers—without even trying—had given up the effort to provide sizes that would really fit.

Take shoes, for example. Before the mid-nineteenth century, even after shoe-making machinery had been invented, the shoes you could buy ready-made in a store were usually "straights." That meant there was actually no difference between the shoe sold for the right foot and for the left foot. If you really wanted your shoes to fit, you had to hire a shoemaker to make a pair especially for you.

The uniform-makers in the Civil War learned a lesson. They found that if they made quite a few different sizes they could provide almost everybody with a reasonably good fit. They noticed that certain combinations of measurements were more common than others. For example, lots of men with a 36-inch waist also had a 30-inch trouser length. They kept track of the sizes of the uniforms they made.

When the War was over in 1865 and hundreds of thousands of veterans suddenly needed civilian clothes, the United States actually had a clothing industry. Manufacturers had learned so much about the commonest measurements of the human body that they could produce ready-made suits which fitted better than most homemade suits and almost as well as the best tailor-made. Merchants now began to open clothing stores for everybody because their assortments of sizes would fit any customer. Americans of all classes and occupations were glad to buy their clothes ready-made.

The age of statistics—a new age of careful measurement—had arrived in the world of clothing. A statistically-minded tailor named Daniel Edward Ryan, after years of collecting facts, in 1880 published *Human Proportions in Growth: Being the Complete Measurement of the Human Body for Every Age and Size during the Years of Juvenile Growth.* The new Science of Sizes gave clothing manufacturers a scientific guide for customers of all ages.

To put this new science to use, and to stock clothing stores with all the different sizes, there had to be a whole factory full of new machinery. The old tedious way of making garments—cutting cloth for one suit at a time and then sewing each seam by hand—was not good enough.

Most of the labor went into sewing. So the most important new machine would be a sewing machine. In 1831 a Paris tailor had made a workable sewing machine, and had begun to use it making uniforms for the French army. But Paris tailors, afraid that they would lose their jobs, smashed the machines and drove the inventor out of the city. Soon afterward, several Americans made sewing machines.

Walter Hunt was one of the most ingenious inventors of the age. Once when he needed money to pay a debt, within the space of only three hours he invented the safety pin, made a model of it, and sold the idea for $400. But he was more interested in making inventions than in making money. Among his new devices were a knife sharpener, a stove to burn hard coal, an ice plow, a repeating rifle, a street-sweeping ma-

chine, and paper collars. The vast new department stores and the catalogs of the new mail-order firms offered ways to show and sell such gadgets to Americans wherever they lived.

Most inventors who tried to make a sewing machine had not got very far, because they tried to make their machines imitate hand sewing. So they put the point of the needle at one end, and the eye, or hole, of the needle at the other. Hunt was more original. He put the hole at the pointed end. The thread was attached there. Then the other end of the needle was attached to a machine that simply pushed it up and down while another thread was thrust through the loop underneath the cloth. Using this original idea, by 1832 he had perfected a machine that sewed a lock stitch which would not unravel. But Hunt was not at all a businessman, and he did not even bother to patent his invention.

A few years later Elias Howe, who had been raised on a Massachusetts farm and then worked as apprentice to a scientific instrument maker in Cambridge, made the same invention on his own. He patented his machine in 1846.

The sewing machine that Howe patented in 1846. The spool at the left held the thread.

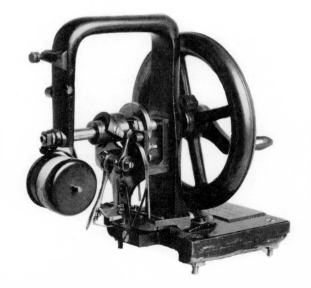

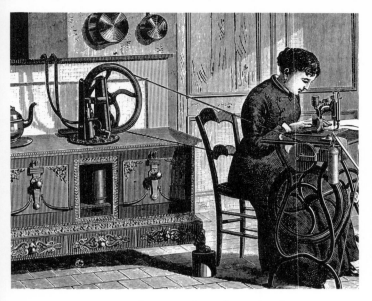

Before Thomas Edison brought electricity into homes, some people used small steam engines (fired by the kitchen stove) to run their sewing machines.

To prove that his machine really worked, Howe staged a public sewing race at the Quincy Hall Clothing Manufactory in Boston. He challenged five of the speediest seamstresses. Ten seams of equal length were prepared. One was given to each seamstress, and five were given to Howe at his machine. To everybody's amazement, before any of the seamstresses had finished her one seam, Howe had finished his *five*. His sewing machine was declared the winner.

But people feared that the sewing machine would put needy seamstresses out of work. As late as 1849 the sewing machine was still so rare that a man carried one around western New York State charging an admission fee of 12½ cents to see "A Great Curiosity!! The Yankee Sewing-Machine." Ladies took home specimens of machine sewing to show their friends.

Not for long would machine sewing remain a curiosity. For a remarkable Go-Getting salesman and organizer had become interested. When Isaac Merrit

Singer saw his first sewing machine in 1850 his main aim—like that of Henry Ford after him—was to make machines so cheap that he could sell them by the hundreds of thousands. When he used Howe's patented designs without permission, the courts eventually made him pay for the right to use Howe's design. But in 1856 Singer persuaded Howe to join a great Sewing Machine Combination to make machines with all the latest improvements.

Singer's dream came true, for by 1871 more than a half-million sewing machines were being manufactured each year. The combination of Howe design and Singer salesmanship sent American sewing machines all over the world. "Every nook and corner of Europe," the advertisements boasted, "knows the song of this tireless Singer."

The women who still had the job of making all the family's clothes were, of course, happy to have a machine to ease their work. And the sewing machine was only one of the first of many new machines—washing machines for clothes and dishes, vacuum cleaners, mixing machines for the kitchen, and many others—which would make the life of the twentieth-century American family both easier and more complicated.

Next to sewing the seams, what took most time in a man's coat or suit was cutting the cloth to the pattern. To cut heavy cloth for one suit at a time was tedious. But it was hard to make a knife that would cut through thick piles of cloth. The knife tended to twist the cloth so that the bottom pieces came out a different shape. This problem was solved in the 1870's when new high-speed, steam-powered cutting machines sliced neatly through twenty or more thicknesses. In the 1880's a Boston inventor perfected a machine that saved more hours by automatically cutting and finishing buttonholes.

Each factory-produced suit had to be neatly pressed. But the old heavy pressing iron (called a "goose" because it was so large and had a long awkward handle) was slow. A clever apprentice, Adon J. Hoffman, who was using a "goose" in a tailor shop in Syracuse, New York, dislocated his shoulder so that he could not handle the cumbersome iron. So he invented a presser he could operate with his feet. A foot pedal controlled the steam pressure which pushed down the top pad. All the operator had to do with his hands was to lay the garment between the pads. Within a few years Hoffman had become rich by selling thousands of his new steam pressers.

As the population grew and the American worker prospered, the demand for good ready-made clothing went up. At the same time, too, near the end of the nineteenth century, the flood of immigrants from Germany, Russia, and Poland included many who had been tailors over there. They naturally went to work in clothing factories here. But the new sewing machine was mak-

In their slum apartment a whole immigrant family (crowded together with their sewing machine) worked at making garments.

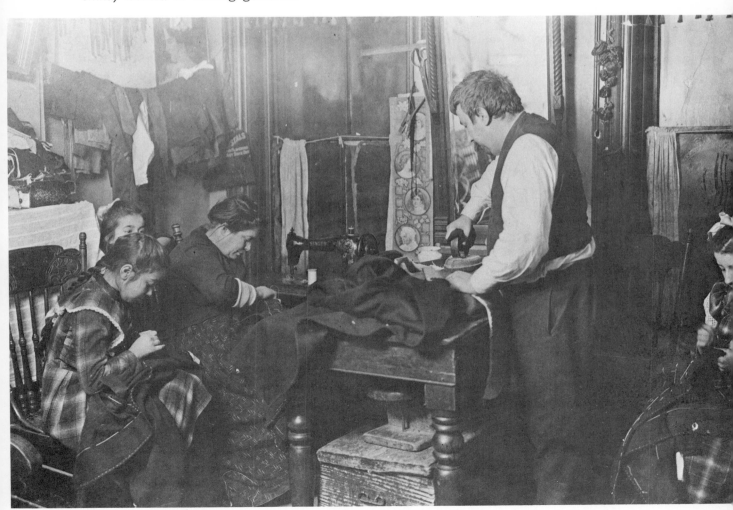

ing the tailor's skill less needed than ever. In the new clothing factories, the wives and children of these immigrants found quick employment.

Some of these factories became "sweatshops," where women and children worked long hours in stuffy rooms for low wages. But soon new laws required the children to stay in school. Meanwhile labor unions, led by enterprising immigrants, organized the clothing workers to demand better wages and shorter hours. Eventually the unions themselves would become rich enough to provide hospitals, clubhouses, and scholarships for their members.

By the end of the nineteenth century the United States saw a revolution in clothing. Here for the first time in history there was beginning to be a democracy of clothing. Here you did not have to be rich to dress well. A new industry was finding ways to make a stylish suit that any man could afford. Before 1900 nine-tenths of the men and boys in the

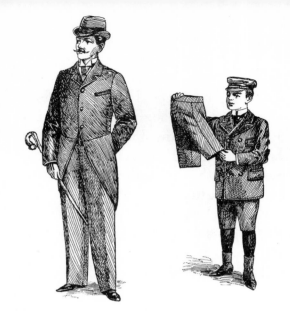

This fashionable man's suit was offered by Montgomery Ward (in 1895) for $7.50. For $2.25 his son could have a suit with extra pants and a cap.

United States were wearing ready-made clothing that they had bought in a store. Even the rich who once hired a tailor found a ready-made suit to fit. Americans dressed more like one another than people in any Old World nation. The new immigrant could go into a clothing store and buy a ready-made outfit that made him an instant American.

CHAPTER 6

Things by the Millions

On July 4, 1876, the nation celebrated its hundredth birthday with a Centennial Exposition held at Philadelphia. On the fairgrounds there were no rifle ranges or roller coasters or freak shows. There was no need for any. American products of all shapes and sizes——from shiny new bicycles to a new machine that sent your voice over a wire——were

themselves quite enough to entertain and amaze.

Visitors from Europe were astonished at how fast the United States had moved ahead. One hundred years before, the country had been thirteen weak and separate colonies—of a few towns and many scattered farms. Even twenty-five years before (when the Great Exhibition

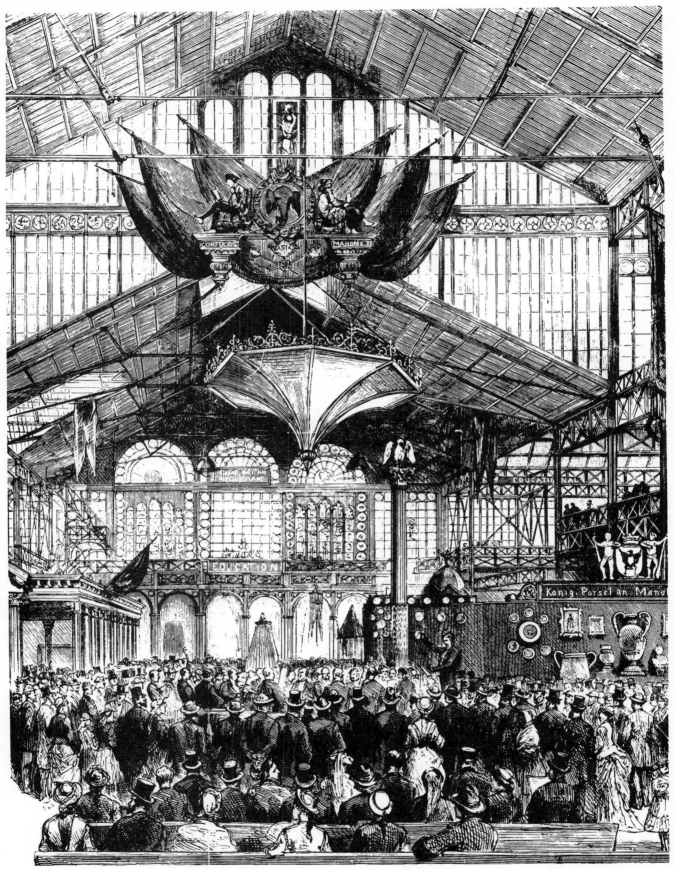

The festivities at the Centennial Exposition in Philadelphia in 1876 included concerts like this one, held in the Music Pavilion.

had been held in London) England was plainly the leading manufacturing nation in the world. But now the United States was already threatening to take her place.

At this Philadelphia Fair, Machinery Hall, which drew the biggest crowds, was dominated by the gigantic Corliss Steam Engine. The largest ever, it was forty feet high, weighed seven hundred tons, and produced over two thousand horsepower.

George H. Corliss, the man who made the great engine, showed how to combine the Go-Getter spirit with American know-how. When timid businessmen would not buy his improved steam engine, he offered it to them free—in return for the money his engine would save them by using less coal. From one engine alone he received in five years nearly twenty thousand dollars, which was several times what the engine cost him to make.

But it was not only size and quality that impressed visitors from the Old World. They were astonished by how cheaply Americans could make so many different things. Early in the nineteenth century one ingenious Connecticut manufacturer, Eli Terry, had already managed to turn out new clocks that sold for so little it was not worth having an old one repaired. Even before the Civil War, American clocks sold for less than fifty cents apiece, and New England factories were producing a half-million clocks each year.

Now in 1876, Europeans who saw the Philadelphia exhibits were convinced that Americans would change the world. The American machines, one Swiss engineer predicted, would "overwhelm all mankind with a quantity of products which, we hope, will bring them blessing."

To make things by the millions, Americans first had to create whole new industries and whole new ways of thinking. Newest and most essential was the industry for making machine tools. Machine tools were the parent machines—the machines for making the sewing machines, the gun-making machines, the clock-making machines, and all the rest. Since all these machines themselves were made of metal, machine tools were mostly metal-cutting tools.

In the early nineteenth century, a number of clever British machinists perfected the art of metal cutting. They invented a new measuring tool called a "micrometer" (from the Greek *meter* for measure and *micro* for small) which could measure thousandths of an inch.

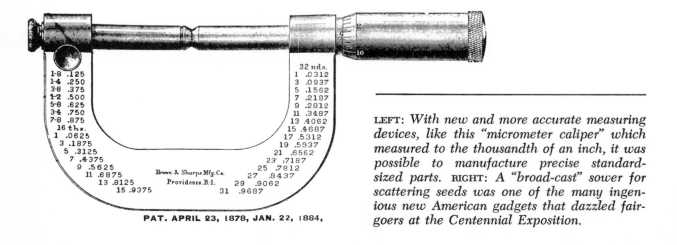

PAT. APRIL 23, 1878, JAN. 22, 1884,

LEFT: *With new and more accurate measuring devices, like this "micrometer caliper" which measured to the thousandth of an inch, it was possible to manufacture precise standard-sized parts.* RIGHT: *A "broad-cast" sower for scattering seeds was one of the many ingenious new American gadgets that dazzled fairgoers at the Centennial Exposition.*

The Englishmen had a head start. But England was an old country, with many craftsmen skilled at making things the old way. In America there were fewer skilled craftsmen, and few craft traditions. Workers here were more willing to try new ways. Soon after the Civil War ingenious Americans were making and improving their own machine tools.

One of the most remarkable of the American machine-tool makers was William Sellers of Philadelphia. By the time of the Centennial Exposition his work was already famous. He had invented machines that could measure and cut metal at the same time. These were essential for making standard-size screws.

And now screws were more important than anyone could imagine before. The millions of metal parts of the new machines were held together by metal screws. In the old days nobody could make one screw exactly like another. Each screw had been specially made to go into one particular hole in one particular machine. Then if you took a piece of machinery apart you had to label each screw so you could put it back in the same place.

Now that would not do. What good was it to make guns or clocks with standard-size parts unless you could hold them together with standard-size screws?

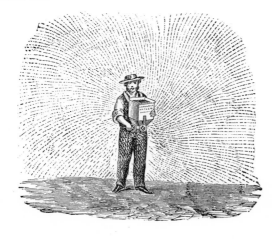

In his *System of Screw Threads and Nuts* (1864), William Sellers offered his own standard designs for the tiny grooves. After that, if you said your machine used a "Sellers Number 6" screw, then everybody knew exactly what you meant. The United States Government officially adopted Sellers' system in 1868. Before the end of the century an international congress in Switzerland made it the standard for Europe too.

Sellers was also interested in the appearance of the large new machines. Earlier machines had been decorated like fancy furniture. They were painted red and green and purple and were prettied up with iron beads and carvings. To Sellers, this made no sense. A machine, Sellers said, ought to look like a machine. He began painting his machines "machine gray"—not for decoration but to prevent rusting and to make cleaning easier. He took off the gimcracks and set the modern machine style which lasted into the twentieth century.

While Sellers was pioneering in new shapes and colors, other Americans were inventing a whole new way of thinking about factories. In the old days, the individual craftsman in his shop would simply do things the way they had always been done before. This was called the "rule-of-thumb." You did the job in a rough, practical way, using your thumb instead of a precise measure.

But the new American factory could not be run that way. If the old gunsmith was crude or inefficient, it meant simply that he made less money, or that people stopped buying guns from him. But in a factory where thousands of men worked elbow-to-elbow, everybody suffered if one man blundered. If your work was not precise, your mistakes were carried all over the country in the thousands of misshapen parts that came off your machine.

Now there was need for a new science —a science of avoiding waste. "Efficiency" was another name for it. The Go-Getting engineer who invented it called it the "Science" of Management.

The efficiency pioneer, Frederick W. Taylor, was born in 1856 in Philadelphia. His mother, a passionate abolitionist, was determined to liberate men from slavery. Taylor hoped to liberate men from waste. He was astonished that people who worried about conserving forests and water power and soil and minerals paid so little attention to conserving human effort.

He believed that there was one best way to do anything. But the one way that was most economical and least wasteful was not necessarily the way it had always been done.

Early in life he experimented to find the most efficient way to walk. He counted his steps and measured his stride. Then he figured out the best way to walk at different times and to different places. He did not drink alcoholic beverages or tea or coffee, and he did not smoke. He said these wasted human energy.

Taylor loved sports and thought they were important in education, not so much because they were fun as because they helped to give a man endurance for his productive work. He designed his own tennis racket, with a curved handle that made it look like a spoon. People laughed at him—until 1881 when Taylor and his partner (with Taylor using his spoon-handle racket) won the United States doubles championship.

The Bethlehem Iron Company hired Taylor to help make their enormous plant more efficient. Every year millions of tons of coal and iron ore were shoveled into furnaces. Paying the men to shovel was one of the largest expenses of making iron. Each man brought his own shovel and shoveled any way he wanted. But wasn't it possible, Taylor asked, that there was actually only one best way to shovel?

Taylor and his crew went into the factory and wrote down exactly what the men were already doing. Each worker was using his one favorite shovel no matter what kind of coal he was shoveling. A shovelful of the extremely light "rice coal" weighed only 3½ pounds, but a shovelful of the heavy iron ore weighed 38 pounds.

"Now," Taylor asked, "is 3½ pounds the proper shovel-load or is 38 pounds the proper shovel load? They cannot both be right. Under scientific management, the answer to the question is not a matter of anyone's opinion; it is a question for accurate, careful, scientific investigation."

Taylor counted the number of shovelfuls of the heavy ore that one man handled in a day. He found that with 38 pounds of ore in each shovel-load, a man in one day handled about 25 tons. Then Taylor cut off part of the metal scoop on the man's shovel so it would hold only 34 pounds. He discovered that this same man now managed to shovel *more* ore in the same length of time. Now the worker handled 30 tons. Yet the worker was less tired. Day after day Taylor kept cutting off a little bit of the shovel.

He found that when the shovel carried 22 pounds in each load, the man moved the most ore in one day.

Taylor had discovered a Science of Shoveling! He designed several different shapes and sizes of shovels and then tested each one to see that it was best suited to the stuff it had to carry. His small flat shovel was for the heavy ore and his immense scoop was for light rice coal. Soon there were 15 kinds of shovels in the Bethlehem tool room. Instead of the 600 men needed to do the shoveling before, with Taylor's Science of Shoveling the same work was done by only 140. Taylor had abolished the waste.

This system, according to Taylor, made it possible to pay each shoveler 60 percent more in wages. The wages of workers actually were increased. But, naturally enough, many workers were afraid they would lose their jobs. Others were afraid that, even if they kept their jobs, they would have to work harder. Many were afraid they would be regimented. They liked their own shovels. They did not like anybody telling them how to do their simple job.

Still, all over the country, "Scientific Management" became more and more popular with employers. They discovered that by making a science of the simplest jobs, they usually could find a better way.

In an astonishingly short time, the American factory took on a new look. Scientific management engineers invented a whole new way of organizing a factory. Instead of having the worker walk around to pick up parts and bring them to his workbench, the manage-

---

One of the last steps in the Ford assembly line. The body (assembled on the second floor) was dropped down onto the chassis and motor (assembled on the ground floor), to be attached and fitted by alert mechanics.

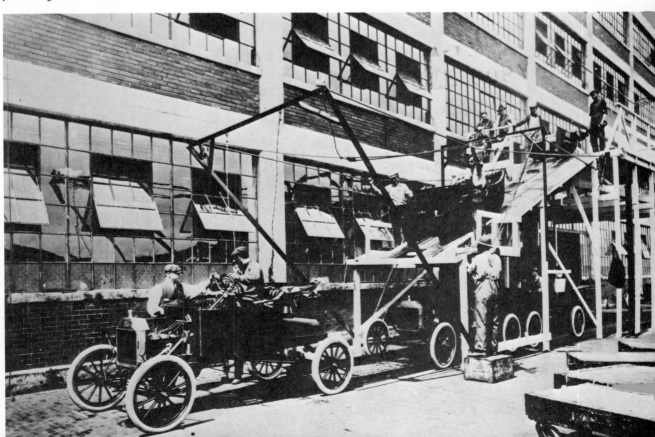

ment engineers designed a workbench that moved. Then each worker could stay in one place and keep his mind on his proper job. The bench (now a moving belt) would carry along the heavy parts from one worker to another.

This new kind of moving workbench was called an "assembly line," because on it the whole machine was put to-gether or "assembled."

In early April 1913 a bold mechanic named Henry Ford decided to try an assembly line for making automobiles. He wanted to make automobiles so cheaply that he could sell them by the millions. He made some improvements of his own in the assembly line. For example, he arranged the moving belt so that it

When Edison's new phonograph was still rare, this man made money by giving programs of recorded music and talk. Here he holds one of his cylinder-shaped records, chosen from a case decorated with Edison's photograph.

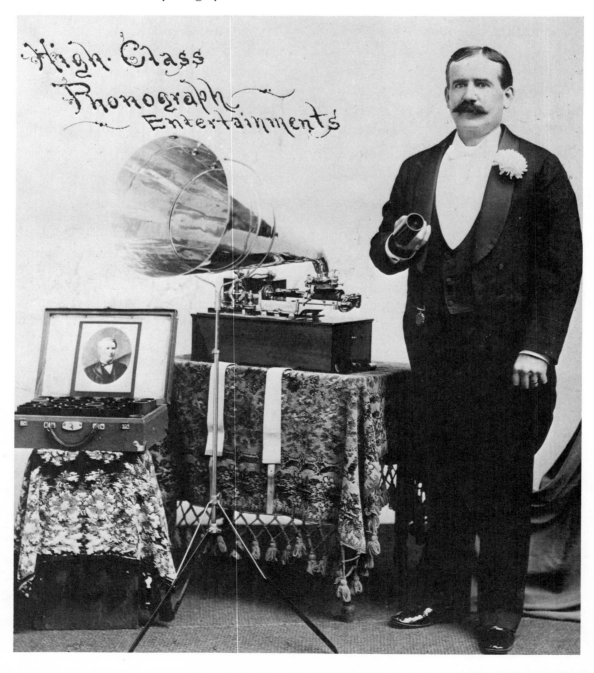

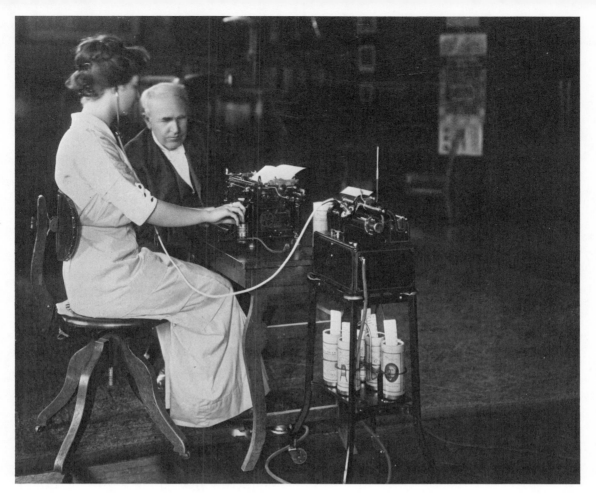

Edison's main interest in the phonograph was not for music but for office use. In this picture Edison watches while a secretary listens to the recorded voice of her employer and copies the words on a typewriter. Like the typewriter and the telephone switchboard, the new device helped to open a whole new world of office work to American women.

---

would always be "man-high." He changed the height according to the job so that nobody had to waste energy bending down or reaching up.

Ford also varied the speed of the belt. He explained:

> The idea is that a man must not be hurried in his work—he must have every second necessary but not a single unnecessary second. . . . The man who puts in a bolt does not put on the nut; the man who puts on the nut does not tighten it. On operation number 34 the budding motor gets its gasoline. . . . On operation number 44 the radiator is filled with water, and on operation number 45 the car drives out.

In the early years when Henry Ford had been trying to perfect a gasoline-driven motor, many people laughed at him. They put him in the same class with crackpots who tried to make perpetual-motion machines. It was hard to imagine a self-propelled machine that would run not on steam but on a liquid fuel.

Luckily, in 1897, Ford met the already famous Thomas A. Edison. Some of Edison's own friends had been working on an electric automobile which worked on storage batteries that had to be recharged frequently. When Ford explained his "gas car," Edison cheered him on. "Young man, that's the thing!

You have it! The self-contained unit carrying its own fuel with it. Keep at it." Edison said the fuel could be a "hydrocarbon"—a chemical name for fluids like gasoline. Although Ford then did not even know the meaning of "hydrocarbon," he was encouraged and later said that the talk with Edison was a turning point in his life.

Ford and Edison became best friends. Even before they had met, Edison (who was sixteen years older) had been an inspiration to Ford, as he was to many other inventors.

Edison had invented a new kind of factory—an "invention factory." It's purpose actually was to invent new kinds of things to make. In the 1870's Edison set up his first "invention factory" with $40,000 he received from his own early inventions.

To his "invention factory" he brought the most ingenious men he could find. He inspired them with loyalty and hope, and built them into a team. Following the example of earlier Go-Getters like Benjamin Silliman and others who had found ways to make "Rock Oil" into fuel to light American homes, these men tried to find new uses for old materials, and also to invent new machines for all sorts of purposes.

Edison and his associates were tireless testers and imaginative mechanics. One of their first feats was to help make electric lighting possible. The most difficult problem had been to find a thread, to put inside the bulb, that would give light when electricity was sent through it and yet would not quickly burn out.

They tried all sorts of materials—carbon, bamboo, hair, platinum, copper, and scores of other substances. They finally discovered that a filament of charred paper served well if it was in a vacuum. This made possible the commercial production of light bulbs, which soon replaced Rockefeller's oil lamps.

Edison and his fellow inventors, looking for a way to record the human voice, invented the phonograph. They worked on a way to use the new art of photography to show "moving" pictures. In 1891 Edison patented a "kinetoscope"— a kind of peep show which showed moving pictures inside a box.

Edison's own ingenuity seemed endless. But he was also a great organizer, and when he could not make an invention of his own to solve a problem, he bought up the patent rights of others. Then he found ways to manufacture the new products cheaply and efficiently. He was most interested in the improvements in daily life that could reach everybody.

Edison fired the imagination, not only of Henry Ford, but of the whole American people. He was nicknamed the "Wizard." When Congress awarded him a special gold medal in 1928 it was announced that his inventions had been worth $15,599,000,000 to humanity! But this was only to say that there really was no way of measuring his enormous contribution to American life. By the time of his death at the ripe age of 85, in 1931, he had become an American hero —a truly democratic hero, because his work benefited every living American.

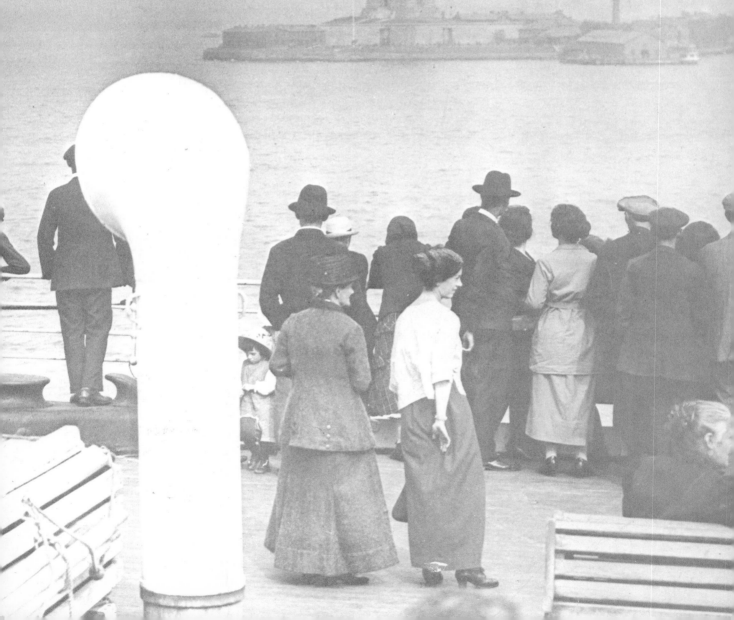

PART TWO

PEOPLE ON THE MOVE

PEOPLE ON THE MOVE

Americans were people on the move. There would have been nobody here except the Indians unless Old World millions had been willing to cross the ocean. The United States might have been only a string of seaboard farms and cities if brave new Americans had not then been willing to risk the move farther west. Going into the half-mapped continent was, of course, traveling into the unknown. But Americans were willing—even eager—to risk new places.

The Civil War, too, meant the moving of peoples. Great battles were fought by thousands of men in armies on the move. The fortunes of war brought Virginians to Gettysburg in Pennsylvania and sent Massachusetts volunteers deep into Georgia. Even while the armies of General William T. Sherman cut their bloody swath through the South, the Union men could not help seeing the beauties of the Southern land. They discovered that Southerners were not so different from themselves. Thousands of Americans pried into far corners of their country.

After the war, many soldiers returned to their old homes. A few stayed where they had fought, and found wives and homes in the new places. Some Northerners went south to teach school or help in the Freedmen's Bureau. From the burnt-over south, hopeful Southerners went north or west in search of opportunity. Negroes, at last free to leave the old plantation, for the first time were able to move about like any other Americans.

"Go-Ahead" became an American motto. Of course, Go-Getting Americans were eager to move up in the world. But they were just as eager to move around. The same spirit that before the Civil War had led Americans to move westward in wagon-towns, that had led them to build railroads even before there were cities to go to, now led Americans to move and keep moving.

After the Civil War, brave and needy men and women were still risking the ocean to come fill the land and crowd the cities. From impoverished European farms, many were drawn by extravagant promises. And thousands already here, who were disappointed by the American land, moved hopefully to the cities.

The Americans already here kept telling themselves: "Go ahead. Move on. Try to find a better place."

As Americans churned about the vast continent, they came to know their land —and to know one another. Most nations of the Old World were rooted to the same spot. Their people were held together because their ancestors had so long lived inside the same boundaries. It was unusual for them to move. They learned to be satisfied with their place.

But Americans would not long let themselves be confined anywhere. Americans were held together by their ways of moving and by their shared desire to move. And the freedom to move to a better place helped build the nation.

CHAPTER 7

To Punish—or to Forgive?

Lee's surrender to Grant at Appomattox brought peace to the nation. But peace brought new problems. How to find jobs for the million men who left the Union and Confederate armies? How to change factories from making cannon and rifles and ammunition to making harvesters and sewing machines?

When the South agreed to unconditional surrender, they put themselves at the mercy of the North. This gave Northerners their most difficult problem —what to do with the South.

Was it more important to punish the former rebels, to teach them a lesson they would never forget, so they never again would try to break up the Union? Or was it better to forgive the rebels, to welcome them back into the Union, so they would feel at home and never again want to leave?

Of course the South had already been punished. A quarter-million Southerners had died in the war. The Confederacy was a land of cinders and desolation —of charred plantation houses, broken bridges, twisted railways, and desecrated churches. An Englishman who traveled halfway across the South said he did not see a single smiling face. But

Ruins of Charleston, South Carolina, by the pioneer Civil War photographer, Mathew Brady. For many people in the South, "Reconstruction" after the Civil War meant clearing away rubble and rebuilding cities.

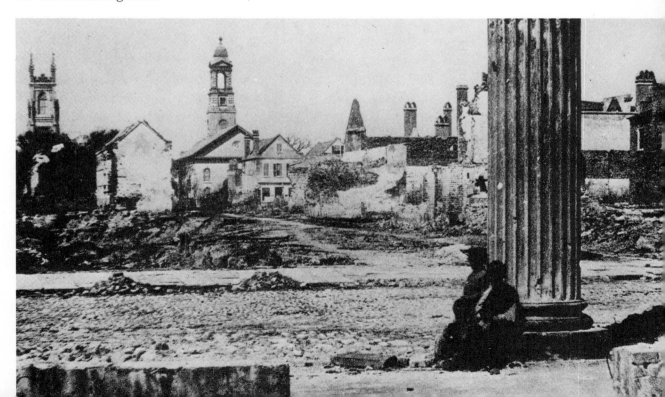

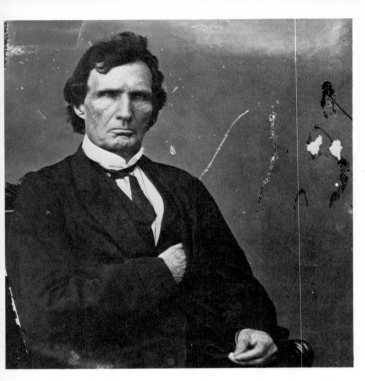

Thaddeus Stevens, Congressman from Pennsylvania (from an old and damaged photograph).

the North had also suffered, with its own quarter-million dead. And for Northerners who had lost fathers, sons, or husbands, no punishment of the South would be enough.

Yet this was not just a question of feelings. Unless the North wanted to feed and house millions of Southerners, it was important to get the South back into working order. This meant getting crops planted, factories built, railroads running, and pupils and teachers into schools. It also meant getting the Southern States organized to govern themselves, to collect their own taxes, to keep the peace, and to protect life and property.

But it was not easy to get people to agree on how to revive the Southern States. There was wide disagreement on what the war had really meant. What the North called "The War of the Rebellion" in the South was still called "The War between the States." The

Southerners argued that their State governments had never been destroyed. Once a State always a State!

Lincoln himself had almost agreed with the Southerners on this point. He also believed, Once a State always a State! But for Lincoln this meant that the Southern States had no power to secede. And if the Southern States had never really seceded, then even after the Civil War the Southern States were still within the Union.

Naturally, once the war was over, Southerners wanted to agree with Lincoln. They said they still had their States and therefore could still run their own affairs. The most, then, that the victorious North could properly ask was that some Confederate leaders be barred from office.

But on the other side were the Northern Avengers. The most powerful of them were in a group of Northern Senators and Congressmen called Radical Republicans. They were bitter against the Southern rebels. They remained suspicious of all white Southerners. They did not want to forgive and forget, but instead wanted to rub salt in Southern wounds. The Southern States, said the Radical Republicans, had actually "committed suicide." By trying to rebel, they had not only violated the Constitution but actually destroyed their own States. They were no longer States at all.

People who thought like this believed that after the war the Southern "States" could claim *no* rights under the Constitution. They had no right to govern themselves or to be represented in the Senate or the House of Representatives. They were nothing but so much territory

—like parts of the sparsely settled West. And, like those Western territories, they could be governed in any way Congress decided.

Congress could treat them as "conquered provinces." They could be ruled by military governors—generals of the Union army. When, if ever, they would be allowed to govern themselves and take part in the national government—this would depend on how they behaved themselves and what the victorious Congress wanted. This offered anything but a cheerful prospect for the Southerners.

The leader of the Radical Republicans was one of the strangest men in American history. Thaddeus Stevens was sometimes called "a humanitarian without humanity." For he seemed to use up all his good feelings on large noble causes and then he had very little left for individuals. Stevens was a sour man. Just as Lincoln inspired love and respect, Stevens inspired fear.

Very early in life he took up the great cause of abolishing slavery. He never gave it up, nor did he ever forgive men who had ever held slaves or who had been entangled in the web of slavery. After Appomattox, Stevens made it his purpose in life to punish all "traitors." Old age never mellowed him. At the age of seventy-five he boasted that he would spend his remaining years inventing new ways to make the Southern rebels suffer.

During the Civil War, Lincoln had shown his greatness—and his forgiving spirit—by his plan for bringing Southerners back to the Union. He was less interested in the past than in the future. Back in December 8, 1863, in his Proc-

lamation of Amnesty and Reconstruction, he had explained his plan. He would pardon almost all Southerners, even if they had fought against the Union.

All Lincoln asked was that Southerners take a solemn oath to support the Constitution of the United States in the future. As soon as enough citizens of a Southern State took the oath, Lincoln would recognize the government of that State and let the people govern themselves. Of course they must agree to abolish slavery. It would be enough, Lincoln said, if a number equal to only one-tenth of the voters in the last election took the oath.

This plan did not satisfy the Radical Republicans. They were busy in Congress making a plan of their own. During the war they concocted their Wade-Davis Bill in quite another spirit. They could not take their eyes off the past. Under their plan each Southern State was to make a list of all its white men. The State could not be recognized or given the power to govern itself until a *majority* of the people on that list took a new oath to support the Constitution. Then (since these Radicals believed that the old Southern States had committed suicide) there would have to be an election to call a convention to make an entirely new constitution for each Southern State.

No one could even vote in that election, much less be a delegate to help make the new constitution, unless he took the "ironclad oath." This oath was not merely a promise of future loyalty but was also an oath of past purity. You had to swear that you had never held office under the Confederacy or fought in the Confederate army. By the end of the war, most white men in the South could not honestly take such an oath.

Under the Radicals' scheme it would be years before any Southern State could set up a majority government for itself. It would have to wait until the whole Civil War generation was dead. But that did not bother the Radical Republicans. They were quite willing to keep the Southern States under military rule by Northern generals. They said they were in favor of liberty, but they were not willing to give it to white Southerners.

This was the Wade-Davis Bill, which passed Congress on July 2, 1864. It could not be law unless Lincoln signed it. What would Lincoln do?

Lincoln refused to sign the bill. But he was shrewd. Instead of attacking it, as he might have, for being evil and vengeful—or instead of saying simply that the plan for the South was the business of the President and not of Congress—he issued a new proclamation. He would not sign the Wade-Davis Bill into law, he said, because he did not think it should be the *only* way a Southern State could get back into working order. Any "seceded" Southern State that wanted to follow the Wade-Davis plan should feel free to do so.

But there were now, Lincoln said, two possible paths. Any Southern State could choose between Lincoln's one-tenth plan and the Radicals' majority-ironclad-oath plan. In the long run, of course, no Southern State would prefer the vengeful Radical plan. But still Lincoln had done his best to avoid a head-on clash with Congress.

On April 14, 1865, Lincoln called his Cabinet together to explain his policy to them. He urged them to use charity. He begged them to help bring the wartime spirit to an end.

That very night when President Lincoln and his wife went to Ford's Theater in Washington to attend a play, there occurred one of the great disasters of the Civil War era—and of all American history. It was less than a week after Lee had surrendered to Grant at Appomattox. The demented actor John Wilkes Booth rushed past the Secret Service men guarding the President's box and shot President Lincoln. The President died the next morning.

We cannot be sure what would have happened if Lincoln had lived. But we do know that Lincoln's combination of qualities was extremely rare. He was, of course, a strong man who would fight for what he believed. Yet he was also a simple, gentle man who understood other people. And, most important for a President, he was a clever politician. He knew how to give up less important things in order to persuade people to support him on what was more important.

Andrew Johnson, the new President, was in many ways like Lincoln. With no schooling, he began as a poor tailor. He, too, was a self-made man. Like Lincoln, he had been born in the South. And though he came from Tennessee, he had been against secession. When he was the Democratic Senator from Tennessee he was the only Southern Senator to support the Union after the Confederates fired on Fort Sumter.

Still, in some important ways, Johnson was no Lincoln. He was not good at persuading. He did not know how to use a joke to make a serious point. Just as Lincoln was gentle, generous, and compromising, so Johnson was crude and obstinate. His weaknesses would not have been serious in an ordinary citizen. But they were disastrous in a President.

When Lincoln was assassinated in April 1865, Congress was not in session. Many Republicans distrusted Johnson because he had been a Democrat. They had added him to the Republican ticket as their candidate for Vice-President in 1864 in the hope that he might draw the seceded States back into the Union.

Now, when the death of Lincoln had brought Johnson to the White House, the Radical Republicans wanted President Johnson to call Congress into special session to make new rules for the South. But he refused. President Johnson would follow the rules already declared by Lincoln. And *he* alone would decide when the Southern States had satisfied Lincoln's requirements so they could govern themselves.

Lincoln's requirements were not too hard for the Southern States to satisfy. By December 1865, when President Andrew Johnson made his first report to Congress, every one of the old Confederate States (except Texas, which soon came along) had done what Lincoln asked for. Each of these now had its own State government in working order. President Johnson reported happily that the Union was restored.

When the Congressmen from these "restored" Southern States came to take their seats in Congress, they were shut out. The Radical Republicans who controlled the House of Representatives told them that they were not really Congressmen at all—because the Southern States were not really States at all. Even if the Confederate States had followed

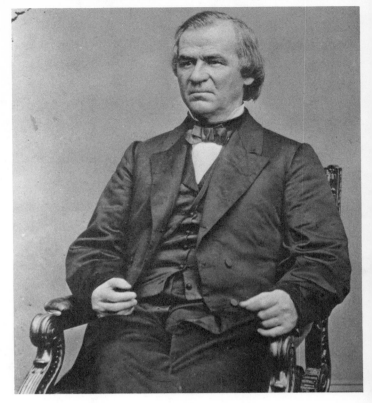

President Andrew Johnson, who had no Vice-President. If he had been removed from office, a Member of Congress (the Speaker of the House) would have become President.

the President's rules, the Radicals said, the President had no power to make the rules. Only Congress (by which they meant, of course, the Radical Republicans themselves) had that power. Their Punishing Bill—the Wade-Davis Bill—had declared what Congress wanted. The South would have to be "restored" by Congress or not at all.

Congress set up its own Committee on Reconstruction led by the Radical Avenger, Thaddeus Stevens, to make its own plan. The watchword of Stevens' Congressional plan was, Force! The South, he said, was a "conquered province" and nobody would be allowed to forget it. Northern troops would be sent to occupy the South.

The committee divided the old Confederacy into five military districts. The boundaries of the eleven seceded States were not to be respected. Each of the five districts would be ruled by a Northern general. The Northern Radical Republicans in Congress laid down new rules for building new Southern States. They wished to see the new States designed so as to keep political control in Republican hands.

Some of the Radical demands, such as abolishing slavery and giving civil rights to Negroes, were of course just and necessary. But others were not.

Worst of all was the Radical refusal to forgive. They denied many leading citizens in the Old South the right to vote, or even to work at their regular jobs. Hungry for power, the Radicals wanted to rule the South through a small group of their puppets. Anxious to hold their Republican majority in Congress, they were afraid the new Southern Congressmen might be against them. Although they said they loved liberty, they really were afraid of it. They were afraid to give political liberty to their old enemies.

What was President Johnson to do? Under the Constitution he was supposed to enforce the laws of Congress. Though he believed these laws unwise, he tried to enforce them. But the Radicals were out to "get" Johnson. They could not bear the idea of a President who was not in their pocket. They passed laws taking away powers which the Constitution had given to the President. For example, even though the Constitution made the President the Commander in Chief of the Army, the Radicals passed a Command of the Army Act taking away his power to command.

They were spoiling for a fight, hoping to tease the President into violating one law so that they could have him removed from office. They hoped that then they could seize the powers of the President.

But Johnson was careful to obey every law, to follow all the instructions of Congress.

Still there was a limit to his patience. When the Radicals passed the Tenure of Office Act which took away the President's control over his own Cabinet, that was too much. Secretary of War Stanton, whom Johnson had inherited in the Cabinet from Lincoln, had become Johnson's enemy and was actually plotting against him. So the President fired Stanton to test the Tenure of Office Act, which he believed to be against the Constitution. This was a small thing, but enough to give the Radicals their chance. They took it.

The framers of the Constitution, being wise men, had provided a way to remove a criminal President. But they saw that if they made it too easy to remove a President, opponents would be tempted to use it to get rid of any President they could not beat at the polls. Then every President would live in terror—afraid to do his duty, for fear some political enemy would make a crime out of it.

The Constitution said (Article II, Section 4) that the President could not be removed except "on Impeachment for, and Conviction of, Treason, Bribery, or other high Crimes and Misdemeanors." First the House of Representatives would have to "impeach" the President. This meant a majority vote to support a list of accusations. Then the President would actually be tried by the Senate. The Chief Justice of the United States would preside. But to remove a President a mere majority of the Senate was not enough. The framers showed their special wisdom when they required a vote of *two-thirds* of the members present.

When the Senate met on March 30, 1868, to try President Andrew Johnson on the impeachment brought by the House of Representatives, the nation was in breathless suspense. Few really believed that Andrew Johnson had been guilty of "Treason, Bribery, or other high Crimes and Misdemeanors."

Johnson, like Lincoln, was a man of rock-ribbed honesty. No one could prove otherwise. Earnestly he had followed his inaugural oath "to preserve, protect, and defend the Constitution of the United States, against all enemies foreign and domestic." Perhaps he had sometimes lost his temper, had shown bad judgment, or had used language that a President should not use. But these were not crimes. His only "crime" had been that he believed it *his* duty to obey the Constitution. And he was determined to follow a policy of forgiveness. He could not have satisfied the Radicals without surrendering all the powers of the Presidency into their hands.

On May 16, 1868, when the vote of the Senate was finally taken, 35 Senators voted "guilty" and 19 voted "not guilty." This was a big majority. But, luckily, it was *one* vote less than the two-thirds which the Founding Fathers required. Andrew Johnson remained President.

CHAPTER 8

A Two-Nation South

Peace and reunion brought an end to slavery. But the roots of slavery ran deep. They reached into every nook and cranny of Southern life.

One of its roots was racism—the belief that one race was naturally better than another. This belief had helped keep slavery alive. At the same time slavery had kept racism alive. Under slavery, nearly all the Negroes in the South did lowly tasks. Therefore, it was easy for white people—and sometimes even for Negroes themselves—to believe that God had meant it that way.

Slavery could be abolished simply by changing laws. But it was much harder to abolish the belief that one race was better than another. Many generations of Southerners had taught that to their children. After the war it was still rooted in their minds and hearts.

And after the war it became clearer and clearer that the South was still split into two "nations." There was a White South and a Negro South. Much of the time these two "nations" lived at peace.

Some of the time they lived in a nervous truce. Occasionally they were actually at war. Obviously the United States could not be truly united until the South ceased to be divided.

Lincoln and Johnson had their eyes mainly on the abolition of slavery. The future they looked to—a South without slavery—seemed not too hard to accomplish. Stevens and the Radicals also wanted to abolish slavery. But for them, abolishing slavery was not enough. They believed that slavery would not really be abolished until the Negro was treated as the equal of the white man. Their hopes were wider and deeper—and much harder to accomplish—than the hopes of Lincoln or of Johnson.

The Radical Republicans saw the wickedness of slavery. But they did not really see its full tragedy. Part of the tragedy was that the roots of slavery could not be removed in a year or two— nor perhaps even in a generation. The Radical Republicans were right when they said that the problem was not *only* slavery. But they were violent and impatient men.

For the deep problem they had no deep solution. They knew what they wanted, but they did not know how to get it. To transform the life of the South, to bring equality to the Negro, to cure both the white man and the Negro of the disease of racism, would take a patience and a charity and a wisdom which the Radicals lacked. They were wrong when they believed that the old cancer of slavery could be ripped out quickly and by force.

The Thirteenth Amendment to the Constitution, which abolished slavery, was proclaimed on December 18, 1865.

But when the legislatures of the Southern States (under the Lincoln-Johnson one-tenth plan) had their first meetings, they promptly adopted "Black Codes." These were supposed to provide for the new situation of the Negro now that he was no longer a slave. They provided, for example, that now the Negro could own property, and they gave him certain other rights.

But, under the Black Codes, the freedom of the Negro was still strictly limited. He could not vote. He was not allowed to marry a white person. He could generally be a witness only in trials against other Negroes. He could not leave the land where he had been a slave. He could not look for a new job. In Mississippi, for example, if a Negro was convicted of being a "vagrant"—a wandering person without a job—he could be fined $50. If he could not pay the fine, he could be hired out against his will to anybody who would pay the fine in return for his labor.

Had Northerners died in a Civil War merely to preserve slavery under a new name?

The Radical Republicans in the North, who anyway expected the worst from the Old Confederates, were not taken by surprise. Even before the war was over they had set up the Freedmen's Bureau. Its purpose was to help war refugees, to get Southern farms back in working order, and to help Negro freedmen make their new start in life.

The Freedmen's Bureau did a great deal of good work that nobody else could do. It handed out millions of free meals to Negroes and to white refugees. It built hospitals. And it brought thousands of Southerners back onto farms

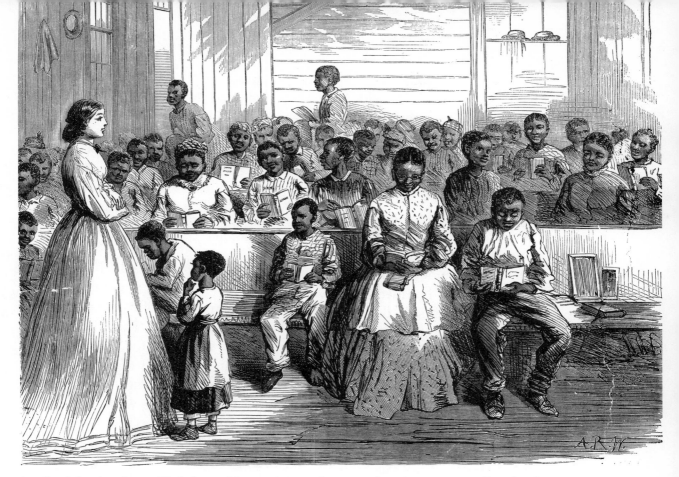

A school for freedmen, Vicksburg, Mississippi, in the year after Appomattox. For the first time, many Negroes had a chance to learn to read.

where they could make a living again. The Bureau also helped Negro freedmen find jobs, and helped protect them against a new slavery.

The Bureau's most important work was in building schools and in providing teachers—to give Negroes the education they had been denied under slavery. Howard University, Hampton Institute, Atlanta University, and Fisk University were set up for Negro students of college age. A quarter of a million Negro children were sent to school for the first time.

Few white Southerners were grateful for this help. They were worried that Negroes were no longer being kept in their "place." And they were especially annoyed at this interference by "outsiders."

It took courage to go south to teach for the Freedmen's Bureau. One young lady teacher who went to North Carolina reported that while the men who passed her on the street only rarely lifted their hats, "the ladies almost invariably lift their noses."

Northern teachers in the South found it hard to survive. In South Carolina, for example, grocers charged them especially high prices hoping to starve them out. One Southern farm woman said she "would not sell milk to Yankees to save her life, she hated the very ground they trod." Some Yankee teachers were afraid to buy the food anyway, because they thought it might be poisoned. Some found that no one would rent them a room to live in. Even in church they were shunned and insulted.

The South was now at war with itself. Many Southerners said they were only fighting against meddling "outsiders." But they were really fighting their fellow Southerners—Negroes who wanted to be free and equal.

Before long, the Old Confederates in the South had organized a secret army. Its purpose was really to carry on the Civil War under another name. Although slavery was abolished by law, the Old Confederates still desperately hoped to preserve as much as possible of their old Southern Way of Life.

Late in 1865 a half-dozen ex-Confederate soldiers in Pulaski, Tennessee, founded an odd new club. It was the first unit in this secretly revived Confederate army. It called itself the Ku Klux Klan—nobody knows exactly why. Soon many branches appeared all over the South.

Almost everything about the Ku Klux Klan was peculiar, and many of its features were ridiculous. Its members met in secret and tried to keep everything about it a mystery to outsiders. Each member swore never to reveal the names of other members—nor even to admit that he was a member himself. At the initiation of a candidate the Grand Cyclops ordered, "Let his head be adorned with the regal crown, after which place him before the royal altar and remove his hoodwink." The "royal altar" was a big mirror, and the "regal crown" was a high hat sprouting donkey's ears.

According to the Klan's constitution:

The officers of this [secret lodge] shall consist of a Grand Wizard of the Empire and his ten Genii; a Grand Dragon of the Realm and his eight Hydras; a Grand Titan of the Dominion and his six Furies; a Grand Giant of the Province and his four Goblins; a Grand Cyclops of the Den and his two Night Hawks; a Grand Magi, a Grand Monk, a Grand Exchequer, a Grand Turk, a Grand Scribe, a Grand Sentinel, and a Grand Ensign.

No wonder some people thought this was only a "hilarious social club."

But there was nothing funny about the Klan's activities. The Klan actually pretended to be (as it said in its constitution) "an institution of Chivalry, Humanity, Mercy and Patriotism." It pretended to protect the weak and the innocent, and to support the Constitution of the United States. It soon became a weapon of violence and terror.

Klan members traveled the countryside flogging, maiming, and sometimes killing Negroes who tried to vote or who in other ways presumed to be the white man's equal. The Klan uniform was a pointed hat with a white hood to conceal the face, and a long robe, either white or black.

In the beginning, Klan members included some respectable citizens. A famous Confederate cavalry general, Nathan Bedford Forrest, was the Grand Wizard. But the Klan's "Invisible Empire" also included many hoodlums. They wanted to frighten Negroes into *not* claiming their rights under the Constitution. The object of these Klan members was to keep the South separated into two *un*equal nations. They could not do their work except by blackmail and bloodshed. In 1869 when the crimes of the Klan became too scandalous, General Forrest resigned as Grand Wizard and pretended to "dissolve" the organization. The Klan then simply went underground.

Nobody knows exactly how many people joined the Klan. In 1868, General Forrest said the Klan had forty thousand members in Tennessee alone and a half-million in all the South. Scores of other organizations joined in the bloody work—the Tennessee Pale Faces, the Louisiana Knights of the White Camelia, the North Carolina White Brotherhood, the Mississippi Society of the White Rose, the Texas Knights of the Rising Sun, the Red Jackets, and the Knights of the Black Cross. In 1871 alone, in a single county in Florida, 163 Negroes were murdered, and around New Orleans the murders came to over 300. Thousands of Negroes were driven from their homes, maimed, or tortured.

Under pressure from Northern Radical Republicans, some Southern State governments passed laws against these crimes. On December 5, 1870, President U. S. Grant—who as general had commanded the Union forces to victory—delivered a special message to Congress. "The free exercise of franchise," he warned, "has by violence and intimidation been denied to citizens of several of the States lately in rebellion." Congress then passed the Ku Klux Klan Acts to outlaw these organizations and to protect the rights of all citizens. But these laws had little effect.

For the State governments set up in the South by the Radical Republican Congress were being replaced by old-fashioned Southern State governments. Confederate heroes were back in charge. The land and the factories were still

owned by white Southerners. The last few Northern troops were not withdrawn from the South until 1877. But by 1875—within ten years after Appomattox—eight of the eleven old Confederate States had already come back under rule of Old Confederates.

The work which only a few years before had been done by disreputable terrorists was now being done "legally" by the State governments. Although the Southern States had approved the Civil War Amendments (Thirteenth, Fourteenth, and Fifteenth) to the Constitution, although they had abolished slavery and their laws "guaranteed" the Negro his rights, all these proved to be

Members of the Ku Klux Klan, hooded and armed, 1868.

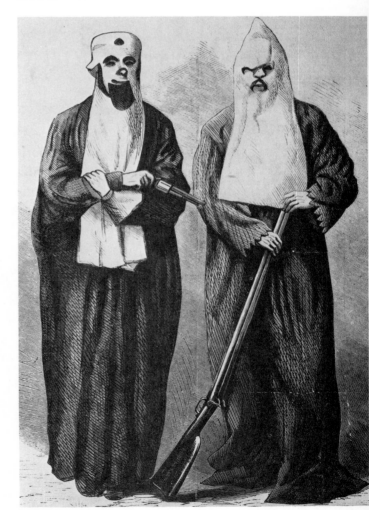

mere technicalities. Before long it was pretty plain that slavery itself was just about the only thing the Civil War had abolished.

Thaddeus Stevens died in 1868, and soon enough his avenging spirit—along with his special concern for the Negro's rights—was dead. Now more and more Northerners were anxious to "leave the South alone." In practice this meant putting the South back in the hands of white Southerners. And the South then remained divided into the same two nations—a "superior" race and an "inferior" race.

The South would not really become united with the rest of the United States until the South itself had become one. And this would take time.

The Two-Nation South was a One-Party South. When the Old Confederates came back into charge of the Southern States, they had no love for the Republican Party. That was the party of the Yankees, the party that had made war on the South and had then held the South under military rule. By keeping their control of the State governments, the Confederate heroes also kept those governments under the control of the new Democratic party. And the Negro was to have no voice in Southern politics for many years.

A divided South remained afraid of equality, afraid of change. This was at the very time when the American people —and newcomers from the whole world —were filling up the land and churning about the rest of the country faster than ever before.

CHAPTER 9

Filling the Land

From the earliest colonial days, America's leading import had been people. Before the Civil War nearly all immigrants arriving in New York or other American ports had come by sail. The passage from the Old World to the New had been a risky adventure lasting as long as two or three months. Sailing vessels depended on the wind, and the old sailing routes went only to certain places. Built mainly for cargo, these vessels stowed their poorer passengers like cattle.

Within a decade after Appomattox nearly all immigrants from across the ocean were arriving by steam. They were coming more speedily and in larger numbers than ever before. During the Civil War the need quickly to import supplies had encouraged the development of steamships. After the war the nation was eager to renew a free-flowing commerce with the world.

Steamships, unlike sailing vessels, could run on a reliable timetable. The uncertainty of the winds was replaced by a ten-day transatlantic schedule. The new steamships were actually planned for passengers. They were a good deal less uncomfortable—even for those who

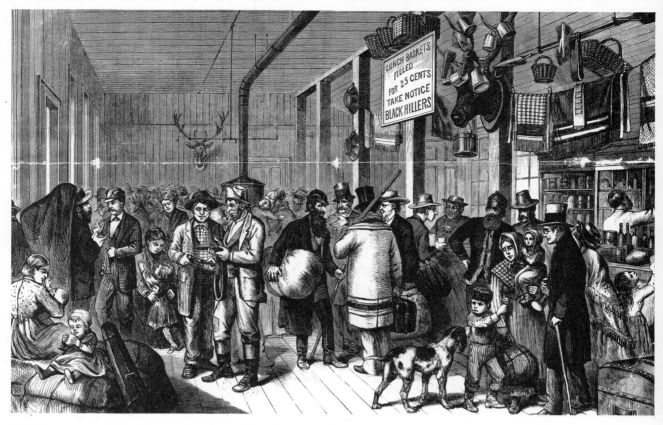

Waiting room of the Union Pacific Railroad in Omaha, Nebraska, in 1877. Here immigrants from many countries, lured by promises of choice land advertised by the States and the railroad companies, could stock up for the journey farther west.

came most cheaply in steerage. Steamships could now pick up new thousands of immigrants in remote ports of the eastern Mediterranean and of Asia.

German and French and Italian and other steamship lines competed for passengers, offering lower rates, better accommodations, and a new easy system of prepaid passage. Prosperous immigrants who had already settled in the United States could pay in advance for the tickets of friends or relatives who wanted to come. The steamship companies opened offices all over the United States. By 1890 the Hamburg-Amerika Line had three thousand of these. More than one-quarter of the immigrants in that year came on tickets that someone in the United States had paid for in advance.

Before the Civil War, revolutions in France and Germany and Italy and famines in Ireland prodded Europeans to leave. So too, in the later years of the nineteenth century, multiplying miseries drove out European peasants by the thousands.

Many of those peasants in western Europe who were lucky enough to own a few acres of land were losing their ancestral plots. The price of wheat in their home countries went down as the new railroads and cargo steamers brought wheat from the United States, from Russia, and even from India. A strange disease (phylloxera) was killing the grapevines in the Balkans. When Americans began raising their own oranges and lemons in the 1880's and when the French began keeping out Italian wines, Italian farmers with orchards and vineyards found themselves on the edge of starvation.

The Jews of Russia were being bar-

barously persecuted, and whole villages were murdered for their religion. Turks were slaughtering Syrian Christians.

Once again, there was plenty to get away from. And now that the United States was at peace, this country seemed more attractive than ever.

To generations of European peasants, owning a piece of land had been the sign of dignity, the beginning of freedom.

When President Lincoln signed the Homestead Act on May 20, 1862, America seemed to offer everybody the chance to be a landowner. The whole American West was begging for people. All you had to do was come. You only needed to be twenty-one years of age and to say that you intended to become a citizen. Then you picked a 160-acre plot of "homestead" land somewhere on the vast Public Domain that belonged to the United States government. If you simply lived on it and cultivated a part, then the whole 160 acres would be yours at the end of five years. You paid nothing but a small registration fee.

This was an Old World dream come true. Every man a landowner!

Before the Civil War, the Southern States had opposed this Homestead Act. They were afraid it would strengthen the anti-slavery forces by increasing the population of the Free States. As soon as the Slave States left the Union it was possible to pass the Act through Congress. Lincoln's simple aim was "settling the wild lands into small parcels so that every poor man may have a home."

But the "free" land was not really as free as it seemed. In the Western plains where most of the best homesteads were found, it cost labor and money to make wild land into a farm. Before anything could be planted, the ground had to be broken. The prairie grass had roots that grew in thick mats, unlike anything known in Europe. The familiar Old World plow would not cut through but was quickly twisted by the heavy sod.

The Oklahoma "Land Rush" which began at noon, April 22, 1889. At the firing of a starter's gun and the sound of a bugle, more than 20,000 people rushed in to stake their claims. Oklahoma was then still called "Indian Territory" because it was supposed to be reserved for Indians removed from the East.

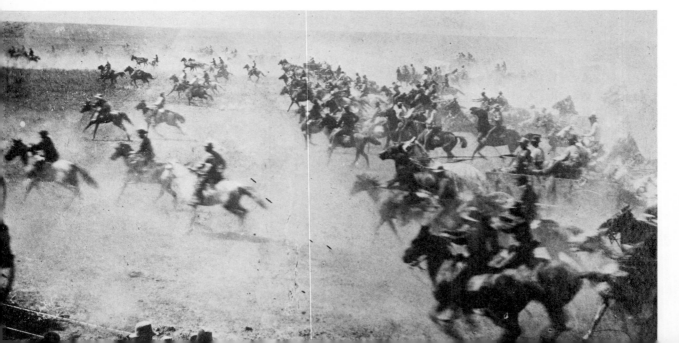

It was slow work to plow up enough land to support a family and it was expensive to hire a man with the right tools to do the job.

Then you needed to find water. Where streams and springs were rare, the only answer was to dig a well. And to pump up the water you had to build a windmill. On the treeless plains you had to buy the lumber for your house. Posts and barbed wire for fencing had to be brought from great distances. All this added up. You needed about $1,000 to make your homestead livable. That was a big fortune for a landless peasant.

Still, if you were healthy, willing to work year round, and not afraid to shiver for a few winters in a crude house of earth or sod, you might manage. The Homestead Act allowed you to be away from your land for six months each year without losing your claim. Some energetic homesteaders used this time to earn money by working as lumberjacks in the pine forests of Minnesota, Wisconsin, and Michigan. Others helped build the short "feeder" railroads that branched off through the countryside. Or they worked as farm laborers for their more prosperous neighbors.

Even if life was hard on the "free" lands of the West in the post-Civil War years, it still was not so bad by comparison with peasant life in Europe. What had been little trickles of immigrants from faraway places now became wide fast-flowing streams. For example, the old Austro-Hungarian Empire in eastern Europe, which had sent only seventeen thousand in 1880, sent over one hundred thousand in 1900, and seven years later, over a third of a million.

Americans worked hard at finding ways to attract the dissatisfied peoples of the world—to persuade them to come here instead of going to those English, French, or German colonies in Africa, South America, or the South Pacific which also wanted new settlers. Even before the Homestead Act, Western States sent their agents abroad. They helped immigrants with information and with loans.

More people in Wisconsin, for example, would mean more business for everybody there. Everybody's land would be more valuable. The State of Wisconsin therefore appointed a commissioner of immigration in 1852. He enlisted the aid of the United States consul in Bremen, Germany, and of other consuls elsewhere. He advertised in European newspapers and in a single year distributed 30,000 pamphlets about the glories of Wisconsin.

The Americans used the empty lands of their vast Public Domain to help pay for building the first railroads here. These were the lands that belonged to the United States government—land given to the new nation by the States at the time of the Revolution, land acquired from Napoleon in the Louisiana Purchase in 1803, land taken from Mexico in 1848.

After all, the government land might be worth very little if there was no way to reach it. The railroad companies would give the land value—in two ways. While they provided the transportation to open up the West, they would also be working as real-estate salesmen.

So the federal government assigned large tracts of land to the States with the understanding that the States would grant these lands to the companies that

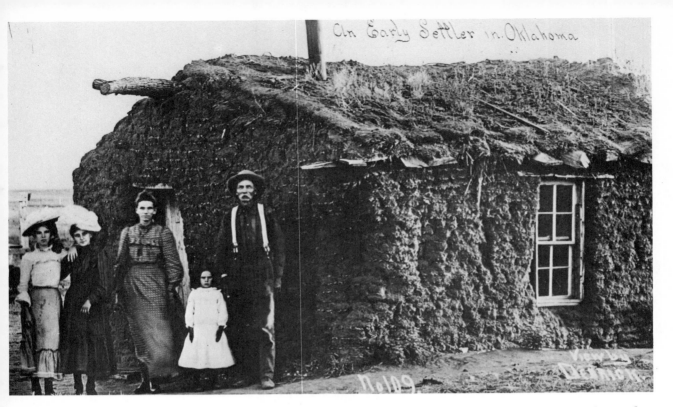

A sod house of the type common in the early West. This family was fortunate to have glass for a window. The teen-age daughters had perhaps been ordering the latest fashions from a mail-order catalog.

built railroads. And the federal government also granted some of its land directly to the railroad companies. These companies suddenly found themselves in the real-estate business.

Like the State governments, the railroad companies themselves became colonizers. They sent their own agents to Europe to attract immigrants to live along their tracks. These agents, too, helped with information and with loans. Sometimes they actually provided newcomers with a house while they were getting settled.

Often the railroad builders were granted the best lands in the West. And, anyway, once the railroads were built, the land near the tracks—since there were no automobiles and few roads—would be the most valuable. While railroad lands sold at higher prices, they were usually much more attractive than the more remote lands left over for dis-

tribution under the Homestead Act.

Land grants to the railroads finally amounted to about 150 million acres—an area almost as big as the whole State of Texas. Nine-tenths went to the companies that built railroads west of the Mississippi.

The first railroad company to receive a land grant from the federal government was the Illinois Central. The land along its future track was divided into a checkerboard pattern extending six miles from the track on each side. Each "section" in the checkerboard was one mile square (640 acres). The railroad was given every other square all along the way. The squares in between were kept by the federal government.

The Illinois Central Railroad extended four hundred miles from Chicago, the whole length of the State of Illinois. When it was completed in 1856 it was the longest railroad in the world.

And the company paid for the construction mainly by selling its two and a half million acres.

"Homes for the Industrious," the Illinois Central land salesmen announced, "in the Garden State of the West!"

> There is no portion of the world where all the conditions of climate and soil so admirably combine to produce those two great staples, Corn and Wheat, as the Prairies of Illinois. . . . Nowhere can the industrious farmer secure such immediate results for his labor as upon these prairie soils, the fertility of which is unsurpassed by any on the globe.

The railroad printed brochures, bought space in newspapers and magazines, and hired "runners" in New York City to mingle with arriving immigrants.

To Norway and Sweden, the railroad sent a super-salesman. Oscar Malmborg was a Swedish immigrant who had succeeded. After serving in the Mexican War, he had helped build the railroad in Illinois. From personal experience he could convince people that the railroad lands were really fertile. He sang the praises of Illinois Central land from Gothenberg at one end of Sweden through all the big cities to Bergen at the other end of Norway. He published 2,500 brochures in Swedish and a thousand in Norwegian. He planned meetings at churches and country fairs until he had covered the countryside of both nations.

Swedish farmers began to fear he would lure away all their laborers. To keep their laborers at home they invented horror stories. The Swedes who

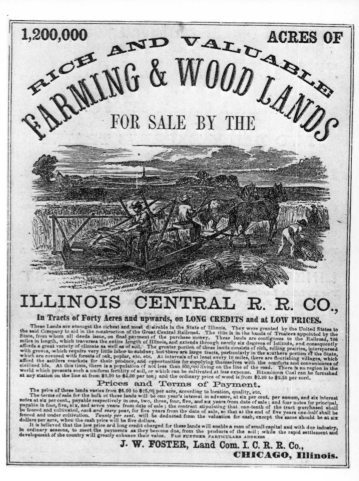

Advertisement by the Illinois Central Railroad to attract settlers to its lands.

arrived in New York, they warned, would be shipped to Siberia or sent as slaves to the Southern States. But in 1861, after Malmborg's successful campaign, nearly ten thousand Norwegians —a third more than in any earlier year —were planning to leave for America. The Swedish exodus was just as large. Even before the end of 1862 substantial new communities of Swedes and Norwegians had taken root near Chicago.

Scandinavia was only one of the immigrant sources. The Illinois Central hired the best-known German-born citizen of Illinois, Lieutenant Governor Francis Hoffmann, to cover Germany with a crew of salesmen. Within four years he settled Germans on eighty thousand acres of Illinois Central land.

To attract settlers from nearby Canada, an Illinois Central booklet claimed that while Canadian farms "are covered with huge boulders of granite, the summers are very hot, and the mosquitoes abound," the Illinois Central lands were a cool, mosquito-free earthly paradise. Colonies of hopeful Canadians were soon settled along the Illinois tracks.

CHAPTER 10

Crowding the Cities

Within the United States during these same years after the Civil War, there was another great movement of peoples —from the country to the cities. When the Civil War began, only one American in five was living in a city. By 1915, cities held half of all Americans. And this was only a beginning.

They came from everywhere. First of all they came from the countryside. While the railroad builders sent abroad their super-salesmen boasting the wonders of American farms, many American farmers were actually moving to the city. Older sections of New England offered visitors the sad spectacle of farms that had lost their farmers.

Many deserted farm villages seemed relics of a departed civilization. A traveler to one such village saw an abandoned church and a school half taken apart for its lumber. There were only two inhabitants, one living on each side of the broad street. Some of these farmers had gone west, but most had gone to the cities. By 1910 more than a third of all people who were living in American cities had moved in from American farms, many from the rural South.

Of the twenty-five million immigrants who came to the United States between the Civil War and World War I, most stayed in the cities. Outside of cities many of them would have felt lonely and lost. They loved the friendly bustle and wanted to be close to people like themselves. And some of them had no choice. They had spent everything to cross the ocean and had no money left for the trip west.

Within the big American cities there grew little immigrant cities. By 1890 New York City held twice as many Irish as Dublin, as many Germans as Hamburg, half as many Italians as Naples. And besides, there were large numbers of Poles, Russians, Hungarians, Austrians, Norwegians, Swedes, and Chinese. Four out of every five New Yorkers either were born abroad or were the children of foreign parents. The Germans and Irish who had come before 1880 were found nearly everywhere in the United States. There were also lots of Canadians in Boston and Detroit, Poles in Buffalo and Milwaukee, Austrians in Cleveland, and Italians in New Orleans.

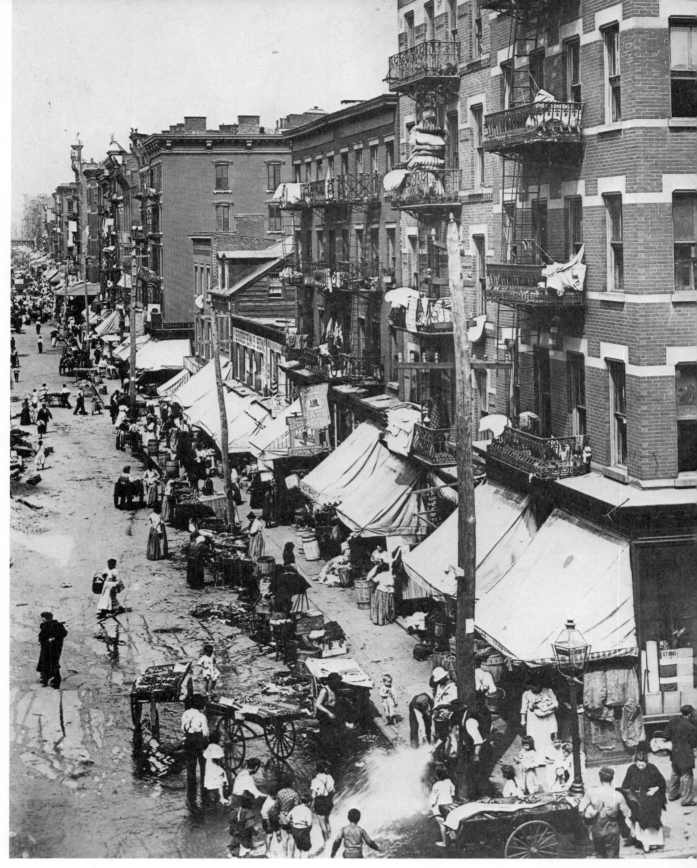

Crowded Hester Street, on the lower East Side of New York City (shown here about 1900), was where many immigrants settled on their arrival. Some who later became famous department-store owners started by selling from pushcarts like these.

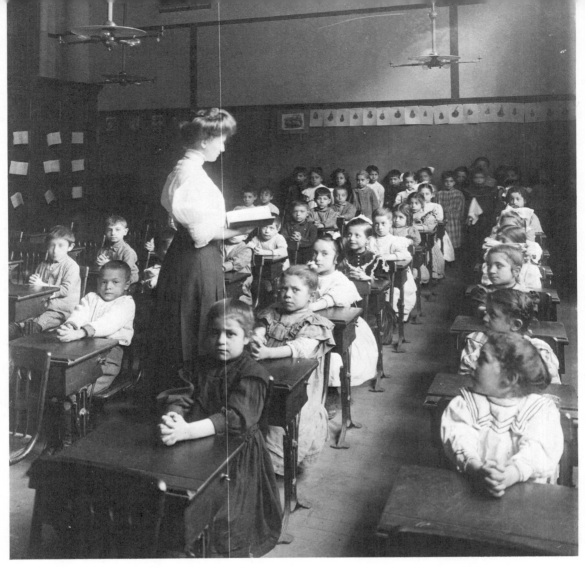

In a public school like this, the children of immigrants from many lands learned to speak and read English—and also learned American ways.

Cities were sometimes called the nation's "melting pots." Perhaps they should have been called "mixing bowls." The individual adult immigrant sometimes became Americanized only slowly. But very quickly his whole colony found its special place in American life. Just as the new United States had first been made from thirteen different colonies, now a great nation was being made from countless colonies of immigrants.

In New York City, for example, there were separate colonies from different parts of Italy. Italians from Naples and Calabria lived around Mulberry Bend,

those from Genoa had settled in Baxter Street, and Sicilians clustered about Elizabeth Street.

Wherever you came from, you could find a neighborhood in New York or in the other big cities where you could feel at home. Whether you were from Germany, Italy, Hungary, or Poland, you could shop in your own old-country language, buy familiar old-country foods, and attend a church offering your old-country services. By 1892 nearly a hundred newspapers in German were published in American cities. And there were dailies in French, Italian, Japanese,

Polish, Yiddish, and a dozen other languages.

In the making of Americans nothing was more important than the public schools. They were free, and the States passed laws requiring all children to attend. There the children of Irish, German, Italian, and all sorts of other families learned and played—and sometimes fought—together. They came to know one another better than their parents knew people from other countries.

At home many families spoke only Polish or Italian, but in school everybody spoke English. Even if the parents spoke English with a foreign accent soon the children sounded like all other Americans. And the children taught their parents. They not only taught them English, but all sorts of American customs. One little girl in New York City who had learned to use a toothbrush brought it home from school. She showed it to her mother, who had been born in a peasant hut in Poland and had never seen such a thing. Her mother, too, was soon brushing her teeth like an American.

Although these immigrant colonies tried to keep separate, they could not stay separate forever. People from the different colonies became more and more alike. Children who stopped speaking their parents' language sometimes stopped going to their parents' church. They were afraid to seem foreign. Then, too, a young man from the Italian colony might marry a girl whose parents spoke German. In the city, people could not help feeling closer to one another.

If the crowds were the joy of the city, crowding was the curse. Old World cities had grown mostly by children being born to the people already living there. The parents put a cradle in the room with the other children. As the family grew larger everybody was more crowded.

The American city was different. It grew by adding not just new children but whole new families.

In the crowded cities after the Civil War land was expensive. Unless you were rich you could not afford a private house. Still the thousands who came pouring in had to be put somewhere.

New York—the nation's biggest city and busiest seaport and the magnet of the world's immigrants—was where the problem was worst. And in New York, American know-how, which at the same time was building grand cast-iron palaces for department stores, produced another, but unlucky, American invention. This was the "tenement house."

New Yorkers, of course, did not invent the slum. European cities had their streets of ancient rickety buildings and evil-smelling hovels where the poor were tumbled together. But in the years after the Civil War, New York City produced a new kind of slum—the tenement-house slum.

Most newcomers to the city could not afford to pay much rent. Back in the early years of the nineteenth century the poorer people of New York had lived in shacks on the swamps at the edge of Manhattan Island. But as the island filled with people, specially designed buildings went up for the city's new poor. A tenement house was a building six or seven stories high designed to hold the largest possible number of families. They were solid blocks of deep buildings whose inside rooms had no windows or ventilation. There were also helter-skelter buildings of many other kinds.

Then in 1878, to help find something better, *The Plumber and Sanitary Engineer,* a builders' magazine, announced a contest for architects. The editors offered a $500 prize for the best plan for tenement apartments for the poor.

The winning plan was the "dumbbell" tenement. The floor plan of the whole building, looked at from above, had the shape of a dumbbell. And it had a good deal to be said for it compared with some of the flimsy firetraps that were common before. The dumbbell tenement, built of brick, was meant to be fireproof.

It was specially designed to fit on a narrow lot twenty-five feet wide and a hundred feet deep. It was six or seven stories high, with the stairway running up the middle. On each floor were four sets of apartments—two in front and two in back. The front and back rooms got some light and air from their windows on the street.

What was new about the plan was that the inside rooms were also supposed to get some light and air. The building was slightly narrower in the middle.

Although the prizewinning tenement design was supposed to provide "light, air, and health" for working people, actually whole families (like this mother and six children) were crowded into little rooms. The new art of photography made it easier for reformers like Lewis W. Hine (who took this picture) and Jacob Riis (who took the picture on page 59 above) to awaken the conscience of other Americans.

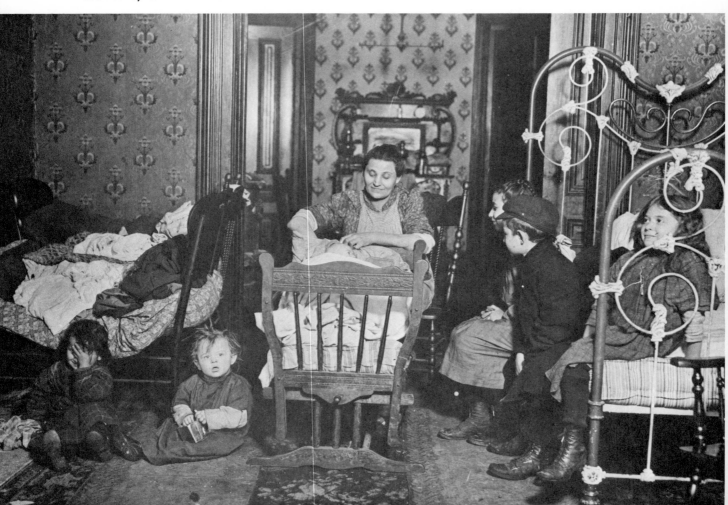

When another tenement like it was built alongside, between them there was a narrow air shaft on which each inside room had a window. This became the standard plan for tenements.

By 1900 the island of Manhattan alone had over forty thousand buildings of this type, holding over 1,500,000 people. A prizewinning plan had produced the world's prize slum!

The air shaft between the buildings was only twenty-eight inches wide—so narrow that it did not really bring in light. Instead the foul air brought up smells from the garbage accumulating at the bottom. If there was a fire, the air shafts became flues which quickly inflamed all the rooms around. Up the air shaft resounded the noise of quarreling neighbors. There was no privacy.

The primitive plumbing in the hallway on each floor was shared by four families. It bred flies and germs. Sometimes the toilets became so disgusting that the tenants would not use them, but depended on the plumbing at work or at school. There were no bathtubs with running water. Nearly every one of these tenement houses had at least one sufferer from tuberculosis, and in some there were twenty or more.

When Theodore Roosevelt was Governor of New York, he appointed a commission in 1900 to report on the tenement-house slums. They were not at all surprised that these buildings festered with poverty, disease, and crime. But they were surprised that in spite of it all, so many of the people raised there managed to become decent and self-respecting. And they reported that the slums were even worse than they had been fifty years before.

Slum neighborhoods were given names like "Misery Lane" and "Murderers' Alley." This was hardly the America that the thousands of hopeful immigrants were looking for.

CHAPTER 11

Whose Country? Oldcomers and Newcomers

The bulging cities and bustling factories were full of men and women who had been raised in the quiet American countryside—or of European peasants who had come across the ocean with high hopes. Here, they had been told, anybody could succeed, if only he was honest enough and worked hard.

But many honest, hard-working immigrants found that they could not get ahead. These disappointed new Americans would not take their disappointment lying down. The United States was the land of help-yourself. It is not surprising, then, that the post-Civil War years became a time of conflict. Workingmen were organizing into labor unions. Their aim was a better life—shorter hours, higher wages—but peaceful means did not always seem strong enough.

Beginning in the 1870's labor battles

became more common. In 1872, nearly a hundred thousand builders and mechanics in New York City went on strike. They refused to work longer than eight hours in any one day. After several months, they won their point.

Miners in the eastern Pennsylvania coal fields organized a secret society called the "Molly Maguires." In 1875, on flimsy evidence that private detectives had gathered for the employers, ten Molly Maguires were hanged for murder. Then in 1877 a railroad strike, beginning with workers on the Baltimore and Ohio, spread across the country. It brought death to nine persons in West Virginia and to twenty-six in Pittsburgh.

In 1886 came the so-called Haymarket Massacre when a bomb killed seven policemen and wounded seventy after they tried to break up a meeting of anarchists and communists. In a fight at the steelworks at Homestead, Pennsylvania, in 1892, seven were killed. The Pullman Strike in 1894 again tied up the railroads. This became a minor civil war when Federal troops began fighting against workers.

A conservative and law-abiding organization of trade unions, the American Federation of Labor, became strong among skilled workers. The Federation's aim was simply better wages and shorter hours. Meanwhile a small number of radicals called "Wobblies," who aimed to take the factories away from their owners, started the International Workers of the World.

All over the country crime showed an alarming increase. In 1890 the prisons held 50 percent more criminals than ten years before. And the murder rate in the

United States, already twice the rate in England or in Germany, was going up every year. National crime "rings" used hideouts in Chicago, Boston, Philadelphia, Detroit, and scores of other cities to help their members escape the police. The city crowds—at the Philadelphia Centennial Exposition of 1876, at the Chicago Columbian Exposition of 1893, and every day on streetcars or in department stores—were a pickpocket's paradise. Young hoodlums terrorized San Francisco with knives and six-shooters.

New expressions had to be invented to describe the assorted new criminals. There were "badger-game experts" and "knock-out drop" artists. "Green-goods" men tricked innocent farmers into exchanging their real money for large bundles of counterfeit. In 1880 one Go-Getting criminal from Springfield, Illinois, went to New York where he made a fortune selling "gold bricks." Before he was killed by a fellow thief,

Two Molly Maguires on trial, 1875.

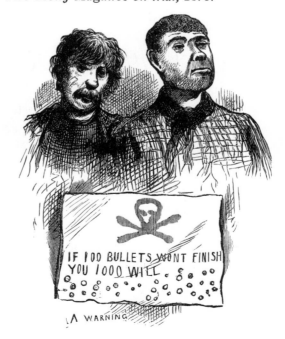

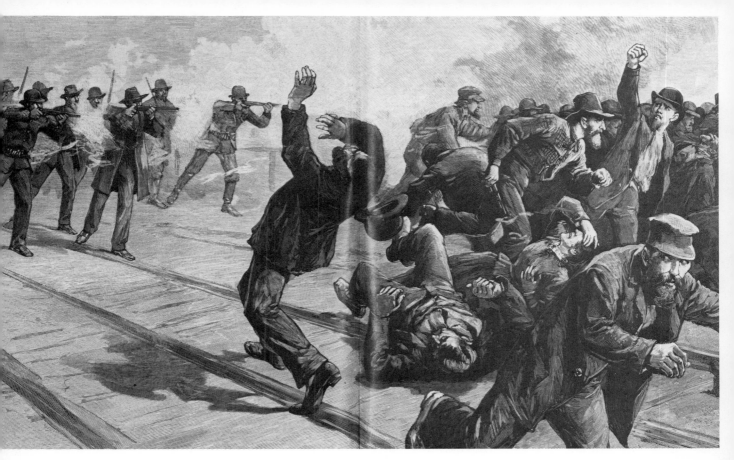

Police firing on strikers in East St. Louis during the railroad strike that began in 1877.

he actually had taken in over a quarter-million dollars from the lead bricks which he had painted gold before he sold them to gullible country boys. Stores with fancy goods on display naturally attracted shoplifters.

A ring working out of New York managed one of the biggest bank robberies in history. In 1878 from a single job they had planned for three years, they got three million dollars.

Meanwhile newspapers, anxious to sell more copies so they could attract more advertising, became more sensational than ever. They found that it paid to feature the worst crimes and to glamorize the worst criminals.

In business and in government too there were notorious scandals. Beginning soon after the Civil War, President U. S. Grant made a bad start. He was

so honest himself that he did not know a crook when he saw one. Some found their way into his Cabinet, and then used their position in the government to make a fortune for their railroads or their banks.

All decent Americans had reason to be worried. Was this the best that could be expected from what Jefferson had so hopefully called an "Empire for Liberty?"

The early American frontier had been a line on the outer edge of settlements. Beyond was the no-man's land where Indians had not yet given up and where settlers had not yet conquered. Out there a man could make a fresh start. In the Centennial Year of 1876, the defeat of Chief Sitting Bull and Chief Crazy Horse and their braves marked the last great battle between the Indians and

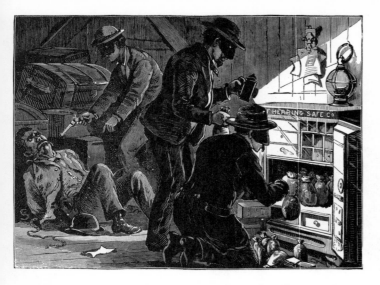

Sensational magazines like the Illustrated Police News *attracted their readers by playing up stories of crimes, such as the Indiana train robbery shown here.*

the invading settlers. Fifteen years later, the Superintendent of the Census reported that the wilderness-frontier had come to an end.

By the end of the nineteenth century, then, the New World had lost much of its newness. One bright young historian, Frederick Jackson Turner, who had been raised in the backwoods of Wisconsin, proposed the theory that this disappearance explained many of the country's troubles.

According to Turner, what had made America the Land of Promise was not its cities but its frontier. The free land out west, he explained, had also been a safety valve. In earlier times if a man in an Eastern city wanted a second chance, he could move to the West. But now that the country was being filled up it was no longer possible to find your second chance by going out to the edge of civilization. If you were unlucky enough to be a newcomer in a slum, there seemed to be no escape. Was it surprising, then, that so many Americans were unhappy? And that so many felt that

they had to fight for a better life?

For a while it seemed that the country might be divided between Oldcomers and Newcomers. Oldcomers themselves, of course, came from immigrant families originally, but their families had been here for a long time. Among them were the rich and famous. Few of them were crowded into slums.

In the older Eastern States that still controlled Congress, the Oldcomers were in charge. They were most of those who had money and education and power. But the Oldcomers did not agree on how to cure the country's ills. Some were simply frightened. They wanted to keep the country the way it was. They blamed the troubles on the Newcomers. Their answer was to slam the door. Simply because *their* families had been here longer they thought the whole nation belonged to them.

At Harvard College, a group of New England bluebloods thought that their world was coming to an end. Three young men in the graduating class of 1889, Charles Warren, Robert De Courcy Ward, and Prescott Farnsworth Hall, had been taught by their professors that there was an "Anglo-Saxon" race superior to all others. The race was supposed to be separated from other races not by color but by what countries the people had come from. The "superior" people were supposed to come from England and Germany. And that just happened to be where Warren's and Ward's and Hall's families had come from.

These young men had been raised near Boston. Their parents were horrified by the hordes of "vulgar" immigrants and especially by those with unfamiliar ways—from Ireland and from southern and eastern Europe. The New England aristocrats said the nation's problems could be solved by keeping out all people who were not like themselves.

Five years after their graduation, Warren and Ward and Hall formed the Immigration Restriction League to persuade Congress to pass laws to keep out all "undesirable" immigrants. In their League they enlisted famous professors and writers. Their real object was to keep out the "new" immigrants—the Newcomers. These "new" immigrants, they argued, were the main cause of the increasing crime, the strikes, and most of the troubles of the country.

To keep out "undesirables" they proposed a "Literacy Test." According to their proposed law anyone over fourteen years of age who wanted to come into the United States would have to prove that he could read and write. He did not have to know English, provided he could read and write the language of the country he came from.

At first sight the test seemed harmless enough. Actually it was aimed against the Newcomers from certain countries, such as Italy and Greece, where poor peasants had no chance to go to school. The Boston bluebloods believed that because Newcomers from such countries were not "Anglo-Saxons" they must be "inferior."

But in their proposed law they did not dare list particular countries. There

Poor Newcomers arriving in America while rich Oldcomers (with their governess) leave for a vacation in Europe. A magazine illustration by Charles S. Reinhart (1878).

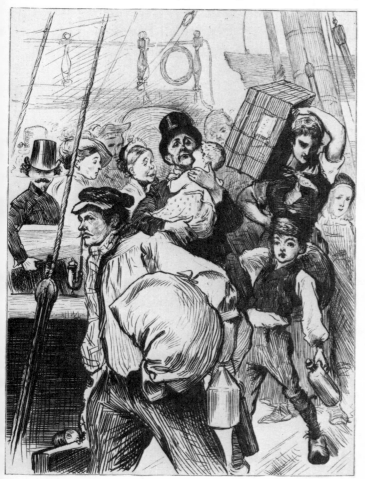
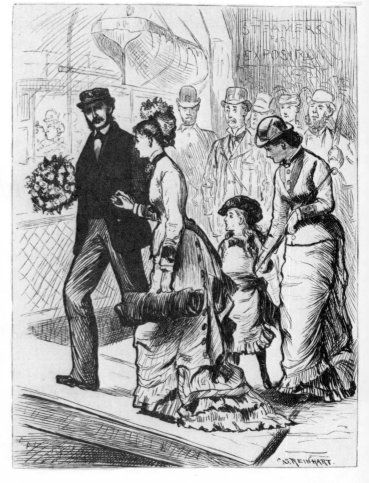

already were many people in the United States from those countries. They would be insulted—and they, too, elected members of Congress.

Year after year the Immigration Restriction League tried to persuade Congress to pass a Literacy Test. But even when they finally pushed their bill through Congress, they did not manage to make it into a law. One President after another vetoed the bill. President Grover Cleveland called the law "underhanded," because it did not say what it really meant. President William Howard Taft said the United States needed the labor of all immigrants and should teach them to read. President Woodrow Wilson agreed.

All three Presidents said the law was un-American. The United States had always been "a nation of nations." It made no sense to keep out people simply because they had been oppressed. America was a haven for the oppressed. Here the starving could find bread and the illiterate could learn to read.

In 1917, however, when the war in Europe was frightening Americans, the Literacy Test finally had enough votes in Congress. The law was passed, over the strong objections of President Wilson, who had already vetoed it twice.

Out on the West Coast, Oldcomers feared Newcomers from Asia. They worried about imaginary hordes that might come across the Pacific. And they had persuaded Congress to pass a Chinese Exclusion Act in 1882. Then, in 1907, President Theodore Roosevelt persuaded the Japanese government to stop their people from emigrating. For some odd reason, this was called a "Gentlemen's Agreement." This became the slang expression for any agreement to discriminate against people on account of their race when you were ashamed to admit what you were really doing. Since there were so few Chinese-American and Japanese-American voters among the Newcomers, the fearful few among the Oldcomers found it easier to have their way.

CHAPTER 12

Reformers and Self-Helpers

Not all the Oldcomers were frightened. Some became Reformers. If the whole country had troubles, they said, it was everybody's fault. If the country had too many strikes and too much crime, it could hardly be blamed on those who had just arrived.

It was mainly the fault, they said, of the Americans who had been here long-

est and who had had the most chance to make the country better. Who had built the very cities and constructed the very slums where the poor were condemned to live? Who were the Congressmen and Senators and businessmen and policemen? It was not the immigrant's fault if the nation was not prepared to receive him.

One of the most remarkable of the Reformers and one of the most original Americans of the age was Jane Addams. She was born with a deformity of the spine which made her so sickly that after graduating from college in 1882 she had to spend two years in bed. Her wealthy family sent her to the best schools and colleges, she traveled abroad whenever she wished. One evening in Spain after watching a bullfight—"where greatly to my surprise and horror, I found that I had seen, with comparative indifference, five bulls and many more horses killed"—she suddenly decided that she could waste her life no longer.

The trouble with people like her, Jane Addams decided, was that they had been caught in "the snare of preparation." To become leaders they needed long years of education. But this meant that they were kept out of action at the very time when they were most anxious to rebuild the world. Jane Addams knew that she and her friends needed more education than they could find in books.

In June 1888, she stopped in London to visit the famous Toynbee Hall. There in the poorest section of the city lived a group of Oxford and Cambridge graduates while they tried to help the people of the neighborhood. She decided to try starting something like it in the United States.

Jane Addams' plan was simple. In the poorest, most miserable city slum she would settle a group of educated young men and women from well-to-do families. Like Toynbee Hall, the place would be called a "settlement house." And the well-bred young men and women newly "settled" in the midst of

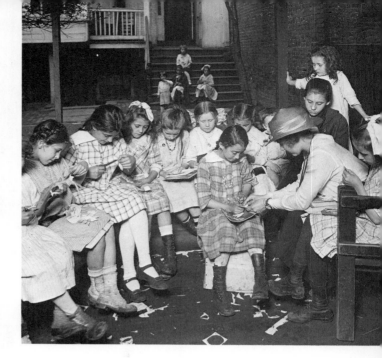

A young woman settlement-house worker with girls of the neighborhood.

a slum reminded her of the early colonial "settlers" who had left the comforts of English life to live in an American wilderness.

The young men and women who came to live in the slum, seeing the struggles of the poor, would learn things they could never learn from books. At the same time, the people of the slum would use the settlement house as a school, a club, and a refuge.

With her purpose clearly in mind, she acted quickly. Since she knew Chicago she decided to do her work there. She looked for the neediest neighborhood. And she persuaded the owner of a large old house to let her have it free. She opened her settlement house between an undertaker's parlor and a saloon. She called it "Hull-House" after the man who had built it for his home years before.

In the neighborhood of Hull-House there were Newcomers from all over Europe—Italians, Germans, Polish and Russian Jews, Bohemians, French Cana-

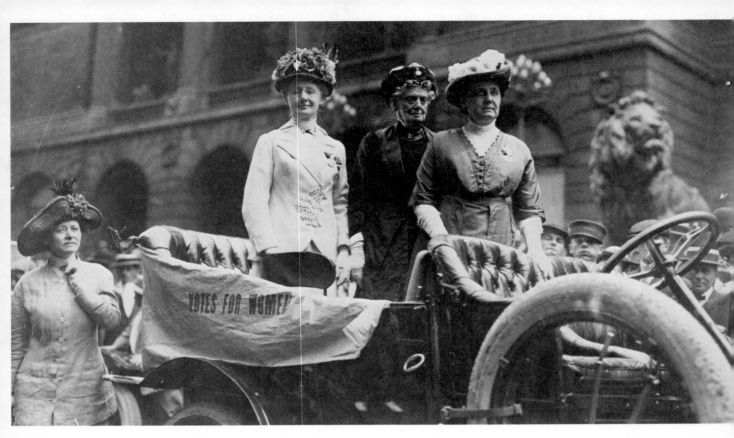

Jane Addams (right) in a parade supporting votes for women. The Nineteenth Amendment to the Constitution, prohibiting the States from depriving women of the vote, was finally ratified in 1920.

dians, and others. For the young, Jane Addams set up a kindergarten and a boys' club. And she paid special attention to the very old people whom nobody else seemed to care about.

One old Italian woman was so delighted at the red roses which Jane Addams displayed for a Hull-House party that she imagined they must have been brought all the way from Italy:

She would not believe for an instant that they had been grown in America. She said that she had lived in Chicago for six years and had never seen any roses, whereas in Italy she had seen them every summer in great profusion. During all that time, of course, the woman had lived within ten blocks of a florist's window; she had not been more than a five-cent car ride away from the public parks; but she had

never dreamed of faring forth for herself, and no one had taken her. Her conception of America had been the untidy street in which she lived and had made her long struggle to adapt herself to American ways.

Jane Addams' work became famous. All sorts of unexpected projects started at Hull-House. The Little Theater movement, of amateur actors putting on plays to entertain themselves and their friends, developed and spread all over the country. She started a book bindery and a music school.

Settlement houses on the Hull-House model appeared in big cities everywhere. Future playwrights, actors, composers, and musicians who had happened to be born into poor slum families now found their chance.

For the first time many thousands of immigrants discovered that somebody else cared about them. Jane Addams—without the aid of governments or politicians—had helped make America the promised land.

America had always been a land of help-yourself. Before long some of the most energetic Reformers came from the immigrants. But it was not easy for Newcomers to become leaders. So many respectable institutions remained in the hands of the Oldcomers—whose families had been here for a century or more. For example, Harvard College—the oldest college in the country, where young bluebloods had learned their ideas of Anglo-Saxon superiority—was run by Oldcomers. It was hard even to become a student there if you were not one of them.

New institutions offered the best chance for Newcomers. Among the most remarkable—and most American—of the new institutions were the scores of new colleges and universities.

At the outbreak of the Civil War there were only seventeen State universities. Then, in 1862 an energetic Congressman, Justin S. Morrill from rural Vermont, secured the passage of the Morrill Act. This act granted government lands from the Public Domain to States—30,-000 acres for each of the State's Senators and for each of its Representatives in Congress—to support new State colleges. There students would be taught to be better farmers. These were called "Land Grant" Colleges.

After the Civil War, hundreds of other colleges and universities were founded. In the later years of the nineteenth century, some of the wealthiest Go-Getters gave millions of dollars to found and endow still more institutions of higher learning. In 1876 Johns Hopkins University was founded by a fortune left by a Baltimore merchant. In 1885 a railroad builder, Leland Stanford, in memory of his son, founded Leland Stanford Jr. University. In 1891 John D. Rockefeller, the Go-Getting oil millionaire, founded the University of Chicago. And there were scores of others.

Many of these college-founders were men who themselves had never gone to college. But they shared the American faith in education. Even before the end of the century, the United States had more colleges and universities than there were in all western Europe. And a larger proportion of the citizens could afford to go to college here than in any other country. The children of poor immigrants, along with millions of other Americans, now had a better chance to rise in the world.

The new labor unions also became centers of new leadership and of self-

Mayor Fiorello La Guardia, during a newspaper strike, reading the comics aloud over the radio.

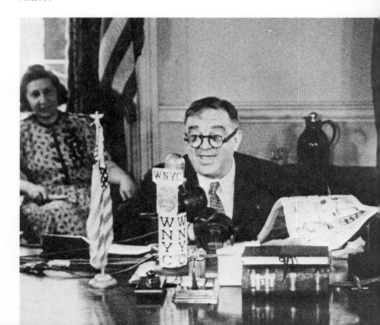

help. Samuel Gompers, who had been born in London, came to New York as a boy. He worked at starvation wages as a cigarmaker before becoming president of his Cigarmakers Union and then the first president of the American Federation of Labor (1886). Sidney Hillman, who came from Lithuania when he was twenty, led the Amalgamated Clothing Workers, the union that did most to help the new immigrants in big-city sweatshops.

In politics the support of your fellow immigrants counted for something. Crowded together in the cities, the immigrants of any one nationality found it easy to stick together to support one of themselves. Soon new political leaders from among the Newcomers themselves were livening up City Hall and even the halls of Congress, which began to sound like a United Nations. The representatives of Italian-Americans and German-Americans, and of the new arrivals from everywhere, gave a new spice to American politics.

One of the most colorful of these was Fiorello La Guardia. His mother and father had come from Italy, and Fiorello was born in New York City only three years after they arrived. His father, a musician, joined the army and soon became the leader of an infantry band. On an army post in Arizona in the 1880's Fiorello saw the pioneer West. He found it "a paradise for a little boy. We could ride burros. Our playground was not measured in acres, or city blocks, but in miles and miles. We could do just about anything a little boy dreams of. We talked with miners and Indians. We associated with soldiers, and we learned to shoot even when we were so small the

gun had to be held for us by an elder."

Out there La Guardia had his first glimpse of corruption. And it was something he would never forget. The men who had been paid to supply wholesome beef to feed the army were supplying diseased beef instead, and then pocketing the money themselves. La Guardia's father became so ill from eating this diseased beef that he had to be discharged from the army and a few years later he died. No wonder Fiorello spent his life fighting corruption.

For several years he worked at United States consulates in eastern Europe. He learned about the problems of the immigrants in their homelands. When La Guardia returned to New York in 1906 he joined the Immigration Service on Ellis Island. There the Newcomers were examined before being admitted to this country. La Guardia knew Croatian as well as German and Italian. While he worked as an interpreter, he learned the immigrants' troubles and the immigrants' hopes.

In 1917 La Guardia went to Congress, where he began his long fearless career of defending the poor and of fighting corruption. He carried on his fight when he became mayor of New York City in 1934. Now the city was his family and all the city's problems were his. With the broad-brimmed cowboy hat he had learned to wear out in Arizona, his familiar figure bounced all over the city. He especially liked to be on hand at trouble spots. Whenever there was a big fire La Guardia somehow arrived with the fire chief. In twelve years as mayor he did more than any New Yorker before him to remove the blot of the slum and to brighten big-city life.

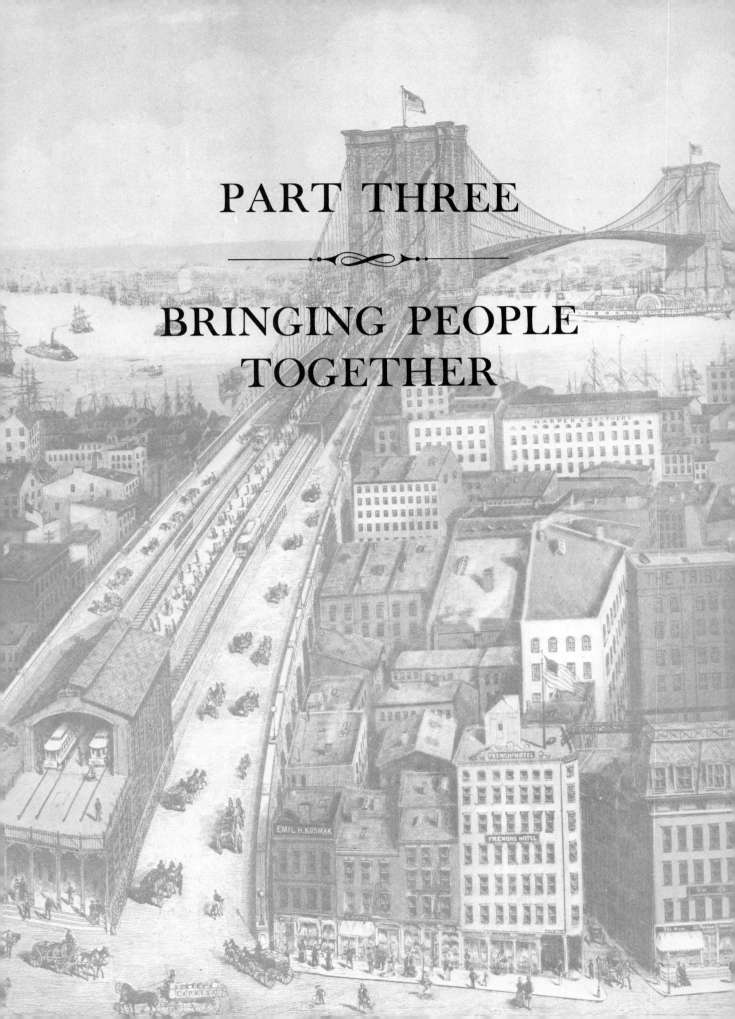

PART THREE

BRINGING PEOPLE TOGETHER

BRINGING PEOPLE TOGETHER

After the Civil War the United States was as large and varied as all western Europe. From the alpine heights of the Rockies and Sierras to the tropical everglades around the Gulf of Mexico there stretched nearly every kind of landscape.

And this variety made the nation more attractive to immigrants from all over. Just as the English could feel at home on the rolling landscape of "New" England, the Swedes felt less strange on the snowy stretches of Minnesota and the Dakotas, and Italians found familiar sunny seacoasts in southern California. The imported people spread across the land.

From Chicago to New York was as far as from London to Rome. And if you traveled all the way from London to Constantinople and back to London you had still not gone quite as far as if you went from New York to San Francisco. How could these spread-out people ever become a nation?

People in the United States wanted and needed new ways to feel closer together. This challenged American know-how. And American know-how—using telegraph wires, rails, and new-style bridges—organized new ways to bind a nation.

The nation of many cities remained a nation of many centers. Chicago and St. Louis and Denver, even before the end of the nineteenth century, were rivaling Boston, Philadelphia, and New York—the capitals of the eastern seaboard. And by mid-twentieth century Los Angeles on the Pacific was one of the nation's fastest-growing big cities.

Even before the continent began to seem overcrowded, American know-how, with materials and techniques borrowed from everywhere, sent skyscrapers high in the air, collecting thousands to live and work in a single towering building. In American cities— in the once-wilderness of open spaces and fresh air—people were close-packed together as never before.

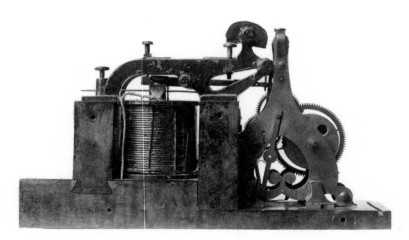

The telegraph instrument patented by S. F. B. Morse.

CHAPTER 13

Everybody Shares the News

Newspapers were not very newsy until nearly the time of the Civil War. They used up much of their space to print stories and poems and essays and the strong opinions of their owners. And they copied much of their "news" from other newspapers which arrived by slow mail. The best-known papers were owned or controlled by political parties. They praised their own side and slandered the other. If you wanted to know what was happening far outside your neighborhood you had to wait for a traveler to come by.

Businessmen and generals organized their own systems to send urgent messages over great distances. One of the oldest was the "semaphore" (from the Greek words meaning "signal-bearer"), sometimes called the "visual telegraph." People arranged in advance what their signals would mean. Then they built fires, sent up smoke, or arranged a pattern of boards on a high tower. All these could be seen at a far greater distance than the voice would carry. The Greeks and Romans and the American Indians had used rows of these semaphore stations to relay messages for many miles. By the mid-nineteenth century a French semaphore system used 556 separate stations to stretch three thousand miles.

In the 1840's a young New England Go-Getter, Daniel Craig, decided to try sending news by carrier pigeons. He ordered pigeons from Europe and trained them for his Pigeon Express. Soon newspapers subscribed to his service. In his boat he would go out into the Atlantic for many miles to meet a ship arriving from Europe. The captain would throw him a watertight canister containing the latest London newspapers. Then Craig would quickly summarize the news on thin pieces of paper. These he would attach to the legs of his pigeons, who swiftly flew to the newspapers.

His pigeons went all the way from Halifax, Nova Scotia, to a newspaper in Washington, D.C. The New York *Sun* even built a dovecote for its own carrier pigeons on the roof of its new building. But the pigeon service, too, was unreliable. And there was a limit to how much news a pigeon could carry.

It was hard to imagine a system that did not depend on seeing signals, or on sending written messages. Samuel F. B. Morse found a way to make an electric current do the job. Morse was a man of many talents. At Yale he painted portraits of his fellow students for five dollars apiece. Then he went to London where he studied at the Royal Academy,

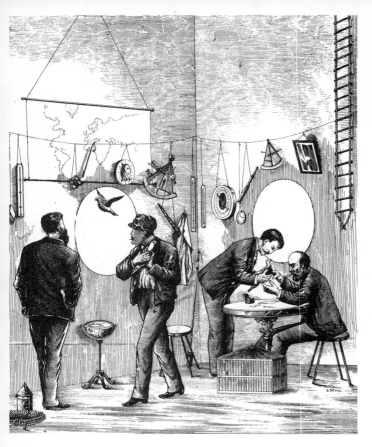

In the days before the telegraph or radio, sending news "by air" meant using carrier pigeons.

the honor society of English artists. When Morse came back in 1815 he was a famous artist but he nearly starved because people would not buy his large paintings. Once again he made a living by painting portraits. At the age of thirty he went to Italy and France, the headquarters for painting at the time.

Among Morse's fellow passengers on the sailing ship *Sully* coming back from Europe in 1832 was a talkative young physician from Boston, Charles T. Jackson. In Paris, Dr. Jackson had learned a great deal about electricity. To while away the six-week ocean trip, Morse asked him lots of questions. Morse was an educated man, but he still knew very little about the new science. Would electricity flow through a long wire?

How fast did it travel? Why, Morse asked, couldn't electricity be used to send messages? Others before him had asked the same question—and got nowhere with their answers. But Morse did not know enough about the subject to be discouraged. He suddenly decided to make an electric "telegraph" (from the Greek words for "far writer").

As an artist Morse had a bold imagination about new shapes of things. Then and there he began to invent his telegraph. In our National Museum of American History in Washington, D.C., we still have the shipboard notebook in which Morse every day wrote his new ideas. Before he reached New York he had drawn a picture of a telegraph instrument very much like that used today. He had even begun to use dots and dashes for his new Morse code.

"Well," Morse told the captain of the ship as they arrived in New York on November 16, 1832, "should you hear of the telegraph one of these days, as the wonder of the world, remember the discovery was made on board the good ship *Sully*."

It took Morse five years to make a telegraph instrument that would work. During that time he supported himself by giving painting lessons.

To build a telegraph line would require a small fortune. Most people thought the telegraph was nothing but a toy—"a thunder and lightning 'jim crack.'" Morse decided to change their minds by a public demonstration. He took his machine with him to Washington, where the Committee on Commerce of the House of Representatives allowed him to demonstrate his telegraph in the Capitol. It was a sensation. "The world is coming to an end," one witness declared. "Time and space are now annihilated." President Martin Van Buren and members of his Cabinet came to see the new electric marvel.

The chairman of the House Committee, Congressman "Fog" Smith of New Hampshire, saw his own chance to make a fortune. When he asked Morse to make him a partner in a firm developing the telegraph, Morse could hardly refuse. For Congressman Smith had the power to persuade the House of Representatives to give Morse the money to build a telegraph line.

The Congressional debate was hilarious. Opponents jokingly proposed that the money be split among Morse's telegraph and the supporters of hypnotism and the crackpots who believed the world was about to end. Finally, in 1843, eleven years after Morse had his first inspiration, Congress appropriated $30,000. With this money Morse was supposed to stretch a telegraph line from Baltimore to Washington.

At first Morse and his partners tried burying the wire. They spent $23,000 before they discovered that, because the wire was defective, the buried line would not work. They then started all over again by stringing a wire on poles. They were in a hurry to get the job done before the whole Congress began to believe the telegraph was a hoax. Mile after mile, they placed 24-foot-high chestnut poles two hundred feet apart. In holes they bored in the poles, they stuck the necks of old bottles which served very well as insulators.

Luckily, at that very moment in May 1844 both the main political parties were holding their national conventions

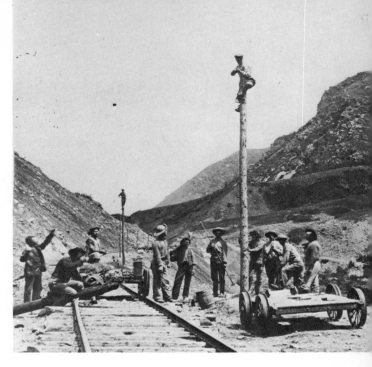

As the railroads pushed westward across the continent, telegraph lines kept pace.

in Baltimore. This gave Morse his chance to impress all the people in Washington who were especially anxious to learn the names of the candidates. But when the candidates were actually selected, Morse's wire still reached only twenty-two miles—from Washington to Annapolis Junction.

To demonstrate his telegraph, Morse had the news brought by train from Baltimore to Annapolis Junction. Then —to beat those who had to carry the news all the way by train—he flashed it over the wire to his telegraph receiving machine in the Capitol. The politicians there were amazed when Morse told them (before anyone else in Washington knew) the names of the Whig Party candidates—Henry Clay for President and Theodore Frelinghuysen for Vice-President. This was the first news ever flashed by electric telegraph.

The telegraph soon impressed people

by other sensational uses. When a thief escaped from Washington by train, his description was telegraphed ahead to the station in Baltimore. There he was arrested as he stepped off the train. Newspaper editors predicted that before long there would be no more crime, since criminals would be too afraid to be "struck" by this telegraphic "lightning."

Morse joined two newspapermen to form the Magnetic Telegraph Company. They built new lines—from Philadelphia to New York, from Philadelphia to Baltimore, and around to all the larger cities. By 1848 the telegraphic network reached northward to Portland, Maine, southward to Charleston, and westward to St. Louis, Chicago, and Milwaukee. Regular newspaper columns offered the latest bulletins under the heading "BY MAGNETIC TELEGRAPH." Newspapermen boasted of the "mystic band" that now held the nation together.

The Mexican War of 1846–48, the Gold Rush beginning in 1848, and the national troubles that foreshadowed a Civil War—all these whetted the Americans' appetite for news. And the more news people had the more they wanted.

Because it was expensive to gather news by telegraph, the newspapers came together in groups. Since they all shared the latest dispatches, each of them had to pay only part of the cost of telegraphing the news. In 1848 six New York daily newspapers formed the first Associated Press. Their man in Boston took the news brought by ships from Europe and put it in one telegram to the New York office. Then the Associated Press sold its speedy and reliable dispatches to newspapers in Boston, Philadelphia, and elsewhere.

Gathering and selling news became a big business. With the news-gathering experience of the Civil War behind them, Go-Getting newsmen extended the Associated Press throughout the nation. Then every member newspaper supplied its own local news to all the hundreds of other members. Since there were so many members, they could also afford to open offices with full-time reporters all over the world. This increased the quantity and improved the quality of news. The Associated Press stories tried not to be prejudiced or one-sided, for their readers were members of all political parties. Papers would not buy the "A.P." news unless it gave the straight facts. By the early twentieth century there was also a United Press and an International News Service.

At the same time many other new inventions were helping to turn out papers fast and by the millions. In the early nineteenth century an ingenious Englishman improved the presses used by big-city newspapers. Instead of using a frame that went up and down he used a cylinder. The blank paper was attached to the cylinder and rolled evenly against the type. This was much faster because the cylinder could be kept going continuously and a new piece of paper put in every time it went around.

Then Richard Hoe, a young New Yorker, had a still better idea. Why not put the *type* itself on a cylinder and roll the type smoothly and rapidly against the paper? By 1855, his Hoe Rotary Press was printing 10,000 newspapers in an hour.

The next step was to manufacture paper in long rolls instead of sheets. In 1865, a Philadelphian, William Bullock, made the first machine that printed on a continuous roll of paper—and it printed both sides of the paper at once. The finishing touch came with a gadget that actually folded the papers as they came off the presses.

Some metropolitan papers soon put out six different editions each day. Newspapers became larger and larger. Sunday newspapers—including advertisements, comics, magazine sections, book reviews, and everything else—became big enough to fill the whole day for Americans who did not go to church.

Richard Hoe's speedy web printing machine was among the new wonders shown in Machinery Hall at the Centennial Exposition in Philadelphia. This new-style press, instead of printing on separate sheets, used a continuous roll of paper, which could be more than four miles long.

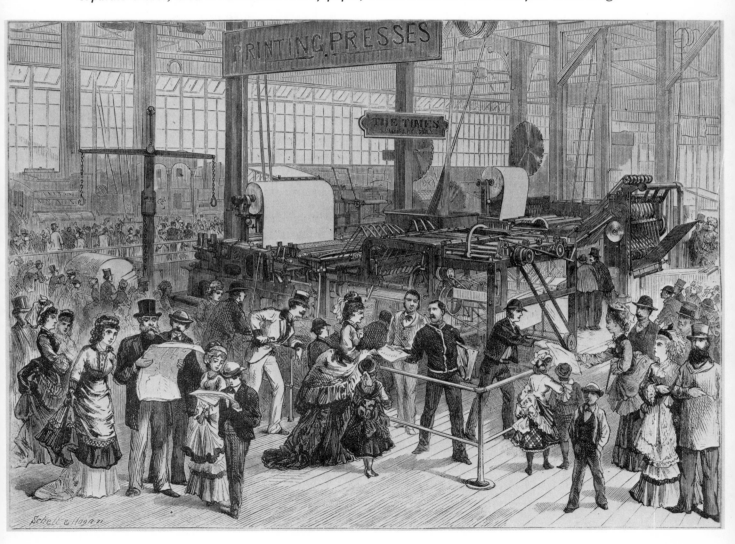

CHAPTER 14

Letters in Every Mailbox

A workable national mail system was slow in coming to the nation. The framers of the Federal Constitution in 1787 had given Congress the power "to establish Post Offices and Post Roads." A Post Road was a main road with special stations to provide fresh horses for the riders who carried the mail. For some years, almost all postal service was on one Main Post Road along the Atlantic coast. People used the mail very little. When George Washington was President the letters in the mail averaged less than *one* for every *twelve* Americans each *year!*

In those early years the postage on a letter was usually paid by the person who received it. If he did not want to pay the postage he never got your letter.

Of course there was no home delivery. To get your mail you had to go to the post office. Even after Philadelphia had a population of 150,000 everybody in the city who wanted his mail had to wait in line at the post office.

Then in 1825 came the dim beginnings of modern mail delivery. The postmaster in each town was allowed to give letters to mail carriers to deliver to people's homes. The carriers still got no government salary. They lived by collecting a small fee from anybody to whom they delivered a letter. If you were not at home to pay they would not leave your letters in your mailbox.

By the 1840's the growing country desperately needed a cheap and efficient postal system. The government service was still so haphazard and expensive that there was widespread demand to abolish the Post Office. People called it an "odious monopoly" and said that private businesses could do much better.

As a result in 1845 Congress passed a law establishing cheap postage and tried to reform the whole system. At first each postmaster printed his own stamps and there was chaos. Then, in 1847, the reformed Post Office Department issued the first national postage stamps—a five-cent stamp showing the head of Benjamin Franklin and a ten-cent stamp with the head of George Washington.

Now the postage would be paid by the person who mailed the letter. Some people objected. They said that if a person really wanted to receive a letter, the least he could do was pay the postage. Before postage stamps, people would simply fold their letters and write the address on the outside. But now letters became more private because everybody began to use envelopes which could be sealed.

With the growth of the railroads just before the Civil War it was possible to carry the mail much faster than on horseback or by stage coach. But when a train arrived at a railroad station and dropped several large bags of mail they had to be sorted all at once. That caused annoying delays. Then in 1865 the Railway Mail Service began using specially designed railway cars to sort the mail while it was in transit.

There were still problems of how to pick up mail from small towns along the track where the trains did not even stop for passengers. With a clever new gadget—the mail-bag catcher—the speeding train, as it passed, could snatch a bag of mail hanging beside the track.

Postage stamps, too, became a way of bringing Americans together. The pictures on stamps reminded the nation of its heroes (like Franklin and Washington) and told of great events, past and present. The first "commemorative" series of American postage stamps appeared in 1893 at the time of the World's Columbian Exposition in Chicago. Sixteen large stamps in different denominations showed scenes of Columbus and the discovery of America. In 1938 the Post Office issued a complete series of Presidents. From the very beginning the Post Office had a rule against using the images of persons still alive.

Even after postage stamps were introduced, at first they paid for delivery only as far as the post office. They did not include delivery to anybody's home. About the time of the Civil War, when private letter-carrying businesses were actually delivering mail to the home address on the envelope, they were often speedier than Post Office mail. To compete with them the Post Office began to provide the same service.

Finally in 1863 Congress provided a regular salary for letter carriers. They took the mail from the post office and delivered it to home addresses. This serv-

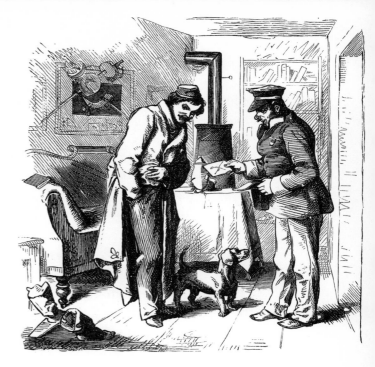

Paying the postman for a letter received.

ice was offered only in the cities. By 1887 a city had to have at least 10,000 people to be eligible for free home delivery. But most Americans still lived on farms or in small towns. As late as 1890 nearly three-quarters of the people in the United States never received a letter unless they went to the post office to collect it.

The old-fashioned system had its points. People did not receive "junk" mail they didn't want. The general storekeeper was commonly the village postmaster. When the post office was in a corner of the general store—between the drygoods and the farm tools—the system brought customers to the general store. There, too, farmers would enjoy meeting friends from the whole countryside who had come for their mail.

But it was also a nuisance. The farmer never received mail unless he came to town. He was out of touch with the news. No wonder the farmer had a reputation for being out-of-date.

In 1889 a Go-Getting department-store pioneer from Philadelphia, John Wanamaker, became Postmaster General. He saw that it was time for a change. The whole nation would profit if *everybody*—not just the city dweller—had mail delivered to his mailbox. Wanamaker's plan would finally bring the mail to the farmer. It would be called "Rural Free Delivery"—RFD for short.

"RFD!" became the farmers' battlecry. And there really was a battle. On one side were the farmers who wanted mail-order catalogs and mail-order packages and newspapers delivered to their doors. They wanted to be in touch with the world every day. On the other side were the village storekeepers. They wanted to keep the farmers coming into their stores to get their mail—and incidentally to do some shopping. If it became too easy to shop by mail, the farmers

might buy all their goods from Sears and Ward's and the country stores would lose their customers.

At the same time, in the 1890's, many American farmers in the West were suffering from drought and hard times. Farmers were organizing in their Grange Clubs (which had supported Ward's) and in their Populist political party. And many city people, too, wanted to help the farmer—especially if it could be done in some way that would help make the cities prosper.

In 1896 Congress adopted RFD. Incidentally, Congressmen were glad to create lots of new jobs—and perhaps win new votes. In one of the great American organizing achievements of the nineteenth century, the Post Office laid out nine thousand new routes in one year. The Postmaster General approved the design for a standard rural mailbox, which ever since has been the trademark of country life.

RFD helped open the world to the farmer. Now when he ordered from Sears and Ward's, his goods came promptly by RFD. Soon farmers insisted on—and were getting—the latest styles and the newest improvements. The farmer was no longer a "back number" as he used to be called.

Now, at last, he shared with other Americans all the news of the world. When his only way of receiving mail had been his weekly trip to the village, no sensible farmer would subscribe to a daily newspaper. Who wanted an armful of stale newspapers once a week? But now the newspaper came to the farmer's mailbox every day. In 1911 over a billion newspapers and magazines were delivered over RFD.

A Railway Mail Service employee aboard a moving train, using the improved "catcher" to snatch a mailbag from a post beside the track.

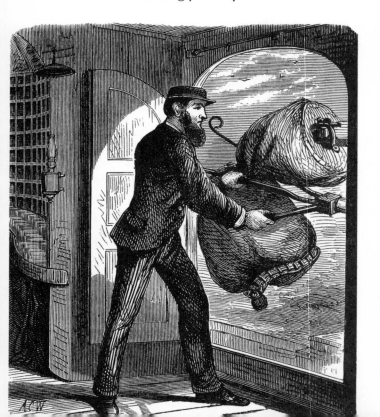

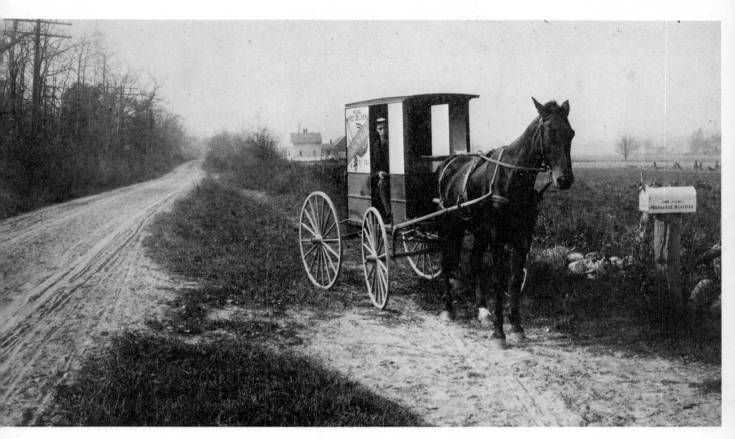

In the days before the automobile, mail wagons like this brought letters and packages by Rural Free Delivery to the farmer's own mailbox.

CHAPTER 15

The Sun Is No Longer Boss ⟡⟡⟡⟡⟡⟡

In the days before the railroad, people did not worry much about being on time. George Washington or Thomas Jefferson did not consider a person late simply because he arrived fifteen or twenty minutes after the time they had agreed on. When Benjamin Franklin listed in his *Autobiography* the thirteen virtues he would practice till he became perfect in them, he included "sincerity" and "cleanliness"—but he did not include punctuality.

In colonial days it was hard to be on time anyway, because watches were expensive and not many people carried them. Most people depended on the clock they saw—or heard—on the town hall or the church steeple. "Grandfather clocks" struck the hour and the half-hour to tell time to people who had no watches. If you took a trip, there was no regular timetable. Stagecoaches left whenever they had arrived from some other place or whenever the driver and

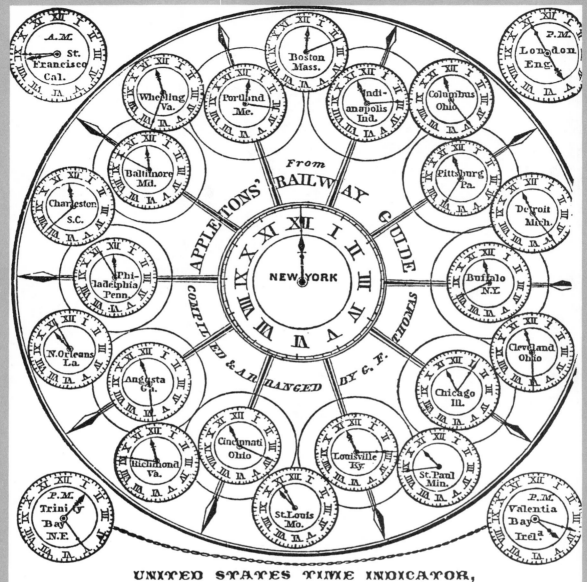

UNITED STATES TIME INDICATOR,

Showing the Difference of Time between the various Cities of the United States : including San Francisco, California ; Trinity Bay, Newfoundland ; Valentia Bay, Ireland ; and London, England.

It will be perceived, by glancing at the "Indicator," that when it is noon at New York, it is 12 minutes past 12 00 at Boston, 25 minutes past 1 00 at Trinity Bay, 24 minutes past 4 00 P. M. at Valentia Bay; when it wants 15 minutes of 9 00 A. M. at St. Francisco, Cal., it wants 5 minutes of 5 00 P. M. at London, England. Thus, by a little calculation, the reader will readily perceive the difference of time between the several points, and obviate the necessity of moving the hands of his watch to be in time.

There is no standard railway time in the Union, each Railway Co. adopting the time where its princ pal office may be located ; we would, therefore, su gest to the traveller the necessity of consulting t "Indicator," and, if possible, to be at the depot son few minutes previous to the departure of the trains

To TRAVELLERS.—As our object is to publish *reliable Guide*, regardless of expense, we woul thank the travelling community if they will notif us of the incorrectness of a Time Table, and we wil not only exclude it from the "Guide," but notit the public of the same.

Before Standard Time. This cover of Appletons' Railway Guide *shows the time in different cities when it was noon in New York.*

the horses were ready.

In a stagecoach on a good road you might average five miles an hour. After the railroads were built you could average forty. And you could travel on schedule. When a single track was used for trains in both directions, the engineer had to know exactly what time the train was due from the other direction so he could be on the siding to let it pass. Trains ran by the minute.

And now, with trains speeding from city to city, there were strange new problems that nobody had ever noticed before. The trouble was that every town had its own clocks set to its own particular time. The astronomers said that it was "noon" when you saw the sun reach its zenith—the highest point in the heavens. Since the earth was constantly in motion, and since the sun rose sooner when you were more to the east, then when it was noon obviously depended on *where* you were. Since you saw the sun rise earlier if you were in New York than if you were in Chicago, and still earlier in Chicago than in San Francisco, the time was different in those places.

There actually was a difference in the "astronomical" time, between any two places if one was to the west of the other —that is, if the places were on different longitudes. When it was precisely noon (that is when the sun had reached its zenith) in Boston, it was still only 11:56 in the morning in Worcester (slightly to the west). And when it was precisely noon in Chicago it was already 12:06 in Indianapolis (slightly to the east).

Cities became as patriotic about their own time as about the splendor of their city hall or the grandeur of their hotel. In every city the people said God had given them their "own" time, when He fixed the sun in the heavens.

Imagine what this meant for a railroad! The Pennsylvania Railroad tried to use Philadelphia time on its eastern lines. But that was 5 minutes earlier than New York time and 5 minutes later than Baltimore time. In Indiana there were 23 different local times, in Illinois 27, and in Wisconsin there were 38.

Even in any one town people disagreed about what the time really was. Each jeweler might have his own special time, which his customers were loyal to. To keep business running smoothly, and so that people would know when the stores would open and close, and when to meet their appointments, each city somehow had to announce its own time. Some used chimes on a town clock. Others blew a whistle or used a ball, called a "time ball" (held up on a pole in a conspicuous place) which was dropped at the precise moment of noon.

Generally the railroads used the local time for their arrival in each station. In between cities there was the greatest confusion. Yet for speeding express trains a few minutes could make the difference between a clear track and a fatal collision.

It is not surprising, then, that railroad men were among the first to try to bring order out of this confusion. But it was not easy. If you began tampering with their time, citizens were as outraged as if you tried to change the name of their city. And, of course, the astronomers really had a point. If you measured time by the sun in the heavens, then it was not man but nature that had made the confusion. And then perhaps nothing could be done about it.

But maybe, others said, this way of handling time was only a matter of habit. Suppose people simply stopped using sun time or astronomical time. And suppose that instead they used a new kind of "Railroad Time"—which could be the "Standard Time."

Suppose you managed to persuade the different cities along the railroad line to set their clocks to the same time. Take, for example, the train which ran west from Boston to Worcester. Although Worcester's astronomical time was 4 minutes earlier than Boston's, the people of Worcester might be persuaded to set their clocks to the same time as those in Boston.

For the United States as a whole, you could mark off on the map a few conspicuous time belts—up and down the whole country. You would need only four—Eastern Time, Central Time, Mountain Time, and Pacific Time— each several hundred miles wide. Standard Time would be exactly the same for all the places within each belt. At the edge of each belt, the time would change by a whole hour. These time belts would be marked on all maps, and then everybody could know exactly what time it was everywhere.

This was a sensible plan. But it took many years to persuade Americans. The leader of the campaign was William Frederick Allen, an energetic man who was not afraid to make enemies. He had seen the confusion when he had been an engineer on the Camden and Amboy Railroad before he joined the staff of the *Official Guide of the Railways*. And he made time reform the main purpose of his life. Allen aimed to provide a railroad timetable that everybody could understand and could rely on. This would help make railroad travel safer and speedier. His plan for Standard Time finally was adopted by the railroads to go into effect at noon, November 18, 1883.

Everywhere people prepared for the dramatic moment. At 11:45 in the morning according to the old Chicago time, conductors and engineers gathered in the lobby of the railroad station in Chicago. With their old-fashioned stem-winding pocket watches in their hands they looked at the clock on the wall. When the official Chicago railroad clock reached noon, it was stopped. The switch instantly connected it by telegraph wire to the new official clock for the whole Central time belt. At what would have been 9 minutes and 32 seconds past noon by the old Chicago time, the clock was started again. The railroad men all set their watches. Now everybody was on Standard Time!

Some people still objected. They thought the railroads were trying to take the place of God. "It is unconstitutional," warned Mayor Dogberry of Bangor, Maine, "being an attempt to change the immutable laws of God Almighty and hard on the workingman by changing day into night." He told churches not to ring their bells according to the new Standard Time. The editor of the Indianapolis *Sentinel* was outraged:

> The sun is no longer boss of the job. People—55,000,000 of them—must eat, sleep and work as well as travel by railroad time. It is a revolt, a rebellion. The sun will be requested to rise and set by railroad time. . . . People will have to marry by railroad time, and die by railroad time. Minis-

ters will be required to preach by railroad time.

One minister in Tennessee was so disgusted at this effort to take the place of God's own sun time that he took a hammer into his pulpit and smashed his watch to pieces just to shock his congregation.

But others found reason to be pleased. "The man who goes to church in New York on November 18th," applauded the New York *Herald*, "will hug himself with delight to find that the noon service has been curtailed to the extent of nearly four minutes, while every old maid on Beacon Hill in Boston will rejoice to discover that she is younger by almost 16 minutes."

Gradually people forgot their outrage. They discovered that it was wonderfully convenient to have Standard Time. One city after another changed its clocks to agree with the clock on the railroad station. In 1918 Congress finally gave the Interstate Commerce Commission the legal power to mark off time belts. The government simply followed the time belts that William Frederick Allen had persuaded the railroads to adopt thirty-five years earlier.

Standard Time helped to draw all the nation's railroad lines together. But other steps were needed too. In 1860 there were about 350 different railroad companies and about 30,000 miles of railroad tracks in the United States. Yet there was not really a national railroad network.

The main reason was that the many railroad lines were not on the same "gauge." The gauge is the distance between the two rails, measured from the inside of one rail to the inside of the other. There were many different gauges. Some railroad builders put their tracks six feet apart but some put them closer together, and there were at least eleven different gauges in general use. A railroad car that would just fit the six-foot gauge would not run on the narrower gauges.

If you wanted to send a package any distance by railroad it had to be taken out of the car that fitted one gauge and moved into a car to fit the gauge of the next railroad. In 1861 a package sent by railroad from Charleston, South Carolina, to Philadelphia, had to change railroad cars eight times.

Moving a package from one railroad to another made work for porters and teamsters. At the same time the passengers, who had to wait in the town while they changed trains, made business for hotels, restaurants, and storekeepers. Naturally enough, then, town boosters were not anxious to have all railroads on the same gauge.

From the beginning, quite a few lines happened to have the same gauge. George Stephenson, the English railroad inventor, had designed his locomotive to measure 4 feet 8½ inches between the wheels—the usual distance between wheels on a wagon. When Stephenson locomotives were imported to the United States, they had this "Standard Gauge." And many early railroad lines naturally built their tracks to fit the imported trains.

By 1861 about half the railroad tracks in the United States were on Standard Gauge. These were mainly in New England and the Middle Atlantic States, where most of the early railroads had

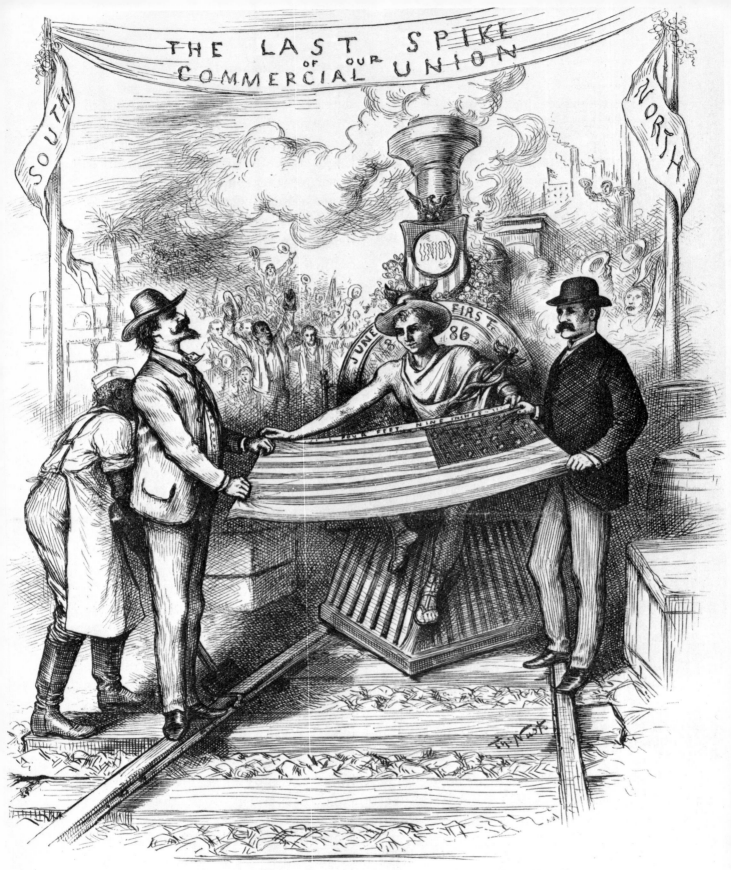

OUR STANDARD (GAUGE) ADOPTED ALL OVER THE UNION.

Thomas Nast, who drew this cartoon, came to New York from Germany as a child. He supported the Radical Republicans, attacked corrupt politicians, and invented the Republican Elephant and the Democratic Donkey.

been built. But the other half of American railroad tracks were on every sort of gauge—from about three feet to about six feet.

The Civil War brought an urgent need to ship arms and men quickly across the country. In the Confederacy, lines which ran into Richmond on Standard Gauge were hastily connected to one another. Now passengers and freight could go straight through. In the North, too, the war hurried progress. For the first time through service connected New York City with Washington, D.C.

At the end of the war Americans, North and South, saw the overwhelming advantages of a uniform gauge. And when the transcontinental railroad was completed with Standard Gauge in 1869, that settled the question. Now if a railroad builder wanted to join the traffic across the continent, he had to set his rails 4 feet 8½ inches apart.

By 1880 about four-fifths of the tracks in the United States had been converted to Standard Gauge. Most of the other gauges were in the Old Confederate South. Finally, in 1886, representatives of Southern railroads decided to change the gauge of all their 13,000 miles of track to the national standard.

A month in advance, crews went along loosening the old track. They measured the distance for the new Standard Gauge and put spikes along the wooden ties. On May 31 and June 1, 1886, the men worked frantically. One record-breaking crew on the Louisville and Nashville Railroad changed eleven miles of track in 4½ hours. June 1, 1886, was a holiday along the Southern tracks. By 4:00 P.M. the Southern railroads had joined the Union.

CHAPTER 16
Company Towns and Garden Cities

The American West was known for its "instant cities." Even before the Civil War, these grew quickly if they happened to be located at way stations where the westward travelers passed—at the joinings of riverways, on lake ports, at railroad terminals, or near new mines. As these cities grew, their boosters competed with one another to attract new settlers who, of course, would also be new customers. Each city hoped to become "bigger and better" than all the others. Some of them—Cincinnati, Chicago, Denver, Omaha, Kansas City, and others—became the great cities of the new Middle West.

But after the Civil War, as the whole country became more citified, there grew up new kinds of instant cities. These had not been way stations on the road west. They were found all over the country. At first their aim was not to grow big, but to stay small—and so escape the troubles of the crowded metropolis. They were actually planned— by businessmen, real-estate developers, and others—and they had common patterns.

Businessmen were looking for new places to put their factories. Workers were anxious to escape the dumbbell tenements and the darkened, crowded cities. Prosperous merchants and lawyers and doctors were eager to raise their families out in the open air.

With the new railroad network there was less reason than ever for factories to stay in big cities. Almost everywhere along a railroad line would do. For raw materials could be brought in from anywhere and finished products could be transported to anyplace.

Then why not build a "Company Town"? If an industrialist built his factory away from a big city, the workers would not have to live in slums. Where land was so much less expensive, each worker could have an attractive little house with his own garden. The employer could provide parks and playgrounds, and workers might be more content. After the Civil War many energetic businessmen had this idea.

In 1881 Andrew Carnegie, a Go-Getting steel industrialist, built a steel plant and a whole new town called Homestead seven miles up the Monongahela River from Pittsburgh. Besides small houses for the workers and their families, Carnegie provided a library and even bowling alleys. Homestead was not beautiful, but at least it lacked the crowds and the filth of the city slums.

George M. Pullman, inventor of the Pullman sleeping car for railroads, also decided to build a new town ten miles outside Chicago. In 1884 he bought a tract of land on the shores of Lake Calumet. He named it after himself and hoped it would be a model for other Company Towns. Pullman's architect designed the whole town, including a central square with town hall, churches, a library, and parks. All the buildings, including the small houses for the workers, were of dark-red brick.

Then in 1893 Granite City was founded outside St. Louis, to manufacture "graniteware" pottery. The Diamond Match Company and the Pittsburgh Plate Glass Company built Company Towns near Akron, Ohio. The United States Steel Company in 1905 built Gary in Indiana (not far from Chicago), named after Elbert Henry Gary, the head of the company.

Company Towns sprang up all over the country. There workers escaped the worst horrors of the big city. But they found some new horrors. Living in a Company Town was something like being a feudal serf in the Middle Ages. The company not only controlled your job, but it also decided where you would live, where (and at what price) you could buy your food. The company controlled your schools, and even hired your police.

Some of the most violent strikes were in these Company Towns. When the Carnegie Steel Company cut wages at its Homestead plant in 1892, the angry workers went on strike. In the resulting violence a dozen men were killed. When the Pullman Company cut wages but kept up its rents during the business depression of 1893, their whole town went on strike against the company and for months the nation's railroads were paralyzed. For Americans who wanted to run their own lives the Company

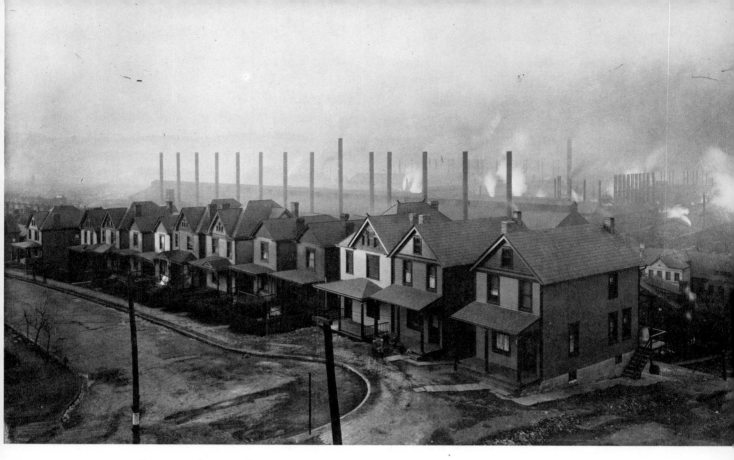

Homestead, Pennsylvania, the company town built by Andrew Carnegie, where workers escaped the city slum but lived in a pall of smoke from the blast furnaces.

Town was a spiritual failure.

But the Company Town was not the only new-style instant city which appeared at the end of the nineteenth century. On the "suburban frontier" there appeared the Garden City. An English reformer, Ebenezer Howard, who had come to America as a young man and had spent five years around crowded Chicago, tried to design a suburban utopia. Howard's *Garden Cities of Tomorrow* (1898) was his blueprint for a better life. He wished to combine the best features of the city and the country. He urged people to group together to build Garden Cities—new small towns out in the country. These towns, he said, should be planned with a garden belt all around. Then, if the Garden City was

connected to the big city by a railroad, it gave its residents the best of both worlds.

Some rich men who owned summer houses in the country near cities began living out in the suburbs year-round. For example, some businessmen who worked in New York City preferred living in Old Greenwich, Connecticut, three-quarters of an hour away on the railroad. Since there was not enough traffic to persuade the railroad to stop there, they would hop on or off the train outside Old Greenwich as it slowed down for a bridge. By the 1880's when enough New York businessmen were living there, they built their own railroad station, and the train stopped for them. These rich suburban pioneers built their own country clubs, and tried to keep their communities "exclusive"—for Oldcomers.

Soon other Americans, following Ebenezer Howard's advice, were building Garden Cities. These were no longer only for the very rich, but they were not yet for people of modest means. Lake Forest outside Chicago and Shaker Heights outside Cleveland showed a special effort to make the Garden City more romantic than the big city. Instead of the monotonous parallel streets of checkerboard city blocks, the Garden City streets wound up and down the hills and by the trees of the countryside. Wide lawns separated the houses from the roads and from one another. Before long, Garden Cities like Radburn, New Jersey, were being specially planned for people of modest income. In 1910 a New York architect made a new design for space-saving "garden apartments" with "kitchenettes" (a new American word for a compact kitchen and pantry). Now you no longer needed to be rich to live out in a garden suburb.

Ebenezer Howard's diagram (1898) of the ideal arrangement of lands in a Garden City. Houses were to be built in a circle around a park. Outside the Circle Railway there were to be farms and forests.

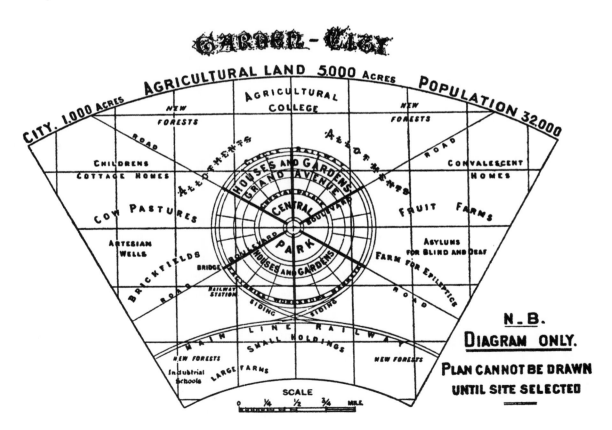

CHAPTER 17

Bridge-Building Heroes

Many fast-growing American cities had started on the banks of wide rivers. To expand, they had to find ways of carrying the railroad—and thousands of daily passengers—out beyond the old city limits. The growth of these American cities, and their ability to hold their citizens together, depended on their ability to span the neighboring waterway. Go-Getting American engineers transformed the ancient art of bridge building to help the cities to reach out to their new frontiers.

Something about bridge building specially attracted the American inventive genius. James Buchanan Eads, the man who built the bridge for St. Louis, had first shown his inventive talents during the Civil War as an adviser to the Union navy. In 1861 he proposed a fleet of ironclad gunboats to control the Mississippi River. When the government took up his suggestion he manufactured the needed ships in sixty-five days. After the war the people of St. Louis, which was on the west bank of the Mississippi, saw that they had to bring the railroad across the wide river and into their city if St. Louis was to grow.

Many different schemes were offered. But all were rejected until Eads appeared. As a boy he had worked on a river steamboat. When only twenty-two years old, he had invented a diving bell to salvage ships that had sunk in the river. And then he had done a lot of walking underwater on the very bottom of the Mississippi. He knew that river bottom almost as well as other men knew the city streets.

What Eads had learned was important. Building a bridge across the Mississippi depended first on finding solid support under the sandy river bottom. As Eads had moved along 65 feet below the surface of the water, he saw the swift currents churning up the sands. He knew that the supports for his bridge would have to go far below those river sands—all the way down to bedrock.

In 1867, when Eads began construction, his first problem was to lay the foundations of the two stone towers which would hold up the arches of the bridge in midstream. The towers would rise 50 feet above water level. The foundation of one would have to go down 86 feet below water level, and the other, where bedrock was deeper, had to go down 123 feet. But was this possible?

Eads's plan was to use his own diving bell together with some new caissons—watertight working chambers—that had recently been perfected in England. The 75-foot-wide caissons would keep out the water while the men dug, and the men would keep digging beneath the river sands until they reached solid rock.

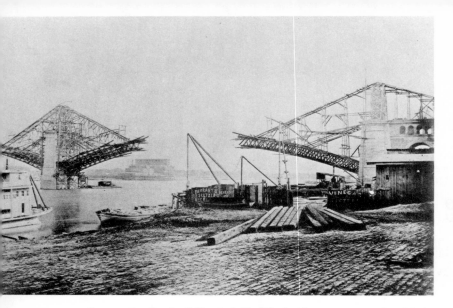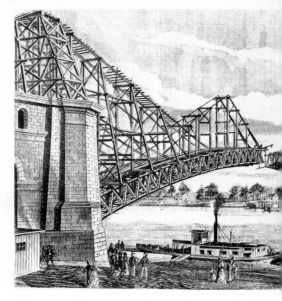

Stages in the building of Eads's bridge to span the Mississippi River at St. Louis. From the two stone towers in midstream, steel arches thrust out to meet arches thrusting from other towers on the shore.

When his men finally reached bedrock, they were working ten stories below the surface of the water! Because of the great pressures at that depth, the men could stay down only 45 minutes at a time. They had to come up slowly. Between shifts they rested long periods. Despite all precautions thirteen men died of "caisson disease" (sometimes called "the bends") from too rapid change in air pressure.

The Mississippi River boatmen and ferrymen feared competition from the new railroad that would cross the bridge. They tried to persuade the Secretary of War to dismantle the towers when they were half built. President U. S. Grant knew St. Louis and he had faith in Eads. He knew the bridge would be important to the future of the city and to the growth of the Middle West. And he saw that it would help bind the nation together. He ordered the engineers in the War Department to keep the project going.

For the three vast arches of the bridge Eads decided to use steel, though it had never been used in such a large struc-

ture. When the usual carbon steel did not meet his tests, he ordered large quantities of the new chromium steel, and then supervised its production. While chromium steel was more costly, it was rustproof and needed no covering.

It took Eads seven years to bridge the Mississippi. Finally in 1874 in a grand ceremony the former Union general, William T. Sherman, pounded the last spike of the double-track railroad crossing the bridge. Then fourteen locomotives, two by two, chugged triumphantly across the river. President Grant came to St. Louis to proclaim Eads an American hero.

And there were other heroic bridge builders who helped open ways to the suburban frontiers. Few other cities were quite so hemmed in by water as New York. Manhattan Island, heart of the city, was surrounded by the East River, the Hudson River, and the Atlantic Ocean. For a half-century there had been proposals for a bridge across the East River, connecting lower Manhattan Island to Brooklyn. When the fierce winter of 1866–67 stopped all ferry

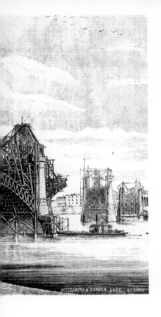

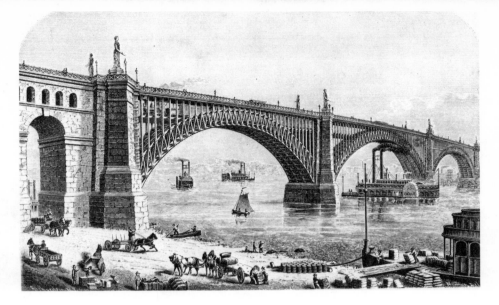

service and isolated Brooklyn from Manhattan for days, it was plain that something had to be done.

John Roebling was ready with a plan. When he came to the United States from Germany as a young man he opened the first factory for making wire rope out of many strands of wire twisted together. This new material was wonderfully suited for reaching over wide rivers where it was difficult or impossible to build masonry towers in midstream. From high towers on both ends you could suspend the strong wire rope to hold up the bridge.

If the Niagara River, for example, was to be spanned near the Falls, it would have to be by such a "suspension" bridge. In 1855 Roebling completed a wire-supported bridge over the Niagara —strong enough to carry fully loaded trains. This feat made John Roebling famous. In 1860 he completed another suspension bridge, just outside Pittsburgh, reaching a thousand feet across the Allegheny River. And by 1867 he had completed still another outside Cincinnati, across the Ohio River.

A suspension bridge, Roebling style, could solve New York's problem. For the bridge from Manhattan to Brooklyn had to stay high above water level in order to allow the sails and smokestacks of large ocean-going vessels to pass underneath. Roebling's ambitious plan in 1867 proposed towers 271 feet above water level, holding up a main suspension span of 1,595 feet.

During the very beginning of construction in 1869, a ferry crushed John Roebling's foot against the dock and he died from tetanus infection in two weeks. John Roebling's son, Washington Roebling, was ready to carry on. He too was a man of courage. He had enlisted in the Union army as a private on the day after President Lincoln's first appeal for volunteers. By the time of the Battle of Gettysburg, young Washington Roebling's services had earned him the rank of colonel. On the second day of the battle, with his own hands he helped drag a cannon up to a strategic hilltop, and so helped to prevent the defeat of the Union Army.

On his father's death, Washington Roebling at once took over the building of the bridge. In 1872, when fire in the Brooklyn caisson threatened the whole project, Roebling stayed below in the

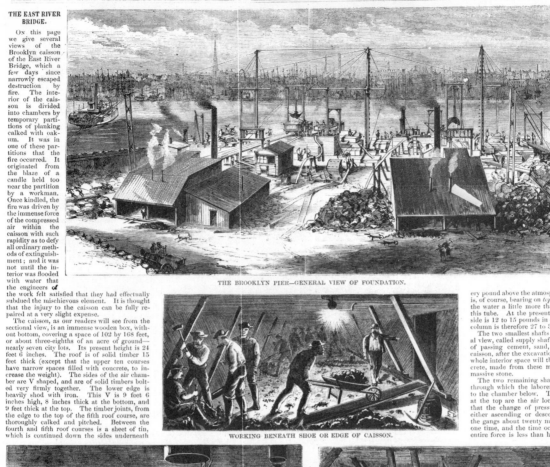

THE EAST RIVER BRIDGE.

ON this page we give several views of the Brooklyn caisson of the East River Bridge, which a few days since narrowly escaped destruction by fire. The interior of the caisson is divided into chambers by temporary partitions of planking called with oakum. It was in one of these partitions that the fire occurred. It originated from the blaze of a candle held too near the partition by a workman. Once kindled, the fire was driven by the immense force of the compressed air within the caisson with such rapidity as to defy all ordinary methods of extinguishment; and it was not until the interior was flooded with water that the engineers of the work felt satisfied that they had effectually subdued the mischievous element. It is thought that the injury to the caisson can be fully repaired at a very slight expense.

The caisson, as our readers will see from the sectional view, is an immense wooden box, without bottom, covering a space of 102 by 168 feet, or about three-eighths of an acre of ground—nearly seven city lots. Its present height is 24 feet 6 inches. The roof is of solid timber 15 feet thick (except that the upper ten courses have narrow spaces filled with concrete, to increase the weight). The sides of the air chamber are V shaped, and are of solid timbers bolted very firmly together. The lower edge is heavily shod with iron. This V is 9 feet 6 inches high, 8 inches thick at the bottom, and 9 feet thick at the top. The timber joints, from the edge to the top of the fifth roof course, are thoroughly calked and pitched. Between the fourth and fifth roof courses is a sheet of tin, which is continued down the sides underneath

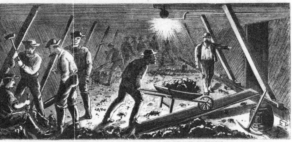

WORKING BENEATH SHOE OR EDGE OF CAISSON.

the outside sheathing; this is intended to prevent all escape of air from the inside.

The air or working chamber is divided by massive timber trusses or frames into six rooms, in each of which fifteen to twenty men are employed. Some are drilling the immense boulders preparatory to blasting, others pulling stone from the trenches by means of tackle; gangs of men are wheeling material that has been excavated and dumping it into the pools under the water-shafts, and here others are constantly shoving the material under the shafts, from whence it is taken by the dredging buckets. The interior is lighted by fourteen calcium lights; the gas

being led into the caisson through pipes connected with receivers placed outside.

The caisson is supported mainly by blocks placed 12 feet apart in the trenches, and wedged tightly up to the frames, and the lowering is effected by clearing material from under the V, and in taking out the blocking and replacing it at a little lower level. The movement downward is imperceptible, but it goes on steadily at an average rate of three inches per day.

The water or excavating shafts are essentially barometers, which measure accurately the pressure of air in the caisson. The shaft is the barometer tube, but is filled with water instead of mercury, and the pool at the bottom is the cistern. Every pound above the atmospheric pressure (which is, of course, bearing on top of the column) forces the water a little more than two feet higher in this tube. At the present time the pressure inside is 12 to 15 pounds in excess, and the water column is therefore 27 to 34 feet high.

The two smallest shafts shown in the sectional view, called supply shafts, are for the purpose of passing cement, sand, and gravel into the caisson, after the excavation is completed. The whole interior space will then be filled with concrete, made from these materials, forming one massive stone.

The two remaining shafts are the air shafts, through which the laborers descend by ladders to the chamber below. The enlarged cylinders at the top are the air locks, and it is in these that the change of pressure is experienced in either ascending or descending. In changing the gangs about twenty men enter each lock at one time, and the time occupied in shifting the entire force is less than half an hour. One of the air pipes from the compressors enters one of these shafts, and the other one of the supply shafts.

The spaces left around the shafts are inclosed by coffer-dams, to prevent water entering from without through the masonry. There are now 18 feet of masonry completed. It is of massive blocks of limestone and granite, weighing from one and a half to six tons each. The arrangement of derricks and railway track is so complete that it is not an uncommon thing to unload and set twenty of these blocks in an hour.

There were used in the construction of the caisson over 3,000,000 feet, board measure, of yellow pine timber, and about 35 miles of bolts.

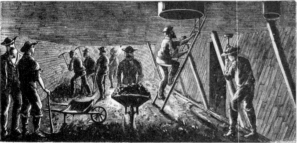

AIR CHAMBERS FOR THE INGRESS AND EGRESS OF WORKMEN.

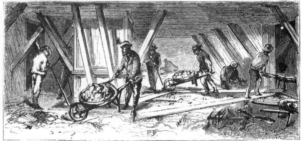

SENDING UP DÉBRIS THROUGH THE WATER SHAFT.

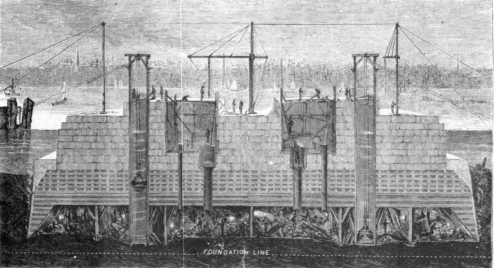

SECTIONAL VIEW OF FOUNDATION, SHOWING CAISSON AND MASON-WORK.

Building Brooklyn Bridge was one of the wonders of the age. The problems of working far underwater were just as challenging as the later problems (brought by the skyscraper) of working far into the air.

compressed-air chamber for seven hours. As a result he acquired "caisson disease."

Washington Roebling never fully recovered. Too weak to supervise the bridge on the spot, he would sit in a wheelchair in his apartment and watch the work through field glasses. Then he would give instructions to his wife, who carried them down to the bridge. All his communications with the world were through her. Efforts were made to remove him from the job, but his mind remained active and he would not give up the command.

At 1:30 on the afternoon of May 24, 1883, fourteen years after John Roebling had begun the job, President Chester A. Arthur and his Cabinet joined with Governor Grover Cleveland of New York for the formal opening of the Brooklyn Bridge. Six warships anchored below the bridge fired a resounding salute, and from the center of the bridge came a dazzling display of fireworks. The orator of the occasion declared that this, the world's greatest bridge, was a triumph of "the faith of the saint and the courage of the hero."

The "saint," Mrs. Roebling, herself attended the celebrations. But Washington Roebling, the heroic bridge-building son of a heroic father, was too ill to leave the room from which he had overseen the work. The President of the United States went to Roebling's simple apartment at No. 110 Columbia Heights to give his congratulations.

CHAPTER 18

Going Up!

Oddly enough, although the growing United States had lots of land to spare, the most distinctive American way for a city to grow was not to stretch *out*. After the Civil War, Americans began using their own know-how—together with materials and know-how from all over the world—to stretch their cities *up*. Although some Americans were moving to the suburbs, more people than ever before wanted to live and work right in the center. Businessmen wanted to be where the action was. And many people who could afford to live in the suburbs, still preferred to live downtown.

With old kinds of construction the tallest buildings had seldom been over five or six stories high. There were two problems which had to be solved before buildings could go higher.

The first problem—how to get the people up and down—was beginning to be solved even before the Civil War. In a few luxury hotels, elevators already carried guests up to the fifth and sixth floors. And in some early department stores the elevator was an attractive curiosity.

But elevators were thought to be dangerous. People feared that if the rope holding up the elevator cage should

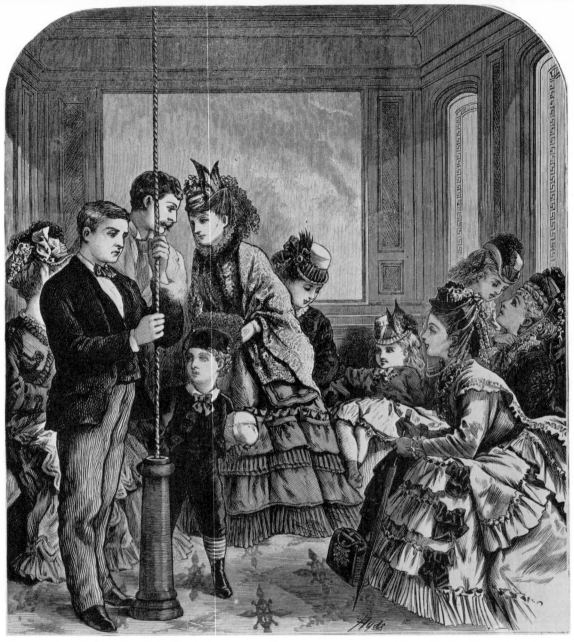

On opening day at Lord & Taylor's, a new department store in New York City, the elevator was one of the chief attractions.

break, the passengers would drop to their death. Elisha Graves Otis found a way to dispel the public fears. He invented a simple automatic safety brake. If the rope broke, instead of the cage plummeting to the bottom, the brake would automatically clamp the cage safely to the sides. Otis staged a demonstration in New York in 1854. He rode the elevator to the top. Then an attendant cut the rope while breathless spectators watched. As the cage was clamped in place, Otis bowed nonchalantly to the crowd.

Otis' early steam-driven elevators moved only 50 feet a minute, which amounted to about half a mile an hour. To Americans, who now could speed along on railroads at forty miles an hour, this steam-driven "vertical railway" seemed to climb like a snail. But before 1880 the improved "hydraulic" elevators (pushed up by water pressure in a long vertical cylinder) were climbing at 600 feet a minute. By 1892 an electric motor was carrying passengers up so fast that it "stopped" their ears.

The second problem—how to hold up the building—began to be solved when James Bogardus and others had used cast iron for their Buyers' Palaces. No longer was it necessary to build a tall building like a pyramid, with thick supporting walls on the lower floors. Cast-iron construction helped the department stores keep the lower floors wide open, with broad vistas and narrow pillars, allowing attractive show windows in between. But iron construction also made it possible to build higher and higher. Soon an eight-story building like Stewart's Cast Iron Palace would seem small.

The time was ripe for the "skyscraper." Of course Bogardus was only dreaming when he forecast buildings "ten miles high." But he was not far wrong when he told American builders that only the sky would be the limit.

Bogardus himself constructed one of the first buildings of true skyscraper design. Its frame was a tall iron cage. If the cage was strong and rigid, and solidly anchored at the bottom, then the building could go up high without needing thick walls at the bottom. This was "skeleton" construction. The building was held up, not by wide foundations at the bottom, but by its own rigid skeleton.

The first time Bogardus actually tried this, his structure did not have any rooms at all. It was a skeleton-framed tower for an ammunition factory. In those days lead shot was made by pouring molten lead through a sieve inside a high tower. The little liquid balls of lead dripped through, a few at a time. As these plummeted down through the air they became naturally rounded. And as they fell into the tank of water at the bottom they hardened into their rounded shape—ready for use in a rifle or a cannon.

In 1855, when the McCullough Shot and Lead Company needed a new shot tower in New York City, Bogardus gave them his radical new design. He built them an octagonal iron tower eight stories high. A tall iron cage, it needed no filled-in, weight-bearing walls to hold it up. Yet it was strong. When the openings in the iron frame were covered with brick, it served just as well as any heavy column of stone.

It was one thing to build a shot tower but quite another to trust the lives of hundreds to such a newfangled way of building. The first real try was in Chicago where the pioneer was William Le-Baron Jenney. An adventurous man of wide experience, he had helped build a railroad across Panama before there was any canal. In the Civil War he served on General Sherman's staff as an engineer.

In 1884 when the Home Insurance Company decided to construct a new office building in Chicago, they gave him the job. Jenney, who had probably heard of Bogardus' shot towers built twenty years before, decided himself to use an iron skeleton. In the next year his building was completed.

Even before Jenney's first skyscraper was completed, a better new material had been perfected. This new material was steel. The first six floors of the Home Insurance Building had been

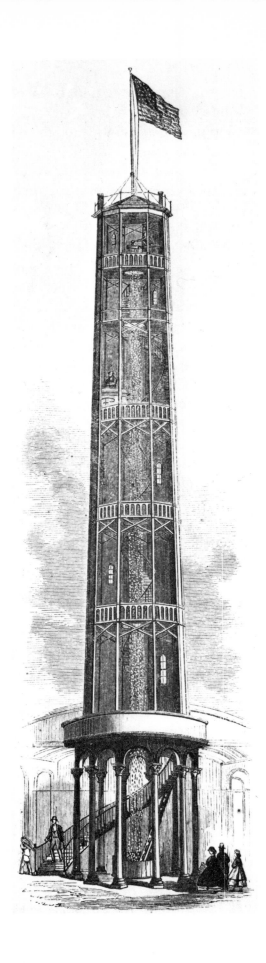

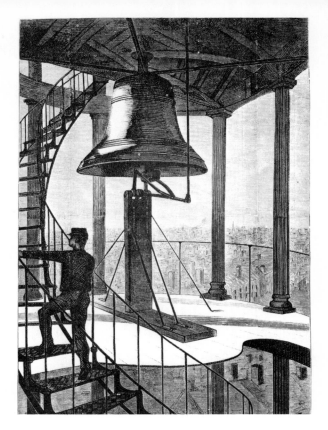

LEFT: *In the Bogardus tower, pieces of lead became rounded as they fell through the hollow center down into a well of water below.* ABOVE: *A New York City fire tower, also designed by Bogardus. The drawing is by Winslow Homer, who first became famous from his Civil War drawings for* Harper's Weekly. *Later he settled on the coast of Maine and had a second career as a painter of fishermen and the sea.*

framed with wrought iron. The top three stories were framed in steel. Steel, like wrought iron, was made almost entirely from iron ore, but steel was far superior. While wrought iron was easily shaped into beams and connecting plates, it bent readily. It was not ideal for a skyscraper frame. Steel was the answer. And it was the material that made higher and higher American skyscrapers possible.

Though men had known how to make steel for centuries, the process had been difficult and time-consuming. Therefore steel was so expensive that it was used only for small objects. The swords used by knights in the Middle Ages were made by endlessly hammering and re-heating and then again hammering the blades. Until the mid-nineteenth century this was the usual way to harden iron to make it into steel.

Then an Englishman, Henry Bessemer, invented his new mass-production steel furnace. By blowing air through the molten iron mass, the carbon in it was burnt out much more quickly. Now it was possible to produce a hundred tons of steel from a single furnace in twelve hours. Before the end of the nineteenth century, the United States—borrowing English methods, improved by American know-how—was producing about twice as much steel as Great

Steel skeleton for a pioneer skyscraper, Chicago's Reliance Building, 1894.

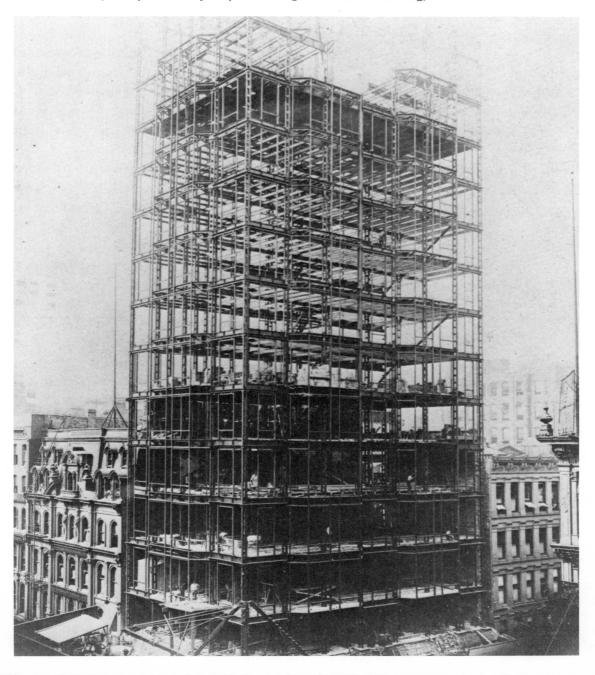

Britain, and now led the world. Better, cheaper steel meant more tall buildings.

Jenney's example in Chicago was followed in New York. The skeleton system was especially useful for building high structures on the tiny lots of crowded Manhattan Island. In 1888 an architect, Bradford Gilbert, was asked to design an 11-story building on Broadway, on a lot that was only 25 feet wide and 103 feet deep. With the old-fashioned heavy masonry the walls would have had to be so thick on the ground floor that there would have been no space for any rooms there. Gilbert designed a true iron-skeleton building— the first in New York City.

At first the building inspectors refused a building permit for Gilbert's Tower Building because they believed that no iron-skeleton building could stay up. Even after the building was completed, Gilbert had to show his confidence by taking the offices at the very top for himself. The age of the skyscraper had arrived.

Twenty-five years later, on the night of April 24, 1913, President Woodrow Wilson pressed a button in Washington to light the tallest habitable building in the world—the Woolworth Building in downtown Manhattan. The Woolworth Building, with its 55 stories rising 760 feet to the base of a towering flagpole, was a monument to the American Go-Getter.

The Woolworth Building was the biggest advertisement in the world. It advertised the success of Frank W. Woolworth, who had begun thirty years before as a poor farm boy in upstate New York. His empire of Five-and-Ten-Cent Stores with their brilliant red-and-gold storefronts now covered the nation. The biggest building in the world had been built from the selling of millions of little things. In that very year the 611 Woolworth stores sold 27,576,000 pairs of hosiery, 12,000 gross (1 gross = 12 dozen) of mousetraps, 300,000 gross of clothespins, 10,000 gross of tin toys, 3,000 gross of baby pacifiers, 368,000 gross of pearl buttons, and 186 tons of hairpins!

The Woolworth Building was a city in itself. With its thirty high-speed elevators it held 15,000 office workers and service employees. Its own power plant generated enough electricity to light fifty thousand homes.

Frank Woolworth wanted an office grand enough to go with the building. On a European tour in 1913 he selected the design of the Empire Room of Napoleon's palace in Paris for "the handsomest office in the country and possibly the world." For the Napoleon of American merchants, why not an office that was truly imperial? And beside his desk he placed a bust of Napoleon.

Skyscrapers still went up and up. Above the Woolworth Building rose the Chrysler Building in 1930. Then in 1931 came the Empire State Building. With its 105 stories reaching up 1,250 feet (almost twice as high as the Woolworth Building), it long remained the highest structure in the world.

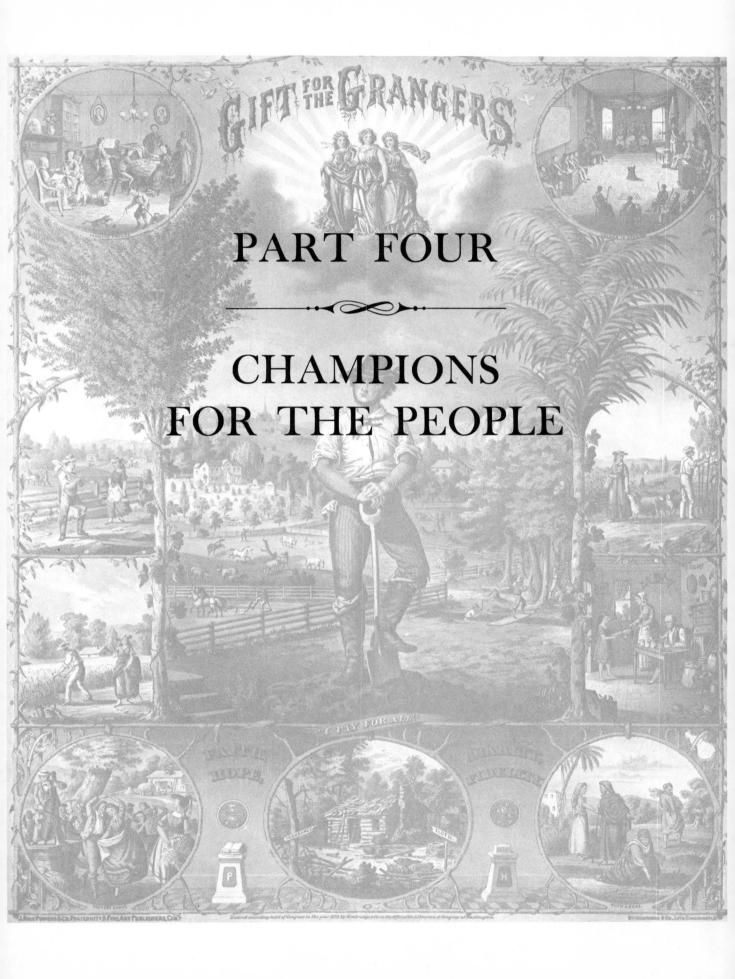

PART FOUR

CHAMPIONS
FOR THE PEOPLE

CHAMPIONS FOR THE PEOPLE

The Old World had long been ruled by aristocracies. In France and England and Germany, men who had inherited their titles and their lands held power over the life of the whole nation. For centuries government was by a privileged few looking after the silent many. Even after the European revolutions of the late eighteenth and early nineteenth centuries the old aristocrats still controlled the government in most countries.

In the United States, while some people were richer than others, there was no old-style aristocracy. If the people did not look after themselves, who would look after them?

In these years after the Civil War, there came a great new test for self-government. Could a nation so vast and varied find national leaders to speak for all its citizens?

The nation was growing strong and rich. It was becoming more and more citified, with bigger and bigger businesses. Could it find loud clear voices to speak for the farmer, for the small businessman, for the individual factory worker—and for all those others who had little wealth or power and who were in danger of being left out?

Grangers' meeting in Illinois. One sign says: "President $50,000 a year. Farmers 75 cents a week."

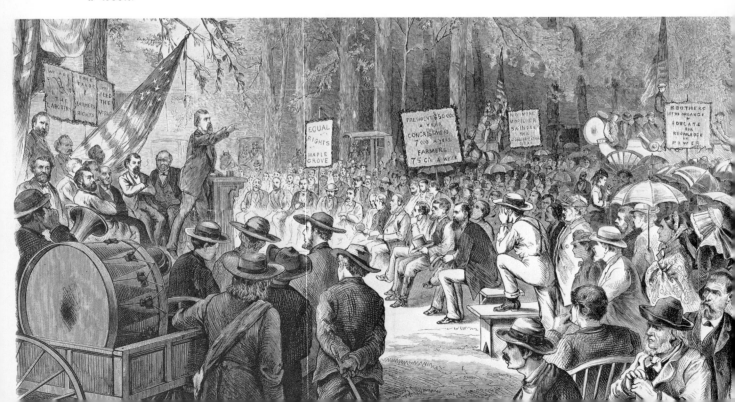

CHAPTER 19

The Farmers Find a Voice

During the Civil War many farmers—in both North and South—prospered. There was a great demand for food to supply the armies, there were fewer people working on farms, and the prices for farm products went up.

But within a few years after Appomattox the farmers' troubles began. A bushel of wheat, which in 1873 still sold for $1.21, twelve years later had gone down to 49 cents. A pound of cotton, in 1873 priced at 21 cents, in twenty years sank to 5 cents. At the same time the farmer's expenses went up.

Millions of farmers—like many homeowners today—were painfully buying their farms on mortgage loans. In good times and bad, the farmer had to make regular payments. The heartless sheriff with a long moustache who threatened to "foreclose" the mortgage was no joke to the poor farmer between about 1870 and 1900.

"In God we trusted," the farmers' saying went, "and in Kansas we busted." In the Depression of 1893 when factories closed, many unemployed workers went back to the farm and added to the farmers' burdens. Banks foreclosed their mortgages. Farm families walked the country roads in desperation.

But they did not take their troubles lying down. As early as 1867 they had begun to organize. Within ten years the Patrons of Husbandry had members all over the country in the 20,000 local lodges they called "Granges." On the Fourth of July, 1873, groups of farmers had met to hear a "Farmers' Declaration of Independence."

Farmers who believed they needed their own political party formed a "Farmers Alliance" and then organized the Populist Party in Omaha, Nebraska, in July 1892. Crusaders like the rabble-rousing Tom Watson of Georgia spoke for them in Congress, and spoke loud and clear. "Before I will give up this fight," Watson warned, "I will stay here till the ants tote me out of the keyhole."

One of the farmers' loudest demands was for "cheap money." That meant a high price for wheat and corn and cotton. For the farmers, who were always in debt, were most worried about how to keep up the yearly payments on their mortgages, so they could hold onto their farms.

Suppose for example, that a farmer owed $500 on his mortgage every year. Then if the price of wheat was $1 a bushel, he would have to raise 500 bushels of wheat to pay the $500. But if there was "cheap money"—say, if the price of wheat went up to $2 a bushel—

then the farmer could pay off his yearly debt by selling only 250 bushels of wheat. Of course the banker, to whom the farmer owed the $500 each year, would rather have seen all prices kept down, so the money he received would buy more things.

"Cheap money" meant finding ways for the government to mint as much money as possible. The more money there was around, the more likely people would pay higher prices for farm produce. On the other hand the bankers were against "cheap money" and wanted "hard money." They wanted the "Gold Standard." This meant keeping gold as the *only* basis for money. Since the amount of gold was extremely limited, and was not likely to increase much, the Gold Standard was one way of keeping prices down.

In the 1860's large new deposits of silver had been found in Nevada, Colorado, and elsewhere in the West. The farmers saw that if the government would be required to mint all this silver into money, then the quantity of money would be much increased. The price of wheat and corn and cotton would go up, and the farmers' problems might be solved. This program for minting silver was called "Free Silver" because it meant the "free," that is the unlimited, coining of silver into dollars.

Free silver, then, had a sure-fire appeal. It appealed to debt-burdened city laborers as well as debt-burdened farmers all over the country. And it appealed also to miners and prospectors in the Western States who wanted a guaranteed market for their silver. When the farmers put together their Populist Party to run their own candidates in the Presidential election of 1892, they demanded Free Silver.

The farmers' colorful leaders were not afraid to shock the comfortable people. The handsome, unladylike Mary Elizabeth Lease of Kansas was the mother of four. "What you farmers need to do," she urged, "is to raise less corn and more *Hell!*" She also said:

> Wall Street owns the country. It is no longer a government of the people, by the people and for the people, but a government of Wall Street, by Wall Street and for Wall Street. The great common people of this country are slaves, and monopoly is the master.

Then, also from Kansas, there was "Sockless Jerry" Simpson. Once when he ran for Congress he accused his well-dressed opponent of wearing silk stockings. A reporter then sneered that Simpson was so crude that he wore no socks at all. Simpson made this into a boast. Always after he was known as "Sockless Jerry."

The famous farmer-orator, Ignatius Donnelly, came to be known as "the Sage of Nininger," after the town he had tried to build. Before the Civil War he had bought some Minnesota land, and hoped to get rich by making it into a boom town. When the town died, he plowed up what were supposed to be city lots and downtown streets, planted them with wheat, and so became a farmer.

Donnelly wrote many books and he loved outlandish ideas. His *Great Cryptogram* (1888) offered a secret code that was supposed to prove that the plays of Shakespeare had really been written by Sir Francis Bacon. Donnelly could attract a crowd anywhere. Some people were afraid to go hear him because they feared he would make them believe things against their will.

When the regular Democratic and Republican politicians saw the appeal of these farm crusaders, they naturally wanted to steal the Populist thunder. The Populist Platform of 1892 demanded many different reforms. But what would appeal most to the farmers was some one cure-all—a single reform that would solve all their problems at once.

It was not hard to believe that the cure-all might be Free Silver. There was something magical and mysterious about money. The amounts of money somehow seemed to change the value of everything else. Money seemed a medicine for everybody's ills.

Many Democrats and Republicans were especially afraid to see the country get into control of a third party. They called Populists the "lunatic fringe."

Inside the regular parties the most successful of the farm crusaders was William Jennings Bryan. Some called him "The Great Commoner" (because he championed the common people). Others called him "The Prairie Avenger," or "The Boy Orator of the Platte" —after the Nebraska river near his home. Born in Salem, Illinois, he studied law in Chicago and then practiced law in small towns. He distrusted rich people and people of "good family."

Bryan had a holier-than-thou way of speaking. He liked to preach against sin. Proud that he did not drink or smoke or gamble, he was always telling others how to behave. He also had a great appetite. One of his Sunday School class-

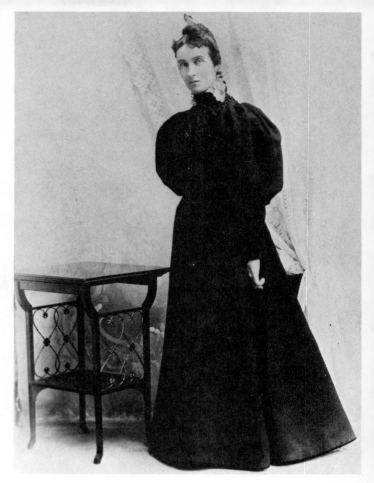

Mary Elizabeth Lease, a founder of the Populist Party, and one of the most colorful political leaders of the day.

mates recalled that Bryan was too good a boy to help steal the watermelons— "but he would enjoy eating them when the other boys had secured the booty." As a boy he would carry around bread in his pockets "for an emergency." His enormous appetite became famous. On his political campaigns it was not uncommon for him to eat six full meals a day.

A tall man of great energy, Bryan loved a political battle. And he had a talent for making every issue seem very simple. After he had explained it, every political battle seemed to be between Bryan and God on one side, and his opponents and Satan on the other. His enemies said Bryan did not really understand how complicated the problems

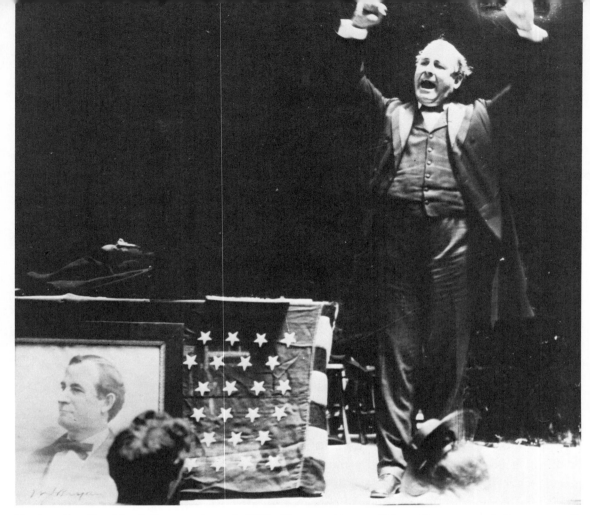

During the Presidential campaign of 1896, Democratic candidate Bryan traveled strenuously about the country carrying his rousing message to anyone who would listen.

were. Even his friends had to admit that what made him famous was not a sharp mind but his loud musical voice.

The "silver-tongued" William Jennings Bryan had decided that "Free Silver" would cure the ills of all mankind. When Bryan arrived at the Democratic Convention in Chicago on July 7, 1896, he was thirty-six years old—one year over the minimum age for a President. He had served only four years in Congress and was barely known outside of Nebraska. Unlike the other leading candidates, he did not have rich supporters.

As the Convention met, it was still not decided whether the Democratic Party would stay with the Gold Standard or whether they would join the farmers for Free Silver. President Grover Cleveland, the Democrat in the White House, was strong for the Gold Standard. But he had lost the support of many laborers and farmers by using federal troops against the railroad workers in the big strike at Pullman. He had a reputation as spokesman for big business.

Until Bryan came to the platform, the speakers at the Chicago convention had been dull and long-winded. Since there was no public-address system most of the speakers could hardly be heard. Bryan was the final speaker for Free Silver.

This was young Bryan's great chance. The first sound of his ringing voice awakened the perspiring audience. They responded to his words with laughter and applause, "like a trained choir" (as he said), down to his last syllable. He spoke without hesitating, for he had given substantially the same speech many times before—to farm audiences all over Nebraska. "We will answer their demand for a Gold Standard," he ended, "by saying to them: You shall not press down upon the brow of labor this crown of thorns. You shall not crucify mankind upon a cross of gold."

The crowd went wild. Their yelling and cheering lasted for an hour. The delegates from Alabama led a "grand march of glory" around the hall. Others reached for Bryan, proud even to touch his coat. They lifted him and marched him in triumph. After they put him back in his seat, admirers sat in his lap, "hugged him until his collar wilted, shook his hand, shouted into his ears, danced all over his feet, and hemmed him in until he could scarcely get his breath." This one speech had transformed a Nebraska small-town lawyer into a front runner for President!

On the next day, the Democratic Convention voted him to lead their ticket.

Bryan was a rousing candidate. From millions of admirers he received all kinds of gifts—ostrich eggs, a stuffed alligator, four live eagles, a cane supposed to have belonged to Andrew Jackson, and lots of rabbits' feet for good luck. "If all the people who have given me rabbits' feet in this campaign will vote for me," Bryan declared, "there is no possible doubt of my election."

The campaign offered one of the most spectacular contrasts in American history. "The Boy Orator of the Platte" went careering about the country by

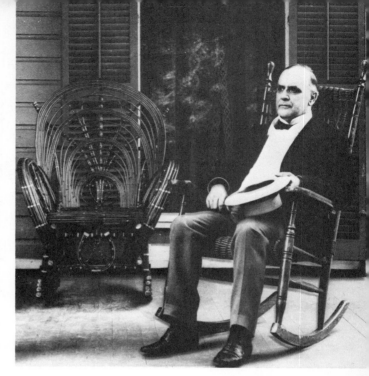

Meanwhile Republican candidate McKinley sat calmly on his own front porch.

train, making speeches far into the night at every little town, and often in between. On some days he made thirty-six speeches. Meanwhile, his conservative Republican opponent, William B. McKinley, remained calmly seated on his front porch in Canton, Ohio. McKinley made almost no speeches. When he did, he was careful to say nothing in particular—except that he was in favor of "sound money" (the Gold Standard) and "restoring confidence."

Mark Hanna, a clever Cleveland businessman and political boss who had secured the Republican nomination for McKinley, managed McKinley's campaign. Hanna counted on letting Bryan talk himself to defeat. And he used every trick to convince voters that Bryan was a dangerous radical. For example, he persuaded some factory owners, as a stunt, to pay their workers in Mexican dollars (worth only 50 United States cents). This was supposed to show the workers what their wages would really be worth if Bryan won.

Hanna's tactics succeeded. The election went to McKinley by a narrow margin. But Bryan had attracted so many votes that the Democratic leaders could not ignore him. Twice again—in 1900 and 1908—he was named the Democratic candidate for President. Bryan never won.

The Age of Reform had arrived. Free Silver, the simple-minded cure-all, was never adopted. But other Populist reforms—the regulation of railroad rates, control of monopolies, limits on the hours of labor, and a federal income tax—all these finally became law. The Populists had done more than anybody else to advertise the farmers' troubles. And the big, old parties—the Democrats, and then the Republicans—got the message. They adopted the main Populist reforms as their own. The Populists, who had lost many noisy battles, finally won a silent victory.

CHAPTER 20

From Umpire to Guardian

Everything seemed to be growing. While at the outbreak of the Civil War, the country had numbered thirty million people, by 1900 there were over seventy-five million. From thirty-four States, the number had grown to forty-five. Before the war the nation's population was mostly between the Mississippi River and the Atlantic Ocean, plus a few sparsely settled States on the Pacific Coast. By 1900 four transcontinental railroads poured people into the great heart of the continent, filling lands between the Mississippi River and the Sierra Nevada Mountains.

There were more cities, more big cities, and the big cities were bigger than ever. In 1860 there were only nine places that contained 100,000 people or more. But by 1900 there were nearly forty. And there were three giant metropolises each with over a million people.

Businesses were growing bigger. Now you bought your clothes and furniture not from a friendly storekeeper, but from a huge mail-order house or a vast department store. In the old days, you dealt with men you knew personally. Now more and more of everybody's needs were supplied by big companies.

Your goods were manufactured in large factories thousands of miles away. Whom would you complain to? Whom could you count on? Many families who had braved the wilderness and had known loneliness, who had faced the horrors of Civil War, were now frightened by the new menace of Bigness.

What had happened to the old neighborly spirit?

The dangers of Bigness were not only imaginary. As the companies that made the things you needed became larger and larger, the number of different companies supplying your needs became

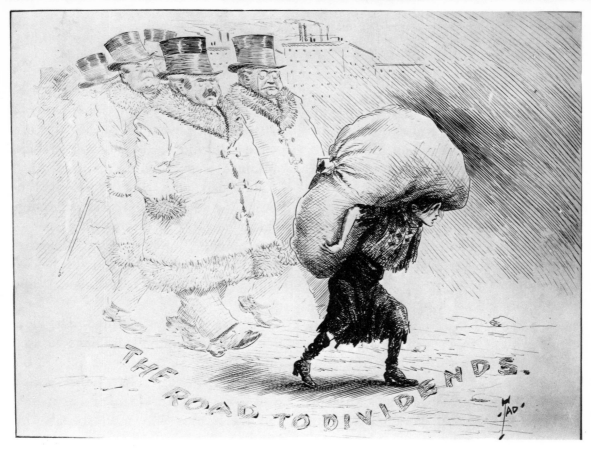

THE ROAD TO DIVIDENDS.

Newspapermen and cartoonists joined in the popular campaign against Big Business. "Muck-rakers" awakened the nation's conscience by accusations, real and imaginary, against all men of wealth.

fewer and fewer. For example, by 1880 the Standard Oil Company controlled over 90 percent of the lamp-oil refining in the United States. In those days before electric light, if you wanted oil to light your house at night you had to pay whatever price that company asked.

Bigness meant monopoly. And monopoly meant that a few men had the power to dictate to everybody.

Everywhere, it seemed, some company was squeezing out its competitors. In the 1890's, if you wanted sugar for your table, you had to buy it from the company that controlled 98 percent of the sugar refining in the whole country. For tobacco, you were in the clutches of the American Tobacco Company. Almost every machine—along with the many new ships and bridges and sky-scrapers—now had to use steel. In 1901

the United States Steel Company became the country's first billion-dollar corporation.

The Go-Getters (with the help of their lawyers) invented new ways to combine small businesses into big. And they found ways to keep their control secret. One new kind of company, whose only business was to own other companies, was called a "trust." The men who owned a trust really (but sometimes secretly) controlled smaller companies that still carried on under their own name.

In these ways ambitious Go-Getters built their businesses into empires. Soon there were Banking Empires and Mining Empires, Steel Empires and Railroad Empires. The men who built them were full of imagination and energy, but some of them were as arrogant and as ruthless as the despots of the Middle Ages. Some believed that the only law they had to obey was the law they made for themselves. Once when J. P. Morgan, the giant of American banking, heard that his company was being prosecuted for violating the laws, he went to see the President. "If we have done anything wrong," he explained, "send your man [the Attorney General of the United States] to my man [Morgan's lawyer] and they can fix it up."

Congress passed a law in 1890 making it a crime for businessmen to combine in order to prevent competition. This Sherman Antitrust Act was supposed to punish "restraint of trade or commerce." But like other laws, the law against trusts would work only if the government enforced it.

Presidents did not want to offend the powerful businessmen who had helped them get elected and who might help again at the next election. They pretended that the law did not exist. In the rare case when a President dared to use the law, the Supreme Court saved the trusts by thinking up technicalities. For example, in 1895 the Attorney General prosecuted the one company that controlled 98 percent of the sugar refining in the whole country. But the Supreme Court said that the company really was *not* guilty of preventing competition under the Sherman Antitrust Act—because it was in "manufacturing" and not in "commerce."

The President who actually started using the power of the national government to protect ordinary Americans was Theodore Roosevelt. He had been elected Vice-President on the Republican ticket with William B. McKinley in 1900. When President McKinley joined

the festivities at the Pan-American Exposition in Buffalo on September 6, 1901, a man he had never seen before walked up and fired two shots at him. Within a week McKinley was dead.

The man who shot President McKinley called himself an anarchist, which meant that he was against all government. But by making Theodore Roosevelt President, he actually helped to give the national government strong powers.

No one who had visited Theodore Roosevelt as a child would have guessed that he would become a champion of the ordinary American. His father was a well-to-do New York banker who owned country houses and used to take his family to Europe for vacations. Among Teddy Roosevelt's early memories were seeing the Pope during a walk in Rome, and visiting the tomb of Napoleon in Paris.

Young Teddy had no worries about money. But he had other worries. He suffered from asthma, which made it hard for him to exercise, and his eyesight was poor. He became seriously interested in nature and began collecting specimens of plants and animals. When he was twelve, his mother told a maid to throw away some dead mice that the boy had stored in a dresser drawer. "The Loss to Science," Teddy lamented. "The Loss to Science!"

His father built a gymnasium at home. There Teddy worked with a punching bag and did pull-ups on the horizontal bars. He also took boxing lessons. By the time he was seventeen he was expert in track events including running, pole vaulting, and high jumping. On his grandfather's country estate at Oyster

Bay on Long Island he became an enthusiastic horseman and a crack shot. All his life Teddy Roosevelt felt that he had to make up for the childhood weakness of his body.

Roosevelt never lost his boyish excitement. He continued his boxing. After he was hit in the eye while boxing with a young army officer, his left eye became completely blind. He managed to keep this secret, and he devised ways to prevent people knowing that he could see in only one eye. He even became world-famous as an explorer and big-game hunter in Africa and South America.

From the White House he preached "The Strenuous Life." Some genteel European diplomats dreaded being assigned to Washington when "TR" was in the White House. They could not do their diplomatic duty by sipping tea and making polite conversation. TR expected them—along with panting Cabinet members and generals—to join his exhausting tramps through the countryside. "You must always remember," a British ambassador once explained, "that the President is about six years old."

TR liked a good fight—not only in the boxing arena, but also in politics. He had been shocked that earlier Presidents had not enforced the laws against monopolies, and he was disgusted by the Supreme Court's technicalities. The growing power of corporations worried him. "Of all forms of tyranny," he complained, "the least attractive and the most vulgar is the tyranny of mere wealth, the tyranny of a plutocracy."

No sooner had TR moved into the White House than he had his chance. The owners of the anthracite coal mines had become reckless about the safety

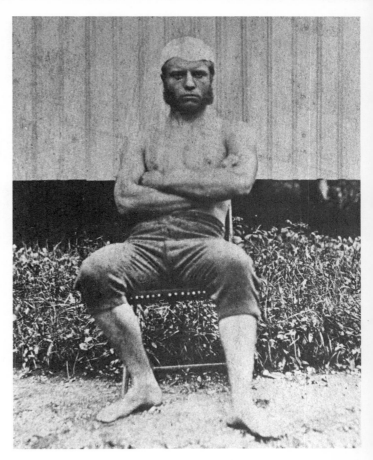

Teddy Roosevelt as a boxer at Harvard.

of their men. Workers were dying needlessly each year. In 1901 alone, 441 men were killed in mining accidents in the anthracite coal fields of Illinois, Ohio, Pennsylvania, and West Virginia.

The men had received no raise in wages in twenty years. They were paid by the weight of the coal they dug, but the companies were not weighing honestly. Sometimes they made a man dig four thousand pounds before giving him credit for a ton. Miners were forced to spend their wages in "company stores" which charged high prices.

By 1902 the miners could endure no more. The union leaders decided to take action. John Mitchell, then the energetic young president of the United Mine Workers of America, was the son of a miner who had lost his life in the mines. Mitchell himself had begun mining at the age of twelve. His union—

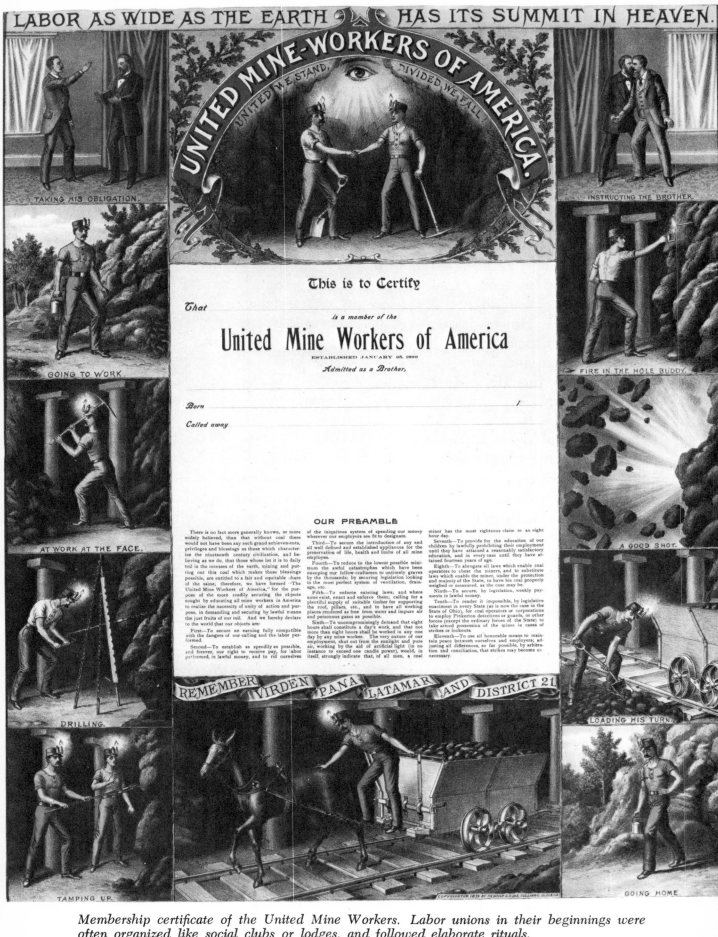

Membership certificate of the United Mine Workers. Labor unions in their beginnings were often organized like social clubs or lodges, and followed elaborate rituals.

150,000 strong—included thousands of Newcomers who spoke over a dozen different languages.

The coal miners went on strike in May 1902. By October, with winter coming, people feared that the railroads would have to stop running and that the nation would freeze.

President Roosevelt came to the miners' rescue. Regardless of who owned the mines, Roosevelt insisted, nobody owned the miners. He shamed the mine owners into granting most of the workers' demands. When the strike ended TR had shown how, in the new age of big business, it was possible for the federal government to help. He had proven himself a champion of the ordinary American.

This was only a beginning. President Roosevelt enforced the law against trusts—even when it offended the richest men in the country. He added to the Cabinet a Secretary of Commerce and Labor, one of whose jobs was to keep an eye out for monopolies. He sponsored a law making it a crime for the railroads to show favoritism (for example, by giving secret refunds or "rebates") to anybody.

It was just as important, Roosevelt saw, to protect future Americans against the greed of living Americans as it was to protect mine workers against greedy mine owners. This was what he meant by "Conservation." As a young man out West he had enjoyed the open spaces. From his Dakota ranch he himself had ridden the range and explored the wilderness. He loved everything about the West—the cowboys, the life of the trail, fishing and hunting. And he was shocked to see lumber companies wast-

ing forests which had taken centuries to grow. He knew that the wilderness could never be put back.

He saw some parts of the country troubled by floods while others lacked water. Saving rivers and streams was just as important as protecting the land or the forests. To the White House he called scientists, Governors, Supreme Court Justices, and others, to plan an inventory of the natural wealth. Soon "Conservation" was a popular word.

During most of American history, the money to run the federal government had been raised by selling lands from the Public Domain in the West, by customs duties on imports, and by "excise" taxes on certain kinds of goods (for example, liquor and tobacco). These taxes were not democratic enough for Roosevelt. Shocked by the "swollen and monstrous fortunes," he wanted the rich to pay a bigger share.

But the Constitution said that the only "direct" taxes Congress could pass were those apportioned according to the *population* of the States. Income was a very different thing from population. During the Civil War the government somehow had got around these technicalities and had actually passed a tax on income. But after the war the income tax was dropped.

Later, when Populists and others demanded an income tax, the Supreme Court stood in the way. The Supreme Court said that an income tax was exactly the kind of tax that the Constitution had prohibited. President Roosevelt then demanded an amendment to the Constitution. Within a few years, the required number of States had passed this income-tax amendment.

Now Congress had the power to tax the rich Americans more heavily than the poor.

Now taxes themselves would protect most Americans by making it harder for any Americans to become monstrously rich. The income tax was a "progressive" tax. The higher you progressed up the ladder of wealth the larger the *proportion* of your income you had to pay. This was a sign that Americans were beginning to think in a new way.

After Theodore Roosevelt, fewer Americans believed it was good enough for the government to be only an umpire. Even in a prosperous democracy, the powers of different citizens and corporations were not equal. In the twentieth century more and more Americans expected their government to be a guardian. They expected it actually to help protect the weak from the strong.

CHAPTER 21

Who Killed Prosperity?

During the twenty years after President Theodore Roosevelt left the White House in 1909, the United States seemed a land of miracles. Never before in history were factories making so many new things. Never before had the daily life of a nation been so quickly transformed.

At the opening of the twentieth century the automobile was still such an oddity that in Vermont the law required the driver to send someone an eighth of a mile ahead with a red flag. But before Herbert Hoover took his oath as President in 1929 the American automobiles made each year came to five million.

Back in 1900 the closest thing to a movie was the crude "nickelodeon." In return for your nickel you looked into a box to see pictures move for a few minutes. But in 1929 one hundred million tickets were being sold to the movies every week, and the movies could actually talk!

Until World War I most Americans had not even heard of the radio. But by 1929 the annual turnout of radio sets numbered over four million. Television was still in the future—but it seemed amazing enough that voices could be sent without wires.

Americans were making the highest wages in history—and working shorter hours.

The American diet was more varied. Most homes had refrigerators, and even city people could have their fill of milk and of fresh fruit and vegetables at all seasons. With advancing medical knowledge, now at last the diseases which most threatened children—typhoid, diphtheria, and measles—were coming under control. Americans were healthier and were living longer than ever before.

Education in the United States was better and reached a larger proportion of the people than in any other country. By 1928 the money that Americans

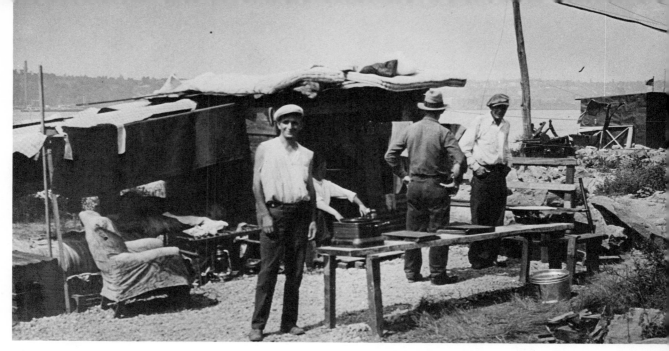

Unemployed New Yorkers in 1932 (at the Hudson River and 75th Street), using old boxes and discarded mattresses for shelter. They entertained themselves with a wind-up phonograph.

spent each year for education was more than that spent by all the rest of the world put together. In most European countries only a grade-school education was free. But in the United States a free high-school education was normal, and millions could hope to go to college.

Progress seemed endless. Then suddenly, in late October 1929, came terrifying signs that the success story might have an unhappy ending.

The first hint was the Great Stock Market Crash. The New York Stock Market was where people bought and sold stocks—"shares" in the largest American corporations. The owner of a share in a company really owned part of the company. If the company grew and made a large profit, then the owner of the share would be paid a dividend as his part of the profit. Then, too, the value of that share went up. Naturally, everybody wanted to own shares in the most profitable companies.

But by 1929 many people who bought shares hoped to make their profits, not from the earnings of the company, but from the higher price that other Stock Market gamblers would pay them for their shares. More and more people began risking their money in the Stock Market. They expected to get rich when the price of their shares would suddenly go up. And with the money they made they would buy other shares, which they hoped would also go up.

Stock Market gambling became a national mania, a contagious disease. Americans who never would have thought of borrowing money to bet on the horse races now were actually borrowing to bet on stocks. The more the stock mania grew, the less connection there was between the real value of a company and the price people were paying for that company's shares on the Stock Market. People came to expect every stock to go *up*.

The "impossible" began to happen on October 24, 1929. All prices seemed to be falling. On that day thirteen million shares were sold. Then, it seemed, *everybody* wanted to sell his stocks—and as fast as possible, before they went further down.

In the months that followed the prices of stocks sank faster than ever. A share in United States Steel which had sold for $262 soon brought only $22, while a share of Montgomery Ward sank from $138 to $4, and a share of General Motors went from $73 to $8.

In the panic, people forgot an important fact. Even though the market price of a share of General Motors went down to nearly zero (simply because Stock Market gamblers no longer bet on it) the automobile factories and the men with know-how were all still there, just as good as ever. The wealth of the land and the energy of the people were still there.

But were they? People who never really understood why American progress had seemed so endless, now, of course, had no better understanding of why prosperity had vanished. In unreasoning fear, Americans who heard of this "impossible" drop in the price of stocks began to wonder. Perhaps this was only the first signal of the collapse of all America. If stocks could so quickly lose their value (they sank by forty billion dollars before the end of 1929), maybe nothing else was worth as much as people thought.

They lost faith in their banks. Of course, one way banks make money is to lend out at interest much of the money that people deposit with them. Usually only a few people at any one time want to draw out their money, and banks keep enough on hand to take care of them.

But during the Crash nearly everybody seemed to want to draw his money out at the same time. By the hundreds, then, banks, which could not suddenly produce all that cash, failed. Many people lost their life savings. Over six hundred and fifty banks failed in 1929, thirteen hundred failed in 1930, twenty-three hundred failed in 1931. Eventually the federal government itself would provide a new kind of insurance guaranteeing the depositors their money in an emergency. But there was nothing like that at the time of the Great Crash.

After the Great Stock Market Crash came the Great Depression. Manufacturers, finding fewer customers for anything they could make, began slowing down their factories, making fewer automobiles, fewer refrigerators, and fewer radios. They laid off their workers. And workers out of a job could not afford to buy things. Then still more factories closed down. Storekeepers went bankrupt. Soon, it seemed, collapse of the prices of stocks on the Stock Market had signaled the collapse of American business and American industry.

By the end of 1932 about thirteen million able-bodied Americans—about one in every four—were out of work. They could not afford to pay their own rent and had to squeeze in with friends or relatives. Young people with no money, no job, and no prospects did not dare marry. Within three years, the number of marriages was down by one-quarter. College enrollments sank.

Millions did not have enough to eat. Children cried for the food their parents could not give them. Hungry, sad Americans were actually wandering down alleys, routing through garbage pails for scraps to keep their families alive.

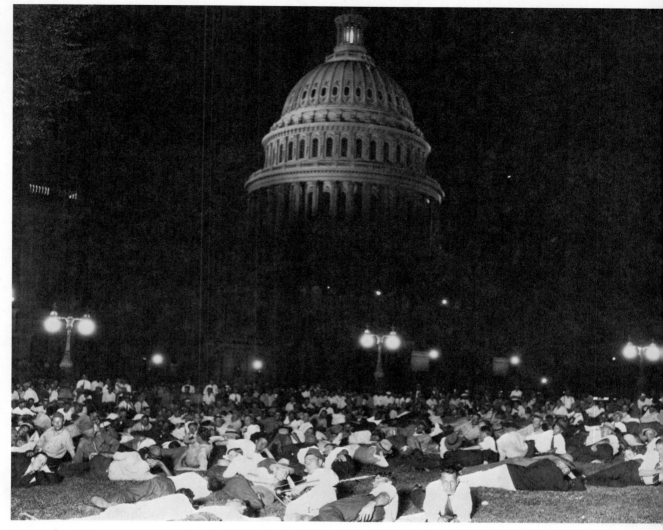

Unemployed war veterans, who had joined the "Bonus March," waiting outside the Capitol as the Senate in a special night session in July 1932 debated the bonus. The Senate voted it down.

Desperate unemployed went on hunger marches. In Henryetta, Oklahoma, three hundred men broke into food stores. In Iowa and Nebraska, farmers, who could no longer pay the money due on their mortgages, used pitchforks to drive off the sheriffs who came to seize their land. In the spring of 1932 thousands of unemployed veterans formed a "Bonus Army." Demanding that the government pay them a bonus for their service fourteen years earlier in World War I, they marched on Washington. President Herbert Hoover called out the army to drive them from government buildings and parklands that they had occupied.

Where would it end?

But before Americans could cure what ailed the country, they had to know what really was the disease. Who —or what—had killed prosperity? In the panic many Americans lost their heads. Everybody wanted to have somebody to blame it on. Crackpot leaders quickly appeared with fantastic explanations and imaginary cure-alls. Abolish banks! Print more money!

The unlucky man in the White House, the Republican Herbert Hoover, had been elected President in November 1928 by the second largest popular majority until then in all American history. But he had the misfortune to be inaug-

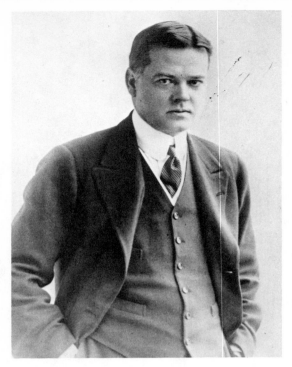

The young Herbert Hoover as a mining engineer.

urated in March 1929, just in time to get the blame for the Great Stock Market Crash.

Never was there a more honest or a more hard-working President. Hoover, a poor boy raised in a small Iowa town, went to Stanford University where he studied engineering. Then he made a fortune working as a mining engineer—in Australia, Africa, China, Latin America, and Russia. He became world-famous during World War I, when he headed the Relief Commission that fed starving Europeans. He was also in charge of conserving food in the United States so Americans could share it with their European allies. He had proven himself a great humanitarian and a remarkable organizer.

But Hoover was no politician. He did not like to try to persuade people. He did not enjoy the arts of compromise. As an engineer, he felt he saw problems clearly. After he had carefully prepared his solution he expected people to follow his instructions without arguing. Wearing a high stiff collar, he was a stiff man who inspired respect but not love. He had none of William Jennings Bryan's eloquence, nor any of Theodore Roosevelt's pep. In ordinary times he might have been a good President to keep America on the familiar road to success.

These were not ordinary times.

President Hoover was the handiest person to blame, even though the Depression had actually begun to happen almost before he had moved into the White House. The shacks made of cardboard and flattened tin cans, where some unemployed lived, were soon called "Hoovervilles." One folk song of the unemployed declared, "Hoover made a souphound out of me." A man's empty pocket, turned inside out, was called a "Hoover flag."

But when the collapse came so unexpectedly, President Hoover did not sit still. He used all the familiar ways to relieve suffering. He called upon cities, States, and all private charities to help feed the hungry. He brought business leaders and labor leaders to the White House, where they promised to try to keep up wages and keep the factories going. At the same time he started an ambitious new plan to use government money to hold up the price of tobacco, cotton, corn, and wheat in order to help the suffering farmers. He actually cut his own Presidential salary by one-fifth.

What Hoover did helped some, but it was not enough. The disaster was more unfamiliar than President Hoover realized. And it required remedies even more unfamiliar than he could imagine.

CHAPTER 22

Nothing to Fear but Fear Itself

When the election of 1932 came around and Herbert Hoover ran for President again, almost anybody could have beaten him. Who wanted to vote *for* the Depression? But the Democrats happened to pick one of the most winning men in American history. He was a distant cousin of Theodore Roosevelt, and his name was Franklin Delano Roosevelt.

Although only a few people in the country realized it at the time, Franklin Delano Roosevelt was a man of heroic character. From his youth he had enjoyed athletics. He had always loved politics and had been the Democratic candidate for Vice-President in 1920. One August day in 1921 he was stricken with polio and left paralyzed. This single, sudden thunderclap of bad luck reduced him from a bouncy, athletic, runabout politician to a bedridden invalid. A man of weaker character might have given up.

Instead, after his misfortune, he became more determined than ever to be an active politician. An old friend who came on a sympathy visit to the hospital was surprised when FDR unexpectedly gave him a strong, good-natured wallop. "You thought you were coming to see an invalid," FDR laughed from his bed. "But I can knock you out in any bout."

People who went to cheer him up found that FDR gave them a lift instead.

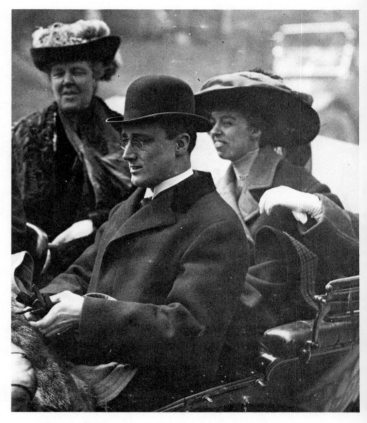

Franklin Delano Roosevelt and his wife Eleanor (right), eight years before his paralysis. Eleanor, who was a niece of the Republican President Theodore Roosevelt, later became world-famous for her humanitarian activities.

Sometimes he joked about his affliction. FDR wrote a friend that he had "renewed his youth" by "what was fortunately a rather mild case of *infantile paralysis.*"

But his case really was far from mild. He was never able to walk again. Only after long and painful exercises and by wearing heavy braces did he learn to use his hips so he could get around on crutches. He told his friends that he had an advantage, because while they were running around he could sit still and think. He used his long period of recovery in bed to write hundreds of letters to politicians all over the country—not about his personal problems, but about politics and how to build a stronger Democratic party. All over the country Democratic politicians valued his advice.

FDR made a fantastic comeback. When the Democratic Convention in Chicago in 1932 nominated Franklin Delano Roosevelt to be their candidate for President, it was really not because of his heroic personal qualities. For he had already proven himself a spectacularly successful politician in New York. In 1928, only a few years after he had been stricken with infantile paralysis, he managed to be elected Governor of his State. After a successful term as Governor he ran again in 1930, and he won by the biggest majority ever.

With his broad, contagious smile, he was a wonderful persuader. He loved people, and could make them love him. People cheered up when they saw his jaunty long cigarette holder and felt his warm firm handshake. He had all the human qualities that Herbert Hoover lacked. And these were what the nation wanted in that dangerous year of 1932.

FDR was no radical. In fact, during his campaign he was careful not to offend anybody. When he made speeches, he sounded more like William McKinley than like William Jennings Bryan. Some people, who thought the nation needed strong medicine, criticized FDR.

They said he was too eager to please everybody. They were afraid that he was simply "a pleasant man who would very much like to be President."

Those critics were wrong. For FDR had courage in politics just as much as in his private life. And as soon as he took office on March 4, 1933, he showed it.

"A New Deal for the American people!" This was what FDR had announced in Chicago when he accepted the nomination. He promised to *experiment*. The nation and all its wealth were still there, he reminded people in his inaugural address. "We are stricken by no plague of locusts. Compared with the perils which our forefathers conquered because they believed and were not afraid, we have still much to be thankful for. Nature still offers her bounty and human efforts have multiplied it. Plenty is at our doorstep." He had faith that there really were lots of new ways that could be tried.

"The only thing we have to fear," he said, "is fear itself." His courage and his optimism, like his smile, were contagious. Americans were encouraged most of all because they believed that their new President really would experiment. He would try one thing, and then another—until ways would be found to put the country back on the track, and to put people back to work.

FDR began trying things from his first day in the White House. In order to preserve people's life savings, he ordered all banks closed for four days while ways were found to restore confidence in them. He called Congress into special session to pass laws for the emergency.

Congress, on his urging, arranged special loans to help people pay their mortgages so they could keep their farms and homes till the crisis was over. A fund of over two billion dollars helped citizens start new construction—of homes, offices, shops, and factories—and thus create new jobs. Over three billion dollars was appropriated for new government buildings, and a half-billion dollars for outright relief. New laws guaranteed workers their right to organize into unions. New laws prohibited child labor, set minimum wages and maximum hours. A new program was passed for the farmer, to keep up the price of his crops.

Some experiments were not so successful. For example, one of FDR's pet projects was a law—the National Recovery Act or NRA—enforcing new "codes" to be made by representatives of business and labor in each industry. These codes aimed to keep up prices and wages. They said what should be manufactured, how many of everything, and at what price. They made many of the kinds of arrangements which big businesses had been punished for making when they fixed prices by monopoly. But the new law said that the antitrust rules did not apply. Small businessmen objected. They said the big businessmen were simply using the law to protect their own monopoly profits.

The Supreme Court declared the NRA codes unconstitutional. Congress, the Court said, was trying to give away the power to make laws. But the Constitution had assigned the lawmaking power only to Congress.

Still, on the whole, FDR seemed to be making headway. By the end of his first term in office, there were fewer people without jobs. The country was looking up. When FDR ran again in 1936, he was reelected by an even bigger majority.

All over the rest of the world, desperate people were handing over their liberty to dictators who promised them food and jobs in return. In Italy, only ten years before FDR was inaugurated, Benito Mussolini and his gang of fascists marched on Rome. They seized the government, abolished democracy, destroyed the liberties of the Italian people —all on the promise that they would provide more and better jobs.

In Germany, too, in the very month when FDR took his oath of office, Adolf

President Franklin D. Roosevelt (seen here by cartoonist Gluyas Williams) reached the American people through the new and democratic devices of the press conference and the radio fireside chat.

Copr. © 1942, The *New Yorker* Magazine, Inc.

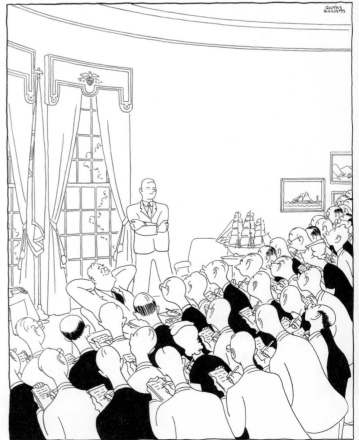

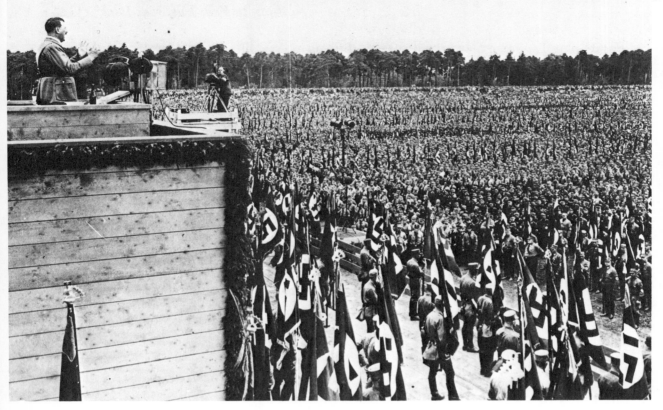

Adolf Hitler addressing the 160,000 Storm Troopers who, by spreading terror, helped "persuade" the German people to become Nazis.

Hitler, with his gang of Nazis, was made dictator. Screaming slogans of race hate and fear, the Nazis destroyed the universities. They used secret police and concentration camps. They murdered, robbed, and tortured. They abolished liberty and decency. And the civilized German people somehow tolerated it all because many of them needed jobs, their children were hungry, and they believed Hitler's promise of prosperity.

FDR had faith that it did not need to happen here. He tried all sorts of experiments—democratic experiments—to restore hope and prosperity, while strengthening American liberties. He consulted with business leaders, labor organizers, university professors, social workers, judges, scientists, lawyers, and doctors. Anybody who had an idea

knew that somebody in the New Deal would listen. Of course some people accused FDR of wanting to be a dictator. But he never lost his faith in democracy and in the ability of Americans to handle the unexpected.

"Happy Days Are Here Again!" had been FDR's campaign song. Many Americans wanted to believe that FDR was a kind of magician who could suddenly bring back prosperity. Of course, FDR did not believe government had a magic formula.

He did believe, though, that there were many helpful things the government could always do, and had to do. And he believed that the government did not need to wait till the next emergency. It ought to promise people help in advance. Then, if Americans felt sure they would get the emergency help they needed, they would be more cheerful and less worried about their future. This itself might help bring back prosperity and keep prosperity alive.

FDR therefore proposed a scheme of insurance. While a person had a job, he paid a small amount every month out of his wages, and his employer paid the same amount. This went into the federal treasury. Then when the worker was out of a job or when he became too old to work, he received back a payment every month. He could be sure that he would never starve.

The people who received their insurance payments did not feel they were charity cases. Since they had been putting in their own money when they were prosperous, they felt they were only getting what they were entitled to when times were bad. This system was called Social Security. It aimed to make everybody in the whole society feel more secure.

Following the lead of the Republican Roosevelt, FDR set up a grand new plan for conservation, to prevent the soil from being used up or washed away, and so to help farmers make a better living. And he found other ways to preserve resources for the future.

FDR enlarged Teddy Roosevelt's idea to include "People Conservation." The government spent millions of dollars encouraging artists by employing them to decorate post offices and other government buildings. Government programs also provided useful work for young people who could not afford to go to college.

One of the most ingenious plans was to "conserve" the people of a whole region. In the mountains of western Kentucky, Tennessee, and Alabama, around the valley of the Tennessee River, there lived about 3,500,000 people. Most of them lived poorly. Their land was exhausted. Electricity was too expensive, yet without electricity they could not modernize their farms or bring in the factories to provide jobs.

FDR's idea was to build a great dam on the Tennessee River. This would protect against floods. At the same time the water flowing through the dam would turn generators to make cheap electricity. And two old munitions plants left over from World War I could be made into factories for fertilizer to improve the farms. These were FDR's plans for the Tennessee Valley Authority (TVA).

The lives of thousands of people in the Tennessee Valley were brightened. Public Health doctors used this chance to rid the countryside of malaria. Librarians sent "bookmobiles" into the farms. Better houses and better schools were built. Again, some people objected that FDR was trying to be a dictator. They accused the government of competing unfairly with private electric and fertilizer companies.

Yet the experiment was a success. Of course, it did not solve all the problems of the poor farmers in the Tennessee Valley. But it showed how much *could* be done if a democratic government was willing to help.

Hope came back to America. FDR had found ways to cure the symptoms of the Great Depression. But had he cured the disease? Many Americans were not sure. Prosperity did not fully return until World War II put the fac-

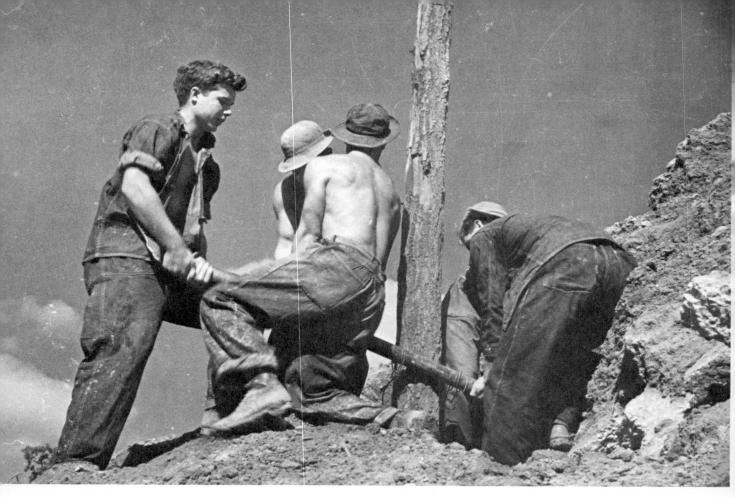

These energetic young men were among the three million members of the Civilian Conservation Corps, one of many New Deal programs to put people to work. The CCC planted more than seventeen million acres of forests, stocked over a billion fish in hatcheries, built trails in the National Parks, fought forest fires, and worked on countless other useful outdoor projects.

tories back to working full steam. Some people said the real end of the Depression did not come till then. But Americans had learned a lot about how to deal with the dangers of unemployment and how to keep the factories working in peacetime.

Americans too had lost many of their old fears of economic Ups and Downs. That itself was a gain. The Great Depression proved that, the more people were frightened, the worse things became.

Americans had discovered a new strength. Through the crisis the federal Constitution proved adaptable, and came out stronger than ever. Americans had proved that they could survive their worst peacetime disaster—without spreading hate, without taking away liberties, without installing a dictator.

This was a great and reassuring discovery. It was as important as anything Americans had ever learned about their land or about themselves.

CHAPTER 23

Who Was Left Out?

When prosperity returned, Americans boasted that this was a land where *every*body had a fair chance. But that still was not quite correct. When you surveyed the whole country and all the people in it you had to wonder. Many Americans were not getting their full fair chance. Some were almost entirely left out.

The United States was, of course, a nation of minorities. Had there ever before been a nation built of so many different groups?

There were many kinds of minorities. Of the religious minorities, for example, in some parts of the country Catholics were commonly discriminated against. It was taken for granted that no Catholic could ever be elected President—until the 1960 election of John F. Kennedy. Although the Jews had a long tradition of learning, even before they arrived in this country, strict quotas in colleges and medical schools kept out all but a few, even if they were the best qualified. The Mormons, who were a distinctive American religion, actually had laws passed against them.

We have seen how the Oldcomers—in New England, for example—had looked down their noses at Newcomers. And it was especially easy to be snobbish when the Newcomers looked different. Mexican immigrants, who came across the border for seasonal farm work, were not allowed to buy land, or to get an education, or to find a better job. The Chinese and Japanese, who had been imported to help build the Western railroads, afterwards in some places were not permitted to live equally among other Americans, or to own land, or to become voting citizens.

The American Indians, of course, were the oldest of the Oldcomers. But they were deprived of their best land and forced onto barren "reservations" of desert wastes and rocky mountain slopes. They were not allowed to become full-fledged Americans. And there were many others.

The largest single group of left-out Americans were the Negroes. This was especially disappointing because the whole nation had fought its most terrible war and had even split families apart so that all Americans would be treated like men. While the Civil War was, of course, a war for Union, it was also emphatically a war to help the Negro. For that cause a quarter-million Union soldiers had given their lives.

Never before in history had so many people fought for the freedom of others. In relation to the Negro, the United States had shown its best and its worst. Some Americans had kept him a slave. But other Americans fought and died to make him free.

After the Civil War, as we have seen,

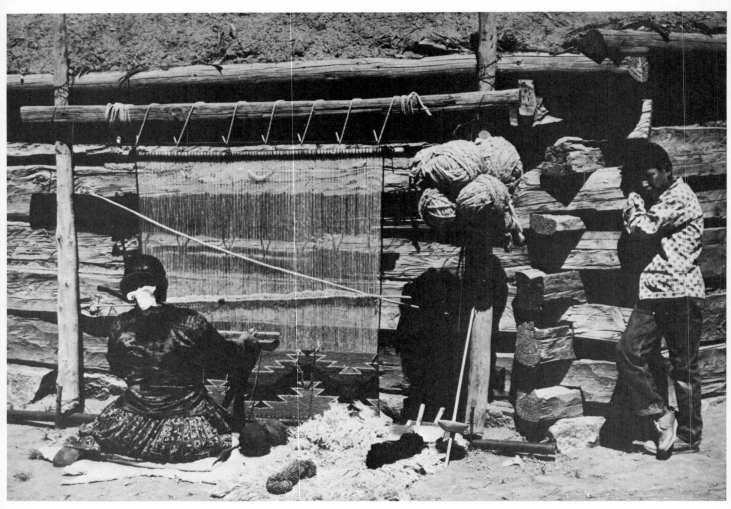

Some American Indians have carried on their traditional crafts. But these Americans, the oldest of the Oldcomers, were sometimes treated as if they were not Americans at all. An Act of Congress in 1924 finally admitted all Indians born in the United States to full citizenship.

the United States had as hard a job as faced any nation. The millions of Americans who had been treated as *things* were suddenly to be given their rights as *people*. They had owned no property and had not even been allowed to go to school. Now they were suddenly to become citizens with the duty to govern themselves and to help govern others. All this had to be done in the shadow of the hateful "peculiar institution," slavery, which had bred fears and hates on all sides. And all this had to be done in the aftermath of a bloody war which had bred still more fears and hates.

The mark of slavery could not be erased by magic. The South—and

Southerners—might take generations to recover. The full tragedy of slavery was only now appearing.

Yet by the early twentieth century there had been progress. When the Freedmen's Bureau ended in 1872, money to educate former slaves and their children then came from churches and missionary associations.

Wealthy men and women, mostly from the North, gave millions of dollars to help educate the Negro. By 1900 there were already about thirty thousand Negro teachers. John D. Rockefeller, for example, had contributed over $50 million of the money he had made from oil, most of it to train more teachers for

Negro schools. Every year more Negroes owned their own farms. And in the long run, better education, better wages, and more property would help the Negro to equality.

But a small number of Americans still actually *wanted* a Two-Nation America. These people were afraid that if Negroes had their share of education and owned their share of property, they really would become equal. And they were especially afraid to let the Negroes vote. Most of these fearful Americans were in the South. Less money was spent there than in other parts of the country for all kinds of education. In the South Negroes had to attend separate, and inferior, schools. There, especially, Negroes found it hard to borrow money in order to buy houses or farms.

The whole South suffered. By 1938 President Franklin Delano Roosevelt called the South "the nation's No. 1 economic problem." Almost any way you measured—by the health of the people, the quality of schools or houses, the number of automobiles, the amount of farm machinery, or the income of the families—the South was the worst-off section of the whole United States. And in the South, the Negroes were generally even worse off than others.

In 1930, 80 percent of American Negroes were still living within the boundaries of the old Confederacy. Yet new forces were working on all America. One of the most important of these was the Negro himself. Emancipation gave him a new power to be heard.

Even before the Civil War, a few eloquent Negroes like Frederick Douglass had managed to speak up loud and clear against slavery. Douglass, the slave son of an unknown white father, had been working on the Baltimore wharves. One day in 1838, at the age of twenty-one, he stowed away on a ship sailing for New York. After that he became one of the best propagandists against slavery. His books described the sufferings of slaves, and urged everybody to help them escape. Beginning in 1847, Douglass' newspaper, *The North Star,* worked for many reforms, including women's right to vote.

As more Negroes were educated and acquired property, more were able to help themselves. But how could they do it best? Negro leaders could not agree.

One way was proposed by Booker T. Washington. Born a slave, Washington was a self-made man. He worked as a janitor and at all sorts of jobs to support

Frederick Douglass helped recruit Negroes for the Union army. After the Civil War he became U.S. Minister to Haiti.

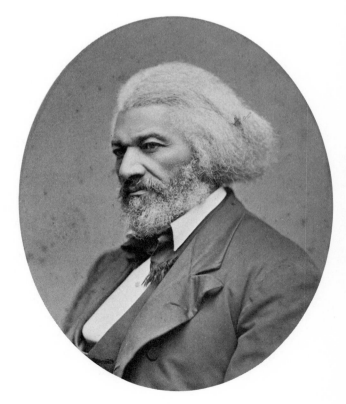

himself in school. Before his death he was famous throughout the world. For his own story of his life, *Up From Slavery* (1901), was read by millions.

"No man," he said, ". . . black or white, from North or South, shall drag me down so low as to make me hate him."

He preached a gospel of love and common sense. He told the Negro to make the most of himself and of his opportunities. He told white Southerners to show new respect for the Negro, to realize that only by bettering the Negro's life could they make a better South for everybody. Self-respect, self-education, and self-help, he said, would bring Negroes the opportunities they deserved. Some people thought he sounded old-fashioned. This might have been Benjamin Franklin speaking!

But Booker T. Washington did not merely talk. In 1881 he founded Tuskegee Institute in Alabama, which became one of the most powerful forces in American education. There he trained thousands of Negroes to be better farmers and mechanics, to make a good living, and to help build their communities.

He believed in a step-by-step way "up from slavery." First, he said, Negroes should get education and get property. But he believed in a special kind of education. Most important for Negroes right away was not a "liberal" education of the kind American college students were getting all over the country. He did not want Negroes to spend their efforts learning history and literature and foreign languages and science and mathematics. Instead, he said, they should train quickly for jobs—and mostly for jobs they could do with their hands. The vote, he said, could wait.

The Negro first should become a free man with a job before he became a free man with a vote.

Many who admired Booker T. Washington still did not agree with his program for the Negro. One-step-at-a-time was not good enough. Americans were quick with their know-how, quick in covering the continent and building cities. Why should they be slow to give *all* Americans *all* their rights?

Twenty-five years after Booker T. Washington started his Tuskegee Institute in Alabama, a group met at Niagara Falls. They demanded for Negroes all the rights of Americans. *Now!*

Their Negro leader was W. E. B. Du Bois. His life had been very different from that of Booker T. Washington. Born in Massachusetts after the Civil War, he studied at the University of Berlin in Germany and then received a Ph.D. degree from Harvard in 1895. While Booker T. Washington's roots were in the South, Du Bois's roots were in abolitionist Massachusetts, and in the whole world. Du Bois was a poet, and a man of brilliant mind and vast learning. Why should anyone try to tell Du Bois and others like him to be satisfied to work with their hands?

In 1905 the Declaration by Du Bois's Niagara Movement expressed outrage. It demanded for Negroes *all* their human rights, all their rights as Americans, and *at once.* It opposed all laws and all customs that treated Negroes as if they were different from other people. And, of course, it demanded the right to vote.

After the Civil War, white Southerners who believed in a Two-Nation South (run by the whites) had used all sorts of tricks to deprive Negroes of their rights

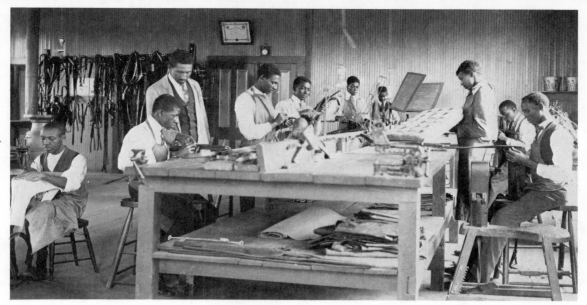

Booker T. Washington's Tuskegee Institute aimed to train its students for skilled and useful jobs. ABOVE: Young men learn upholstering. BELOW: Young women learn nursing.

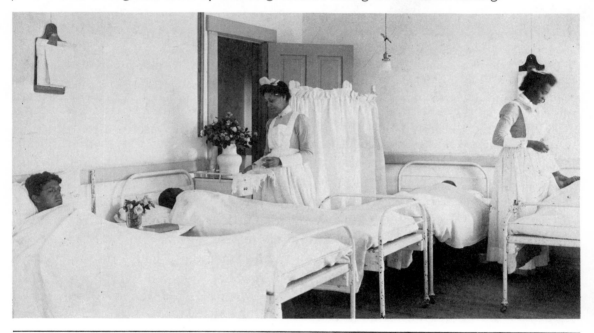

as citizens. The Fifteenth Amendment, adopted during Reconstruction, plainly declared that the right of citizens to vote should not be denied "by the United States or by any State on account of race, color, or previous condition of servitude." This set a real puzzle for the Two-Nation Southerners.

They tried using the "grandfather clause." They simply passed a law in the State Legislature giving the right to vote to those persons who *did* have the right to vote on January 1, 1867 (before the Fifteenth Amendment had been passed) and to those persons' descendants. Anybody else who wanted to vote had to pass all sorts of impossible tests. Of course that included Negroes. *They* would not be allowed to vote simply because their *grandfathers* did not have the right to vote! Beginning in 1895, seven Southern States passed "grandfather" laws. Not until 1915 did the United States Supreme Court declare

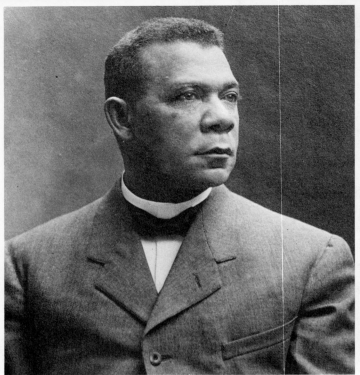 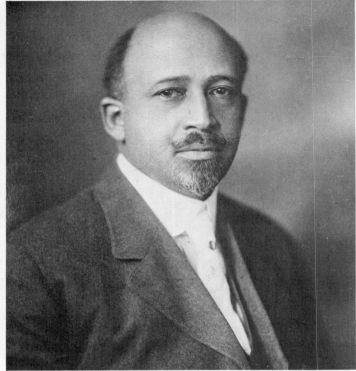

Booker T. Washington (left) believed that permanent progress must come slowly. W. E. B. Du Bois, himself a scholar, feared that Booker T. Washington's "gradualist" program would keep Negroes in lowly jobs.

that these laws violated the Constitution.

Another trick was the so-called Literacy Test. It was as dishonest as the Literacy Test which Oldcomers had tried to use to keep out immigrants from certain countries. It pretended to limit the vote to people who could read. But prejudiced election judges gave ridiculously complicated tests (which they themselves probably could not have passed) whenever Negroes came to vote. They would ask a Negro to explain the most difficult part of the Constitution. But a white person only had to read out a simple sentence.

Some Southern States also used the Poll Tax. That was a tax that everybody was required to pay before he could vote (or go to the "poll"). Most Negroes in the South were so poor they really could not afford the few dollars for the tax. And even if a Negro paid his tax, the election judge could always find some technical mistake in his tax receipt, and

so keep him from voting.

The craftiness of Two-Nation Southerners seemed endless. They even went so far as to pretend that the great political parties in the South were not political parties at all, but only private clubs. Therefore, they said, nobody except the white "members" had a right to vote in the primary election when their "club" picked its candidates.

Since the Democratic Party was in complete control in most of the South, whoever won in the Democratic primary automatically won the office. By keeping a person from voting in the primary, then, you would actually be taking away his vote. Finally, in three separate decisions—in 1944, 1947, and 1953—the United States Supreme Court declared that these laws violated the Fourteenth Amendment to the Constitution. But it took a special Twenty-fourth Amendment to the Constitution, adopted in 1964, to outlaw the Poll Tax.

CHAPTER 24

"A Triumph for Freedom" ༄

Intelligent citizens all over the country were beginning to be ashamed and disgusted that the nation had been so slow to give all Americans their simple rights. The Niagara Movement, sparked by Du Bois and aided by white Americans who gloried in the anti-slavery tradition, became stronger. To help prevent shameful race riots like the one in Springfield, Illinois (Lincoln's birthplace) in 1908, a new organization, the National Association for the Advancement of Colored People (NAACP), was founded in 1909 on Lincoln's birthday.

Americans of all races and religions, from all parts of the country, joined hands. People like Jane Addams, who already were working for the poor of all races in the northern city slums, gave money to pay for lawyers to help Negroes secure their rights in the South. The president of the NAACP, a famous Boston lawyer, argued the case before the Supreme Court in 1915 when the "grandfather" laws were declared unconstitutional. The NAACP also won other important cases. One of these declared that no trial of a Negro could be a fair trial (as the Constitution required) if Negroes were kept off the jury. During the next years the NAACP was the most important group trying to awaken all Americans to the rights of Negroes.

Things were getting better for the Negro. But the progress was painfully slow—even considering the long distance the Negro needed to rise from slavery.

For millions of Negro Americans—especially in the South and in the big city slums in the North—there still seemed almost no change. Negro workers were the last hired and the first fired. Negro children still had less money spent on their education. Negroes were not allowed to live wherever they could afford, but had to live in special neighborhoods. Even under the New Deal, Negroes were not always given their share. For example, they were not allowed to live in the model towns built with government money in the Tennessee Valley. Most of the Negroes whom Du Bois called the "Talented Tenth" still had to take lowly jobs.

Some, in fact, gave up. Du Bois, for example, joined the Communist Party and then renounced his United States citizenship. In 1961 at the age of 93 he moved to the new African country of Ghana, which before 1957 had been a British colony. Others kept their faith in America and struggled for new ways to keep the nation true.

During two World Wars, Negro Americans fought for their country. In World War I, Negro soldiers numbered over a third of a million. In World War II they numbered a million. In both wars they proved their bravery and their loyalty. The wars gave them other chances, too—to move outside the South, away from their farms and villages, into the larger world.

They discovered that the prejudices which some white Southerners had inherited from the days of slavery were not found everywhere. They mixed with other Americans from all over the country, and they went abroad. They had new experiences and new adventures.

Yet, even in the army and navy and air force, Negro Americans still were not given equal rights. In World War I, Negroes found it difficult to become officers. They were not allowed at all in the Marines, and in the navy they had no hope for promotion. Even in uniform, they were often insulted. It took great faith and patriotism, then, for a Negro American to risk his life for a country that was not yet giving him his full rights as a citizen.

President Woodrow Wilson was leading the country in a war "to make the world safe for democracy." Yet President Wilson himself, born in Virginia before the Civil War, had never outgrown the feelings of the Two-Nation South. Though elected on the slogan of the "New Freedom," after he came to Washington he actually segregated Negroes working in the government. And he took government jobs away from Negroes in the South.

In World War II things were better for the Negro soldier. The Marines no longer kept him out, and before the war was over there were 17,000 Negro "Leathernecks." It became easier for qualified Negroes to become officers. Even the navy, which before had taken in Negroes only for kitchen work and as waiters, began to open up. The air force trained Negro officers and pilots, and more than eighty won the Distinguished Flying Cross.

But the long shadow of the Two-Nation South remained. Negroes, once more fighting for democracy, were usually still segregated.

Finally, though, the stain of slavery was washed away in the armed services. President Harry S Truman in 1946 appointed a national committee to recommend action. By 1949 the army, navy, and air force had all abolished racial quotas. They made it their policy to give all Americans an equal chance. By the time of the Korean War in 1950–1953 *all* Americans were fighting for democracy side by side.

During these later wars, even more than during the Civil War, Americans moved all around the country. Many went to new war jobs. Returning soldiers settled in new places. Before World War I only about 10 percent of Negro Americans lived outside the South. After that war the number rose to 20 percent. And after World War II about one-third of all Negro Americans were living outside the Old Confederacy.

Negro Americans, like other Americans, were becoming more and more citified. Outside the South nearly all of them were living in cities. Even in the South they too were moving off the countryside. Many Americans—including, of course, more Negroes—were churning quickly and easily around the whole country. It was harder than ever for the South to keep its old ways.

In Africa, new republics were declaring their independence from the old colonial powers. First came Ghana in 1957, and by 1965 there were over thirty new African members of the United Nations. When they sent their ambassadors to the United States, the discrimination against Negroes here was more embarrassing than ever.

Then, too, the United States Supreme Court began to wake up. In a series of decisions it began to outlaw those Southern practices and laws which had taken from the Negro his full rights as an American. Back in 1896 the Court actually had declared that laws which required Negroes to stay separate—to use separate washrooms, separate schools, and separate railroad cars—did *not* violate the Fourteenth Amendment. It was all right, the Court said, for any services to be separate so long as they were "equal." But this was a trick argument.

Anyone who knew the South could have known that the white Southerners who ran the government would *say* they were providing "equal" schools. But who had the power to complain if the schools were not really equal? Negroes, who still were not allowed to vote, had no way of forcing government officials to listen. The Supreme Court had okayed the Two-Nation South.

In the South, Negroes continued to have the worst of everything. Their schools and hospitals, and even their washrooms and water fountains, were inferior.

Anyway, the whole idea of "separate but equal"—even if it could have been enforced—was wrong. It was not only wrong, it was nonsense. Because, in a democracy, people who are forced to be separate, forced to use washrooms and water fountains and schools not used by other Americans, are not being allowed

Segregated water fountain.

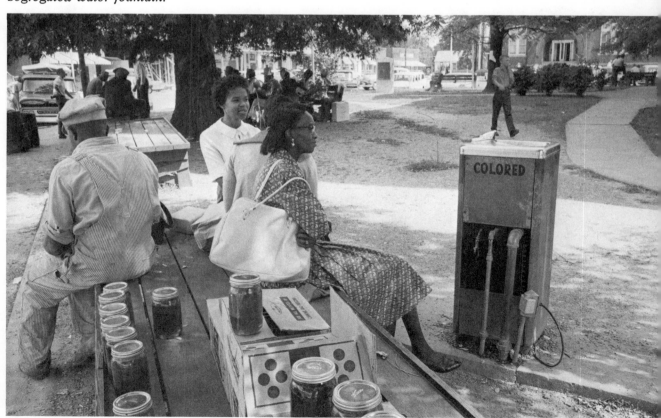

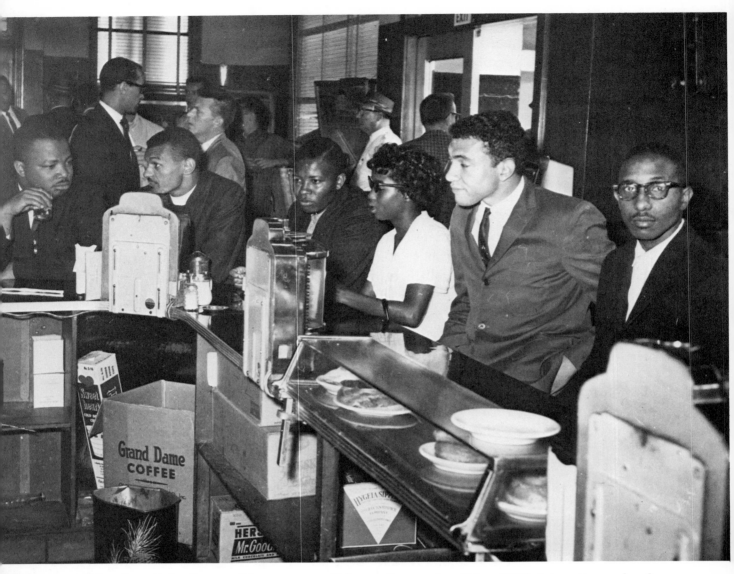

"Freedom Riders" in a Montgomery, Alabama, bus station (May 1961) integrating a lunch counter with a nonviolent "sit-in."

---

to be equal. The special separate schools for Negroes could not possibly be equal —simply because they were separate.

Finally in 1954, in one of the most important decisions it had ever made, the Supreme Court ordered that, under the Constitution, public schools could not be separate. Americans had a right to go to school with all other Americans of their age and grade. This was a part of their education. No American should be deprived of that right. The opposite of separation was "integration"—bringing together into one. And the Supreme Court ordered that all public schools in the United States had to be "integrated."

These changes in American life, in American thought and feeling all over the country, made the time ripe for the work of Martin Luther King, Jr. His work began in a small way and in one place. Within only a few years his message had carried to the world.

Born in Atlanta in 1929, son of a minister, he attended Morehouse College and received a doctor's degree from Boston University. He was a natural leader, American to the core. He combined the common sense of a Booker T. Washington with the impatient visions of a Du Bois.

On December 1, 1955, a tired Negro seamstress returning from work boarded a crowded bus in Montgomery, Alabama. She took a seat. But the seat she took was in the part of the bus reserved for white passengers. When she was asked to give up her seat to a white person, she refused. The police arrested her for violating the law.

Martin Luther King, who was then a Baptist minister in Montgomery, decided it was time for action. It was time to stop any Americans from being degraded.

Although King was indignant and saddened, he was not angry. He was a thoughtful man, and a Christian, and he decided to try a new way. He called it the only true Christian way. It was the way of nonviolence.

He did not tell people to burn the buses or to fight the police. No, he said. All people need to be educated in the ways of peace and decency. If you fight your enemies with violence, you are using their weapons and brutalizing yourself. But if you are peaceful and simply do not go along with them, you will eventually prevail. And if you win this way, your victory will not merely be the truce in a running battle. It will actually be peace. Your enemies then

will understand, and they will begin to be decent, too.

So he preached to the Negroes in Montgomery. He told them to stop using the buses until the buses gave them their place as Americans. Of course many Negroes were angry. But Martin Luther King begged and pleaded with them to keep their heads, and to keep love in their hearts, even while they joined the bus boycott.

For 381 days the Negroes of Montgomery refused to ride the buses. It was inconvenient. Some formed car pools. Many were given rides by friendly white neighbors. Many walked miles to work. Others simply did not get to their jobs and had to lose their wages.

And the bus company was about to go bankrupt.

In the end the Negroes and all the decent people of Montgomery won. When the buses ran again, every passenger was treated like all the others. Martin Luther King called this a "Stride Toward Freedom." And he was right.

It was not only a stride toward freedom. It was a step along a new path. Many Americans were encouraged to walk along that path in the years that followed. By 1960 many Negroes in the South were using this new way to fight segregation. They sat down at lunch counters where they had not been allowed to sit. They swam in public swimming pools that had been denied to Negroes. And they worshiped in churches that had kept out Negroes. They did not fight the police or strike out at anyone. Quietly and peacefully, they simply acted like decent Americans who knew their rights.

The movement spread. In 1963—a

full century after the Emancipation Proclamation—there came a climax. In February, the season of Lincoln's birthday, President John F. Kennedy sent a Civil Rights Bill to Congress. The bill would guarantee the vote to all Americans, outlaw segregation in all public places, and protect the right of all Americans to use motels and hotels and barber shops and restaurants. But Congress did not act. The Two-Nation Southerners and a few of their Northern supporters blocked the law. They acted as if the Civil War had never been fought—or as if it had been won by the South.

Americans of all races became impatient. Members of all religious groups—Catholics, Protestants, and Jews—leaders of labor unions and many others decided to show Congress how strongly Americans felt. They planned a "March on Washington." The purpose of their march was peaceful, entirely in line with Martin Luther King's ideas. They did not want to fight the police or take over the government. They simply wanted to use their democratic right to show their representatives in Congress how many Americans were demanding equality for everybody.

On August 28, 1963, nearly a quarter-million Americans gathered at the Lincoln Memorial in Washington, D.C., within sight of the White House and the Capitol where Congress met. The meeting was orderly and eloquent. It was the largest number of Americans until

The March on Washington, August 1963. Americans of all faiths and races and several labor unions joined hands in demanding equal rights for all. In the center of the front row was Dr. Martin Luther King.

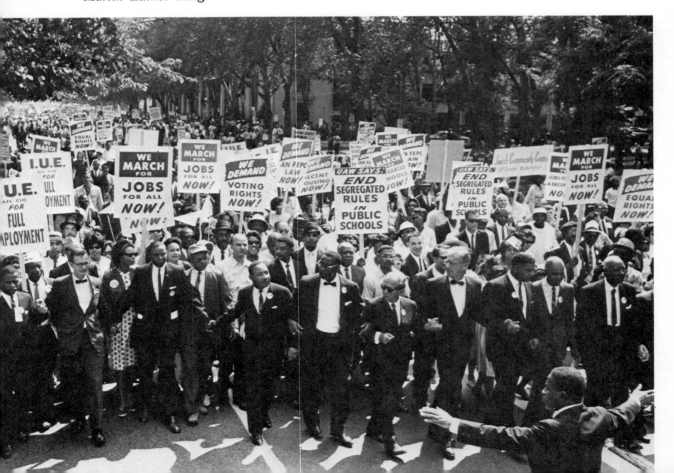

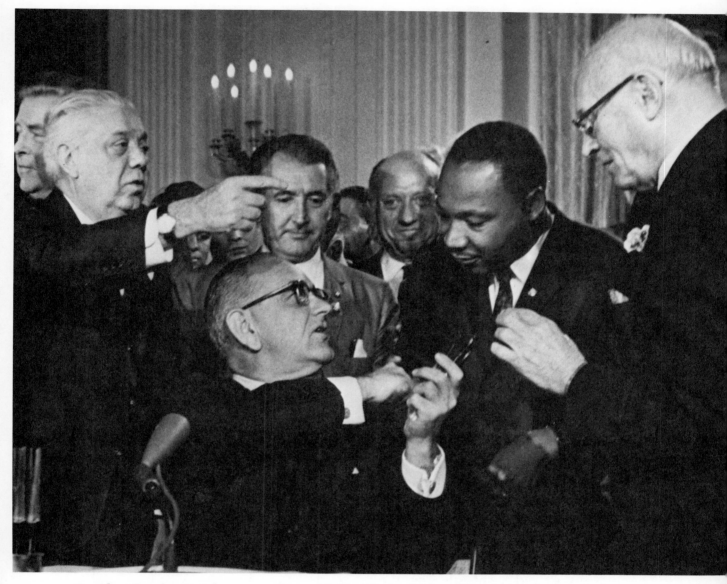

President Lyndon B. Johnson speaking with Dr. Martin Luther King during the televised ceremony at the signing of the Civil Rights Act of 1964.

that time ever gathered in one place for any purpose in peacetime.

Some were afraid there might be trouble. But trouble did not come. Americans could ever after be proud that so many of their countrymen cared enough for the rights of all Americans to make that meeting possible, and to keep it peaceful.

Congress still delayed. They did not want to act when it might seem they were acting under threat. Then, on November 22, 1963, the nation was shaken by tragedy. While riding in an open car in Dallas, Texas, President Kennedy was shot. He died within minutes. But the spirit of all who believed in America, and in the promise of equality, lived on.

The new President was Lyndon B. Johnson. His first act was to address

Congress demanding immediate passage of the Civil Rights Bill. He also offered a new Voting Rights Act, with effective new ways of protecting the right of everybody to vote—even in the South.

These acts meant business. The day of legal trickery had passed. "Today is a triumph for freedom," President Johnson declared when these acts became law, "as huge as any victory that's ever been won on any battlefield. . . . Today the Negro story and the American story fuse and blend." He could have called this peaceful victory even bigger than the victories in war.

Still, the forces of hate and fear—of a Two-Nation America—were not yet dead. Martin Luther King himself was shot while he stood on the balcony of a Memphis motel on April 4, 1968. No American who knew history could be surprised that the spirit of hate still walked the land—and it found new preachers of hate in all races.

The twentieth-century battle for rights left new wounds, stirred new fears and hates. The future of the nation would depend on the ability of all Americans to remember the long struggle which *all* Americans shared. And also on their ability to forget harsh words and old insults. The nation needed a renewal of the generous, forgiving spirit of Lincoln.

The next years showed that the spirit of Lincoln was alive and well. There was a long way to go to make up for the years of slavery. Even after the Civil War, Negroes were only half-free, for in many parts of the country and for many kinds of jobs, they had no chance.

Now the nation's conscience was awake. Some of the most important new opportunities were in education. The old segregated classrooms were changed by school busing. Now white and Negro children sat happily together. Colleges that had never seen a Negro in the lecture hall opened their minds and their doors. The best colleges, law schools, and medical schools in the land, instead of finding reasons to keep them out, went in search of qualified Negroes. Special scholarships were offered to Negro students. Negro professors who once could find jobs only in Negro colleges could take their rightful place in any university. These great changes were going on behind the scenes.

Out front, too, there were great changes that no one could miss. Thurgood Marshall, a Negro appointed by President Lyndon Johnson, now sat on the Supreme Court. And when you turned on your TV set, you saw Negroes not only as maids or chauffeurs, but as police captains, businessmen, news reporters, priests, doctors, and lawyers.

The civil rights movement was contagious. If Negroes should have a new chance, why not others? What about women? It had taken a long time for women to get the right to vote, to be admitted to universities with men, and to have their fair chance to study law, medicine, and business administration. Now a woman, Sandra Day O'Connor of Arizona, had been appointed by President Ronald Reagan to sit on the Supreme Court. And by the 1980's there were six women governors of States of the Union. On TV, too, women were seen not only as wives and mothers but as people who could handle any kind of job—from truck driver to airplane pilot. Once the nation's eyes were opened, they would never be closed again.

PART FIVE

———❦———

TO THIS
WHOLE WORLD
—AND BEYOND

TO THIS WHOLE WORLD—AND BEYOND

Until the Civil War the United States had seemed a world of its own. It had been easy for Americans to imagine that they really did not need the rest of the world. The continent was so large. It offered so many different climates. Almost every needed crop or animal, almost every mineral, was found somewhere within the nation and its territories. When the first settlers had called this a New World they were speaking the sober truth.

Then after the Civil War, more and more Americans discovered that America needed the world. The nation still wanted to import people by the millions. And it needed the outside world for many new reasons.

The prosperity of American farmers and factory workers and businessmen now depended on faraway customers and on the ability of Americans to deliver their goods overseas. American consumers were coming to rely on silk from Italy and China, on rubber from the Congo and Sumatra, on coffee from Brazil, on tin from Malaya, on gold from Rhodesia—and on a thousand other items from across the oceans.

The United States became the world's know-how center—for trying new ways of making and doing.

And people everywhere expected to learn from America. Americans began to feel it their duty to help make the whole earth into a New World.

But could the United States preach democracy and help other nations become democratic without trying to choose other peoples' governments for them?

Could Americans take their place in the world competition for customers and for raw materials without making remote peoples into a new kind of colonies?

Could the most powerful nation on earth resist the temptation to run the affairs of mankind?

Could the nation do its duty in the battles of the Old World and yet stay free of the Old World curse of endless wars?

Could the nation become the most modern, most intricately organized people on earth, and yet preserve self-government and the spirit of adventure?

CHAPTER 25

Ocean Paths to World Power

After the Civil War, Americans realized that the United States had become a two-ocean nation. The Atlantic seaboard looked eastward toward Europe and Africa. The Far Western States looked across the Pacific toward Australia and Asia.

Some Americans were beginning to think differently about their place in the world. An Annapolis graduate, Admiral Alfred T. Mahan, wrote a powerful book called *The Influence of Sea Power Upon History* (1890). What *Uncle Tom's Cabin* was to the Civil War, Mahan's *Sea Power* would be to the Spanish-American War.

Sea Power, Mahan said, was the key to all history. A nation became great and kept its greatness only if it ruled the waves. Americans, he said, had long shown "the instinct for commerce, bold enterprise in the pursuit of gain, and a keen sense for the trails that lead to it." Yet these were not enough. The nation also needed to be rich in all kinds of ships. Then, of course, she would need colonies in faraway places where her ships could refuel and find protection.

A few years after Mahan began preaching Sea Power he found one of his strongest allies in Theodore Roosevelt, whom President McKinley appointed Assistant Secretary of the Navy in 1897. Even before he had finished at Harvard,

Teddy had begun writing *The Naval War of 1812*, which was published in 1882, only two years after he graduated. He remained fascinated by ships. And he was especially intrigued by the puzzle of power. What really made a nation strong? He was delighted by Mahan's writings.

At that time trouble was brewing only a few miles off the coast of Florida. The island of Cuba had been a colony of Spain ever since it was first sighted by Columbus. In the nineteenth century Spain was tyrannizing over the inhabitants. And the Cuban rebels declared their independence in February 1895.

The Spanish government sent out troops and put the island under a ruthless general, Valeriano "Butcher" Weyler. On February 10, 1896, General Weyler ordered that "all the inhabitants of the country" who were still outside the towns should "concentrate themselves in the towns." Anybody found outside a town would be shot. This made Cuban towns into "concentration camps." The whole island became a prison. Men, women, and children were herded together. Some were tortured, others died of disease and starvation—including some United States citizens.

American newspapers splashed the stories of "Butcher" Weyler's atrocities on the front pages of papers which went out in six editions a day to the cities and at least once a day (by RFD) even to remote farms. Joseph Pulitzer, an energetic Hungarian immigrant who had bought the New York *World*, was anxious to make his paper popular. The more copies he sold, the more he could charge for advertising—and advertising supported the paper.

Pulitzer was brilliant at finding new ways to attract readers. For example, he hired a clever cartoonist, Richard F. Outcault, to make the first color comic strip. It showed the adventures of a bad boy called the "Yellow Kid" who ap-

in whether they were true. Because they featured the Yellow Kid these newspapers—and others like them—were soon called the "Yellow Press."

The United States had a long-standing interest in Cuba. Back in the early nineteenth century Thomas Jefferson himself had said he hoped to see Cuba become part of the United States. Now American businessmen had invested over fifty million dollars in Cuban sugar. In 1895 the rebels destroyed sugar plantations and mills, hoping to prod the United States to intervene. Then, in 1896, William McKinley was

Sensational headlines in Hearst newspaper.

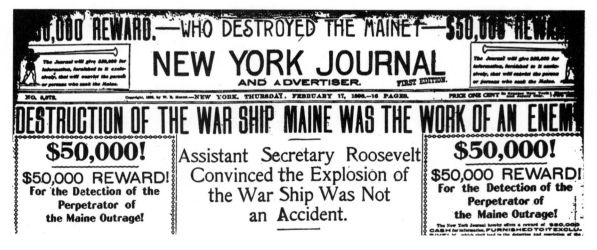

peared regularly in the Sunday edition. Outcault's cartoons were so successful that Pulitzer's leading competitor, the Go-Getting William Randolph Hearst, hired the same cartoonist to do another Yellow Kid series for the Sunday edition of *his* paper, the New York *Journal*.

While on Sundays both papers used the Yellow Kid to attract readers, every day they competed by printing shocking stories. They were more interested in whether the stories were shocking than

elected President with a promise to help Cuba become independent.

When Spain began to negotiate with the United States about freedom for the Cubans, it seemed there would be no need to fight. But on February 9, 1898, the New York *Journal* printed a stolen letter in which the Spanish ambassador called President McKinley a coward and other nasty names.

To protect American lives and property, the United States battleship *Maine* had been sent to Havana harbor. At 9:40 P.M. on the night of February 15, 1898, the *Maine* was shattered by an explosion, and 260 officers and men were killed. The navy's court of inquiry reported that the cause was an underwater mine, but they could not say for sure whether the Spanish were to blame. Anyway the Yellow Press called for war against Spain, and headlined the slogan, "REMEMBER THE MAINE!"

When the excitable Assistant Secretary of the Navy, Theodore Roosevelt, heard that McKinley was hesitating, he said the President "had no more backbone than a chocolate éclair." On February 25 the Secretary of the Navy made the mistake of taking the afternoon off. That left impatient Teddy as Acting Secretary—in charge of the whole United States navy. Without consulting anyone, he instantly cabled his friend Admiral George Dewey, who commanded the United States fleet in Asiatic waters. Make sure, he ordered, that Spanish ships do not leave the coast of Asia. Begin "defensive operations" against the Spanish colony out there— the Philippines!

When the Secretary of the Navy returned to his office next day, he was astonished. "Roosevelt," he wrote in his diary, "has come very near causing more of an explosion than happened to the *Maine*." But it was too late to change the order. And even *before* war had begun in nearby Cuba, Teddy had arrayed the United States fleet for war on the other side of the world.

If President McKinley had been a stronger man he would not have been afraid to keep the peace. The government of Spain now actually told him

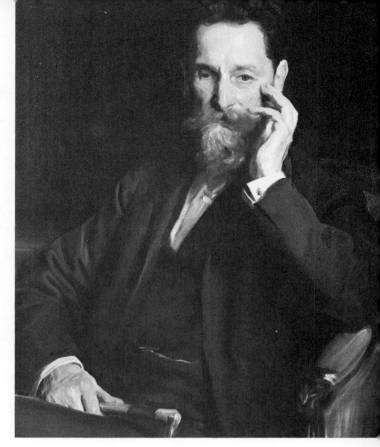

Joseph Pulitzer, a painting by John Singer Sargent, who was famous for his portraits of notable Americans.

they would give Cuba her independence. But the Yellow Press was still demanding Spanish blood. The "jingoes" —the people who loved to see a fight— wanted war. On April 11, the day *after* President McKinley learned that Spain would agree to do everything Americans said they wanted, he asked Congress to declare war.

The war lasted only a few months— but that was long enough to create the greatest confusion. At the training camp in Tampa, Florida, commanding officers could not find uniforms, while for weeks fifteen railroad cars full of uniforms remained on a siding twenty-five miles away. The commander of United States troops in Cuba, Major General W. R. Shafter, weighed three hundred pounds and was therefore "too unwieldy to get to the front." Unprepared for combat,

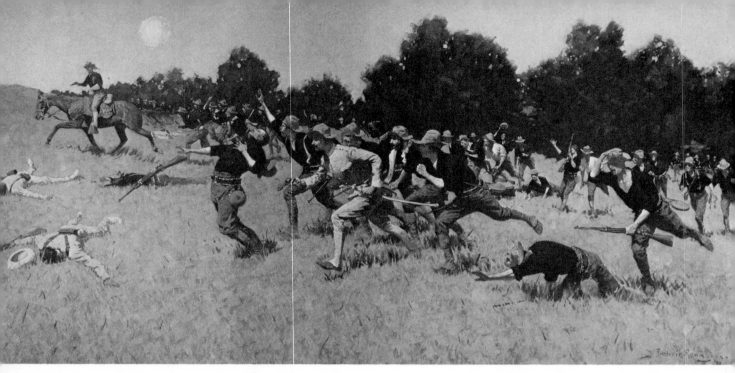

"Charge of the Rough Riders at San Juan Hill," a painting by Frederic Remington, who went to Cuba as an artist-correspondent. The "Rough Riders" had to run up the hill on foot. Teddy Roosevelt, leading them on horseback, made himself the most conspicuous target.

the army committed every foolishness known to man.

The navy was in better shape. On May 1, when Admiral Dewey, following Roosevelt's impulsive orders, attacked the Spanish warships in the Philippines, he finished off the Spaniards in seven hours. The remnant of the Spanish fleet, which was in North American waters, then sneaked into Santiago harbor on the southeastern tip of Cuba.

Meanwhile Teddy Roosevelt had himself appointed lieutenant colonel of a new regiment of cavalry. At a training camp in San Antonio, Texas, he gathered cowboys, sheriffs, and desperadoes from the West, and a sprinkling of playboy polo players and steeplechase riders from the East. They came to be known as Roosevelt's Rough Riders.

Roosevelt himself was preparing for serious combat. What worried him most was his bad eyesight. If he broke or lost his glasses he could not see where he was going, much less find the Spaniards

to shoot. He ordered a dozen extra pairs of steel-rimmed eyeglasses. He then stowed them separately all over his uniform and even put several extra pairs inside the lining of his campaign hat.

On June 22, Roosevelt's Rough Riders arrived in Cuba. They were given the job of storming San Juan Hill, which overlooked Santiago bay. To capture the steep hill his "Rough Riding" cavalry (who had been selected for their horsemanship) actually had to dismount. "I waved my hat and went up the hill with a rush," Roosevelt recalled. After a bloody fight, they reached the top.

Theodore Roosevelt never suffered from modesty. When Roosevelt published his book *The Rough Riders*, the humorist "Mr. Dooley" said Teddy should have called it "Alone in Cuba."

The decisive naval battle occurred even before the Americans could place their big guns on San Juan Hill to bombard the enemy navy below. When the Spanish fleet tried to run for the open sea the United States navy exterminated every last warship of Spain. All over the United States, enthusiastic Americans celebrated their victory.

By the standards of American history, this had not been a full-size war. There were 385 battle deaths—less than one-tenth the deaths in the American Revolution, and only one-twentieth the deaths at the Battle of Gettysburg alone. While the American Revolution had lasted nearly eight years and the Civil War had lasted four years, the Spanish-American War lasted only four *months*. Even this "little" war cost a quarter-billion dollars and several thousand deaths from disease.

And the little war marked a big change in the relationship of the United States to the world. The tides of history were turned. Cuba, given her independence, became an American protectorate.

The defeated Spain forfeited to the United States an empire of islands. This nation, born in a colonial revolution, would now have her own colonies. All were outside the continent, some were thousands of miles away. The United States acquired Puerto Rico at the gateway of the Caribbean, along with Guam, important as a refuelling station in mid-Pacific. The Philippine Islands (there were seven thousand of them, of which over one thousand were inhabitable) off the coast of China were sold to the United States for the bargain price of twenty million dollars.

These new American colonies added up to one hundred thousand square miles, holding nearly ten million people. That was not much, compared to the vast empires of England, France, or Germany. But for the United States it was something quite new.

The meaning of this Spanish-American War in American history, then, was actually less in what it accomplished than in what it proclaimed. The American Revolution had been our War of Independence. Now the Spanish-American War at the threshold of the twentieth century, was our first War of Intervention. We had joined the old-fashioned race for empire—on all the oceans of the world.

Many Americans were worried. Some were saddened, and even angry. They called themselves "Anti-Imperialists," for they hated to see the United States become an empire. To be an empire, they said, meant lording it over people in faraway places. Anti-Imperialists included Democrats and Republicans, of all sections and classes—labor leader Samuel Gompers, industrialist Andrew Carnegie, President Charles W. Eliot of Harvard and President David Starr Jordan of Stanford, the philosopher William James, the social worker Jane Addams, and the popular writer Mark Twain.

Theodore Roosevelt, however, believed that the United States could accomplish her mission only if she was a great world power. We must be willing to have colonies, he said, while we help the people learn to be democratic.

He built a great navy. In the Spanish-American War we had only five battleships and two armored cruisers. But before Roosevelt left the White House in 1909, we had twenty-five battleships and ten heavy cruisers. We had become, next to the British, the strongest naval power in the world.

President Roosevelt foresaw some grand accomplishments which would never have been done by stay-at-homes. For years Americans going westward had tried to find ways to shorten the voyage to California. Now, as a world power, the United States had to be able to move its navy speedily from one ocean to another. This was an urgent new reason to cut a waterway through Central America.

When TR came to the White House, a French company had already been working on a canal for twenty years. But they were stymied by tropical disease. Their progress was slow and international complications seemed to make the whole enterprise hopeless.

TR would let nothing stop him. First he tried to make a treaty with the little Republic of Colombia, which then included the part of the Isthmus of Panama where the canal had to be built. When the government of Colombia blocked Roosevelt's treaty in 1903, a revolution suddenly occurred in Panama. A lucky coincidence for the United States! But there was evidence that American money had helped the "coincidence" to happen. Immediately, the new "independent" Republic of Panama made a treaty granting the Canal Zone to the United States.

Within only ten years after construction began, ships were actually passing through the canal. The canal cost over a half-billion dollars.

Building the canal had produced some world-wide benefits that even TR had never dreamed of. In order to build the canal through the fever-infested swamps, the Americans had to conquer tropical diseases. When Americans occupied Havana after the Spanish-American War, Dr. Walter Reed had discovered the mosquito that carried the deadly yellow fever. Then Dr. William Gorgas, who had worked with Reed in Cuba, applied this discovery in Panama. His work finally made the canal possible —and incidentally helped conquer that tropical disease all around the world.

CHAPTER 26

How Submarines Killed the Freedom of the Seas

With world power and an island empire came a greater need to use the ocean highways. Ever since the eighteenth century, the civilized nations had agreed on certain rules. Since wars were always going on somewhere in the world, the purpose of these rules was to allow the neutral countries to carry on their commerce in peace.

The countries that were not fighting had certain Neutral Rights. The most important was their right to send their ships anywhere, and to have their citizens be safe wherever they traveled.

Warring nations were allowed to seize certain war materials ("contraband"— explosives, guns, and ammunition) even from a neutral ship. But they were not supposed to seize the other goods carried by neutrals. Before sinking any

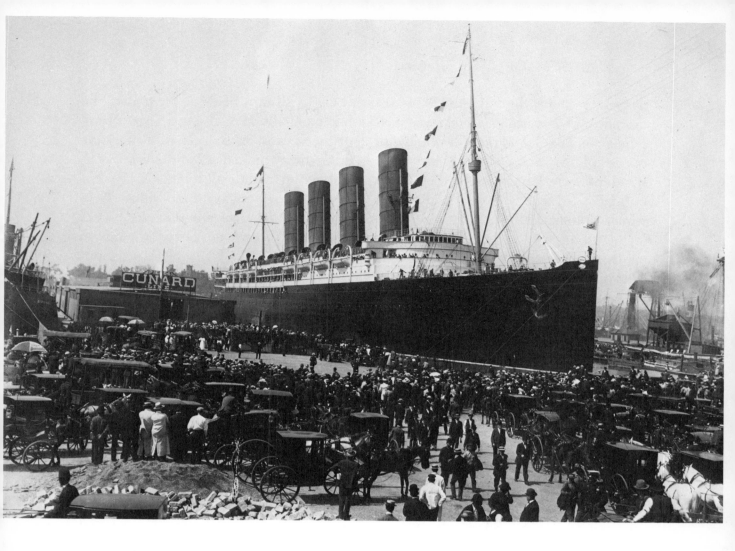

ABOVE: *The luxury liner* Lusitania *at the dock in New York. When launched in 1907 it was the largest steamship in the world.* BELOW: *A German submarine in World War I. Posing a new threat to warships and passenger vessels, it was too small and crowded to rescue its victims.*

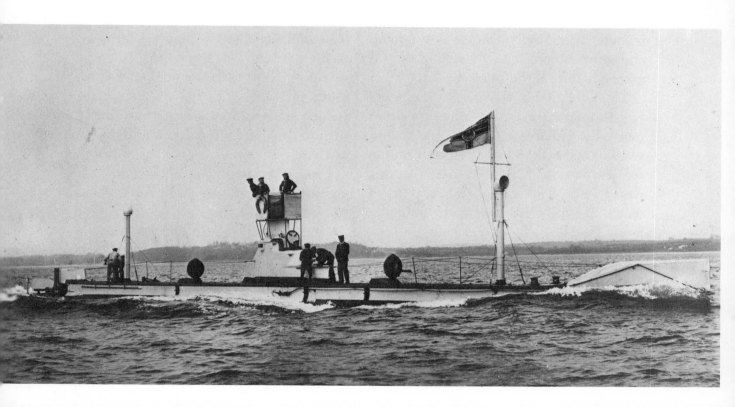

passenger ship, the attacker was required to give warning, to take the passengers on board, and do everything else reasonable to save civilian lives. Since warships were large vessels, they could normally be seen at a great distance, which automatically gave some warning. And anyway it was not too inconvenient for large warships to carry some extra passengers.

Such rules as these were what people meant by International Law. There was no court or police force to make nations obey. But the rules were still called "Law" because so many people believed they ought to be obeyed. The special rights of neutrals were also called Freedom of the Seas.

In 1914, when World War I broke out in Europe, these rules were still substantially the same as they had been for about two centuries. But the navies had changed. Most important was a new kind of ship—the submarine. The submarine's great strength was its new power to surprise. At the same time, however, the submarine was a crowded, tight-packed little vessel. With barely enough room for its own crew and food and ammunition, it had nowhere to put passengers from the ships it sank.

To say that all warring nations still had to follow the old rules would automatically outlaw the submarine. This would not have bothered Great Britain, for she had the greatest navy in the world. She commanded the seas anyway. But for Germany, with her relatively small navy, submarines would make all the difference. To forbid the submarine, then, was only another way of saying that Britain must forever rule the waves.

Great Britain made it plain that she had no intention of giving up her control of the oceans. She declared a blockade of Germany and enlarged the list of contraband to include all sorts of goods that neutrals had always been allowed to carry. Britain declared that she would even stop ships from carrying goods to neutral countries if any of those goods would eventually get to Germany. None of this was according to International Law.

Germany could hardly be expected to sit still and let herself be strangled. Her submarines could do their deadly work only if they, too, disobeyed International Law. Germany therefore decided to use the submarine for all it was worth, and to let others worry about the old rules. The Germans advertised in American newspapers urging Americans not to travel on British ships.

Then, on the night of May 7, 1915, the British luxury liner *Lusitania* was sunk without warning off the coast of Ireland by the German submarine U-20. Of nearly two thousand persons on board, 1,198 died, including 128 Americans. The ship sank within eighteen minutes of the time she was torpedoed. She was carrying 4,200 cases of small-arms ammunition and 1,250 shrapnel cases (which under International Law made the whole ship contraband and liable to be sunk).

President Woodrow Wilson sent a strong protest to Germany. He insisted on Neutral Rights. And he said this meant the right of Americans to travel wherever they pleased—even on the ships of the fighting nations, and right into the war zone. Wilson said this was a matter of national honor.

Woodrow Wilson's family background had not aroused his interest in naval or military affairs. His father, a Presbyterian minister who taught in a seminary, wanted young Woodrow to train for the ministry. Although Woodrow Wilson decided against becoming a minister, in some ways he always thought and talked like an old-fashioned minister.

Like Theodore Roosevelt, Wilson was a literary President, the author of many books. But in almost every other way he was TR's opposite. While TR's first book was on sea power, young Wilson wrote about moral questions for the North Carolina *Presbyterian*. While TR adored "The Strenuous Life," Wilson lived in the world of ideas, "longing to do immortal work." At the age when TR was learning to ride broncos and was bunking with cowboys, Wilson was sitting in post-graduate seminars on political science at Johns Hopkins University.

Wilson was an indoor sort of man. After a bright career as a professor he was elected president of Princeton University, where his educational reforms made him nationally famous. Then in 1910 he was elected Governor of New Jersey, and in 1912 he received the Democratic nomination for President. He could inspire people in large groups or from the printed page. But face to face he was stiff and stand-offish.

While Wilson had some of William Jennings Bryan's religious appeal, his tone was very different. Bryan sounded like the preacher at a country tent meeting, but Wilson could have been the minister of the best church in town. Both could persuade voters that they were joining the Army of the Lord. Wilson, like Bryan, championed the

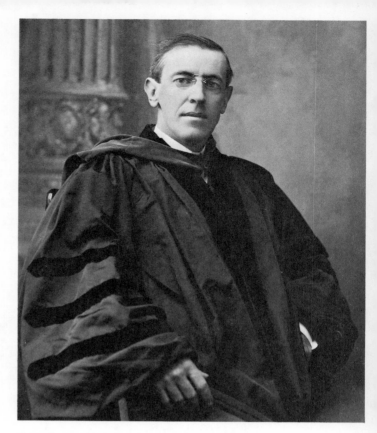

Woodrow Wilson as president of Princeton University.

struggling farmers and underprivileged workers. As a more moderate kind of Bryan, Wilson had a wider appeal.

In 1916, two years after the outbreak of war in Europe, Wilson was reelected on the slogan, "He Kept Us Out of War!" But one thing after another was taking Americans further down the road. The German foreign minister, Arthur Zimmermann, sent a foolish message to the German ambassador in Mexico. Zimmermann asked Mexico to join the German side, and in return Germany promised to help the Mexicans recapture from the United States all of Texas, Arizona, and New Mexico. The message was intercepted and decoded by the British, who then eagerly relayed it to the United States.

Meanwhile, powerful unseen forces were drawing Americans naturally like a magnet toward the British. After all, we spoke the English language, our laws were built on English foundations, and we had fought our American Revolution to preserve our rights as Englishmen. Early in the war, the British succeeded in cutting the transatlantic cable that brought news to America direct from Germany. After that, all news from Europe was channeled through England. This gave the British a great advantage that very few people noticed.

Even before we declared war the United States was already supporting the British side. Because of the British blockade against Germany and her allies, the value of American goods sent to Germany and Austria plummeted from nearly $170,000,000 in 1914 to about $1,000,000 in 1916. During the same two years, American trade with Britain and her allies rocketed from $800,000,000 to over $3,214,000,000. While the United States was still technically neutral, American bankers had actually loaned the British allies $2,300,000,000 to buy war supplies.

On April 2, 1917, within a month after the Zimmermann Note was published, President Wilson went to Congress to demand a declaration of war against Germany. He no longer spoke only about Neutral Rights. He would not ask Americans to die for a technicality. "The world," Wilson said, "must be made safe for democracy." Americans must fight "for the rights and liberties of small nations," to "bring peace and safety to all nations and make the world itself at last free."

There was, in fact, a good reason why the United States did not want to see the British lose. While European nations had spent their treasure on armies and navies, Americans had put their own wealth into schools and factories and railroads, into a better life for all citizens. Why had Americans been allowed to go about their business in peace? One reason was that the United States had the good luck to be protected by British Sea Power.

While the friendly British ruled the waves, they let us carry our cargoes and our people all over the world. The British, like the Americans, did not want to see other European nations build new empires in North or South America. The Monroe Doctrine—that European countries should not make new colonies in America and should not interfere in American affairs—had actually been enforced by the British navy. It had been very economical and extremely convenient, then, for Americans to have the British control the seas. But no one could predict what might come from a victorious Germany, with its new imperial ambitions.

In January 1918, President Wilson went before Congress again—to explain the American program for the future of the world. He listed Fourteen Points. They were a noble list. And if they could have been lived up to, there would never have been any more wars. All secret diplomacy was to be abolished—to make statesmen ashamed to barter away other people's lives and liberties. Freedom of the Seas would be restored. National boundaries would be adjusted so that all peoples could govern themselves. And, finally, there would be a League of Nations to preserve peace and insure justice.

The Fourteen Points impressed the world. They meant more to people outside the United States than any American statement since the Declaration of Independence or the Emancipation Proclamation.

President Wilson had proved himself one of the greatest preachers in modern history. He had lifted the spirits of the battle-worn, and he expressed the hopes of millions everywhere. But to make even half his dreams come true required a master politician. Could Wilson do the job?

CHAPTER 27
Winning a War, Losing a Peace

When the United States entered the war in April 1917, our Allies had almost lost.

In Europe the land war was in a new style. The trench warfare was like nothing ever seen before. When the war broke out in 1914, both German generals and French generals had their own plans for a knockout blow to end the war in a hurry. But the new automatic weapons were deadly and accurate against attack. The advantages of the defensive had so increased that *both* armies immediately went on the defensive.

This was Stationary Warfare. Both armies dug their trenches, lived underground, and fired at each other from fixed positions. For three and a half years, the trenches stretched from the Swiss border to the North Sea. The battle lines had hardly moved.

On both sides the trenches became elaborate systems. There was usually a line of front trenches, held as outposts. Behind were networks of supply and command trenches, sometimes stretching back as far as five miles. These were connected by complicated tunnels, and sometimes even by specially designed railways. Soldiers became human moles, hiding by day and digging by night. As soon as darkness fell, they went to work, digging new trenches, stringing barbed wire, and connecting telephone lines.

Instead of the higher officers leading their men into battle, these officers often stayed far back in command posts located in comfortable chateaus. Men in the front trenches had a terrible feeling of isolation. They were threatened not only by enemy gunfire, but by darkness, cold, and mud. Out of the filth and fatigue arose new ailments, which came to be called "trench fever," "trench foot," and "trench mouth."

In this kind of warfare, a "battle" was when large numbers of men from one set of trenches rushed out and tried to break through the enemy's trenches. The hope was always to force a big gap so your troops could pour through and then attack the whole enemy line from the rear. But advancing soldiers were tangled in barbed wire and mowed down by deadly machine-gun fire.

In the opening battles in 1914, even before the trenches were dug, each side lost a half-million men, which was more men than had been in the entire German army fifty years before. Then, during the whole year of 1915, the British and French did not advance more than three miles at any point. Still the French lost nearly a million and a half men in 1915, and a million in 1916. At the Battle of the Somme alone, the Germans lost more men than had been killed during the whole four years of the American Civil War.

Never before had so many men been slaughtered so rapidly or so senselessly. Before the war was over, the soldiers killed on both sides would number ten million, and another ten million civilians would die from disease, starvation, and the revolutions that grew out of the war.

When the United States finally plunged in, both sides were weary and sick of the bloodshed. In May 1918, the Germans had pushed their trenches to within fifty miles of Paris. They aimed at all costs to reach Paris and so force the surrender of the Allies before American troops could make a difference.

But the Americans came just in time. In July, 85,000 Americans arrived to help save Paris and to join a new counter-offensive. By August an American army of a half-million under General John J. Pershing advanced against the Germans on the southern front. Before the end of September a million and a quarter Americans were fighting in France.

After a bloody battle in October, the Americans advanced to Sedan, fifty miles behind the trenches which the Germans had held for three years. The Americans then cut the railroad line that

"Battle of the Marne," an eyewitness drawing by an artist-reporter. In the days of Stationary Warfare armies advanced on foot with fixed bayonets, hoping to break through the enemy's entrenchments.

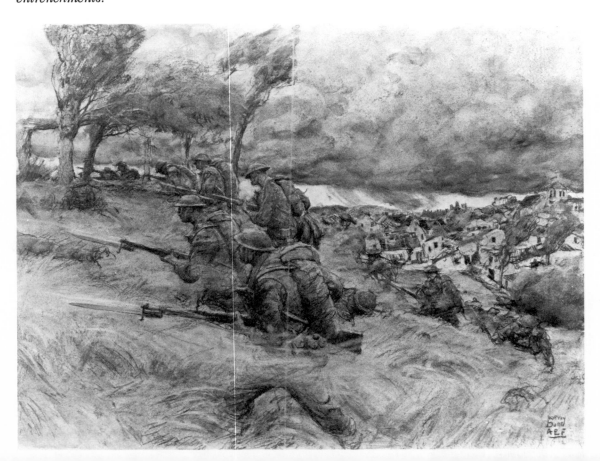

had supplied the German army, and the whole German defense disintegrated. With this American encouragement, the French and the British were advancing too.

The German generals and the German Emperor had badly miscalculated. They had thought they would win the war before the United States came in. They could not imagine that American help at the last moment could possibly turn the tide. Though the Americans arrived late in the battle, they actually made the difference that decided the war. The United States lost 50,280 men in action.

That bloodiest war yet in history ended with the Armistice on November 11, 1918. In New York and San Francisco and Dallas and Chicago and Atlanta, Americans danced in the streets.

The Germans, in agreeing to an Armistice in November, believed that the peace would be based on Wilson's generous Fourteen Points.

When President Wilson himself decided to go to a Peace Conference in Paris, he gave ammunition to his critics. They said he was more anxious to be the Preacher to the World than to be the Protector of the United States. No President while in office had ever before gone to Europe.

In Paris, the three Allied leaders whom Wilson had to bargain with—the Prime Ministers of Great Britain, France, and Italy—were clever and tough. Each of them remembered the enormous cost of the war to his country during the four bloody years. Each wanted to get as much as possible in lands and wealth

"Blitzkrieg," Hitler's new technique of warfare in World War II, sent motorcycles and tanks speeding over highways to get behind the enemy's lines before he knew what was happening. Support by airplanes (not shown here) was crucial. This scene: Poland, 1939.

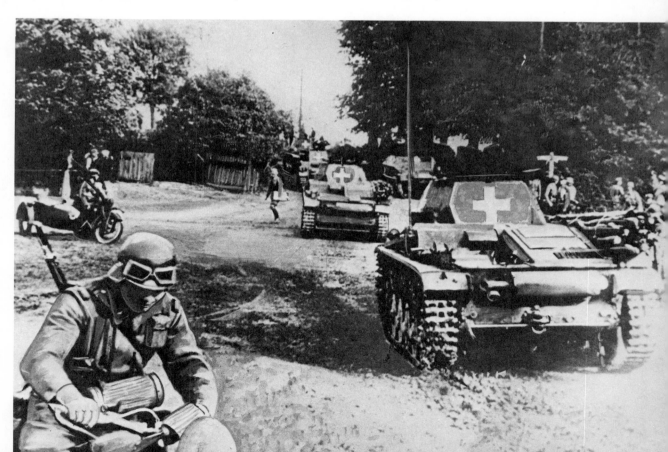

and power for his own country, and hoped to punish the enemies so they would never rise again.

The victorious European statesmen were irritated by the self-righteous American President who always said he was worrying about "all mankind." They compared the Points that Wilson had announced from Washington with the Commandments given to Moses on Mount Sinai. "Mr. Wilson bores me with his *Fourteen* Points," the French Prime Minister, Georges Clemenceau, sneered. "Why, God Almighty has only *ten!*"

The treaty that came out of the Paris conference rooms was not as selfish or as vengeful as the European leaders would have wished. Nor was it nearly as just and noble as President Wilson might have hoped. Each victorious power got territories it had been promised in secret treaties. The German colonies were parceled out among the Allies. At the same time, some new smaller republics—like Czechoslovakia and Poland—were created so that at last these people could govern themselves.

The provisions most poisonous for the future of Europe had to do with "reparations." These were payments the Allies demanded from Germany to "repair" all the war damage. When the Germans signed the Armistice they did understand they might have to pay for the damage to civilians.

But the British and the French raised the damages to include the *total* cost of the whole war to all the Allies. This meant not only the homes and farms and factories destroyed, but also the cost of guns and ammunition, the uniforms and pay for soldiers, and even the pensions to wounded Allied soldiers and to their relatives. This sum was so vast and so hard to estimate that the Allies refused to name a figure—or even to name a time in the future when the Germans would be allowed to stop paying.

President Wilson did manage to put his own scheme for permanent peace— the League of Nations—in the very same package with all those things the other Allied powers really wanted. He believed that, even if the whole treaty was not perfect, his new League of Nations could correct the mistakes later.

When President Wilson returned to the United States, he was greeted like a returning hero. An escort of festive warships accompanied him into New York harbor. Ten thousand people welcomed him at the Union Station in Washington.

His triumph was short. Now his political mistakes came home to roost. When Wilson had appointed the American Peace Commissioners to go to Paris, he snubbed both the Republican Party and the Senate. Yet the Republicans held the majority in the Senate. And before any treaty became law, the Senate would have to approve it by a two-thirds majority.

President Wilson simply could not believe that there were reasons why sensible Americans might not want to approve his treaty. What frightened Americans most was the plan for a League of Nations—but especially Article 10. Wilson, with typical obstinacy, said that Article 10 was the heart of the whole League, and that the League was the heart of the treaty.

In Article 10 each League member promised to respect and preserve all the other members of the League against "external aggression." At first sight that looked harmless enough. But the real purpose of the Article was to make each member of the League regard an attack on any other member as an attack on itself. And in that case, each League member would be expected to prepare for war.

To agree to this would overturn one of the oldest American traditions. Should the United States let herself be *required* to plunge into some future European war?

Two able, contrasting Republican statesmen led a relentless battle against allowing the United States to join Wilson's League. One was William E. Borah, Senator from the Far Western State of Idaho. Borah, like President Wilson himself, was the son of a Presbyterian minister, who wanted him also to go into the ministry. A graduate of the University of Kansas, he was as eloquent as Wilson, but had more experience in politics. Although technically a Republican, he supported many Democratic measures when he happened to agree with them. He had worked for the income tax and had fought against trusts and monopolies.

Just as Senator Borah's own personal rule in politics had been to stay independent, and then support whatever measures were best, so he believed the United States should always stay independent in her relation to other countries. He bitterly opposed our joining the League of Nations, for fear it would take away our independence.

The other leader of the anti-League forces was the learned Senator Henry Cabot Lodge of Massachusetts. He, too, had had a long career as a politician.

But he came from a wealthy and aristocratic New England Oldcomer family. After attending Harvard, he wrote many books on American history. At the time of the World War he was chairman of the Senate Committee on Foreign Relations, which had the power to recommend to the Senate whether or not they should adopt the treaty. Unlike Senator Borah, he was a man of strong personal hates. He distrusted Woodrow Wilson and so he feared Wilson's League.

Then President Wilson made his fatal decision to appeal direct to the American people. In early September 1919, though already in ill health, he traveled eight thousand miles, visited twenty-nine cities, and gave forty speeches in twenty-two days. At Pueblo, Colorado, he collapsed and had to be taken back to the White House. For nearly eight months President Wilson could not even meet his Cabinet. His wife carried messages back and forth from everybody else to the President—and it was never quite clear which messages actually reached him.

Before the election of 1920 Wilson made another grave political blunder. If he had been willing to work with Senator Lodge, he might still have found some compromise and so might have passed the Treaty and the League through the Senate. Instead Wilson once again became the preacher. "Shall we," he asked "or shall we not, redeem the great moral obligation of the United States?" He declared that the Presidential election of 1920 would be a "solemn national referendum" on the League of Nations.

The Democratic candidate for President, Governor James M. Cox of Ohio, stood up for the League. The weak but likeable Republican candidate, Senator Warren G. Harding of Ohio, opposed the League and said vaguely that he favored some sort of "association of nations." Americans chose the Republican Harding by a resounding majority of seven million votes.

The United States never joined Wilson's League of Nations. Wilson was saddened that the American people chose a "barren independence." But he did not give up hope that what a union of States had accomplished in North America, a union of nations might someday accomplish for the whole world.

CHAPTER 28

The Battlefield Is Everywhere

When Franklin Delano Roosevelt moved into the White House in March 1933, the world prospects once again were grim. Italy, Russia, and Japan—three former American allies in the war "to make the world safe for democracy"—had become threats both to democracy and to peace. Germany, the leading enemy in that war, had risen from defeat, was building an enormous new army, was manufacturing weapons at frightening speed, and soon proclaimed her intention to rule the world. Any one of the new military powers had a bigger army and was beginning to have stronger armaments than the old democracies. Each proclaimed its intention to fight.

In the United States the national slogan had become, "Never Again!" Many Americans were becoming pacifists, saying they would never go to war for *any* reason. Others were becoming Isolationists, looking for ways to fence off the New World. And others refused to give up the old-fashioned hope that the country could always stay neutral. But by

1935 the idea that neutrals had rights which everybody would respect was more unrealistic than ever.

Each of the new warlike powers wanted not just a bigger empire for itself. It wanted its own kind of world —Communist, Fascist, or Nazi. All were battling for the minds of men. The winner aimed to take all.

This meant that, whether Americans liked it or not, the battlefront was everywhere. Now the airplane had made nearly all traditional thinking about war out-of-date. What the submarine had done to Freedom of the Seas, the airplane was doing to almost all the other rules of warfare.

Just as Admiral Mahan had once argued for the decisive influence of Sea Power on history, so during World War I the brilliant and energetic Billy Mitchell began to advertise Air Power.

Air Power was still so new that few took it seriously. In the Spanish-American War one light observation balloon had actually been used in Cuba. But "military ballooning" (as it was

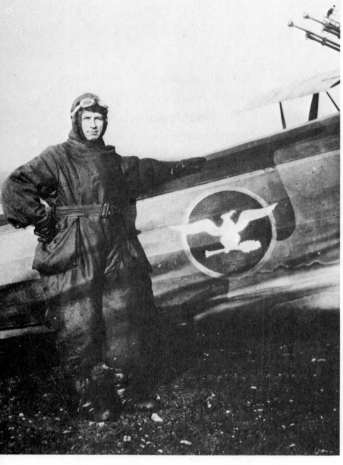

Billy Mitchell, commander of United States aviators in France during World War I, was a bold and enthusiastic pioneer of Air Power.

called) was considered mostly a sport or a hobby. In 1913 when Mitchell was a young officer in the Signal Corps he began to be intrigued by the airplane's military possibilities. Then, during World War I, as General Pershing's Chief of Air Service he was impressed by the effectiveness of British and French warplanes.

At the end of the war, American generals and admirals still considered the airplane at most merely another new weapon. Like a new machine gun, it was to be used by either the army or the navy in their own regular operations.

Billy Mitchell had other ideas. His experience as a flyer and his other wartime observations persuaded him that airplanes really ought to be organized into an entirely new military unit, under a command all their own. So long as Americans thought of airplanes as only helpers in traditional army and navy maneuvers, he argued, Americans were sure to be left behind. They would lose the next war to nations who recognized that Air Power was something new and world-shaking.

Air Power, Mitchell said, had actually shifted the main targets. No longer were they the enemy *armies*. Now the most important targets were the "vital centers"—the centers of industry, the centers of supply, and the centers of the enemy's will to resist. "Armies themselves can be disregarded by air power," he explained, "if a rapid strike is made against the opposing centers."

Americans could not bear the thought of a new warfare that was so horrible. They hated to believe that whole cities might have to be destroyed.

Mitchell was an expert at getting publicity. He wrote magazine articles and books, and made speeches to alert all citizens to the importance of Air Power. Many of his fellow officers disliked him for it. Some called him "General of the 'Hot Air' Force."

But Mitchell was not discouraged. To prove that airplanes were an effective and economical force against battleships, he planned a spectacular demonstration. He arranged to have the German battleship *Ostfriesland*, which had been surrendered at the end of World War I, hauled to a position sixty miles off the Virginia coast. The battleship had a reputation for being "unsinkable." Now it was a ghost ship, with not a soul on board.

Just before noon on July 21, 1921, a flight of Mitchell's army bombers left Langley Field eighty-five miles away. As they arrived over the battleship, they dropped six 2,000-pound bombs. Within twenty minutes the "unsinkable" battleship was at the bottom of the ocean. It was the first time a battleship had ever been sunk by planes.

When admirals and generals still refused to grasp the full meaning of Air Power, Mitchell tried other tactics. He publicly denounced "the incompetency, criminal negligence, and almost treasonable administration of the National Defense by the Navy and War Departments." This was the sure road to court-martial—and that seemed to be his purpose. On December 17, 1925, a panel of generals found Brigadier General Billy Mitchell guilty of "conduct which brought discredit upon the military service." They sentenced him to a five-year suspension from active duty.

But his publicity campaign had already forced President Calvin Coolidge to take some action. The committee he appointed did not support all of Mitchell's demands, but they did urge the buildup of an American air force.

Then, on May 21, 1927, a young airmail pilot named Charles A. Lindbergh surprised and delighted the world by flying his light monoplane, *The Spirit of St. Louis,* nonstop from New York to Paris. Americans were proud of his courage and his modesty. He called his book *We* (meaning his plane and himself).

Charles Lindbergh at Curtiss Field, New York, before beginning his solo flight across the Atlantic. When he arrived at Le Bourget Airport outside Paris, to his astonishment he was greeted by 100,000 people.

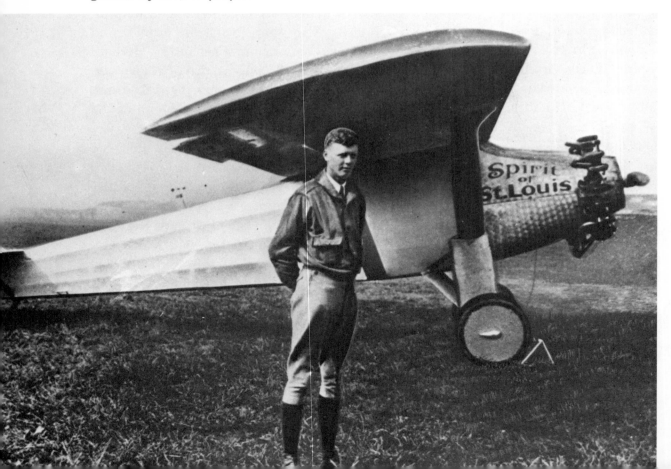

As the military meaning of Lindbergh's feat sank in, Americans began to realize that Billy Mitchell's "wild" ideas no longer were so wild. Now it seemed quite possible that some day the United States might be attacked by airplanes which came nonstop across the ocean. The nation began to take Mitchell, and Air Power, seriously.

In 1935 the new American long-range B-17 bomber (soon called the "Flying Fortress" and equipped with the super-accurate Norden bombsight) first went into the air. Now it was hard for Americans to doubt that Air Power would change the meaning of war. Air war against "vital centers" would be as different as possible from the old stationary trench warfare.

Adolf Hitler's shocking new strategy depended on Air Power. The German name for it was *Blitzkrieg*, which means "lightning war." The idea was to strike with lightning speed. Using the fastest new vehicles (airplanes, tanks, trucks, and even motorcycles) the Nazis would rush quick and deep into enemy territory. The sluggish, unprepared enemies would be overwhelmed.

Blitzkrieg also meant war that struck like lightning—from the sky. Air Power made it possible. Leaping over "standing" armies, over water barriers and coastal fortifications, the Nazi air force would strike abruptly at the heart of the defenseless nations.

On September 1, 1939, Hitler invaded Poland, which fell before the end of the month. Then, on April 9, 1940, he horrified the world by invading Denmark and Norway. One month later he rushed into the Netherlands, Belgium, and Luxembourg, and then lunged deep into France around the "impregnable" Maginot Line. On June 14 his Nazis marched into Paris. Thousands of weeping Frenchmen lined the streets, helpless against this lightning barbarian invasion.

Luckily, President Franklin Delano Roosevelt recognized the Nazi menace. Even before the Nazis had overrun France he had sent a special message to Congress warning the nation to rearm. He announced his plan to turn out fifty thousand planes in the next year and every year until the Nazis were beaten. In one of his most effective "fireside chats" over the radio, he alerted the nation:

> The Nazi masters of Germany have made it clear that they intend not only to dominate all life and thought in their own country, but also to enslave the whole of Europe, and then to use the resources of Europe to dominate the rest of the world. . . . We cannot escape danger, or the fear of danger, by crawling into a bed and pulling the covers over our heads. . . . No nation can appease the Nazis. No man can tame a tiger into a kitten by stroking it. . . . Let not the defeatists tell us that it is too late. It will never be earlier.

But still there were those who believed they could ward off the Nazi menace by the old-fashioned magic word, "Neutrality!"

The Isolationists had passed a Neutrality Law requiring that all military supplies sent abroad had to be "cash-and-carry." This law required all the warring countries to pay for the goods they bought here before the goods left our shores and then also required them to carry the goods in their own ships. The Isolationists hoped this would keep the United States out of the war.

The British had run out of cash and were running out of ships. If this law was not quickly changed the United States might not be able to get help to the British before they were defeated by the Nazis.

President Franklin Delano Roosevelt showed his usual genius for compromise and for persuasion. He offered a clever plan called "Lend-Lease." We would "lend" or "lease" to the British—or any other country whose defense the President considered vital to the defense of the United States—whatever war supplies we could make. In that way the British would not need cash, and the hesitating Congressmen might be per-

suaded that we were getting value in return.

At the same time, in January 1941, in his annual message to Congress, President Roosevelt proclaimed the Four Freedoms. After the war he hoped for "a world founded upon four essential human freedoms"—freedom of speech, freedom of religion, freedom from want, and freedom from fear. Later that year, after a secret meeting with British Prime Minister Winston Churchill on a warship off the coast of Newfoundland, the two men issued the Atlantic Charter. This was an up-to-date version of Woodrow Wilson's Fourteen Points.

Meanwhile Hitler made his fatal blunder. In his maniac belief that all battlefields were alike and that *Blitzkrieg* could conquer all, on June 22, 1941, only

The bombing of Pearl Harbor by Japanese war planes helped convince all Americans that the age of Air Power had arrived.

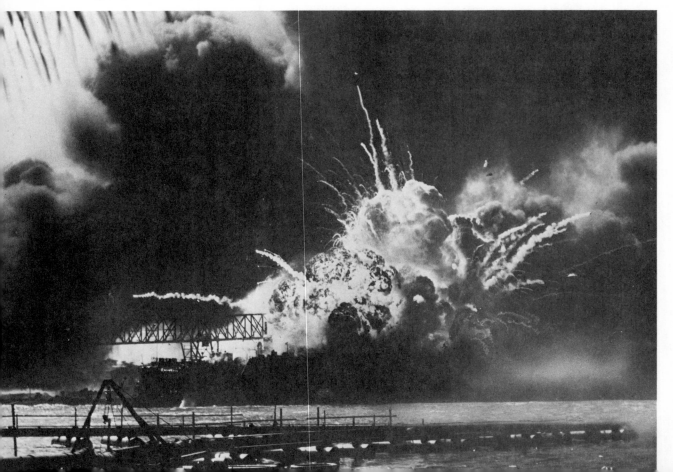

a year after mastering France, he suddenly invaded Russia. But Russia was bigger—and colder—than Hitler had imagined. When the Russian winter arrived, the fingers of Nazi soldiers became numb. Frozen oil paralyzed the motors of his tanks. The Russians counterattacked and Hitler's *Blitzkrieg* was buried in the snow.

At the same time, halfway around the world, the Japanese suddenly forced even the most Isolationist of Americans to realize that Air Power had already put them on the battlefield. On the morning of December 7, 1941, while Japanese diplomats were pretending to discuss peace at the White House, a fleet of 189 Japanese warplanes attacked American airfields at Pearl Harbor in Hawaii. Then they attacked the ships of the United States navy anchored in the harbor. An hour later came a second fleet of 171 Japanese warplanes.

The surprise had been perfect. 150 American warplanes—the bulk of our air force in the Pacific—were destroyed on the ground. It was a better demonstration than Billy Mitchell could have imagined, and the fulfillment of his direst prophecies. There were eighty-six American ships in Pearl Harbor at the time. The most powerful of these, the eight battleships, were put out of action, together with three cruisers and three destroyers, and one battleship was actually sunk. 2,323 men were killed. This was the worst naval catastrophe in American history.

The very next day Congress announced that we were at war.

CHAPTER 29

The Exploding World of the Atom

As soon as Americans had been plunged into battle by this lightning stroke of Air Power, it was plain that the new kind of war was even newer than anyone had imagined. Now the battlefield was everywhere—but especially in the hearts of civilians. Warplanes sometimes flew so high they could not be seen and could barely be heard, to strike at homes and factories.

At first the bombing of Germany followed an American plan of "pinpoint" daylight attacks. Since daylight bombers could actually see their targets they could focus their bombs on the crucial factories. But at the same time the Germans could see the approaching planes, and they downed a disastrous number. The damage to the whole German war machine was slight.

By contrast with the American scheme of "precision" bombing, the British bombers went over at night and bombed whole areas. Incendiary bombs set fire to entire cities. Since these attacking bombers could not be seen, the British losses were much lower. And the damage to the "vital centers"—to the enemy's production, communication, and transportation and the enemy's will to

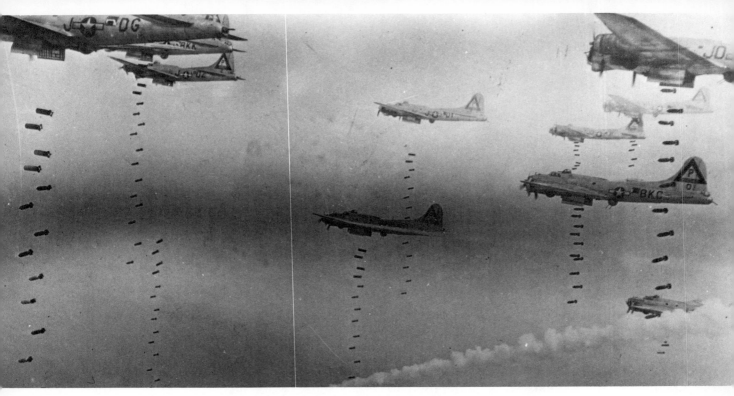

Massed United States bombers attacking a target in Germany in World War II.

---

resist—was far greater.

Now the war came home to the people on both sides. Never before in the history of warfare was there so much suffering by civilians. The Germans sent their bombers over London and other British cities, killing thousands. The Americans and British sent their bombers back over Germany. Finally it was the destruction of factories and cities behind the lines that broke the Nazi will to war. Allied planes had killed nearly a third of a million Germans and had destroyed over five million homes.

When the defeat of the Nazis appeared to be in sight, in February 1945, President Roosevelt met with the Allied leaders, British Prime Minister Churchill and Russian Dictator Josef Stalin. They met at Yalta, a Russian summer resort on the Black Sea. There they agreed on their plans for the Nazi surrender. Germany was to be taken apart. The Germans once again would have to

pay enormous "reparations," with Russia receiving half.

At first Stalin demanded that Poland, on the Russian border, be put under a Communist puppet government. Then when Roosevelt and Churchill objected, Stalin promised to let the Polish people choose their own government by free elections.

The Russians agreed to declare war against Japan soon after the defeat of Germany, and they agreed that they would join the United Nations. In return the Russians gained certain Japanese islands and would be allowed to conquer Outer Mongolia—a vast area twice the size of Texas—on the Russian border in central Asia. At the same time, Stalin solemnly promised not to interfere in the countries along the Russian border in eastern Europe. He promised to let those countries choose their own governments.

Of course Churchill and Roosevelt

knew that for years the communist leaders had called democracy a fraud. But since the Russian armies still had unrivaled power in eastern Europe, the British and American leaders did not have much choice. From their Russian ally all they could expect was promises. They considered themselves lucky to get those. Soon enough they would discover what Stalin's promises were really worth.

Within one short month the Nazi armies crumbled—caught between the Russian communist armies speeding westward and the Anglo-Americans speeding eastward.

General Dwight D. Eisenhower was Supreme Commander of Allied forces. Now his decision could change the history of Europe. If he wanted, he could quickly move his forces into Berlin, the capital of Germany, and also into Prague, the capital of Czechoslovakia.

In Anglo-American hands, Berlin and Prague would be strongholds to help the democracies enforce the Russian agreement to let eastern Europe decide its own fate.

On the other hand General Eisenhower could wait to mop up the German troops behind his own lines—meanwhile letting the Russians overrun more of eastern Europe and consolidate their positions in the capitals. In communist hands, those capitals would help the Russians to foist their dictatorship on all the surrounding peoples. The Russians could make Poland, Czechoslovakia, Hungary, Rumania, and Bulgaria into "satellites" revolving around Moscow.

The far-sighted Winston Churchill saw the threat. "I deem it highly important," he warned General Eisenhower, "that we should shake hands with the Russians as far to the east as

General Eisenhower talking to American paratroopers in June 1944 just before "Operation Overlord"—the successful landing on D-Day of Allied troops on the German-held coast of France. The paratroopers were assigned to drop behind enemy lines before the Allied landing.

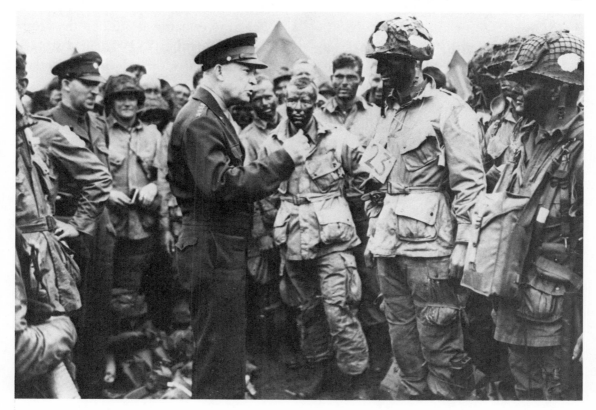

possible." But General Eisenhower was anxious to avoid the loss of more American soldiers. Instead of rushing his democratic forces eastward, he decided to halt fifty miles west of Berlin at the River Elbe. Stalin applauded this decision, for now both Berlin and Prague were left to the Russians.

Until the last minute, Churchill was still trying to warn President Roosevelt. The new "mortal danger to the free world," he said, was our "ally," Russia. It would be tragic, after the long struggle against the Nazi tyranny, to hand over half of Europe to a communist tyranny.

Before Churchill's wisdom could prevail in Washington, President Roosevelt was dead. Worn down by wartime burdens, he had gone for a rest to Warm Springs, Georgia, where he often went for treatment of his paralyzed limbs. On April 12, 1945, he complained of a bad headache, and within a few hours a blood vessel had burst in his brain. The cheerful leader, who had helped raise his fellow Americans from the depth of their Great Depression and who had organized their battle against Nazi barbarism, finally did not have the satisfaction of receiving the Nazi surrender.

The nation grieved as it had grieved for few Americans since Lincoln. Men and women wept in their offices, at home, and in the streets. They felt they had lost not only a national leader, but a personal friend.

To the White House in his place came the courageous, peppery Vice-President, Harry S Truman. He was destined to make some of the most fateful decisions in the history of modern warfare. But when he solemnly took his oath of office and asked the nation to pray for him, he could not have imagined what was in store. He still had not even heard of the super-secret project that was already nearing completion—to build an atomic bomb.

Those who made the American bomb possible (in addition to many American scientists) were a "Who's Who" of world science. From Germany came the greatest physicist of the age, Albert Einstein. Because he was a Jew, the Nazis had taken away his German citizenship and seized his property. From Italy, as a refugee from Mussolini, came the brilliant Enrico Fermi, who was one of the first to propose an atomic bomb as a practical possibility. Scientists, engineers, and mathematicians came also from Hungary, Austria, Denmark, and Czechoslovakia—refugees from all the enslaved parts of Europe.

To build the atomic bomb certain theoretical questions first had to be answered. Was it really possible to achieve "the controlled release of atomic energy"?

The answer came at 3:25 on the afternoon of December 2, 1942, in a squash court on the campus of the University of Chicago. Professor Enrico Fermi supervised the experiment. When everything was prepared, he gave the signal to pull out the control rod. Suddenly the Geiger counters resounded with telltale clicks from the radiation made by the successful breaking up of uranium atoms. The dignified scientists let out a cheer. They had produced a chain reaction that transformed matter into energy! The Atomic Age had begun.

One of the physicists hurried to the long-distance telephone and gave the code message to be relayed to the President of the United States.

"You'll be interested to know," he reported with mock casualness, "that the Italian navigator has just landed in the New World. The Earth was not as large as he had estimated, and he arrived in the New World sooner than he had expected."

"Is that so?" he was asked. "Were the natives friendly?"

"Everyone landed safe and happy." This meant that Professor Fermi (the "Italian navigator") had succeeded even ahead of schedule. The "New World" was, of course, the uncharted world of Atomic Power.

In May 1942, seven months before the Fermi experiment succeeded, President Roosevelt had set up the super-secret "Manhattan Project" to be prepared to build a bomb. Within less than three years and at a cost of two billion dollars, "Manhattan Project" did its job.

At 5:30 on the morning of July 16, 1945, in the remote desert near Alamogordo, New Mexico, the moment came to prove that the bold thinking of the scientists could be matched by the practical know-how of engineers. The answer required no delicate Geiger counter to detect it. The world's first atomic bomb exploded—with a blinding flash and a mushroom cloud such as had never been seen before.

By the time the bomb was perfected, the Germans and Italians had already surrendered. Of the enemies now only Japan remained. On July 26, the Allied leaders gave the Japanese a solemn warning that "the alternative to surrender is prompt and utter destruction."

Still they did not surrender.

Should the United States use the atomic bomb? President Truman alone had to decide. No one knew how long Japan would hold out. Despite the terrifying fire raids of March 1945, when much of Tokyo was destroyed, the Japanese militarists showed no signs of giving up. If the war dragged on and Americans had to invade Japan, it might cost a million lives. The atomic bomb, President Truman knew, might kill hundreds of thousands of innocent Japanese. But life for life, the odds were that it would cost less.

Devastation at Nagasaki, Japan, after the dropping of the second United States atomic bomb on August 9, 1945.

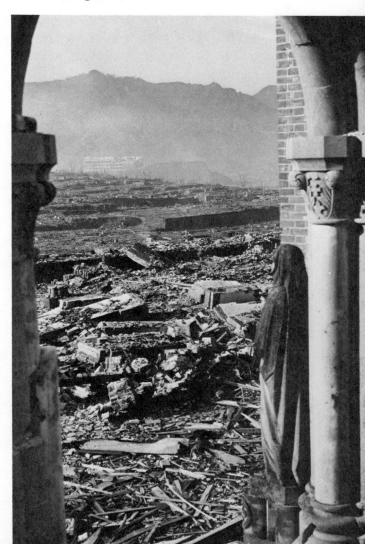

On August 6, 1945, three weeks after that first blinding blast on the New Mexico desert, a single American plane dropped an atomic bomb on Hiroshima. About eighty thousand people were killed. The Japanese still held on. A few days later another plane dropped an atomic bomb on Nagasaki. The Japanese caved in. They announced their surrender on August 14, 1945.

CHAPTER 30

"Little" Wars and Big Risks

World War II was over. The menace of Nazi barbarism and of Japanese militarism was destroyed. But the world was haunted by new fears. Could democracy survive in a world where the Russian communists were more powerful than ever before—and more determined than ever to conquer the world?

By now the United States had joined a modernized version of Wilson's League of Nations. The United Nations had been organized in San Francisco in 1945 even before the German surrender. President Truman hoped the United Nations would help keep the world at peace. But he had fought in France in World War I and he remembered the letdown after that war. Therefore he scaled down his hopes and made plans to fit. He did not promise perpetual peace or freedom for all men on earth.

Instead President Truman offered a simple two-pronged plan. People weakened by the war would receive American machinery and food and money. This would make them stronger to resist tyranny. He would also use American force, wherever it was needed, to help any particular country fight off a takeover by the communists from the outside. This was called "Containment" because it aimed to "contain" the communists and prevent them from taking over the world.

The Truman Doctrine was not as inspiring as Wilson's dream of an entirely democratic world. It was a country-by-country approach. It aimed to help free people stay strong and to help weak people stay free.

And, on the whole, it worked. The exhausted countries of western Europe —Great Britain, France, West Germany, and Italy—which might have been easy pickings for the Russian communists, became stronger in these postwar years. On the shaky borderlands of Greece and Turkey, the communist threat was held back.

The first armed test of the Truman Doctrine came in far-off Korea. The communists set up a puppet government in North Korea—like the puppets they had already set up in eastern Europe— and they claimed the right to rule the whole country. The United Nations (supported by the United States) proposed free elections so all the Koreans could choose their own government. But the Russians objected. And on June

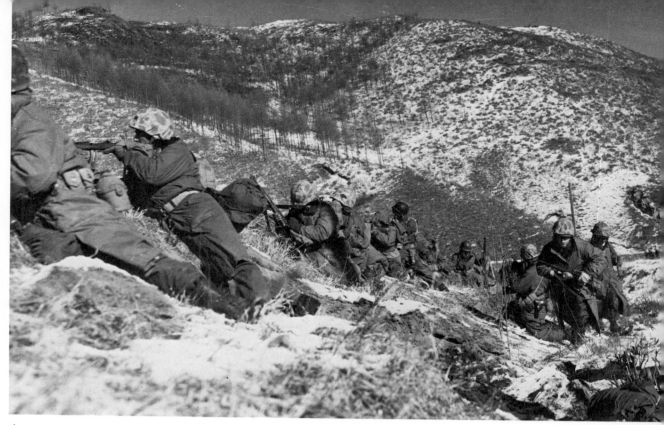

American troops like these, fighting in Korea under the United Nations command, struggled over a hilly country, often barren and frigid.

25, 1950, an army of 100,000 men, who had been armed and trained by the Russian communists, swooped down to take possession of South Korea.

President Truman instantly sent in American troops. The United Nations condemned North Korea as an aggressor. And a United Nations army was organized with troops drawn from fifty-three member nations, commanded by the American General Douglas MacArthur. At first the United Nations forces drove back the invading North Korean communists.

Then suddenly the whole picture changed. Communist China, aided by the Russians, poured in masses of its own troops against the United Nations. They came down from north of the Yalu River. Now the Chinese communists threatened a third World War—if the United Nations forces stepped over the Yalu River into Chinese territory.

On March 24, 1951, General MacArthur, supreme commander of American forces in Korea, publicly warned that he would attack communist China if her forces did not withdraw from South Korea. Unlike President Truman, General MacArthur was willing to risk World War III.

But President Truman had not forgotten the powers of the President. The Constitution said that the President was Commander in Chief of all the United States armed forces. And the general had disobeyed the President's orders by refusing to keep the war inside Korea. President Truman called a surprise press conference at one o'clock in the morning on April 11, 1951, to announce that General MacArthur had been removed.

When the picturesque General MacArthur returned to the United States, admiring crowds greeted him in San Francisco, Chicago, and New York. In

Washington on April 19, he gave an oration to Congress. "In war," he urged in his deep baritone voice, "there can be no substitute for victory."

But even as the sound of the general's voice died away, more and more Americans saw that President Truman was talking common sense. You could no longer talk about "victory" in the general's simple phrase. Communist Russia now had its own atomic bomb. If there was another World War both "winners" and "losers" would go up in atomic blasts. The only hope for mankind, said President Truman, was to keep the fighting limited. Now even "little" wars carried big risks.

When General Eisenhower cam-

paigned for President in 1952, he promised that if he was elected he would go to Korea to find a way to end the war. And the Korean War ended in a compromise, arranged by President Eisenhower, on July 27, 1953. The American dead numbered thirty-five thousand. The Korean peace was no "victory" for the United States. But since it removed the most immediate threat of an atomic war, it was a kind of victory for mankind.

The expanding forces of communism had been warned that any attempt to conquer their neighbors would be extremely costly. They had not been defeated, but they had been held back. It was not all that Americans really wished

An American military adviser in Viet Nam (third from right) with South Vietnamese Marines at the edge of a rice paddy. At far left are two enemy (Viet Cong) prisoners.

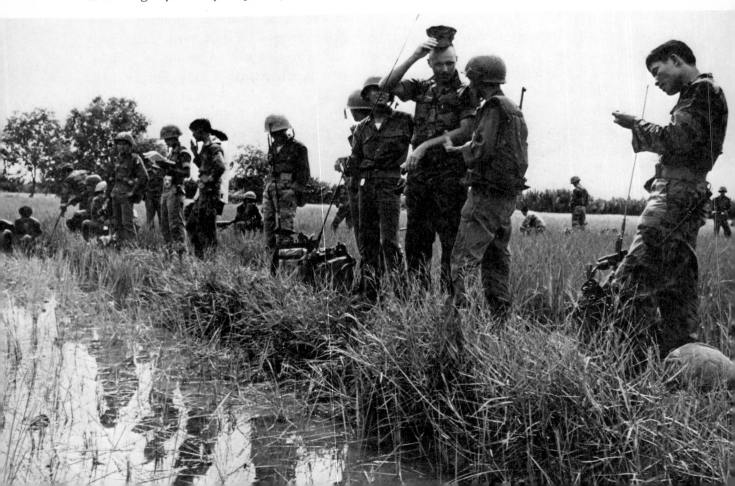

but it was probably the best that could be expected for some time to come.

Within a few years after the Korean truce, again on a peninsula which bordered on communist China, came another test of Containment. In April 1954 the United States met at Geneva with communist Russia, communist China, and countries that once had colonies in Southeast Asia. They agreed that Indochina, the old French colony, should be divided into new independent nations. The people in the area called "Viet Nam" were already split between the communists in the north (on the border of communist China) and the anti-communists in the south. It was therefore agreed to set up *two* Viet Nams.

But then, as in Korea a few years before, communist forces from the North began invading the South.

Would the United States again try to hold back the expanding forces of communism?

In October 1961, President John F. Kennedy made the decision to intervene. Then, after the assassination of President Kennedy in November 1963, Congress on President Lyndon B. Johnson's request voted to use American forces. By 1967 there were nearly a half-million American soldiers in Viet Nam.

This new War of Containment was in many ways similar to the war in Korea. But there were some important differences. Now it was not the whole United Nations but the United States forces with only a few allies who were fighting.

This was the most unpopular war in American history. College students and others objected to being drafted to fight in a strange far-off country. Why, they asked, should the United States be trying to settle Viet Nam's problems? They were told that the countries in Asia were like dominoes standing in a row. If one fell over to communism, the others could not help falling.

On television Americans saw our young soldiers dying and our bombs killing thousands of Vietnamese villagers. Hard-fighting American forces could not win, but they did not quite lose. This undeclared war was unlike any other war in American history. It was not fought on the battlefield but in steamy jungles against communist guerrillas who knew every inch of their own territory.

It was clear after years of fighting that the war in Viet Nam could not be won. Never before had Americans lost a war. After his election in 1968, President Nixon promised to bring our troops home. This was easier said than done. While he began bringing the Americans back, he kept up the bombing attacks to force the communists to come to the conference table. Not until January 1973, after long and tiresome negotiations, was a cease-fire declared.

The war was a great tragedy for the people of Viet Nam, and for Americans, too. At least two million Vietnamese had died. More than 46,000 Americans lost their lives, 1,200 were missing, and 300,000 were wounded. The war had shown the patriotism of young Americans. But it had also shown that the American people would not support a war whose purpose they did not understand.

CHAPTER 31

Windows to the World

By 1960 there were many more automobiles in the United States than in all the rest of the world put together. Two-thirds of American households had at least one automobile.

Perhaps more than anything else that Americans had made by the millions, the automobile expressed their new civilization. All American wealth and ingenuity and organizing ability had been required to give Americans their cars.

The automobile was democratic. Just as ready-made clothing had made it harder in the United States than anywhere else to tell a man's occupation or social class by what he wore, so it was harder than anywhere else to guess an American's bank account by the car he drove.

The automobile was a symbol of freedom. A man who owned a car was free to live at a considerable distance from where he worked. He could take his family to the country on weekends, and to far parts of the continent on vacations.

The automobile was a symbol of speed. With it a man could go as fast as the fastest locomotive, and he could make his own timetable. Americans had always valued their ability to go where and when they wanted. In the twentieth century it was the automobile that helped make this possible.

While automobiles took Americans all around their own country, they no longer had to be rich to vacation abroad. In 1930 less than a half-million Americans traveled overseas, but in 1970 the number reached three million. Jet airplanes took them on three-week holidays to all the continents. And the enormous jumbo jet began to carry four hundred passengers from New York City to London in less time than a farmer used to spend on his weekly drive to the village post office.

Each American felt closer to others, too, when messages came to him more quickly and more easily. But it was almost the time of the Civil War before the U.S. mail had begun to be speedy and reliable. Before Lincoln came to the White House, Morse's telegraph had made it possible for Americans to share the news, which reached newspaper readers throughout the whole nation within a day after it happened. In 1866 the transatlantic cable, which had taken twelve years to complete, brought messages instantly from the Old World.

Then came the telephone. Alexander Graham Bell was twenty-three when he immigrated from Scotland with his family in 1870. Young Bell, following his father's interests in helping the deaf, studied acoustics (the science of sound) and electricity.

Bell determined to find a way to use

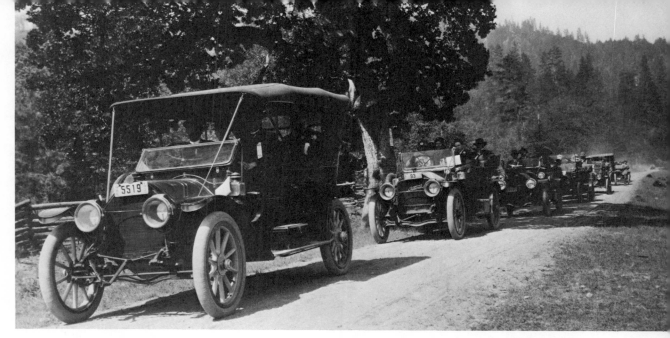

American automobiles, about 1913, on a group excursion to the Great Oregon Caves. Some critics feared that Americans would stop going to church and instead would spend Sundays in their automobiles.

electricity to carry the human voice. For Morse's telegraph would carry nothing but dots and dashes.

By 1876 Bell's new electromagnetic telephone was being displayed at the Centennial Exposition in Philadelphia as a great curiosity. Bell, like Edison, was a skillful organizer, and in the early twentieth century his telephone company had overtaken U. S. Steel to become the largest corporation in the United States.

On remote farms and ranches, medical-care-by-telephone saved the life of many a child—and incidentally saved the doctor a long ride. New businesses were started by new-style Go-Getters who sold their goods exclusively by telephone. The telephone (like the typewriter, which was perfected about the same time) provided new jobs for women.

Within a century after Bell made his invention, it was unusual for any American family to be out of reach of a telephone. The nation's hundred million telephones were more than half of all those in the world. By 1970 three hundred million separate phone conversations were carried on in the United States each day.

Back in the 1880's it was hard enough for people to imagine that a voice could be sent on a wire. But how much harder to imagine that messages could be sent even *without* a wire!

Before 1890 a German physicist, Heinrich Hertz, had discovered the existence of radio waves. At first people called them "Hertzian waves." These had the amazing quality of being able to pass through solid objects—even through wooden and brick walls.

In 1894 a young Italian named Guglielmo Marconi, still in his teens, happened to see a magazine article on "Hertzian waves." The idea fascinated him. He retreated to his room on the third floor of the family home near Bologna, locked the door, and experimented with "Hertzian waves" for hours

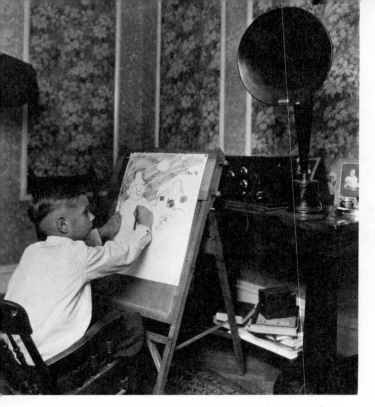

A boy learning to draw by listening to lessons broadcast over the newfangled invention, the radio (about 1924). The term "broadcast" (used on page 32) now had a new meaning.

on end. His first success was to use these waves to ring a bell across a room or downstairs. The very next year, when he was still only twenty-one, he succeeded in sending these waves outdoors (the distance of a twenty-minute walk) and even across the neighboring hill.

In 1896 Marconi and his mother went to England with a "little black box" containing his invention. Encouraged by the chief of telegraph in the British Post Office, he pursued his experiments and soon was sending messages nine miles. In 1897 Marconi received a British patent for his "wireless telegraph" and founded Marconi's Wireless Telegraph Company in London. His company was a great success.

His wireless equipment was installed in three British battleships in 1899. And in that year Marconi came to the United States.

Americans, with their new colonial empire, had special reasons to want news quickly from everywhere. During the Spanish-American War, when Admiral Dewey reported his victory at Manila Bay, he first had to send dispatch boats to Hong Kong. There the news was telegraphed westward (on British-controlled cables) by way of the Indian Ocean, the Red Sea, the Mediterranean, and then across the Atlantic, before it finally reached the President in Washington. Now wireless might make it possible (without depending on cables owned by the British or by anyone else) to get messages to Washington instantly from anywhere. The American Marconi Company prospered.

But Marconi's wireless still sent only dots and dashes. It would not send voices or music. The next step was taken by Reginald Aubrey Fessenden, a Canadian who had worked with Edison in his "invention factory" in the 1880's.

Fessenden had a simple but revolutionary idea. Marconi, using wireless waves, had sent out dots and dashes by stopping and starting electrical signals. Suppose, said Fessenden, the wireless message was sent out in a *continuing* wave of radio rays. Then, by making the waves correspond to the vibrations made by sounds, you could actually transmit speech and music. Fessenden experimented with this idea at the laboratory of the General Electric Company, which had grown out of Edison's invention factory.

The startling result occurred on Christmas Eve, 1906. That night, wireless operators on ships at sea, wearing their earphones, were listening for the usual stream of dots and dashes. To their amazement, they suddenly heard a human voice. A woman sang a Christmas carol, someone played a violin, then someone read a passage from the Bible, and finally Fessenden's own voice wished them Merry Christmas.

The very word broadcast took on a new meaning. In the 1901 dictionary it usually meant "the act or process of scattering seeds." But by 1927 *broadcast* usually meant "to scatter or disseminate, specifically, radio messages, speeches, etc."

Within the twenty years after Fessenden's first Christmas broadcast in 1906, events moved with a peculiarly American speed. Many other Go-Getters, inventors, and adventurous businessmen joined in.

One of the most remarkable of these Go-Getters was Lee De Forest, born in Council Bluff, Iowa, in 1873. His father went to Alabama, to be president of Talledega College, which had been founded by missionaries just after the Civil War to help educate the Negro freedmen.

Like Marconi, young De Forest began to read about the new "Hertzian waves." His summer job pushing a chair for sightseers at the World's Columbian Exposition in Chicago in 1893 gave him the opportunity to study the electrical exhibits. He worked his way through Yale College, sometimes rising at 4:00 A.M. to mow lawns. And he studied hard. But he was not popular with his classmates, who voted him both the "nerviest" and the "homeliest" of their year.

After graduation—and for the rest of his life—De Forest gave his enormous energies to inventing ways to improve radio. His new radio tube which he patented in 1906 was called the Audion. It was based on a tube that Edison had made in his laboratory when working on the incandescent lamp. With the Audion tube it was easier to tune in, all reception became louder and clearer, and the broadcast of voice and music was much improved. Before his death De Forest had received over three hundred patents.

The man who did more than anyone else to bring radio and then television into American homes was David Sarnoff. He showed that the Go-Getting spirit was as alive in the mid-twentieth century as it had been in the days of the trailblazer John Iliff or the merchandising giants, Montgomery Ward and Richard Sears.

David Sarnoff's life was an American saga. He was born in southern Russia in 1891, to a poor family who intended him to become a rabbi. Even before he was nine he was reading the sacred texts in Hebrew. Then his father, who had gone to America a few years before, sent back money for the family's transatlantic passage.

When the Sarnoffs settled in a crowded immigrant section of New York City, David still did not know a word of English. But he went to public school and soon spoke like an American. When his father became too sick to earn a living, David at the age of ten began supporting the whole family with the profits from his newsstand on Tenth Avenue.

David was ambitious. Deciding to become a wireless operator, he taught himself the Morse code and was hired by the American Marconi Company.

Then, by luck, Sarnoff happened to be the only operator at a New York wire-

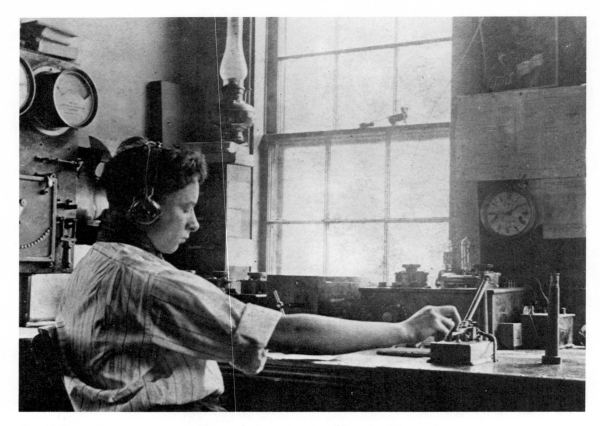

David Sarnoff as a teen-age telegraph operator working for Marconi.

less receiver when word came dimly through on the afternoon of April 15, 1912, that the luxury liner *Titanic* had struck an iceberg and was sinking in mid-Atlantic. He gave the news to the press, and stayed at his instrument (while all other stations were ordered off the air) to alert other ships to send help. The name of David Sarnoff reached everyone who read the newspapers.

When the American Marconi Company was taken over by the Radio Corporation of America (RCA), Sarnoff joined the new firm. By 1921 Sarnoff was running the large company, making plans to sell the new "radio music boxes" by the millions.

During World War I the soldiers hidden in trenches had needed the radio to keep in touch with their units. And radio sets improved in wartime, when the different manufacturers had been

required to pool their know-how. After the war, radio entered American homes. With the new sets listeners no longer had to wear earphones. Now they could receive the program over a loudspeaker.

In 1920 the Department of Commerce issued the first license for a regular commercial broadcasting station to KDKA in Pittsburgh. Within two years there were over five hundred licensed commercial broadcasting stations, and over a half-million radio sets were being produced annually. Before World War II, the annual production of radio sets numbered ten million.

Sarnoff was just as bold in forecasting the success of television. He invested large sums in the RCA television research laboratory where another Russian immigrant, Vladimir Zworykin, was making remarkable progress.

While Zworykin was collaborating

with a large staff in the costly RCA laboratory, another inventor was working quietly by himself. Philo Taylor Farnsworth, born to a large Mormon family on a farm near Beaver, Utah, in 1906, began studying electronics on his own when he was still in high school. Encouraged by his science teacher, he tried to make a television set. Then a businessman furnished a small laboratory for him in California. Philo worked alone and in secret, with the blinds drawn. Once the police (suspecting he was building a still to make illegal whiskey) raided his laboratory. At the age of only twenty-four, Farnsworth had patented his own new system for television.

World War II delayed the manufacture of television for the home. But out of wartime needs came "radar"—a word made up from *ra*(dio) *d*(etecting) *a*(nd) *r*(anging). Radar used radio waves to locate enemy planes and ships. The many returning servicemen with radar experience were well prepared to work on television.

By 1948 television was booming. Sarnoff's foresight had paid off. In that year alone nearly one million television sets were produced. In the very next year production reached three million, and in the year following 7,500,000. By the mid-1960's it was hard to find an American household without a television set.

When people could see a movie at home for free, why should they go to the movie theater? Thousands of movie theaters closed. Fewer new movies were made for the theater each year, yet old movie spectaculars (like *Gone With the Wind*) were still successful.

Old movies, especially Westerns, found a new life on television. There was a new interest in experimental movies. Though shown in small theaters, they aroused widespread interest. And now it was possible to rent or buy cassettes of new movies, too, and play them through your television set at home.

Television gave everybody a window to the world. Now everyone—whether he lived on a farm or in the city, whether his neighborhood was rich or poor, whether in Oregon, New Mexico, Maine, or Florida, whether young or old, sick or well—could look through the television window at the very same world. Now, as never before, Americans shared their experience.

Even in the days before television, when President Franklin Delano Roosevelt broadcasted his first inaugural address on radio he received in response a half-million pieces of mail. During the Great Depression and World War II he skillfully used his radio "fireside chats" to bring all Americans together.

Now with television all Americans could not only hear their candidates. They could actually see them in action. They could watch the expression on a candidate's face and could follow his gestures. In this new way, American voters could feel personally acquainted with their leaders.

In 1948, for the first time, the National Party Conventions were telecast. While sitting in the White House, President Truman saw the nomination of his Republican rival, Governor Thomas E. Dewey, in Philadelphia. During the campaign President Truman seemed relaxed and homey on television while

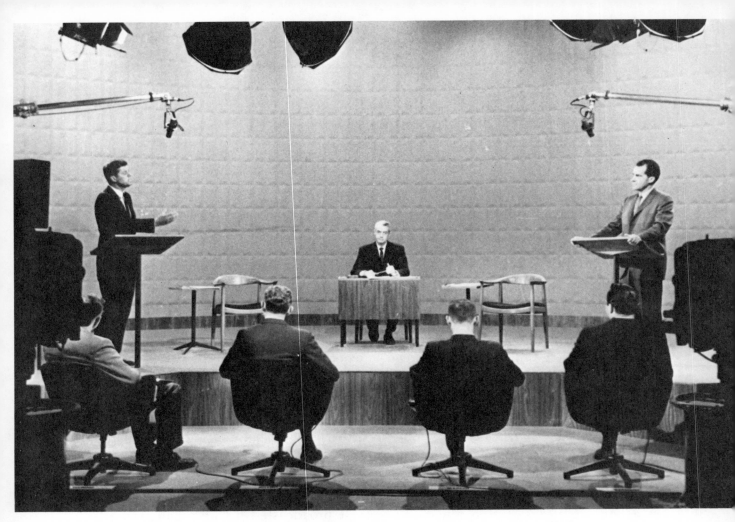

One of television's "Great Debates" in 1960. LEFT: *John F. Kennedy.* RIGHT: *Richard M. Nixon. Presiding: Howard K. Smith of ABC. William Jennings Bryan's strenuous campaigning had brought his voice to a few million Americans; each of the Great Debates reached about seventy million.*

Governor Dewey (his opponents said he looked like the bridegroom on a wedding cake) appeared stiff and formal. This new opportunity for American voters to size up the personalities of the candidates on television helped explain why President Truman won reelection.

In the Presidential campaign of 1960 the two candidates appeared together on television. In the "Great Debates"—a series of four one-hour programs—John F. Kennedy, the Democratic candidate, and Richard M. Nixon, the Republican candidate, discussed the issues. These were not really "debates" like the old-fashioned Lincoln-Douglas Debates a

century earlier. For now newspaper reporters put the questions. Each Presidential candidate had 2½ minutes in which to give his answer. Then he had 1½ minutes for reply after the other candidate had made his brief statement.

These "Great Debates" probably reached the largest audience in history up to that time. Seventy million people were watching each program. Television's new window to the world had made American life more democratic. Television showed more Americans more about everything and everybody in their country. American technology—drawing on the know-how of Americans and of the whole world—had come to the service of American democracy.

But there were dangers. The man who showed up best on television was bound to be the man who was the best "performer." He was the man who could give the cleverest response in 2½ minutes to questions he had just heard. But was that the best test of a President?

"Telstar," an American satellite, made it possible to exchange television programs between continents. With television Americans could even reach out beyond this world. And by looking through the window in his living room every American would join the nation's adventures to the New Worlds of outer space.

CHAPTER 32

Footprints on the Moon

When the first Europeans came to America, they came in their familiar ships "over the vast and furious ocean." They feared the ocean, but they knew its perils. When the first Americans pushed off into outer space, they had to invent new kinds of ships. And they had to brave the unknown perils of a new kind of ocean.

By the time of World War II, of course, a great deal was known about airplanes. But airplanes would not work in outer space. For every airplane engine then known—whether an internal-combustion engine like an automobile's that used gasoline to turn a propeller, or a jet engine that pushed ahead by burning gases—depended on the air. From the air came oxygen to explode the gasoline or to burn the gases. But in outer space there is no air. Out there you would need a very special kind of engine.

The pioneer American space scientist, Robert H. Goddard, proposed propelling spacecraft by rocket. A rocket carries its own fuel, and also carries its own "air"—usually in the form of liquid oxygen—which it uses to burn the fuel. The shooting of the rocket behind pushes the spacecraft forward.

In 1914 Goddard received a patent for his liquid-fuel rocket engine. In 1920 he wrote a technical report for the Smithsonian Institution in Washington explaining how his rocket engine worked. He said it might even be possible someday to reach the moon by rocket. The New York *Times* and other respectable newspapers wrote editorials ridiculing his idea. For the rest of his life Goddard distrusted newspapers. Unlike Billy Mitchell he kept his work secret and hated publicity. And he went ahead perfecting his rocket engine. He finally secured 214 patents on rocket improvements.

When he died in 1945, few Americans yet believed that man would ever travel through interplanetary space.

The people of London, however, already had sad reason to know that rock-

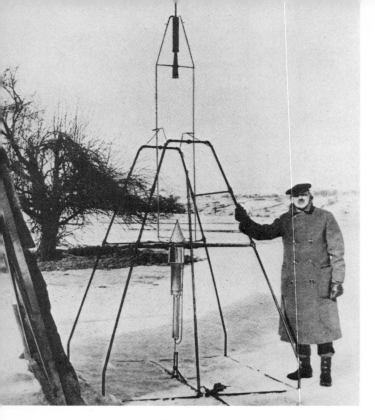

Robert Goddard with his first successful rocket. His imaginative experiments with small rockets laid the groundwork for later American achievements in space.

ets provided a fantastic new source of Air Power. Raining down from the skies in 1944 came thousands of German V-2 rockets. Aimed from distant launching pads in Germany they did not carry pilots but still reached their English targets with terrifying accuracy. They traveled at a speed of 3,500 miles an hour and each dropped a ton of explosives.

The V-2 rockets were the work of a group of German scientists who had been experimenting since 1932. When the Nazis came to power and plunged the world into war, the Nazis had provided these scientists with a secret new laboratory in Peenemuende, a little fishing village on the Baltic Sea in northeastern Germany.

By 1944, about twelve thousand Germans were engaged in making the V-2 rockets which were pouring down

on England every day. The name "V-2" came from a German term meaning "Vengeance Weapon, No. 2." It was the most terrifying weapon of the war because no defense against it had been found. If the Nazis had only perfected this weapon earlier, they might have won the war. But by mid-1944 Germany was near collapse.

When the Russians speeded westward across Europe in their final triumphal march, they hastened to Peenemuende to capture the German rocket factory— for their own future use. When they arrived they were dismayed to find that the most valuable resource, the rocket scientists themselves, had already fled westward.

"This is absolutely intolerable," Dictator Stalin complained in a rage. "We defeated the Nazi armies; we occupied Berlin and Peenemuende; but the Americans got the rocket engineers!" Stalin was especially irritated because the Russian communists were not strong in big bombing planes. Their only weapon, then, for a possible long-distance attack on the United States was transatlantic rockets.

Some far-sighted American generals organized a new project under the code name "Operation Paperclip." They collected 118 of the best German rocket scientists (including Wernher von Braun), and signed them up to work on rockets and space travel for the United States. Wernher von Braun became head of the U.S. Army rocket research.

The United States and communist Russia began a competition in rockets. By 1956 the chief of the Russian Communist Party boasted that soon Russian military rockets would be able to hit any target on the earth. The Russians had improved the old V-2 into a new weapon called the T-1.

Then, on October 4, 1957, the Russians sent up the first man-made earth satellite. It was a package of instruments weighing 184 pounds. They called it "Sputnik" which in Russian meant "fellow traveler" (of the earth). One month later they launched a much heavier satellite, Sputnik II. It weighed 1,120 pounds and for experimental purposes carried a dog named Laika.

The Space Race was on!

Early American efforts were not always successful. The White House announced that on December 6, 1957, the United States would launch its own satellite with a Vanguard rocket. While the whole nation watched on television this much-advertised rocket collapsed on the wet sand around the launching pad.

The next try did succeed. Two months later Explorer I, the first American satellite, went into orbit. And it made some important scientific discoveries.

But Americans still worried about the "Space Gap." Within the next few years, both Russia and the United States performed spectacular feats in space.

On April 12, 1961, the Russians sent up Yuri Gagarin, the first man in space. He went whirling around the earth in a satellite, and made nearly a full orbit —in 89 minutes. A year later the United States sent John H. Glenn, Jr., into orbit in the American spaceship called Friendship 7. Probably Russia and the United States each would have lagged if it had not been for the competition of the other.

President John F. Kennedy at first had doubts about space exploration. He doubted whether man could survive outside the earth's atmosphere. He feared another Vanguard fiasco. And he thought that the enormous sums of money might be better spent on earth. But his persuasive Vice-President Lyndon B. Johnson was a great space enthusiast. After the Russians had sent Yuri Gagarin into orbit, President Kennedy announced that the United States would aim to land a man on the moon before 1970. When President Johnson came to office, he gave space exploration his strong support.

The moon-landing project did need all the support it could find. For there were great risks and vast expenses. When a fire exploded in 1967 during tests of a spaceship, three of the most experienced astronauts were killed. The costs of preparing for the moon shot came to over $25,000,000,000. But this meant new industries, new products, and employment in new jobs for a third of a million people all over the country.

"We work in a place," boasted someone at the Manned Spacecraft Center in Houston, Texas, "where 13,000 men can feel like Columbus."

Finally, after nine years of preparation and two voyages around the moon and back, on July 16, 1969, Americans set out to land on the moon. Neil Armstrong commanded the mission, Michael Collins piloted the command ship Apollo 11, and Edwin E. Aldrin, Jr., was to work with Armstrong when they landed on the moon.

None of them was a great scientist. None came from a family that was rich or famous. They all had a passion for

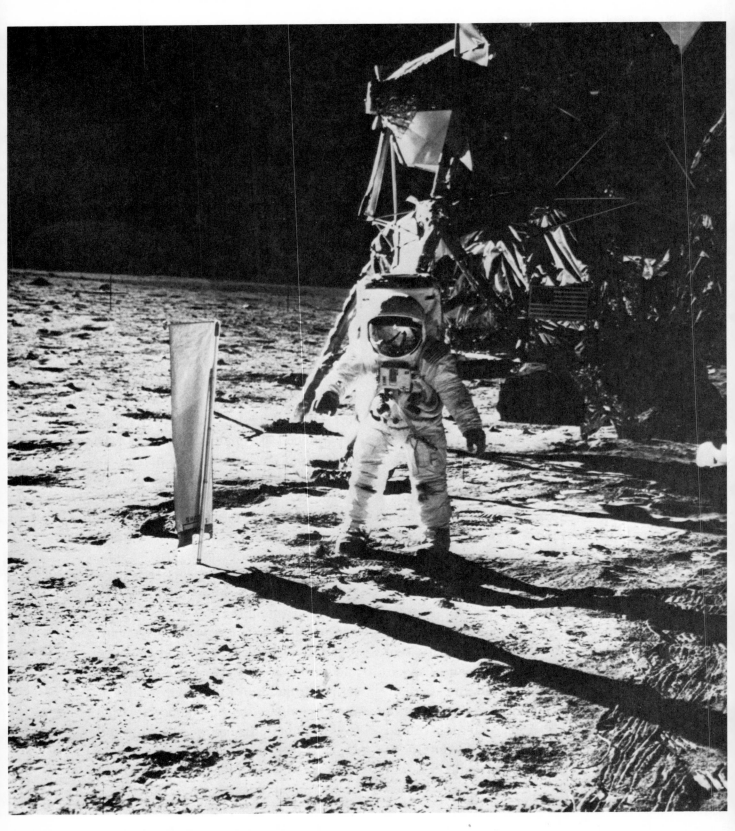

American on the moon, July 20, 1969.

flying. Armstrong had made a reputation as a daring yet reliable test pilot. Aldrin's father, an army colonel, had studied with the space pioneer Goddard. Aldrin himself, after graduating from West Point in 1951, piloted a Sabrejet in the Korean War, and then earned a doctor's degree in aeronautics at Massachusetts Institute of Technology. Collins had been born in Rome while his father, a professional army officer, was stationed there. He graduated from West Point, joined the Air Force, and became a test pilot. As an astronaut, he had taken a 5½-hour space walk, the longest ever. All three men were athletes, in top physical condition. They were all modest men, who had practiced working together.

The moon trip was unlike earlier explorations of unknown lands. For this voyage was watched on television by the whole world—including the explorers' own families. Hundreds of millions of people could share the adventure and the suspense.

The three astronauts shot up in the command ship Apollo 11, which took them orbiting around the earth. Then, after 2½ orbits, they steered Apollo 11 off toward the moon, over two hundred thousand miles away. After a three-day journey through interplanetary space, they arrived in their moon orbit. Armstrong and Aldrin climbed into a small "lunar module" attached at the nose of Apollo 11. They called this little ship "Eagle."

They separated Eagle from the mother ship. After orbiting the moon to the agreed position, they landed Eagle on the moon at 4:17 P.M. Eastern Daylight Time on July 20, 1969.

There were risks till the last instant of the landing. As the computer guided them down, Armstrong noticed they were about to settle in a deep crater about the size of a football field, filled with large boulders. He seized the controls and guided Eagle to a safe, smoother site.

By the original plan, Armstrong and Aldrin were supposed to take a long nap within their Lunar Module before risking the strain of the moon walk. But they were impatient and in no mood for napping. After receiving permission from the Mission Control Center in Houston and putting on their complicated space suits, they opened their hatch, six and a half hours after landing.

The first man, an American, stepped out on a heavenly body. For that moment the whole world, except those whose dictators forbade them to know, watched proudly together.

Surrounded by the footprints of the first earthlings on the moon is the launching stand from which Armstrong and Aldrin took off from the moon, in their Lunar Module. And on it is a plaque that may remain forever. For on the moon there is no oxygen to rust and no water to erode. The message on the plaque boasts an American achievement and proclaims the hope of the world. "Here men from the planet earth first set foot upon the moon, July 1969, A.D. We came in peace for all mankind."

But already—long before American dreams to make the world safe for democracy could come true, long before world-wide peace was in sight—Americans back on earth were asking the familiar American question, "Where next?"

Chapter 33

No More Secrets: The World Is Watching

Because travel on the sea was so much easier than travel on land, the Puritans had managed to cross the three-thousand-mile ocean to this mysterious New World in only seven weeks. That was how they escaped the government that was persecuting them. Back home in England people could not really know what the Puritans were doing and even whether they were still alive.

Our world of airways is a whole new world. There are no more secrets. The three American astronauts in the *Apollo 11* were jammed into a spacecraft. But the whole watching world heard their voices. Their success depended on the Mission Control Center in Houston, Texas, where thirteen thousand people were joining the adventure. The whole nation in front of their television sets on July 16, 1969 felt *they* were somehow going along in the tiny *Apollo 11*. All across the country the people who had supplied materials, and with their taxes provided the billions of dollars for the voyage, watched anxiously.

Space voyages and the new triumphs of air travel would depend on inventions never imagined by the astronauts' grandfathers. When a vehicle sped through outer space to the moon—more than 238,000 miles in only three days—it had to be steered precisely and kept on its lightning-fast course. The slightest delay or tilt in the wrong direction might send the *Apollo 11* and its three passengers into the nowhere of outer space.

What made this speedy control possible was the computer. It was based on the ideas of a brilliant refugee from Hungary, John von Neumann, who had helped design the atomic bomb and then turned to making computers to work with fantastic speed. These miraculous machines could in the wink of an eye make computations that before had taken days. New ways were found to make computers smaller and smaller. Some were on the *Apollo 11*, and there were many at the space center. It was von Neumann's idea that made possible the computers we now use in homes, factories, businesses, and classrooms.

Travelers through the ocean of outer space could not have the privacy of *Mayflower* passengers. They could not sneeze without the controllers at home base knowing it and without making the nation's television watchers worry. Houston had to guide them, and without Houston's help they would be lost.

The trip to the moon was only a beginning. The astronauts had been picked up by navy vessels 940 miles southwest of Hawaii in the Pacific Ocean, where the *Apollo 11* splashed down. But the *Apollo 11* could not be used again for another space flight.

The next step was a space shuttle. This was an old word but a new idea. *Shuttle* is a word for the reel used in weaving to carry the thread to the woof back and forth between the threads of the warp. It has come to mean anything that goes back and forth—for example, the bus between a suburban parking lot and downtown. The new idea was a space shuttle unlike the *Apollo 11:* one that could come back and land at an airport like any other airplane. It could be used again and again and save millions of dollars.

The first space shuttle took off from Kennedy Space Center in Florida on April 12, 1981, and landed at Edwards Air Force Base in California two days later. Then shuttle trips became routine. They served many purposes. Some had military uses. One tested the effect of outer space on human blood. Another carried cages with two monkeys and twenty-four rats to learn more about life processes during space travel. All took spectacular photographs of earth.

For the twenty-fifth shuttle it was decided to include a teacher in the crew. After a nationwide search Christa McAuliffe, a social studies teacher from Concord, New Hampshire, was chosen. And she took off with the six other crew members from Kennedy Space Center on January 28, 1986. That morning was bitter cold, unusually cold for Florida. But the *Challenger* took off anyway. To the horror of the nation, 73 seconds after takeoff the *Challenger* exploded in full sight of the world watching on television. There had been failures in the American space efforts before, but none so terrible. All seven astronauts were killed on that day of tragedy. President Reagan ordered a prompt public study of the causes. And on television he led the nation's memorial service for these soldiers on our newest frontier. Before the *Challenger* the nation had begun to take for granted the courage of the astronauts. Now the nation saw with its own eyes the mortal risks of space heroes.

Before the year 1986 was out, the saddened nation would have its spirits lifted—not by another voyage into outer space but by a more familiar kind of adventure.

For nearly five hundred years seafarers had planned voyages circling our planet earth. The bold Portuguese Ferdinand Magellan started from Spain with five ships in 1519. After a horrendous voyage through the Strait of Magellan (later named after him) at the tip of South America, he sailed his ships into the Pacific. That ocean proved much vaster than he had imagined. The starving crew desperately chewed the pieces of leather that held the sails in place, and even ate the rats they found on board. Magellan himself was killed by natives in the Philippines, but one of his ships did manage to reach home. This first round-the-world trip had taken three years and had cost four of the five ships and the lives of all but eighteen of the more than two hundred fifty men who had begun the voyage.

Other adventurers have kept trying to find a speedier, safer way to circle our globe. The French writer Jules Verne's fantastic tale *Around the World in Eighty Days*, published in 1873, followed the breathless hero on ships, trains, and balloons to complete his journey to win a bet. Astronauts in outer space orbited beyond the atmosphere, but that was not the same as circling through the earth's air and weather.

Americans had always been in a hurry to set records. The story of the *Voyager* is another chapter in this wonderfully American quest. One day in March 1981 test pilot Dick Rutan and his friend and fellow pilot Jeana Yeager were having lunch with Dick's brother Burt Rutan, an airplane designer, near Burt's airplane factory in Mojave, California. Dick and Jeana were looking for adventure. Burt described a new carbonfiber featherweight material for making a light aircraft which could carry more fuel; thus it could go farther without needing to refuel.

Jeana urged that they build a plane of this new material. Then and there on a restaurant napkin Burt sketched a plane to fly around the world nonstop without refueling. Instantly they agreed to "do this thing or die trying." Burt would design the plane and they would all help build it. Dick and Jeana, good persuaders, would raise the two million dollars needed and secure donations of costly equipment from manufacturing companies. They spent three years along with a few volunteers building the plane with their own hands.

The plane they finally put together was like none ever seen before. With propellers front and back it resembled sketchy plans for a kite. It really was a flying fuel tank, designed to carry four times its own weight in fuel. The two pilots were squeezed into a cockpit three and a half feet wide by seven and a half feet long. They were so close to the engine that earphones for them had to be specially designed to cancel out the engine sounds to avoid permanent damage to their hearing.

With Dick and Jeana wedged inside, the *Voyager* took off from Edwards Air Force Base on the edge of the Mojave Desert in California on December 14, 1986. The plane's seventeen fuel tanks would keep the plane perfectly balanced by allowing fuel to flow from one tank to another as it was consumed. But the fuel load was so heavy on takeoff that the sagging wing tips were damaged by scraping the runway. The *Voyager* went westward across the Pacific, South Africa, and the Atlantic, then across the southern United States and back to Edwards. As the trip advanced, the plane used fuel and became lighter. But the less the *Voyager* weighed, the slower it flew. At the end it was going only 75 miles an hour. For the whole trip the speed would be about what Charles Lindbergh averaged on his way to Paris, 107 miles per hour.

Brother Burt Rutan was at mission control, nervously watching this proof of his design while the whole world, with television glimpses of the plane tumbling through African storms, followed the trip moment by moment. This trip that Dick and Jeana could not wait to make was no picnic. They carried only twenty-two pounds of food and ten and a half gallons of water. Each day they ate one hot meal specially packaged like the food for astronauts. In between they chewed peanut butter crunch or other dry food. The weather was especially rough, because they traveled at eight thousand to twelve thousand feet above the earth—much lower than the forty thousand feet where passenger liners fly. They did not want to waste fuel to pressurize the plane for the higher altitude. And they did not have enough oxygen to fly high. Juggled by turbulence, Jeana suffered severe bruises. Once the front engine scared them by quitting. Another time the rear engine stopped for a terrifying five minutes. Luckily, Dick was able to get fuel to that engine, and the outside flow of air turned the propeller and started the engine again.

An autopilot, working automatically by computer, operated the controls. This saved the energy of the two live pilots, who had many tasks and had to work frantically to see that the fuel flowed from one tank to another to keep balance. Each pilot took a turn at the controls while the other slept. It was a rocky trip. Dick, who had been shot down in combat in Viet Nam, finally said, "Compared to this flight, I felt a lot safer in combat."

Just nine days, three minutes, and forty-four seconds after takeoff, Jeana Yeager and Dick Rutan had covered the

---

Voyager on its first test flight in 1984.

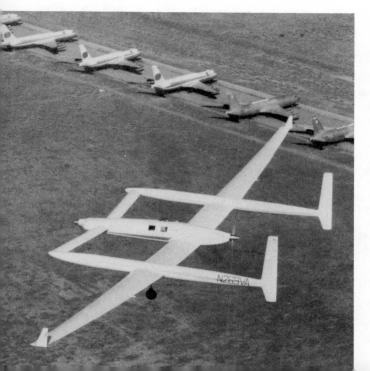

25,012 miles around the earth—without ever stopping to take fuel. They landed back at Edwards Air Force Base before cheering thousands while the world shared their joy and relief on the television screen.

When before had a sketch on a napkin made so much history? Both Dick and Jeana had risked their life's savings and their lives on what aviators called "the last plum" to be picked. "What kind of world would there be," Dick asked, "if there were no daring?"

How many of the thousands in 1927 in New York City who had welcomed Lindbergh from his sensational nonstop flight to Paris could have imagined that just sixty years later Americans on the other side of the continent would be celebrating a two-person nonstop voyage around the world? American technology and daring were no longer merely links between New York and Paris, ties to the Old World from which Americans had come. Now Americans were circling the whole world with the whole world watching!

* * *

The land that began as the best-kept secret had become the best-known land in the world. Everybody shared the adventures of astronauts and round-the-world pilots. Television, added to movies and radio and newspapers and books, now made it possible for Americans to know more about the world and themselves. The world had become one big television screen. Now all could share the suspense. American history had been a story of surprises. Like the past, the future was sure to be full of the unexpected. And these surprises were just another name for America.

INDEX

DANIEL J. BOORSTIN, the Librarian of Congress Emeritus, is one of our nation's most eminent and widely read historians. He is the author of the best-selling book *The Discoverers*, now translated into thirteen languages. And his celebrated earlier trilogy, *The Americans*, was awarded the Bancroft, Parkman, and Pulitzer prizes.

Prior to his twelve-year tenure at the Library of Congress, Dr. Boorstin served as director of the National Museum of American History of the Smithsonian Institution. Earlier he had been the Morton Distinguished Service Professor at the University of Chicago, where he taught for twenty-five years.

Born in Georgia and raised in Oklahoma, he received his B.A. from Harvard University and his doctorate from Yale. He has spent a good deal of his life viewing America from the outside, first in England as a Rhodes scholar at Balliol College, Oxford, and more recently as a professor in Rome, Paris, Kyoto, Cambridge, and Geneva.

His wife and collaborator, Ruth Frankel Boorstin, is a graduate of Wellesley College and holds a master's degree in social science from the University of Chicago. She has contributed as an editor to all of her husband's books.

The Boorstins live in Washington, D.C. They have three grown sons and four grandchildren.

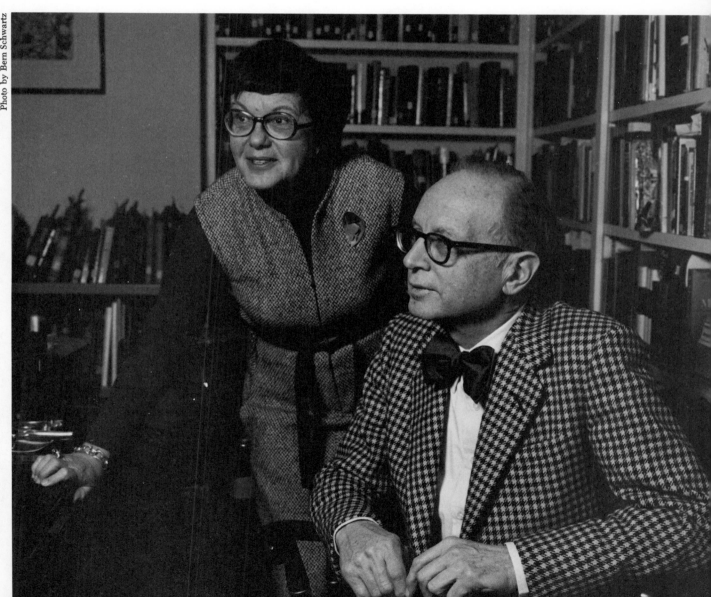

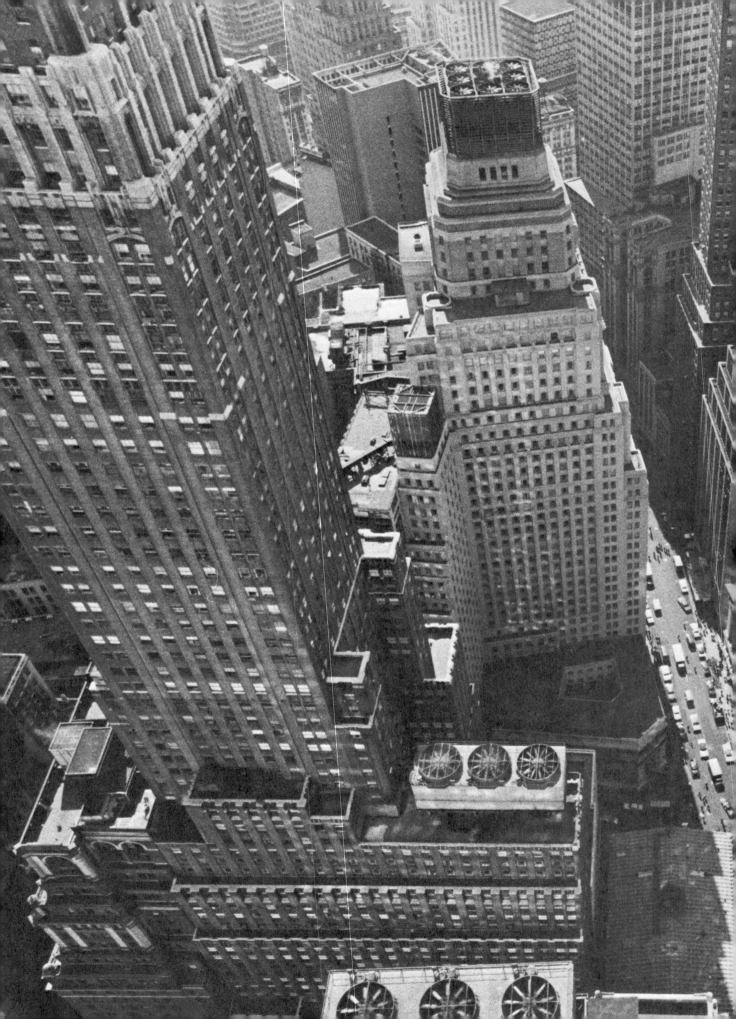

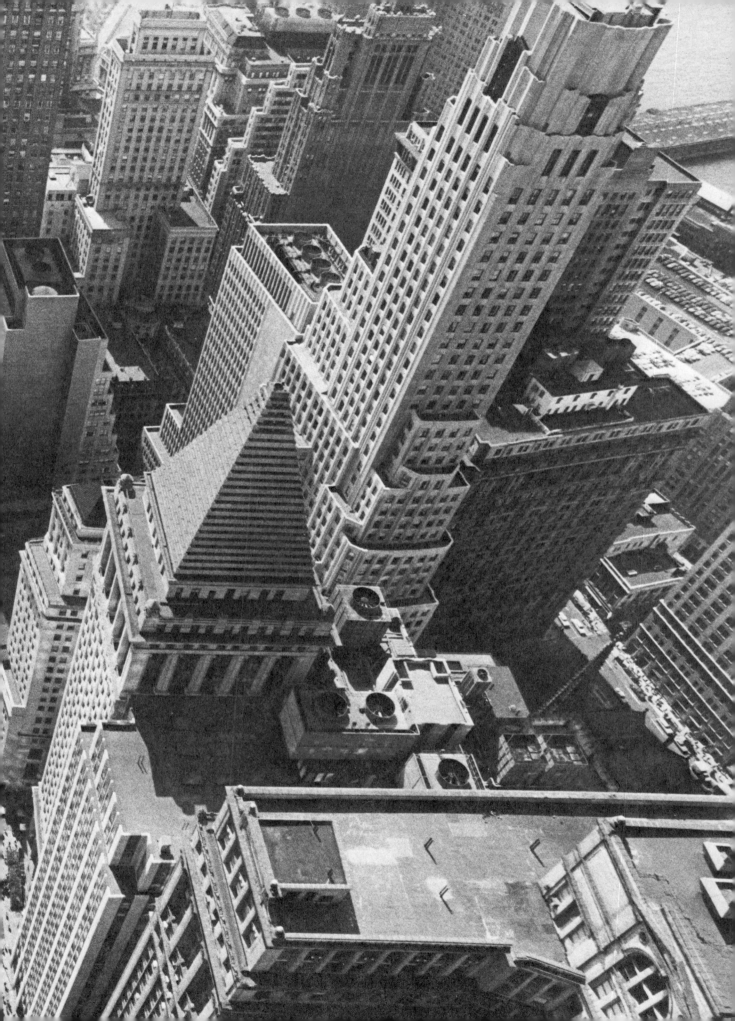